Clinical Anaesthetic Pharmacology

Clinical Anaesthetic Pharmacology

John W. Dundee OBE MD PhD FFARCS FFARCSI
Emeritus Professor of Anaesthesia,
The Queen's University, Belfast, N. Ireland, UK

R. S. J. Clarke BSc MD PhD FFARCS FFARCSI
Professor of Anaesthetics,
The Queen's University of Belfast, Belfast, N. Ireland, UK

William McCaughey MD FFARCS FFARCSI
Consultant Anaesthetist,
Craigavon Area Hospital, Co. Armagh, N. Ireland, UK
Lecturer, The Queen's University of Belfast, Belfast, N. Ireland, UK

CHURCHILL LIVINGSTONE
EDINBURGH LONDON MELBOURNE NEW YORK AND TOKYO 1991

CHURCHILL LIVINGSTONE
Medical Division of Longman Group UK Limited

Distributed in the United States of America by Churchill
Livingstone Inc., 1560 Broadway, New York, N.Y. 10036,
and by associated companies, branches and representatives
throughout the world.

First published 1991

ISBN 0-443-02073-6

British Library Cataloguing in Publication Data
Anaesthetic Pharmacology.
  1. Anaesthetics
  I. Dundee, John W. (John Wharry) II. Clarke, R. S. J.
  III. McCaughey, William
  615.781

Library of Congress Cataloging in Publication Data
Dundee, John W. (John Wharry)
    Anaesthetic pharmacology/John W. Dundee, R. S. J.
  Clarke, William McCaughey
        p. cm.
    Includes index.
    ISBN 0-443-02073-6
    1. Anesthetics. 2. Neuropharmacology. I. Clarke,
  R. S. J.
  (Richard Samuel Jessup) II. McCaughey, William. III.
Title.
        [DNLM: 1. Anesthetics — pharmacology. QV 81
        D914a]
    RD85.5.D86 1991
    617.9′6 — dc20
    DNLM/DLC
    for Library of Congress   90-15079
                                                    CIP

Printed and bound in Great Britain by
Butler & Tanner Ltd, Frome and London

Preface

The principle on which this book was conceived is that it should be an authoritative text on the pharmacology of drugs used by anaesthetists, having a strong scientific foundation while also relating to everyday practice. It is written largely by anaesthetists, and largely by those associated with the Belfast Anaesthetics Department, but individual chapters which are on topics of basic science or are in areas on the fringe of anaesthetic practice have been covered by authors whose experience lies in these.

Anaesthetists do not confine their activities to the operating theatre, and the scope of this book is intended to be wide enough to include areas of pre- and post-operative care as well as the intensive therapy unit.

The first section of this book describes the basic principles on which the understanding of the pharmacology of anaesthetic and other drugs must be based. Drugs have long been used empirically, the rationale for their use being observation of the results of their administration. A major advance occurring mainly in the past two decades has been the rational application of pharmacokinetic principles, especially important in anaesthesia where the time-course of the onset and termination of effect of drugs must be so closely controlled. Although pharmacokinetic data may be scarce for some older drugs, continuing research and improved detection methods mean that the kinetics of most newly introduced drugs are well studied. An emphasis is placed throughout the book on the pharmacokinetics of the drugs described.

Less well known in many cases are the mechanisms underlying the actions of drugs — general anaesthesia itself is a case in point.

However this is an area in which probably the most rapid advances in basic knowledge are occurring at present and beginning to influence rational use of the drugs as well as guide development of new drugs. An attempt has been made throughout to examine the current position with regard to each drug, but often it is not possible to discuss all recent data, not least because much recently published material may be controversial.

We aim that this book should fulfil a role as a practical guide as well as being a basic text. Thus the sections on individual drugs as well as discussing basic chemical, pharmacokinetic and pharmacodynamic properties, include details of the clinical use of the drug, methods of administration and dosage, adverse effects, and where relevant drug interactions. Separate chapters deal with special aspects of drug therapy, such as adverse responses, management of drug overdose, and the special features of drug action in pregnancy.

In the fields outside anaesthesia, hard decisions about exclusions have had to be taken. Thus in microbiology we have retained the anti-tuberculous drugs but largely omitted anti-viral agents. Nevertheless it is hoped that the anaesthetist will find most of the drugs which his or her patient is likely to be receiving from physicians or which he will need to administer in the intensive therapy unit (including a discussion of the controversial 'selective decontamination').

The original concept was a book written from one department, with a single editor, but what was to be the work of the senior editor alone became possible only by the addition of two colleagues. The source of authorship also was expanded to include people with whom the editors have worked and a few colleagues from other disciplines. All of us acknowledge the long-term secretarial assistance of Mrs Noelle Collins who was involved from the first attempt to the final manuscript. Her knowledge of this type of work was invaluable.

John W. Dundee
Richard S. J. Clarke
William McCaughey

Belfast 1991

Contributors

J. P. Alexander MD FRCPI FFARCS
Consultant Anaesthetist, Belfast City Hospital,
Belfast, N. Ireland, UK

J. G. Bovill MD FFARCSI
Professor of Experimental Anaesthesia, University
Hospital, Leiden, The Netherlands

J. R. Carpenter BSc PhD
Lecturer in Pharmacology, Department of
Physiological Sciences, University of Manchester, UK

R. S. J. Clarke BSc MD PhD FFARCS FFARCSI
Professor of Anaesthetics, The Queen's University of
Belfast, N. Ireland, UK

D. L. Coppel MB FFARCSI
Consultant Anaesthetist, Regional Intensive Care
Unit, Royal Victoria Hospital, Belfast, N. Ireland, UK

H. J. L. Craig MD FFARCS FFARCSI
Consultant Anaesthetist, Royal Victoria Hospital,
Belfast, N. Ireland, UK

Ciaran C. Doherty MD MRCP
Consultant Nephrologist, Regional Nephrology Unit,
Belfast City Hospital, Belfast, N. Ireland, UK

J. W. Dundee MBE MD PhD FFARCS FFARCSI
Emeritus Professor of Anaesthesia, The Queen's
University of Belfast, N. Ireland, UK

J. P. H. Fee MD FFARCSI
Consultant Anaesthetist, Royal Victoria and
Musgrave Park Hospitals, Belfast, and Senior
Lecturer in Anaesthetics, The Queen's University of
Belfast, N. Ireland, UK

J. A. S. Gamble MD FFARCSI
Consultant Anaesthetist, Belfast City Hospital, N.
Ireland, UK

J. N. Halliday MB FFARCSI
Associate Professor of Clinical Anesthesiology,
University of Miami, Florida, USA

A. R. Hunter MD FRFPS FRCS FFARCS
Emeritus Professor of Anaesthetics, University of
Manchester, UK

J. R. Johnston MD FFARCSI
Consultant Anaesthetist, Regional Intensive Care
Unit, Royal Victoria Hospital, Belfast, N. Ireland, UK

J. Kelly PhD
Senior Lecturer, Department of Clinical
Pharmacology, Royal College of Surgeons in Ireland,
Dublin, Eire

G. Gavin Lavery MD FFARCSI
Consultant Anaesthetist, Regional Intensive Care
Unit, Royal Victoria Hospital, Belfast, N. Ireland, UK

W. B. Loan MD FFARCSI
Consultant Anaesthetist, Belfast City Hospital,
Belfast, N. Ireland, UK

Kenneth G. Lowry MB FFARCSI
Consultant in Anaesthetics and Intensive Care
Medicine, Royal Victoria Hospital, Belfast, N.
Ireland, UK

S. M. Lyons BSc MD FFARCS
Consultant Anaesthetist, Royal Victoria Hospital,
Belfast, N. Ireland

W. McCaughey MD FFARCS FFARCSI
Consultant Anaesthetist, Craigavon Area Hospital,
Co. Armagh and Lecturer, The Queen's
University of Belfast, N. Ireland, UK

P. J. I. McIlroy BSc PhD
Managing Director, Project Managing Resource,
London, UK

A. C. McKay MD FFARCSI
Consultant Anaesthetist, Belfast City Hospital,
Belfast, N. Ireland, UK

J. S. Millership BSc PhD CChem FRCS
Lecturer, School of Pharmacy, The Queen's
University of Belfast, N. Ireland, UK

Rajinder K. Mirakhur MD PhD FFARCS
Senior Lecturer in Anaesthetics, The Queen's
University of Belfast, N. Ireland

J. Moore MD PhD FFARCS
Consultant Anaesthetist, Belfast City and Musgrave
Park Hospitals, Belfast, and Honorary Professor of
Anaesthetics, The Queen's University of Belfast, N.
Ireland, UK

Samuel D. Nelson BA MB FRCPI FRCPath
Consultant Haematologist, Craigavon Area Hospital,
Co. Armagh, N. Ireland

Ian A. Orr MD DRCOG FFARCS
Consultant Anaesthetist, Craigavon Area Hospital,
Belfast, N. Ireland, UK

Barbara J. Pleuvry B Pharm MSc PhD MRPS
Senior Lecturer in Anaesthetics and Pharmacology,
University of Manchester, UK

T. S. Wilson MB FRCPI FRCPath
Consultant Bacteriologist, Belfast City Hospital and
Honorary Lecturer in Microbiology, The Queen's
University of Belfast, N. Ireland, UK

Contents

Basic principles

1. Chemistry

John G. Kelly   Paul J. McIlroy

INTRODUCTION

With the exception of nitrous oxide, all clinically used anaesthetic agents are organic in nature, that is, they belong to the class of compounds containing carbon. In general, then, the study of the chemical structures and properties of substances used in anaesthesia is a study of organic chemicals. As well as a knowledge of their chemical properties, some knowledge of the physical characteristics of substances used in anaesthetic practice is essential in order to understand something of their modes of action and their formulation, and to assist in their administration.

Most drugs used currently as anaesthetics or in combination with anaesthetic agents are synthetic, and this is particularly so for newer drugs. Some older drugs of relatively complex chemical structure are still derived from plant materials, for example morphine and atropine. These compounds are often complex nitrogenous bases (alkaloids) and even though a laboratory synthesis may be possible it may often not be commercially feasible. Sometimes a substance derived from a plant may be modified chemically to change a particular action, for example the acetylation of morphine to produce heroin.

Chemical structures of anaesthetic agents range from the simplest types of organic molecules to compounds of considerable complexity, and physically they range from gases and volatile liquids to compounds of fairly high melting point.

ORGANIC CHEMISTRY (ALIPHATIC SUBSTANCES)

Alkanes

These form a homologous series; that is, each member of the series differs from the next by a constant amount. For the alkanes the general formula is $C_n H_{2n}+2$. Each member, a homolog, differs from the next by a CH_2 unit and they have common names derived from the Greek prefix for the number of carbon atoms in the molecule.

Thus:

CH_4	$H—CH_2—H$	methane
C_2H_6	$H—CH_2—CH_2—H$	ethane
C_3H_8	$H—CH_2—CH_2CH_2—H$	propane
C_4H_{10}	$H—CH_2—CH_2—CH_2—CH_2—H$	butane

In homologous series there is a gradation in chemical reactivity and in physical properties. Physically the alkanes range at room temperature from gases to liquids, to solids, as the molecules grow in size.

As alkanes (or indeed any such long-chain substances) grow in size, the possible structures become more complex; for example the structure for propane (C_3H_8) is illustrated in Figure 1.1.

However, the alkane of formula C_4H_{10} may be written in two ways (Fig. 1.2). These two materials are structural isomers, compounds with the same molecular formula but with different structural formulae. As the number of carbon atoms increases so the possible number of isomeric structures increases. For pentane, three structures can be drawn, and for decane ($C_{10}H_{22}$), 75 isomeric structures can be constructed.

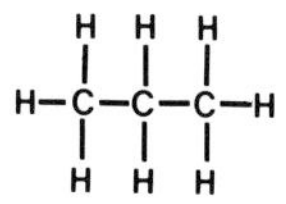

Fig. 1.1 Structure of propane.

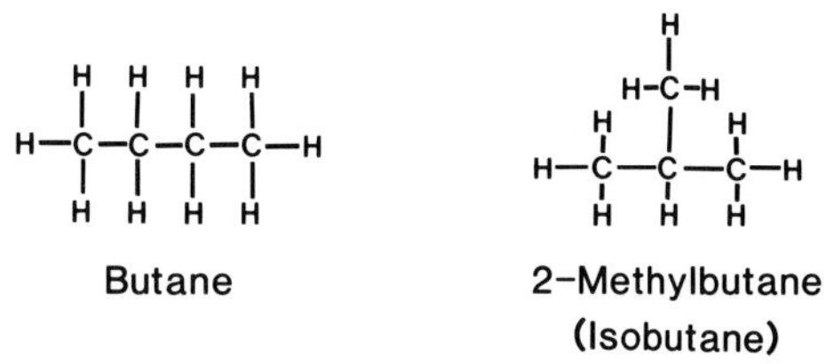

Fig. 1.2 Structural isomers of C_4H_{10}.

3

A rational system of nomenclature for these is to select the longest continous chain as the parent structure, to sequentially number the carbon atoms on this chain and to indicate by these numbers the carbon to which other substituents are attached.

Physical properties depend on molecular shape as well as size, and structural isomers may have different physical characteristics such as melting or boiling points.

Chemically, alkanes are characterized by relative inertness. However, they are the 'backbone' of aliphatic organic chemistry; addition of a halogen atom produces an alkyl halide, or of an OH group produces an alcohol, or of an NH_2 produces an amine, and so on.

No anaesthetic agent is a continuous chain alkane.

Alkyl halides

As mentioned previously, these are formed from alkanes by adding one or more halogen atoms. They are then derivatives of alkanes and are named by indicating the presence and position of a halogen by a prefix.

These substances are of higher boiling point than their parent alkanes. As with alkanes they are insoluble in water and, if they are liquids, they form discrete layers above or below water, depending on their densities.

Reactions can involve substitution of the halogen atom to form, for example, alcohols or ethers. Many general anaesthetics are halogenated substances, usually alkyl halides or halogenated ethers. The simplest example of these is chloroform (trichloromethane; Fig. 1.3). A good example of a commonly used halogenated alkane is halothane (2-bromo-2chloro-1,1,1-trifluoroethane; Fig. 1.3). Halothane is generally not explosive when mixed with oxygen at normal atmospheric pressure.

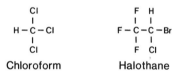

Chloroform   Halothane

Fig. 1.3   Halogenated hydrocarbons.

Unsaturated hydrocarbons

These are the alkenes and alkynes. They are hydrocarbons since they contain only carbon and hydrogen. However, the bonding is different from that of alkanes. Alkenes contain at least one double bond in which two carbon atoms form bonds with each other by sharing two pairs of electrons (instead of one pair). Alkynes con-

tain at least one triple bond in which two carbon atoms share three pairs of electrons.

The simplest alkene is ethylene and the next is propylene (Fig. 1.4). The simplest alkyne is acetylene. The unsaturated hydrocarbons are named systematically by replacing the -ane ending of the corresponding alkane by -ene for alkenes and -yne for alkynes. The position of double or triple bonds is described by numbering the carbon atoms in the carbon chain and arranging this so that the position of the unsaturated bond has the lowest number.

As the carbon chain lengthens there are various opportunities for isomerism. As well as possible differences in positions of double bonds we can have the structural isomerism described for alkanes. Figure 1.5 shows the various structures possible for a hydrocarbon composed of four carbon atoms and one double bond.

With alkenes we meet for the first time *geometric isomerism*. The double bonds hinder free rotation about the carbon–carbon bond and result in two possible spatial arrangements of the terminal methyl groups (Fig. 1.6). Geometric isomers have different properties, for example the boiling point of *cis* but-2-ene is higher than that of *trans* but-2-ene.

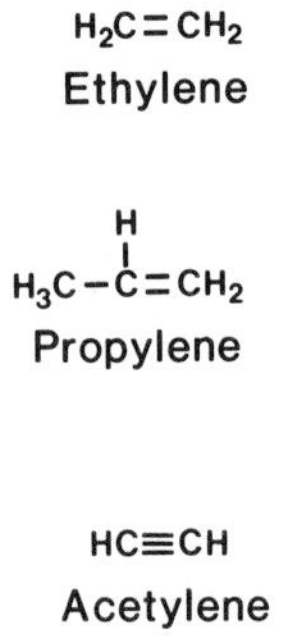

$$H_2C = CH_2$$
Ethylene

$$H_3C - \overset{\overset{\displaystyle H}{|}}{C} = CH_2$$
Propylene

$$HC \equiv CH$$
Acetylene

Fig. 1.4   Unsaturated hydrocarbons.

$$CH_3 - CH_2 - CH = CH_2$$
But–1–ene

$$CH_3 - CH = CH - CH_3$$
But–2–ene

$$CH_3 - \overset{\overset{\displaystyle }{|}}{\underset{\underset{\displaystyle CH_3}{|}}{C}} = CH_2$$
2-Methyl prop–1–ene

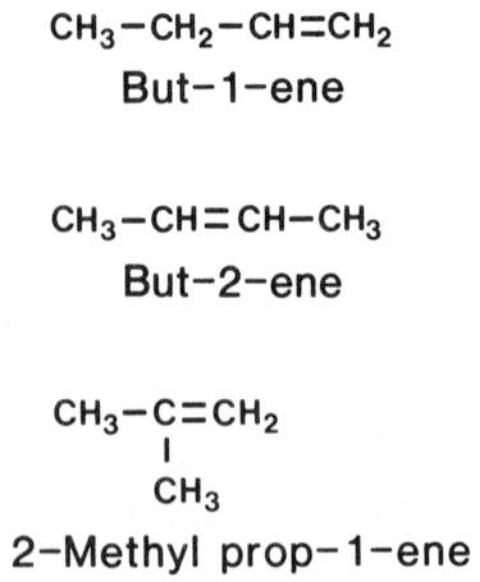

Fig. 1.5   Structural isomers of C_4H_8.

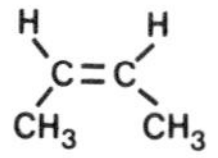

$$\underset{CH_3}{\overset{H}{C}}=\underset{CH_3}{\overset{H}{C}}$$

cis But-2-ene

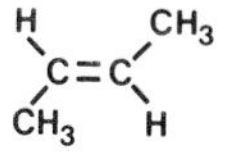

$$\underset{CH_3}{\overset{H}{C}}=\underset{H}{\overset{CH_3}{C}}$$

trans But-2-ene

Fig. 1.6 Geometric isomerism.

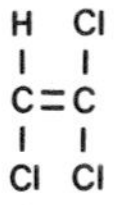

$$\underset{Cl}{\overset{H}{C}}=\underset{Cl}{\overset{Cl}{C}}$$

Trichloroethylene

Fig. 1.7 Structure of trichlorethylene.

In their physical properties the alkenes and alkynes resemble the alkanes. Simpler members are gases. Boiling points increase with carbon chain length. They are insoluble in water but are soluble in non-polar organic solvents and in fat.

Chemically, the characteristic reactions of alkenes and alkynes is addition of reagents to the double bonds. They are chemically reactive.

Trichloroethylene (Fig. 1.7) is a halogenated alkene. Fluroxene is an unsaturated ether.

Ethers

Ethers have the general formulae R—O—R. They are most easily named by giving the two alkyl groups as prefixes before the word 'ether'.

Physically, ethers are only slightly soluble in water. Boiling points are of the same order as alkanes of comparable molecular weight. Chemically ethers are relatively unreactive. It is important to note that ethers are potentially very flammable, and their vapours form explosive mixtures with air, oxygen or nitrous oxide. Free-radical oxidation of ethers results in formation of peroxides. These can explode if heated. Use of a non-volatile antioxidant (added to the ether) will avoid this.

Diethyl ether is the oldest inhalational anaesthetic in use after nitrous oxide. It is very flammable and decomposes readily. It is the most water-soluble of the ethers, resulting in slower induction of anaesthesia. Many other ethers have been introduced as inhalational anaesthetics over the years. The alkyl portions are almost always composed of one or two carbon atoms (methyl or ethyl).

$C_2H_5-O-C_2H_5$
Diethyl ether
$CH_2=CH_2-O-CH_2=CH_2$
Divinyl ether
(Vinyl ether)

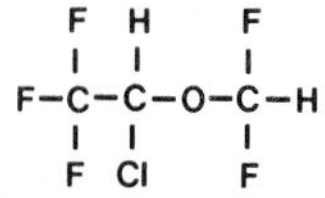

$$F-\overset{\overset{\displaystyle F}{|}}{\underset{\underset{\displaystyle F}{|}}{C}}-\overset{\overset{\displaystyle H}{|}}{\underset{\underset{\displaystyle Cl}{|}}{C}}-O-\overset{\overset{\displaystyle F}{|}}{\underset{\underset{\displaystyle F}{|}}{C}}-H$$

1-Chloro-2,2,2-trifluoryethyl
difluoromethyl ether
(Isoflurane)

Fig. 1.8 Anaesthetic ethers.

The structural variations lie in the presence of unsaturation, halogen groups or both. While many of these are flammable, newer ethers containing halogen atoms may not be so prone to this.

Representative ethers used as inhalational anaesthetics are shown in Figure 1.8.

Alcohols

All alcohols contain the hydroxyl (—OH) group which is the functional group in alcohol, and which determines the characteristics of this group of substances. Alcohols can be primary, secondary or tertiary, depending on the number of other carbon atoms attached to the carbon bearing the hydroxyl group (Fig. 1.9).

Alcohols contain the polar —OH group and in the smaller molecular weight alcohols this results in miscibility with water. As the carbon chain lengthens then the contribution of the hydroxyl group lessens. Thus ethanol, C_2H_5OH, is very water-soluble, but octanol, $C_8H_{17}OH$, is practically insoluble. The —OH groups also cause intermolecular interactions, resulting in rela-

$R-CH_2-OH$
Primary alcohol

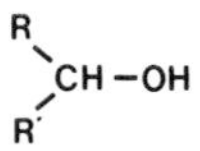

$$\underset{R'}{\overset{R}{>}}CH-OH$$

Secondary alcohol

$$R'-\overset{\overset{\displaystyle R}{|}}{\underset{\underset{\displaystyle R''}{|}}{C}}-OH$$

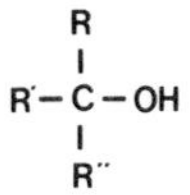

Tertiary alcohol

Fig. 1.9 General structures of alcohols.

tively high boiling points. Primary alcohols are oxidized to aldehyde or acids. Secondary alcohols are oxidized to ketones. Tertiary alcohols are not oxidized.

Alcohols are named by considering the longest chain containing the hydroxyl group to be the parent compound and this chain is named by replacing the 'e' of the alkane named by '-ol.' The position of the —OH group is indicated by the lowest possible number, and the positions of substituent groups indicated by numbers. Alcohols are depressants of the central nervous system and of course ethanol is widely used socially. Ethanol is flammable. Ethanol and isopropyl alcohol are used as skin cleansing and disinfectant agents.

Aldehydes and ketones

These possess the group —C=O, called a carbonyl group (Fig. 1.10). The carbonyl group is mainly responsible for the properties of these substances.

Physically these compounds are polar, because of the carbonyl group. Lower members are water-soluble. Solubility decreases with increasing carbon-chain lengths. Oxidation of aldehydes and ketones produces primary and secondary alcohols respectively.

For an aldehyde the name is derived by placing the -e of the corresponding alkane by -al, the positions of substituents are indicated by numbers with the carbonyl carbon atom being considered as the first carbon. Ketones are named by replacing the -e of the alkane by -one. The position of the carbonyl atom is indicated by a number (Fig. 1.11).

Paraldehyde is a polymer of acetaldehyde.

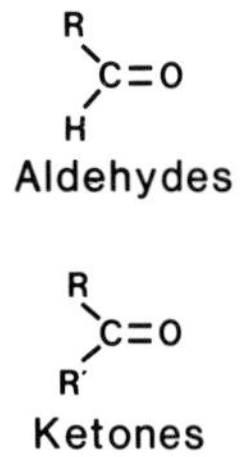

Fig. 1.10   Carbonyl compounds.

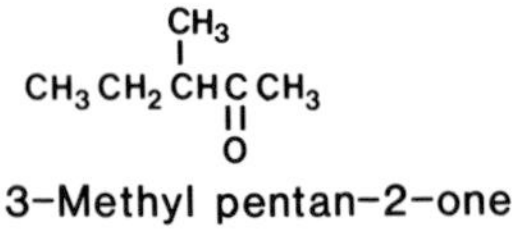

3-Methyl pentan-2-one

Fig. 1.11   Naming a ketone.

Carboxylic acids and their derivatives

These substances also contain the carbonyl group but with the addition of —OH to produce the carboxyl group (Fig. 1.12). Functional derivatives are α compounds in which the —OH of their carbonyl group has been replaced by one of a variety of other groups to produce the structures shown in Figure 1.12.

Physically, carboxylic acids are very polar and lower members are miscible with water. The liquids have relatively high boiling points because of intermolecular bonding.

These acids are systematically named by replacing the terminal '-e' of the corresponding alkane by '-oic acid'. The carbon atom of the —COOH group is regarded as the first atom when a numbering system is used. Many of these acids have specific names, such as acetic acid for $CH_3 COOH$ or stearic acid for $CH_3 (CH_2)_{16} COOH$.

The fatty acids are long-chain carboxylic acids (such as stearic acid). They may be saturated or unsaturated. Prostaglandins are a group of long-chain polyunsaturated fatty acids. Lipids are esters in which at least one of the acid components is a fatty acid.

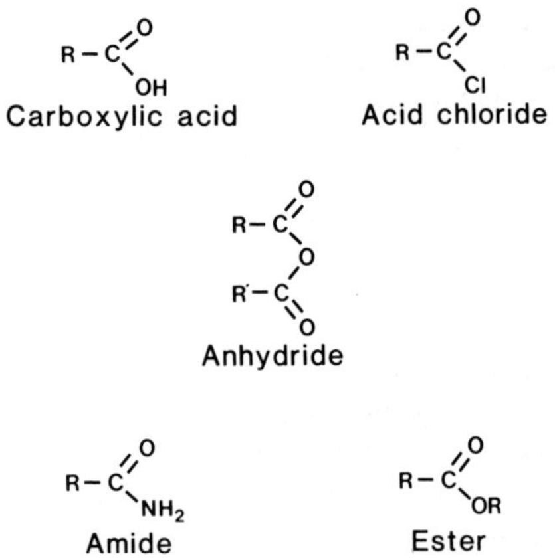

Fig. 1.12   General structures of carboxylic acids and derivatives

Amines

These can be considered as derivatives of ammonia where one or more of ammonia's hydrogen atoms are replaced by a carbon atom. They can be primary, secondary or tertiary amines in a fashion similar to alcohols (Fig. 1.13).

Amines are polar and basic. Smaller amines may be gases or liquids at room temperature and are soluble in water. The simplest method for naming amines is to

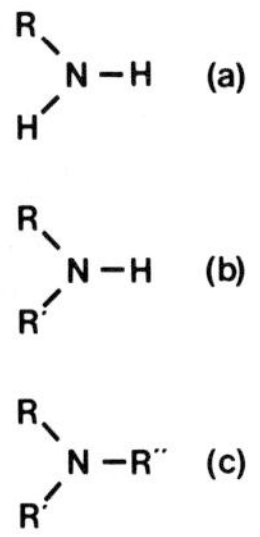

R
\
 N – H (a)
/
H

R
\
 N – H (b)
/
R'

R
\
 N – R'' (c)
/
R'

Fig. 1.13 General structures of amines.

CH₃NHCH₂CH₃
Ethylmethylamine

H₂NCH₂CH₂OH
2–Aminoethanol

Fig. 1.14 Naming amines.

name the alkyl group or groups attached to nitrogen and to follow these by '-amine'. They can also be named by adding 'amino-' to the parent chain (Fig. 1.14).

Most substances of pharmacological interest contain nitrogen. 'Alkaloid' is a general name given to nitrogen-containing, naturally occurring substances. Thus atropine and morphine are alkaloids. The amine group (primary, secondary or tertiary) is a very common feature of alkaloids and also of many drugs. Lignocaine, for example, is a tertiary amine; prilocaine has a secondary amine and an amide group. Neurotransmitter substances are often amines. Noradrenaline, dopamine and histamine are primary amines, adrenaline is a secondary amine. Many drugs acting at α- and β-adrenoceptors are amines.

Amines will react with alkyl halides (alkylation) to form a mixture of compounds but exhaustive alkylation produces compounds of general formula $R_4N^+X^-$, and these are known as quaternary ammonium salts (Fig. 1.15). Four organic groups are bonded to nitrogen, and the resulting positive charge is balanced by one negative ion. These are also important pharmacologically. Acetylcholine is a quaternary ammonium compound. Many other substances having actions at

CH₂ COOCH₂CH₂Ṅ(CH₃)₃
|
CH₂ COOCH₂CH₂Ṅ(CH₃)₃

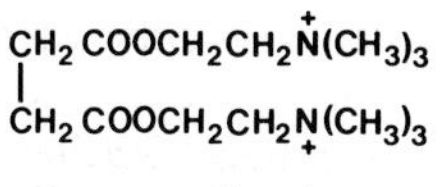

Suxamethonium

Fig. 1.15 A quaternary ammonium compound.

autonomic ganglia, at the postganglionic parasympathetic receptors and at the neuromuscular junction, are quaternary ammonium compounds, including neostigmine, propantheline, suxamethonium and tubocurarine.

Cyclic compounds

So far most substances discussed have had their carbon atoms linked to form chains. Carbon atoms can also join to form rings, producing cyclic compounds. In the simplest case a carbon chain, for example hexane, can be considered as having adopted a ring structure to form cyclohexane. The substances are named by prefixing 'cyclo-' to the name of the corresponding straight-chain alkane. The positions of substituents are numbered and the lowest combination of numbers used. Usually the cyclic compounds are represented by a corresponding figure, for example a hexagon for cyclohexane (Fig. 1.16).

Physically these substances have properties similar to the open-chain hydrocarbons. They are non-polar and do not dissolve in water. The only compound here of (mainly historical) anaesthetic interest is cyclopropane. Cyclopropane is highly flammable and forms explosive mixtures with air and oxygen.

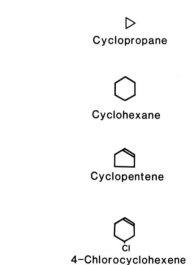

Cyclopropane

Cyclohexane

Cyclopentene

4–Chlorocyclohexene

Fig. 1.16 Structures of cyclic compounds.

AROMATIC SUBSTANCES

Benzene, of course, is the starting point of aromatic chemistry. Most drugs contain an aromatic nucleus in their structure.

Benzene

Benzene has a cyclical structure containing six carbon atoms. It also contains six hydrogen atoms, one per carbon atom, in contrast to cyclohexane which contains two hydrogen atoms per carbon atom. Benzene is then a highly unsaturated compound. In fact the structure of benzene is such that each carbon atom has a 'spare' electron, not involved in binding to another carbon or hydrogen. These occupy sequential orbitals above and below the plane of the carbon ring. The benzene ring is then a flat, hexagonal structure.

Naming of simple benzene derivatives is relatively easy, although common names are often used, such as phenol for hydroxybenzene and toluene for methylbenzene. Where more than one substituent is present then the positions of these must be indicated, and there are several ways of doing this. One is to use the words *ortho*, *meta* and *para* (abbreviated to *o*, *m* and *p*, respectively). Another is to number the positions in the benzene ring. If one substituent results in a special name for the molecule then this may be considered as the parent compound for numbering purposes (Fig. 1.17).

Obviously, while many drugs have benzene rings in their structure, as a molecule becomes larger, naming it systematically becomes extremely complicated, since several functional groups or complicated, fused ring structures may be present.

Fused ring compounds

The simplest aromatic fused ring substance is naphthalene, which is two benzene rings fused together.

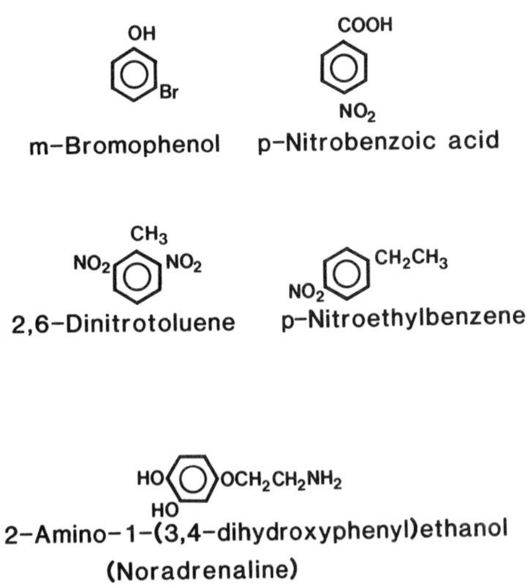

Fig. 1.17 Naming benzene derivatives.

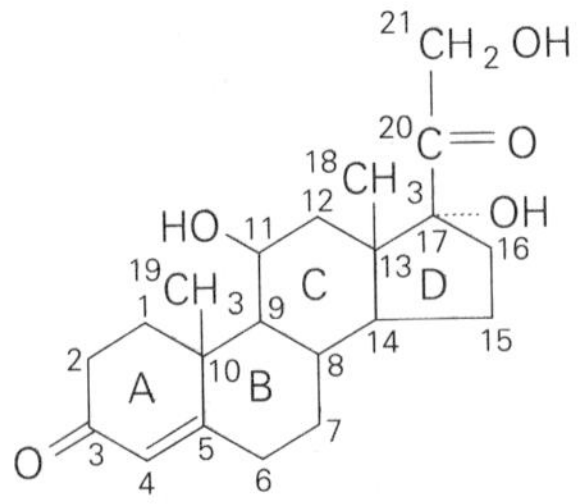

Fig. 1.18 Numbering a steroid.

Anthracene is three benzene rings fused together. There are also, of course, heterocyclic fused ring compounds, an example being the steroid nucleus present in digitalis glycosides and althesin (Fig. 1.18). Some drugs contain mixed aromatic/aliphatic heterocyclic fused rings (for example the ergot alkaloids).

Heterocyclic compounds

These are ring structures made up of more than one kind of atom. Most commonly these are nitrogen, oxygen or sulphur. Heterocyclic systems can be very complex, and there are many pharmacological examples such as nicotine (containing saturated and unsaturated heterocyclic rings, Fig. 1.19), quinidine, phenothiazines and opioid analgesics.

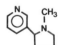

Fig. 1.19 A heterocyclic alkaloid, nicotine.

Stereochemistry

Although chemical structures are generally given a two-dimensional shape on paper, it is very important to realize that in reality their shape is three-dimensional. A knowledge of shape is important in understanding, for example, the mechanism of a chemical reaction or the reason for a drug–receptor interaction. That branch of chemistry which deals with chemical structure in three dimensions is called stereochemistry. Stereoisomers are molecules which are like one another in respect of which atoms are joined to each other, but differ in the way the atoms are oriented in space.

Optical isomerism is probably the most common type of isomerism encountered in pharmacology. When carbon is bound to four hydrogen atoms (methane), the bonds formed point towards the four corners of a tetrahedron with carbon in the centre and the angle between each bond is 109.5°. Substitution of one hydrogen atom always leads to the same compound, substitution of two hydrogen atoms by different substituents also always leads to the same compound. No matter which two hydrogen atoms are replaced, simple reorientation of the molecule always produces compounds which are superimposable. However, when three hydrogen atoms have been replaced by three different substituents, then the situation changes. The substituent atoms can be placed in two different ways so that the two possible isomers are not superimposable no matter how the molecules are placed. However, they are mirror images of each other. Figure 1.20 illustrates this for warfarin. A carbon atom showing this type of isomerism is called an asymmetric or chiral carbon atom. In the illustration the asymmetric carbon atom is represented by the central circle. The dotted lines are bonds going into the page, and the wedges are bonds coming out from the page. Such a subtle difference results in only very small differences in physical properties; indeed it is not usully possible to separate optical isomers on the basis of differing physical properties. However, the two isomers differ in that when a beam of polarized light is passed through a solution of them, each isomer rotates the plane of the light by the same amount but in different directions. Isomers like this are called enantiomers, and mixtures containing equal parts of the enantiomers are known as racemic mixtures. Such mixtures are not optically active. Synthetically produced compounds containing an asymmetric carbon atom are usually racemic mixtures, but enantiomers can be separated by chemical means. Biological processes, however, often result in the synthesis of isomers. An enantiomer rotating polarized light to the right is known as the (+) or d (for 'dextro') iso-

mer, and an enantiomer rotating polarized light to the left is known as the − or l (for 'levo') isomer. In pharmacology, where a substance is optically active, the pharmacological activity is almost always chiefly possessed by the l-isomer. Thus l-isoprenaline is orders of magnitude more potent in its actions on β-adrenoceptors than d-isoprenaline. The terms d- and l- should be distinguished from D- and L-, which do not necessarily indicate the direction of rotation of light. A rational system for indicating the absolute orientation of groups around a chiral carbon uses the prefixes (R) and (S) from the latin "rectus" and "sinister". The group of lowest priority (on a systematic scale) is placed going away from the observer at the rear of the chiral carbon. The other three groups will be facing the observer. If an arrow connecting these from lowest to highest priority is going in a clockwise direction then the molecule is given the prefix (R); if anticlockwise then the prefix (S) is used. This draws no conclusions about the direction of rotation of polarised light.

Other types of stereoisomerism are revealed when carbon atoms are joined together. Geometric isomerism for carbon–carbon double bonds has already been mentioned. For carbon–carbon single bonds there are two possible extreme arrangements (see Fig. 1.21). These two extreme arrangements are known as the eclipsed (a) and staggered (b) conformations. While a molecule can exist in either of these arrangements, or in any intermediate arrangement, it will spend most of its time in the most stable staggered conformation. While geometric isomers can be separated, conformational isomers cannot, because of the free rotation about the carbon–carbon bond.

The situation obviously becomes more complicated with increasing molecular size where other possibilities of molecular folding become possible. Cyclic structures will also fold into optimally stable configurations, although of course aromatic rings are flat structures. Cyclohexane, however, can arrange itself into 'chair', 'boat' or 'twist' forms, and substituents can be parallel to the plane of the carbon atom or be above or below this plane.

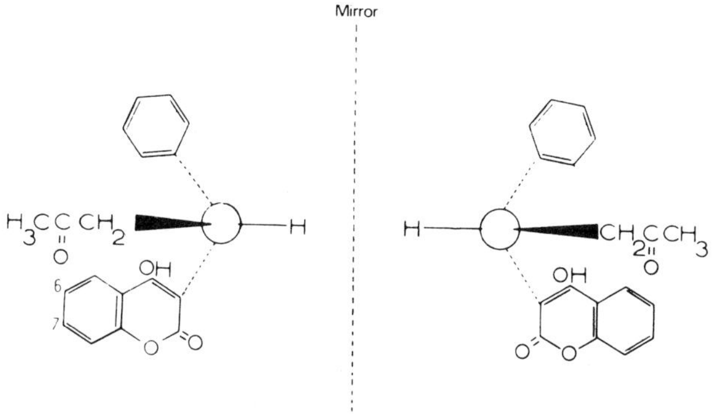

Fig. 1.20 Structure of warfarin, illustrating optical isomerism.

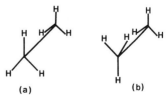

Fig. 1.21 Conformational isomers.

ASPECTS OF PHYSICAL CHEMISTRY

The general gas equation

The fundamental physical and chemical laws concerning gases and vapours are of importance in general anaesthesia. The two principal laws for an ideal gas are Charles's Law (the volume of a fixed mass of gas at constant pressure, is directly proportional to the temperature) and Boyle's Law (the volume of a fixed mass of gas at constant temperature is inversely proportional to the pressure). These two laws may be summarized in the single equation

$$PV/T = \text{a constant (for a fixed mass of gas)}$$

where P is the pressure, V is the volume and T is the temperature on the Kelvin scale of absolute temperature. On this scale, absolute zero, ($0°K$, $-273.15°C$) is the lowest temperature theoretically possible, corresponding to the temperature at which an ideal gas would have zero volume.

The pressure exerted by the gas may be considered to be due to the force of the molecules of the gas striking the walls of the container. In a mixture of gases the total pressure will be due to the collisions of the various gas molecules in the mixture with the container walls, and will therefore be the sum of the individual partial pressures exerted by each of the component gases of the mixture. This is Dalton's Law of partial pressures, where the partial pressure is defined simply as the pressure that one component of a gas mixture would exert if it occupied alone the same volume at the same temperature. An important definition is that a gram molecular weight, a mole, of any gas at standard conditions (1 atmosphere pressure and $0°C$, $273°$ K) will contain the same number of molecules (Avogadro's number) and occupy the same volume, 22.4 litres, the gram molecular volume. As the volume of each gas in a mixture is the total volume, the partial pressure of a gas will be directly proportional to the concentration of the gas in the mixture. The general gas equation for an ideal gas can be rewritten:

$$PV = nR/T$$

where n is the number of moles of the gas present and R is a constant (the gas constant) whose value depends on the units of pressure and volume used. This equation indicates that the pressure of a fixed mass of gas at constant temperature will be proportional to the concentration (in moles per unit volume) of the gas. Dalton's Law of partial pressures states that the pressure exerted by a mixture of ideal gases is the sum of the pressures exerted by the individual gases occupying the same volume alone. As the mole fraction of a gas is the amount (in moles) of that gas relative to the total number of moles of gas in the mixture, it can be deduced that the mole fraction of a gas will be proportional to its partial pressure.

The general gas equation for an ideal gas disregards the mutual attractions of the gas molecules and also the volume of the actual molecules. Van der Waals proposed the relationship

$$\left(P + \frac{a}{V^2}\right)(V - b) = RT$$

where a accounts for the attractive forces between the molecules and b for their volume. This second constant has been shown to be related to the activity of certain anaesthetic drugs. This is consistent with the view that their mode of action is related to the physical size of the gas molecule which fits into the cell membrane and so lowers the membrane's permeability.

Van der Waals' equation roughly fits the behaviour of real gases above their critical temperature (that is the temperature below which it is possible to liquefy a gas by increasing the pressure; a gas below the critical temperature is conventionally referred to as a vapour).

As a vapour is compressed it becomes saturated — the pressure reaches the saturated vapour pressure. If the volume is further reduced, condensation will occur, and pressure will rise sharply above the saturated vapour pressure. Any further small changes in volume will result in very high pressure due to the incompressibility of liquids (Fig. 1.22).

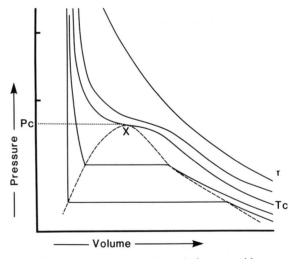

Fig. 1.22 Pressure–volume isothermals for a gas with critical temperature, Tc, critical pressure, Pc and critical point, X.

Inhalational anaesthetic drugs are usually volatile liquids whose vapours possess anaesthetic properties. When a liquid is placed in a closed container, molecules within the liquid moving with sufficiently high velocity towards the surface are able to escape and become vapour. As these fast-moving molecules escape from the surface of the liquid, the average kinetic energy of the remaining liquid falls. The molecules in the vapour phase, if they are unable to escape from the container, may eventually collide with the surface and become liquid again. When the number of molecules leaving the liquid equals the number returning in the same time (a dynamic equilibrium being set up) the vapour is said to be saturated. If the temperature of the liquid is increased the average kinetic energy of the molecules will be increased, with the result that more will be able to escape into the vapour phase (the concentration of molecules in the vapour phase, and the saturated vapour pressure will increase). When the kinetic energy of the molecules is high enough so that their vapour pressure is equal to the atmospheric pressure, bubbles of vapour form within the liquid — the liquid boils at the temperature at which its saturated vapour pressure is equal to atmospheric pressure.

The saturated vapour pressure of a liquid depends on the kinetic energy of the molecules in the vapour, and therefore on the temperature, but is independent of the volume of the liquid remaining or the volume of the vapour. The pressure of a cylinder containing a gas liquefied under pressure — such as nitrous oxide or carbon dioxide — cannot be used to estimate the quantity of liquid in the cylinder, because as long as any liquid remains, the pressure will be that of saturated vapour. The amount therefore remaining is usually determined by weighing the cylinder, the weight of the empty cylinder being known.

CHEMICAL BONDING

The action of drugs at the molecular level involves a reaction between the drug molecule and the molecules of the living organism. It is therefore important to understand the binding forces involved between atoms and molecules of both the drug and the molecular sites with which it interacts.

There are two possibilities when atoms come together: the formation of a stable combination, or the failure to combine. If the electron clouds of the two atoms produce an increasing repulsion as the atoms come together, there will be no bonding between them. When, however, the electrons are attracted not merely to their own nucleus, but also to that of the other atom,

there will be an attraction between the two atoms with the overlap of their electron clouds and the formation of a bond.

When two atoms share a pair of electrons, a covalent bond is formed. This is the familiar strong bond that holds together the atoms of organic molecules. It is not readily broken in biological systems unless a catalytic agent — an enzyme — intervenes. The covalent binding of a drug to the site of action, unlike most drug-receptor interactions, will result in a long-lasting effect, such as the inhibition of the cholinesterase enzymes by organic phosphates and carbamates.

Should both electrons of the electron pair forming the bond be donated by the same atom, a dative covalent or co-ordinate bond is formed. This type of bond binds metal atoms in biological complexes where the donor atom is frequently nitrogen, oxygen or sulphur. The four nitrogen atoms in the porphyrin nucleus, for example, can co-ordinate many different metal atoms, such as iron in the haem proteins, magnesium in chlorophyll or cobalt in vitamin B_{12}.

When two atoms in a bond have different electron affinities there will be unequal sharing of the electrons. In the hydrogen halides HF, HCl, HBr and HI, for example, the displacement of the electrons is from the electropositive hydrogen atom towards the electronegative halide atoms. The bond is therefore polarized, one end of the molecule having a small positive charge and the other a small negative charge — a dipole is formed.

$$\overset{\delta^+}{H}\text{———}\overset{\delta^-}{F}$$

In the extreme case the electron can be detached from one atom leaving a positive ion — an anion — and placed on the other atom forming a negative ion — a cation. The resultant ionic bond is due to the electrostatic attraction between the oppositely charged ions. This type of bond is found in inorganic compounds such as sodium chloride or other metal salts.

The distinction between a covalent bond and an ionic bond is not clear-cut. Unless the molecule formed is symmetrical about the covalent bond there will always be a non-uniform distribution of electron density between the two atoms concerned. Polar bonds, therefore, where there is a partial charge transfer from one atom to the other, could be regarded as having both covalent and ionic character.

When a dipole is formed one end of it can attract the opposite charge on a third atom, and so give rise to a dipole ion or dipole–dipole interaction. These weak interactions caused by dipoles are often known collectively as Van der Waals' forces, and are often responsible for the high degree of selectivity of a drug molecule for a specific receptor.

If a hydrogen atom is bonded to a strongly electronegative atom, X, it can be attracted to another electronegative atom, Y, forming a hydrogen bond

$$\overset{\delta^-}{X}\ \overset{\delta^+}{H}\text{————————}\overset{\delta^-}{Y}$$

This bond is considered to be more than the electrostatic dipole interaction already mentioned as the close approach of the two electronegative atoms, X and Y, would indicate that not only the X—H bond but also the H ——— Y bond has some degree of covalent character. The additive effects of several hydrogen bonds can stabilize an interaction considerably, as is demonstrated in DNA where specific hydrogen bonding between complementary base pairs gives rise to the double-helix configuration. In fact the hydrogen bond, although very much weaker than a covalent or ionic bond, could be considered to be one of the most important forces in nature.

SOLUTIONS AND SOLUBILITY

The solubility of a solute in a solvent can be understood in terms of intermolecular forces. In any pure liquid or solid the attractive forces are quite strong (otherwise vaporization would readily occur). When different compounds are mixed, different molecules are forced to come into contact and, if a true solution is to be formed, intermolecular forces must be overcome both in the solute and in the solvent.

As a general rule a solute dissolves most readily in a solvent of comparable polarity. Nonpolar solvents — for example benzene, hexane or carbon tetrachloride — dissolve non-polar compounds such as greases and oils, whereas polar solvents — for example water, methanol or ethanol — will dissolve polar and ionic substances such as sucrose or sodium chloride.

The introduction of an ionic group into what would otherwise be a non-polar molecule will greatly increase the water-solubility of a drug and this may have implications for its use. For example sodium pentobarbitone is water soluble and can be used in injectable form. Pentobarbitone is only slightly soluble in water. There are many other examples.

Large molecules possessing a polar end group such as sodium stearate, $CH_3(CH_2)_{14}COO^-Na^+$ are used in soaps, since their non-polar, hydrophobic (Greek: water-hating), portion aggregates to dissolve non-polar compounds, having their ionic hydrophilic (water-loving) carboxylate end, ---COO$^-$ to the outside surface.

The aggregate may then be dispersed in a polar solvent as tiny colloidal spheres with the carboxylate end at the surface and the hydrocarbon, non-polar chains pointing towards the centre.

PARTITION COEFFICIENT

When a solute, X, dissolves in two solvents, A and B, which are immiscible, the solute particles are in random motion in both solvents and are capable of passing through the interface from one solvent to the other. The rate at which the solute passes from the first solvent, A, to the second, B, depends on its concentration in the first solvent, $[X_A]$. Similarly the rate at which X passes from B to A depends on $[X_B]$. An equilibrium will be set up when the amount of solute passing from one solvent equals the amount of solute returning from the other, the overall concentration of the solute in each solvent remaining constant.

The ratio of the two concentrations of the solute in the two solvents will be a constant, called the partition or distribution coefficient for that solute in that solvent system

$$K = [X_A]/[X_B]$$

The solvent system need not of course be two liquids, but simply two phases which are immiscible — such as a gas and a liquid — and in which the substance, X, will dissolve.

The distribution of a substance between two phases is important in many circumstances such as the understanding of chromatographic separations or in the uptake and distribution of drugs throughout the body.

By the end of the nineteenth century it had been reported that the potency of an anaesthetic agent corresponded with its partition coefficient between olive oil and water. A better correlation of anaesthetic potency; the octanol/water partition coefficient, has been demonstrated, suggesting that the potency of general anaesthetics is less dependent on their molecular shape, size or chemical nature than the solubility of the anaesthetic molecule at some amphiphilic site in the brain.

EQUILIBRIA

The unusual physical properties of water are a result of extensive hydrogen bonding. Water dissociates to form two ions — the hydronium ion, H_3O^+ and the hydroxide ion, OH^-. An equilibrium is set up

Although it has become the convention for brevity to use the symbol H^+ for the hydronium ion, it must be emphasized that protons do not exist 'bare' in water, but occur only in hydrated form. Indeed the hydronium ion, as also the hydroxide ion and water molecule itself, is further hydrated through additional hydrogen bonding.

In the above reaction, equilibrium is set up when the two reactions, the dissociation and recombination, occur simultaneously. In theory every chemical reaction is reversible; the equilibrium of some reactions, however, lies too far to one side for the reverse reaction to be detectable. When reactions attain equilibrium no further net change in the composition of the reaction mixture occurs. In the general equation

$$A + B \rightleftharpoons C + D$$

the equilibrium constant, K, is defined,

$$K = [C][D]/[A][B]$$

where the brackets indicate concentration (in moles per litre, M).

In many reactions the molecular concentrations of the reactants can be considered to approximate to the effective concentration, or the active concentration, taking part. The active mass of a substance is only equal to its molecular concentration if there is no interaction or interference between the molecules concerned. In chemical systems which do not approach the 'ideal' state, and where there is an appreciable degree of interaction, the molecular concentration has to be multiplied by an activity coefficient to obtain the effective active mass. In principle, therefore, the activity of a substance should be considered and not the concentration. However, in the following discussion the activity coefficient will be regarded as unity — the activity will be taken as being equal to the molecular concentration.

The equilibrium constant for the dissociation of water is therefore

$$K = [H_3O^+] [OH^-]/[H_2O]^2$$

As the concentration of water in pure water is obviously very high (number of grams of H_2O in a litre divided by its gram molecular weight, or $1000/18 = 55.5$ M) and the concentration of H_3O^+ and OH^- ions are very low in comparison (1×10^{-7} M at 25°C) the molar concentration of H_2O is not significantly changed by the slight ionization, and therefore

$$(55.5)^2 K = [H_3O^+][OH^-]$$

This expression can be further rewritten by replacing the term '$(55.5)^2 K$' by a new constant, K_W, the ionic product of water,

$$K_W = [H_3O^+] [OH^-]$$

The value of K_W at 25°C is 1.0×10^{-14}. In an acid solution the H_3O^+ activity is relatively high and the OH^- activity correspondingly low; in a basic solution the situation is reversed.

The pH of a solution is defined as the negative logarithm (to the base 10) of the hydronium ion activity,

$$pH = -\log_{10} [H_3O^+]$$

similarly for the hydroxide ion activity

$$pOH = -\log_{10} [OH^-]$$

for water at 25°C the ionic product can be written,

$$K_w = 1.0 \times 10^{-14} = [H_3O^+][OH^-]$$
Taking logs,
$$\log_{10} 1.0 \times 10^{-14} = \log_{10} [H_3O^-] + \log_{10} [OH^-]$$
$$14 = pH + pOH$$

In a precisely neutral solution at 25°C,

$$[H_3O^+] = [OH] = 1.0 \times 10^{-7}$$
$$pH = pOH = 7.0$$

It is important to note that the pH scale is logarithmic and not arithmetic — a solution of pH 2 has ten times the hydrogen ion activity of a solution of pH 3.

ACIDS AND BASES — THE HENDERSON–HASSELBALCH EQUATION

There are many definitions of acids and bases applicable to non-aqueous and aqueous solutions. According to the Bronsted–Lowry concept an acid is a donor of hydrogen ions (protons) and a base is a proton acceptor. Ammonia (NH_3) and the acetate ion, CH_3COO^- are bases, whereas the ammonium ion, NH_4^+, and acetic acid, CH_3COOH, are Bronsted–Lowry acids. Most acids and bases are weak electrolytes, being only partially ionized in aqueous solution

$$CH_3COOH, \rightleftharpoons CH_3COO^- + H^+,$$
$$NH_4^+ \rightleftharpoons NH_3 + H^+$$
$$Acid \rightleftharpoons Base + Proton$$

A weak acid of the type HA will dissociate to produce a hydrogen ion and its conjugate base A^-

$$HA \rightleftharpoons H^+ + A^-$$

The equilibrium constant will in this case also be the ionisation or dissociation constant of the acid, Ka

$$Ka = [H^+] [A^-]/[HA]$$
$$\log Ka = \log_{10} [H^+] + \log_{10} [A^-] - \log_{10} [HA]$$
$$pKa = pH - \log_{10} [A^-] + \log_{10} [HA]$$

where pKa is defined as the negative logarithm to the base 10 of the dissociation constant of the acid. It reflects the degree of ionization of an acid, being small for strong acids and large for strong bases. As A^- is the proton acceptor (base) and HA is the proton donor (acid) the above equation may be rewritten in the more general form

$pKa = pH - \log_{10}$ [proton acceptor] $+ \log_{10}$ [proton donor]

$$pH = pKa + \log_{10} \frac{[\text{proton acceptor}]}{[\text{proton donor}]}$$

This is known as the Henderson–Hasselbalch equation, and is fundamental to quantitative calculations of acid–base equilibrium in biological systems.

When a system is in equilibrium it will resist any attempt to change the position of equilibrium (Le Chatelier's Principle). This can be understood by considering the general equilibrium.

$$A + B \rightleftharpoons C + D$$
$$\text{and } K = [C][D]/[A][B]$$

If the activity of 'C' should be increased, 'D' will react with it to form more 'A' and 'B' so that the overall value of 'K' and the position of the equilibrium will be unchanged.

BUFFERED SOLUTIONS

Buffered solutions resist changes in $[H^+]$ that would result from the addition of an acid or base. A buffer solution contains a weak acid (or weak base) and its salt

formed from a strong base (or strong acid), for example acetic acid and sodium acetate.

$$CH_3COONa \rightleftharpoons CH_3COO^- + Na^+$$
$$CH_3COOH \rightleftharpoons CH_3COO^- + H^+$$

Sodium acetate is a strong electrolyte, being completely ionized in solution, whereas acetic acid will be only partially dissociated. If a strong acid is added to this buffer system its hydrogen ions will react with acetate ions (of which the main source is sodium acetate) until the equilibrium conditions are again reached. The overall effect will be that the hydrogen ion activity will change only slightly. The pH of the buffer solution can be calculated using the Henderson–Hasselbalch equation if the pKa value of the weak acid is known. The proton acceptor would be the acetate ion and the proton donor the acetic acid, which may be assumed to be undissociated and contributing very few acetate ions — even less than in the absence of sodium acetate. The Henderson–Hasselbalch equation for buffered solutions may then be rewritten,

$$pH = pK_a + \log_{10} \frac{[\text{salt}]}{[\text{acid}]}$$

The relationship between the degree of ionization of a drug, its pKa value and the pH of the solution in which it is dissolved can be written:

$$pH = pKa + \log_{10} \frac{[\text{unionized drug}]}{[\text{ionized drug}]}$$

and is important in pharmacokinetics in determining the rates of passage of drugs across body membranes.

2. Pharmacodynamics

W. McCaughey

The major goal in clinical pharmacology is to understand how the administration of a drug in a particular way may lead to a particular therapeutic action. The study of this has led to the development of two disciplines — pharmacokinetics, and pharmacodynamics.

Study of the absorption, distribution and metabolism of a drug (pharmacokinetics) can often predict remarkably well how the drug concentration at its site of action will vary. This, however, will still not predict the magnitude or time-course of the effect, and the study of how the concentration of drug at its site of action is related to its therapeutic effect is known as pharmacodynamics. In brief, pharmacokinetics is the effect of the patient on the drug, while pharmacodynamics is the effect of the drug on the patient.

In this chapter the basic mechanisms of drug action — the pharmacodynamics — will be considered, and the principles of pharmacokinetics will be described in Chapter 3.

THE CELL MEMBRANE

An understanding of the structure of cell membranes is important, as most of the vital processes of the cell occur at membranes, either the plasma membrane (often simply called the cell membrane) or one of the internal membranes, for example in mitochondria. Virtually all sites at which drugs or endogenous hormones act are at these membranes. Among other functions, the plasma membrane contains structures which actively maintain a difference in concentration of electrolytes such as sodium, potassium and other ions between the intracellular and extracellular spaces, and others responsible for the electrical excitability necessary for nerve conduction, etc.

The membrane is a complex structure which is not simply a container, but is able and necessary to actively maintain the differences in concentration of substances between the inside and outside of the cell, as well as having other functions. It is composed of proteins, lipids and carbohydrates, in what may be described as a fluid mosaic (Singer & Nicholson 1972). The lipids (phospholipids in all cells, together with cholesterol in mammalian plasma membranes) form a bilayer in which the hydrophilic ends of the molecules, containing polar and ionic groups, are outward, while the hydrophobic, non-polar fatty acid chains are inward, away from contact with water (see also Ch. 6, p. 87 and Fig. 6.2). Lipids are by far the most numerous molecules in the membrane, but proteins, being much larger molecules, make up roughly an equal part by mass, while carbohydrate is a minor constituent. Proteins are of two types. Integral proteins are embedded in the phospholipid bilayer, and extend through both surfaces, so that part of the molecule is exposed on each side. As with lipids they have hydrophilic and hydrophobic regions; the hydrophilic ends are exposed, while the hydrophobic regions are hidden in the hydrophobic core of the membrane.

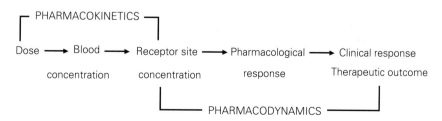

Fig. 2.1 Schematic representation of principal factors involved in drug dosage and response. (Togoni et al 1980.)

Peripheral proteins, which make up 30% of the membrane proteins, are water-soluble, and each is bound to an integral protein. The membrane is asymmetrical, both in terms of lipids and proteins. Thus the integral proteins are inserted into the membrane the correct way round during assembly of the membrane (Lodish & Rothman 1979) — obviously necessary if ion pumps, etc., are to function correctly; while the differences in composition of the two parts of the lipid layer may be simply due to a passive thermodynamic equilibrium.

The integral proteins have several functions — for example they may serve as antigens, as receptors, as channels for movement of water-soluble substances, etc.

Protein molecules consist of many thousands of atoms, but they are made up of a small number of basic modules — the 20 naturally occurring amino acids, which are joined end-to-end to form the protein macromolecule. The protein chain folds into a more compact shape, which is determined by the sequence in which the amino acids occur. This shape is well defined, and it controls the biological properties of the molecule because of the way in which it brings certain crucial parts of the macromolecule into close juxtaposition. Such complex protein molecules can be very specific in their interaction with small molecules whose structure is in some way complementary to that of a region of the protein molecule.

When the interaction is an essential link in a natural control mechanism, the macromolecule is commonly termed a 'receptor'. When the interaction is coincidental, although it may still be very specific, the macromolecule is said to provide a 'binding site'. When the interaction is part of a metabolic or degradative or synthetic process, the macromolecule is an enzyme (Goodford 1981).

Receptors

The concept that drugs might act at specific receptor sites has been familiar since it was first expressed by Langley in 1905. In the past decade it has changed from hypothesis to scientific fact, as receptor molecules begin to be identified and their structure analysed. It is now believed that all endogenous hormones or neurotransmitters act through their own receptors, and an increasing range of exogenous substances — drugs — are being found to act by mimicking or modifying these actions.

In its full sense a receptor must have two properties. Firstly it must react fairly specifically with a small effector molecule — hormone or drug, and secondly it must have the ability to respond to this interaction in such a way as to influence the biological system in which it is situated — to pass on a message. Most of the receptor sites which fulfil these criteria are found in cell plasma membranes. There are also some sites (defined above as binding sites) which bind with the drug or other substance without initiating any action — an example is the binding of drugs to plasma proteins for transport — and these sites may be called secondary or silent receptors, or storage sites. Binding of substances to such sites can often be distinguished from binding to specific receptors because it lacks the stereospecificity of the latter.

The purpose of receptors is intercellular communication. The majority of receptors are integral proteins in the cell membrane. On arrival at the surface of a responsive cell, most intercellular messages, including those from neurotransmitters, antigens and many hormones (other than steroids and thyroid hormones which are lipid-soluble and enter the cell directly), are read and interpreted by receptor sites exposed on the surface of the cell membrane. A mechanism then exists to translate this message into a language understandable within the cell.

Receptor structure

Several receptors have now been isolated. They are protein structures of MW approximately 250 000–400 000, but made up of a number of smaller subunits of MW 25 000–60 000. The subunits are not identical, although there may be more than one of each type. Presumably each subunit has a different function.

Although the three-dimensional shape of a protein is clearly defined and fairly rigid, it is capable of conformational change when it interacts with another molecule, or in some cases when there is a change in electrical charge. Thus when a message is received at the receptor site, which is on the outer surface of one of the protein subunits of the receptor group, there is a change in the shape of this molecule, and this leads to changes in the other members of the group.

In some cases the receptor site is directly coupled to an ionophore — a channel in the membrane through which ions may pass. An example of this is the nicotinic acetylcholine receptor, which forms part of the endplate channel, a fairly large and relatively unselective opening which allows sodium and other cations to enter the cell rapidly, thus depolarizing the membrane.

In most cases, however, the signal is relayed to the mechanisms within the cell by a 'second messenger' (Nathanson & Greengard 1977).

The ultimate effect of the signal following this pathway is to regulate a cellular process such as secretion, contraction, metabolism or growth. The second messenger may sometimes act directly, by binding to a protein and changing its shape — for example in skeletal muscle calcium binds to troponin-C and leads to muscle contraction. More often the second messenger molecule binds to an enzyme, and this phosphorylates a protein, which causes it to change its shape to an active form.

Such a system in which one enzyme catalyses the modification of another enzyme or protein is described as an enzyme cascade. A cascade may be unidirectional (e.g. the clotting cascade), or cyclic. In cyclic cascades two opposing cascades are coupled, one catalysing the modification and the other the 'demodification' of an interconvertible enzyme. In fact the entire spectrum of cellular activities is regulated by cyclic cascade systems, including hormonal and neurotransmitter responses, protein synthesis, energy metabolism, muscle contraction and many others (Schacter et al 1988).

Communication within the cell

The details of the 'second messenger' systems which serve to link the action of a ligand binding to a receptor on the cell surface, to changes within the cell, are complicated and still poorly understood (Berridge 1985, Rasmussen 1986).

Three main types of response are known, and these are often interrelated.

1. Calcium

A common response is the opening of calcium channels in the plasma membrane. For example in the synaptic terminal of a nerve this occurs in response to the voltage change caused by a nerve signal arriving. As the intracellular Ca^{2+} concentration is approximately 10 000 times lower than the extracellular, influx of extracellular calcium rapidly raises the intracellular Ca^{2+} level and initiates a response — in this case the release of acetylcholine. Calcium may also be released from the sarcolemma of muscle cells in the same way, or from the internal stores of the endoplasmic reticulum as related below. Calcium passes on its message by binding to the specific receptor protein calmodulin, or in muscle to troponin-C.

2. Adenyl cyclase

This is a major pathway used by many hormones — for example catecholamines. When the drug or hormone — e.g. isoprenaline — arrives at the cell surface, it attaches to its receptor site. This is a protein subunit which protrudes from the outer surface of the membrane, and the receptor area may be composed of a grouping of glycosylated amino acids (i.e. with sugars attached), toward the amino-terminal end of the integral membrane protein. At the cytoplasmic surface of the membrane is a part of a protein subunit which includes the enzyme

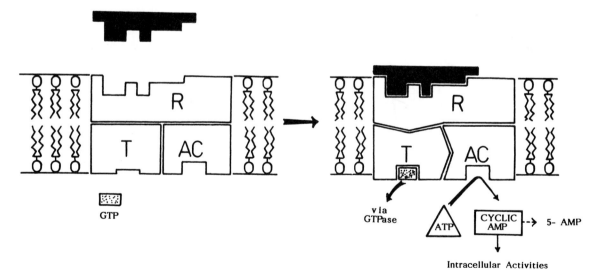

Fig. 2.2 Schematic representation of the components of a typical receptor complex. Binding of the transmitter molecule (dark shape) to the receptor (R) results in a conformational change. This leads through an intermediate GTP-dependent component (T) to activation of adenylate cyclase (AC), which is on the inner surface of the cell membrane. The enzyme then converts some of the ATP in the cytoplasm into cyclic AMP, which relays the signal from the membrane to the interior of the cell.

adenylate cyclase. These two parts are coupled by a third protein subunit (a G-protein), which is dependent on GTP in the cytoplasm for its function. Binding of the drug or hormone to its receptor site causes the protein to change its shape as it folds around the drug molecule. This in turn changes the shape of the intermediate G-protein (provided that it has been 'switched on' by GTP), and in turn this leads to activation of adenylate cyclase and formation of cyclic AMP. This process is probably terminated by removal of GTP by GTPase (Fig. 2.2). The adenylate cyclase is also linked to inhibitory receptors by a similar pathway through an inhibitory G-protein. Thus the first result of the interaction of a drug or hormone with the receptor site on the outside of the cell membrane is an increase (or decrease) in cyclic AMP within the cell. The cAMP then initiates the next stage — for example by binding to a cytoplasmic protein known as A-kinase, it activates this, which then carries out phosphorylation of enzymes.

The cycle is then completed as cAMP is degraded by phosphodiesterase to adenosine monophosphate (AMP). cAMP levels may be affected by drugs which inhibit the action of phosphodiesterase. These may be selective for PDE in one particular tissue, (for example methylxanthines are used as bronchodilators, enoximone as a cardiac inotrope). Four major classes of phosphodiesterase exist with different specificities for cAMP and cGMP, and different allosteric regulators. These are known as Type I, II, III and IV phosphodiesterase respectively (Kincaid and Manganiello 1988).

3. Inositol triphosphate

The lipids of the cell membrane are not simply inert structural components. Phosphatidylinositol is a minor lipid existing mainly on the inner leaflet of the bilayer. Receptors are, as in the adenyl cyclase system, coupled by G-protein intermediates to an enzyme, phosphodiesterase in this case, on the inner surface of the membrane. Phosphodiesterase cleaves the phosphorylated form of the lipid, phosphatidylinositol, to produce inositol triphosphate (IP_3) and diacylglycerol (DG). IP_3 then acts as a second messenger, releasing calcium from the endoplasmic reticulum and so raising the intracellular Ca^{2+} concentration. In many cells this then binds to calmodulin, and this process then leads to activation of a phosphorylase enzyme.

However, some cells have a sustained response to a stimulus; for example the regulation of aldosterone production by angiotensin II. When angiotensin II binds to its receptor there is a rise in intracellular IP_3 and in Ca^{2+} as described above. However, the intracellular Ca^{2+} level soon returns to normal, yet the cell continues to secrete aldosterone. The changes associated with this involve the diacylglycerol released with IP_3. This associates with a membrane protein known as C-kinase,

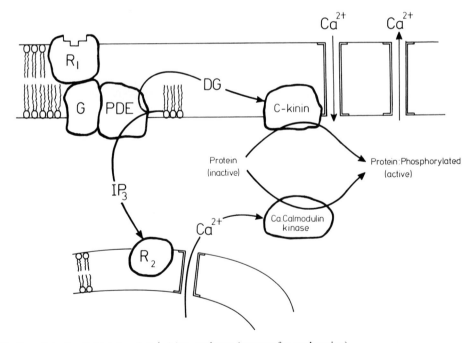

Fig. 2.3 Outline of the inositol triphosphate/calcium pathway (see text for explanation).

which controls aldosterone production. During the sustained phase of cellular response, calcium continues to enter the cell rapidly, although efflux is equally rapid so that the Ca^{2+} level is not raised, and the C-kinase is in some way activated by this calcium flow — not by a raised Ca^{2+} level.

These three second messenger systems can operate independently, but in many cases more than one may regulate one cellular activity. This may involve one modulating the activity of another, or the simultaneous action of two or more in parallel.

Ion channels

Central channels occur in many of the integral proteins, or more accurately between the individual subunits of the protein group, and these form pores through which ions or other substances in aqueous solution may pass when the channel opens in response to the appropriate stimulus. Some respond to changes in membrane potential, and are described as voltage gated, others are regulated by extracellular neurotransmitter molecules and hormones, and many indirectly by intracellular second-messenger systems as described above.

Figure 2.4 shows the functional components of a voltage gated ionic channel. This is a large glycoprotein molecule extending through the membrane. A constriction, narrow enough to touch ions and so distinguish between them, acts as a selectivity filter. However it may not be completely selective – for example the sodium channel with a constriction to 3 nm × 5 nm (Armstrong 1981) will also admit other small cations such as lithium. A 'gate' at the inner end of the channel is opened and closed by a conformational change in the molecule, caused in this case by movement of electrical charges. The channel can be either open or closed — there is no intermediate state. When opened the sodium channel remains open for about 1 millisecond, during which about 100 sodium ions flow through (Keynes 1979). The channel is then closed by a further change at an 'inactivation gate' deeper within the channel, and it then remains in an inactive or refractory state until returning to its original closed conformation. The inactivation receptor deep within the channel may also be acted on by substances such as local anaesthetics or pancuronium. The potassium channel differs in that there is a delay before opening. The voltage-dependent permeability of the membrane, which is the physical basis of cell electrical excitability, is due to these events at sodium and potassium channels.

Because only a few ions need flow through the

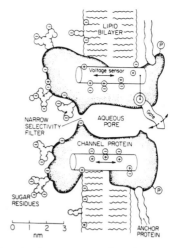

Fig. 2.4 Functional components of a voltage-gated ionic channel. The channel is a large glycoprotein molecule, containing a narrow selectivity filter which touches ions and can distinguish between them. Voltage sensors have collections of charges that are moved by the electric field to open and close the pore — 'gating'. This drawing which is reproduced with permission from Hille (1988), is fanciful and mostly represents ideas obtained by electrophysiological approaches.

channel to cause a depolarisation, many action potentials can be propagated before the normal ionic gradients are affected and need to be replenished by Na^+ and K^+ active transport.

The calcium channel (Lai et al 1988) is, as described in the previous section, a vital component of many communication processes in the body. Opening of an ion channel may also occur in response to the interaction of a molecule with the receptor site which is coupled to the ionophore. For example, within the CNS, GABA receptor sites are linked to chloride channels, and the action of GABA is to increase chloride conductance. These receptor sites are also linked to sites at which benzodiazepines act (Ch. 11).

Other channels may be less selective. For example endplate channels at the neuromuscular junction, whose opening is 6.5 × 6.5/nm (Adams et al 1980) are permeable to several different cations. These channels which form part of the acetylcholine receptor, are proteins of MW 250 000–270 000 (Raftery et al 1980).

All these ion channels allow a passive movement of ions along the concentration gradient. The difference in Na^+ and K^+ concentration between extracellular and intracellular fluids is maintained by a Na^+, K^+ pump which is energy-dependent, and which actively exchanges Na^+ and K^+ ions across the membrane, in approximately the ratio of a 3 Na : 2 K. This pump is also an integral protein structure of the cell membrane. Its action may be depressed by the action of digitalis and other cardiac glycosides.

DRUG ACTION AT RECEPTORS

Receptor sites are designed for intercellular communication, and are acted on by endogenous substances. They become drug receptors when an exogenous substance, a drug, is found which also has an affinity for the site. This implies a similarity in structure between the drug and its natural counterpart, at least in the region which interacts with the receptor site, but the rest of the molecules may be very different. A good example is the contrasting chemistry of the enkephalins which are polypeptides, and morphine, an unrelated plant alkaloid. Here the benzene ring A of morphine and a benzene ring in the tyrosine group of enkephalin are in exactly the same orientation (Snyder 1977; see Ch. 13), so that their molecules can fit the same protein template.

When the drug or endogenous transmitter binds to a pharmacologically active receptor site, then it changes the receptor, and this initiates a sequence of events leading to the drug's characteristic action. Usually binding is reversible, and so an equilibrium is set up. This can be represented as:

$$\text{Drug (D)} + \text{receptor (R)} \underset{K_2}{\overset{K_1}{\rightleftharpoons}} \text{drug–receptor complex (DR)} \rightarrow \text{effect}$$

where K_1 and K_2 are rate constants for the association and dissociation of drug and receptor. In this simple model, drug effect is proportional to the fraction of receptor occupied, and maximal effect will occur when all the receptors are occupied.

Affinity

Affinity is the ability of the drug to bind to the receptor site and form a stable complex. The relative affinity (R_A) of the drug for the receptors may be defined as the concentration required to produce half the maximal effect. However, this is a simplification as other steps — e.g. second messengers, may be involved, and be the limiting factor in the initiation of action.

Affinity is often represented by an IC_{50} value, which is the concentration producing 50% inhibition of the binding of a highly selective ligand. There is a high correlation between the IC_{50} of a drug and its potency.

Dose–response curves

When the dose of a drug is plotted against the effect obtained, as shown in Figure 2.5(a), then a dose-response curve can be constructed. This is approximately a rectangular hyperbola. It is more usual to graph log dose versus effect, which allows a greater range of doses to be represented, and this gives the familiar sigmoid curve, shown in Figure 2.5(b).

Efficacy or intrinsic activity

The efficacy, or maximal efficacy, of a drug is simply the maximum effect which it is capable of producing, and it is represented by the plateau of the dose–response curve (although in some cases it may be limited by other factors, such as the ability to deliver a sufficient drug concentration to the receptor sites). The use of these terms is restricted to drugs with agonist actions.

Potency

The potency of a drug is an expression of the position of the dose–response curve along the dose axis. Thus two drugs (for example morphine and fentanyl) might have similar efficacy, but the potency of one — expressed as mg kg^{-1} required to produce a given effect — might be many times greater than that of the other.

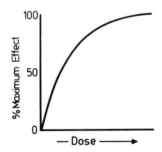 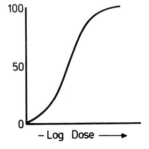

Fig. 2.5 Dose–response curves for a drug plotted on (a) linear and (b) semilogarithmic scales.

A difference in potency of two drugs is of itself not important, unless the actual mass of drug to be given is so large that it causes problems in administration.

It is often useful to compare two drugs by their relative potency — the ratio of equi-effective doses. This apparently simple concept will work well for similar drugs, which have parallel dose–response curves, but if this is not so, as in some of the cases described below, then the relative potencies of the two drugs will be different at different dose levels (Fig. 2.7).

Agonists and antagonists

When a drug binds to a receptor, the subsequent sequence of events may be complex, but for the sake of the following argument it will be assumed that the important change is that the receptor moves from an inactive to an active state. An equilibrium state exists (Fig. 2.6). When no drug is present, the receptor tends to be in the inactive state (R). If the drug (D) binds to the receptor and has a higher affinity for the active (R_a) than the inactive configuration of the receptor (which is another way of saying that it activates the receptor), then the equilibrium moves toward the active state — towards the bottom right-hand corner in Figure 2.6. Thus the drug, by associating with the receptor, will

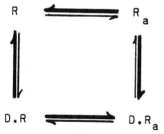

Fig. 2.6 Drug–receptor equilibria.

activate it and initiate a response in the effector tissue. This is described as agonist activity. Pure agonist drugs have high intrinsic activity or efficacy.

Partial agonists

If a drug binds to the receptor, but has only slightly greater affinity for the active than the inactive state of the receptor, then even in high concentration it will not cause all the receptor sites to be activated, and thus the maximal effect of the drug will be less. Such a drug may be referred to as a partial agonist, in contrast to the drug whose affinity is strongly in favour of the active receptor, and which is referred to simply as an agonist. It may also be said that the partial agonist has a lower intrinsic activity or efficacy than the agonist drug.

Antagonists

A drug which has no preference for R or R_a, or one which encourages the inactive state, will act as an antagonist, by competing with an agonist for receptor sites.

This type of antagonism is known as competitive antagonism. Antagonism may also be non-competitive, where the antagonist inactivates the receptor so that an agonist cannot combine with it in such a way as to cause activation. Such competition may be reversible or irreversible.

A partial agonist, by binding to receptors but failing to produce a maximal response, can act as a competitive antagonist to a full agonist, and for this reason some such drugs are also referred to as agonist–antagonists. The opioid agonist–antagonists are discussed in Chapter 13.

Dose–response curves are useful in determining some of the characteristics of a drug. Two drugs of similar efficacy but differing in potency will have parallel

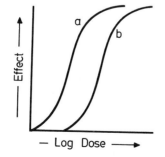
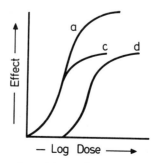

Fig. 2.7 and 2.8 The effects of differing potency and of partial agonist activity on dose–response curves (see text for explanation).

curves, as in Figure 2.7, where drug (b) is of lower potency. A common example would be morphine and fentanyl, each capable of producing the same degree of analgesia, but at very different milligram doses. The same displacement of the dose–response curve to the right would be seen in the presence of a competitive antagonist. In this case, the potency of the drug (a) is reduced, so that it follows curve (b), but it is still able to achieve its maximum effect if given in sufficient concentration.

A different situation occurs if the drug is unable to obtain the maximum effect from the system. This might occur if a non-competitive antagonist had removed some of the receptor potential from the system (for example by binding irreversibly with them), or if the drug is by nature a partial agonist. In this case, as compared with the normal response to a full agonist (curve a), the maximal response is depressed (Fig. 2.8c). Thus the potency of the drug, at least over the lower part of the dose range, is relatively unchanged, but the maximal efficacy is reduced. A useful quantifiable parameter in studying drug–receptor interaction, particularly when several receptors may be involved, as with the opioids, is the pA_2. This is the negative logarithm of the concentration (in vitro), or dose (in vivo), of antagonist (usually naloxone) which doubles the concentration of drug necessary to produce a particular level of response. If a series of agonists acts on the same receptor, then, though a different concentration of each may be required to produce the same effect, the pA_2 will be the same. Studies examining the antagonism by naloxone of the analgesia produced by a wide variety of μ-agonist opioids including morphine and β-endorphin give uniform pA_2 values of approximately 7. In contrast the pA_2 value with DADL, a δ-receptor agonist, is approximately 6, that is it takes ten times more naloxone to antagonize DADL than does morphine. This suggests that these two classes of agents act on different receptor populations for which naloxone has differing affinities.

OTHER FACTORS IN DRUG RESPONSE

Drugs do not all act as has been implied in this simplified description of drug action, by a single action occurring at a single receptor site. More than one receptor type or subtype may be involved, and many other factors come into play, so that actual dose–response curves may differ widely from those shown above. The opioids again provide a good example of drugs which produce similar and also different effects at different receptors, and the several opioid receptor types are discussed in Chapter 13.

Some drugs act by mechanisms not involving active receptor sites, for example by competing for transport systems, or by purely physical effects, like osmotic diuretics.

The clinical usefulness of the drug may be influenced by some other features of its action.

Selectivity

Selectivity, the ability of the drug to produce its desired effect with a minimum of other undesired or side-effects, is important in this context.

Therapeutic index

Therapeutic index is a measure of the safety of the drug in normal use. It is a ratio of the dose of the drug which produces the desired effect, to the dose which produces an important toxic effect. If the slope of the dose–response curve is steep, then increasing the dose will more easily raise the effect to levels where toxic effects can arise, so that the drug must be treated more carefully.

VARIATION IN RESPONSE

Normal distribution

Individual patients vary in their response to a drug, and the same patient may exhibit a different response on different occasions. This can be seen either as different responses to the same dose, or as different doses being required to produce the same response. In either case the variation between individuals can be seen almost always to follow the usual normal distribution or Gaussian curve of variation (Fig. 2.9a) when, for example, the number of individuals having each degree of response is plotted. This simply represents the random differences between people, as would be found with height, weight, etc.

ED_{50}, LD_{50}

When different doses of the drug are given, and a certain endpoint sought, a dose can be found when half the individuals produce the effect sought. The dose at which 50% of individuals show a specified effect is the median effective dose, or ED_{50}. The dose to produce an effect in a different percentage of individuals could also be estimated. In animal testing of drugs the dose to produce a toxic effect in 50% of individuals is also used — if the endpoint is death, this is the median lethal dose or LD_{50}. The therapeutic index can then be defined as the ratio of these:

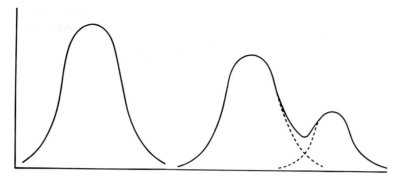

Fig. 2.9 (a) Continuous or Gaussian distribution; (b) discontinuous or bimodal distribution.

$$\text{Therapeutic index} = \frac{LD_{50}}{ED_{50}}$$

In some situations another toxic effect might be used to define toxicity – for example in testing a respiratory stimulant, the ratio of the dose to produce a therapeutic degree of stimulation, and that to cause convulsions. The therapeutic index of a drug is important in determining its safety in use, and is a useful comparison between drugs.

Pharmacogenetics

Some of the variation between individuals is genetically determined. This may be pharmacodynamic in origin — a variation in responsiveness to the drugs, leading to the normal Gaussian distribution curve described above (Fig. 2.9a). More of the important variations are pharmacokinetic — there is an altered handling of the drug by the body. When the distribution of responses is examined in some of these cases, it can be seen that there exist two (or more) distinct populations, which behave differently in response to the drug, and which also have a normal variation within each population (Fig. 2.9b).

Such different populations are likely to be due to genetic polymorphism — and the different populations are maintained from one generation to the next by inheritance of different genes. A common example of this is that drug acetylation in the liver may proceed at a slow or a fast rate, and that patients can be divided into two populations of 'slow acetylators' and 'fast acetylators'. This is of clinical significance with a drug such as isoniazid, which is metabolized in this way, and which must be given in very different doses to the two groups of patients.

A classical example in anaesthetic practice is the rare occurrence of an abnormal response to suxamethonium,

resulting in abnormally prolonged paralysis and apnoea. There are several variants of the cholinesterase enzyme which breaks down suxamethonium, and these are genetically determined. Among individuals who are homozygous for the normal enzyme (Ch_1^u, Ch_1^u), i.e. who are apparently genetically normal people, about 1 in 3200 is moderately sensitive to suxamethonium, and these are probably individuals whose response is near the extreme limit of the normal range of distribution. Of those who are homozygous for the commonest abnormal cholinesterase (Ch_1^D, Ch_1^D) — 1 in 2800 of the population, all are markedly sensitive to suxamethonium, and these form a separate group (Fig. 2.9b). Those who are homozygous for other abnormal variants of the enzyme, and the various heterozygotes, all form separate, though probably overlapping, populations in terms of their response to suxamethonium.

While the last two examples are of altered pharmacokinetics, a dramatic instance of genetically determined alteration in response to drugs is the malignant hyperthermia syndrome. In this the inheritance is more complicated; it is inherited as an autosomal dominant trait with variable expression and incomplete penetrance. Due probably to an abnormality of calcium binding to muscle cell membranes, certain drugs including halothane and suxamethonium trigger off a massive and often fatal hyperthermic response.

Other clinically relevant examples of genetically determined conditions in which there is an altered response to drug therapy include the porphyrias, and some of the conditions due to haemoglobin variants.

Factors modifying the degree of response to drugs

While there is inherently a variability in the response of patients to drugs, some factors can be identified, and when they are taken into account, the dosage of drug can be better tailored to the patient's needs. Not all are relevant to anaesthetic practice, but some are described in the following section.

Psychological factors

These include the willingness and ability of the patient to take the prescribed drug, and of the nurse or doctor to prescribe and administer the drug appropriately and accurately. These medication errors are in practice extremely common.

The placebo response is also important in many cases, the response to the drug being modified by the patient's mental attitude, so that a response can be obtained from an inert substance, or an exaggerated response obtained from an active drug. For this reason many clinical trials to test the efficacy of a drug must use a protocol which assesses or eliminates the placebo response. A variant of this type of response is seen in the fact that it has been shown that a preoperative visit to a patient by his anaesthetist has an equal anxiolytic effect to that produced by administration of a barbiturate (Egbert et al 1963).

Age

The young, particularly the neonate, may differ profoundly from the adult in handling of and response to drugs. In the elderly, too, there are differences, partly due to changes in physiological variables, and partly due to an increased incidence of disease. The influence of age on drug therapy is discussed in Chapter 4.

Body weight and volume of distribution

These are essentially pharmacokinetic factors and are considered elsewhere.

Time of administration

The effect of an orally administered drug may vary considerably depending on whether it is given before, with or after food.

Body rhythms

The influence of circadian or other rhythms on drug treatment is not well known, but may be important — for example the anticoagulant effect of a constant dose of heparin may vary by as much as half between night and morning (Decousus et al 1985), and other drugs might theoretically vary in their effect and toxicity depending on the time of administration.

Physiological and pathological variables

There are marked variations in the response to drug therapy caused either by physiological variations in respiration, cardiac output, blood flow and distribution of blood flow, renal function, etc, or by changes in these and similar variables caused by acute or chronic disease. Some of these are discussed in Chapter 4.

Tolerance, addiction and sensitivity

The response to a drug does not always remain the same. In some cases a greater response is achieved initially than later – the body becomes tolerant to the effects of the drug. This may take several days or months to occur, or may occur very rapidly in a few seconds or minutes. In the latter case it is known as acute tolerance or tachyphylaxis. Conversely, situations exist in which the response is exaggerated — there is a state of sensitivity or supersensitivity to the drug (the term hypersensitivity is used only to describe conditions of an allergic nature).

Altered sensitivity to a drug may occur by one or several mechanisms. Continued administration may lead to a change in its absorption, or to an increase in its rate of elimination, or there may be a change in its passage to its site of action. Homeostatic mechanisms may compensate for its action — patients taking thyroid hormone may become tolerant to its effects because of feedback effects involving pituitary and thyroid glands. Antibodies may develop, as in some cases of insulin resistance. Some cases may be mixed — tolerance to chronic use of barbiturates or alcohol is partly due to increased drug metabolism, but tolerant individuals will show less response to the drug even when brain levels are identical to those in non-tolerant individuals. There may be cross-tolerance between drugs of similar pharmacological classes.

Altered sensitivity at a cellular level must be the mechanism in many cases, and details are largely speculative. Tolerance, dependence and addiction to opiate drugs occur, related to their mechanism of action on receptors normally occupied by enkephalins. Occupation of the receptor by an opiate may activate a feedback mechanism to reduce the amount of enkephalin, either by reducing the quantity released — for which there is some evidence, or by increasing its rate of breakdown — there is a considerable increase in the enzyme which degrades enkephalin. Thus with lack of endogenous enkephalin at the receptor site, more opiate is needed to replace it — tolerance has occurred. Also when opiate is withdrawn the lack of the inhibitory effect, which activation of the enkephalin receptor causes, is seen as the withdrawal syndrome. This may be due mainly to increased activity of certain noradrenergic neurones in the locus coeruleus region of the brain. The activity of these can be reduced, and the withdrawal syndrome suppressed, by low doses of the antihypertensive drug clonidine.

Some cases of altered sensitivity might be due to a change in the events which occur after the receptor is activated, such as an increase in adenylate cyclase activity. Opioids inhibit the action of adenylate cyclase in normal cells, but after a few days this activity returns to normal. If the opioid is now withdrawn there is a rebound increase in adenylate cyclase activity and of concentrations of cyclic AMP, which could cause the hyperexcitability and other manifestations of a withdrawal syndrome (Sharma et al 1975). Increased sensitivity to a drug or natural transmitter substance may also be due to an increase in the number of receptor molecules. Following denervation of a muscle, it can be shown that the muscle endplate region expands to cover virtually the whole of the muscle fibre, leading to increased sensitivity (and also to the danger of excessive release of intracellular potassium when suxamethonium is administered). An increase in the number of receptor sites can also be found as a result of drug therapy. Long-term treatment with β-adrenergic blocking drugs in rats has been shown to cause an increase in the number of adrenergic receptor sites, and abrupt cessation of these drugs in patients can sometimes lead to cardiac dysrhythmias or myocardial infarction.

Tolerance which develops very rapidly to a drug, so that there is a decreasing response to repeat doses given within a short time, is known as tachyphylaxis. This occurs with several drugs including local anaesthetics. The mechanism of this effect is different with different drugs — for example it occurs to indirectly acting sympathomimetic amines like ephedrine because stores of noradrenaline become depleted. Another phenomenon which develops in an extremely short time, and presumably is due to a change at cellular level, is the acute tolerance seen with barbiturate anaesthetics (Dundee 1956). Patients who receive thiopentone regain consciousness while the blood concentration of thiopentone is still higher than that at which they lost consciousness.

REFERENCES

Adams D J, Dwyer T M, Hille B 1980 The permeability of endplate channels to monovalent and divalent metal cations. Journal of General Physiology 75: 493–510

Armstrong C M 1981 Sodium channels and gating currents. Physiological Reviews 61: 644–683

Berridge M J 1981 Receptors and calcium signalling. In: Lamble J W (ed) Towards understanding receptors Elsevier/North Holland, Amsterdam, pp 122–131

Berridge M 1985 The molecular basis of communication within the cell. Scientific American 253(4): 124–134

Decousus H A, Croze M, Levi F A, Jaubert J G, Perpoint B M, DeBonadona J F, Reinberg A, Queneau P M 1985 Circadian changes in anticoagulant effect of heparin infused at a constant rate. British Medical Journal 290: 341–344

Dundee J W 1956 Thiopentone and other barbiturates. Livingstone, Edinburgh

Egbert L D, Battit G E, Turndorf H, Beecher H K 1963 The value of the preoperative visit by an anaesthetist. Journal of the American Medical Association, 185: 553–555

Goodford P 1981 The haemoglobin molecule: is it a useful model for a drug receptor. In: Lamble J W (ed) Towards understanding receptors. Elsevier/North Holland, Amsterdam, pp 205–216

Hille B. 1988 Ionic channels: Molecular pores of excitable membranes. Harvey Lectures 82: 49–69.

Jakobs K H, Schultz G 1981 Actions of hormones and neurotransmitters at the plasma membrane: inhibition of adenylate cyclase. In: Lamble J W (ed) Towards understanding receptors. Elsevier/North Holland, Amsterdam

Keynes R D 1979 Ion channels in the nerve cell membrane. Scientific American 240(3): 98–107

Kincaid R L, Manganiello V C 1988 Assay of cyclic nucleotide phosphodiesterase using radiolabelled and fluorescent substrates. Methods in Enzymology 159: 457–470

Lai F A, Erickson H P, Rosseau E, Lin Q Y, Meissner G 1988 Purification and reconstitution of the calcium release channel from skeletal muscle. Nature (London) 331: 315–319

Lodish H E, Rothman J E 1979 The assembly of cell membranes. Scientific American, 240(1): 38–53

Marchesi V T 1979 Functional components of surface membranes: potential targets for pharmacological manipulation. Pharmacological Reviews 30: 371–381

Nathanson J A, Greengard P 1977 Second messengers in the brain. Scientific American 237(2): 108–119

Putney J W, Askari A 1980 Modification of membrane function by drugs. In: Andreoli T E, Hoffmann J F, Fanestil D D (eds) Membrane physiology. Plenum Press, New York, pp

Raftery M A, Hunkapiller M W, Strader C D, Hood L E 1980 Acetylcholine receptor: complex of homologous subunits. Science 208: 1454–1457

Rasmussen H 1986 The calcium messenger system. New England Journal of Medicine 314: 1094–1101, 1164–1170

Schacter E, Stadtman E R, Jurgensen S R, Chock P B 1988 Role of cAMP in cyclic nucleotide regulation. Methods in Enzymology 159: 3–19

Singer C J, Nicholson G L 1972 The fluid mosaic model of the structure of cell membranes. Science 175: 720

Snyder S H 1977 Opiate receptors and internal opiates. Scientific American, 236: 44–56

Sharma S K, Klee W A, Nirenberg M 1975 Dual regulation of adenyl cyclase accounts for narcotic dependence and tolerance. Proceedings of the National Academy of Science of the USA 72: 3092–3096

Togoni G, Bellantuono C, Bonati M et al 1980 Clinical relevance of pharmacokinetics. Clinical Pharmacokinetics 5: 105–136

3. Pharmacokinetics

W. McCaughey   J. A. S. Gamble

BASIC PHARMACOKINETIC CONCEPTS

The fate of a drug in the body — its absorption, distribution, biotransformation or metabolism and excretion, is dealt with by the branch of pharmacology known as pharmacokinetics. The main aim of the study of pharmacokinetics is to predict the concentration of a drug at its site of action, and the time-course of changes in this.

The concentration of drug in plasma is the most frequently used guide to concentration at the site of action, and to the clinical effect of the drug. In fact there may be significant differences both in the concentrations in plasma and at the site, and in the time-course of changes in these, but in most cases the concentration at the site of action cannot in practice be measured, and plasma level is the best available estimate.

To produce its desired effect the drug must be absorbed from its site of administration and transported to its site of action. The concentration of drug here will depend on many factors: the extent and rate of absorption, the route of transport and the effect of binding to proteins in the blood or tissues, the rate of metabolic degradation and excretion, as well as any other interactions with other drugs or body constituents.

Figure 3.1 summarizes the processes involved in the movement of the drug through the body. The body is a complex structure, and in order to reduce this complexity to an understandable level it is usually regarded as composed of a number of 'compartments'. A picture can then be built up of the movement of the drug between compartments, and the changes in measured drug concentration explained with reference to an arbitrary model.

Pharmacokinetic models

Attempts to apply mathematical analysis to the processes of absorption, distribution, and elimination of drugs have led to the practice of regarding the body as made up of one, two, three or more compartments, depending

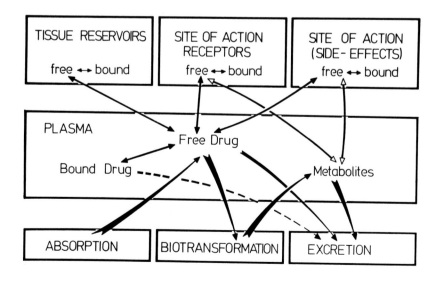

Fig. 3.1

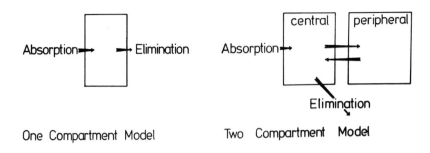

One Compartment Model   Two Compartment Model

Fig. 3.2

on the drug studied and the sophistication of the mathematics applied, and thus constructing mathematical models of the rate of transfer of drug from one to the other, which can be matched with actual measured values. Although the 'central' compartment is composed largely of the plasma and richly perfused tissues, and the 'peripheral' or tissue compartment of the less well-perfused tissues, the compartments do not represent accurately any anatomical or physiological reality. In practice it has turned out that too-complex models have been less successful than simpler ones, because the quality of information available as to the exact constants involved in various intercompartmental movements is insufficient.

The two-compartment model is that of which most general use is made.

A multiple-compartment model which is familiar to anaesthetists is the division of the body tissues in terms of tissue perfusion into a vessel-rich group (VRG), a muscle group (MG), and a fat or vessel-poor group (VPG). This is used in particular in describing the disposition of intravenous induction agents (Ch. 9).

Several basic concepts must be grasped in order to understand the way in which drugs are dealt with by the body. The factors determining the transfer of drugs between body compartments are summarized in Table 3.1, p. 34 (Hug 1978).

1. Lipid solubility and ionization

In order to be distributed within the body a drug must be soluble in water. However, as described in Chapter 2, the composition of biological membranes which separate body compartments is largely lipid in nature, and the ability of a drug to cross these membranes is largely dependent on lipid solubility, although some small (i.e. MW below 100) hydrophilic molecules may cross reasonably readily, probably through small aqueous channels. Lipid solubility is a property which may be

quantified as a partition coefficient (λ) by measuring how a drug in solution will divide itself between a water and an oily phase, which has been chosen to simulate the lipids of body membranes. In the early work by Overton and Meyer (Ch. 6), olive oil was used, but more commonly used now are other substances such as butanol, octanol or heptane. These different substances may each be more appropriate as models of different body membranes (Albert 1979).

Many drugs are weak electrolytes; acids or bases, which can exist in an ionized or an unionized form, the degree of ionization depending on the pH of their surroundings. Usually only the unionized form of the drug is sufficiently lipid-soluble to diffuse through biological membranes — lipophilicity falls by a factor of about 10 000 when ionization occur — and the ionized drug can cross only if it is of sufficiently low molecular size to penetrate the aqueous channels in the membrane.

The ionized and unionized drug are in equilibrium. From the Henderson–Hasselbalch equation (Ch. 1, p. 13), it can be seen that when the pH is close to the pKa of the drug (the pH at which the drug is 50% ionized), then small changes in pH will result in large changes in the degree of ionization of the drug, and in its behaviour. Strong acids have low pKa values and strong bases have high values, so that both are highly ionized at the range of pH found in the body. However, the degree of ionization of weak acids and weak bases with pKa values close to body pH (6.5–8.5) will be markedly affected by pH changes. Increased acidity, i.e. a decrease in pH, will cause a weak acid to become less ionized and therefore more highly lipid-soluble — thus phenobarbitone, for example, will be readily absorbed from the acidic surroundings of the gastric juice. The reverse situation will occur with weakly basic drugs, in which acidification will increase ionization, and decrease lipid solubility.

As an example of how these factors interact, thiopentone has a fat : plasma partition coefficient of 11 : 1. the chemical energy of the thiopentone molecules in each phase, and thus the force tending to make them cross between fat and plasma or vice-versa, is proportional to the concentration multiplied by the partition coefficient (λc). thus at equilibrium (other factors considered being equal), fat will contain 11 times as much thiopentone as plasma.

2. Zero-order and first-order kinetics

The Law of Mass Action states that the rate at which a chemical reaction proceeds is proportional to the active masses of the reacting substances. This law leads to several principles fundamental to drug disposition.

Normally when a substance is being changed into another, $X \rightarrow Y$, then the rate at which the reaction occurs depends on the concentration of the substance present. This is simply because the rate of reaction is proportional to the rate at which the molecules involved collide with each other and react. Thus rate of reaction concentration of X, or rate = $K_x \cdot [X]$, where K_x is a constant known as the rate constant or velocity constant of the reaction. A constant proportion of the remaining substance X disappears in any given time, independent of the initial concentration, and so it is customary to quote a half-life ($t_{\frac{1}{2}}$) for the process — the time required for the amount to fall to half its initial value.

The concentration of drug in fact falls exponentially, and so the concentration at any time can be calculated using the equation:

$$C = C_0 \, e^{-kt}$$

where C_0 is the initial concentration, and e = 2.718.

The time constant (τ) is the time which it would have taken for the concentration to drop to zero if the rate of decay had continued at its initial rate (in fact it falls to 1/e or 36.8% of its initial value in one time constant.) One half-life is equal to 0.698 τ.

A graph of concentration of X against time is an exponential curve, but log concentration is proportional to time, and so if plotted on semilogarithmic paper the curve is transformed into a straight line. A reaction of this type is known as a first-order reaction, or as a process following first-order kinetics.

This concept applies not only to reactions in which substances react chemically, but also to processes such as diffusion between compartments of the body. Again the rate can be described in terms of a rate constant. Often movement is bidirectional, and in this case a different rate constant may apply to movement in each direction.

$$\underset{K_2}{\overset{K_1}{\rightleftharpoons}}$$

It must be remembered in considering the movement of drugs between compartments, and the eventual establishment of equilibrium, that as well as the difference in concentration in the compartments, the partition coefficient for the drug between the compartments must also be taken into account. (At equilibrium 1 g of fat contains 11 times as much thiopentone as 1 g of blood.)

Occasionally processes occur in which a constant amount of substance is changed per unit time, independent of the concentration of the substance present. These are known as zero-order reactions, or reactions following zero-order kinetics (Fig. 3.4).

It is obvious that there will also be some drugs which at clinically used doses will fall into an intermediate position. These are said to have dose-dependent kinetics. Phenytoin is an example of such a drug, but this phenomenon is relatively rare. A different type of dose-dependent variability in drug response can be due to the effect of a drug on, for example, cardiac output.

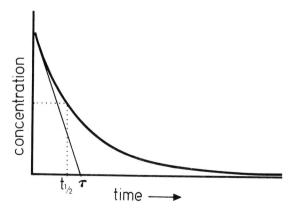

Fig. 3.3 Exponential decay.

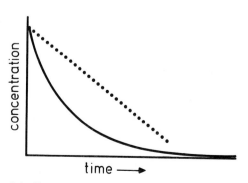

Fig. 3.4 Zero-order (. . .) and first-order (———) kinetics.

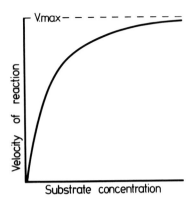

Fig. 3.5   Kinetics of enzyme reactions.

Second-order and higher-order reaction kinetics occur in chemistry, where rate of reaction is proportional to the concentration of two or more substances reacting together, but in pharmacology usually one is in such excess that the rate of the process in effect depends only on the concentration of the least abundant substance.

To see why processes in the body should be zero- and first-order it is useful to look superficially at the kinetics of reactions involving enzymes acting on a substrate. From a mathematical treatment known as the Michaelis–Menten equation, it can be shown that a graph of velocity of reaction vs. substrate concentration is a rectangular hyperbola (Fig. 3.5). In the majority of cases the substrate concentration is relatively low, so that the lower, straight part of the graph is used, and in the presence of an excess of enzyme the concentration of substrate is the controlling factor, and first-order kinetics prevail. Occasionally the enzyme system is easily saturated, for example in metabolism of alcohol, and thus the reaction is occurring at its maximum rate, and a zero-order reaction results.

Often reactions proceed by several steps, and in these cases the step which proceeds most slowly is known as the rate-limiting step. If the rate-limiting stage is not the first, there may be a build-up of intermediate substances, which can be an important factor in drug toxicity.

3.   Volume of distribution (Vd)

When a drug is injected into the body the plasma concentration found should, in the simplest case, be the dose given, divided by the volume through which it distributes itself — or Vd = dose/concentration. However, because drugs do not all cross membranes equally easily, some may distribute into a volume less than the whole

body. On the other hand some may give a low plasma concentration, having apparently distributed into a volume larger than that of the whole body. This is possible because some tissues may be able to take up large amounts of drug — e.g. into fat if the partition coefficient for fat is high, or by binding to tissue proteins. Because of these factors, the Vd is described as the apparent volume of distribution, but although it is an artificial concept it is useful in allowing correct prediction of the relationship between total drug content of the body and plasma concentration of the drug.

The volume of distribution of many drugs is reduced in the elderly, partly because of reduced binding of the drug to proteins. Some disease states may also be important — for example decreased cardiac output from heart failure or haemorrhage, by reducing perfusion of tissues, may lead to a reduced volume of distribution, and thus an increased plasma level of the drug.

Because drugs and other substances do not distribute equally rapidly to all compartments of the body, it is possible to have more than one measurement of the volume of distribution, depending on whether it is measured early, when the drug is largely in the hypothetical 'central' compartment, or later, when it has equilibrated further. These different values may be expressed as Vd_1 and Vd_{ss}, and more sophisticated models of drug kinetics may require even further definitions.

4.   Kinetics of drug disposition

If a drug is given rapidly into the bloodstream, i.e. into the central compartment of the body, its initial plasma concentration will approximate to the dose distributed within the central compartment; i.e.

$$C = \text{Dose}/V_1$$

The concentration will then begin to fall as the drug leaves the central compartment, both by elimination from the body and by distribution to the peripheral compartment (Fig. 3.2). The rate of elimination of the drug from the body, by metabolism or excretion, will be proportional to the concentration in the central compartment. However, initially most of the transfer of drug out of the central compartment is to equilibrate with the peripheral compartment. The rate of this transfer is proportional to the difference between drug concentrations in central (C_1) and peripheral (C_2) compartments. As distribution and elimination continue, C_2 will increase to equal C_1 and then as elimination continues to lower C_1, C_2 will exceed it, and drug is thereafter moving from peripheral to central compartments and thence to elimination (Fig. 3.6).

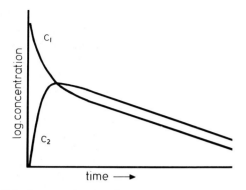

Fig. 3.6 Log concentrations in both compartments of a two-compartment open model after an intravenous dose.

The result of these interrelated processes is that an initial rapid distribution phase is succeeded by a slower elimination phase. The curve of plasma (central compartment) concentration after such a bolus intravenous injection is the algebraic sum of two exponential curves (commonly described as a bi-exponential curve), and can be expressed as:

$$C = Ae^{-\alpha t} + Be^{-\beta t}$$

α and β are the rate constants for the two exponential components, and half-lives can be calculated for each of the components. These are described as distribution or alpha phase with a half-time $t_{\frac{1}{2}}\alpha$ and elimination or beta phase with a half-time $t_{\frac{1}{2}}\beta$.

On a graph of log concentration vs. time these phases can be separated. As in the later phases elimination is the dominant process, and is a first-order process, the later part of the graph is approximately a straight line (Fig. 3.7). By extrapolating this line back to intercept the Y axis, and subtracting it from the original combined plot, a second straight line can be derived which

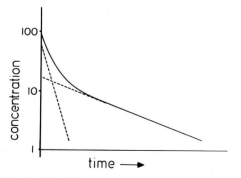

Fig. 3.7 Semilogarithmic plot of bi-exponential decline in plasma concentration.

represents the component due to drug distribution. The intercepts A and B of these lines are the constants which appear in the equation for the curve.

In studies of drug pharmacokinetics an attempt is made to find the mathematical model which best parallels the actual measurements made. A two-compartment model may give a reasonable fit, or it may be necessary to use a more complicated model. Any such descriptions, as fitting two- or three-compartment models for example, must be approximate for reasons already stated.

If a model with more than two compartments is used, then other terms may be introduced. In a three-compartment model it is usual to use π as the constant for the first, most rapid phase of distribution, followed by a slower alpha phase and by a beta elimination phase. Thus:

$$C = Pe^{-\pi t} + Ae^{-\alpha t} + Be^{-\beta t}$$

However, terminology is not entirely constant, and the idea of a late 'gamma' phase following α and β has been used in describing, for example, the very slow terminal elimination of a drug such as gentamicin which is only slowly released from tissue binding sites.

5. Clearance

A further useful concept in describing the pattern of drug elimination is that of clearance. If the amount of drug eliminated per unit time is proportional to the plasma concentration of the drug, then it follows that the equivalent of a constant volume of plasma is completely cleared of drug in a unit of time. This volume is the clearance (Cl).

Rate of elimination (mg min^{-1}) = Clearance (ml min^{-1}) × Concentration (mg ml^{-1})

The total clearance of the drug from plasma may be due to contributions by different organs — e.g. total clearance = hepatic clearance + renal clearance.

Extraction ratio

In general, drugs are not completely cleared from the plasma in one passage through the eliminating organ. The proportion which is removed is the extraction ratio, which is the ratio of clearance to total blood flow through the organ. For example if an opioid drug eliminated by the liver has a clearance of 1200 ml min^{-1}, and the total hepatic blood flow is 1500 ml min^{-1}, then the extraction ratio for this drug will be 80%. It could be predicted from such figures that this drug would be relatively ineffective by the oral route, because of the high rate of first-pass metabolism.

AUC

The drug concentration–time curve may be used as a measure of the total amount of drug in the body. Modifying the equation above, for a small interval of time, dt,

Amount eliminated = Clearance × Concentration × dt

Concentration × dt is the corresponding small area under the curve (AUC) for the time interval dt. The total amount eventually eliminated will be the sum of all these small increments, and so will be the total area under the curve (AUC) × clearance. For an intravenous dose this will be equal to the total dose administered, and so Dose = Cl × AUC.

The AUC may be used in several ways. For example in determining the contribution of renal and other routes to the total clearance of a drug, the total clearance may be calculated from the dose administered and the area under the plasma concentration–time curve, while the renal clearance is estimated from the total amount eliminated in the urine, and the urinary excretion rate.

If a drug is given other than directly intravenously, then the total amount administered may not enter the circulation in an active form. After oral administration, not only may absorption be incomplete, but metabolism of the drug to a different form may occur in the gut wall or liver before the drug reaches the systemic circulation. AUC for the plasma concentration–time curve following oral administration may be used to estimate the amount of the drug absorbed, and compared with the dose administered (or with the AUC after an intravenous dose), to estimate the oral bioavailability of the drug as a percentage.

Multiple dosing

Anaesthetic practice is unusual in that a majority of drugs are given as a single dose, and by the intravenous route. Where repeated doses are given, then the principles described above can be used to calculate the effect of later doses of drug. Usually the aim is to maintain the plasma level of the drug at a certain therapeutic level, or within a therapeutic range.

Using the simplest, one-compartment model, if a drug is given intravenously then the plasma concentration C = Dose/Vd. Following administration, the concentration declines exponentially, and so if a second equal dose is given before elimination is complete, a

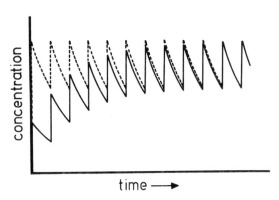

Fig. 3.8 One-compartment model of drug accumulation with multiple dosing: (**a**) —— no loading dose, (**b**) ----- correct loading dose given.

higher peak plasma drug will be reached. This will occur with each succeeding dose, but eventually a steady state will be reached (Fig. 3.8a) as the tendency to accumulate is balanced by the increased rate of elimination at higher plasma concentrations. The rate at which the steady state is reached will depend on the elimination half-life of the drug — 50% of steady state is reached in one half-life, and 97% in five half-lives. There will, of course be a fluctuation between peak and trough values with each dose, even when the steady state has been reached, and this will be more marked if the dosage interval is relatively long in comparison to the half-life of the drug, and vice-versa. The steady state reached will depend on the dose and interval between doses, as well as the half-life and volume of distribution of the drug.

In order to avoid the delay between starting treatment and achieving therapeutic drug concentrations, a loading dose may be given, followed by appropriate maintenance doses of the drug (Fig. 3.8b).

Intravenous infusions

The fluctuation of plasma levels between peak and trough values may be minimized by giving smaller doses of drug at more frequent intervals, and the logical conclusion of this process is to use a constant intravenous infusion. During a steady-state infusion the plasma concentration will rise exponentially towards a steady-state value. This curve (Fig. 3.9a) is often referred to as a 'wash-in' curve, as opposed to the more familiar 'wash-out' curve. Again the steady state will be achieved in approximately five half-lives, while it could be achieved immediately by giving a loading dose equal to the desired steady-state concentration × volume of distribu-

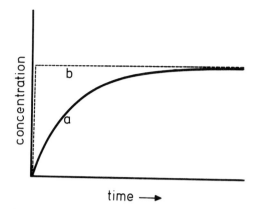

Fig. 3.9 One-compartment model of (**a**) infusion and (**b**) loading dose and infusion.

tion and maintained by a constant infusion at a rate equal to the rate of elimination (Fig. 3.9b).

In practice, of course, the one-compartment model described falls far short of describing what actually occurs, as redistribution must be taken into account as well as elimination, and this is to one or more peripheral compartments. In the real-life situation the rate of infusion for maintenance is still as described, but the idea of a loading dose must be modified because of the time taken for diffusion into various compartments. Figure 3.10 shows the pattern of change in plasma concen-

tration with different approaches to this problem. From this diagram, it would seem that 'e', a combination of bolus + loading infusion + maintenance infusion, would achieve the ideal, but in practice the difficulty in obtaining the numerical values needed, and inter-individual variation, make this difficult to achieve.

DRUG TRANSFER ACROSS MEMBRANES

For a compound to be effective it must reach its site of action in adequate concentration and remain there for a suitable period of time, and this is dependent on the influence of the body on the drug.

To reach its site of action a drug must cross a series of membranes, for example the gastrointestinal epithelium, the blood–brain barrier, membranes surrounding individual cells, and finally subcellular boundaries. Thus a knowledge of how compounds penetrate biological membranes is helpful in forecasting the action of a specific drug.

Kruhoffer (1961) has defined a membrane as any structure or complex of structures through which substances or ions pass at rates significantly different from that at which they would pass through a similar layer of water.

There are three main types of body membranes:

1. those made of several layers of cells, for example skin;

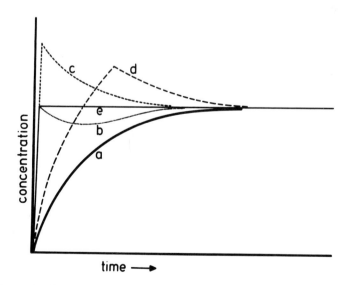

Fig. 3.10 Theoretical changes in plasma concentration of drug with various intravenous infusion techniques: (**a**) maintenance infusion alone; (**b**) loading dose ($C \times Vd_{initial}$) + maintenance infusion; (**c**) loading dose ($C \times Vd_{ss}$) + maintenance infusion; (**d**) loading infusion + maintenance infusion; (**e**) loading dose + exponentially reducing loading infusion + maintenance infusion.

Table 3.1 Rate and capacity of tissue uptake of drugs (Reproduced with permission from Hug 1978)

Rate of tissue uptake of drug is determined by:
  Blood flow
  Concentration gradient of diffusible form of drug
  Permeability coefficient of drug
    Membrane characteristics
      Capillary
      Cellular
    Physicochemical properties of drug
      Lipid solubility
      Ionization
      Molecular size
      Protein binding
    Special features
      Blood–brain barrier
      Membrane transport systems
      Metabolism of drug in tissues
      Maternal–placental–fetal relationships

Capacity of tissue to take up drug is determined by:
  Tissue/plasma partition coefficient
    Dissolution in lipids
    Binding to macromolecules
    pH-dependent partitioning
    Active transport
  Mass of tissue
  Non-reversible processes removing drug from equilibrium
    Covalent binding
    Metabolism
    Excretion

---

2. those consisting of a single layer of cells, for example the intestinal epithelium;
3. those consisting of a boundary less than one cell in thickness, for example the membrane of a single cell.

Except for the boundaries around intracellular structures, all body membranes are composed of a fundamental structure, the cell membrane or plasma membrane (Schanker 1962). The structure of the cell membrane has been described in Chapter 2.

Membrane transport mechanisms

Solutes pass through membranes in two ways: either by passive transfer or by specialized transport mechanisms.

Passive transfer

Passive transfer processes can be subdivided into three groups: (a) simple diffusion, (b) filtration, (c) osmosis.

Simple diffusion. Many substances move across membranes by simple diffusion, their rate of transfer being directly proportional to their concentration gradient. Some penetrate the membrane as though it were a layer of lipoid material, the rate of transfer being governed also by their lipid solubility. A number of lipid-insoluble substances cross the membrane as though it were a fine sieve, the smaller molecules or ions crossing faster than the larger ones. With ions, however, the speed of transfer may be determined more by their charge than by their size.

A difference in pH on the two sides of a membrane affects the distribution of a partly ionized substance. This is due to the preferential permeability of membranes to the lipid-soluble unionized form of a compound. At equilibrium the concentrations of the unionized form on both sides of the membrane will be equal, whereas the concentrations of the ionized form will be unequal, as these are dependent on the pH on either side of the membrane and on the dissociation constant (pKa) of the compound. This may have important clinical consequences, as for example in an acidotic fetus which may accumulate a concentration of bupivacaine which is higher than that in the maternal circulation.

Filtration. Filtration is the process by which fluid is forced through a membrane due to a difference in the hydrostatic pressure on the two sides. Solutes dissolved in the fluid pass through the pores of the membrane provided that their molecular diameters are smaller than the membrane pores.

Osmosis. Unlike filtration, where molecules move from an area of high concentration to an area of low concentration, osmosis describes the movement of solvent molecules across a membrane into a compartment where there is a higher concentration of a solute, the membrane being impermeable to the latter.

Specialized transport mechanisms

Specialized transport mechanisms can be divided into three subgroups: (a) active transport, (b) facilitated diffusion, (c) exchange diffusion. In all of these groups the concept of membrane carriers is used to explain the permeability of cell membranes to certain lipid insoluble solutes.

Active transport. Active transport processes have the following characteristics:

1. the solute moves against a concentration or electrochemical gradient;
2. the transport mechanism can become saturated at high solute concentrations;
3. carriers are specific for particular types of chemical structure;
4. when two substances are transported by the same carrier one will competitively inhibit the transport of the other;

5. the transport mechanism is inhibited by chemicals which interfere with cell metabolism.

Facilitated diffusion. This term is used to describe carrier transport mechanisms in which the solute does not move against a concentration gradient but which are similar in other respects to active transport processes.

Exchange diffusion. In this process a carrier is thought to transport the solute from one surface of the membrane to the other. Here it releases the solute and after picking up another solute molecule returns to the original side.

ABSORPTION OF DRUGS

Drugs are generally absorbed by passive diffusion; thus absorption is largely governed by lipid solubility, water solubility, molecular weight, molecular shape and degree of ionization of the drug. The exceptions are those drugs that resemble natural body substrates (for example antimetabolites), which are transferred by specialized carrier processes.

Drugs are generally given either via the alimentary tract or by parenteral injection. Complete entry into the general circulation is possible only when the drug is given by intravenous or intra-arterial injection. Other routes of administration may permit only a fraction of the administered drug to reach the general circulation, and this results in a decrease in its bioavailability. An understanding of the factors which influence the absorption of drugs, and thus their bioavailability, enables one to predict more accurately the intensity and duration of their pharmacological effects.

Gastrointestinal absorption of drugs

Absorption from the gastrointestinal tract is mainly dependent on:

1. the physicochemical state of the substances;
2. the structure of the absorbing surface;
3. the non-absorptive functions and state of the gastrointestinal tract.

The physicochemical properties of the substance

Factors influencing solution of the drug. Most drugs are given in the solid state. However, absorption usually results only after the drug is in solution, thus absorption must be preceded by disintegration of the dosage form and dissolution of the drug. If a drug is not fully dissolved by the time it passes its absorptive site, absorption must also become incomplete.

Disintegration of tablets is governed by their hardness, presence or otherwise of protective coatings, surface area and the agitative forces of the bowel. In addition to the active ingredient, tablets also contain other substances which may influence the release of the drug from its initial dosage form.

Dissolution. As most drugs are passively absorbed they depend upon an adequate concentration gradient at the site of absorption, the rate of absorption being proportional to the concentration gradient. Thus the absorption rate is greatly influenced by the dissolution rate. The dissolution rate is dependent upon several factors:

1. *Solubility.* The solubility of a drug in the gastrointestinal juices depends on the chemical nature of the drug in that some salts are more soluble than others. A drug which is soluble at neutral pH could be precipitated as an insoluble salt in the acid environment of the stomach.
2. *Adsorbents.* As the dissolution process progresses the concentration of the drug in solution increases. The resultant decrease in the solid–liquid concentration gradient reduces the dissolution rate. Incorporation of inactive ingredients in pharmaceutical preparations which adsorb drug molecules following dissolution helps to maintain the initial concentration gradient and thus maintain the dissolution rate.
3. *Agitative forces.* The greater the agitative forces the faster the dissolved drug is removed, thus the initial solid–liquid concentration gradient and dissolution rate are maintained.
4. *Particle size.* Smaller particles have larger surface areas in relation to their masses than larger particles. A large number of small particles have a greater surface area than a small number of large particles of equal mass, and thus have a larger area in contact with the dissolving medium.

Absorption of dissolved drug. Once in solution the drug factors which influence its absorption rate are mainly its lipid solubility, water solubility, molecular weight and degree of ionization.

Solubility and molecular weight. Lipid-soluble drugs are absorbed at rates roughly parallel to their oil:water partition coefficients. Water-soluble drugs are absorbed at rates inversely proportional to their molecular weights. Since the rates of intestinal absorption of numerous drugs are dependent on the proportion of lipid-soluble, unionized, drug molecules, and not on their molecular weights, it appears that the main pathway of absorption is through lipoid areas in the intestinal boundary rather than through small aqueous pores (Schanker 1962). For most drugs with molecular weights greater than 100, penetration through pores is relatively unimportant.

Degree of ionization. The influence of ionization has been described earlier.

Structure of the absorbing surface

Rapidity of absorption through a membrane is directly related to the surface area of the membrane. In humans the small intestine is the main site for absorption of most compounds, including drugs.

The surface area of the small intestine decreases rapidly from proximal to distal end, with almost half of the total mucosal area being in the proximal quarter whose surface area is greatly increased by numerous folds and villous processes in its mucous membrane. The proximal part of the small intestine has the greatest capacity for absorption.

Although weak acids are more rapidly absorbed from the stomach than are weak bases, and weak bases more rapidly from the small intestine than are weak acids, the small intestine is the main site for absorption of both basic and acidic compounds. The greater surface area of the intestinal mucosa more than compensates for any decrease in the rate of absorption per unit area.

The non-absorptive functions and state of the gastrointestinal tract

Gastrointestinal motility. The rate of gastric emptying markedly influences the rate at which drugs are absorbed, whether they be acidic, basic or undissociated compounds. Gastric motility may be considered to be the result of three components; namely, gastric peristalsis, gastric tonus and the state of the pylorus, the last being the most important factor in gastric emptying.

No matter how vigorous the gastric peristaltic waves, or the degree of gastric tonus, gastric emptying cannot occur without the pylorus relaxing. However, with a relaxed pylorus the first two components are important in emptying the stomach.

The rate at which the stomach empties into the duodenum is regulated by a variety of mechanisms operating either through autonomic reflexes or through a hormonal link between the duodenum and the stomach.

The following have all been shown to influence the rate of gastric emptying:

(a) *Physical composition and volume of gastric contents.* Solid meals do not affect the transit time through the small intestine; nor do they depress the total amount absorbed. However, the presence of solids almost doubles the stomach emptying time (Marcus & Lengemann 1962a,b). Distension of the duodenum initiates a neurally mediated decrease in gastric motility, the enterogastric reflex. This may account for the longer time taken by solids to leave the stomach.

The stomach empties in an exponential manner, gastric emptying becoming progressively slower as the volume in the stomach decreases in such a way that a constant fraction of the gastric contents, 1–3%, empties per minute (Hunt & Knox 1968).

(b) *Chemical composition of gastric contents.* The stomach usually acts under powerful inhibition from the duodenum, the rate of gastric emptying being usually much less than the maximum that the stomach could achieve. This is due to inhibition of gastric peristalsis following stimulation of receptors in the walls of the duodenum and small bowel. Solutions of high osmotic pressure empty more slowly than those of lower osmotic pressure. Similarly solutions of low pH empty more slowly than solutions of higher pH. When the pH of the duodenum falls below 6, duodenal receptors reflexly inhibit further gastric emptying until the secretions of the pancreas and duodenum neutralize the effluent acid.

The reflex inhibition of gastric motility by the duodenum may be neurally mediated (the enterogastric reflex), or chemically mediated. The chemical agents, enterogastrone and secretin, are produced by the duodenal mucosa and are carried in the circulation to the stomach where they inhibit gastric motility.

(c) *Nervous control.* Gastrointestinal motility and secretion are under the control of the autonomic nervous system, the vagus being the chief nerve supply. Increased vagal tone hastens gastric emptying and vice-versa. Excitement is said to hasten gastric emptying, and fear and depression to slow it.

(d) *Drugs.* Many drugs have intrinsic effects on gastrointestinal motility and can modify the absorption of other drugs taken at the same time. Thus compounds with anticholinergic activity such as atropine can slow down or reduce the absorption of other drugs. Similarly drugs which increase gastrointestinal activity and speed up the rate of gastric emptying will increase the rate of absorption of orally administered drugs. Histamine H_2 antagonists inhibit gastric acid production and may alter the rate of gastric emptying, and hence the rate of drug absorption (Houghton and Read 1987, Smith and Kendall 1988).

Although increasing the rate of gastric emptying generally results in an increased rate of drug absorption, Levine (1970) points out that the crucial factor in determining how much of a drug is absorbed in a particular segment is not the absorptive capacity of that segment in isolation, but rather how long the material remains in contact with the segment. Since the proximal end of the small intestine has the greatest capacity for absorption, increased intestinal activity may decrease drug absorption rate by reducing the time the drug remains in the area favouring rapid absorption. The rate of passage of material along the small intestine decreases as the material progresses towards the large intestine, and thus the distal portions of the small intestine usually become the sites in which the greater amount of drug is absorbed (Marcus & Lengemann 1962a,b).

Intestinal blood flow. The intestinal mucosa is generally overperfused in relation to its nutritional demands, and blood flow is generally not a rate-limiting factor in drugs absorbed by passive diffusion. However, a decrease in blood supply may retard the absorption of actively transported drugs (Levine 1970). Passive absorption of drugs is not affected until the decrease in blood supply causes actual mucosal structural damage. Congestive heart failure causes congestion in the liver and gut, and leads to delay in drug absorption (Shammas and Dickstein 1988).

Intestinal contents. A reduction in the amount of drug absorbed may occur if the drug forms a complex with another substance within the bowel lumen. Food or mucus may also form complexes with drugs and reduce their absorption.

In summary the following are the main factors influencing the absorption of drugs following oral administration: (a) formulation, (b) lipid solubility, (c) water solubility, (d) molecular weight, (e) degree of ionization, (f) stomach emptying time, (g) mucosal area, (h) intestinal motility.

Parenteral absorption of drugs

A parenteral preparation is one which is intended for administration through or under one or more layers of skin. Absorption is not involved when the drug is given by intravenous or intra-arterial injection. However, with other types of parenteral administration, for example subcutaneous or intramuscular, a depot of some type is formed and the drug must leave the depot and reach the blood or lymph systems by some process or processes.

Parenteral administration is generally used when the oral route is unsuitable, or when rapidity of action is required. Although it is generally assumed that intramuscularly or subcutaneously injected drugs are completely bioavailable, this has been found not to be true for digoxin (Greenblatt et al 1973) and diphenylhydantoin (Wilensky & Lowden 1973). An understanding of the factors involved in absorption of parenterally administered drugs may enable one to make forecasts regarding their bioavailability.

It has been shown that drugs disappear from parenteral depots according to pseudo-first-order rates, i.e. in an approximately exponential manner (Wagner 1961). Hence the rate of absorption from a parenteral depot is most rapid immediately following the injection of a drug, and slows down with increase in time following administration. Many pharmaceutical and biological factors, however, determine the rate at which absorption occurs.

Pharmaceutical factors

Many of the factors which control the rate of dissolution of a solid and/or its transfer from one phase to another influence the rate of release of a drug from a parenteral depot (Wagner 1961). The following have all been shown to be important factors in the absorption of drugs following parenteral administration.

Solubility. Drugs may be injected either as solutions or suspensions. In the case of the latter the drug must first dissolve in the tissue fluids prior to absorption, and its rate of dissolution will largely determine its rate of absorption. In the discussion on gastrointestinal absorption of drugs the factors influencing the dissolution of drugs have already been mentioned, and the same factors apply for parenteral administration.

Concentration. Following parenteral injection, the drug will diffuse along the concentration gradient between the depot and the tissue fluid, the greater the gradient the quicker the rate of absorption.

Surface area. Absorption takes place at the interface between the depot and the surrounding body fluids; thus the surface area of a preparation, rather than its volume, determines the diffusion rate. It follows that if a given volume is divided and injected into several sites the absorption will be the more rapid.

Solvent. The solvent in which a drug is dissolved is of prime importance in determining the rate at which it is absorbed. The solvent may be either water-miscible or immiscible. When a water-miscible solvent is used, the injection will be generally rapidly diluted by the tissue fluid. In the case of a water-insoluble drug contact with tissue fluid may cause precipitation of the drug at the site of injection, giving much the same effect as the injection of an aqueous suspension of the drug (Eastland 1951). When the solvent is immiscible with water, such as an oil, the rate of diffusion from the depot will be governed by the solvent : tissue fluid partition coefficient for the drug. The more this is in favour of the oil, the slower will be the release of the drug from the depot.

Viscosity. Highly viscous injections spread slowly, resulting in a smaller area of contact between the injected solution and tissue fluids. This results in a reduction in their absorption rate. They are thus often used in the preparation of injections for prolonged action.

pH. The pH of the injection solution has been shown to influence the absorption of sodium chloride in rats following subcutaneous administration and the absorption of organic bases following intraperitoneal administration in mice (Ballard 1968). In both cases low pH delayed absorption, while high pH increased absorption.

Biological factors

A number of biological factors have been shown to influence the rate of drug absorption following parenteral administration, including body movement, the site of administration and the tissue blood flow.

Body movement. When a molecule is absorbed primarily via the lymphatic route, body movement or exercise can often have a profound effect on how rapidly it reaches the general circulation (Ballard 1968). Barnes & Trueta (1941), using snake venom and bacterial toxins, found that more rapid absorption occurred in active rabbits than in those immobilized by a plaster cast.

Site of administration. It is generally accepted that intramuscular injections are absorbed more quickly than subcutaneous injections (Eastland 1951). However Nora et al (1964) found that injections into the upper arm produced more rapid absorption of insulin than those given into the thigh, irrespective of whether they were intramuscular or subcutaneous. Intramuscular administration of lignocaine has resulted in higher plasma levels following injections into the deltoid region than those given in the thigh, the latter site in turn producing higher levels than injections in the buttock (Cohen et al 1972, Schwartz et al 1974). Similarly Gamble et al (1975) found that diazepam when given intramuscularly was absorbed more rapidly from the thigh than from the buttock.

Tissue blood flow. Evans et al (1975) have demonstrated that there is a higher blood supply to the deltoid muscle than to the lateral rectus or gluteus maximus muscle. It is thus likely that variations in blood supply between these sites account for the variations in drug absorption. The inclusion of a vasoconstrictor in an injected solution causes a reduction in the blood flow to the site of injection. By slowing its rate of absorption the local action of a drug may thus be prolonged. Adrenaline is often used for this purpose, to prolong the action of local anaesthetics.

Histamine release. Certain drugs cause local histamine release following injection, and Schou (1958) demonstrated in rats that this may be the cause of delayed absorption, particularly immediately after injection.

In summary, the following are the main factors influencing the absorption of drugs following parenteral administration: (a) solubility of drug, (b) concentration of drug, (c) nature of solvent, (d) pH of solution, (e) site of injection, (f) tissue blood flow.

BLOOD–BRAIN BARRIER

The blood–brain barrier separates two of the major compartments of the central nervous system (CNS) — the brain and the cerebrospinal fluid (CSF) — from the third compartment, the blood. It exists to regulate the access which substances in the blood have to the nervous system. The essential feature of the blood–brain barrier is that, at these sites, cells are connected by 'tight junctions', with the result that they act almost like a continuous layer of cells. The endothelial cells of capillaries within the CNS are separated by only about 12 nm, in comparison to a distance of 100 nm or more in most other tissues, where these gaps form fenestrations or a 'small pore system' through which molecules in aqueous solution can exchange. At barrier sites, substances which can most easily cross are those which are highly lipid-soluble, so that they are able to pass directly through the layer of cells. The barrier is highly impermeable to ions and macromolecules such as proteins, although they can still cross at a very slow rate, probably through the tight junctions (Fig. 3.11).

The blood–brain barrier is situated at the interface between the blood and the other compartments — at the choroid plexus and the blood vessels of the brain and subarachnoid spaces, and also at the arachnoid membrane. Peripheral nerves have a barrier at the blood vessels of the endoneurium and at the perineurium, which surrounds nerve bundles. The eye, being derived directly from nervous tissue, also has a barrier. The blood–brain barrier is not complete, and there are certain sites where normal fenestrated capillaries exist. These sites are required for, and involved in, transfer of

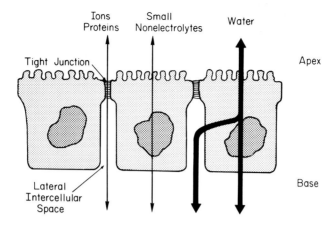

Fig. 3.11 Routes of transfer of different substances across epithelial cells connected at their apical ends by tight junctions. (Reproduced with permission from Rapoport 1976.)

hormones between blood and nervous tissues. Peripherally, olfactory receptor cells, terminal endings of peripheral nerves, and sensory ganglia also have no barrier.

CSF is produced at the choroid plexus. Here the choroidal epithelial cells are joined by tight junctions, and passive exchange of water and solutes between blood and CSF is restricted. In a current model (Rapoport 1976), sodium is actively transported into the CSF, accompanied by Cl^- and HCO_3^-, and water follows passively down the osmotic gradient. Many other substances cross the choroid plexus by processes such as facilitated diffusion and active transport. These include mono- and divalent ions, glucose, amino acids, and various organic acids and bases, some of which are drugs. The purpose of this activity is to maintain an environment around neurons and glia which is homeostatic and distinct from plasma.

The CSF may be considered together with the brain, as there is no barrier to diffusion between these two compartments, so that drugs which do not have ready access to the brain may sometimes be given by injection into the CSF.

The blood–brain barrier, as well as some other aspects of brain development such as myelination, seems to be incomplete at birth, and the penetration of drugs in the neonate may differ from what happens in adults (see Ch. 4)

Drug transfer across the blood–brain barrier

The major feature of the blood–brain barrier is that, as described above, it behaves mainly like a continuous lipid membrane. Many of the drugs used in anaesthetic practice are weak acids or bases, and are largely unionized at body pH, so that they readily penetrate the blood–brain barrier. Some of the factors involved are shown in Table 3.2.

Thiopentone, which is largely non-ionic at plasma pH and has a very high partition coefficient, penetrates rapidly into the brain, while pentobarbitone, which is also highly unionized, and less protein-bound than thiopentone, has a very low partition coefficient; it thus penetrates the blood–brain barrier slowly and has a slow onset of action (Dundee and Wyant 1974). Substances which are highly ionized, such as strong acids or bases, or quaternary ammonium compounds, would by this theory not be expected to be able to cross in any detectable quantity. In fact ions also have a finite though small lipid solubility, and may be able to cross in amounts which are pharmacologically significant.

The permeability of the blood–brain barrier may be increased if the tight junctions between cells are opened up. This may be caused by inflammation, as in menin-

Table 3.2. Some physical properties of thiopentone and pentobarbitone Taken from survey by Lant (1982) and based on the work of Hogben et al (1959) and Brodie et al (1960).

	Thiopentone	Pentobarbitone
pKa	7.6	8.1
Fraction non-ionized at pH 7.4	0.61	0.83
Fraction bound to plasma protein at pH 7.4	0.75	0.40
Partition coefficient (n-heptane/water) of non-ionized form	3.30	0.05

gitis or encephalitis or in other pathological situations, such as hypertensive encephalopathy, cerebral ischaemia, or head injury. It may also be caused by osmotically active substances, for example contrast media used in cerebral angiography. If this occurs, then drugs or other substances may enter the brain more readily. The dangers of this are obvious, but it may also be useful in allowing better access of antibiotics in treatment of meningitis, or antimitotic drugs in tumour therapy.

PROTEIN BINDING

During transport of the drug in the circulation, some drugs are simply dissolved in serum water, but many are partly associated with blood constituents such as albumin, globulins, lipoproteins and erythrocytes. Binding to albumin is for most drugs by far the most important of these, and often accounts for almost the entire drug binding in plasma. This method of transport has important effects on the fate of drugs in the body. Only the free, unbound drug can diffuse through the capillary walls and reach the sites of drug action, or sites of biotransformation and excretion. However the drug–albumin binding is easily reversible, and thus the complex forms a reservoir of drug, smooths out peaks and troughs in the intensity of drug action, and in most cases delays excretion and prolongs the action of the drug. Drugs also bind to proteins in the tissues, and this may constitute a large reservoir of drug, and delay its final elimination.

The extent of binding of drug to albumin varies widely, from very low values to 98–99% binding in the case of warfarin or diazepam. The drug binds to specific sites on the albumin molecule, and for different drugs there may be one or several sites. There may also be non-specific sites. The type of bond formed varies, but will be covalent only where irreversible bonds form. The more usual reversible bond obeys the law of mass action, and thus an equation can be written:

$$\text{(Unbound drug)} + \text{(Albumin)} \underset{K_2}{\overset{K_1}{\rightleftharpoons}} \begin{array}{l} \text{(drug–albumin} \\ \text{complex)} \end{array}$$

where K_1 and K_2 are the rate constants for the forward and reverse actions. This equation can be written:

$$\frac{[\text{Bound drug}]}{[\text{Unbound drug}] \times [\text{Albumin}]} = \frac{K_1}{K_2}$$

and the affinity of the drug for albumin expressed as an affinity constant, which is the ratio of bound drug concentration to the product of albumin and unbound drug concentrations.

This constant, $K_a = K_1/K_2$. More commonly used is a dissociation constant, K_d.

$$K_d = 1/K_a = K_2/K_1.$$

Thus a drug with a high affinity for albumin has a low value of dissociation constant. As there may be more than one binding site on each molecule, and each may have a different dissociation constant, the concentration of the drug left unbound will depend on the total drug concentration, the albumin concentration, the number of binding sites, and the dissociation constant(s).

A high degree of binding of the drug to albumin will have several important effects. These could be anticipated from the facts that only free drug diffuses into, and is in equilibrium with, the water of the extracellular fluid and other body compartments, and that the drug–albumin binding is easily reversible. Firstly, the plasma concentration of the drug as commonly measured is an estimate of the total amount of the drug, bound and unbound, and will often be much higher than the concentration of drug dissolved in body fluids and available to produce a therapeutic effect. The level of free drug in body fluids can be measured using a physical separation technique such as ultrafiltration of plasma, or by measuring levels in a relatively protein-free body fluid such as saliva, and such values should correlate better with biological effects than do plasma total drug levels. When a bolus injection of the drug is given, much of this will bind to albumin, so that the tendency to produce an instantaneously high blood level and pharmacological effect is smoothed out. However, occasionally if a very rapid intravenous injection is given, which does not have time to mix with the whole blood volume, then the binding capacity of albumin molecules in the limited volume of blood with which the drug mixes initially may be exceeded, and a higher level of free drug and pharmacological effect will result.

Secondly, there may be an influence on the metabolism and excretion of the drug. In the glomeruli, ultrafiltration occurs, and only free drug passes into the tubules. As there is no concentrating effect there is no tendency for the bound drug to dissociate, and thus only the free drug is exposed to excretion processes, while that part which is bound to albumin is protected from excretion. However, if a drug is actively excreted by the kidney tubules, this process reduces the concentration of free drug in plasma, bound drug dissociates immediately to replace this and is excreted — so albumin binding has little effect on the rate of elimination of the drug. Therefore drugs which are excreted by passive filtration through the glomeruli, and which are highly albumin-bound, will have long half-lives, as much as a year for some iodinated contrast media. When excretion is by active tubular secretion, as in the case of penicillins, then even if the drug is highly albumin-bound, rapid excretion may occur; in fact the rate of excretion may be increased by albumin binding, as this acts in effect as a transport mechanism carrying more drug to the site of excretion.

The same situation obtains in the liver, where some drugs reach their sites of metabolism in the hepatocytes by passive diffusion while others are actively transported. Albumin binding will also hinder removal of drug from the circulation by haemodialysis or peritoneal dialysis.

When more than one drug is given to the patient, then the drugs may compete for protein-binding sites, and this can result in the displacement of one or other drug from its binding sites and lead to an increase in the concentration of free drug, and an increase in the pharmacological effect of the drug. This interference of one drug with the binding of another may be due to competitive inhibition, in which the drugs simply compete for binding to the same site on the albumin molecule, or to non-competitive inhibition in which the binding of the drug to albumin results in a change in the tertiary conformation of the albumin, and thus alters the number or affinity of the sites accessible to the second drug.

Endogenous compounds such as bilirubin or fatty acids also bind to serum proteins, and may be displaced by drugs competing for the same sites. In the newborn with jaundice this may lead to development of kernicterus, while administration of heparin by raising free fatty acid levels causes an increase in free diazepam fraction by several-fold (Desmond et al 1980). Similar interaction may take place with drugs such as diazepam or tricyclic antidepressants, which are extensively bound to tissue proteins, but the clinical importance of this is unknown.

Drug competition for binding sites is most likely to occur to a significant degree if both drugs are highly albumin-bound, and if high concentrations of the drug are reached either by rapid administration of a large dose, or by repeated administration. The potentiation of the effect of one drug by another by this process is likely to be transient, as an increase in the concentration of the free drug results in an increase in its rate of elimination, and a new state of equilibrium is soon reached. The converse will occur when the competing drug is stopped (Fig. 3.12). However, although the effect is short-lived, if the drug has a narrow range of therapeutic concentrations, or if the therapeutic and toxic doses are close, it may be clinically important. This compensating safety factor may not apply in drugs with high extraction ratios, where protein binding is helping to accelerate elimination, and adverse reactions will be more likely in these cases. Some examples of these interactions are discussed in Chapter 34.

BIOTRANSFORMATION

Drugs are modified by the actions of enzyme systems within the body. Most drug metabolism occurs in hepatic microsomes, but biotransformation also occurs elsewhere in the body, including the plasma, gastrointestinal tract, lungs, and non-microsomal systems in the liver. The main useful purpose of biotransformation is to rid the body of the drug. Highly polar substances may easily be excreted by the kidney, and are often excreted unchanged, at least in part. Those which are non-polar and highly lipid-soluble are rapidly reabsorbed from the kidney tubules after filtration by the

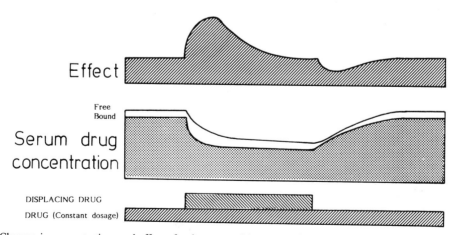

Fig. 3.12 Changes in concentrations and effect of a drug caused by a second drug which competes for binding sites.

glomeruli, and thus not easily excreted. Biotransformation to more polar and less lipid-soluble metabolites will make excretion more easy. Metabolic degradation will also often change the drug to an inactive form before it is excreted, and lead to a termination of its action — suxamethonium is metabolized rapidly by plasma pseudocholinesterase — but metabolic change may have different effects. In some cases an active drug is metabolized to a still-active metabolite (diazepam to desmethyldiazepam) or an inactive 'prodrug' to an active metabolite (codeine to morphine) which is responsible for its therapeutic effect. A metabolite may also be responsible for the toxic effects of a drug; for example fluoride ion causes the nephrotoxicity associated with prolonged methoxyflurane administration.

These metabolic processes have evolved both to deal with substances produced by the body, often degraded by specific enzymes, and to deal with toxic chemicals introduced into the body, which in evolutionary terms were mainly from plants in the diet, but now include drugs. These are usually metabolized by non-specific 'general-purpose' enzymes.

It is also possible for a drug to be degraded by purely chemical reactions. The recently introduced neuromuscular blocking agent atracurium becomes unstable at the relatively alkaline pH of the body, and breaks down partly by a process known as Hofmann elimination, and partly by ester hydrolysis.

Phase 1 and 2 metabolism

Drug metabolism may be divided into two phases. Phase 1, or non-synthetic reactions, involve inactivation of the drug by oxidation, reduction, hydrolysis, dealkylation or similar modifications of the administered molecule in which a polar group is added. A majority of these are carried out in the liver by a versatile group of enzymes known as mixed-function oxidases, a system in which one of the most important components is cytochrome P450. (This is an enzyme, or group of enzymes, whose name is derived from the fact that light of wavelength 450 nm is absorbed.)

Phase 2, or synthetic reactions, are also known as conjugation reactions. These involve coupling of endogenous compounds with the drug, or with the products of phase 1 reactions. The endogenous substance is usually a carbohydrate or amino acid, or a derivative of these, or acetic acid or inorganic sulphate. The common conjugation reactions are therefore: glucuronidation, other glycosylations, sulphation, acetylation, conjugation with amino acids or with glutathione, and methylation.

Glucuronidation, most oxidation reactions and some other non-synthetic reactions are catalysed solely by liver microsomal enzymes, but all other reactions may occur both in liver microsomes, and at non-microsomal sites in the liver and elsewhere.

A drug is often metabolized simultaneously along several pathways. This is illustrated here by morphine, some of whose pathways of metabolism are shown in Figure 3.13. Glucuronidation at the 6 position gives rise to a still-active metabolite, while conjugations at the 3 position account for about 60% of morphine elimination, and the products are inactive. N-demethylation, a phase 1 reaction, gives normorphine, which is then conjugated to a glucuronide. As well as these, other pathways such as methylation to codeine exist, and also 10% of morphine is excreted unchanged.

The relative importance of different pathways changes under different circumstances. For example, halothane metabolism is normally mainly oxidative, but under hypoxic conditions an alternative reductive pathway becomes more important, and in this case reactive intermediates may be formed (Ch. 7, Black 1982). Reactive intermediates formed in this way by phase 1 reactions are usually made harmless by inactivation of their reactive groups in a phase 2 or synthetic reaction. Because the phase 2 reactions may depend on an available supply in the liver of, for example, glutathione, it is possible for the capacity of this pathway to be over-

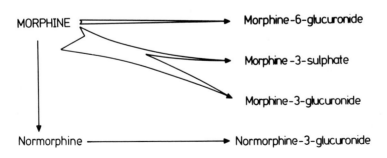

Fig. 3.13

whelmed if a large amount of the toxic intermediate compound is made. This might occur with halothane, as described above, or with paracetamol (acetaminophen) in overdose, and liver damage can then occur as irreversible binding to macromolecules in the liver cells occurs. In the case of paracetamol this may to some extent be prevented by administering a glutathione precursor such as acetylcysteine to the patient.

Modification of metabolism

There are genetically determined differences in drug metabolism which may result in up to a six-fold difference in the rates of metabolism in different individuals. Much of this difference can be accounted for by the normal Gaussian distribution of any property between individuals. There are, however, also some specific genetic differences in metabolic processes. An example is metabolism of drugs by acetylation — patients may belong to one of two populations, 'fast' or 'slow' acetylators, and the dose regime of a drug eliminated by this pathway — for example isoniazid — must be greatly modified depending on its rate of metabolism. A similar example of genetic polymorphism in suxamethonium is described in Chapter 2.

The rate at which an enzyme system carries out its activity is largely dependent on the amount of substrate present, as described above (Fig. 3.5). However, certain substances are able to stimulate enzyme activity without a change in the amount of enzyme present — enzyme stimulation or enzyme activation. More importantly, it is also possible to increase the amount of enzyme in the system. Enzymes are proteins which, like other proteins, are assembled from amino acids according to instructions transferred by messenger RNA from a structural gene. This process is controlled by the influence of a second, repressor, gene. Whereas this system is presumably intended to maintain a constant level of metabolism, depression of the repressor action will lead to an increase in the amount of enzyme present. This is known as induction of metabolism, or enzyme induction, and can be caused by many drugs and other substances. All these do not act through exactly the same mechanism; indeed in some cases different inducing agents may induce different molecular forms of the enzyme. Induction of enzymes by a drug leads to an increase not only in its own metabolic degradation, but often also that of other drugs. This is one of the most important mechanisms of drug interaction. The mixed-function oxidases of the liver microsomes are involved in the biotransformation of many different drugs. Barbiturate drugs are among those which are particularly

effective in causing induction of oxidation enzymes. Thus, for example, if a patient maintained in a steady state of anticoagulation by warfarin then starts barbiturate treatment, an increase in warfarin metabolism will ensue, and with a fall in plasma warfarin levels there will be a decrease in anticoagulation effect. If a metabolite is toxic, then induction of metabolism may result in increased toxicity — for example the nephrotoxic potential of methoxyflurane may be potentiated.

Inhibition of metabolism may also occur, but is much less important clinically. It will usually be due to competition between drugs for the same metabolic pathway. With most drugs, which are eliminated by processes obeying first-order kinetics, competition rarely causes significant inhibition of metabolism, but competition is more important in those eliminated by zero-order kinetics, where the enzyme system is easily saturated.

Inhibition may also be due to temporary or permanent inactivation of enzymes. The most important example in anaesthetic practice is inhibition of cholinesterase. Similarly, inactivation of hepatic enzymes can occur.

The breakdown of drugs which depend on hepatic metabolism may be greatly influenced by changes in liver blood flow. In general a reduction in hepatic blood flow will lead to a reduction in metabolism of the drug, but this may not always be so.

First-pass metabolism

First-pass metabolism occurs to a significant extent after absorption of many drugs from the gastrointestinal tract. Since the drug is absorbed into the splanchnic circulation it must pass through the liver before it can reach the systemic circulation and its target. It may therefore be metabolized both in the liver and, usually to a lesser extent, by enzymes in the gut wall. If a significant proportion is metabolized by the liver (i.e. the hepatic clearance of the drug is relatively high), then the amount reaching the systemic circulation will be greatly reduced. Thus the drug, even if it is absorbed well, will be relatively ineffective when given orally — as with, for example, morphine. Where the drug is used by the oral route, the dose administered will be much larger than when given parenterally. When the rate of metabolism of the drug by the liver is high, then hepatic blood flow may be the limiting factor. Thus any situation where hepatic blood flow is reduced will result in a reduction in hepatic clearance of the drug.

If the drug is metabolized according to zero-order kinetics, an increase in hepatic blood flow will allow more of the drug to pass through the liver unaffected, and in this case increased hepatic blood flow can result in an increase in drug action, in contrast to the general rule described above.

Newborn babies have immature metabolic processes. However, their capacity to carry out phase 1 processes such as oxidation is relatively well developed, although the situation is different in many other animal species.

Phase 2 processes of conjugation are not carried out well in human newborn, and therefore there is a reduced capacity to deal with drugs which are detoxified by these processes. There may also be a reduced capacity to metabolize drugs in the elderly. These topics are covered in more detail in Chapter 4.

REFERENCES

Albert A 1979 Selective toxicity. The physico-chemical basis of therapy, 6th edn. Chapman & Hall, London

Ballard B E 1968 Biopharmaceutical considerations in subcutaneous and intramuscular drug administration. Journal of Pharmaceutical Sciences 57: 357–378

Barnes J M, Trueta J 1941 Absorption of bacteria, toxins and snake venom from the tissues. Lancet 1: 623–626

Black G W 1982 Metabolism and toxicity of volatile anaesthetic agents. In: Atkinson R S, Hewer C L (eds) Recent advances in anaesthesia and analgesia, 14th edn. Churchill Livingstone, Edinburgh, pp 31–44

Brodie B B, Kurtz H, Schanker L S 1960 The importance of dissociation constant and lipid-solubility in influencing the passage of drugs into the cerebrospinal fluid. Journal of Pharmacology and Experimental Therapeutics 130: 20–25

Cohen L S, Rosenthal J E, Horner D W, Atkins J M, Matthews O A, Sarnoff S J 1972 Plasma levels of lidocaine after intramuscular administration. American Journal of Cardiology 29: 520–523

Desmond P V, Roberts R K, Wood A J J, Dunn G D, Wilkinson G R, Schenker S 1980 Effect of heparin administration on plasma binding of benzodiazepines. British Journal of Clinical Pharmacology 9: 171–175

Dundee J W, Wyant G M 1974 Intravenous anaesthesia, 1st edn. Churchill Livingstone, Edinburgh

Dutton G J 1978 Developmental aspects of drug conjugation, with special reference to glucuronidation. Annual Review of Pharmacology and Toxicology 18: 17–35

Eastland C J 1951 Some aspects of modern formulation. Journal of Pharmacology and Pharmacy 3: 942

Evans E F, Proctor J D, Fratkin M J, Velandia J, Wasterman A J 1975 Blood flow in muscle groups and drug absorption. Clinical Pharmacology and Therapeutics 17: 44

Gamble J A S, Dundee J W, Assaf R A E 1975 Plasma diazepam levels after single dose oral and intramuscular administration. Anaesthesia 30: 164–169

Gelehrter T D 1976 Enzyme induction. New England Journal of Medicine 294: 522–526, 589–595, 646–651

Greenblatt D J, Duhme D W, Koch-Weser J, Smith T W 1973 Evaluation of digoxin bioavailability in single-dose studies. New England Journal of Medicine 289: 651

Hogben C A M, Tocco D J, Brodie B B, Schanker L S 1959 On the mechanism of intestinal absorption of drugs. Journal of Pharmacology and Experimental Therapeutics 125: 275–282

Houghton L A, Read N W 1987 A comparative study of the effect of cimetidine and ranitidine on the rate of gastric emptying of liquid and solid meals in man. Alimentary Pharmacology and Therapeutics 1: 401–408

Hug C C 1978 Pharmacokinetics of drugs administered intravenously. Anesthesia and Analgesia, Current Research, 57: 704–723

Hunt J N, Knox M T 1968 Control of gastric emptying. American Journal of Digestive Diseases 13: 372–375

Koch-Weser J, Sellers E M 1976 Binding of drugs to serum albumin. New England Journal of Medicine 294: 311–316, 526–531

Kruhoffer P 1961 The pharmacology of membranes. Journal of Pharmacy and Pharmacology 13: 193–203

Lant A F 1982 Factors affecting the action of drugs. In: Scurr C, Feldman S (eds) Scientific foundations of anaesthesia. 3rd edn. Heinemann, London, pp 425–450

Levine R R 1970 Factors affecting gastrointestinal absorption of drugs. American Journal of Digestive Diseases 15: 171–188

Marcus C S, Lengemann F W 1962a Use of radioyttrium to study food movement in the small intestine of the rat. Journal of Nutrition 76: 179

Marcus C S, Lengemann F W 1962b Absorption of Ca^{45} and Sr^{85} from solid and liquid food at various levels of the alimentary tract of the rat. Journal of Nutrition 77: 155

Nora J J, Smith W D, Cameron J R 1964 The route of insulin administration in the management of diabetes mellitus. Journal of Paediatrics 64: 547–551

Rapoport S I 1976 Blood–brain barrier in physiology and medicine. Raven Press, New York

Schanker L S 1962 Passage of drugs across body membranes. Pharmacological Reviews 14: 501–530

Schou J 1958 Self-depression of the subcutaneous absorption of drugs due to release of histamine. Nature 182: 324

Schwartz M L, Meyer M B, Covino B G, et al 1974 Antiarrhythmic effectiveness of intramuscular lidocaine. Influence of different injection sites. Journal of Clinical Pharmacology 14: 77–83

Shammas F V, Dickstein K 1988 Clinical pharmacokinetics in heart failure. An updated review. Clinical-Pharmacokinetics 15: 94–113

Smith S R, Kendall M J 1988 Ranitidine versus cimetidine. A comparison of their potential to cause clinically important drug interactions. Clinical-Pharmacokinetics 15: 44–56

Wagner J G 1961 Biopharmaceutics: absorption aspects. Journal of Pharmaceutical Sciences 50: 359–389

Wilensky A J, Lowden J A 1973 Inadequate serum levels after intramuscular administration of diphenylhydantoin. Neurology 23: 218

4. Influence of age and disease

I. A. Orr   J. W. Dundee   W. McCaughey   J. P. Alexander

PART 1
AGE: PAEDIATRIC RESPONSE
I. A. Orr

PHYSIOLOGICAL CONSIDERATIONS

Physiological variation, due to age, complicates the aim of achieving the correct dose of a drug at its receptor in a child. 'A child is not a small adult' is an aphorism which is useful, but disguises the variation amongst children. The children's age group can be further divided into subgroups: the perinate (0–1 week in a term baby or 0–2 weeks if premature — premature being defined as < 37 weeks gestation or < 2.5 kg birthweight); the neonate (1–4 weeks in a term baby, 2–8 weeks in a premature baby); the infant (remainder of first year); and the older child (1–16 years). Variation in drug efficacy may be due to differences in drug absorption, distribution, metabolism and excretion, or to immaturity of anatomical pathways and receptors. Thus drug half-lives vary markedly in the different age groups (Table 4.1).

Absorption

Absorption from the gastrointestinal tract is governed by the factors which apply to passage of a drug through a membrane. Gastric pH is close to neutral at birth, but pH drops to below 3 within 8 hours of birth, followed by a slight decrease in pH during the second week (Smith & Nelson 1976). Active transport mechanisms are immature in neonates. Gastric emptying takes longer in neonates and attains adult levels at 6–8 months, so oral drugs such as paracetamol are absorbed more slowly (Levy et al 1975). Hypoxia in perinates and neonates causes reduced blood flow to skin and muscle, so satisfactory blood levels will be achieved most reliably by intravenous drug administration. In the well-perfused infant, absorption of intramuscular drugs depends largely on regional blood flow, which varies between muscles (Evans et al 1975).

The small doses of drugs required for neonates often mean that they can be given intravenously much more quickly than a similar surface area related dose could be given to an adult. Dilution of a drug, such as thiopentone, or slow injection must be used if cardiovascular depression is to be avoided.

Distribution

Variation of distribution of drugs in children is caused by variation in protein binding, body composition, cardiac output and tissue permeability. Serum albumin concentration in term infants is usually 35 g l^{-1}, rising to the adult value of 45 g l^{-1}, around the end of the first

Table 4.1 Comparative apparent plasma drug half-life (hours) for different development ages

Drug	Perinate		Neonate	Infant	Older child	Adult
	Premature	Term				
Ampicillin	3.6–6.2	2.0–4.9	1.7–2.8			1–1.8
Gentamicin	5.1–5.9	3.8–5.5	2.3–3.9	2.3–3.9		(2–3)
Paracetamol		3.5–4.9			4.4–4.5	3.6
Diazepam	75	31			18	(20–42)
Phenobarbitone	(41)–380	102–250	(67–99)	44–86	53–64	(53)–118

Values indicated are means except those in parentheses, which are ranges of means or individual values (Data from Done et al 1977).

year, thus giving higher serum concentration of protein-bound drugs and a lower therapeutic range in infants. The high serum bilirubin level in jaundiced infants leads to displacement of protein-bound drugs, though conversely the drugs themselves can also displace bilirubin, potentially causing kernicterus in neonates, who have an immature blood – brain barrier. Marked changes in the size of body compartments take place between infancy and adulthood. Total body water as a percentage of body weight decreases from 96% in the 12-week fetus to 70% in neonates and 60% in adults (Houston 1979). The distribution of this fluid between intracellular and extracellular compartments also varies (Fig. 4.1). This variation in compartment size has most relevance when dealing with a drug such as sodium bicarbonate, which is distributed in the extracellular fluid, so neonates may require 0.45 to 0.50 × body weight (kg) × base deficit in mmol l^{-1} in comparison to adults who only require 0.3 × body weight (kg) × base deficit in mmol l^{-1} to give a total correction of metabolic acidosis though in clinical practice a full correction is rarely undertaken. Similarly, water-soluble drugs, without extensive tissue binding, such as benzylpenicillin, will require higher dosage levels if a weight-related scale is used, to produce similar plasma concentrations. However, extracellular fluid volume is more directly related to surface area, and dosage scales related to surface area are in general much more accurate.

Adipose tissue comprises 1% of body weight in pre-term infants, 16% in neonates and 25% in adults, thus affecting the redistribution volume of fat-soluble drugs. In the neonate the brain is 12% and muscle 25% of body weight, whereas in adults the brain is 2% and muscle 25% of body weight. These variations must be

considered when a drug is being directed at individual organs. Maturation of the blood – brain barrier and myelination is incomplete in the newborn. Thus drugs such as opioids and barbiturates can enter the neonatal brain more easily. Morphine has a greater respiratory depressant effect in neonates when compared with adults (Way et al 1965), and animal work has shown that thiopentone has a lower LD_{50} in young guinea pigs compared with old guinea pigs (Carmichael 1947).

When the respiratory distress syndrome or low cardiac output occur, distribution time may be prolonged. Relative tissue hypoxia can cause a reduction of cerebral blood flow, but with preservation of brainstem perfusion, in the face of systemic hypotension. This can affect brain distribution of lipophilic drugs and cause general alteration of absorption and excretion rates. The metabolic acidosis found with poor tissue perfusion may cause changes in the plasma and tissue levels of drugs such as phenobarbitone which have a pKa near the pH values of blood.

Metabolism

Neonatal metabolic pathways are often immature when compared with adults, but rapidly mature during the first month of life (Done et al 1977) (Fig. 4.2). Reductive pathways and oxidative pathways are particularly slow, hence prolonging the elimination half-life of diazepam to 75 h in premature infants and 31 hours in neonates. The glycine and glucuronide conjugation pathways take 2–3 months to mature, and those involving acetylation take 2 months (Gladtke & Heimann 1975). However, the sulphate pathway is not depressed at birth, and can conjugate drugs such as paracetamol, which would normally be shared with the glucuronide pathway, so effectively as to give an elimination half-life equal to that in adults (Levy et al 1975). The rate of hydrolysis of esters is reduced at birth. There is reduced activity of acetylcholinesterases, pseudocholinesterases and arylesterases, with adult values being attained at about 1 year of age (Ecobichon & Stephens 1973). Recovery from suxamethonium in infants is similar to that in adults, suggesting that the volume of distribution compensates for the lower pseudocholinesterase activity (Cook & Fischer 1975).

Excretion

Glomerular filtration rate may be as low as 3 ml min^{-1} at birth, but both it and tubular function mature with age (Fig. 4.2). In the low birthweight infant drug elimination may be hampered not only by renal imma-

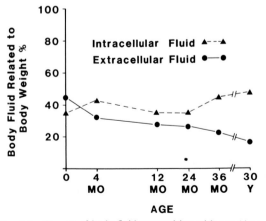

Fig. 4.1 Change of body fluid composition with age (data from Friis Hansen, 1957).

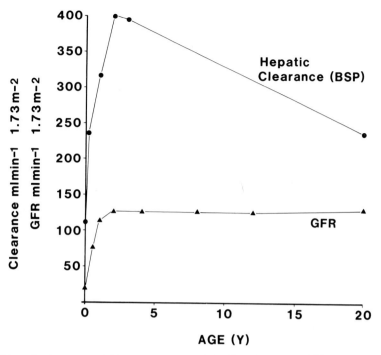

Fig. 4.2 Change of hepatic clearance and GFR with age (data from Chantler 1979 and Habersang 1980).

turity but also by hypoxaemia (Myers et al 1977). Neonates have a lower urinary pH so there is increased tubular reabsorption of weakly acidic compounds. The expected faster clearance of basic compounds is not seen, because of the low glomerular filtration rate. Neonates are less able to excrete barbiturates due to renal immaturity, and excretion of drugs such as aminoglycosides and pethidine, which depend on glomerular filtration rate, is reduced (Axline et al 1967). Elimination half-lives of drugs, such as penicillin, which are actively secreted by the tubules, are 2–3 times longer in the newborn than in older children, but this function usually matures by 2–3 months (Gladtke & Heimann 1975). Because of the rapidly changing renal function it is important to monitor blood levels of drugs, such as aminoglycosides, which are frequently used in the paediatric intensive care unit.

Dosage rules

When dosage is based on weight:

$$\text{Dose paed} = \text{Dose adult} \times \frac{\text{Weight paed}}{\text{Weight adult}}$$

children tend to be underdosed with the adult dose as

standard. It is more appropriate to adjust dosages in relation to surface area, which can be evaluated from a simple nomogram if both height and weight are known. Failing this a close estimate of surface area can be made from the formula:

$$\text{Surface area (m}^2) = \frac{\text{Weight (kg)} \times 4}{\text{Weight (kg)} + 90}$$

and if the weight is unknown it can be estimated from the formula:

$$\text{Weight (kg)} = \text{Age} \times 2 + 8$$

though these formulae only hold good for the age group 1–10 years. Perhaps a compromise is to assume that surface area follows weight to the 0.7 power (Dawson 1940) and use the formula:

$$\text{Dose paed} = \text{Dose adult} \times \left(\frac{\text{Weight paed}}{\text{Weight adult}}\right)^{0.7}$$

Despite this theoretical consideration most anaesthetists find it simple to remember a drug dose on a mg kg^{-1} basis, adjusting dosage according to response, so this dosage regime will be used in the remainder of this chapter.

A number of factors can give rise to inadvertent administration of the incorrect dose to a child. Incorrect weighing or recording of weight, ignorance of the variability of drug effect in the very young, or incorrect dilution or measurement of a dose must all be guarded against. However, dilution of concentrated solutions is recommended as excessive amounts of drug are more easily administered from the small syringes used with children.

COMMON DRUGS USED IN PAEDIATRIC ANAESTHESIA

Inhalational anaesthetic agents

Inhalational agents are taken up more quickly by children than by adults (Salanitre & Rackow 1969). This is caused by greater alveolar ventilation, relative to the functional residual capacity, and to a greater proportion of vessel-rich tissues in the child. Inhalational agents are also more rapidly excreted by neonates. After discontinuing administration of 70% nitrous oxide, the alveolar concentration falls to 10% in 2 min with infants, and in 10 min with adults (Steward & Creighton 1978). Lerman and colleagues (1983) have now shown that the minimum alveolar concentration (MAC) of halothane is 0.87% in neonates, rising to 1.2% in infants, whereas the adult value is 0.78%, contradicting previous thinking that all children required increased amounts of inhalational agents. The lower neonatal values may be due to increased plasma endorphin concentrations, and the higher value for infants may be related to different concentrations of neurotransmitters in the brain.

Halothane

Halothane is still the inhalational agent of choice for children. It is suitable for inhalational induction as it has minimal irritant properties and its potency allows rapid deepening of anaesthesia. When normal anaesthetic concentrations are used cardiovascular depression is not marked. Neonates are not more prone to cardiovascular depression, provided notice is taken of their lower MAC relative to infants and children (Lerman et al 1983). Care must be taken when controlled ventilation is used, as overdosage is easier. Nodal rhythm is frequently found in children during halothane anaesthesia.

In the absence of surgical stimulation halothane anaesthesia may cause a rapid rate of ventilation with a decreased tidal volume, emphasizing the need for specially designed paediatric equipment with minimal dead space. Alveolar ventilation may be further compromised as halothane appears to selectively depress intercostal muscle action while sparing diaphragmatic activity (Tusiewicz et al 1977).

Laryngospasm may occur at extubation after halothane anaesthesia, and can be dangerous in small children with low oxygen reserves. Laryngospasm can be avoided by extubation during deep anaesthesia or by awaiting full recovery. Shivering and muscle rigidity are found as frequently as in adult anaesthesia.

Children recover quickly from halothane anaesthesia, nausea and vomiting being minimal in the absence of opioid administration (O'Neill et al 1982). Despite its high level of usage and frequent repeated administration, the incidence of hepatitis after halothane anaesthesia in children is extremely low. However, cases of hepatitis in children confirmed serologically by the presence of antibodies to halothane altered liver cell membrane antigens have now been reported (Kenna et al 1987). The problem has been reviewed by Walton (1986), who points out that no child who has previously demonstrated jaundice or (perhaps) late unexplained pyrexia after halothane, should be re-exposed to the drug. However, he supports the repeated use of halothane in children as safe anaesthetic practice in view of the potential problems with alternatives.

Enflurane

This agent offers no significant benefit for children when compared with halothane. Inhalational induction times are similar for the two agents but enflurane can give more difficulty with troublesome coughing or laryngospasm (Steward 1977). Enflurane causes significantly more hypotension and respiratory depression tends to be greater (O'Neill et al 1982). There is a small increase in fluoride levels in the urine but this increase is much less than that found after methoxyflurane anaesthesia (Chase et al 1971).

Isoflurane

Isoflurane is more irritant to the respiratory tract than halothane. This can lead to a difficult induction (Pandit et al 1983) and laryngospasm with secretions can be a disturbing problem (Friesen & Lichtor 1983). This problem can be partially attenuated by raising the isoflurane concentration steadily (Joseph et al 1985) to give a reasonably swift induction in keeping with the rapid uptake demonstrated in pharmacokinetic studies in children (Gallagher & Black 1985). As with halothane the MAC is decreased in the neonate (1.6%) compared with older infants (1.87%), but is similar to the value for older children (1.6%) (Cameron et al 1984). Cardiovascular stability is maintained with isoflurane with a reduction in blood pressure, less than that produced by halothane when used to induce anaesthesia in infants

(Friesen & Lichtor 1983), though MAC values for isoflurane were not established at the time of this study. When a volatile agent has to be used without nitrous oxide, isoflurane makes a suitable alternative to halothane as cardiac muscle depression, as documented in adults (Hickey & Eger 1981), is less.

Recovery from isoflurane is rapid, but differences in recovery from halothane are difficult to detect clinically, despite its low blood gas solubility (Kingston 1986). There are no significant differences in the occurrence of nausea and vomiting when isoflurane, halothane or enflurane are used with nitrous oxide for anaesthesia for procedures in children with malignancies (Fisher et al 1985).

Intravenous anaesthetic agents

Thiopentone

Thiopentone is the most commonly used intravenous induction agent for children. The dosage of 4–6 mg kg^{-1} (Cote et al 1981) is slightly higher than with adults but it must be used cautiously in neonates, who are particularly sensitive. Induction is smooth and recovery rates are rapid with minimal postoperative morbidity. Because children have a shorter elimination half-life, repeat doses will be required more frequently if it is used as a sole anaesthetic (Sorbo et al 1984). It can produce sleep in a dose of 40 mg kg^{-1} rectally, but this mode of administration should be carried out only when the child is constantly supervised.

Methohexitone

This agent has similar characteristics as an intravenous induction agent for adults and children. It can be given rectally in a dose of 25 mg kg^{-1} producing sleep in 8–12 minutes and normal recovery times after a $\frac{1}{2}$ hour operation (Goresky & Steward 1979). However, the potentially long induction time after this route of administration limits its usefulness. Intravenous induction frequently causes hiccoughs and abnormal muscle movements, though this can be partly overcome by heavy premedication. Pain on injection can be minimized by the addition of 2% lignocaine, 1 mg ml^{-1} of solution.

Ketamine

Ketamine is a satisfactory induction agent for children when specifically indicated. The cardiovascular effects are similar to those found in adults (Saarnivaara 1977) and it is sometimes used with less hesitation for children because the incidence of hallucination and dysphoric reactions, which is high in adults, is thought to be lower, though evidence for this belief is scanty. Children require more ketamine in relation to their body weight than do adults (Lockhart & Nelson 1974).

Etomidate

This agent has been used in children but the high incidence of side-effects, such as pain on injection and myoclonia, with no major clinical advantages over other agents, has reduced its acceptability (Kay 1976).

Propofol

Early reports on this agent suggest that it will have a place in paediatric anaesthesia. An induction dose of 2.8 mg kg^{-1} in unpremedicated children and 2.0 mg kg^{-1} in those premedicated with trimeprazine has been found satisfactory by Patel et al (1988). Mirakhur et al (1987) found a dose of 2.9 mg kg^{-1} to be required for induction using a 20–30 s injection up to loss of eyelash reflex, compared with 6.9 mg kg^{-1} for thiopentone, but with a more rapid recovery. The incidence of pain on injection was found to be high, but was reduced by the addition of lignocaine (1 mg per 1 ml of propofol).

Muscle relaxants

Although paediatric dosage schedules are generally more accurate when adult dosages are scaled down using a surface area comparison, muscle relaxant dosages are best based on body weight comparisons (Goudsouzian et al 1975), despite the fact that muscle mass is 25% of an infant's weight and 40% of an adult's weight. Early studies of non-depolarizing muscle relaxants in children were often carried out before the advent of suitable equipment for measuring twitch height after electrical stimulation, but more recent work indicates that infants and children require similar amounts of these agents compared with adults (Goudsouzian et al 1975). However, these workers showed a high degree of variability of relaxation in neonates given tubocurarine (0.15–0.62 mg kg^{-1}) as opposed to infants and children (0.25–0.47 mg kg^{-1}). For this reason the correct dose of relaxant is best given by slow administration of aliquots until satisfactory relaxation is achieved, or nerve stimulation indicates paralysis. The neuromuscular junction exhibits different properties in neonates from adults, but approaches maturation during the first 2 months of age (Goudsouzian, 1980). Hypothermia in infants receiving muscle relaxants is associated with an increased requirement for assistance with ventilation postoperatively, though this may be partly due to more complex surgical procedures being more likely to produce hypothermia (Rackow & Salanitre 1969). Tubocurarine is frequently used with children and neonates. Children below 5 years of age show less hypotension after this drug than those above 5 (Nightingale & Bush 1973). Similar age-related differences were found with pancuronium, with hypertension being more common in the under-5-year age group. Other non-depolarizing agents such as alcuronium, metocurine, atracurium and vecuronium have been used satisfactorily with children with minimal differences from adult experience.

When suxamethonium dosage requirements are evaluated on a weight-related scale, infants have higher requirements, 1.0 mg kg^{-1}, compared to children, 0.5 mg kg^{-1}, to achieve similar relaxation. However, this is mainly due to the relative large extracellular fluid volume in the infant, a compartment which is more closely related to surface area; and when surface area-related scales are used, differences are reduced. Intragastric pressure falls in most children after suxamethonium, but in the older age group, when fasciculation is more common, a rise in intragastric pressure is found (Salem et al 1972). The fall in heart rate associated with large doses or repeated administration is counteracted by administration of atropine (0.02 mg kg^{-1}). The incidence of afterpains is reduced, being found in 3% of 5–9-year-olds and 23% of 10–14-year-olds (Bush & Roth 1961).

Opioids

Morphine and pethidine are satisfactory drugs for the relief of pain in children, and may also be used as part of a balanced anaesthetic technique. Use of a less potent drug such as codeine may give the prescriber a false sense of safety, as it too has respiratory depressant properties if given in excessive dosage. Neonates are reported to be particularly sensitive to morphine, perhaps due to immaturity of the blood–brain barrier or of the liver and kidney (Way et al 1965), but in children over 3 weeks of age rates of metabolism are similar to those found in adults (Chinyanga et al 1983). High-dose fentanyl may be used for induction of anaesthesia in high-risk children undergoing corrective cardiac surgery under cardiopulmonary bypass, but a dose of 30 μkg^{-1} is adequate compared with 50 μg kg^{-1} frequently used for adults (Crean et al 1983).

REFERENCES

Axline S G, Yaffe S J, Simon H J 1967 Clinical pharmacology of antimicrobials in premature infants: 11 ampicillin, methicillin, oxacillin, neomycin and colistin. Pediatrics 39: 97–107

Bush G H, Roth F 1961 Muscle pains after suxamethonium chloride in children. British Journal of Anaesthesia 33: 151–155

Cameron C B, Robinson S, Gregory G A 1984. The minimum anesthetic concentration of isoflurane in children. Anesthesia and Analgesia 63: 418–420

Carmichael E B 1947 The median lethal dose (LD$_{50}$) of pentothal sodium for both young and old guinea pigs and rats. Anesthesiology 8: 589–593

Chantler C 1979 The kidney. In: Godfrey S, Baum J D (eds) Clinical paediatric physiology, Blackwell, Oxford, p 356

Chase R E, Holaday D A, Fisherov A, Bergerova V, Saidmann L J, Mack F E 1971 The biotransformation of ethrane in man. Anesthesiology 35: 262–267

Chinyanga H M, Vandenberge H, Bohn D, Macleod S, Soldin S 1983 Pharmacokinetics of morphine in young children following cardiac surgery. Anesthesiology 59: A447

Cook D R, Fischer C G 1975 Neuromuscular blocking effects of succinylcholine in infants and children. Anesthesiology 42: 662–665

Cote C J, Goudsouzian N G, Letty M P, Liu M D, Dedrick D F, Rosow C E 1981 The dose response of intravenous thiopental for the induction of general anesthesia in unpremedicated children. Anesthesiology 55: 703–705

Crean P, Goresky G, Koren G, Klein J, McCleod S M, Roy W L 1983 Fentanyl pharmacokinetics in children with congenital heart disease. Anesthesiology 59: A448

Dawson W T 1940 Relation between age and weight and dosage of drugs. Annals of Internal Medicine 13: 1594–1615

Done A K, Cohen S N, Strebel L 1977 Pediatric clinical pharmacology and the 'therapeutic orphan'. Annual Review of Pharmacology and Toxicology 17: 561–573

Ecobichon D J, Stephens D S 1973 Perinatal development of blood esterases. Clinical Pharmacology and Therapeutics 14: 41–47

Evans E F, Proctor J D, Fratkin M S, Velandia J, Wasserman A J 1975 Blood flow in muscle groups and drug absorption. Clinical Pharmacology and Therapeutics 17: 44–47

Fisher D M, Robinson S, Brett C M, Perin G, Gregory F A 1985. Comparison of enflurane, halothane and isoflurane for diagnostic and therapeutic procedures in children with malignancies. Anesthesiology 53: 647–650

Friesen R H, Lichtor J L 1983 Cardiovascular effects of inhalation induction with isoflurane in infants. Anesthesia and Analgesia 62: 411–414

Friis Hansen B 1957 Changes in body water compartments during growth. Acta Paediatrica, Stockholm, Suppl 46: 110

Gallagher T M, Black G W 1985 Uptake of volatile anaesthetics in children. Anaesthesia 40: 1073–1077

Gladtke E, Heimann G 1975 The rate of development of elimination functions of kidney and liver of young infants. In: Mariselli P L, Garattini S, Seremi F (eds) Basic and therapeutic aspects of perinatal pharmacology, Raven Press, New York, p 393

Goresky G V, Steward D J 1979 Rectal methohexitone for

induction of anaesthesia in children. Canadian Anaesthetic Society Journal 26: 213–215

Goudsouzian N G 1980 Maturation of neuromuscular transmission in the infant. British Journal of Anaesthesia 52: 205–214

Goudsouzian N G, Donlon J V, Savarese J J, Ryan J F 1975 Re-evaluation of dosage and duration of action of d-tubocurarine in the pediatric age group. Anesthesiology 43: 416–425

Habersang F 1980 Dosage. In: Shirkey H C (ed.) Paediatric therapy. Mosby, St Louis, p 17

Hickey R F, Eger E I 1981 Circulatory pharmacology of inhaled anaesthetics. In: Miller R (ed) Anaesthesia. Churchill Livingstone, New York, p 331

Houston I B 1979 Fluid and electrolyes. In: Godfrey S, Baum J D (eds) Clinical paediatric physiology. Blackwell, Oxford, P

Joseph M M, Win K K, Nelson D H, Warner D L, Steen S N 1985 Mask induction responses to a predetermined technique and recovery characteristics of isoflurane anesthesia in children. Anesthesia and Analgesia 64: 234

Kay B 1976 A clinical assessment of the use of etomidate in children. British Journal of Anaesthesia 48: 207–211

Kenna J G, Neuberger J, Mieli-Vergani G, Mowat A P, Williams R 1987 Halothane hepatitis in children. British Medical Journal 294: 1209–1210

Kingston H G G 1986 Halothane and isoflurane anesthesia in pediatric outpatients. Anesthesia and Analgesia 65: 181–184

Lerman J, Robinson S, Willis M M, Gregory G A 1983 Anesthetic requirements for halothane in young children 0–1 month and 1–6 months of age. Anesthesiology 59: 421–424

Levy G, Khanna N N, Soda D M, Tsuzuki O, Stern L 1975 Pharmacokinetics of acetaminophen in the human neonate. Paediatrics 55: 818–825

Lockhart C H, Nelson W L 1974 The relationship of ketamine requirement to age in pediatric patients. Anesthesiology 40: 507–510

Mirakhur R K, Elliott P, Crean P M 1988 Induction characteristics of propofol in children: comparison with thiopentone. Anaesthesia 43: 593–598

Myers M G, Roberts R J, Mirhij N J 1977 Effects of gestational age, birthweight and hypoxemia on pharmacokinetics of amikacin in serum of infants.

Antimicrobial Agents and Chemotherapy 11: 1027–1032

Nightingale D A, Bush G H 1973 A clinical comparison between tubocurarine and pancuronium in children. British Journal of Anaesthesia 45: 63–69

O'Neill M P, Sharkey A J, Fee J P H, Black G W 1982 A comparative study of enflurane and halothane in children. Anaesthesia 37: 634–639

Pandit U A, Leach A B, Steude G M 1983 Induction and recovery characteristics of halothane and isoflurane anesthesia in children. Anesthesiology 59: A445

Patel D K, Keeling P A, Newman G B, Radford P 1988 Induction dose of propofol in children. Anaesthesia 43: 949–952

Rackow H, Salanitre E 1969 Modern concepts in pediatric anesthesiology. Anesthesiology 30: 208–234

Saarnivaara L 1977 Comparison of thiopentone, althesin and ketamine in anaesthesia for otorhinolaryngological surgery in children. British Journal of Anaesthesia 49: 363–370

Salanitre E, Rackow H 1969 The pulmonary exchange of nitrous oxide and halothane in infants and children. Anesthesiology 30: 388–394

Salem M R, Wong A I, Lim Y H 1972 The effects of suxamethonium on the intragastric pressure in infants and children. British Journal of Anaesthesia 44: 166–170

Smith C A, Nelson N M 1976 Physiology of the newborn infant, 4th edn. Thomas, Springfield,

Sorbo S, Hudson R J, Loomis J C 1984 Pharmacokinetics of thiopental in pediatric surgical patients. Anesthesiology 61: 666–670

Steward D J 1977 A trial of enflurane for paediatric outpatient anaesthesia. Canadian Anaesthetic Society Journal 24: 603–608

Steward D J, Creighton R E 1978 The uptake and excretion of nitrous oxide in the newborn. Canadian Anaesthetic Society Journal 25: 215–217

Tusiewicz K, Bryan A C, Froese A B, 1977 Contributions of changing ribcage–diaphragm interactions to ventilatory depression of halothane anesthesia. Anesthesiology 47: 327–337

Walton B 1986 Halothane hepatitis in children. Anaesthesia 41: 575–578

Way W L, Costley E C, Way E L 1965 Respiratory sensitivity of the newborn infant to meperidine. Clinical Pharmacology and Therapeutics 6: 454–461

PART 2
AGE: RESPONSE IN THE ELDERLY
J. W. Dundee

The differing response of ageing patients to drugs given in the anaesthetic period is assuming increasing importance. We have rising numbers of elderly patients in the population and also an increasing chance that these elderly patients may have had a previous anaesthetic, up to 77–80% in patients aged 60 and over (Fee et al 1980). While the relationship of repeat administration of halothane and the time between administration and development of liver damage is not quite clear (Editorial 1986) this is an important point to consider in elderly patients. These factors are important when one considers that major surgery in the elderly is increasing in frequency.

While elderly patients have a high chance of having been previously exposed to general anaesthesia, this applies to a number of other drugs, some of which could affect cerebral tolerance to anaesthetics. Generally this will be in the form of resistance, and it can occur in patients whose cardiovascular and respiratory systems respond poorly to high doses. Some other drugs could induce hepatic enzymes; these will be discussed later.

THE AGEING PROCESS

It is difficult to separate the disease processes which occur more frequently in the elderly, from the ageing process, but it is important to realize that even healthy elderly patients react differently to the stress of operation and to the drugs given in the perioperative period, and also have less efficient compensatory and reparative processes than younger patients. A good example of this is the marked decrease in total elastase in the plasma in the seventh decade of life (Hall 1979). Although the clinical significance of this is not known, it is typical of many other changes which extensively contribute to organ failure (Crooks & Stevenson 1979).

For the anaesthetist the most dramatic effects are the changes in factors which influence the pharmacokinetics of drugs in the elderly; these will be reviewed later. Some are of only minor importance, e.g. the anatomical dead space increases as the diameter of the larynx and trachea increase in the elderly. The dead space–tidal volume ratio (V_d/V_t) and alveolar–arterial oxygen tension differences also increase with age.

There is a tendency for body temperatures to be related to environmental temperatures in the elderly, and there may be an undetected degree of hypothermia on exposure to even a moderately cold environment.

As a side issue we are aware that the elderly are more at risk of developing drug reactions. Surveying a hospital population Hurwitz (1969) found adverse reactions occurring in 3% of patients aged 20–29, and in 21% of those between 70 and 79 years. While part of this was due to inappropriate prescribing and poor compliance, both pharmacokinetic and pharmacological factors contribute to the altered drug response in the elderly. Many drugs have been marketed with inadequate information on their side-effects in the elderly, but since the 'Opren' incident, this has been tightened up.

Replacement of active haemopoietic tissue in bone marrow by fat and fibrous tissue in healthy elderly patients leads to a tendency to lower haemoglobin levels, and Lloyd (1971) found one-fifth of the patients admitted to a geriatric assessment unit were anaemic. Although plasma electrolytes tend to remain normal in the healthy elderly plasma albumin levels may fall. This can decrease protein binding of some drugs and lead to increased levels of free, pharmacologically active, drug.

RESPONSE OF THE ELDERLY TO DRUGS

It is possible to consider the response of the elderly patients under three headings:

1. differing type of response;
2. pharmacokinetic alterations;
3. altered pharmacodynamic (or end organ) response.

This is an over-simplification as it is unusual to get an abnormal response which involves only one of the above. As an example the restlessness which elderly patients sometimes exhibit after benzodiazepines might not be noticed if there were not a concomitant increase in the drugs' duration of action in the elderly. Most examples of sensitivity to drugs in the elderly are the result of alterations in pharmacokinetics rather than a true age-dependent difference in response, but the two may exist together.

Differing type of response

True age-dependent differences in response to drugs used by the anaesthetist are rare, and may be more anecdotal than proven. Elderly patients often develop mild restlessness and anxiety after barbiturates or hyoscine, and these drugs should be avoided or used sparingly.

The rise in intraocular pressure induced by atropine, while of little consequence in normal subjects, may induce acute glaucoma in the elderly. Extended venous thrombosis following intravenous diazepam is much more likely to occur in elderly patients (Hegarty & Dundee 1978). These latter two may be examples of an exaggeration of a normal response rather than a differing type of response; however, their clinical importance is obvious.

Pharmacokinetic alterations

The main pharmacokinetic changes which affect the response to anaesthetic drugs in the elderly are summarized in Tables 4.2 and 4.3. For a more detailed discussion readers are referred to Crooks et al (1976) and Crooks & Stevenson (1979.)

The arm–brain circulation time is frequently prolonged in the elderly, and this is the main factor in determining the rate of onset of action of thiopentone and similar drugs; if a fixed rate of injection is used there is an increased risk of giving an overdose. One frequently notices a delay in the occurrence of muscle fasciculations following suxamethonium in the elderly; this is likewise due to a slow circulation time. Since fasciculations precede relaxation, a second (unnecessary)

Table 4.2 Main pharmacokinetic changes in the elderly

Reduced body weight	Standard dose gives greater mg kg^{-1}
Reduced body water	Water-soluble drugs have a higher blood level and lower volume of distribution
Increased body fat	Lipid-soluble drugs have lower blood levels and greater volume of distribution
Reduced plasma albumin	Protein binding of some drugs is reduced
Metabolism	Oxidative processes reduced: some reduction in first-pass metabolism
Excretion	Glomerular filtration and tubular secretion decline with age

(From Ramsay & Tucker 1981).

Table 4.3 Factors influencing the onset of action of anaesthetic drugs in the elderly.

Slow circulation time
Decreased pulmonary function
Poor absorption from injection sites
Delayed oral absorption

From Dundee (1979.)

travenously during anaesthesia, but this is of less clinical importance than with drugs given during induction.

Although most important pulmonary functions decline with age this does not markedly affect the response to inhalational anaesthetics. Increases in residual volume result in a slower rate of change of alveolar and arterial blood levels, but this is not of great clinical importance. However, the additive effects of smoking and age can make an inhalational induction both slow and stormy.

Recent work has shown the important influence of plasma binding on the onset of action of midazolam (Halliday et al 1985). This is a highly bound benzodiazepine and small alterations in binding result in large changes in free drug which are sufficient to hasten its onset of action in the elderly (Fig. 4.3) and make it more acceptable as an induction agent.

dose of relaxant could readily be given if the importance of the prolonged circulation time is not appreciated. A slow circulation time will also affect the rate of onset of effect of opioid analgesics and of other drugs given in-

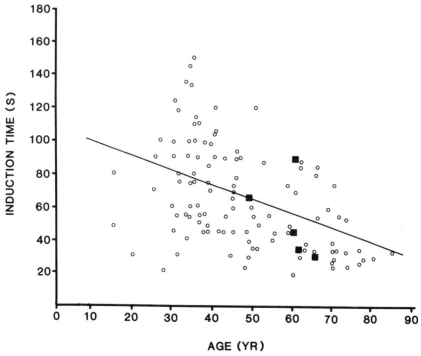

Fig. 4.3 Induction time following 0.3 mg midazolam given over 20 s related to the age of patients (Dundee et al 1985): ○, single patient; ■, more than one patient.

The reduction in plasma proteins, which is not uncommon in the elderly, may also affect the action of other intravenous anaesthetics, with more free drug reaching the target organ. This will produce not only a deeper level of narcosis but also a more profound depression of vital centres. A vicious circle is quickly established (Table 4.4), with reduced regional blood flow and tissue perfusion further decreasing redistribution and prolonging the clinical effects. This is undoubtedly the most serious type of sensitivity to anaesthetic drugs in elderly patients. It occurs in those who are not well able to tolerate sudden cardiovascular depression, and the eventual outcome may be disastrous.

Table 4.4 Sequence of events which can modify the action of thiopentone in the elderly and lead to prolonged hypotension

Decreased binding to albumin
Increased free-drug concentration
Exaggerated pharmacodynamic action
Hypotension and reduced tissue perfusion
Decreased redistribution in the body
Prolonged clinical effect
Possible cerebral hypoxia

Pharmacokinetic disturbances do not have such a marked effect on the action of inhalational agents. In contrast, paralysis from myoneural blocking drugs may be prolonged because of decreased tissue perfusion and slower removal from their site of action. Plasma protein derangements affect both their intensity and duration of action. This, and the influence of decreased renal function, will be discussed later.

There is one interesting pharmacokinetic finding in relation to local anaesthetics. Bromage (1954) found an inverse relationship between the dose of local anaesthetic required for epidural anaesthesia and the age of the patient. With increasing age the intravertebral foramina become less permeable and so hinder the escape of solutions, so that a given volume travels further up the spinal canal and causes a wider area of block.

The altered ability of elderly patients to eliminate drugs which are entirely metabolized in the body is not of great importance in anaesthesia. The fact that patients with liver disease may be unable to detoxicate repeated doses of pethidine has led to problems in the postoperative period (Dundee & Tinckler 1952) when its effects became exaggerated, yet this analgesic is widely used in geriatric practice with no reports of adverse reactions. Renal excretion of relaxants will be discussed later.

Klotz et al (1975), investigating the effect of age on the disposition and elimination of diazepam in man, found the plasma half-life ($t_{\frac{1}{2}}\beta$) to be approximately 20 h at 20 years of age, increasing linearly with age to about 90 h at 80 years. This prolongation appeared to be due to an alteration in the distribution of the drug, since total plasma clearance was not found to be a function of age. This is probably of little clinical importance in relation to its use as a premedicant or an intravenous sedative, as its repeated administration has largely been replaced by midazolam. However, Harper et al (1985) have demonstrated a decreased rate of elimination of this drug with age (Fig. 4.4) and when it is given by infusion or intermittent injection as a sedative in the intensive-care situation, there may be a prolonged effect in elderly patients.

There are no clinically important pharmacokinetic factors influencing the use of inhalational drugs in the elderly. Long-acting opioids will have a greater cumulative effect on repeat administration, and methadone is better avoided in these patients. Because of impaired vasomotor function postural hypotension is more likely to follow the use of phenothiazines in the elderly. This also applies to a lesser extent to some opioids, particularly pethidine.

ALTERED END ORGAN RESPONSE

Reference has already been made to the profound hypotension which may follow the use of thiopentone in the elderly. This is not all due to altered pharmacokinetics, but in part to the increased sensitivity of the myocardium to its depressant action and to the lesser ability to compensate for peripheral vasodilation. This sensitivity applies to all intravenous anaesthetics and to a lesser extent to inhalational drugs. It is also seen with some opioids, particularly pethidine, and occasionally with the histamine-releasing tubocurarine. Phenothiazines, droperidol and other vasodilator drugs may also produce marked hypotension in the elderly. The increased tendency to postural hypotension must also be remembered in this age group.

While arrhythmias are relatively common during anaesthesia in the elderly patient, it is difficult to say whether this is a true accompaniment of the ageing process or whether it is associated with coronary artery disease.

Altered respiratory responses to anaesthetics in the elderly may be due to disturbance of ventilation–perfusion ratio, but also in part associated with concomitant disease such as emphysema and chronic bronchitis. In addition, increased irritability of the tracheobronchial tree may occur, with tendency to breath-holding,

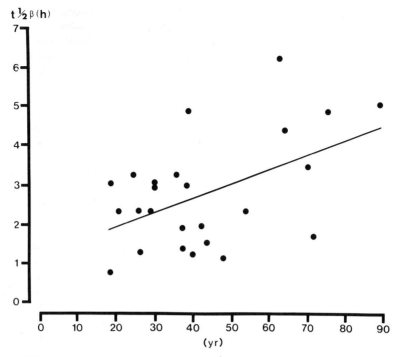

Fig. 4.4 Midazolam half-life related to age of patients (0.3 mg kg^{-1} given i.v.). (Harper et al 1985).

coughing, etc. Many elderly patients have a higher Pa CO_2 level than normal, and difficulty may occur in re-establishing normal respiration after relaxants or opioids.

A diminished respiratory exchange, with a decrease in tidal volume, may lead to an exaggeration of the depressant effects of opioids, particularly in the postoperative period, and minor degrees of persistent curarization can have serious effects in the elderly.

There is increasing evidence that differences in cerebral receptor sensitivity may account for some of the increased drug sensitivity seen in the elderly. As an example, Belville and his colleagues (1971) found a greater than expected degree of analgesia in elderly patients given morphine or pentazocine for postoperative pain relief. The increasing sensitivity to benzodiazepines in the elderly (Castleden et al 1977) can only partly be explained on a pharmacokinetic basis (Klotz et al 1975 Wilkinson 1979). Bender (1979) and Castleden & George (1979) have shown that cognitive function is depressed to a greater degree by nitrazepam in the elderly, perhaps reflecting the general deterioriation in speed of performance which accompanies ageing. The widely publicized increased incidence of side-effects from benzodiazepines in the elderly found by the Boston Col-

laborative Drug Surveillance Program (1973) falls into this class.

For many years clinicians have known that elderly patients require lower doses of thiopentone to induce anaesthesia than the young (Andreasen & Christensen 1977, Dundee et al 1982). Is this due to concurrent pathology or to age alone? The findings of a controlled study are shown in Fig. 4.5. Here we see not only a reduction in thiopentone requirements in the elderly, but also the effects of alcoholism, which markedly increase the dose of this drug required to induce anaesthesia irrespective of age. Toxic effects from these large doses are not uncommon, and pretreatment with an opioid is recommended in the alcoholic. This will reduce the induction dose to safe levels.

Figure 4.6 shows some of the results of a controlled dose-finding study with propofol (Dundee et al 1986). There was an obvious reduction in dosage over the age of 60. When given as a bolus over 20 s to unpremedicated fit patients those under 60 years required 2.25 mg kg^{-1} to reliably induce anaesthesia as compared with 1.50 mg kg^{-1} in those aged 60 and over. More important than dose requirement was the response of the cardiovascular and respiratory system to propofol in the two age groups. When the drug was administered slowly

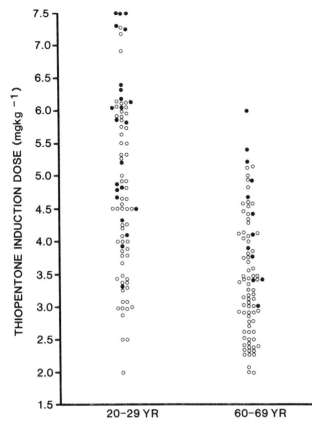

Fig. 4.5 Individual requirements of thiopentone for induction of anaesthesia, when administered according to a fixed plan in two age groups: ○, patients with no or small alcohol intake, ●, patients with moderate to marked alcohol intake.

in the dose-finding study there was minimal hypotension, even in the elderly, while the 20 s bolus administration of moderate doses resulted in marked hypotension and apnoea.

Hypothyroidism and hypothermia, which are not uncommon, will also induce sensitivity to depressant drugs in the elderly. From the clinical point of view, one must not forget that the aged patient is unduly susceptible to the adverse effects of hypoxia, whether this be of the hypoxic or stagnant form. A degree of hyperventilation which in younger patients will produce no adverse effects from cerebral vasoconstriction may cause persistence of minor degree of personality changes, confusion, urinary upset or other undesirable cerebral sequelae.

There are no grounds for believing that the response of the liver or kidney to exposure to general anaesthesia is per se altered in the elderly patient. An increased toxic action on these organs results mainly from an exaggerated cardiovascular depression reducing their blood supply. This, in turn, will alter their ability to detoxicate or excrete certain drugs. One must not forget the potentially nephrotoxic action of large amounts of methoxyflurane — whether from short administration of a high concentration or long administration of a low concentration — which might have serious consequences in elderly patients who already have some impairment of renal function. Nephrotoxicity will be potentiated by tetracyclines, and this combination is better avoided in the elderly.

The action of drugs on the myoneural junction may be very different in the elderly, and this is such a major topic that the neuromuscular blocking drugs will be considered separately.

NEUROMUSCULAR BLOCKING DRUGS

Table 4.5 lists some of the factors which influence the response of the elderly to these drugs. Since they are bound to a variable degree to plasma proteins, the alteration in plasma protein levels or in the ratio of individual proteins which occurs commonly in the elderly will affect the response, and increased sensitivity to all relaxants can be expected where there is a low level of plasma protein. Patients with a low albumin level are particularly sensitive to alcuronium (Stovner et al 1971a).

Table 4.5 Factors influencing the response to myoneural blocking drugs in the elderly

Altered plasma proteins
Liver dysfunction
Hypothermia
Electrolyte and acid–base disturbance
Impaired renal excretion

Tubocurarine is bound to gamma-globulin (Aladjemoff et al 1958) and studies by Baraka & Gabali (1968) and by Stovner et al (1971a) showed a positive correlation between tubocurarine requirements during anaesthesia and plasma gamma-globulin level. This agrees with reports of resistance to tubocurarine in patients with an altered A/G ratio (Dundee & Gray 1953). Surprisingly, one may encounter this resistance in elderly patients with liver disease or an increased gamma-globulin from other causes. Theoretically, these patients would be expected to react normally to other non-depolarizing relaxants (Stovner et al 1971b, 1972).

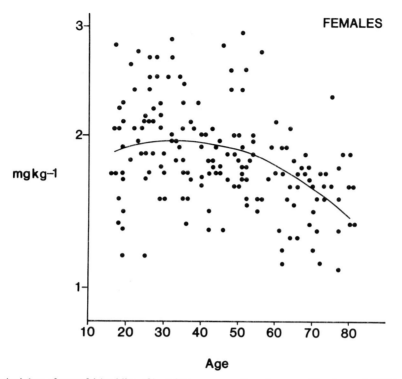

Fig. 4.6 'Induction' dose of propofol (and line of best fit) in women of varying ages. (Dundee et al 1986.)

Liver dysfunction, malnutrition and general debility may be accompanied by a low level of plasma pseudo-cholinesterase of sufficient degree to prolong the action of suxamethonium and possibly produce a 'dual' block.

Impaired temperature homeostasis is not uncommon in the elderly (Collins et al 1977). On coming to surgery, particularly for emergency operations, many elderly patients may have an undetected low body temperature. Even moderate degrees of hypothermia will decrease the effectiveness of tubocurarine and other non-depolarizing relaxants. This can produce problems of reversal if patients are warmed during the operation, at the end of which they may have received a very large dose of relaxant. There is an enhancement of the action of depolarizing relaxants at low body temperature.

Although the problem is not confined to the elderly, there may be difficulty in establishing adequate respiration after non-depolarizing relaxants in patients with electrolyte and acid–base disturbances. Acidaemia and a low serum potassium influence the response to these drugs, but hypovolaemia may be a contributory factor. One must hesitate to incriminate a specific pharmacological action in this syndrome of 'neostigmine-resistant curarization' in elderly patients. In the absence of relax-

ants, metabolic acidaemia can cause confusion or unconsciousness, and even inadequate respiration (Brooks & Feldman 1962), and the term 'moribundity' has been applied to this situation.

Some degree of renal dysfunction is common in the elderly, and this could prolong the action of gallamine, which is solely dependent on the kidneys for removal from the body. Although tubocurarine is largely excreted in the urine, its action is seldom prolonged in patients with renal disease. There is no evidence to suggest that the new shorter-acting non-depolarizing drugs, vecuronium and atracurium, show a sensitivity in the elderly.

SUMMARY

While there is a great variation in the age at which patients can be classed as 'elderly' and respond differently to drugs, the age at which end-organ sensitivity was demonstrated is earlier than might be expected. With the benzodiazepines this appeared to be 50 years, and with thiopentone and propofol this was at about 60 years. On looking at Figure 4.6 one sees a lower scatter of dose requirements in the elderly. This applies to all agents,

Table 4.6 Some problems associated with non-anaesthetic drugs in elderly patients

Drug	Problems include	Reason
Digoxin	Toxicity	Reduced clearance
K-sparing diuretics	Hyperkalaemia	
Renal excreted β-adrenoreceptor blockers	Overdosage	Reduced clearance
Warfarin	Many drug interactions	
Diazepam/nitrazepam	Daytime drowsiness	Increased sensitivity Reduced metabolism
Some phenothiazines	Extrapyramidal effects	Increased sensitivity
Opioids	Dysphoria, sedation	Increased sensitivity
(Long-acting opioids)	(Increased toxicity)	(Decreased metabolism)
Potassium supplements	Hyperkalaemia	Reduced clearance
Non-steroidal anti-inflammatory drugs	Na retention	
	Greater toxicity	

Modified from *Drugs and Therapeutics Bulletin* 1984.

and a reduced margin of safety is one of the features of the response of the elderly to drugs.

In clinical practice with adequate knowledge of the factors which alter the response to drugs, and with careful handling and prompt treatment of emergencies, the anaesthetist can safely use most of our available drugs in the elderly patient. True age-dependent differences in response to such drugs are rare.

A slower circulation time and decreased respiratory function may prolong the onset of action of injected or inhaled drugs. Impairment of normal processes of redistribution in the body can increase the toxicity of thiopentone, and this is probably the greatest problem which crops up in clinical practice. Slower detoxication is not important with most drugs used in anaesthesia.

The elderly patient is relatively sensitive to the depressant effects of most drugs given by the anaesthetist. This can be manifested by more marked and more prolonged hypotension and respiratory depression, and also by a delay in return of full consciousness. The additional adverse effects of hypoxia may contribute to this. However, on occasions, elderly patients may show unexpected resistance to cerebral depressants.

The response of the geriatric patient to neuromuscular blocking drugs is complex, and will be affected by reduction or alteration in plasma protein, liver dysfunction, hypothermia, electrolyte imbalance and renal impairment. With these drugs in particular adequate knowledge of the overall condition of the patient can prevent problems which may well endanger life.

NON-ANAESTHETIC DRUGS

One can only summarize the important alterations in response to or effects of non-anaesthetic drugs which the anaesthetist may encounter in the perioperative period. Table 4.6 shows that these are mainly due to pharmacokinetic alterations in the elderly. Awareness of the potential problem can reduce the likelihood of accidents.

REFERENCES

Aladjemoff L, Dikstein S, Shafrir E 1958 The binding of d-tubocurarine chloride to plasma proteins. Journal of Pharmacology and Experimental Therapeutics 123: 43–47

Andreasen F, Christensen J H 1977 Individual variation in response to thiopentone. British Journal of Clinical Pharmacology 4: 64OP

Baraka A, Gabali F 1968 Correlation between tubocurarine requirements and plasma protein pattern. British Journal of Anaesthesia 40: 89–93

Belville J W, Forrest H W, Miller E, Brown B W 1971 Influence of age on pain relief from analgesics. Journal of the American Medical Association 217: 1835–1841

Bender A D 1979 Drug sensitivity in the elderly. In: Crooks J, Stevenson I H (eds) Drugs and the elderly. Macmillan, London, pp 147–153

Boston Collaborative Drug Surveillance Program 1973

Clinical depression of the central nervous system due to diazepam and chlordiazepoxide in relation to cigarette smoking and age. New England Journal of Medicine 288: 277–280

Bromage P R 1954 Spinal epidural analgesia. Livingstone, Edinburgh

Brooks D K and Feldman S A 1962 Metabolic acidosis: a new approach to 'neostigmine resistant curarisation'. Anaesthesia 17: 161–169

Castleden C M, George C F 1979 Increased sensitivity to benzodiazepines in the elderly. In: Crooks J, Stevenson I H (eds) Drugs and the elderly. Macmillan, London, pp 169–178

Castleden C M, George C F, Marcer D, Hallett C 1977 Increased sensitivity to nitrazepam in old age. British Medical Journal 1: 10–12

Collins K J, Dore C, Exton-Smith A N, Fox R H, MacDonald I C, Woodward P M 1977 Accidental hypothermia and impaired temperature homoeostasis in the elderly. British Medical Journal 1: 353–356

Crooks J, O'Malley K, Stevenson I H 1976 Pharmacokinetics in the elderly. Clinical Pharmacokinetics 1: 280–296

Crooks J, Stevenson I H 1979 Drugs and the elderly. Perspectives in geriatric clinical pharmacology. Macmillan, London,

Drugs and Therapeutics Bulletin 1984 Medication for the elderly. Vol 23, pp 49–52

Dundee J W 1979 Response to anaesthetic drugs in the elderly. In: Crooks J, Stevenson I H (eds) Drugs and the elderly. Macmillan, London, pp 179–187

Dundee J W, Gray T C 1953 Resistance to d-tubocurarine chloride in the presence of liver damage. Lancet 2: 16–17

Dundee J W, Tinckler L F 1952 Pethidine and liver damage. British Medical Journal 2: 703–704

Dundee J W, Hassard T H, McGowan W A W, Henshaw J 1982 The 'induction' dose of thiopentone. Anaesthesia 37: 1176–1184

Dundee J W, Halliday N J, Loughran P G, Harper K W 1985 The influence of age on the onset of anaesthesia with midazolam. Anaesthesia 40: 441–443

Dundee J W, Robinson F P, McCollum J S C, Patterson C C 1986 Sensitivity to propofol in the elderly. Anaesthesia 41: 482–485

Editorial 1986 Halothane-associated liver damage. Lancet 1: 1251–1253

Fee J P H, McDonald J R, Dundee J W 1980 Frequency of atopy, allergy and previous general anaesthesia in surgical specialties. Annals of the Royal College of Surgeons 62: 125–128

Hall D A 1979 Biochemical background to current theories of ageing. In: Crooks J, Stevenson I H (eds) Drugs and the elderly. Macmillan, London, pp 3–14

Halliday N J, Dundee J W, Collier P S, Loughran P G, Harper K W 1985 Influence of plasma proteins on the onset of hypnotic action of intravenous midazolam. Anaesthesia 40: 763–766

Harper K W, Collier P S, Dundee J W, Elliott P, Halliday N J, Lowry K G 1985 Age and nature of operation influence the pharmacokinetics of midazolam. British Journal of Anaesthesia 57: 866–871

Hegarty J E, Dundee J W 1978 Local sequelae following the i.v. injection of three benzodiazepines. British Journal of Anaesthesia 50: 78–79

Hurwitz N 1969 Predisposing factors and adverse reactions to drugs. British Medical Journal 1: 536–539

Klotz U, Avant G R, Hoyumpa A, Schenker S, Wilkinson G R 1975 Effects of age and liver disease on the distribution and elimination of diazepam in man. Journal of Clinical Investigation 55: 347–359

Lloyd E L 1971 Serum iron levels and haematological status in the elderly. Gerontological Clinics 13: 246–255

Ramsay L E, Tucker G T 1981 Drugs and the elderly. British Medical Journal 282: 125–127

Stovner J, Theodorsen L, Bjelke E 1971a Sensitivity to tubocurarine and alcuronium with special reference to plasma protein pattern. British Journal of Anaesthesia 43: 385–391

Stovner J, Theodorsen L, Bielke E 1971b Sensitivity to gallamine and pancuronium with special reference to serum proteins. British Journal of Anaesthesia 43: 953–958

Stovner J, Theodorsen L, Bjelke E 1972 Sensitivity to dimethyltubocurarine and toxiferine with special reference to serum proteins. British Journal of Anaesthesia 44: 374–380

Stevenson I H, Salem S A M, Shepherd A M M 1969 Studies on drug absorption and metabolism in the elderly. In: Crooks J, Stevenson I H (eds) Drugs and the elderly. Macmillan, London, pp 51–63

Wilkinson G R 1979 The effect of ageing on the disposition of benzodiazepines in man. In: Crooks J, Stevenson I H (eds) Drugs and the elderly. Macmillan, London, pp 103–110

PART 3
INFLUENCE OF CARDIAC DISEASE
W. McCaughey

THE INFLUENCE OF CARDIAC DISEASE

A normally healthy heart adjusts, with the aid of other nervous and hormonal mechanisms, to changes in demand made of the circulation. When the output of the heart is no longer able to meet the requirements of the peripheral tissues for oxygen and nutrients, then the heart is failing. As the heart fails, the forward, arterial pressure tends to fall, while backward pressure on the venous system tends to rise. Compensatory mechanisms come into play, which may be viewed as defending the arterial pressure and the perfusion pressure in critical organs such as the heart and brain (Cannon 1977). These adaptations may succeed in maintaining a normal blood pressure, and blood flow to these vital organs, but they do so at the expense of changes in intracardiac pressures, and of reduced perfusion of other organs and peripheral tissues. These changes may affect the uptake and distribution of drugs, as well as their elimination in some cases.

Absorption

Gastrointestinal absorption. In cardiac disease, several factors may lead to impaired absorption of drugs. These include oedema of the gut wall, decreased splanchnic blood flow, reduced gastric emptying and reduced intestinal motility. The interaction of all these factors is unpredictable; thus it will be difficult to forecast the overall effect on absorption, but for most drugs which have been studied, absorption is reduced (Benet et al 1976). Thus the time taken for an orally administered drug to reach its peak effect will be longer. However, as considered below, a fall in the volume of distribution may mean that the plasma levels may not be any less than in patients with normal cardiac function.

Splanchnic blood flow is reduced as a result of both a reduction in cardiac output and a redistribution of blood flow and in some cases a direct relationship can be found between cardiac output and systemic bioavailability (Dunselman et al 1989). The effect of reduced splanchnic blood flow on absorption is most marked with drugs which penetrate the gut wall readily — those which are highly lipophilic or those whose small molecules diffuse readily through pores, and where therefore the rate of perfusion of the gut is the limiting factor in removing drug from this situation.

The rate of absorption from intramuscular, subcutaneous and fat sites is also reduced due to reduction in perfusion of these tissues.

Distribution

Reduced perfusion of the more 'peripheral' organs means in pharmacokinetic terms that the central compartment of the body is smaller. The drug is also slower at penetrating to the limits of its distribution, and so the ultimate or steady-state volume of distribution (Vd_{ss}) may be somewhat reduced, but the initial volume of distribution, which represents distribution into well-perfused regions, will often be markedly reduced (Woosley 1987). For example the volume of the central compartment for quinidine is reduced to about 60% in patients with cardiac failure, thus resulting in a higher plasma level of the drug, and necessitating a reduction in dose of about one-third (Ueda and Dzindzio 1978).

More relevant to anaesthetic practice are drugs such as lignocaine where plasma levels in patients with congestive heart failure may be double those normally expected (Thompson et al 1973), or intravenous agents such as thiopentone, where similar principles apply.

If, on the other hand, a drug normally has a small volume of distribution, i.e. it does not spread readily beyond the central compartment, then cardiac failure will have little effect on its distribution. Frusemide (furosemide) is an example of this type of behaviour (Benet et al 1976).

If a drug is given relatively rapidly, then as the circulation is relatively slow, mixing of the drug with all the blood of the central compartment will occur more slowly. Thus with rapid intravenous injection it will be easy to have a 'slug' of highly concentrated drug passing through the circulation, and this will be directed preferentially to the vital organs, making rapid cardiovascular depression by an intravenous anaesthetic agent, or by lignocaine, for example, much more likely. This would, of course, be accentuated by saturation of binding sites and higher free drug levels within the 'slug'.

Inhalational drugs

The uptake and distribution of inhalational anaesthetic drugs is also markedly affected by changes in blood flow. The changes in situations with a hyperdynamic circulation are essentially opposite to those in conditions with reduced cardiac output, such as heart failure or shock. An additional factor which comes into play in pulmonary absorption is the rate of supply of drug to the alveoli, limited by ventilation. With increased blood flow, drug is removed rapidly from the alveoli, thus reducing the rate at which alveolar concentration can rise and delaying the establishment of equilibrium. Conversely, in shock or cardiac failure, slow circulation results in slow removal of drug from alveoli, but this allows time for the alveolar concentration to build up, and time for full equilibration with the blood. Thus the concentration of drug in the pulmonary blood will rise rapidly. Poor perfusion of peripheral tissues such as muscle which normally take up drug rapidly (i.e. reduced Vd) will also contribute to rapid development of a high tension of the anaesthetic drug. This change will be more marked with the more soluble drugs, while less soluble substances such as nitrous oxide will be relatively less affected. The circulatory depressant effect of drugs such as halothane or enflurane may exert a positive feedback on this mechanism, thus further increasing the rate of rise of blood concentration towards inspired concentration, with a risk of anaesthetic overdose and cardiovascular collapse (Gibbons et al 1977).

Elimination

Most drugs are eliminated mainly by renal or hepatic routes. Both of these are affected by the condition of the heart. Reduction in splanchnic blood flow includes reduction in hepatic blood flow, and thus affects the removal of drug by this organ. As described later, this effect will depend on the extraction ratio of the drug, so that elimination of a drug with a high hepatic extraction ratio will be much influenced by changes in blood flow, while a drug with a low extraction ratio may be flow-independent.

In some cases the rate of metabolism by the liver may also be reduced because there is less enzyme activity. This may be as a result of congestion and consequent hepatocellular hypoxia and damage.

Despite such a reduction in clearance of the drug in cardiac failure, there is in many cases little or no increase in its plasma half-life, because not only is clearance reduced, but so is the volume of distribution, in approximate proportion. Nevertheless, the dosage requirement will often be much less — for example the infusion rate for lignocaine should, as a first approximation, be reduced to 50% (Benowitz and Meister 1976). In other cases, the half life is significantly Prolonged (Cavalli et al 1988).

Renal clearance of drugs is also likely to be impaired in patients with cardiac failure, and this will make any changes in hepatic metabolism more important than they might otherwise be, especially in drugs which are normally mainly excreted by the renal route. The importance of metabolites of the drug will also be greater.

Cardiopulmonary bypass

Cardiopulmonary bypass represents an extreme situation of alteration of normal cardiovascular dynamics. The main changes at commencement of bypass are: hypotension and altered regional blood flow, hypothermia, haemodilution, lung isolation, and heparin administration. During bypass the body's response to non-pulsatile flow differs from that to pulsatile flow, while hormonal responses occur to stress, and electrolyte shifts occur. Formal studies of changes in drug kinetics related to these have been relatively few, and have been reviewed by Holley and colleagues (1982).

The most dramatic changes in drug distribution are those caused by haemodilution, but as well as a simple dilutional effect, changes occur in plasma protein binding at the same time, probably partly due to competition by free fatty acids released by heparin, and it may be difficult to unravel the two effects. For example, plasma fentanyl concentration has been found to fall by 53%, 5 min after initiating bypass (Bovill and Sebel 1980), but the free fraction increases from 20 to 43% with dilution and acidosis (McClain and Hug 1980). Propranolol concentrations follow a similar pattern.

Drug elimination is not usually an important consideration during the short period of the bypass, but in the case of some drugs, e.g. fentanyl, the elimination half-life is increased, probably due to reduced hepatic perfusion during and after bypass.

REFERENCES

Benet L Z, Greither A, Maister W 1976 Gastrointestinal absorption of drugs in patients with cardiac failure. In: Benet L Z (ed) The effect of disease states on drug pharmacokinetics. American Pharmaceutical Association, Washington, P

Benowitz N L, Meister W 1976 Pharmacokinetics in patients with cardiac failure. Clinical Pharmacokinetics 1: 389–405

Bovill J G, Sebel P S 1980 Pharmacokinetics of high dose fentanyl. British journal of Anaesthesia 52: 795–801

Cannon P J 1977 The kidney in heart failure. New England Journal of Medicine 296: 26–32

Cavalli A, Maggioni A P, Marchi S, Volpi A, Latini R 1988 Flecainide half-life prolongation in 2 patients with congestive heart failure and complex ventricular arrhythmias. Clinical Pharmacokinetics, 14: 187–188

Dunselman P H, Edgar B, Scaf A N, Kuntze C E, Wesseling H 1989 Pharmacokinetics of felodipine after intravenous and chronic oral administration in patients with congestive heart failure. British Journal of Clinical Pharmacology, 28: 45–52

Gibbons R T, Steffey E P, Eger E I (II) 1977 The effect of spontaneous versus controlled ventilation on the rate of rise of alveolar halothane concentration in dogs. Anesthesia and Analgesia: Current Research 56: 32–34

Holley F O, Ponganis Katherine V, Stanski D 1982 Effect of cardiopulmonary bypass on the pharmacokinetics of drugs. Clinical Phamacokinetics 7: 234–251

McClain D A, Hug C C 1980 Intravenous fentanyl kinetics. Clinical Pharmacology and Therapeutics 28: 106–114

Thompson P D, Melmon K L, Richardson J A et al 1973 Lidocaine pharmacokinetics in advanced heart failure, liver disease and renal failure in humans. Annals of Internal Medicine 78: 499–508

Ueda C T, Dzindzio B S 1978 Quinidine kinetics in congestive failure. Clinical Pharmacology and Therapeutics 23: 158–164

Woosley R L 1987 Pharmacokinetics and pharmacodynamics of antiarrhythmic agents in patients with congestive heart failure. American Heart Journal 114: 1280–1291

PART 4
INFLUENCE OF LIVER DISEASE
W. McCaughey

The liver is the site of the majority of the body's metabolic processes, whether detoxification of drugs or other substances; those concerned with energy provision, or other processes. Its arterial blood supply is from the hepatic artery, but more than four-fifths of the total hepatic blood flow of approximately 100 ml 100 g^{-1} min^{-1} comes from the portal vein. The cells of the liver, hepatocytes, are arranged in acini grouped around each portal tract – the portal tract being a grouping of branches of hepatic artery, portal vein and bile duct. The acini drain into the central veins. Within the cells the rough endoplasmic reticulum is mainly concerned with protein synthesis, and the smooth endoplasmic reticulum with synthesis of lipids, accumulation of glycogen and the metabolism of drugs and endogenous hormones. These metabolic processes have been described in more detail in Chapter 3.

Liver blood flow

As liver blood flow accounts for approximately one-quarter of the total cardiac output, factors which change it are obviously of importance, as they may modify the supply of oxygen, the delivery of drugs or other substrates of metabolism, or both. A number of factors associated with anaesthetic practice do reduce hepatic blood flow by a variety of mechanisms. These include:

1. spinal or epidural anaesthesia — flow drops in proportion to fall in mean arterial blood pressure;
2. inhalational anaesthetic agents;
3. intravenous agents;
4. sympathetic nervous activity;
5. mechanical ventilation.

Functions of the liver: changes in disease

The primary function of the liver is to metabolize drugs to more polar and water-soluble metabolites, whilst that of the kidney is to excrete water-soluble drugs and water-soluble metabolites. The basic concepts of metabolism, and of enzyme induction and inhibition, have been described in Chapter 3.

The complexity of the processes in the liver makes study of changes in disease difficult, and current knowledge is incomplete. Much of the work has been in chronic cirrhosis, often alcoholic in origin. In such hepatic disease, several factors may be identified which influence the elimination of drugs by the liver.

The first of these is hepatic blood flow. As well as changes in total blood flow, in hepatic disease there may be shunting of blood so that it is not delivered to functioning hepatocytes. Shunts may be intrahepatic or extrahepatic — mesenteric or splenic shunts may divert more than 50% of blood flow in chronic hepatic disease (Groszman et al 1972).

Secondly, the intrinsic function of the hepatocytes may be reduced. In cirrhosis, drug conjugations with glucuronic acid, i.e. phase II reactions, remain relatively efficient as compared to drug oxidation, i.e. phase I reactions, which are impaired.

Thirdly, enterohepatic recycling of drugs may be altered in hepatic disease, and finally the degree of protein binding of the drug may be altered.

These will all have different influences on different drugs. The major factor which is of help in differentiating the ways in which the handling of various drugs will be changed in liver disease, is the extraction ratio of the drug, and on this basis drugs can be classified as low or high extraction compounds.

The extraction ratio of a drug is the proportion of the drug removed from the blood on one passage through an organ. It may vary between 0 and 1. When a drug is efficiently extracted, as in the case for example of propofol, lignocaine (lidocaine) or propranolol, then the extraction ratio approaches unity, and the hepatic clearance approximates to the hepatic blood flow. Such drugs have a low systemic bioavailability as they are removed by this first-pass hepatic metabolism. In fact the bioavailability (F) is related to the extraction ratio (ER) as:

$$F = 1 - \text{ER}.$$

This means that, for a highly extracted drug, a small change in extraction ratio — from, for example, 0.95 to 0.90 — would cause a doubling in bioavailability from 5% to 10%. This increase in bioavailability of highly extracted drugs may be seen most dramatically where there are large portosystemic shunts, due either to the disease process or to surgical management.

Reduction in clearance of these drugs is accompanied by a matching increase in the half-life of the drug. However, there is not generally any notable change in volume of distribution in chronic liver disease. The clinical implication is that there is no change expected in the initial dose of drug required to achieve the required therapeutic level, but that subsequent dosage needs to be reduced, frequently by around 50%.

The hepatic clearance of a drug (Cl_H) may be related to the factors which influence it: the hepatic blood flow (Q), the intrinsic activity of the hepatocytes ($Cl_{intrinsic}$) and the free fraction of drug in the blood (f_b) by the following equation (Williams 1983)

$$Cl_H = Q \; \frac{f_b \times Cl_{intrinsic}}{Q + f_b \times Cl_{intrinsic}}$$

For highly extracted drugs $Cl_{intrinsic}$ is much higher than Q, so the equation approximates to

$$Cl_H = Q$$

Thus these drugs show *flow-dependent* kinetics, metabolism being affected by those factors noted above which influence hepatic blood flow, while they are relatively unaffected by drugs which cause enzyme induction or inhibition.

However, for poorly extracted drugs the reverse situation applies, and the equation approximates to

$$Cl_H = f_b \times Cl_{intrinsic}$$

For such drugs, the hepatic clearance is sensitive not to liver blood flow but to the intrinsic ability of the cells to metabolize it. These drugs, e.g. theophylline, warfarin, show *capacity-limited* metabolism. The rate of metabolism is also related to the free drug concentration in the blood, which in turn is influenced by the degree of protein binding of the drug. A further corollary of these is that the elimination of these drugs is relatively unaffected by route of administration, in contrast to the high ER drugs which undergo extensive first-pass metabolism.

Because these factors are interrelated in this way, changes in disposition of low extraction drugs will be more variable and harder to predict than is the case with high ER drugs. Some examples (Williams 1983) may help to illustrate these factors.

1. Pattern of metabolism. Benzodiazepines which are eliminated primarily by glucuronidation (e.g. lorazepam and oxazepam) are unaffected by chronic liver disease, whereas those which require phase I non-synthetic pathways (e.g. diazepam, chlordiazepoxide) have reduced elimination.
2. Protein binding. The influence of protein binding is complex, because it influences both the elimination of the drug and also its distribution. Reduced plasma binding will increase the volume of distribution by making more of the drug available for equilibration with extracellular tissues, while at the same time there is an increase in the free fraction of the drug (Shand 1977).

Clearance of tolbutamide is increased in acute viral hepatitis (Williams et al 1977), because of reduced protein binding — but this example introduces another complicating factor in interpretation of results.

Clearance as described above, and as used in this report, is based on total plasma drug concentration, which is the measurement most commonly made and quoted. If calculation of clearance were based on measurement of free drug, then an increase would not be found for tolbutamide clearance in the case of viral hepatitis. This is because, although total drug concentration may be reduced, free drug concentration is unchanged, and the liver is still eliminating the drug equally efficiently, so no adjustment in drug dosage is required.

If both binding and intrinsic clearance of the drug (based on free drug) were reduced (e.g. naproxen), then total clearance of the drug would remain unchanged; in these circumstances, to maintain a steady concentration of free drug (which determines pharmacological effect), the dose of drug needs to be reduced.

REFERENCES

Groszman R, Kotelanski B, Cohn J N, Khatri I M 1972 Quantitation of portosystemic shunting from the systemic and mesenteric beds in alcoholic liver disease. American Journal of Medicine 53: 715–722

Shand D G 1977 Drug disposition in liver disease. New England Journal of Medicine 296: 1527–1528

Williams R L, Blashke T R, Meffin P J, Melmon K L, Rowland M 1977 Influence of acute viral hepatitis on disposition and plasma binding of tolbutamide. Clinical Pharmacology and Therapeutics 21: 301–309

Williams R L 1983 Drug administration in liver disease. New England Journal of Medicine 309: 1616–1622

PART 5
KIDNEY DISEASE
J. P. Alexander

INFLUENCE OF RENAL DISEASE

Even the healthy kidney may have its capacity to excrete normally occurring substances overwhelmed under certain circumstances. Many ions and molecules accumulate in the body fluids of patients with reduced renal function. Simple substances such as water, H^+, Na^+, K^+, and more complex molecules such as urea, creatinine, uric acid, methylguanidine, guanidino-succinic acid, other guanidines, aminoacids, amines both aliphatic and aromatic, phenols, indoles, aromatic oxyacids, pseudouridine, oxalic acid, magnesium, arsenic, myoinositol, 'middle molecules', glucagon, growth hormone, and parathyroid hormone. All these have been suspected of being uraemic toxins (Anonymous 1977).

PHARMACOKINETICS
ESTIMATION OF RENAL FUNCTION

Drugs are cleared by passive glomerular filtration and by active tubular excretion, and may return to the circulation by passive reabsorption from the renal tubule. Clearance of endogenous creatinine gives a reasonable indication of glomerular filtration, the normal value for a 70 kg person being 100–130 ml/min.

Drug clearance is the sum of renal and non-renal clearances, and the latter is often proportional to creatinine clearance, and may be estimated from it, as discussed further in the appendix to this chapter.

As renal function deteriorates, the concentration of endogenous substances in urine increases. Blood urea is a poor index of renal drug elimination, being influenced by protein uptake, metabolism, hepatic function, heart failure, gastrointestinal haemorrhage and urine output. Plasma creatinine depends on age, sex and muscle mass, but can be determined without urine collection. It is of direct value only for drugs such as gentamicin which are cleared unchanged solely through the kidneys (see Appendix).

DRUG DISTRIBUTION AND METABOLISM

Little is known about changes in metabolism in uraemia, but there is a great deal of evidence that drug distribution changes, and there may be concentration in the central compartment at the expense of the peripheral compartment. The apparent volume of distribution of digoxin is reduced considerably. Conversely, increased apparent distribution volumes have been found for many drugs including phenytoin, diazoxide, penicillin G, and some cephalosporins. These changes in distribution are associated with decreased plasma protein binding which will increase the apparent volume of distribution and decrease the plasma levels of the drug. The clinical consequences of these effects are difficult to predict. A higher fraction of unbound drug may lead to more intense effects and a higher incidence of adverse effects, but also increase drug clearance and decrease half-life. Decreased binding may also accentuate peak concentrations so that increased pharmacological effects and increased incidence of unwanted effects are seen.

The precise nature of these changes in protein binding in uraemic patients is not understood. The defective binding is not corrected by dialysis but is corrected by successful renal transplantation. It would appear more likely that altered albumin synthesis and structure are involved. Protein binding of some drugs (quinidine, trimethoprim, chloramphenicol) is unchanged in renal failure.

TUBULAR FUNCTION

In the proximal renal tubule many organic acids, bases and metabolites are excreted by active tubular secretion. The carrier systems can be bidirectional so that some drugs are both secreted and reabsorbed.

In the proximal and distal tubules, non-ionized forms of weak acids and bases undergo passive reabsorption and the concentration gradient is determined by reabsorption of water, sodium and other inorganic ions. Passive reabsorption of some substances is pH-dependent. Alteration of urine pH can result in significant change in drug elimination if pH-dependent passive reabsorption can be influenced. Thus alkalinization of urine can produce a four- to six-fold increase in excretion of a relatively strong acid such as acetylsalicylic acid (pKa = 3.5) and of phenobarbitone (pKa = 7.2) when urinary pH is changed from 6.4 to 8.0. Excretion of bases (pKa > 7.5) such as amphetamine and quinine is enhanced by acidification of urine, but has no practical application. The proximal renal tubules receive the brunt of drug-induced injury. There is progressive concentration of toxic drugs and metabolites as water is absorbed during passage down the nephron. Proximal tubular damage is common, although mild injury may not be obvious. Some drugs concentrate in cells during repeated administration (e.g. gentamicin) while ischaemia and vasoconstriction may lead to extensive damage and acute renal failure.

DIALYSIS

The patient with complete absence of renal function requires some form of dialysis, and this will affect removal of drugs from the body. As the molecular weight of a solute increases, diffusiveness through a given membrane decreases and when molecular weight exceeds 500 daltons, conventional haemodialysis is unlikely to effectively remove a drug. Drugs which are insoluble in water cannot be expected to move from blood to aqueous dialysate. Highly protein-bound drugs such as atropine, propranolol and some of the semisynthetic penicillins (cloxacillin, flucloxacillin), are also not dialysable. Peritoneal dialysis is less effective in removing dialysable drugs than is haemodialysis, although the peritoneal membrane may be more permeable to large molecules than is the artifical kidney. Water solubility, plasma protein binding, and molecular weight do not limit the effectiveness of haemoperfusion, which will rapidly remove phenobarbitone, which is moderately (about 50%) protein-bound. Since each molecule of absorbed solute occupies a binding site on the column, the latter will become saturated and may require periodic replacement.

Dialysis will, of course, further complicate the elimination of drugs from the body, depending on their dialysability. Account must also be taken of the effect of impaired renal function on drug metabolites. Most drugs are lipid-soluble and are metabolized to water-soluble compounds before excretion in urine or bile. If the metabolites are pharmacologically active, drug action will be prolonged.

Altered ratio of metabolite to active drug may lead to confusion if plasma concentrations are measured by non-specific methods which detect metabolites as well, so that falsely high plasma concentrations are obtained.

DRUG THERAPY

When the glomerular filtration rate is greater than 30 ml/min, it is seldom necessary to modify usual doses except perhaps for certain antibiotics and cardiovascular drugs. As already mentioned, the initial or loading dose is essentially unaltered for patients with renal dysfunction. Maintenance doses are adjusted by either lengthening the interval between doses or by reducing the size of individual doses. In practice a combination of both methods is used. Serum concentrations may be an invaluable guide to therapy, but allowances must be made where electrolyte disturbances are present. Serum levels are only of value if the time from administration of the last dose and the elimination half-life is known. For best estimate of peak concentration, blood samples should be taken 1–2 h after an oral dose and $\frac{1}{2}$–1 h after an intravenous or intramuscular dose.

In patients undergoing dialysis, consideration must be given to adjustments for drug removal. Small molecules unbound to protein are most easily removed by haemodialysis. Lipid-soluble drugs with large distribution volumes have low blood levels and removal by haemodialysis is poor. Protein binding will also restrict drug clearance. For drugs which are significantly dialysable it may be wise to omit a dose just prior to dialysis, and to administer the drug when dialysis is completed. A further consideration is the rapid shifts of electrolytes which may occur during dialysis, and which can influence drug toxicity (for instance, digitalis). The pharmacological consequences attached to peritoneal dialysis are similar to those related to haemodialysis, although losses are less significant in spite of the longer durations of treatment.

Drugs which may impair renal function

More than 70 drugs have been listed that can produce acute renal failure. Among those incriminated have been the penicillins, thiazides, sulphonamides, paracetamol, frusemide, co-trimoxazole, phenobarbitone, phenylbutazone and rifampicin. Sudden deterioration of renal function is seen when plasma creatinine concentrations reach 200–300 μmol l^{-1} (2.2–3.3 mg dl^{-1}).

Table 4.7 lists the non-anaesthetic drugs most commonly associated with deterioration of renal function, although the list is not exhaustive.

Non-steroidal anti-inflammatory drugs

Isolated cases of renal failure have been reported, but recognition of renal problems has been slow. Prostaglandins are synthesized in the kidney, and the principal prostaglandins E$_2$, D$_2$ and I$_2$ (prostacyclin) are powerful vasodilators. In normal conditions these prostaglandins do not play a big part in the maintenance of the renal circulation, and drugs such as indomethacin have little effect on the kidney. In a patient with increased amounts of vasoconstrictor substances such as angiotensin II, noradrenaline or antidiuretic hormone, however, vasodilatory prostaglandins become important in maintaining renal blood flow. Clinical conditions such as congestive cardiac failure, cirrhosis of the liver with as-

Table 4.7 Drugs considered to have occasional nephrotoxicity (Porter and Bennett 1981)

Group	Drug	Comments
Antibiotics		
Sulphonamides		crystal formation with earlier members; sulphadimidine in normal dosage
	acetazolamide	worsens acidosis
	co-trimoxazole	deterioration in renal function; trimethoprim preferred
Penicillins		occasional interstitial nephritis
		injectable preparations contain Na$^+$ or K$^+$ reduce dosage in renal failure
Cephalosporins	cephaloridine	toxic, particularly with aminoglycoside or diuretic
	cephalothin	occasionally toxic
	second and third generation	reduce dosage except with cefotaxime
Aminoglycosides		all toxic; tobramycin and netilmicin preferred to gentamicin: monitor levels
Tetracyclines	tetracycline	
	oxytetracycline	toxic; anti-anabolic effect may produce fatal uraemia
	doxycycline	safe — can be used in normal dosage
Anti-fungal	amphotericin B	distal tubular dysfunction
Antituberculous	rifampicin	occasional nephropathy — may colour urine red
Analgesics		
	phenacetin	should never be prescribed
	aspirin	can cause nephropathy
	non-steroidal anti-inflammatory	isolated reports of renal damage; cyclo-oxygenase inhibition
	penicillamine, gold	nephropathy
Sedatives, hypnotics		
	barbiturates	acidosis increases tubular reabsorption
	phenytoin	toxic effects and drug interactions common — monitor plasma levels
Cardiovascular	digoxin	increased sensitivity with electrolyte disturbances
	beta-blockers	reduce dosage
	antihypertensive	adjust dosage according to therapeutic response
Diuretics	thiazides	not effective if GRF < 20 ml/min
	frusemide	effective when GFR < 20 ml/min but occasional nephropathy or dehydration
Cytotoxic, uricosuric		
	sulphinpyrazone	urate crystals deposited in urinary tract
	allopurinol	preferred in renal failure
	cis-platinum	nephrotoxic in one-third of treated patients
Others	radiological contrast	occasional deterioration, probably undeserved reputation but may be dose-related or associated with volume depletion
	cimetidine	accumulates in renal failure, affects metabolism of other drugs
	K$^+$deficiency	leads to nephropathy

cites, diuretic-induced volume depletion, salt restriction and the nephrotic syndrome will cause the release of vasoconstrictor substances to maintain blood pressure. In these circumstances inhibition of prostaglandin synthesis (cyclo-oxygenase inhibition) by non-steroidal anti-inflammatory drugs may cause unopposed renal arteriolar constriction, leading to acute renal insufficiency or renal tubular necrosis.

Another form of renal toxicity that may be induced by these drugs is hyperkalaemia. Prostaglandins directly stimulate the release of renin, and the resulting inhibition of cyclo-oxygenase leads directly to a hyporeninaemic hypoaldosteronism with subsequent hyperkalaemia. Stopping the drug quickly reverses the hyperkalaemia, but serum potassium may need to be monitored in patients having potassium supplements or potassium-sparing diuretics (Orme 1986).

Renal papillary necrosis, acute interstitial nephritis and the nephrotic syndrome have also been described. Any clinical situation in which elevated circulating levels of anigiotensin II and catecholamines exist must be considered a high-risk setting for the development of non-steroidal anti-inflammatory drug-induced renal failure. Since an activated renin — angiotensin system characterizes the anaesthetized state, the implications for anaesthetists are obvious (Clive and Stoff 1984). The widespread use of non-steroidal anti-inflammatory drugs suggests that it would seem prudent to monitor both well-established and newer agents of this type (Bennett and DeBroe 1989).

DRUGS USED IN ANAESTHESIA IN THE RENAL FAILURE PATIENT

The importance of over- and under-hydration, electrolyte shifts and acid–base disturbances on the pharmacokinetics of drug action have already been discussed. Drugs which act mainly on the central nervous system must be fat-soluble and hence are normally reabsorbed during passage through the kidneys. The duration of action of such agents therefore depends on redistribution, metabolism or excretion via the lungs, and not on renal function. This applies to the intravenous induction agents, narcotic analgesics and inhalational agents, but not to the water-soluble non-depolarizing relaxants which are highly ionized at body pH.

Preoperative medication

Virtually all the standard premedicant drugs have been used, although dosage schedules may need to be modified in view of the increased sensitivity to the undesirable effects of medication that is seen in renal failure patients.

Induction agents

The dose of thiopentone necessary to induce sleep has been shown to be about half that required in the normal subject (Dundee and Richards 1954). Since hypoproteinaemia was rare, increase of the unbound form of the drug could not have been an important feature, nor defective renal excretion during the few minutes following injection in which the major effects are seen. These results may have been due to the bolus injection techniques fashionable at that time. With a decreased rate of drug administration in line with modern anaesthetic practice, the dose required for induction will remain unaltered from that required in healthy patients, because the underlying free drug volume of distribution and free drug clearance are unchanged (Sear 1987). The

induction dose of other agents, and of hypnotic and sedative drugs, may need to be reduced. The response to neuroleptic agents appears to be normal.

Choice of muscle relaxant

Although gallamine has been used successfully in renal failure patients, there have been a number of reports of prolonged curarization and its use cannot be recommended. Tubocurarine has been widely used in renal failure patients. Although normally excreted by the kidneys, an alternative excretory pathway exists via the liver and biliary systems. However, postoperative respiratory failure due to recurarization can occur. Both alcuronium and pancuronium have been satisfactory in clinical practice. Normally 50% of a given dose of the latter can be recovered from the urine, but in renal failure its mode of excretion is similar to that of tubocurarine. There have been isolated reports of prolonged curarization following the use of pancuronium in renal failure; it should be noted that acidosis slows down the metabolic degradation of non-depolarizing relaxants. Since only 15–20% of a dose of vecuronium is excreted by the kidney, and atracurium does not require either renal or hepatic routes for elimination, either should be suitable for the patient with little or no renal function (Hunter et al 1984). Although the majority of non-depolarizing muscle relaxants have been used safely in renal failure patients, atracurium is probably the best drug available at present (Hunter 1987). Laudanosine, a major metabolite of atracurium, has central nervous system stimulant properties in animals; Fahey and co-workers (1985) found higher plasma concentrations of laudanosine in renal failure patients but firm evidence that this can produce toxic effects in man has yet to be produced. Parker and co-workers (1988) considered that even prolonged infusions of atracurium in renal failure patients did not produce levels of laudanosine which were likely to be epileptogenic. Our personal observations are contrary to this view. New neuromuscular blocking drugs still under investigation include pipecuronium and doxacurium. These are long-acting agents which are primarily eliminated in the kidney unchanged. It is as yet too soon to comment on the potential of three short-acting drugs, mivacurium, ORG 9426 and ORG 9616 (Miller 1989).

Renal failure prolongs the duration of action of the anticholinesterase agents neostigmine, pyridostigmine and edrophonium at least 100% since they are excreted mainly by the kidney. Patients with chronic renal failure have normal serum cholinesterase unless there is atypical cholinesterase inheritance, so that there is no contra-indication to the use of suxamethonium, provided serum potassium levels are not greater than 5.5 mmol l^{-1}.

Inhalation agents

Diethyl ether and cyclopropane are unlikely choices. Fluoride ion, one of the metabolites of methoxyflurane, is known to be nephrotoxic, and oxalate crystals have been found in transplanted kidneys following methoxyflurane anaesthesia. A metabolite of trichlorethylene, trichloracetic acid, requires a renal pathway for excretion. There have been isolated reports of acute renal failure following enflurane anaesthesia in patients with pre-existing renal disease. Although peak inorganic fluoride levels in blood do not produce clinically significant postoperative impairment of renal function in normal patients, there may be a transient impairment following enflurane anaesthesia. This is evident where the duration of anaesthesia exceeds 2–4 MAC hours. The possibility of enzyme induction or a genetic variation in the metabolism of enflurane in some humans producing higher fluoride levels has been mooted.

Anaesthesia with all inhalational agents temporarily depresses renal blood flow, glomerular filtration rate and urine production, but there are usually no lasting effects.

Halothane, in low concentration, has been widely used in renal failure and transplant patients. Patients given isoflurane demonstrate no renal impairment following anaesthesia. Either drug can be recommended (Brown and Gandolfi 1987). These volatile agents have the additional advantage of potentiating the neuromuscular blocking action of many non-depolarizing muscle relaxants, especially vecuronium and atracurium, so that dosage of the latter can be reduced (Halsey 1987). This effect is particularly noticeable with isoflurane, and similarly with enflurane, although for reasons already stated, use of enflurane should be restricted or perhaps avoided. Bennett and Hahn (1985) found a similar potentiation of a combination of pancuronium and metocurine when halothane or isoflurane was used.

Analgesic drugs

Nearly all the major analgesic drugs cause a fall in urine production and a rise in circulatory ADH levels. Fentanyl or derivates may be the analgesics of choice in renal failure, although respiratory failure due to unexpected high levels of sufentanil has been described. Norpethidine, the metabolite of pethidine, accumulates in renal failure and has an excitatory effect on the nervous system (Sear 1987). Prolonged effects of narcotic analgesics in anuric patients have been described and accumulation of the narcotic or its metabolites or enterohepatic recirculation postulated. Evidence that the kidney has an important role in the elimination of opioid narcotics is accumulating. The pharmacokinetics of a single oral dose of dihydrocodeine is altered in renal failure patients. Uraemic patients appear to be exceptionally susceptible to the effects of intrathecal narcotics.

The precise reason for morphine intoxication in renal failure was eventually explained by Osborne and colleagues (1986). Although morphine may not be present in plasma in measurable quantities, the active metabolite morphine-6-glucuronide, which relies on renal excretion, accumulates. Previous reports of morphine accumulation during renal failure probably resulted from the use of radio-immunoassays which did not distinguish between morphine and morphine-6-glucuronide.

Immunosuppression

Patients undergoing renal transplant require long-term immunosuppression with azathioprine, which inhibits purine synthesis. A dose of 5 mg/kg is given intravenously during the operation, together with a loading dose of hydrocortisone (3 mg kg^{-1}) and both are continued in reduced dosage orally post operatively. Rarely cyclophosphamide, an alkylating agent with less hepatotoxicity, is used in preference to azathioprine. Cyclosporin A is an effective immunosuppressant but nephrotoxicity is a problem, while hepatotoxicity, altered glucose tolerance, reduced prednisolone metabolism and increased serum cholesterol and triglyceride levels have been described. It may be that the ideal dose of this drug has not yet been realized (Carpenter 1990).

Local and regional anaesthesia

The local anaesthetic esters procaine, 2-chloroprocaine and tetracaine, undergo enzymatic hydrolysis with plasma cholinesterase. The toxicity of these agents is inversely proportional to their rate of degradation. The metabolism of the amide-type drugs (bupivacaine, etidocaine, lignocaine, mepivacaine, and prilocaine) is more complex. Inactive metabolites formed in the liver are normally excreted by the kidney. Accumulation of metabolites is minimized by the use of the longer-acting bupivacaine and etidocaine, which are both highly bound to protein when in the blood stream. Gould and Aldrete (1983) reported a case of bupivacaine cardiotoxicity in a patient with renal failure. Although renal failure will delay excretion of the metabolites of lignocaine, problems are unlikely to arise unless significant hepatic dysfunction is also present.

Collodial plasma substitutes

Kohler et al (1978) compared the effects of infusing commercially available preparations of hydroxyethyl starch, dextran 40 and gelatine on plasma volume in healthy patients and those with terminal renal failure on chronic maintenance haemodialysis. As would be expected, increases in plasma volumes were greater in the renal failure patients, and lasted twice as long. Although low molecular weight dextrans do not appear to be nephrotoxic if given in recommended doses to patients with normal hydration and normal renal function, acute renal failure may be precipitated if shock or hypovolaemia is present. The renal tubular cells become grossly swollen with vacuoles containing dextran. With current knowledge of the fate of these substances in the body, their use in patients with poor renal function or those receiving a kidney transplant cannot be recommended.

APPENDIX: DRUG KINETICS IN RENAL DISEASE

When we consider the elimination of a drug which distributes in the body according to a linear one-compartment model, the apparent first-order elimination rate constant k is the sum of k_r, the rate constant for renal elimination, and k_{nr}, the rate constant for non-renal elimination, so that

$$k = k_r + k_{nr} \qquad (1)$$

If renal elimination is proportional to creatinine clearance, and a is the proportionality constant, then

$$k_r = aCl_{cr} \qquad (2)$$

and this by substitution into equation (1) yields

$$k = aCl_{cr} + k_{nr} \qquad (3)$$

which is the equation of a straight line for a plot of k against creatinine clearance with a slope of a, and y- intercept of k_{nr}.

Using this relationship, three types of drug behaviour may be recognised (Fig. 4.7).

Type A: Drug elimination is almost entirely via the renal route
$(k_{nr} = 0; a > 0)$

Type B: Drug elimination is almost entirely extrarenal and independent of renal function
$(k_{nr} > 0; a = 0)$

Type C: Drug elimination occurs by both renal and non-renal routes
$(k_{nr} > 0; a > 0)$

If the slope of the line is known for a Type A drug, a simple calculation will determine changes in drug elimination with alteration in renal function. For example, it has been shown in the case of gentamicin that for a regression line $y = a + bx$ where y is the percentage hourly loss, the values a, b and x are 0.2, 0.25 and Cl_{cr} respectively. In other words, the percentage hourly loss of gentamicin $= 0.2 + (0.25 \times Cl_{cr})$ and is approximated by dividing endogenous creatinine clearance by four.

Equation (3) can be expressed in terms of elimination half-life $(t_{\frac{1}{2}})$ where

$$t_{\frac{1}{2}} = \frac{0.693}{k} = \frac{0.693}{k_{nr} + aCl_{cr}} \qquad (4)$$

It is apparent from Figure 4.7 that marked changes in $t_{\frac{1}{2}}$ do not occur until renal function is considerably depressed, but for practical purposes the linear relationship of creatinine clearance with k is more useful than the relationship with elimination half-life. If normal values of k and values in anephric patients (k_{nr}) are obtained (Table 4.8), estimation of k for other subjects can be obtained by drawing a straight line between the two points. Thus in Figure 4.8 the value of k for gentamicin has been determined for a patient with a creatinine clearance of 10 ml/min.

When k_{nr} for the anephric patient is not known, an approximate value can be calculated if one assumes a simple one-compartment model, since

$$t_{\frac{1}{2}} = \frac{0.693}{k} = \frac{0.693}{k_r + k_{nr}} \qquad (5)$$

The fraction f of the absorbed dose excreted unchanged in the urine is given by

$$f = \frac{k_r}{k_r + k_{nr}} \qquad (6)$$

and provided f and $t_{\frac{1}{2}}$ are known from normal subjects, k_r and k_{nr} can be found.

Plasma creatinine concentration C_{cr} is related to endogenous creatinine production K_0 and creatinine clearance by

$$C_{cr} = \frac{k_0}{Cl_{cr}} \qquad (7)$$

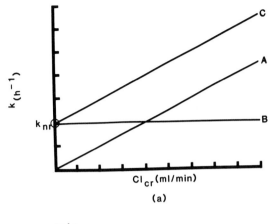

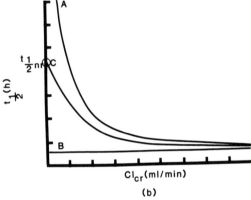

Fig. 4.7 (a) The Dettli diagram illustrates the dependence of elimination rate constant k on the endogenous creatinine clearance Cl_{cr} for drugs of type A, B and C (see text; Dettli 1976); (b) dependence of elimination of half-life $t_{\frac{1}{2}}$ on creatinine clearance for drugs of type A, B and C. (After Rodgers et al 1981, with permission.)

Solving for Cl_{cr} and substitution in equation (3) gives

$$k = \frac{ak_0}{C_{cr}} + k_{nr} \qquad (8)$$

A linear relationship therefore exists between K $1/C_{cr}$, and can be used to determine k in renal failure patients, but would require determination in each individual. Additional problems arise if the drug demonstrates multi-compartment characteristics. Also, although creatinine production falls in the aged, plasma levels remain constant due to diminished clearance, so that dosage regimens should not be based on data obtained from a younger population. Changes in plasma creatinine levels also lag behind acute fluctuations in renal function, so that similar strictures apply to their use in ill patients.

Table 4.8 Calculated elimination rate constants ($k = 0.693/t_{\frac{1}{2}}$) for drugs in patients with normal renal function (k_N) and in anephric patients (k_{nr}). The quotient $k_{nr}/k_N \times 100$ (%) is the relative amount of drug excreted extrarenally. Other examples are given by Dettli (1976)

	k_N	k_{nr}	$k_{nr}/k_N \times 100$ (%)
	(h^{-1})	(h^{-1})	
Chlortetracycline*	0.1	0.1	100
Cefoperazone	0.35	0.33	94
Chloramphenicol	0.26	0.19	73
Ceftriazone	0.08	0.058	73
Pancuronium	0.32	0.16	50
Procainamide	0.16	0.06	38
N-acetylprocainamide	0.10	0.01	10
Flucloxacillin	0.87	0.31	36
Bretylium	0.09	0.03	33
Acetbutolol	0.09	0.017	19
Solatol	0.09	0.012	13
Moxalactam	0.32	0.032	10
Cefotaxime	0.69	0.069	10
Desacetyl cefotaxime	0.43	0.033	8
Cefuroxime	0.53	0.046	9
Cephamandole	0.99	0.069	7
Cephaloridine*	0.51	0.03	6
Gentamicin	0.30	0.015	5
Tobramycin	0.32	0.01	3

* Should not be used in renal failure.
† Active metabolite.

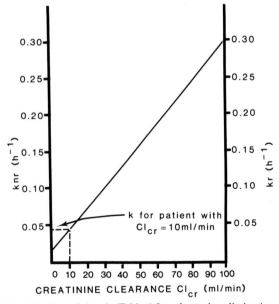

Fig. 4.8 Use of data in Table 4.8 to determine elimination rate constant for gentamicin in a patient with a creatinine clearance of 10 ml min^{-1}.

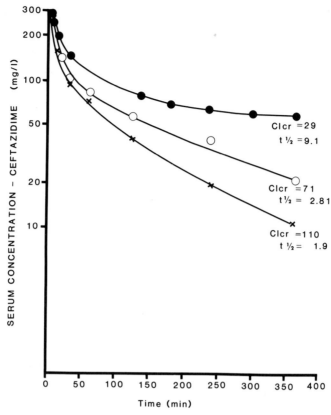

Fig. 4.9 Serum levels of ceftazidime after 2 g i.v. in three patients with varying degrees of renal function (after Gozzard et al (1982), with permission).

Figure 4.9 shows a plot of plasma levels against time of the cephalosporin, ceftazidime, in patients with normal renal function, and mild and moderate impairment. About 90% cent of ceftazidime is excreted by the kidneys. It is generally assumed that the loading dose, L, is the same for the renal failure patient as for the normal.

Plasma steady-state concentration is not reached until at least five half-lives elapsed. If an immediate therapeutic effect is desired in the renal failure patient where plasma half-life is going to be prolonged, a loading dose will be required. This can be calculated from

$$L = \frac{X_0}{1 - e^{-KT}} \qquad (9)$$

where X_0 is the normal 24 h requirement, and T is the dosing interval. Thus taking the case of gentamicin once again, where the normal dose is perhaps 480 mg/24 h, $k_N = 0.3 \text{ h}^{-1}$ and $k_{nr} = 0.015 \text{ h}^{-1}$ (Table 4.8). From Figure 4.8 we find that for a patient with a creatinine

clearance of 10 ml/min, $\widehat{K} = 0.35 \text{ h}^{-1}$ ($\wedge$ denotes the renal failure patient). Then

$$\widehat{X}_0 = \frac{480 \times 0.035}{0.3} = 55 \text{ mg/24 h} \qquad (10)$$

This will not be enough to achieve therapeutic concentrations with one dose, so

$$\widehat{L} = \frac{56}{1 - e^{-0.035 \times 24}} = 98.5 \qquad (11)$$

For obvious practical reasons (the drug is marketed in 2 ml vials containing 40 mg/ml), the loading dose would be 80 mg followed by 40 mg at 24 h intervals, and getamicin levels would be monitored during therapy, since patients are not exact pharmacokinetic models and certain factors such as metabolism and drug distribution may cause variability in response. Matzke and others (1983) discuss the calculation of peak (Cp_{max}) and trough (Cp_{min}) serum concentrations of gentamticin and tobramycin. Since the maintenance dose X_o and the dosing intervals T are known

$$Cp_{max} = \frac{X_0}{Vd\,k} \frac{(1-e^{-kt})}{(1-e^{-kt})} \quad (12)$$

$$Cp_{min} = Cp_{max} \quad (e^{-k(T-t)}) \quad (13)$$

Vd is normally $0.2\,l\,kg^{-1}$ but can vary from 0.15 to $0.3\,l\,kg^{-1}$ depending on under or over-hydration; t is the infusion duration. The elimination rate constant (k) is calculated from a series of three serum concentrations obtained at suitable intervals after a loading dose. The time interval over which these samples are drawn should encompass approximately one half-life, and creatinine clearance can be used as a guide. Recommended values for trough levels are $1.5\,mg\,l^{-1}$, amd for Gram-negative infections, peak levels of $5\,mg\,l^{-1}$. Serum levels should be monitored to assess the accuracy of the pharmacokinetic model. Burn patients may require very large doses of aminoglycosides to achieve therapeutic serum concentrations.

Critically ill patients have significantly larger volumes of distribution and may require larger doses per kilogram of aminoglycoside to achieve therapeutic concentrations. The use of standard doses or dosing normograms is not recommended (Beckhouse et al 1988).

REFERENCES

Anonymous 1977 What causes toxicity in uraemia? British Medical Journal 2: 143–144

Beckhouse M J, Whyte I M, Byth H L, Napier J C, Smith A J 1988 Altered aminoglycoside pharmacokinetics in the critically ill. Anaesthesia and Intensive Care 16: 418–422

Bennett M J, Hahn J F 1985 Potentiation of the combination of pancuronium and metocurine by halothane and isoflurane in humans with and without renal failure. Anesthesiology 62: 759–764

Bennett W M, De Broe M E 1989 Analgesic nephropathy—a preventable disease. New England Journal of Medicine 320: 1269–1271

Brown B R, Gandolfi A J 1987 Adverse effects of volatile agents. British Journal of Anaesthesia 59: 14–23

Carpenter C B 1990 Immunosuppression in organ transplantation. New England Journal of Medicine 322: 1224–1226

Clive D M, Stoff J S 1984 Renal syndromes associated with non-steroidal anti-inflammatory drugs. New England Journal of Medicine 310: 563–571

Dettli L 1976 Drug dosage in renal disease. Clinical Pharmacokinetics 1: 126–134

Dundee J W, Richards R K 1954 Effect of azotemia upon the action of intravenous barbiturate anaesthesia. Anesthesiology 15: 333–346

Fahey M R, Rupp S M, Canfell C et al 1985 Effect of renal failure on laudanosine excretion in man. British Journal of Anaesthesia 57: 1049–1051

Gould D B, Aldrete J A 1983 Bupivacaine cardiotoxicity in a patient with renal failure. Acta Anaesthesiologica Scandinavica 27: 18–21

Gozzard D I, Geddes A M, Farrell I D et al 1982 Ceftazidime — a new extended-spectrum cephalosporin. Lancet i, 1152–1156

Halsey M J 1987 Drug interactions in anaesthesia. British Journal of Anaesthesia 59: 112–123

Hunter J M 1987 Adverse effects of neuromuscular blocking drugs British Journal of Anaesthesia 59: 46–60

Hunter J M, Jones R S, Utting J E 1984 Comparison of vecuronium, atracurium and tubocurarine in normal patients and in patients with no renal function. British Journal of Anaesthesia 56: 941–952

Kohler H, Kirch W, Klein H, Distler A 1978 Die volumen — wirking von 6% Hydroxyäthylstarke 450/0.7, 10% Dextran 40 and 3.5% Isozyanatvernetzter Gelatine bei patienten mit terminaler Niereninsuffizienz (The effect of 6% hydroxyethyl starch 450/0.7, 10% dextran 40 and 3.5% gelatine on plasma volume in patients with terminal renal failure). Anaesthetist 27: 421–426

Matzke G R, Burkle W S, Lucarotti R L 1983 Gentamicin and tobramycin dosing guidelines: an evaluation. Drug Intelligence and Clinical Pharmacy 17: 425–432

Miller R D 1989 New muscle relaxants. International Anesthesia Research Society 1989, review course lectures 84–86

Orme M L'E 1986 Non-steroidal anti-inflammatory drugs and the kidney. British Medical Journal 292: 1621–1622

Osborne R J, Joel S P, Slevin M L 1986 Morphine intoxication in renal failure; the role of morphine-6-glucuronide. British Medical Journal 292: 1548–1549

Parker C J R, Jones J E, Hunter J M 1988 Disposition of infusions of atracurium and its metabolite, laudanosine, in patients in renal and respiratory failure in an ITU. British Journal of Anaesthesia 61: 531–540

Porter G A, Bennett W M 1981 Nephrotoxic acute renal failure due to common drugs American Journal of Physiology 10: F1–F8

Rodgers H J, Spector R G, Trunce J R 1981 A textbook of clinical pharmacology. Hodder & Stoughton, London, Ch. 5, p 121

Sear J W 1987 Toxicity of i.v. anaesthetics. British Journal of Anaesthesia 59: 24–45

Drugs acting on the central nervous system

5. The pharmacology of the central nervous system

B. Pleuvry

The ingestion of drugs which cause changes in the activity of the central nervous system (CNS) has been a characteristic of man since before the dawn of history. Ethanol was probably the first drug to achieve widespread usage, mainly in the form of beers and wines, and there is some evidence that opium was known to the Sumerians as early as 4000 BC

Despite this, it is only in recent years that we have achieved even the remotest understanding of what the brain does, let alone how drugs may affect it.

The concept that the nervous system is composed of discrete units or nerve cells was not proposed until 1886. The terms 'neuron' and 'neuron theory' were coined in 1891 and a 'synapse', defined as a site of contact between two neurons, was first described just before the turn of the century.

The CNS consists of about 10 billion neurons, each of which may receive thousands of synaptic connections. The neuronal cell bodies are organized into groups, and areas of the brain concerned with one type of activity are linked together. It is possible to identify a number of functional systems. The autonomic nervous system is regulated from centres situated in the hypothalamus and medulla oblongata. Efferent fibres descend from the hypothalamus and synapse with cells in the medulla and lateral horns of the spinal cord. These cells send out efferent fibres which emerge from the CNS to synapse with sympathetic and parasympathetic postganglionic nerves. Mood changes appear to originate in the limbic system. Mood-associated autonomic changes also originate in the limbic system via the hypothalamus. Central control of respiration occurs in the medullary and pontine reticular formation, and pain pathways are associated with the substantia gelatinosa, spinoreticular and spinothalamic tracts and the thalamus.

None of these systems operates independently, and considerable interaction occurs. Neuronal systems may produce either excitatory or inhibitory effects on other areas. Excitation is usually direct excitation of a postjunctional neuron but inhibition occurs by at least two mechanisms. Postsynaptic inhibition is associated with direct reduction of the activity of the postjunctional cell, whilst presynaptic inhibition involves the inhibition of the release of an excitatory transmitter from a prejunctional neuron.

It is now clear that both excitatory and inhibitory transmissions at synapses within the CNS are accomplished by specific chemical transmitters. However, the identification of a specific transmitter at a particular synapse is strewn with difficulties and this identification has been made with any degree of confidence only at a minute percentage of sites. The situation is further complicated by the observation that many of the neuroactive peptides coexist with other neurotransmitters in the same neuron (Cooper et al 1986).

DRUG ACTIVITY

It is likely that most centrally acting drugs interfere with neurotransmission. The evidence for this comes from structure–activity relationships, known interactions with transmitter substances in the periphery and the drug effects on stereospecific binding in the brain of putative neurotransmitter substances. A possible exception to this is the group of general CNS depressants. These drugs, which include the anaesthetic gases and vapours and the sedative hypnotic drugs, are capable of depressing the excitability of tissues throughout the CNS. However, the state of anaesthesia is not synonymous with only depression of neuronal activity. Neurophysiological studies have provided evidence that the state of general anaesthesia involves both depression and excitation of the CNS (Chapter 10). Although the complete lack of a common chemical structure among anaesthetics suggests that anaesthesia is not mediated via a specific receptor site, it is possible that the end-product of their action, anaesthesia, may be achieved through a variety of mechanisms (Roth 1980, Halsey et al 1980). In order to try and classify drug activity in the CNS the major likely neurotransmitters will be examined in turn. Much of the evidence for the physiological role of each of these substances comes either from disease states, in which excess or lack of a particular substance has been recorded, or from the end-result of drug-induced modification of transmitter function. It will also be necessary to consider neuromodulators which influence neurotransmission but are of non-synaptic origin, e.g. prostaglandins and neuromediators which participate in the production of a postsynaptic response to a neurotransmitter. The clearest example of neuromediation is the involvement of cyclic adenosine 3,5-monophosphate (cyclic AMP) and possibly cyclic guanosine 3,5-monophosphate (cyclic GMP) as second messengers at specific sites of synaptic transmission (Bloom 1975). The synthesis of the second messenger is triggered by the activation of neurotransmitter sensitive enzymes such as adenylcyclase.

NEUROTRANSMITTERS IN THE CNS (Table 5.1)

Acetylcholine

Acetylcholine is a neurotransmitter at the neuromuscular junction, ganglia and postganglionic parasympathetic nerve endings in the periphery. In the CNS acetylcholine has been proved to be the transmitter at the α motor neuron collateral synapsing with the Renshaw cell in the dorsal horn of the spinal cord. At this site acetylcholine is excitatory on the Renshaw cell via a nicotinic receptor. The Renshaw cell in turn inhibits the activity of the α motor neuron, thus preventing repetitive firing.

Although difficult to prove conclusively, it is highly likely that acetylcholine is a transmitter in other areas of the CNS (Krnjevic 1974). Acetylcholine evokes responses in a varying proportion of neurons in different brain areas. The response is usually excitatory, although some show depression and some a biphasic effect. Acetylcholine receptors of both the muscarinic and nicotinic type are found within the CNS. The sure identification of cholinergic tracts is made difficult by the lack of a specific staining technique for acetylcholine. Thus it has been necessary to rely on acetylcholine esterase staining in the hope that this is associated with only cholinergic nerves. Studies of this nature suggest that the ascending reticular arousal systems and primary afferent fibres from the auditory and visual systems are cholinergic.

Some degenerative conditions of the CNS appear to involve cholinergic neurons. Presenile dementia (Alzheimer's disease) is associated with decreased acetylcholine synthesizing ability, especially in the hippocampus. The levels of choline acetyltransferase at

Table 5.1 Neurotransmitters in the Central Nervous System

Neurotransmitter	Receptors	Drugs affecting transmission	
		Enhance or mimic	Reduce or antagonise
Acetycholine	muscarinic	physostigmine	hyoscine, atropine
	nicotinic	physostigmine	dihydro-erythroidine
Monamines			
Dopamine	D_1	L-dopa	phenothiazines
	D_2	L-dopa, bromocryptine	all neuroleptics
Noradrenaline	α_1	chronic antidepressant treatment	phentolamine
	α_2	clonidine	yohimbine
	β	isoprenaline	propranolol, chronic antidepressant treatment
Adrenaline	See Noradrenaline		
5-Hydroxytryptamine	5-HT_1	LSD	
	5-HT_2	LSD (but greater) affinity for 5-HT_1) methysergide	
	5-HT_3	morphine	methysergide, LSD
Diamines			
Histamine	H_1	—	antidepressants, mepyramine
	H_2	—	cimetidine
Amino acids			
GABA		benzodiazepines barbiturates other G.A.s?	bicuculline picrotoxin

both autopsy and biopsy are significantly lower than matched controls (White et al 1977). Memory deficits are symptomatic of this disease and since hyoscine, muscarinic antagonist to acetylcholine, causes amnesia and physostigmine, a centrally active anticholinesterase agent, can enhance memory, a role for acetylcholine in memory has been proposed. However, it must be appreciated that Alzheimer's disease is associated with deficiencies in many other neurotransmitter systems (Dunnett et al 1982).

Physostigmine has been used clinically to treat the anticholinergic syndrome induced by either overdose or unusual reactions to phenothiazines, anti-histamines and tricyclic anti-depressants (Aquilonius, 1977). It has been suggested that enhancement of CNS cholinergic activity by physostigmine may be useful in treating the somnolence induced by other agents such as diazepam (Di Libertie et al 1975) and morphine (Weinstock et al 1982). In these circumstances it is important to administer a peripherally acting anticholinergic agent such as N-butyl-hyoscine hydrobromide prior to the physostigmine. Weinstock et al (1982) reported that physostigmine reversed the respiratory depressant actions of morphine when used for postoperative pain, and tended to enhance morphine-induced analgesia. Centrally acting cholinomimetics have been reported to have significant analgesic activity in their own right and the analgesic activity of meptazinol, at least in the experimental animal, may have a cholinergic component (Green 1983).

Centrally acting antagonists at the muscarinic receptor for acetylcholine are useful in the treatment of Parkinsonian tremor and motion sickness. This suggests that activation of cholinergic systems is important in these disorders.

Catecholamines

Histochemical and immunochemical techniques have demonstrated that the brain utilizes three catecholamines – dopamine, noradrenaline and adrenaline – in separate and distinct neuronal systems. Dopaminergic neurons lack dopamine hydroxylase, the enzyme which converts dopamine to noradrenaline, and adrenaline-containing neurons can be mapped by the presence of phenylethanolamine N-methyl transferase, which converts noradrenaline to adrenaline.

Dopamine

More than 50% of the catecholamine-containing neurons are dopaminergic. The anatomical distribution of the dopaminergic system is widespread (see Moore & Bloom 1978); the highest concentrations of dopamine occurring in the basal ganglia, limbic system and hypothalamus. On balance the literature suggests that local application of dopamine to receptive neurons usually results in inhibition of activity, although there are a number of well-documented if controversial exceptions (Siggins 1978). Experiments with dopamine agonists and antagonists have implied various types of dopamine receptor with differing properties (Fluckiger & Vigouret 1981). These may be grossly divided into D_1 receptors, which mediate adenyl cyclase activity, and D_2 receptors, which do not regulate cyclic AMP synthesis. There is no evidence that either type of receptor has a restricted presynaptic or postsynaptic localization, although inhibition of prolactin release from the anterior pituitary is brought about by a D_2 receptor on the prolactin-producing cell itself. Bromocriptine, which is used to suppress lactation, is a selective agonist at D_2 receptors.

Parkinson's disease is associated with a massive depletion of dopamine from the striatum (Hornykiewicz 1966) and drugs which are antagonists at dopamine receptors, the neuroleptic drugs, produce extrapyramidal disturbances similar to the symptoms of Parkinson's disease. This suggests a role for dopamine in normal motor function. Replenishment of dopamine with L-dopa is the standard treatment for this condition, and is effective in 75% of cases (Langrall & Joseph 1972). Bromocriptine is also an effective treatment for parkinsonism and parkinsonism-like side-effects can be obtained with the dopamine antagonists, metoclopramide and salpiride. These two agents have selectivity for D_2 dopamine receptors which are not linked to adenyl cyclase activation (Kebabian & Clane 1979). Thus activation of D_2 receptors by dopamine appears to be important for motor control.

Antipsychotic activity appears to correlate closely with D_2 receptor antagonism although the development of an improvement in psychoses is slower than the development of other manifestations of D_2 antagonism such as prolactin release (Silverstone & Cookson 1983). It may be that chronic D_2 receptor blockade leads to other biochemical changes leading to antipsychotic activity. At present it seems that most of the behavioural effects of dopamine agonists and antagonists are mediated via D_2 dopamine receptors.

The development of selective D_1 receptor agonists and antagonists, however, has demonstrated interesting functional links between the two types of dopamine receptors (Waddington and O'Boyle 1989).

Noradrenaline

Noradrenergic neurons are less widespread than

dopaminergic neurons. Cell bodies arise in the pons and medulla, and the highest concentrations of noradrenaline are found in the hypothalamus and limbic system (Iversen & Iversen 1975). Local application of noradrenaline produces inhibitory responses in many neurons. These are usually mediated via β-adrenoceptors linked to adenyl cyclase (Bloom 1980). The brain also contains α-adrenoceptors and both the sedative and hypotensive effects of centrally acting α-agonists such as clonidine are mediated via this receptor. It is unclear whether α_1 or α_2 activation or both is important for the hypotensive action of these drugs (Clough & Hatton 1981), although an increase in blood pressure has been reported in man after treatment with a selective α_2-adrenoceptor antagonist (Elliott et al 1983). Sedation appears to be closely allied to α_2-adrenoceptor activation as the selective α_2-agonist, azepexole, has been shown to be highly sedative (Pleuvry & Redpath 1982). α_2-Receptor activation also has a role in activating descending analgesic pathways (Fitzgerald 1986).

No diseases in man have definitely been attributed to noradrenaline lack or excess. However, a subgroup of depressed patients have been shown to have low urinary levels of the major metabolite of noradrenaline, and these patients respond better to drugs which acutely enhance noradrenergic systems than do depressed patients without this abnormality. The latter group respond better to drugs which enhance tryptaminergic systems (Matussek 1979). However, antidepressant activity, like antipsychotic activity, is slow to develop, and thus the acute pharmacological effects of the drugs may not be their primary mechanism of antidepressant activity. Chronic treatment with the tricyclic antidepressants result in complex changes in the sensitivity or number of several neurotransmitter receptors. β-Adrenoceptors become less responsive whilst α_1-adrenoceptors become more responsive. The latter change may be more important for antidepressant activity (van Praag 1983). The biochemical theories of affective disorders have been reviewed by Baker & Dewhurst (1985).

Adrenaline

The adrenaline-containing cell bodies are found in the reticular formation of the medulla and send descending axons to the sympathetic lateral column, and ascending fibres to many areas including the hypothalamus. Within the mesencephalon the adrenaline-containing neurons innervate the nuclei of the visceral efferent and afferent systems, including the dorsal motor nucleus of the vagus nerve. It has been suggested that the adrenaline-containing system constitutes a vasodepressor system (Bolme et al 1974) and that clonidine might act by stimulating central adrenaline receptors. Furthermore the use of phenylethanolamine N-methyl transferase inhibitors suggests that adrenaline neurons may have a role in behaviour and neuroendocrine regulation (Fuller 1982).

5-Hydroxytryptamine (5-HT)

5-HT is localized within neurons in the mammalian CNS. The distribution of 5-HT-containing cell bodies is largely restricted to a group of neurons known as the raphe nuclei, situated dorsally near the midline of the brainstem. Ascending 5-HT fibres are found in the medial forebrain bundle and descending fibres enter the spinal cord (Iversen & Iversen 1975). 5-HT can produce both inhibitory and excitatory effects within the CNS, and there is evidence for at least three 5-HT receptors (Haigler 1981). $5\text{-}HT_1$ receptors are found on the 5-HT-containing neurons of the midbrain raphe, and they mediate an inhibition of firing. Both 5-HT and lysergic acid diethylamide (LSD) are agonists at this receptor and classical 5-HT antagonists (e.g. methysergide) are without effect. Inhibition of firing is also brought about by activation of $5\text{-}HT_2$ receptors located in areas where 5-HT nerve terminals are dense. LSD is only a weak agonist at this receptor and 5-HT antagonists actually enhance the inhibition brought about by 5-HT. The closest correlation with peripheral 5-HT receptors is the $5\text{-}HT_3$ receptor which mediates excitation and is located in areas where 5-HT terminals are sparse. LSD and 5-HT antagonists all block this excitatory response to 5-HT. The above classification of 5-HT receptors is based on Haigler's (1981) review of the subject, but it must be appreciated that there is no consensus about a precise classification. More recent proposals are described by Bradley et al (1986) and include subdivision of the $5\text{-}HT_1$ receptors into $5\text{-}HT_{1A}$ and $5\text{-}HT_{1B}$. A selective $5\text{-}HT_{1A}$ agonist, buspirone, is being marketed as an anxiolytic (McGowan et al 1988).

It is likely that part of the analgesic activity of morphine is mediated by stimulation of descending tryptaminergic tracts causing release of 5-HT onto the $5\text{-}HT_3$ receptors (Haigler 1981). A number of substances capable of modifying tryptaminergic systems are currently being evaluated as potential analgesics; in addition $5\text{-}HT_3$ receptor antagonists are proving useful in the treatment of nausea and vomiting associated with cytotoxic treatment (Cooper and Abbott 1988). There is evidence that 5-HT may be involved in sleep and the reduction of aggression (Seiden and Dykstra 1977). There is now good evidence that a subgroup of depressed patients have some deficiencies in turnover of 5-HT (Matussek 1979). However, evidence is now accumulating that the long-term effects of all antidepressants, including ECT and the 'atypical' drugs such as mianserine, consistently enhance postsynaptic responses to 5-HT as well as α_1-agonists, as mentioned previously (Charney et al 1981). Thus derangements of either noradrenergic or tryptaminergic systems, or both, may contribute to manic depressive illness.

Histamine

Histamine is unevenly distributed in the brain, the highest concentrations being found in the hypothalamus and the lowest in the medulla, pons and cerebellum. There are two pools of histamine, a slow turnover pool associated with mast cells and a fast turnover pool associated with nerve endings. The latter probably represents histamine with a neurotransmitter function (Hirschowitz 1979, Calcutt 1976). Local applications of histamine to neurons are usually inhibitory, and a histamine-sensitive adenyl cyclase is present in brain (Bloom 1975). Binding sites showing the characteristics of H_1 and H_2 receptors have been demonstrated in brain. Procedures which raise brain histamine have a number of behavioural effects, and brain histamine turnover is increased by stress. Anaesthesia, on the other hand, reduces histamine turnover in the brain. A close correlation between central histamine H_1 antagonism and sedation has been observed for both the tricyclic antidepressants and the classical antihistamines (Schwartz et al 1981). These observations have led to the proposal that histamine may be a 'waking amine' (Pollard & Schwartz 1987).

Gamma aminobutyric acid (GABA)

There is considerable evidence that GABA is an inhibitory transmitter within the CNS. In the spinal cord GABA is largely confined to nerve terminals in the dorsal horn, but within the brain itself, substantial amounts of GABA are found in nearly all grey matter. It may be neurotransmitter in up to one-third of CNS synapses (Iversen & Iversen 1975). It is likely that the Purkinje cells of the cerebellum use GABA as their transmitter, and lesion studies suggest GABA systems originating from the globus pallidus and other striatal regions and terminating in the substantia nigra, which contains the highest density of GABA terminals. Inhibition associated with GABA is associated with a rapid increase in membrane conduction of chloride ions to make the interior of the cell more negative and thus less easily depolarized. This suggests that the GABA receptor is closely associated with the chloride channel (Olsen 1982). Subsequent studies have identified a separate receptor (GABA$_B$), which is not linked to chloride

channels but may be linked to calcium channels. Baclofen, a centrally acting muscle relaxant, is an agonist at GABA$_B$ receptors but not GABA$_A$ receptors (Bowery 1984).

Depletion of GABA and the enzymes which synthesize it has been associated with postmortem brains from patients with Huntington's disease. This effect is variable, some patients showing almost normal levels, and others showing more than 50% depletion. The basal ganglia, cerebellum and dentate nucleus are more affected (Iversen et al 1979). The decrease in GABA appears to be associated with an increase in the concentration of dopamine and 5-hydroxytryptamine in the basal ganglia. Many of the symptoms of Huntingdon's disease are due to the increase in dopamine, and dopamine antagonists are some of the few useful agents in this condition. Drug-induced enhancement of GABA transmission has not proved beneficial, probably because the condition is diagnosed late after significant loss of GABA neurons and receptors has occurred (Bird 1980).

It is difficult to determine what physiological or pharmacological changes in behaviour involve GABA systems, as it is not yet possible to measure GABA turnover in vivo. Nevertheless, there are some drugs which appear to interact with GABA systems. Picrotoxin has been shown to antagonize the inhibitory actions of GABA in invertebrates and subsequently at a number of sites in the mammalian CNS. Picrotoxin has been shown to block both presynaptic inhibition and strychnine-resistant postsynaptic inhibition within the CNS, as well as being a potent stimulant and convulsant. Picrotoxin is not a very selective GABA antagonist and cannot compete with GABA for putative receptor binding. Much greater selectivity is obtained with bicuculline, which does compete with GABA for GABA$_A$ binding sites (Iversen 1978). However, bicuculline is also a powerful convulsant in mammals, thus supporting the proposed key role of GABA in controlling seizure activity (Gale 1989).

The involvement of benzodiazepines with GABA transmission has been discussed (Costa & Guidotti 1979). Benzodiazepines specifically relieve convulsions due to partial inhibition of GABA transmission. Some of the behavioural effects of the benzodiazepines are specifically blocked by picrotoxin, and benzodiazepines seem to have agonist actions in a number of postsynaptic GABA$_A$ systems. However, the benzodiazepine receptor is not identical to the GABA$_A$ receptor and the benzodiazepines are active only when GABA systems are functional. Evidence suggests that the benzodiazepines increase the sensitivity of GABA$_A$ receptors or enhance the binding of GABA to its receptors. Not all GABA binding sites are associated with benzodiazepine binding sites, the high-affinity GABA binding sites in the cerebellum being a notable exception (Olsen 1982).

The sedative and anaesthetic actions of the barbiturates have been ascribed to enhancement of GABA transmission (Ho & Harris 1981). This appears to be an indirect action involving neither GABA nor benzodiazepine receptors. Indeed Cheng & Brunner (1980) hypothesized that the actions of all general anaesthetics could be explained by a functional excess of GABA, although the mechanism by which each agent achieved this excess differed. A whole range of agonist, antagonists and contra-agonists have now been described for the benzodiazepine receptor (Martin 1984). A benzodiazepine antagonist, flumazenil, was marketed in 1988 and its place in clinical practice is presently being assessed.

A number of endogenous ligands have been proposed, some having agonist and some contra-agonist profiles (Costa & Guidotti 1985, De Blas et al 1985, De Robertis et al 1988). The terms 'agonist' and 'contra' (or 'inverse') agonists have been used to describe two classes of compounds which bind to the same receptor site but produce diametrically opposite effects. A contra-agonist at a benzodiazepine receptor, for example, causes anxiety and even panic.

Glycine

There is some evidence that glycine is an inhibitory transmitter in the spinal cord. When applied locally it hyperpolarizes motor neurons in a manner similar to postsynaptic inhibition. Glycine is found in highest concentrations in the spinal cord associated with interneurons like the Renshaw cells. Strychnine blocks the action of glycine and also blocks postsynaptic inhibition of motor neurons (Kuno & Weakly 1972). Furthermore, stimulation of dorsal roots causes release of glycine from perfused spinal cord. However, as yet the release of glycine from interneurons has not been demonstrated, and thus the evidence remains circumstantial. Glycine has been shown to facilitate depolarization produced by excitatory transmitters at N-methyl-D-aspartate receptors (see below). However, at this site the receptor for glycine is not strychnine-sensitive (Wroblewski and Danysz 1989).

Other amino acids

Both *glutamate* and *aspartate* occur in high concentrations in the brain and have powerful excitatory effects. However, since both compounds are also involved in neuronal metabolism it has not been possible to differentiate neuronal tracts where the amino acids exert transmitter rather than metabolic roles. Iontophoretic application of glutamate and aspartate increases the rate of neuronal firing and glutamate release is reduced during sleep. Three receptor sites have been described for these excitatory amino acids and they have been named NMDA (N-methyl-D-aspartate), AMPA (α-amino-3-hydroxy-5-methyl isoxazole-4-proprionate) and KA (kainate) to indicate agonist selectivity. All these agonists are neurotoxins and excessive activation of their receptor has been suggested as a cause of degenerative diseases such as Huntington's disease (Rothman & Olney 1987). The dissociative anaesthetics, e.g. ketamine, are non-competitive antagonists at the N-methyl-D-aspartate receptor (Kemp et al 1987). Receptors for excitatory transmitters have been reviewed by Monaghan et al (1989).

Opioid peptides

In 1975 Hughes et al isolated a small peptide from porcine brain with morphine-like activity in peripheral pharmacological assays. The peptide was called enkephalin, and was subsequently found to be two pentapeptides sharing a common tetrapeptide sequence varying only in the terminal position. The two peptides were called [Leu]-enkephalin and [Met]-enkephalin. Since 1975 a number of longer chain peptides have been extracted from brain fragments and these fall into three main groups: the enkephalins, the endorphins and the dynorphins. The enkephalins are found in diffuse short neurons and are concentrated in the striatum and hypothalamus. Enkephalins are also found outside the CNS, particularly in the adrenal medulla and gastrointestinal tract. The endorphin family consists of larger, more stable peptides found in the anterior and intermediate pituitary endocrine cells and discrete neurons, mainly in the hypothalamus. The dynorphins are peptides containing the [Leu]-enkephalin sequence at the amino terminus and are found in neurons of the posterior pituitary, hypothalamus and gastrointestinal tract. Dynorphin$_{1-13}$ has been described as 'an extraordinarily potent opioid peptide' (Goldstein et al 1979).

Hand-in-hand with the discovery of multiple opioid peptides was the discovery of multiple opioid receptor types. At the time of writing five main subtypes of the opioid receptor have been described, μ, κ, σ, δ and Σ of which there is evidence that the first four exist in human brain (Itzhak et al 1982). The Σ receptor, at which β-endorphin is a selective agonist and most other opioids have no effect or are antagonists, has so far been described only in the rat vas deferens preparation (Schulz et al 1981). Some opioids and opioid peptides appear to have selectivity for one or other of these receptor sites (Table 5.2). However, this selectivity is poor, and intensive research is being directed into assigning a pharmacological action to a particular receptor subtype in the hope that higher receptor selectivity might produce a powerful analgesic with reduced side-effects. There is evidence that this is a fruitful approach. Pasternak (1982) found that the analgesic activity of both proposed μ-receptor and δ-receptor agonists could be inhibited by naloxazone, a compound which irreversibly inhibits high-affinity μ binding sites. Thus the analgesic activity of these opioids resides in the high-affinity μ-receptor (also known as the μ_1-receptor). Subsequently both Ling et al (1983) and Ward and Takemori (1983) found that animals treated with irreversible μ_1 antagonists responded to μ- and δ-agonists with respiratory depression, but no analgesia. This indicates that respiratory depression is not associated with the μ_1-receptor, but may be mediated by either the low-affinity μ-receptor (μ_2) or the δ-receptor. Unfortunately the picture is not as clear-cut as these preliminary observations had suggested. The presence or absence of stress appears to influence the opioid receptor profile of agonist compounds, and different receptors may mediate separate aspects of respiratory depression, e.g. tidal volume and frequency changes (Marin-Surun et al 1984).

The dynorphins have some selectivity for the κ-receptors which appear to mediate analgesia with quite separate characteristics from that produced by μ-receptor agonists. κ-Agonists have little activity in analgesic tests using heat as the noxious stimulus (Tyers 1982) and the analgesia that they do produce is less readily antagonized by naloxone than that of μ-agonists. Binding studies have also demonstrated that naloxone has less affinity for κ binding sites than it does for μ

binding sites (Hutchinson et al 1975). κ analgesics do not substitute for morphine in the dependent animal. Intrathecal administration of δ-agonists also mediates analgesia, even in patients tolerant to morphine (Moulin et al 1985). In the experimental animal the characteristics of analgesia differ from μ and κ analgesia (Yaksh & Noveihed 1985).

The hallucinatory actions of the opioids has been ascribed to the σ-receptor and many κ-agonists exhibit this property. There is some debate as to whether the σ-receptor is truly an opioid receptor as naloxone antagonism is uncertain (see Miller 1982). The hallucinogenic effects of the phencyclidine/ketamine group also appears to be mediated via the σ-receptor (Zukin 1982).

The advent of more selective and potent antagonists such as naltrindole for the δ receptor and nor-binaltorphimine for the κ receptor (Haynes 1988) will lead to a reappraisal of the physiological role of opioid peptides.

Substance P

Substance P is a undecapeptide which is present in small neuron systems in many parts of the CNS and appears to be associated with intraneuronal vesicles. Particularly large quantities of substance P are found in neurons entering the substantia gelatinosa from the spinal cord. It has been proposed that substance P is the transmitter for the primary afferent sensory fibres (Wright & Roberts 1978).

Substance P is also found in high concentrations in the substantia nigra, hypothalamus and cerebral cortex and other brain areas. A role for substance P in pain perception in many of these areas has been discussed (Snyder 1980), together with interactions with the enkephalin/endorphin system (Takahasi et al 1987).

Other neuroactive peptides

A number of peptides, many of which are well known for their hormonal activity, have been localized in neurons within the CNS. Some of these may be transmitters and others may perform regulatory roles (Gregory 1982). The distribution of *neurotensin* in the CNS closely parallels enkephalin and thus a role in pain perception has been proposed (Snyder 1980). *Angiotensin II* was thought to be mainly a peripheral modulator of blood pressure; however, modern techniques demonstrated that angiotensin and the enzymes necessary for its synthesis were present in the brain, mainly in the periventricular zone. When injected into the brain in minute quantities, angiotensin II induces a profound drinking behaviour (Fitzsimons 1975). Originally isolated as a potent releaser of growth hormones,

Table 5.2 Opioid receptor subtypes and their agonists

Receptor type	Agonists
μ	morphine fentanyl group
κ	dynorphins ketocyclazocine, bremazocine pentazocine (also a μ-antagonist)
σ	SKF 10,047 phenylcyclidine
δ	Dala^2 D-Leu^5-enkephalin*
Σ	β-endorphin

* Stable derivative of [Leu]-enkephalin.
NB: agonist receptor selectivity is generally poor.

somatostatin has been found in many other brain regions besides the hypothalamus. When injected into the cerebral ventricles, somatostatin produced depression and a general pharmacological profile reminiscent of phenytoin (Cooper et al 1986).

Luteinizing hormone releasing hormone is found in both the hypothalamus and midbrain. Local injections of the hormone into the hypothalamus of oestrogen-primed, ovariectomized females produces mating behaviour (Moss 1977). Both *oxytocin* and *vasopressin* have been proposed as inhibitory transmitters regulating neurons projecting into the neurohypophysis, and *thyrotrophin-releasing hormone* has complex interactions with other neurotransmitters, enhancing some and inhibiting others. *Cholecystokinin, Vasoactive intestinal polypeptide* (VIP) and *neuropeptide Y* are receiving attention particularly for their co-transmitter role (Cooper et al 1986). In addition *Corticotrophin Releasing Factor (CRF)* has neuronal actions which suggest a more widespread control of response to stress than simply hormone release.

Prostaglandins

Prostaglandins are fatty acids widely distributed in biological tissues including the CNS. The brain contains mainly prostaglandins of the F series but has tremendous capacity for the rapid synthesis of other prostaglandins, particularly PGEs. There is a fairly uniform distribution of prostaglandins throughout the brain, which suggests that they are not associated with any particular neuronal system. The rapid production and breakdown of prostaglandins makes them ideal candidates for a local modulator role in the CNS.

The prostanoids mediate their effects through a variety of receptors. It has been suggested that they are termed P receptors (for prostanoid) preceded by a letter to denote the active prostaglandin, i.e. $PGF_{2\alpha}$ would act at FP receptors (Coleman et al 1984).

A wide variety of both stimulant and depressant effects of prostaglandins on the CNS have been reported (Coceani 1974). Perhaps the most interesting is the fever production in response to PGEs but not PGFs. During fever, a rise in endogenous PGE_1 has been demonstrated, the time-course of which closely follows the time-course of the temperature elevation. Furthermore antipyretic drugs, which are known to prevent prostaglandin synthesis, prevent the rise in temperature due to pyrogens and also prevent the rise in PGE1.

Inhibition of prostaglandin synthesis usually occurs by inhibition of the enzyme cyclo-oxygenase, which converts arachidonic acid to the cyclic endoperoxide precursors of the prostanoids. Cyclo-oxygenase inhibition is also associated with anti-inflammatory and analgesic activity. The former is brought about by a purely peripheral action as paracetamol inhibits cyclo-oxygenase in the brain only, and has negligible anti-inflammatory activity. The selectivity of paracetamol for brain cyclo-oxygenase may depend upon the presence of co-factors which seem important for this drug's inhibitory effects on cyclo-oxygenase, at least in vitro (Robak et al 1978).

In the preceding pages the effects of a few drugs on specific transmitter systems have been discussed, as well as drugs which do not appear to interact with stereospecific receptor sites. However, the vast majority of these drugs interact with more than one transmitter system and may also have non-specific actions. An extreme example is chlorpromazine, which antagonizes, to a lesser or greater degree, the actions of dopamine, the α effects of noradrenaline, some actions of 5-HT, the muscarinic actions of acetylcholine and H_1 receptor effects of histamine. It is only with the development of more selective drugs that we have been able to relate neuroleptic and anti-psychotic activity to dopamine antagonism, although whether this is a primary or a secondary phenomenon is still uncertain.

A further complicating factor is that the same pharmacological response can result from several different mechanisms. Inhibition of parkinsonian tremor can be achieved by enhancing dopaminergic systems and by antagonizing cholinergic systems. Reduction in sympathetic outflow can be achieved by stimulating central α-receptors and by β-receptor blockade.

It is with these factors in mind that the basic pharmacology of the individual groups of drugs, described in the following chapters, should be considered.

REFERENCES

Aquilonius S M 1977 Physostigmine in the treatment of drug overdose. In: Jenden D J (ed) Cholinergic mechanisms and psychopharmacology. Plenum Press, New York, vol 24, pp 817–825

Baker G B, Dewhurst W G 1985 Biochemical theories of affective disorders. In: Dewhurst W G, Baker G B (eds) Pharmacology of affective disorders. Croom Helm, London, pp 1–59

Bird E D 1980 Chemical pathology of Huntington's disease. Annual Review of Pharmacology and Toxicology 20: 533–551

Bloom F E 1975 The role of cyclic nucleotides in central synaptic function. Reviews of Physiology, Biochemistry and Pharmacology 74: 1–103

Bloom F E 1980 Neurohumoral transmission and the central nervous system. In: Gilman A G, Goodman L S, Gilman A (eds) The pharmacological basis of therapeutics, 6th edn. Macmillan, New York, p 235–257

Bolme P, Corrodi H, Fuxe K, Hohfelt T, Lidrrink P, Goldstein H 1974 Possible involvment of central adrenaline neurons in vasomotor and respiratory control. Studies with clonidine and its interactions with piperoxane and yohimbine. European Journal of Pharmacology 28: 89–94

Bowery N G 1984 Baclofen: 10 years on. In: Lamble J W, Abbott A C (eds) Receptors, again. Elsevier, Amsterdam, pp 195–202

Bradley P B, Engel G, Feniuk W et al 1986 Proposals for the classification of functional receptors of 5-hydroxytryptamine. Neuropharmacology 25: 563–575

Calcutt C R 1976 The role of histamine in the brain. General Pharmacology 7: 15–25

Charney D S, Menkes D B, Heniger G R 1981 Receptor sensitivity and the mechanism of action of antidepressant treatment. Archives of General Psychiatry 38: 1160–1180

Cheng S C, Brunner E A 1980 Is anaesthesia caused by excess GABA? In: Fink B R (ed) Molecular mechanisms in anaesthesia. Progress in Anaesthesiology. Raven Press, New York, vol 2, pp 137–144

Clough D P, Hatton R 1981 Hypotensive and sedative effects of α-adrenoceptor agonists: relationship to α_1- and α_2-adrenoceptor potency. British Journal of Pharmacology 73: 595–604

Coceani F 1974 Prostaglandins and the central nervous system. Archives of Internal Medicine 133: 119–129

Coleman R A, Humphrey P P A, Kennedy I, Lamley P 1984 Prostanoid receptors – the development of a working classification. In: Lamble J W, Abbott A C (eds) Receptors, again. Elsevier, Amsterdam, pp 263–269

Cooper J R, Bloom F E, Roth R H 1986 The biochemical basis of neuropharmacology, 5th edn. Oxford University Press, New York

Cooper S J, Abbott A 1988 Clinical psychopharmacology may benefic from new advances in 5-HT pharmacology. Trends in Pharmacological Sciences 9: 269–271

Costa E, Guidotti A 1979 Molecular mechanisms in the receptor action of benzodiazepines. Annual Review of Pharmacology and Toxicology 19: 531–545

Costa E, Guidotti A 1985 Endogenous ligands for benzodiazepine recognition sites. Biochemical Pharmacology 34: 3399–3403

De Blas A L, Sangameswaran L, Haney S A, Park D, Abraham C J, Rayner C A 1985 Monoclonal antibodies to benzodiazepines. Journal of Neurochemistry 45: 1748–1753

De Robertis E, Pena C, Paladini A C, Medina J H 1988 New developments on the search for the endogenous ligand(s) of central benzodiazepine receptors. Neurochemistry International 13: 1–11

Di Liberti J, O'Brien M L, Turner T 1975 The use of physostigmine as an antidote in accidental diazepam intoxication. Journal of Pediatrics 86(1): 106–107

Dunnett S B, Low W C, Iversen S P, Stenevi U, Bjorklund A 1982 Septal transplants restore maze learning in rats with fornix-fimbria lesions. Brain Research 251: 335–348

Elliott H L, Jones C R, Vincent J, Reid J L 1983 α-Adrenoceptor antagonist actions of RX 81094 in man: selective effects on α_2-adrenoceptors. British Journal of Clinical Pharmacology 15: 598P

Fitzgerald M 1986 Monoamines and descending control of nociception. Trends in Neuroscience 9: 51–52

Fitzsimons J T 1975 The renin–angiotensin system and drinking behaviour. Progress in Brain Research 42: 215–233

Fluckiger E, Vigouret J M 1981 Central dopamine receptors. Postgraduate Medical Journal 57(S1): 55–61

Fuller R W 1982 Pharmacology of brain epinephrine neurons. Annual Review of Pharmacology and Toxicology 22: 31–55

Gale K 1989 GABA in epilepsy: The pharmacologic basis. Epilepsia 30 (Suppl. 3) S1–S11

Goldstein A, Tachibana S, Lowney L I, Hunkapiller M, Hood L 1979 Dynorphin-(1–13), an extraordinarily potent opioid peptide. Proceedings of the National Academy of Sciences of the USA 76: 6666–6670

Green D 1983 Current concepts concerning the mode of action of meptazinol as an analgesic. Postgraduate Medical Journal 59(S1): 9–12

Gregory R A (ed) 1982 Regulatory peptides of gut and brain. British Medical Bulletin 38: 219–309

Haigler H J 1981 Serotonergic receptors in the central nervous system. In: Yamamura, H I, Enna S J (eds) Neutrotransmitter receptors, Part 2: Biogenic amines. Chapman & Hall, London, pp 3–70

Halsey M J, Green C J, Wardley-Smith B 1980 Renaissance of non unitary molecular mechanisms of general anaesthesia. In: Fink B R (ed.) Molecular mechanisms of anaesthesia. Progress in anaesthesiology, 2. Raven Press, New York, vol 2, pp 273–283

Haynes L 1988 Opioid receptors and signal transduction. Trends in Pharmacological Science 9: 309–311

Hirschowitz B I 1979 H-2 Histamine receptors. Annual Review of Pharmacology and Toxicology 19: 203–244

Ho I K, Harris R D 1981 Mechanism of action of barbiturates. Annual Review of Pharmacology and Toxicology 21: 83–111

Hornykiewicz O 1966 Dopamine (3-hydroxytyramine) and brain function. Pharmacological Reviews 18(2): 925–964

Hughes J, Smith T W, Kosterlitz H W, Fortherg M L A, Morgan B A, Morris H R 1975 Identification of two related pentapetides from the brain with potent opiate agonist activity. Nature 258: 577–579

Hutchinson M, Kosterlitz H W, Leslie F M, Terenius L, Waterfield A R 1975 Assessment in the guinea pig ileum and mouse vas deferens of benzomorphans which have strong antinociceptive activity but do not substitute for morphine in the dependent monkey. British Journal of Pharmacology 55: 541–546

Itzhak Y, Bonnet K A, Groth J, Hillier J M, Simon E J 1982 Multiple opiate binding sites in human brain regions: evidence for κ and σ sites. Life Sciences 31: 1363–1366

Iversen L L 1978 Biochemical psychopharmacology of GABA. In: Lipton M A, Di Mascio A, Killam K F (eds) Pyschopharmacology — a generation of progress. Raven Press, New York, pp 25–38

Iversen L L, Spokes E, Bird E 1979 GABA systems in human brain in Huntington's disease and schizophrenia. In: Simon P (ed) Neurotransmitters, advances in pharmacology and therapeutics. IUPHAR, Paris; Pergamon, Oxford, vol. 2, pp 3–10

Iversen S D, Iversen L L 1975 Behavioural pharmacology. Oxford University Press, New York

Kebabian J W, Clane D B 1979 Multiple receptors for dopamine. Nature 277: 93–96

Kemp J A, Foster A C, Wong E H F 1987 Non competitive antagonists of excitatory amino acid receptors. Trends in Neuroscience 10: 294–298

Krnjevic K 1974 Chemical nature of synaptic transmission in vertebrates. Physiological Reviews 54: 418–540

Kuno M, Weakly J N 1972 Quantal components of the inhibitory synaptic potential in spinal mononeurones of the cat. Journal of Physiology 224: 287–303

Langrall H M, Joseph C 1972 Evaluation of safety and efficacy of levodopa in Parkinson's disease and syndrome; results of a collaborative study. Symposium on levodopa in Parkinson's disease, June 1971. Neurology, Minneapolis 22(5ii): 3–16

Ling C S F, Spiegel K, Nishimura S L, Pasternak G W 1983 Dissociation of morphine's analgesic and respiratory depressant actions. European Journal of Pharmacology 86: 487–488

Marin-Surun M P, Boudinot E, Gacel G, Champagnat J, Rogues B P, Denavit-Saubie M 1984 Different effects of, μ and δ opiate agonists on respiration. European Journal of Pharmacology 98: 235–250

Martin I L 1984 The benzodiazepine receptor: functional complexity. In: Lamble J W, Abbott N C (eds) Receptors again. Elsevier, Amsterdam, pp 214–220

Matussek N 1979 Biochemical mechanisms of depressive states: evolution of ideas. In: Dumont C (ed) Neuropsychopharmacology, advances in pharmacology and therapeutics. Pergamon Press, Oxford vol 5, pp 147–156

McGowan G, Napoliello M, Alms D 1988 Buspirone for the management of anxiety in patients with concomitant medical conditions: a retrospective preliminary evaluation. Current Therapeutic Research 43: 481–486

Miller R J 1982 Multiple opiate receptors for multiple opioid peptides. Medical Biology 60: 1–6

Monaghan D T, Bridges R J, Cotman C W 1989 The excitatory amino acids receptors: their classes, pharmacology, and distinct properties in the function of the central nervous system. Annual Review of Pharmacology and Toxicology 29: 365–402

Moore R Y, Bloom F E 1978 Central catecholamine neuron systems: anatomy and physiology of the dopamine systems. Annual Review of Neuroscience 1: 129–169

Moss R L 1977 Role of hypophysiotropic neurohormones in mediating neural and behavioural events. Federation Proceedings 36: 1978–1983

Moulin D E, Max M B, Kaiko R F et al 1985 The analgesic efficacy of intrathecal D-Ala^2-D-Leu^5 enkephalin in cancer patients with chronic pain. Pain 23: 213–221

Olsen R W 1982 Drug interactions at the GABA receptor–ionophore complex. Annual Review of Pharmacology and Toxicology 22: 245–77

Pasternak G W 1982 High and low affinity opioid binding sites: relationship to mu and delta sites. Life Sciences 31: 1303–1306

Pleuvry B J, Redpath J B S 1982 Ventilatory and cardiovascular effects of BHT 933 in volunteers. British Journal of Clinical Pharmacology 14: 559–561

Pollard H, Schwartz J-C 1987 Histamine neuronal pathways and their function. Trends in Pharmacological Sciences 10: 86–89

Robak J, Wieckowski A, Gryglewski R 1978 The effect of 4-acetamidophenol on prostaglandin synthetase activity in bovine and ram seminal vesicle microsomes. Biochemical Pharmacology 27: 393–396

Roth S H 1980 Differential effects of anaesthetics on neuronal activity. In: Fink B R (ed) Molecular mechanisms of anaesthesia. Progress in anaesthesiology. Raven Press, New York, vol. 2 pp 119–127

Rothman S M, Olney J W 1987 Excitotoxicity and the NMDA receptor. Trends in Neuroscience 10: 299–302

Schulz R, Wüster M, Herz A 1981 Pharmacological characterization of the Σ-opiate receptor. Journal of Pharmacology and Experimental Therapeutics 216: 604–606

Schwartz J C, Garbarg M, Ouach T T 1981 Histamine receptors in brain as targets for tricyclic antidepressants. Trends in Pharmacological Science 2: 122–125

Seiden L S, Dykstra L A 1977 Psychopharmacology: a biochemical and behavioural approach. Van Nostrand Reinhold, New York

Siggins G R 1978 Electrophysiological role of dopamine in striatum: excitatory or inhibitory? In: Lipton M A, Di Mascio A, Killam K F (eds) Psychopharmacology – a generation of progress. Raven Press, New York, pp 143–158

Silverstone T, Cookson K 1983 Examining the dopamine hypotheses of schizophrenia and mania using the prolactin response to antipsychotic drugs. Neuropharmacology 22: 539–541

Snyder S H 1980 Peptide neurotransmitters with possible involvement in pain perception. In: Bonica J J (ed) Pain. Raven Press, New York, pp 233–243

Takahasi K, Sakurada T, Sakurada S et al 1987 Behavioural characterization of substance P-induced nociceptive responses in mice. Neuropharmacology 26: 1289–1293

Tyers M B 1982 Studies on the antinociceptive activities of mixtures of μ and κ opiate receptor agonists and antagonists. Life Sciences 31: 1233–1236

van Praag H M 1983 In search of the mode of action of antidepressants. Neuropharmacology 22: 433–440

Waddington J L, O'Boyle K M 1989 Drugs acting on brain dopamine receptors: A conceptual re-evaluation five years after the first selective D_1 antagonist. Pharmacology and Therapeutics 43: 1–52

Ward S J, Takemori A E 1983 Determination of the relative involvement of μ-opioid receptors in opioid-induced depression of respiratory rate by use of β funaltrexamine. European Journal of Pharmacology 87: 1–6

Weinstock M, Davidson J T, Rosin A J, Schnieden H 1982 Effect of physostigine on morphine-induced postoperative pain and somnolence. British Journal of Anaesthesia 54: 429–434

White P, Hiley C R, Goodhardt M J et al 1977 Neocortical cholinergic neurons in elderly people. Lancet I: 668–671

Wright D M, Roberts M 1978 Supersensitivity to a substance P analogue following dorsal root section. Life Sciences 22(1): 19–24

Wroblewski J T, Danysz W 1989 Modulation of glutamate receptors: molecular mechanism and functional considerations. Annual Review of Pharmacology and Toxicology 29: 441–474

Yaksh T L, Noveihed R 1985 The physiology and pharmacology of spinal opiates. Annual Review of Pharmacology and Toxicology 25: 433–462

Zukin S R 1982 Differing stereospecificities distinguish opiate receptor sub types. Life Sciences 31: 1307–1310

6. Mechanisms of general anaesthesia

A. C. McKay

INTRODUCTION

At the clinical level, anaesthesia is a drug-induced, reversible disruption of some as yet largely unknown aspects of central nervous system (CNS) activity. A complete theory of anaesthesia would explain how this occurs in terms of the molecular and neurophysiological changes involved, but because the underlying mechanisms of consciousness and related processes are so poorly understood this kind of comprehensive description is not within sight at present. Instead the actions of anaesthetics have to be studied separately at several different levels of CNS function. For example, sophisticated techniques can now be applied to the study of anaesthetic effects on membrane lipid and protein, but these molecular effects cannot be made to relate to changes in the functions of higher-level structures such as axons and synapses except in the most general terms. Anaesthetic modifications in these larger functional units are investigated using techniques appropriate to their size and function, but again, such findings, in turn, are not applicable to complex neurological functions that depend on the integrated activity of billions of axons and synapses and require study at their own level. We thus have at least three disciplines at work on these different aspects of the same process.

There is also the difficulty that anaesthetics have many effects at all these levels which may be unrelated to the production of anaesthesia in the intact organism.

Fortunately, however, all types of study are linked by the common thread which relates them to the observed phenomenon of anaesthesia in the intact animal or man. So, for example, if any experimentally demonstrated effect of an anaesthetic, whether molecular or neurophysiological, is to be regarded as relevant to the anaesthetic state it must occur at the same concentration range of the agent as that which produces anaesthesia. To be comparable with anaesthesia in the intact organism it must also be produced very rapidly on exposure to the agent, be sustainable in a steady state over a prolonged period, and be quickly and readily reversible by removal of the agent. It is also generally accepted that different agents should show the same rank order of potency for the effect as for anaesthesia, although since any experimental effect is probably only a part of a much more complex process, it is possible that this may not always hold. The same applies to the property of reversibility by pressure (see below).

A question which is fundamental to this whole line of inquiry is whether or not a single mechanism of anaesthesia exists or whether, at the other extreme, all agents have different modes of action. Broadly, the long history of this subject has shown a gradual movement away from unitary theories towards explanations involving greater complexity and diversity among agents.

ANAESTHETIC ACTION AT MOLECULAR LEVEL

Two lines of approach are used in the study of the molecular mode of action of anaesthetics. The first, which has a long history and has been very fruitful, involves finding correlations between the relative anaesthetic potencies of different agents and various physical properties in order to characterize the probable molecular nature of the site or sites of anaesthetic action. The second method, which has been possible only with sophisticated modern techniques, involves the study of anaesthetic interactions with experimental biological or artificial model systems.

A number of readily observable features of anaesthetics as a group suggest that they are unusual among pharmacologically active substances. As molecules they are comparatively small and simple, but they vary widely in size and structure with, for example, a 10-fold difference in size between xenon and the halogenated hydrocarbons and ethers. At least among the inhalational agents, optical isomers are usually equipotent, but as a group the potency of anaesthetics is low, so that the concentrations necessary to produce an effect are some 10–100 times greater than those of, for example, opioids (Miller 1987). Thus, anaesthesia is an effect produced by high concentrations of a chemically heterogeneous group of substances, which led the first investigators to suppose that their mode of action is essentially non-specific rather than depending on occupation of specific receptors.

Lipid solubility

The discovery, at the turn of the twentieth century, of the remarkable correlation between anaesthetic potency and olive oil/water partition coefficient lent support to this view (Meyer 1901, Overton 1901). It led to the first physical theory of anaesthesia, which hypothesized that anaesthesia was due to the action of the drug on an olive oil-like, i.e. lipid, site in the CNS. The onset of anaesthesia would occur when the molar concentration of the agent at the site reached a critical level which would be the same for all agents, regardless of their molecular size, shape or chemical nature.

Modern work has confirmed that the relationship between anaesthetic potency and lipid solubility holds over five orders of magnitude of anaesthetic potency (Fig. 6.1). Two advances in methodology have enabled the correlation to be tested more rigorously. First, the introduction of the minimal alveolar concentration (MAC) (Eger et al 1969) gave an accurate measure of anaesthetic potency in mammals. Secondly, Miller et al (1972) improved the correlation by relating potency to solubility of agents in solvents of different polarity, and concluded that the site of action is relatively, but not completely, non-polar in character.

The molecular nature of the site of anaesthetic action is thus reasonably well established, but this in itself does not contribute any explanation of how the interaction of the anaesthetic with the hydrophobic site could bring about a functional change.

Pressure reversal of anaesthesia and the critical volume hypothesis

A possible clue to the mechanism is provided by the fact that, in animal preparations, anaesthesia can be antagonized or reversed by the application of high pressures of up to 200 atmospheres absolute (ATA). Pressure reversal was first demonstrated with inhalational agents (Johnston et al 1942) and has since been shown with intravenous anaesthetics as well as narcotics and tranquillizers (Halsey & Wardley-Smith 1975). The actual change in potency produced by application of pressure is less than a factor of 2 (Miller & Wilson 1978).

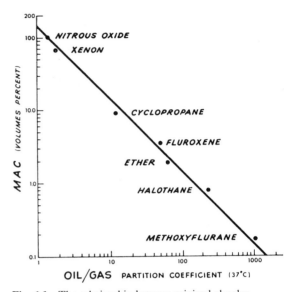

Fig. 6.1 The relationship between minimal alveolar concentration and oil/gas partition coefficient for several inhalational anaesthetics. (Reproduced with permission from Saidman et al 1967.)

The observation of pressure reversal led to the idea that absorption of anaesthetic molecules would cause the site of action to expand, an effect which would be directly antagonized by pressure, assuming that the site of action of the anaesthetic and pressure are the same. This was expressed in the critical volume hypothesis (Mullins 1954), which states that 'anaesthesia occurs when the volume of a hydrophobic region is caused to expand beyond a certain critical amount by the absorption of molecules of an inert substance'. In this way the lipid solubility hypothesis has been given added explanatory power by the introduction of the concept of volume expansion.

Membrane structure

What is the cellular location of this hydrophobic site? Since the information-transmitting function of the CNS, which is disrupted by anaesthesia, is a property of neuronal membranes, which are largely lipid structures, it is logical to assume that anaesthetics disrupt membrane function. Mammalian cell membranes (Fig. 6.2) consist of a phospholipid–cholesterol bilayer, with the lipids arranged so that their polar head groups are oriented outwards towards the aqueous phase and the non-polar hydrocarbon chains meet in the hydrophobic interior. Proteins of many different types are embedded in the bilayer, some contributing to structural stability while others pass through the membrane and function as ion

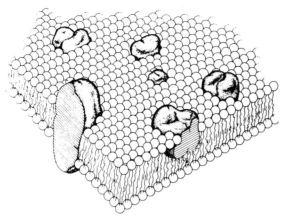

Fig. 6.2 The lipid-globular protein mosaic model with a lipid matrix (the fluid mosaic model); schematic three-dimensional and cross-sectional views. The solid bodies with stippled surfaces represent the globular integral proteins, which at long range are randomly distributed in the plane of the membrane. At short range some may form specific aggregates, as shown. Reproduced with permission from Singer & Nicholson 1972.

channels. These are capable of changing their tertiary structure in response to electrical or chemical stimuli. The detailed structure of some of these ion channels, for example the nicotinic acetylcholine receptor, is now known (Noda et al 1983). It consists of groups of α-helices, largely hydrophobic in nature, which transcend the lipid bilayer and project well beyond it. The structural integrity of these large intrinsic proteins depends greatly on the state of the surrounding lipid. These protein channels with their finely balanced structure and function would be expected to be particularly susceptible to disruption by anaesthetics, but the question of whether this occurs primarily through an action on one or more of the hydrophobic sites on the protein itself, the lipid–protein interface, or the surrounding lipid is more difficult to resolve. General theories like the critical volume hypothesis are of no help in making this kind of distinction.

Anaesthetic action on membranes

The effects of anaesthetics on membranes have been widely studied using model preparations. Artificial lipid bilayers can be prepared by adding phospholipids to an aqueous medium, and have been extensively used as model systems to study anaesthetic effects by means of such techniques as nuclear magnetic resonance (NMR) and electron spin resonance (ESR). A large number of studies have confirmed the correlation between anaesthetic potency and solubility in lipid bilayers and, using

this as a starting point, various hypotheses have been developed to explain how the presence of the anaesthetic in the membrane leads to a perturbation of protein function.

Simple expansion of the membrane, as predicted by the critical volume hypothesis, is clearly one possibility. Work on lipid bilayers and erythrocytes has shown that exposure to anaesthetics does cause expansion of these structures, and that anaesthesia occurs when the expansion is in the order of 0.2–0.6% (Kita & Miller 1982). However, there is some doubt whether the extent of these changes would be sufficient to produce the degree of functional disruption seen in anaesthesia (Franks & Lieb 1978).

This criticism also applies to theories based on the disordering of lipid membranes. ESR studies have shown that the addition of anaesthetic to a membrane usually results in increased fluidity, or disorder, among the lipid molecules. The effect is most marked and widespread in membranes with a phospholipid and cholesterol composition corresponding to that of excitable membrane, and the effect is pressure-reversible (Trudell et al 1973). However, in some situations fluidity may be decreased rather than increased, especially by intravenous agents.

Another group of theories of anaesthetic action in membranes is based on the ability of anaesthetics to lower the phase transition temperature at which membrane lipid changes from a 'solid' or gel phase to a 'liquid' or fluid phase. Trudell (1977) proposed that neuronal membrane lipids normally exist in both gel and fluid phases, and that when a membrane protein such as an ion channel undergoes a conformational change the increase in volume is normally compensated by the conversion of some of the membrane lipid from the higher volume fluid phase to the lower volume gel phase. The action of anaesthetics might be to disrupt function by preventing these phase changes. This property of anaesthetics has been demonstrated in model membranes and is reversible by pressure (Trudell et al 1975).

Thus, anaesthetics have been shown to interact with lipid membranes in a number of ways, any or all of which could theoretically lead to a disruption of the function of membrane protein. However, there is a lack of hard evidence that any of these mechanisms, which are generally associated with structural changes of less than 1%, do actually account for such changes.

Anaesthetic–protein interactions

Since membrane and other proteins contain many hydrophobic regions within their molecular structure, it is not surprising that a considerable number of studies have demonstrated interactions between anaesthetics and proteins. Due to the difficulties of studying membrane proteins directly, many experiments have used soluble proteins, and binding sites for anaesthetics have been identified on many of these. NMR studies of the action of halothane, methoxyflurane, ether and chloroform on the haemoglobin molecule show that these agents, at clinical concentrations, can produce specific conformational change in the molecule, the extent of which are related to the anaesthetic potency and lipid solubility of the agents (Brown & Halsey 1980). The perturbing effects of these agents in hydrophobic regions of the molecule are transmitted to non-hydrophobic regions.

Anaesthetics competitively inhibit luminescence in certain bacteria and in fireflies through an interaction with the luciferase enzymes. This inhibition correlates with anaesthetic potency for a wide range of volatile agents (Franks & Lieb 1984) and in some cases is pressure-reversible. Such observations have led some workers to the conclusion that anaesthetic action is specific, involving direct binding to a site on a particularly sensitive protein. However, such a theory is difficult to reconcile with the structural diversity and low potency of anaesthetics, without postulating a large number of such binding sites.

Experimental studies of anaesthetic action on lipid membranes and on proteins, whose original aim was to uncover a supposedly single mechanism of anaesthesia, have thus in fact shown that a number of different kinds of interaction take place, none of which emerges as more likely than the others to be of key significance.

Multiple sites of anaesthetic action

The critical volume hypothesis predicts that the relationship between anaesthetic potency and pressure should be linear and of equal slope for all agents. However, in detailed comparative studies in rats, Halsey and colleagues (Halsey & Wardley-Smith 1975, Halsey et al 1978) (Fig. 6.3) found non-linearity with inhalational, and especially with intravenous, anaesthetics.

These results led them to formulate the multi-site expansion hypothesis (Halsey et al 1978) in which the concept that anaesthetics act by expansion is retained, but it is assumed that they may affect more than one molecular site, each of which may have different physical properties, and also that pressure need not necessarily act at the same site as the anaesthetic. This would account for the different pressure/potency relationships that are seen with different agents, and possibly also for other anomalous results. For example, as is described below, depression of synaptic trans-

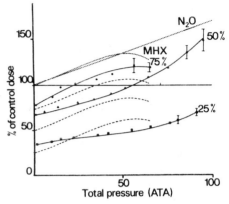

Fig. 6.3 Pressure reversal data for mixtures of methohexitone (MHX) and nitrous oxide (N_2O) in the rat: percentage control anaesthetic dose required at 1 ATA (AD_{95}) (vertical axis) with varying total pressure (horizontal axis). . . . . . ., Pressure reversal characteristics of each agent; —, results for three different mixtures (in each case 25%, 50% or 75% of the control anaesthetizing dose of N_2O was added: MHX was then adjusted until AD_{95} for the mixture was reached. This was expressed as a percentage of MHX required alone at 1 ATA). – – – –, Pressure reversal data curves calculated assuming simple additivity at both ambient and increased pressures. (Reproduced with permission from Wardley-Smith & Halsey 1981.)

mission is probably a major neuronal mechanism of anaesthesia, yet it can be facilitated, rather than antagonized, by high pressure (Kendig et al 1975). However, if the predominant effect of pressure in the whole animal was in the opposite direction at a different molecular site this might account for the discrepancy.

The hypothesis assumes that sites have a finite size and can be saturated by anaesthetic, and also that the site itself can be altered by pressure or anaesthetic. This would explain why pressure/potency curves are non-linear and also why pressure reversal is found to level off at a maximum with some agents.

This model of anaesthetic action represents a marked divergence from the critical volume hypothesis, which is based on a unitary model of anaesthetic action. Although the different sites are regarded as having the same solubility characteristics, in accordance with the lipid solubility rule (Halsey 1980), the limited occupancy of some of the sites suggests that they share some of the properties of specific receptor sites and are probably located on membrane proteins, while other sites have the characteristics of homogeneous bulk solvents. Some features of anaesthesia which are difficult to explain on the basis of a unitary theory of action may be accommodated by the multi-site expansion hypothesis, such as the observed differences in the actions of various agents at clinical and at neurophysiological level. Also, some workers have noted that some mixtures of anaesthetics, especially intravenous agents, are non-additive in their effects — for example, mixtures of alphaxalone and methohexitone show synergism (Archer et al 1977) and the potencies of Althesin/nitrous oxide and methohexitone/nitrous oxide mixtures are non-additive at high pressure (Wardley-Smith and Halsey 1981) (Fig. 6.3). The multi-site expansion hypothesis can explain these observations by assuming that these agents have different sites of action.

It would seem intuitively likely that specific drug–protein interaction would be more important in the case of the larger, intravenously administered molecules such as barbiturates, which exhibit stereospecificity and marked structure–activity relationships (Dundee 1988). Barbiturates have been shown to interact with specific sites on the acetylcholine (ACh) and γ-aminobutyric acid (GABA) receptors and on voltage-sensitive sodium channels in vivo (Miller et al 1986), acting as allosteric modulators or inhibitors at these sites by binding selectively to the resting conformation of the receptor, thereby reducing the proportion of receptor which is in the active state and can bind the transmitter ligand with high affinity. This finding thus provides evidence at molecular level of a direct effect of an anaesthetic on a structure with a precisely understood neurophysiological function.

Summary

A theory of anaesthetic action, such as the multi-site expansion hypothesis, based on the concept of a spectrum of molecular effects ranging from perturbation of membrane lipid to occupation of specific sites on specialized membrane proteins, probably best fits the findings at present. The potency/lipid solubility data enable the molecular nature of the site of action to be defined quite precisely in terms of its polarity, but it is likely that anaesthetics interact within the molecular environment in a number of different ways and at different sites in the neuronal membrane.

ANAESTHETIC ACTION ON THE NEURON AND SYNAPSE

Anaesthetics disrupt the information-carrying functions of the CNS, and these functions depend upon the integrated conduction and transmission of electrically and chemically mediated messages by many millions of neurons. It follows that anaesthetics must affect these processes, but it does not necessarily follow that all neurons and synapses are affected in a similar way, or that all anaesthetic agents have similar effects. It is quite possible that some functions are not simply depressed but may be disrupted in more complex ways or even augmented.

As mentioned above, a direct interaction can now be demonstrated between barbiturates and some neurotransmitter receptors and ion channels. However, the difference in scale between these structures and axons and synapses, which contain many different types of receptors, channels, and other potential sites of action, means that such demonstrations can give only general clues as to how axonal conduction and synaptic transmission might be affected.

Anaesthetic action on the axon and synapse can, however, be studied by direct neurophysiological techniques, mainly using preparations chosen for their experimental suitability, on the assumption that the findings will to some extent reflect the overall mechanism.

One of the fundamental problems has been to establish which part of the information-carrying process is affected. The most obvious distinction is between axonal conduction, which is electrically mediated, and synaptic transmission, which is chemically mediated. Since both these functions are based structurally on the neuronal membrane and its associated proteins, each would theoretically be susceptible to the molecular effects of anaesthetics described in the previous section. Allosteric modification by barbiturates appears to occur at both neurotransmitter receptor sites and voltage-sensitive ion channels, and thus might affect both types of transmission.

Axonal conduction

Information is conducted along axons in the form of trains of action potentials, which reflect transient changes in the ionic and especially sodium ion permeability of the axonal membrane. These permeability changes are due to the effects of an alteration in transmembrane electrical potential on the configuration of the membrane-embedded protein ion channels. When a sufficient electrical stimulus arrives, depolarizing the membrane, the sodium channel changes from a resting to an active or open configuration, during which there is a free flow of ions. It then passes to an inactive configuration for a period corresponding approximately to the refractory period of the membrane, while local current flow leads to depolarization of the next segment of membrane.

Larrabee and Posternak (1952) showed that ether, pentobarbitone and chloroform depressed axonal conduction only at higher concentrations than those required to block synaptic transmission through synaptic ganglia, although short-chain alcohols and urethane showed the opposite pattern. The selectivity of an agent for synaptic rather than conduction blockade correlates strongly with its lipid solubility (Barker 1975) and the particular susceptibility of synapses to the effects of general anaesthetics has been well demonstrated (see below). Findings of this kind have led to the general acceptance of the view that general anaesthetics exert their effects almost entirely on synaptic transmission.

However, supra-clinical concentrations of anaesthetics, of the order of twice MAC, do block conduction in large-diameter fibres, and the possibility exists that lower concentrations might affect conduction in small-diameter pre-terminal fibres in the CNS, with the effect of reducing transmitter release at the synapse. It has been shown that conduction in cortical fibres as narrow as 0.3–0.5 μm is not blocked by high concentrations of barbiturates or halothane (Richard 1980), but, on the other hand, phenobarbitone-induced depression of ACh release in the guinea pig ileum does not occur when the preparation is pretreated with the conduction-blocking agent tetrodotoxin, which implies that the action of the barbiturate on transmitter release is itself partially due to an effect on axonal conduction (Little et al 1980).

It is also notable that, unlike their synaptic effects, the effects of anaesthetics on conduction are partially antagonized by high pressure (Kendig & Cohen 1977). If, as the multi-site expansion hypothesis asserts, anaesthesia and pressure act at different sites, this raises the possibility that the action of pressure on axons may contribute to its ability to reverse anaesthesia in the whole animal.

Synaptic transmission

The arrival of an action potential at an axon terminal causes the release of a quantity of transmitter into the synaptic cleft. This is probably achieved by an electrically induced increase in the permeability of the terminal axonal membrane to calcium ion, causing an influx of calcium which promotes the fusion of transmitter-containing vesicles with the membrane and the release of transmitter. The transmitter then diffuses across the synaptic cleft to interact with a specific receptor protein on the postsynaptic membrane. This interaction changes the configuration of the receptor, causing the opening of ion channel gates in the membrane, so that a transient flow of ions occurs and there is a local change in the postsynaptic membrane potential. The direction of the change depends on the type of ion channel activated. Excitatory changes are mainly brought about by an increase in sodium ion permeability, causing a local

depolarization (excitatory postsynaptic potential, EPSP), while at inhibitory synapses, channels permeable to chloride and potassium are activated and the postsynaptic membrane is locally hyperpolarized (inhibitory postsynaptic potential, IPSP). There is a variety of anatomical types of synapse in the CNS, and increasing numbers of neurotransmitters are being discovered (see Ch. 5). The postsynaptic neuron will discharge, sending an action potential along its own axon, if the algebraic sum of the effects of the hundreds or thousands of synapses impinging on it produce sufficient total depolarization.

There is also a presynaptic mechanism of inhibition, whereby inhibitory fibres impinge on the terminal axon of an excitatory neuron and produce chronic partial depolarization. This has the effect of reducing the amplitude of action potentials passing along the axon, which greatly diminishes the quantity of transmitter released at the excitatory synapse. This very sensitive process may be enhanced or depressed by anaesthetics (Eccles et al 1963).

Anaesthetics and transmitter release

At many synapses in the CNS the transmitter has not been identified and initial work in this field was mainly on peripheral nerve preparations. At sympathetic ganglia, amylobarbitone decreases the quantity of ACh released in response to afferent stimulation (Matthews & Quilliam 1964). In the CNS pentobarbitone decreases release of the excitatory transmitters aspartate and taurine, and enhances release of the inhibitory transmitter GABA (Collins 1980). Weakley (1969) used intracellular recording techniques to show that barbiturates decreased transmitter release in spinal motor neurons. On the other hand a number of gases, including nitrous oxide, increase ACh release in the guinea pig ileum (Little et al 1980), and this effect is not blocked by pretreatment with tetrodotoxin, implying that the action is on the transmitter release process rather than on axonal conduction.

There is no evidence that anaesthesia affects the synthesis, storage or transport of neurotransmitter. It appears likely that most of these presynaptic effects of anaesthetics at excitatory and inhibitory synapses are due to a direct effect on the transmitter release process, although the possibility that conduction blockade makes some contribution cannot entirely be excluded.

Anaesthetics and the postsynaptic neuron

The effects of anaesthetics on postsynaptic mechanisms are usually studied by the iontophoretic technique of applying a putative transmitter to a single neuron from a micropipette and studying the effects of various agents on the response. The results of in vivo studies using this method can be inconsistent, partly because of the unknown effects of the drugs on the many synapses that influence each neuron.

However, in isolated series of guinea pig olfactory cortex, in which unwanted synaptic effects may be minimized by manipulating the ionic composition of the surrounding medium, iontophoretically applied glutamate produces neuronal discharges which are depressed by clinical concentrations of pentobarbitone, alphaxalone, ether, methoxyflurane and trichloroethylene (Richards & Smaje 1976). Thus these agents have a postsynaptic action at this site. Halothane, on the other hand, does not significantly alter glutamate sensitivity in this preparation, although, like the other agents, it blocks synaptic transmission in response to afferent nerve stimulation, which implies that its action here is presynaptic.

In the hippocampus, afferent tract stimulation gives rise to synaptic field potentials which may be analysed into a component due to the effect of EPSPs and a component due to the actual firing of neurons. Richards & White (1975) showed that the relationship between these two components remains unchanged under the influence of three volatile agents, although both components were depressed. Thus, it appears that the electrical response of the neuron as a whole is not altered; therefore the effects of these anaesthetics must be at the postsynaptic membrane.

In contrast to their effects on glutamate-mediated transmission, the muscarinic excitatory effects of iontophoretically applied ACh are enhanced by inhalational agents in olfactory cortical neurons (Smaje 1976). ACh sensitivity was depressed by alphaxalone, while pentobarbitone had no consistent effect.

Anaesthetics and ion channels

It has already been mentioned that barbiturates have been shown to bind allosterically to ACh and GABA receptors and to voltage-sensitive sodium channels. Paralleling these developments, recent refinements in neurophysiological technique have allowed the ionic conductance changes that accompany postsynaptic membrane stimulation to be studied in detail, although at present this is usually feasible only in invertebrates and at neuromuscular endplates.

There is evidence that ion channels which mediate the same ionic conductances may be identical regardless of the receptor they are associated with, and hence of the neurotransmitter (Judge 1983). In the crustacean neuro-

muscular junction, several agents, including pentobarbitone, selectively depress depolarizing responses which depend on increased sodium conductance, while responses involving changes in the conductance of other ions are unaffected (Barker 1975). On the other hand, at inhibitory synapses in cultured mammalian neurons, pentobarbitone acts synergistically with GABA to increase chloride ion conductance (Barker & Ransom 1978). In the molluscan nervous system, approximately similar concentrations of barbiturates depress both chloride-dependent inhibitory responses and sodium-dependent excitatory responses to iontophoretically applied ACh and GABA, while potassium-dependent inhibitory responses to ACh are minimally affected (Cote & Wilson 1980).

Studies of the mechanisms of these effects on ion conductances have shown that, in the mammalian neuromuscular junction, a range of volatile and intravenous agents increase the rate of decay of miniature endplate currents, thus decreasing the average open time of ion channels (Gage & Hamill 1976, Torda & Gage 1977). The potency of agents for this effect is closely correlated with their clinical potency and hence with their lipid solubility.

Summary

The mass of often-conflicting data on the actions of anaesthetics at neuronal, axonal and synaptic level suggests that, as with their action at molecular level, the picture in the whole animal represents the result of a spectrum of complex effects. The overall effect on axonal conduction is one of depression, though its significance for the state of anaesthesia is unclear. The presynaptic and postsynaptic components of both excitatory and inhibitory synaptic transmission may be either enhanced or depressed depending on the agent, the transmitter, and the experimental preparation, while presynaptic inhibition may be enhanced.

This variety of effects is not unexpected when one considers that anaesthetics have been shown to affect all the molecular components of these neurological structures in ways ranging from membrane lipid perturbation to complex and specific interaction with specialized proteins.

ANAESTHETIC ACTION IN THE CENTRAL NERVOUS SYSTEM

Anaesthetic effects, such as those described above, on the basic functional units of the nervous system, are in one sense ultimately responsible for the neuropharmacological and clinical state of general anaesthesia.

However, the human brain contains upwards of 20 billion neurons, many of which may have thousands of synapses, and it is not just the sheer number but also the complex interplay of these myriads of connections that forms the physical substrate of the phenomena of sensation, behaviour and conscious awareness which are temporarily obtunded by anaesthesia. Obviously it is at the integrated level of function that the effects of anaesthetics on the whole CNS and its subsystems must be studied.

Sensory pathways

Sensory information entering the CNS from the periphery travels up the neuraxis by three specific pathways: the comparatively fast dorsal columns and spinocervical tracts and the slower spinothalamic tract. The latter two are particularly involved in transmission of pain sensation, and arise from cells in the dorsal horn laminae of the spinal cord. These three pathways all terminate in the ventrobasal thalamus, from which information is relayed to the somatosensory cortex, and hence spreads to other parts of the cortex. Information is modulated at each level as it ascends, and is influenced by descending pathways.

In addition to these sensory pathways, special sense information is conveyed to the brain in certain of the cranial nerves. For example, auditory information travels from the cochlea in the auditory nerve to the cochlear nuclei in the lower pons, thence to the superior olives and then via the inferior colliculi and thalamic medial geniculate body to the auditory cortex in the superior temporal lobe.

These pathways have only a few synapses along their route, but the neurons comprising them have side connections with the multi-synaptic ascending reticular formation, in which information is also conveyed. The reticular formation influences the general state of arousal of the organism, although full consciousness depends also on the integrated functioning of the cortex, and its complex synaptic arrangement enables it to act as an extremely intricate modulator of the transmission of sensory information.

The study of the effects of anaesthetics on these systems has mainly been based on stimulation, either electrical or direct, and recording, either from within the brain or over the cortical surface, and has tended to look specifically at individual subunits such as the spinal cord, reticular formation and cortex, as well as the intact CNS.

Spinal cord and ascending tracts

The first central relay for afferent information, the spinal cord dorsal horn, has an important role in modulating afferent input. Spontaneous and evoked activity in cat dorsal horn cells is depressed in a dose-dependent way by a number of anaesthetics at clinical concentrations, including ether, halothane and thiopentone (Heavner & de Jong 1974) and ketamine (Kitahata et al 1973). In most studies the cells most affected by anaesthetics were those of lamina V, which are concerned with the integration of noxious stimuli, but this does not appear to be related to the analgesic component of anaesthesia since it was produced to a comparable extent by agents with and without analgesic properties. Nevertheless these studies show that anaesthetics affect the processing of afferent stimuli at cord level, and this must contribute to the total neurological state of anaesthesia.

On the other hand, the bulk of evidence suggests that the dorsal column pathway through the cuneate nucleus is little affected by anaesthetics. The monosynaptic response of rat cuneate neurons to peripheral stimulation was not depressed by a number of different agents (Angel 1977), which may reflect the greater efficiency of transmission built into the arrangement of these synapses.

Ascending reticular formation, thalamus and cortex

The relationship of the reticular activating system to cortical arousal, and early observations that its activity could be directly depressed by anaesthetics, led originally to the view that reticular activating system depression was the key neuropharmacological feature of general anaesthesia.

The effects of sensory stimulation or direct stimulation of the ascending reticular system are reflected, partially via the non-specific thalamic projection system, in the long-latency 'non-specific' component of the cortical evoked response of the EEG. Anaesthetic doses of thiopentone depress the effects of median nerve stimulation upon this component, while leaving the short-latency component intact (Abrahamian et al 1963). Most inhalational agents, however, abolish the long-latency component of the response at sub-anaesthetic concentrations (Hosick et al 1971). Cyclopropane also abolishes the short-latency component at sub-anaesthetic concentrations, while nitrous oxide and ether do so only at higher concentrations (Clark & Rosner 1973).

The ventrobasal group of thalamic nuclei relay somatosensory information to the post-central cortical gyrus. King et al (1957) showed that barbiturates depress transmission through this relay, and this was later confirmed for a variety of anaesthetics using direct recording from rat ventrobasal thalamic cells in response to peripheral stimulation (Angel 1977). While the response of the somatosensory cortex to peripheral stimulation is depressed by urethane, trichloroethylene and pentobarbitone (Angel et al 1973), the response of these cells to microstimulation of thalamocortical afferents is unaffected by urethane. Thus, it would seem that this agent blocks sensory pathways to the cortex at thalamic level, and this was attributed (Angel 1977) to the effect of the drug on control of ventrobasal thalamic transmission by the thalamic reticular nuclei. This action of urethane is antagonized by high pressure (Angel et al 1980).

Angel (1980) has proposed that disruption of the modulation of transmission across the thalamic relay nuclei, via an effect on the balanced inhibitory and excitatory actions of the reticular formation, is a fundamental mechanism of anaesthesia in the intact CNS. This may involve effects on descending fibres originating in the cortex itself.

The auditory evoked response

Recent clinically based work on the effects of anaesthesia on the auditory evoked response (AER) of the EEG gives more consistent results than earlier work on somatosensory evoked response (Jones et al 1985). The human AER contains a series of waves representing transmission of the auditory stimulus through the brainstem and up to the auditory cortex, with waves originating in the brainstem occurring up to about 5 ms following the stimulus and later components after 25 ms representing the effect on the auditory cortex.

Commonly used volatile agents all produce graded, predictable, potency-related changes in both the brainstem and auditory cortical components of the AER. Interestingly, the intravenous agents Althesin, etomidate (Jones et al 1985) and propofol (Savoia et al 1988) have no effect on the brainstem AER while affecting the cortical component similarly to volatile agents. This appears to suggest that there is a fundamental difference in mode of action between the volatile agents and these newer intravenous agents at the level of the intact CNS in man.

SUMMARY

In the past it was often assumed that the large number of synapses in the reticular formation made it more vulnerable to anaesthetic effects than direct pathways containing two or three synapses between the periphery and the cortex. However, it now appears more likely (Angel 1980) that it is the security of synapses, rather than their number, that affects their susceptibility to an-

aesthetics. Since this security is under the control of various components of the reticular formation, it appears likely that this system will eventually be found to have a key role in the mechanism of anaesthesia. However, it also appears that there is wide inter-agent variation in anaesthetic action on the CNS. The findings at spinal cord level, and the marked differences between the effects of volatile and intravenous agents on the brainstem AER, suggest that anaesthetics can affect not only the thalamus but other levels of the CNS, perhaps by disrupting modulatory activity.

CONCLUSION

The study of the mode of action of anaesthetics is still necessarily carried on at the various levels of function more or less in isolation. Nevertheless, research at the different levels has reached the point at which the outline of an integrated picture may be glimpsed. There is ample evidence that anaesthetics act in largely non-polar environments which may include membrane lipids and/or non-polar regions in membrane-embedded proteins which may be so precisely structured as to constitute specific receptor sites. Interactions at these sites cause disruptions of cellular function including, in the CNS, effects on various aspects of synaptic transmission and possibly also axonal conduction. These neuropharmacological effects, in turn, are reflected in the intact CNS by a disruption of function, probably affecting primarily the neuromodulatory systems, and resulting in the observed changes of general anaesthesia.

There has been a movement away from unitary theories of anaesthetic action. As one ascends through the hierarchical levels of CNS function it becomes increasingly clear, firstly, that anaesthetics have many different kinds of action, and secondly that there are wide and significant differences between agents. This is most marked in the differences between the low molecular weight volatile agents and more complex substances such as etomidate, alphaxalone and propofol. Barbiturates appear to have features in common with both groups, but have been shown to have specific binding sites in certain receptors and ion channels.

Knowledge about the mode of action of anaesthetics necessarily depends on advances in molecular biology, neuropharmacology and other disciplines. Clinical anaesthesia has been an empirically based science right from its origins in the 1840s, with the theory of anaesthesia always lagging far behind, but this may not always remain true if further advances, especially in neuropharmacology, eventually permit a more rational approach to drug development.

REFERENCES

Abrahamian H A, Allison T, Goff W R, Rosner B S 1963 Effects of thiopental on human cerebral evoked responses. Anesthesiology 24: 650–657

Angel A 1977 Modulation of information transmission in the dorsal column–lemniscothalamic pathway by anaesthetic agents. In: Hulsz E, Sanchez-Hernandez J A, Vasconcelos G (eds) Anaesthesiology: Proceedings of the VI World Congress of Anaesthesiology. Excerpta Medica, Amsterdam, p p 82–89

Angel A 1980 Effects of anaesthetics on nervous pathways. In: Gray T C, Nunn J F, Utting J E (eds) General Anaesthesia, 4th edn, vol 1, Butterworth, London, pp 117–139

Angel A, Berridge D A, Unwin J 1973 The effect of anaesthetic agents on primary cortical evoked responses. British Journal of Anaesthesia 45: 825–836

Angel A, Gratton D A, Halsey M J, Wardley-Smith B 1980 Pressure reversal of the effect of urethane on the evoked somatosensory cortical response in the rat. British Journal of Pharmacology 70: 241–247

Archer E R, Richards C D, White A E 1977 Non-additive anaesthetic effects of alphaxolone and methohexitone. British Journal of Pharmacology 59: 508P

Barker J L 1975 CNS depressants: effect on post-synaptic pharmacology. Brain Research 92: 35–55

Barker J L, Ransom B R 1978 Pentobarbitone pharmacology of mammalian central neurones grown in tissue culture. Journal of Physiology 280: 355–372

Brown F F, Halsey M J 1980 Interactions of anesthetics with proteins. In: Fink B R (ed.) Molecular mechanisms of anesthesia. Progress in Anesthesiology, vol 2. Raven Press, New York, pp 385–388

Clark D L, Rosner B S 1973 Neurophysiologic effects of general anaesthetics. I: The electroencephalogram and sensory evoked responses in man. Anesthesiology 38: 564–582

Collins G G S 1980 Release of endogenous amino acid neurotransmitter candidates from rat olfactory cortex: possible regulatory mechanisms and the effects of pentobarbitone. Brain Research 190: 517–528

Cote I L, Wilson W A 1980 Effects of barbiturates on inhibitory and excitatory responses to applied neurotransmitters in Aplysia. Journal of Pharmacology and Experimental Therapeutics 214: 161–165

Dundee J W 1988 Barbiturates: chemistry and drugs. In: Dundee J W, Wyant G M (eds) Intravenous anaesthesia, 2nd edn. Churchill Livingstone, London, pp 60–68

Eccles J C, Schmidt R F, Willis W D 1963 Pharmacological studies on presynaptic inhibition. Journal of Physiology (London) 168: 500–530

Eger E I, Lundgren C, Miller S L, Stevens W C 1969 Anesthetic potencies of sulfur hexafluoride, carbon tetrafluoride, chloroform and Ethrane in dogs. Anesthesiology 30: 129–135

Franks N P, Lieb W R 1978 Where do general anaesthetics act? Nature (London) 274: 339–374

Franks N P, Lieb W R 1984 Do general anaesthetics act by competitive binding to specific receptors? Nature 310: 599–601

Gage P W, Hamill O P 1976 Effects of several inhalation anaesthetics on the kinetics of postsynaptic conductance changes in mouse diaphragm. British Journal of Pharmacology 57: 263–272

Gage P W, Hamill O P 1981 Effects of anesthetics on ion channels in synapses. In: Porter R (ed) Neurophysiology IV: International Review of Physiology, vol 25. University Park Press, Baltimore, pp 1–45

Halsey M J 1980 Renaissance of nonunitary molecular mechanisms of general anesthesia. In: Fink B R (ed) Molecular mechanisms of anesthesia. Progress in Anesthesiology, vol 2. Raven Press, New York, pp 273–283

Halsey M J, Wardley-Smith B 1975 Pressure reversal of narcosis produced by anaesthetics, narcotics and tranquillisers. Nature (London) 257: 811–813

Halsey M J, Wardley-Smith B, Green C J 1978 Pressure reversal of anaesthesia — a multi-site expansion hypothesis. British Journal of Anaesthesia 50: 1091–1097

Heavner J E, De Jong R H 1974 Modulation of dorsal horn throughout by anesthetics. Advances in Neurology 4: 179–185

Hosick E C, Clark D L, Adam N, Rosner B S 1971 Neurophysiological effects of different anesthetics in conscious man. Journal of Applied Physiology 31: 892–898

Johnson F H, Brown D E S, Marsland D A 1942 Pressure reversal of the action of certain narcotics. Journal of Cellular and Comparative Physiology 20: 269–276

Jones J G, Heneghan C P H, Thornton C 1985 Functional assessment of the normal brain during general anaesthesia. In: Kaufman L (ed) Anaesthesia review 3. Churchill Livingstone, London, pp 83–98

Judge S E 1983 Effects of general anaesthetics on synaptic ion channels. British Journal of Anaesthesia 55: 191–200

Kendig J J, Cohen E N 1977 Pressure antagonism to conduction block by anesthetic agents. Anesthesiology 47: 6–10

Kendig J J, Trudell J R, Cohen E N 1975 Effects of pressure and anesthetics on conduction and synaptic transmission. Journal of Pharmacology and Experimental Therapeutics 195: 216–224

King E E, Naquet R, Magoun H W 1957 Alterations in somatic afferent transmission through thalamus by central mechanisms and barbiturates. Journal of Pharmacology and Experimental Therapeutics 119: 48–63

Kita Y, Miller K W 1982 The partial molar volumes of some n-alkanols in erythrocyte ghosts and lipid bilayers. Biochemistry 21: 2840–2847

Kitahata L M, Taub A, Kosaka Y 1973 Lamina-specific suppression of dorsal horn unit activity by ketamine hydrochloride. Anesthesiology 38: 4–11

Larrabee M G, Posternak J M 1952 Selective actions of general anaesthetics on synapses and axons in mammalian sympathetic ganglia. Journal of Neurophysiology 15: 91–114

Little H J, Paton W D M, Smith E B 1980 Effects of anesthetics and of helium pressure on acetylcholine release. In: Fink B R (ed) Molecular mechanisms of anesthesia. Progress in Anesthesiology, vol 2. Raven Press, New York, pp 457–461

Matthews E K, Quilliam J P 1964 Effects of central depressant drugs upon acetyl choline release. British Journal of Pharmacology 22: 415–440

Meyer H H 1901 Zur Theorie der Alkoholnarkose. Naunyn-Schmiedeberg's Archiv fur experimentelle

Pathologie und Pharmakologie 46: 338–345

Miller K W 1987 General anaesthetics. In: Feldman S A, Scurr C F, Paton W D M (eds) Drugs in anaesthesia: mechanisms of action. Edward Arnold, London, pp 133–159

Miller K W, Wilson M W 1978 The pressure reversal of a variety of anesthetic agents in mice. Anesthesiology 48: 104–110

Miller K W, Paton W D M, Smith R A 1972 Physico-chemical approaches to the mode of action of general anesthetics. Anesthesiology 36: 339–351

Miller K W, Braswell L M, Firestone L L, Dodson B A, Forman S A 1986 General anaesthetics act both specifically and non-specifically on acetylcholine receptors. In: Roth S H, Miller K W (eds) Molecular and cellular mechanisms of anaesthetics. Plenum Medical, New York, pp 125–137

Mullins L J 1954 Some physical mechanisms in narcosis. Chemical Reviews 54: 280–323

Noda M, Takahashi H, Tanabe T 1983 Structural homology of Torpedo Californica acetylcholine receptor subunits. Nature 302: 528–532

Overton E 1901 Studien uber die Narkose. Fisher, Jena

Phillips G H 1974 Structure-activity relationships in steroidal anaesthetics. In: Halsey M J, Millar R A, Sutton J A (eds) Molecular mechanisms in general anaesthesia. Churchill Livingstone, London, pp 32–46

Richards C D 1980 The mechanisms of general anaesthesia. In: Norman J Whitman J G (eds) Topical reviews in anaesthesia, vol 1. John Wright and Sons, Bristol, pp 1–84

Richards C D, Smaje J C 1976 Anaesthetics depress the sensitivity of cortical neurones to L-glutamate. British Journal of Pharmacology 58: 347–357

Richards C D, White A E 1975 The actions of volatile anaesthetics on synaptic transmission in the dentate gyrus. Journal of Physiology (London) 252: 241–257

Saidman L J, Eger E I, Munson E S, Babad A A, Muallem M 1967 Minimal alveolar concentrations of methoxyflurane, halothane ether and cyclopropane in man. Correlation with theories of anaesthesia. Anesthesiology 28: 994–1002

Savoia G, Eposito C, Belfiore F, Amantea B, Cuocolo R 1988 Propofol infusion and auditory evoked potentials. Anaesthesia 43: supplement, 46–49

Singer C J, Nicholson G L 1972 The fluid mosaic model of cell membranes. Science 175: 720

Smaje J C 1976 General anaesthetics and the acetylcholine sensitivity of cortical neurones. British Journal of Pharmacology 58: 359–366

Torda T A, Gage P W 1977 Postsynaptic effect of i.v. anesthetic agents at the neuromuscular junction. British Journal of Anaesthesia 49: 771–776

Trudell J R 1977 A unitary theory of anesthesia based on lateral phase separations in nerve membranes. Anesthesiology 46: 5–10

Trudell J R, Hubbell W L, Cohen E N 1973 Pressure reversal of inhalation anesthetic induced disorder in spin labelled phospholipid vesicles. Biochimica et Biophysica Acta 291: 328–334

Trudell J R, Payan D G, Chin J H, Cohen E N 1975 The antagonistic effect of an inhalational anesthetic and high pressure on the phase diagram of mixed dipalmitoyl-dioxyristoylphosphatidicholine bilayers. Proceedings of the National Academy of Sciences, USA 72: 210

Wardley-Smith B, Halsey M J 1981 Behaviour of mixtures of anaesthetics at pressure: support for the multi-site expansion hypothesis of anaesthetic action. British Journal of Anaesthesia 53: 187P

Weakley J N 1969 Effect of barbiturates on 'quantal' synaptic transmission in spinal motoneurones. Journal of Physiology (London) 204: 63–67

7. Volatile inhalational agents

J. P. H. Fee

INTRODUCTION

The idea of administering anaesthetic agents by the pulmonary route grew out of an ancient tradition of the inhalation of fumes and vapours either as cures or as a means of intoxication. In the case of opium, for example, inhalation provided a rapid, intense effect unmatched by the oral route and unrivalled until the invention of the hypodermic needle and syringe. The rapid development of science in the early and middle years of the nineteenth century saw both the synthesis of new chemicals and the rediscovery of forgotten ones. A few of these were intoxicants, notably nitrous oxide and ether, and these were initially abused as such, their potential as a means of alleviating pain being overlooked or at least underestimated.

Ether and chloroform were the first of two series of lipid-soluble, volatile ethers and hydrocarbons which are still being evaluated nearly 150 years after their first use as anaesthetic agents.

PHARMACOKINETICS

Absorption, distribution and elimination

The vast majority of drugs are administered orally or by injection, and general pharmacokinetic texts tend to ignore drug uptake by the pulmonary route. In common with the intravenous and sublingual routes, drugs administered through the lungs are not subject to first-pass hepatic metabolism. Quite uniquely, this route of administration presents the agent to the heart in the first instance so that it, initially, is subject to higher tensions of volatile agent than other tissues.

Modern anaesthetic practice dictates that all potent volatile agents such as halothane and isoflurane be administered through a temperature-compensated calibrated vaporizer. In this way volatile agents in oxygen-containing mixtures can be delivered at a predetermined inspiratory concentration. The safe administration of volatile anaesthetic agents requires a good understanding of their pharmacokinetics. These potent drugs exert their anaesthetic effect in a way which is not fully understood, but the depth of anaesthesia is directly proportional to the tension (or partial pressure) of the agent in the brain or in arterial blood. The speed of induction and recovery are similarly related to the rate at which arterial or brain tensions rise and fall.

The tension or partial pressure of volatile anaesthetic agents is, like other blood gas measurements such as oxygen tension, measured in units of pressure, i.e. fractions of an atmosphere, or more commonly kPa or mmHg. The *concentration* of agent — measured variously in units of volume or weight per unit volume — e.g. ml l^{-1}, mg l^{-1}, mmol l^{-1} — or in the gaseous phase as percentage volume — will be different in different compartments and tissues when these are in equilibrium at the same *tension*. The relationship depends on the differing solubility of the gas or vapour in different tissues with differing composition of lipid and aqueous compartments, and is expressed usually in terms of the partition coefficient between different phases — e.g. blood/gas, tissue/gas; and partition coefficients for individual tissues can also be measured. These are discussed in more detail below.

As with drugs given by other routes, the process of uptake and absorption of an inhalational agent is occurring simultaneously with its transport and distribution to the tissues, and later recovery is associated with redistribution, metabolism and excretion. The process must be seen as a cascade where movement from each compartment to another is dependent on the tension gradient between them, and where this gradient depends not only on the rate of delivery to the compartment but also on the rate at which the agent is transferred from it.

The tension of anaesthetic vapour in the brain and in arterial blood is dependent on:

1. alveolar ventilation;
2. concentration (or tension) of the agent in the inspired gas mixture;
3. transfer of vapour from alveoli to blood in the lungs;
4. transfer of vapour from arterial blood to body tissues.

Alveolar ventilation

Each breath transfers some anaesthetic vapour to the lungs. If alveolar ventilation is high the alveolar and arterial tensions rise relatively quickly. On the other hand, an increase in physiological dead space due to pulmonary embolism, emphysema or other ventilation–perfusion inequalities will result in an increased shunt and reduce the amount of volatile agent absorbed. Respiratory depression due to drugs may similarly reduce alveolar ventilation and delay the rise in alveolar and arterial vapour tensions.

Inspired tension

The tension of a vapour in the anaesthetic mixture is directly proportional to its concentration. In clinical practice the inspired tension changes but high inspired percentage concentrations are used during induction to ensure that alveolar and then arterial tensions increase quickly. As anaesthesia deepens the inspired percentage concentration can be reduced to a maintenance value.

During the inhalation of a constant percentage concentration of anaesthetic vapour, the tension in arterial blood is related to that of the inspired mixture as shown in Figure 7.1. In the case of nitrous oxide the arterial tension reaches 90% of the inspired tension in about 20 min compared with about 60% for isoflurane and 45% for halothane. The differences are determined by the solubility of the agents in blood.

Alveolar–blood transfer

As with the majority of drugs movement of an inhalational anaesthetic agent across body membranes is along a concentration gradient.

The transfer of a volatile agent from the alveoli to blood is dependent on four factors:

1. the condition of the respiratory membrane;
2. the solubility of the agent;
3. cardiac output;
4. the tension of vapour in the alveoli and in blood.

1. Respiratory membrane. The respiratory membrane is completely permeable to the passage of anaesthetic vapours and gases. The amount transferred across it will depend on the cross-sectional area and thickness of the membrane. Certain pulmonary diseases may impair the transfer of vapour; emphysema will reduce the cross-sectional area of respiratory membrane available. Thus induction of, and recovery from, anaesthesia will be delayed. Other causes of ventilation–perfusion inequality will similarly alter the rate at which vapour passes into the circulation. An increase in the thickness of the respiratory membrane such as might occur in pulmonary fibrosis will also tend to delay the transfer of vapour.

2. Solubility. The true solubility of a particular agent in blood is expressed as its partition coefficient, representing the ratio of anaesthetic concentration in blood to anaesthetic concentration in a gas phase when the two are in equilibrium (Table 7.1). When an agent has a low blood-gas partition coefficient, then the concentration in the blood needed to achieve any given tension will be low, and so the mass of drug which needs to be transferred into the blood is also low. This also means that the agent is removed from the alveoli at a lower rate and so the alveolar–blood gradient in partial pressure is maintained. Thus, blood and alveolar concentrations approach equilibrium rapidly and induction is rapid (Fig. 7.1). In practice other factors may com-

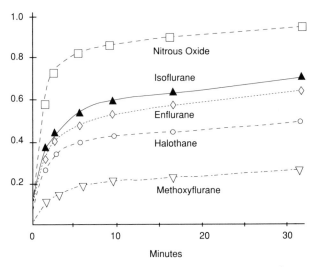

Fig. 7.1 Ratio of inspired to alveolar concentrations (F_A/F_I) of some inhalational agents (Cromwell et al 1971 Munson et al 1978). With permission of Anaquest (Eger 1982).

promise this advantage. For instance, the pungency of isoflurane, an agent which is fairly insoluble, may provoke coughing or breath-holding, particularly when administered in high concentrations. The rapidity of induction may, in the end, be no greater or may even be less, than that achievable with halothane, despite the latter's higher blood–gas partition coefficient (Sampaio et al 1989). The solubility of anaesthetic vapours is much greater in fat than in blood or vessel-rich tissues such as the brain (Table 7.1). Thus the anaesthetic tension of an agent in fat approaches equilibrium with that of the alveoli only after many hours. In most clinical situations the tension of volatile agents in fat does not reach equilibrium with alveolar tensions.

3. Cardiac output. A fall in cardiac output such as may occur in shocked states will cause a more rapid rise in the pulmonary arterial concentration of a volatile agent and permit inspired and arterial tensions to equalize sooner. Thus the speed of induction will be increased. Since many volatile agents cause a drop in cardiac output these drugs may themselves facilitate their own uptake. Similarly, most intravenous induction agents reduce cardiac output, further aiding gaseous uptake and induction.

The tissues with the highest blood flow — brain, kidney, heart (vessel-rich group) — will have a rapid increase in their anaesthetic tension compared with low-flow tissues such as fat and bone. Thus the brain anaesthetic tension approaches the inspired tension quickly, resulting in rapid induction of anaesthesia.

4. Tension in blood. Anaesthetic vapours are taken up by the blood in the lungs and are delivered to all body tissues. Tissue uptake reduces blood anaesthetic tension, and only when the tissues become saturated does the tension of mixed venous blood approach that of the inhaled anaesthetic vapour. Thus the mass of volatile agent taken into the circulation decreases with time (Fig. 7.2).

Blood–tissue transfer

The uptake of volatile anaesthetic agents into tissues is dependent on the blood/tissue partition coefficient (Table 7.1), tissue blood flow per unit volume, and the inspired concentration. The most important factor is tissue blood flow, and those tissues with high unit flows will take up volatile agents relatively quickly. Mapleson (1963) has devised a system whereby tissues are grouped according to their flow per unit volume and solubility coefficients. This simplifies the problem of how to assess the combined effect of all body tissues on the tension of volatile agent in mixed venous blood. The brain, heart and kidney comprise the vessel-rich group (VRG) with high perfusion per unit volume, and the tensions in

Table 7.1 Partition coefficients and MAC values for inhalational anaesthetic agents

	Partition coefficients (37°C)			MAC[a] (% atm)	
	Blood/gas	Brain/blood	Oil gas	100% O_2	70% N_2O
Halothane	2.3	6.7	224	0.75	0.29
Isoflurane	1.4	2.6	98	1.15	0.50
Enflurane	1.8	1.4	98	1.68	0.57
Diethyl ether	12	1.0	65	1.92	–
Nitrous oxide	0.47	1.1	1.4	–	–
Trichloroethylene	9.15	1.7	714	–	–
Chloroform	8.4	1.4	394	–	–
Methoxyflurane	12	1.7	970	0.2	–
Sevoflurane	0.69	–	47[c]	1.7[d]	0.6 (64%)[d]
Desflurane (I-653)[b]	0.42	–	18.7	6.0[e]	–

[a] MAC values for middle-aged humans.
[b] Eger (1987)
[c] Strum & Eger (1987)
[d] Katoh & Ikeda (1987)
[e] Rampil et al (1989)

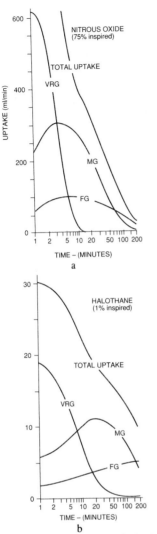

Fig. 7.2 Total uptake is the sum of uptake by individual body tissues. The uppermost curve for each anaesthetic is the sum of the three curves beneath it (with a slight time lag). The curves for nitrous oxide and halothane are identical in shape to those for all anaesthetics. Uptake progressively decreases with duration of anaesthesia and with saturation of the tissue depots. The order of saturation is always vessel-rich group (VRG) first then muscle group (MG), and fat group (FG) last. As noted in the illustration, the inspired concentration is constant at 75% nitrous oxide or 1% halothane. (Eger, 1974.)

these tissues rapidly achieve equilibrium with that of arterial blood.

In contrast, adipose tissue requires a longer time to equilibrate on account of the high fat/blood partition coefficients of the volatile agents and relatively poor blood flow. Muscle and skin also differ from the VRG in hav-

ing a much lower rate of perfusion per unit volume; consequently equilibration is prolonged. This group occupies an intermediate position in terms of anaesthetic uptake. In general the tissues of the VRG may approach equilibrium with arterial blood during the course of routine clinical anaesthesia, in contrast to both the muscle and fat groups (Fig. 7.2).

Similarly, the rate of elimination is based on tissue perfusion and solubility. The anaesthetic tension in tissues of the VRG falls much more quickly than that of the muscle group. The fat group is the slowest to release volatile agent on account of its high solubility.

MAC

MAC is the minimum alveolar concentration of anaesthetic (at one atmosphere ambient pressure) that produces immobility in 50% of those patients or animals exposed to a noxious stimulus (Eger 1974). It is a measure of anaesthetic potency and serves as a means of comparing the potencies of different gaseous and volatile agents. Since it is measured after steady-state conditions have been achieved, MAC is not the sole determinant of the concentration of inspired anaesthetic required for surgical anaesthesia. This latter value is also related to the duration of anaesthesia, the uptake and distribution characteristics of the anaesthetic concerned and the degree of surgical stimulation. In general, to achieve a steady alveolar concentration, high inspired concentrations are required at the commencement of the anaesthetic with a gradual reduction as tissue tensions come into equilibrium with those of blood.

MAC is determined by maintaining a constant endtidal (or alveolar) concentration for at least 15 minutes to ensure equilibration between the alveoli, arterial blood and the central nervous system. It is reasonably assumed that at that point the anaesthetic tensions in the alveoli and at the site of action in the brain and spinal cord are the same, although the concentration in these and in other tissues may differ.

To make the determination in man, the alveolar concentration is adjusted to one of several predetermined values both above and below the one estimated to allow a response to skin incision. Several patients are anaesthetized at each concentration, and the percentage moving are recorded. Using a line of best fit, the concentration (MAC) which prevents movement in 50% of the patients is estimated.

MAC is relatively constant within species and, even more surprisingly, between species there is little variability; MAC for halothane in man, cat and goldfish is 0.75, 0.82 and 0.76 respectively. MAC appears to be unaffected by duration of anaesthesia, gender, acid–base status and induced hypertension. Induced hypotension, hypothermia, hypoxia and anaemia will reduce halothane MAC, although in the case of the latter two this only occurs in the presence of a gross fall in oxygen delivery. MAC values for a particular anaesthetic agent are highest in neonates and lowest in the elderly, although the explanation for this is uncertain. It is perhaps not surprising that opiates, benzodiazepines and other gaseous or volatile anaesthetics all lower MAC (Quasha et al 1980, Melvin et al 1982, Murphy & Hug 1982) but of increasing interest is the role of the α_2-adrenergic receptor in anaesthesia. In animal studies a number of α_2-adrenergic agonists have been shown to reduce MAC (Maze et al 1987, 1988, Segal et al 1988).

The clinical usefulness of MAC might seem doubtful in view of the fact that, by definition, 50% of patients move in response to skin incision. Various other measures have been developed from the concept of MAC, notably the median anaesthetic dose required to prevent

movement in 50% of patients, AD_{50}, and in 95% of patients, AD_{95} (De Jong & Eger 1975). The dose–response curve for halothane is shown in Figure 7.3 (De Jong and Eger 1975). The AD_{50} corresponds to MAC and is on the steepest part of the curve, thereby allowing accurate measurement of the dosage value. The fact that at this dosage half the patients move, makes it a value of limited usefulness to the practising anaesthetist. The AD_{95}, on the other hand, is on a flatter part of the curve and the precision with which this dose can be expressed is somewhat limited. Unfortunately, an AD_{100} representing the minimum concentration applicable to all patients cannot be determined from the dose–response curve, on account of the asymptotic behaviour of the curve at both ends. In general the AD_{95} values are 5–40% greater than MAC.

Another limitation of the concept of MAC, AD_{50}, AD_{95} is that these terms are applicable only to the non-paralysed patient. One of the advantages of blocking neuromuscular function is to enable much lower in-

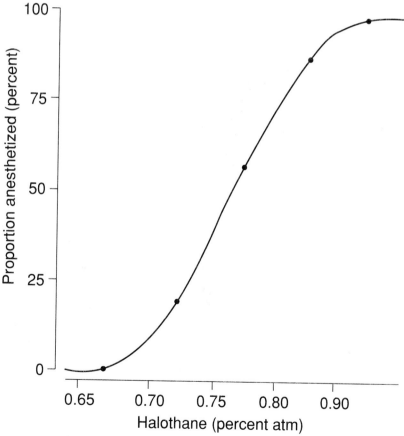

Fig. 7.3 Dose–response curve for halothane.

spired concentrations of volatile agents to be used. In order to prevent awareness with this technique the alveolar concentration must be maintained somewhere between MAC and a value at which the patient would be awake — 'MAC awake'. This was defined by Stoelting et al (1970) as an anaesthetic concentration midway between the value when patients could open their eyes on command and the value just preventing this response in 50% of patients during recovery. 'MAC awake' values are about 0.4% for halothane and 0.08% for methoxyflurane, and are in general about 50% of the MAC values.

In the paralysed patient, therefore, a lower concentration than MAC may safely be used to prevent awareness, particularly when anaesthesia is supplemented with nitrous oxide, opioids, or other CNS depressants.

THE ETHERS

Diethyl ether

History

The discovery of what is now called ether goes back to the thirteenth-century alchemist, Raymond Lilly, who discovered in his laboratory a 'white fluid' which he called 'sweet vitriol'. It was to be 300 years before its analgesic properties were recognized by Paracelsus and documented by his assistant Valerius Cordus in 1542 in Nuremburg. For another two centuries 'sweet vitriol' lay forgotten, until in 1792 a German apothecary, Frobenius, unearthed it and named it 'ether'. It became popular as a treatment for asthma and other respiratory disorders, but it was not until 1842 that Crawford W. Long used it as an anaesthetic for the removal of a small tumour from the neck of a friend. Unfortunately he did not publish his experiences, and it was William Morton who first demonstrated in public the use of ether for a surgical operation in 1846 at the Massachusetts General Hospital, Boston.

Subsequently, diethyl ether became the most widely used anaesthetic agent. With some types of apparatus it was possible to give high concentrations of oxygen and this, together with the complete ablation of pain, revolutionalized surgical techniques. Only with the introduction of halothane in 1956 did its popularity in the West decline, although general anaesthesia for a large proportion of the world's population still means ether anaesthesia.

Chemical and physical properties

Diethyl ether ($C_2H_5OC_2H_5$) is a colourless, highly vol-

atile liquid with a boiling point of 35°C. It is a potent agent with a MAC of 1.92% but the speed of induction is slow on account of its high blood gas partition coefficient (Table 7.1) and its irritant effect on the airway.

Ether is a versatile agent in that it can be administered in any of three ways: the open method using a Schimmelbusch mask, semi-closed, or closed with carbon dioxide absorption. A detailed description of administration techniques is given by Lee (1953), and Conway (1965) has written a very comprehensive review.

The principal disadvantage of ether is its flammability in air, oxygen, or nitrous oxide at all clinically used concentrations. Being about two and a half times as heavy as air, ether is carried downwards in the operating theatre. The open method of administration is less likely to result in serious accidents than the closed method, in which the use of ether in oxygen or nitrous oxide promotes the rapid propagation of flames and violent detonation. Consequently, cautery should not be used for operations on the head and neck. During prolonged operations enclosed body cavities such as the urinary bladder may contain ether vapour; the use of cautery or hot-wire devices in these circumstances may have disastrous consequences. With appropriate precautions, however, the actual incidence of serious fires or explosions can be kept extremely low (Dodd 1962, Price & Dripps 1970).

Cardiovascular system

Ether has a direct depressant action on the heart, but increased sympathetic nervous activity during light anaesthesia ensures that changes in myocardial contractility are minimal (Shimosato 1964). There is also a dose-related increase in heart rate, again mainly due to heightened sympathetic nervous activity, although the mechanism is obscure. Both systemic arterial pressure and total peripheral resistance decline with increasing anaesthetic depth and may remain depressed for some time after discontinuation of ether.

Ether does not sensitize the heart to the effects of catecholamines and standard haemostatic doses of adrenaline can be infiltrated subcutaneously without precipitating ventricular arrhythmias.

Respiratory system

Ether is irritant to the airway and stimulates salivary and bronchial secretions. This may provoke coughing and spasm in unpremedicated patients. Both the tidal volume and respiratory rate are increased when ether is inhaled and alveolar carbon dioxide tension may remain in the normal range or slightly less during planes 1 and 2 of stage III. In the absence of opiates, spontaneous breathing may be satisfactory even at deeper levels of anaesthesia. Larson and his colleagues (1969) have shown that ether reduces the respiratory response to elevated Pa_{CO_2} and so it may stimulate breathing through sensory receptors outside the main respiratory centre. It is a powerful bronchodilator and has been used with success in the management of status asthmaticus where more conventional treatments have failed (Robertson et al 1985).

Neuromuscular blockade

At moderate and high concentrations ether has a specific neuromuscular blocking action. It will potentiate the effects of d-tubocurarine and may itself be potentiated by antibiotics such as neomycin and streptomycin. The neuromuscular blockade induced by ether is not effectively antagonized by neostigmine or edrophonium (Karis et al 1966, Katz 1966). This block, like those caused by other inhalational agents, appears to take place at a site distal to the acetylcholine receptor, perhaps by impeding the passage of ions through membrane channels (Waud & Waud 1975).

Liver and gastrointestinal tract

Ether has no serious toxic effects on the normal liver (Fairlie et al 1951) although short-term changes in bromsulphthalein clearance have been shown (Stevens et al 1973), and long-term exposure in animals is associated with increased liver size (Stevens et al 1975a). Neither of these would appear to be of clinical importance. Nausea and vomiting are common during recovery from ether anaesthesia (possibly as a result of swallowing ether-laden mucus at induction). Vomiting may also occur during the induction phase.

Absorption and excretion

Ether is absorbed rapidly across the respiratory membrane. Less than 10% of a given dose is metabolized to CO_2 and a number of non-volatile substances; the rest is exhaled unchanged.

Methoxyflurane

When halothane was introduced in 1956 it was expected to behave as a non-reactive agent which would be excreted unchanged through the lungs. In fact the halothane molecule was specifically designed to be chemically inert (Suckling 1957). Unfortunately reports of liver dysfunction raised doubts about its supposed reactivity and it has been shown subsequently to undergo extensive biotransformation. As a result of this and other shortcomings, attempts were made to find an alternative.

Methoxyflurane, a halogenated ether, was introduced in 1961, but has never proved a serious threat to the dominance of halothane. Its high lipid solubility makes induction and recovery slow. However, the drug has certain advantages. It is a good analgesic, a good muscle relaxant, it does not sensitize the myocardium to adrenaline and it does not cause uterine relaxation. Unfortunately, methoxyflurane can cause polyuric renal failure if given in high concentrations over a lengthy period of time. In the context of hepatotoxicity, methoxyflurane appears to be capable of cross-sensitization with halothane and so is not a suitable alternative for repeat administration (Inman & Mushin 1978).

Chemical and physical properties

Methoxyflurane (Penthrane) is 2,2-dichloro-1,1-difluoro ethyl methyl ether. Its formula is compared with enflurane and isoflurane in Figure 7.4. It is a clear colourless liquid with a characteristic pungent, mildly unpleasant smell. It is only flammable in high concentrations: 7.0% in air, 5.4% in oxygen, 4.6% in nitrous oxide — concentrations which are very unlikely to occur during clinical anaesthesia.

Methoxyflurane is very soluble in rubber and up to 35% of the vapour can be absorbed by the anaesthetic tubing. Conversely, when the vaporizer concentration is returned to zero near the end of surgery, the tubing re-

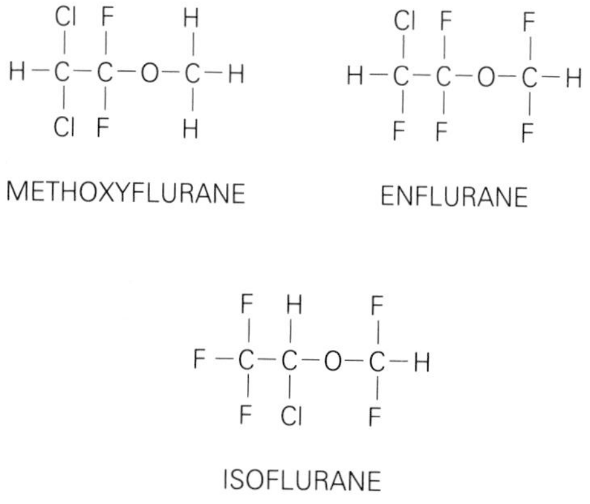

Fig. 7.4 Chemical structure of methoxyflurane compared with enflurane and isoflurane.

Table 7.2 Physical properties of volatile anaesthetic agents

	Ether	Chloroform	Trichloro-ethylene	Halothane	Isoflurane	Enflurane	Methoxy-flurane	Sevoflurane[a]
Molecular weight	74.1	119.4	131.4	197.4	184.5	184.5	165	200
Density at 20°C g/ml	0.72	1.50 (15°C)	1.46	1.86	1.50	1.52	1.43	1.51
Boiling point °C at 1 atm	34.6	61.3	86.7	50.2	48.5	56.5	104.7	58.5
Latent heat of vaporization KJ/mol	27.6	–	31.3	28.9	–	32.3	33.9	–
Vapour pressure at 20°C kPa (mmHg)	59.1 (442)	21.3 (160)	7.7 (58)	32.1 (241)	31.8 (240)	23.3 (175)	3.0 (22.5)	21 (160)
Flammability in air (vol %)	1.9–48	N	N	N	N	N	7.0–	N
O₂	2.0–82	N	N	N	N	N	5.4–	11
N₂O	1.5–24	N	N	4.75	N	5.75	4.6–	10

Modified from Halsey, 1989
N = Non-flammable.
[a] Wallin et al (1975).

leases methoxyflurane vapour into the stream of gases. This effect, together with its high solubility, makes recovery from methoxyflurane anaesthesia slow.

Methoxyflurane is stable in the presence of soda-lime and so can be used safely in closed-circuit anaesthesia. The physical properties are listed in Table 7.2 with those of the other anaesthetic ethers.

Cardiovascular system

Methoxyflurane reduces cardiac output, stroke volume and systemic vascular resistance. Normal sinus rhythm is characteristic of anaesthesia with the drug, and the evidence suggests that there is little myocardial sensitization. Even in the presence of gross hypercarbia, ventricular arrhythmias do not appear (Black 1967). On this basis subcutaneous adrenaline can be used for haemostasis, providing care is taken to minimize other adrenergic influences. Methoxyflurane has been used successfully to maintain normal cardiac rhythm in the presence of high plasma concentrations of catecholamines, e.g. during the surgical removal of

phaeochrome tumours. However, a serious interaction occurs with beta-blockers in the presence of which methoxyflurane, unlike halothane (but in common with ether, trichloroethylene and enflurane), noticeably depresses cardiac output and myocardial contractility (Saner et al 1975).

Respiratory system

Methoxyflurane has a more pronounced depressant effect on respiration than does halothane. As the dose increases the tidal volume becomes progressively reduced and hypercarbia ensues; for this reason it is often best used during controlled ventilation. It does not stimulate salivary or bronchial secretions and, although somewhat pungent, is non-irritant to inhale.

Comparative studies have been made of the effects of diethyl ether, cyclopropane, halothane and methoxyflurane on ventilation (Larson et al 1969). These show that the ventilatory response to carbon dioxide progressively decreases with increasing depth of anaesthesia and that, at equipotent concentrations, halothane and methoxyflurane are the more potent respiratory depressants.

Renal effects

There is ample evidence that serum and urine inorganic fluoride concentrations increase significantly after methoxyflurane anaesthesia (Dobkin & Levy 1973). This is associated with nephrotoxicity when large doses of methoxyflurane have been administered. The ensuing polyuric renal failure is vasopressin-resistant. The critical serum fluoride concentration above which nephrotoxicity is likely to occur is 50 μmol l^{-1}, but this level is unlikely to be reached when exposure is less than 2 MAC hours (Cousins & Mazze 1973). Toxicity is increased by other potentially nephrotoxic drugs such as the aminoglycoside antibiotics and tetracycline. Treatment with drugs such as phenobarbitone which induce the drug metabolizing enzymes may, by enhancing the metabolism of methoxyflurane, result in elevated serum inorganic fluoride concentrations and increase the risk of renal damage (Berman et al 1973). Some 45% of the drug is metabolized in man (Holaday et al 1970), other metabolites being carbon dioxide, oxalic acid, methoxy-difluoroacetic acid and inorganic chloride. In view of the toxic potential of methoxyflurane it is inadvisable to use the drug if renal function is already impaired. Renal blood flow, glomerular filtration rate and urine flow are all reduced during methoxyflurane anaesthesia.

Liver function

There is no firm evidence that methoxyflurane causes adverse effects on the liver. Inman & Mushin (1978) conclude that 'cross-sensitization' may occur with halothane, and since there now exist better alternatives to halothane than methoxyflurane this agent should not be used as a means of avoiding the repeat administration of halothane. Liver blood flow is reduced by 50% during methoxyflurane anaesthesia (Libonati et al 1973) and this reduction is greater than that due to halothane (Price & Pauca 1969).

Obstetrics

Methoxyflurane has been used successfully for obstetric analgesia and as an adjunct to the nitrous oxide–oxygen–muscle relaxant technique in obstetric anaesthesia. Major et al (1966), in comparing it with trichloroethylene, found it to be as effective as an analgesic, and that overall it produced better conditions. Bodley and his colleagues (1966) also used it for analgesia in labour. Pain relief was rapid, safe and without untoward side-effects. They also suggested that there was no increase in blood loss. Increasing anxiety about the drug's nephrotoxicity, together with its slow onset of action and delayed excretion in mother and infant, have led to a decline in its popularity in this field.

Enflurane

Largely as a result of the possible risks of liver damage with halothane and nephrotoxicity with methoxyflurane the search for the 'ideal' volatile anaesthetic agent continued during the 1960s. Enflurane ('Ethrane') was introduced into clinical practice in the UK in 1978 after initial clinical evaluation (Dobkin et al 1968, Black et al 1977). Enflurane is now commercially available in many countries, and is generally regarded as a satisfactory inhalational agent for a wide range of surgical procedures. The enflurane molecule differs from its predecessors in being less reactive, and is thus not extensively metabolized. For this reason it, and its structural isomer, isoflurane, are increasingly the preferred volatile agents for both single and repeat administration.

Chemical and physical properties

Enflurane is 2-chloro-1,1,2-trifluoroethyl-difluoromethyl ether. Its chemical structure and some physical properties are given in Figure 7.4 and Table 7.2. Although resembling methoxyflurane chemically its physical properties are more akin to those of halothane.

Enflurane is a pleasant-smelling colourless liquid, stable in the presence of metals, alkali, indirect natural light and soda-lime. It does not require a preservative. Like halothane it is soluble in rubber, and this may prolong induction and recovery. It is not flammable in oxygen–nitrous oxide mixtures at clinically used concentrations. Enflurane is a potent agent and should be administered only by means of a calibrated temperature-compensated vaporizer.

The minimum alveolar concentration (MAC) of enflurane in 100% oxygen is 1.68% in adults (Gion & Saidman 1971) and the drug is thus only half as potent as halothane (0.8%). In 70% nitrous oxide MAC decreases to 0.6%. Anaesthesia may be induced using 3–5% inspired enflurane, vaporized either in oxygen or nitrous oxide–oxygen, and can usually be maintained using vapour concentrations of 0.4–3.0%. Induction of, and emergence from, anaesthesia are rapid due to the low blood-gas solubility coefficient of 1.8, compared with 2.3 for halothane and 12 for methoxyflurane. It is thus a useful agent for outpatient anaesthesia (Korttila et al 1977).

Cardiovascular system

In common with other halogenated agents, enflurane produces a dose-related fall in systemic arterial blood pressure. The validity of comparing the haemodynamic effects of enflurane with those of halothane is sometimes questionable; variations in species, pre-anaesthetic medication, MAC values and surgical procedures make true comparisons difficult.

Early clinical reports indicated that circulatory changes were minimal during enflurane anaesthesia, and a study of the inotropic effects of enflurane on cat papillary muscle suggested that this agent caused less myocardial depression than halothane (Shimosato et al 1969). Subsequent work indicated that the degree of impairment of myocardial contractility during light enflurane anaesthesia was mild or moderate, and that cardiac output was maintained by increased heart rate. When high concentrations are inhaled, however, there may be pronounced depression of cardiac function.

Calverley and colleagues (1978a) found that cardiac

output, stroke volume, arterial blood pressure and systemic vascular resistance were markedly reduced in volunteers during controlled ventilation with 1 MAC enflurane in oxygen, 2 MAC inducing unacceptable hypotension (Fig. 7.5). The effects were less marked during spontaneous breathing of 1 MAC with associated hypercarbia. Under these conditions, cardiac output rose due to an increase in heart rate, but both mean arterial blood pressure and systemic vascular resistance fell by 52 and 38% respectively (Calverley et al 1978b). In a clinical study Black et al (1977) showed a 10% reduction in mean arterial blood pressure 10 minutes after the commencement of 3–4% enflurane anaesthesia in a group of 150 surgical patients. Although the onset of surgery reduced the frequency of hypotension, it remained a prevalent feature throughout the operative period in 51% of patients.

The fall in arterial blood pressure induced by enflurane may be comparable to or greater than the concurrent decrease in cardiac output, so that total peripheral resistance may be unchanged or decreased.

Heart rate and rhythm

Enflurane causes a slight increase in heart rate (Fig. 7.6) (Heiberg et al 1978), and although sensitizing the myocardium to the effect of catecholamines, it is much less likely to cause cardiac irregularities when adrenaline is injected than is halothane (Reisner & Lippmann 1975). The likelihood of cardiac irregularities during

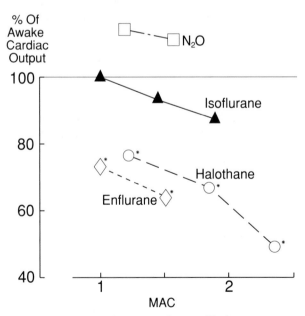

Fig. 7.5 Neither isoflurane nor nitrous oxide depresses cardiac output below awake levels in volunteers. In contrast, both halothane and enflurane decrease output significantly (asterisks) and do so to a greater extent at deeper levels of anaesthesia. (Winter et al 1972, Calverley et al 1978a, Eger et al, 1970.) With permission of Anaquest (Eger 1982).

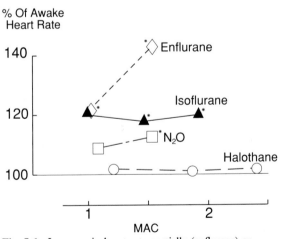

Fig. 7.6 Increases in heart rate partially (enflurane) or completely (isoflurane) compensate for any falls in stroke volume. (Data from Winter et al 1972, Calverley et al 1978a, Eger et al 1970.) Asterisks denote significant changes from awake values. With permission of Anaquest (Eger 1982).

ENT or dental procedures is considerably reduced by using enflurane rather than halothane (Sigurdsson et al 1983, Willatts et al 1983). Thus enflurane is particularly useful when there is likely to be an excess of circulating catecholamines such as infiltration of adrenaline for haemostasis, or during surgery for phaeochromocytoma (Kopriva & Eltringham 1974, Kreul et al 1976).

Respiratory system

Enflurane is non-irritant to the respiratory tract at clinically used concentrations and the use of antisialogogue drugs is not necessary (Dobkin et al 1968). It is a more potent respiratory depressant than isoflurane or halothane. There are marked falls in the tidal and minute volumes and increases in Pa_{CO_2} but the frequency of respiration does not change (Calverley et al 1978b, Wahba 1980, Wren et al 1987). Enflurane depresses respiration, both by inhibition of the respiratory centre and by a marked curare-like action on the respiratory musculature (Wahba 1980). It has a bronchodilating effect comparable to that of halothane, and in common with all volatile anaesthetic agents it depresses the ventilatory responses to both carbon dioxide and hypoxia.

Central nervous system

A characteristic of enflurane is its capacity to induce seizure complexes in the electroencephalogram (EEG). Several clinical studies confirm that episodes of paroxysmal activity and periods of burst suppression are features of EEG tracings during deep enflurane anaesthesia, being most marked at low Pa_{CO_2} levels (Neigh et al 1971). Tonic–clonic twitching of the facial muscles may also appear at deep levels in the presence of passive pulmonary hyperventilation. These responses can be rapidly abolished by permitting a return to normocarbia and reducing the enflurane concentration. Patients recover from anaesthesia without apparent ill-effects, and there is no evidence from animal or human investigations that enflurane causes any permanent upset of the central nervous system. In fact postoperatively there may be less abnormal EEG activity than after halothane anaesthesia (Burchiel et al 1977, 1978). Furthermore, enflurane does not exacerbate pre-existing susceptibility to seizure activity in epileptic patients during normocarbia (Opitz & Oberwetter 1979). In children, however, cerebral sensitivity is greater and this, coupled with the higher concentrations required and hypocarbia, may induce generalized epileptic activity of the grandmal type (Rosen & Soderberg 1975).

In addition to its epileptogenic properties, enflurane alters intracranial dynamics. At normocarbia 1 MAC enflurane or halothane abolishes cerebral autoregulation (Miletich et al 1976) and increases cerebral blood flow (Murphy et al 1974). Hypercarbia potentiates these effects and mask induction of anaesthesia with enflurane produces unacceptable increases in intracranial pressure (Stullken & Sokoll 1975). In general, enflurane increases cerebral blood flow and intracranial pressure (ICP) except during hyperventilation when mild hypocarbia is said to reduce the effect (Moss et al 1983).

The ability of the drug to increase ICP and its epileptogenic potential, particularly during hypocarbia, make enflurane a poor choice both for neurosurgery and for epileptic patients in general.

Effects on other organs

Liver. In contrast to halothane, there has been a notable absence of case reports of jaundice following enflurane anaesthesia. A review of 24 isolated case reports of 'enflurane hepatitis' (Lewis et al 1983) has been strongly criticized on the grounds of inadequate criteria for hepatotoxicity and the questionable validity of at least two of the cases (Dykes 1984). Extensive clinical studies have failed to detect any significant effects of enflurane on liver function even when given repeatedly (Allen & Downing 1977, Fee et al 1979). Evidence is accumulating, however, that volatile anaesthetic agents may share a common immunological mechanism for hepatic damage (Christ et al 1988), the potential of each being related to the extent to which they are metabolized (Hubbard et al 1988a). In spite of the lack of direct evidence, and in the absence of other considerations, enflurane should be avoided if previous exposure to the agent has been associated with postoperative jaundice.

Kidney. Enflurane, like halothane and isoflurane, causes a transient fall in renal blood flow, glomerular filtration rate and urinary output, but there is no evidence that these changes are harmful to the healthy kidney (Cousins et al 1976).

Fluorinated ethers such as methoxyflurane and enflurane are broken down in the liver to produce non-volatile end-products which are then excreted in the urine. The extent of this breakdown is directly related to nephrotoxicity. In the case of enflurane only 2% of an inhaled dose can be recovered in the form of urinary metabolites compared with 50% for methoxyflurane, 20% for halothane and 0.2% for isoflurane (Cascorbi et al 1970; Holaday et al 1970; Chase et al 1971; Holaday et al 1975). In general, serum fluoride concentrations after enflurane anaesthesia are unlikely to reach nephrotoxic levels (50 μmol l^{-1}) and so the danger of enflurane-induced renal damage is slight. However, impairment of urine-concentrating ability has been reported when the average serum fluoride concentration was only 15 μmol l^{-1}) (Mazze et al 1977). Such findings may be inconsequential when renal function is normal, but should not be overlooked when choosing an agent for use in patients with pre-existing renal impairment. Enflurane is an acceptable alternative to halothane or isoflurane for renal transplantation (Cronnelly et al 1984).

Uterus. Enflurane produces a dose-related relaxation of uterine smooth muscle. Concentrations of more than 3% may inhibit oxytocin-induced contractile activity. Several studies have demonstrated the effectiveness of small doses of enflurane or other volatile agents in reducing maternal awareness during caesarian section, and Warren and his colleagues (1983) used 1% enflurane in 50% nitrous oxide–oxygen mixture without any increase in operative blood loss or adverse effects on neonatal condition.

Skeletal muscle. Enflurane produces a dose-related depression of neuromuscular transmission and marked muscular relaxation. Non-depolarizing neuromuscular blocking drugs are potentiated and smaller doses of tubocurarine and pancuronium are required than when equi-MAC concentrations of halothane are used (Fogdall & Miller 1975, Ali & Savarese 1976). This effect is less marked with atracurium, the potency of which does not differ during halothane–nitrous oxide and enflurane–nitrous oxide anaesthesia (Rupp et al 1985).

Isoflurane

Isoflurane was synthesized in 1965. Exhaustive studies in animals and man showed it to be a good agent with minimal side-effects and toxicity, and it was introduced into clinical practice in the UK in 1983.

Chemical and physical properties

Isoflurane is 1-chloro-2,2,2-trifluoroethyl difluoromethyl ether, a halogenated methyl ethyl ether like its structural isomer, enflurane. Its chemical structure and some of its physical properties are shown in Figure 7.4 and Table 7.2.

Isoflurane is a clear, colourless liquid with a pleasant if slightly pungent ethereal odour. It is stable in the presence of daylight and soda-lime and it does not require the addition of a preservative. Isoflurane is non-flammable in air, nitrous oxide or oxygen. In theory its low blood-gas partition coefficient should make induction more rapid than with halothane, but in practice its

pungency tends to offset this advantage, particularly in children.

Although an ether, the physical properties of isoflurane are akin to those of halothane. In particular the vapour pressures of the two drugs are virtually identical, making it possible, although not desirable, to administer isoflurane from a halothane-calibrated vaporizer (Steffey et al 1983).

The minimum alveolar concentration (MAC) for isoflurane is 1.15% in 100% O_2, decreasing to 0.5% in 70% nitrous oxide (Stevens et al 1975b), thus lying between that of halothane and enflurane. Anaesthesia can be induced with isoflurane in nitrous oxide using concentrations of 1.5–3.5%. However, the pungency of the vapour limits the rate at which the concentration can be increased without respiratory upset. Maintenance can usually be achieved with concentrations of 0.75–2.0%. Recovery from isoflurane anaesthesia is rapid and it is suitable for use in outpatient anaesthesia (Azar et al 1984). Partition coefficients are shown in Table 7.1

Cardiovascular system

In a carefully controlled study in human volunteers, Stevens and his colleagues (1971) showed that during 1.0–2.0 MAC isoflurane anaesthesia cardiac output was minimally affected although systemic arterial blood pressure and peripheral resistance fell. This contrasts with halothane and enflurane both of which cause marked falls in cardiac output (Fig. 7.5). Both volunteer and clinical studies show that isoflurane tends to increase heart rate and this may explain the preservation of cardiac output. (Tachycardia with isoflurane is more likely to occur in young patients and other predisposing factors such as the concurrent use of vagolytic drugs, hypercarbia, 'light' planes of anaesthesia and hypo- or hypervolaemia may play a part.) Some workers have failed to demonstrate increases in heart rate in patients over 50 years of age (Bastard et al 1984, Tarnow et al 1976). Increasing the concentration of isoflurane during upper abdominal surgery causes a significant increase in heart rate, a response not obtained in the absence of surgery (Fig. 7.6).

Isoflurane appears to reduce systemic arterial pressure by reducing systemic vascular resistance. The magnitude of the effect is increased by high inhaled concentrations and the absence of nitrous oxide or surgical stimulation (Fig. 7.7). It follows that, by reducing arterial blood pressure, isoflurane, like halothane and enflurane, decreases cardiac work and this must decrease myocardial oxygen consumption. Isoflurane reduces vascular tone in the skin, muscle, kidney, heart,

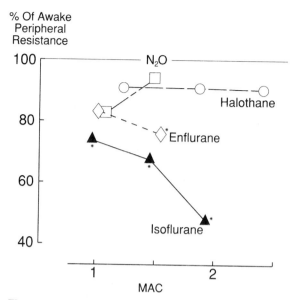

% Of Awake Peripheral Resistance

Fig. 7.7 Isoflurane and, to a lesser extent, enflurane cause peripheral vasodilation while halothane and nitrous oxide do not. (Asterisks denote significant changes from awake values.) (Data from Calverley 1978a, Eger et al 1970.) With permission of Anaquest (Eger 1982).

brain and gastrointestinal tract, and of these, skin and muscle in particular may enjoy increased blood flow. The increased skin perfusion may result in more rapid cooling of the body, which is particularly important in the very young or during long operations.

In the brain and heart any tendency to increased flow is balanced by reduced perfusion pressure. It has been suggested by Reiz and his colleagues (1983) that coronary vasodilatation might produce a 'steal' phenomenon in patients with coronary artery disease. This is analogous to the 'steal' phenomenon seen in the cerebral circulation where areas of ischaemia due to local vasoconstriction may be further deprived of blood and oxygen by vasodilatation elsewhere in the brain. Other studies have failed to substantiate this theory (Moffitt et al 1984, Tarnow et al 1986). Eger (1984) made a detailed analysis of the arguments for and against the phenomenon and concluded that in practice most patients who have coronary artery disease and who are given isoflurane appear not to suffer from myocardial ischaemia. A large amount of confusing and conflicting data has been produced since then. The relevance of some of the animal work to the human coronary circulation is doubtful, and overall the evidence against isoflurane is flimsy (Tinker, 1988). Particular care should be taken to avoid hypotension and tachycardia in patients with myocardial ischaemia.

Isoflurane does not induce premature ventricular beats, nor does it sensitize the myocardium to the effects of adrenaline. During anaesthesia for outpatient dental surgery isoflurane is associated with a lower frequency of arrhythmias than either halothane or enflurane (Willatts et al 1983, Cattermole et al 1986) but it may be less satisfactory overall. It would seem to be a suitable agent for use during surgery for phaeochromocytoma (Suzukawa et al 1983, Fay & Holzman 1983). The dose of adrenaline which will induce premature ventricular contractions in 50% of patients has been calculated by Johnstone and his colleagues (1976) as 2.1 μg kg^{-1} for halothane, 3.7 μg kg^{-1} for halothane–lignocaine, 10.9 μg kg^{-1} for enflurane and 6.7 μg kg^{-1} for isoflurane.

The differences between the volatile agents regarding their cardiac stability can be explained by their effects on conduction and on automaticity. Slowing of atrioventricular, His–Purkinje and ventricular conduction occurs maximally with halothane and least with isoflurane, with enflurane in an intermediate position. Such slowing provides conditions during which re-entry of the cardiac impulse can take place, thereby permitting premature ventricular contractions or supraventricular arrhythmias. Halothane has been shown to inhibit in vitro guinea-pig sino-atrial node driving rate more than enflurane or isoflurane (Bosnjak & Kampine 1983).

Reduced automaticity coupled with prolonged phase 4 depolarization is a feature of halothane and these factors, coupled with slowed conduction, explain the increased likelihood of arrhythmias with this drug. Arrhythmias are certainly less likely during isoflurane anaesthesia, and this is an important advantage, particularly where there are elevated plasma catecholamines, be they endogenous or exogenous in origin.

Respiratory system

Isoflurane would appear to be a slightly more potent respiratory depressant than halothane, although less so than enflurane (Eger 1984). It depresses respiration and the ventilatory responses to carbon dioxide. Oxygen consumption is reduced in all vital organs during anaesthesia with isoflurane, enflurane and halothane (Theye & Michenfelder 1975a,b), amounting to a decrease of about 30% in whole-body oxygen consumption at 2 MAC (Fig. 7.8). It is not clear whether general metabolic activity is depressed by increasing concentrations of volatile agents or whether functional requirements become less, due to reduced physiological activity (e.g. myocardial work).

Surgical stimulation increases both rate and depth of

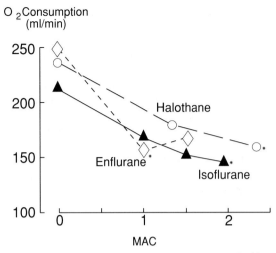

Fig. 7.8 Baseline oxygen consumption was measured with the Fick technique in awake volunteers whose ventilation was controlled. Oxygen consumption again was measured during anaesthesia with the indicated anaesthetics in oxygen while the volunteers were ventilated to maintain a constant Pa_{CO_2}. Enflurane (Calverley et al 1978a), halothane (Eger et al 1970) and isoflurane (Stevens et al 1971) decreased oxygen consumption (asterisks indicate significant decreases), the greatest changes occurring in the transition from wakefulness to sleep. With permission of Anaquest. (Eger 1982).

respiration during isoflurane or halothane anaesthesia. Despite this, end-tidal CO_2 concentration rises due partly to diminished alveolar ventilation and partly to increased CO_2 production through stimulation of the sympathetic nervous system. Bronchomotor tone appears to be reduced during isoflurane anaesthesia, although the effect is less pronounced than with halothane (Heneghan et al 1986).

Effects on other organs

Brain. There is no electroencephalographic or clinical evidence that isoflurane has any of the epileptogenic potential of enflurane (Eger et al 1971, Pauca & Dripps 1973). This applies even when the drug is used in high concentrations and in the presence of hypocarbia. Cerebral blood flow and intracranial pressure increase to a lesser extent with isoflurane than with halothane or enflurane. The rise in intracranial pressure can be prevented by the simultaneous introduction of hyperventilation (Adams et al 1981) although it is probably best to establish hypocarbia initially. The use of isoflurane for neurosurgical anaesthesia is still controversial,

and some feel it may be no safer than halothane (Azar & Thiagarajah 1984).

Kidney. In common with halothane and enflurane, isoflurane reduces renal blood flow, glomerular filtration rate and urine production. It is not toxic to the kidney either in clinical concentrations in man or during very prolonged administration in animals. Minimal biotransformation to inorganic fluoride and speedy elimination explain its very low toxic potential and this has been confirmed in many studies (Stevens et al 1973, Mazze et al 1974). It would appear acceptable for use in renal transplantation.

Liver. The minimal metabolism of isoflurane also explains the absence of toxic effects in the liver, although there is some evidence that all volatile agents may have the potential to induce liver damage (Hubbard et al 1988a). There is no evidence at present that repeat administrations of isoflurane are likely to be harmful to the liver, and in this respect isoflurane is safer than halothane.

Uterus. Isoflurane reduces uterine contractility in vitro to about the same extent as halothane or enflurane (Munson & Embro 1977). A clinical study by Abboud and his colleagues (1989) indicates that 0.4% isoflurane in oxygen is as effective and safe as 33% nitrous oxide in relieving pain in labour. Its disadvantages compared with Entonox are its pungent odour, its high cost and its sedative properties at high concentrations (McLeod et al 1975). When used for Caesarean section 0.75% isoflurane in 50% O_2–N_2O prevents awareness, and would appear not to cause appreciable neonatal depression or to increase intraoperative blood loss (Ghaly et al 1988).

Muscle. Modern volatile anaesthetic agents produce relaxation of skeletal muscle and tend to potentiate the effects of neuromuscular blocking drugs. Isoflurane has a more marked effect than halothane, both by itself and when combined with d-tubocurarine, pancuronium, gallamine, suxamethonium and vecuronium (Miller et al 1971a,b, Rupp et al 1984).

Sevoflurane

Clinical studies are currently in progress on this fluorinated ether. Its physical characteristics and chemical structure are shown in Table 7.2 and Figure 7.9. Wallin and co-workers (1975) reported that anaesthesia could be produced rapidly at vapour concentrations of 5–8% and anaesthesia was well maintained at 4–5%. MAC values and partition coefficients are shown in Table 7.1. Induction of anaesthesia with sevoflurane is smooth and rapid. The drug does not sensitise the

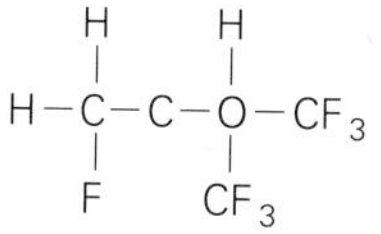

H—C—C—O—CF₃ with H, H, F, CF₃ substituents

SEVOFLURANE

Fig. 7.9 Chemical structure of sevoflurane.

myocardium to catecholamines and is non-irritant. Its metabolism has been studied and whilst some defluorination takes place, this does not appear to cause harmful effects. Unfortunately, sevoflurane reacts with soda-lime although the products are not thought to be toxic. It is flammable in oxygen at 11 vol. % and in nitrous oxide at 10 vol. %.

Desflurane (I-653)

A new fluorinated ether, difluoromethyl 1-fluoro-2,2,2-trifluoroethyl ether has undergone preliminary trials. Its chemical structure is similar to that of isoflurane and its partition coefficients and MAC are shown in Table 7.1. Desflurane is a potent agent of low solubility which produces more rapid induction and recovery than other volatile agents (Eger & Johnson 1987, Jones et al 1990). The drug is suitable for use in closed-circuit anaesthesia, being more stable in soda-lime than any of the current volatile agents (Jones 1990).

A disadvantage is its relatively high saturated vapour pressure of 700 mm Hg (22–23° C) indicating high volatility. Standard design vaporizers are unlikely to be suitable for administration of desflurane.

Animal studies indicate that its effects on the cardiovascular system are indistinguishable from those of isoflurane. Its likely place in the nineteen-nineties has been assessed by Miller & Greene (1990).

THE HYDROCARBONS

Chloroform

Chloroform ($CHCl_3$) is a chlorinated hydrocarbon with the physical characteristics shown in Table 7.2. It was first prepared in 1831 and was introduced into clinical practice by James Simpson of Edinburgh in 1847 as an alternative to ether. It is a colourless, sweet-smelling, volatile liquid with a non-flammable vapour and when formulated with 1% ethyl alcohol is said to be safe with soda-lime (Churchill-Davidson 1978).

In the early years of general anaesthesia it established a superiority over ether, chiefly because of its better in-

duction characteristics. Other advantages were its non-flammability, its analgesic qualities, and the ease with which it could be administered using an open-mask technique. Sudden deaths during chloroform anaesthesia were not uncommon, and were probably the result of crude methods of administration, ignorance of the pharmacological actions and lack of even simple monitoring. Furthermore, surgery was often undertaken in severely ill patients as the last resort, and without any form of resuscitation.

In most of its anaesthetic properties chloroform resembles halothane and it has similar disadvantages, notably its toxic effects on the heart and the liver. A detailed review of its pharmacology is given by Armstrong-Davison (1965). It is a very potent agent and must be accurately administered through a calibrated vaporizer if overdosage is to be avoided. Whitaker & Jones (1965) using a semi-open circuit with nitrous oxide (67%) in oxygen administered chloroform to 1500 cases using a precision vaporizer. The highest inspired chloroform concentration was 3.3%. Before the Second World War, vapour concentrations were calculated by vaporizing a known volume of liquid in a given space. Clover's chloroform apparatus, when properly used, contained a concentration of 4.5% in the reservoir bag which could be further diluted with air at the facepiece (Duncum 1947). Clover believed that less than 1.5% was necessary for maintenance. This was broadly in agreement with the views of a Special Chloroform Committee (1903), which pronounced that the safe range for induction and maintenance in man was 2.0–0.5% in air. When given by the open-drop method, or with an uncalibrated vaporizer, cardiac arrhythmias and sudden arrest may occur, even in the presence of adequate breathing. Like halothane, chloroform sensitizes the ventricular conducting system of the heart to the effects of adrenaline, and catecholamines should not be used to control bleeding during chloroform anaesthesia. It is a myocardial depressant and both cardiac output and arterial blood pressure fall with increasing depth of anaesthesia. Sudden bradycardia may occur at very deep levels.

Chloroform depresses respiration and the minute volume diminishes as anaesthetic depth increases. A popular mixture contained 2 parts chloroform by volume with 3 parts diethyl ether and 1 part ethyl alcohol (Harley's ACE mixture) to reduce this depressant effect. In theory, ether, by virtue of its irritant effects on the airway, acted as a respiratory stimulant.

The first two cases of jaundice and death following exposure to chloroform occurred in 1848 and were described by Defalque (1968). Similar case reports were published between 1892 and 1896 and were reviewed by Bourne (1936). Heintz, in 1896, stated that 'idiosyncrasy' appeared to be a factor in the development of hepatic damage associated with the administration of chloroform — a term more recently resurrected to explain the hepatic effects of halothane. In one week in 1899 no less than nine deaths with chloroform were reported in the *Lancet*.

In more recent years chloroform has been investigated in modern circumstances using calibrated vaporizers (Waters 1951, Smith et al 1970). Liver function studies were carefully conducted by the Waters group, and they found that in comparing chloroform with cyclopropane, tribromoethanol, ether and other agents, the incidence of one or more abnormal liver function tests was only slightly greater in the chloroform group than in the control group (52% and 44% respectively). Smith and his colleagues (1970) found no significant increase in postanaesthetic ALT, AST or alkaline phosphatase. Waters's study was extended by Siebecker and his colleagues (1960): between 1948 and 1957 an additional 1210 cases of chloroform anaesthesia were undertaken. Only one fatal case of hepatotoxicity occurred, in a patient who had a prolonged period of hypoxia. In a study to compare the hepatic effects of chloroform and halothane, Griffiths (1964) reported no differences between the groups in serum bilirubin, ALT, AST or bromsulphthalein retention test results.

Dykes (1970) used chloroform as a supplement to nitrous oxide anaesthesia in more than 25 000 cases, without a single case of clinical liver damage. In offering guidelines for its use he emphasizes the importance of administering a minimum dose of the drug, of ensuring adequate hydration and of preventing hypoxia and hypoglycaemia.

Trichloroethylene

Trichloroethylene (Trilene) was introduced to anaesthetic practice in the early 1940s at a time when ether was the standard inhalational agent. The non-flammability of trichloroethylene was its greatest asset, and despite having a weak anaesthetic action it enjoyed a period of popularity until after the introduction of halothane in 1956. Since then its use has declined in the western world.

Trichloroethylene is a good analgesic with only mild sedative properties, and on this account it earned a useful place in obstetric analgesia and anaesthesia. Muscle tone is scarcely affected and other major disadvantages are its slow induction characteristics, tachypnoea, delayed recovery and postoperative nausea (Dundee 1953).

Chemical and physical properties

Trichloroethylene is an unsaturated chlorinated hydrocarbon the chemical structure of which is given in Figure 7.10. It has been comprehensively reviewed by Parkhouse (1965). The industrial chemical is colourless but the pharmaceutical preparation is distinguished by a blue dye (waxoline blue 1 : 200 000). Trichloroethylene is decomposed by strong light and requires the addition of thymol as a stabilizing agent.

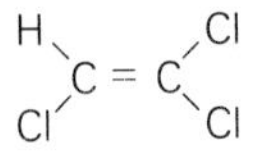

TRICHLOROETHYLENE

Fig. 7.10 Chemical structure of trichloroethylene.

At high temperature trichloroethylene breaks down to form phosgene, dichloroacetylene, hydrochloric acid and other toxic compounds. Suitable conditions may occur in soda-lime canisters or when cautery or diathermy are being used, particularly during ENT or facial surgery. In these circumstances cranial nerve damage may occur and trichloroethylene should be avoided when using closed-circuit techniques. This incompatibility probably accounts for the unpopularity of the drug in the United States where closed-circuit anaesthesia is widely employed. The other physical properties of the drug are given in Table 7.2.

Cardiovascular system

Like methoxyflurane and halothane, trichloroethylene does not increase plasma catecholamine concentrations (Unni et al 1970), but cardiac output and peripheral vascular resistance are unchanged. Inhaled in moderate concentrations trichloroethylene is associated with a considerable degree of cardiovascular stability. Only when attempts are made to achieve deep planes of anaesthesia do arrhythmias occur, and these may in part be due to hypercarbia secondary to tachypnoea. Adrenaline should be avoided during trichloroethylene anaesthesia. McArdle and his colleagues (1968) found no significant alteration in forearm vascular resistance, mean arterial pressure or heart rate.

In common with all the volatile anaesthetic agents, trichloroethylene should be administered only through an appropriate calibrated vaporizer, thus minimizing the risk of accidental overdosage.

Respiratory system

Trichloroethylene is pleasant and non-irritant to inhale at concentrations of up to 3%. At high concentrations tachypnoea may occur, particularly in the absence of opiates, causing reduced alveolar ventilation, with the possibility of hypercarbia and hypoxaemia.

Other effects

Jennett and his colleagues (1969) found that trichloroethylene anaesthesia causes a rise in intracranial pressure during normocarbia, and that this is accompanied by increased cerebral blood flow and vasodilatation. It is therefore unsuitable for neurosurgical anaesthesia.

Trichloroethylene has been widely used as an analgesic in obstetrics. In the past midwives received training in the use of draw-over vaporizers such as the Emotril or Tecova, which were capable of delivering 0.5–0.35% of the vapour. It can be used very successfully as a supplement to nitrous oxide in patients having Caesarean section, preventing awareness in the mother without depressing the baby (Crawford 1978).

Approximately 20% of inspired trichloroethylene is metabolized to form trichloroacetic acid (10%) which is excreted by the kidneys and trichloroethanol (10%), the active metabolite of chloral hydrate, which is conjugated and excreted in the bile (Greene 1968). Enzyme induction may result in even more extensive metabolism of the drug and produce high levels of sedative metabolites. Liver function appears not to be affected by trichloroethylene.

The drug is still widely used in Third World countries, and Prior (1972) has produced a useful review of the use of trichloroethylene in air with non-depolarizing relaxants. The same author makes the point that analytical and industrial-quality trichloroethylene is perhaps even purer than the anaesthetic preparation (1979).

Halothane

Introduced to clinical practice in 1956, halothane has, in the western world at least, gradually displaced ether and other agents, and is now the standard against which all new inhalational agents must be judged. It was synthesized by Suckling (1957) and its pharmacology was investigated by Raventos (1956). It is a versatile, easily controllable, non-irritant, halogenated hydrocarbon of very low toxicity, and has been the subject of intense investigation and sometimes bitter controversy. Undeniably halothane has some disadvantages, notably the sensitization of the myocardium to the effects of adrena-

line, the relaxation of uterine muscle and a rare propensity to cause liver damage.

Chemical and physical properties

Halothane ('Fluothane') is a halogenated hydrocarbon with the chemical name 1-bromo-1-chloro-2,2,2-trifluoroethane. Booth & Bixby (1932) tested two fluorinated paraffins on mice, and were the first to suggest that this type of compound ('Arcton') might have anaesthetic properties. Although their experiment was unsuccessful, research and synthesis of other fluorinated compounds continued after the Second World War. The objective was to find a molecule which, in addition to its anaesthetic properties, would be non-flammable and chemically inert. Fluorocarbons are inert, chemically, because of the strong bond between carbon and fluorine; in particular the CF_3 group in halothane was considered highly stable and likely to be of very low toxicity. Halothane's chemical structure and physical properties are compared with those of enflurane, isoflurane and methoxyflurane in Figure 7.11 and Table 7.2.

It is a colourless liquid with a pleasant, sweet smell. Slightly unstable on exposure to light, halothane must contain 0.01% w/w thymol as a preservative and should be stored in amber glass bottles. It reacts with soda-lime to produce very small amounts of a toxic decomposition product, 2-bromo-2-chloro-1,1-difluoroethylene (CF_2CBrCl) (Sharp et al 1979) but it is widely and apparently safely used for closed-circuit anaesthesia. It is non-flammable and non-explosive in all clinical concentrations.

The minimum alveolar concentration for halothane is 1.08% in infants, reducing to 0.64% over 80 years of age. Nitrous oxide (70%) in the breathing mixture can

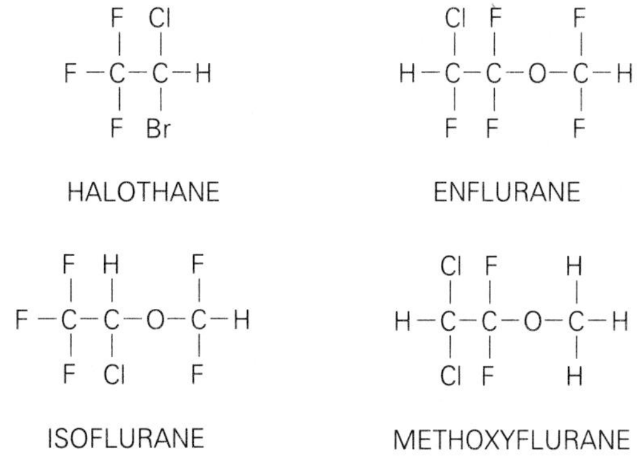

Fig. 7.11 Chemical structure of halothane compared to isoflurane, enflurane and methoxyflurane.

reduce MAC by as much as 60% (Table 7.1). Intrathecal morphine analgesia has also been shown to reduce the MAC from 0.81% to 0.46% (Drasner et al 1988). Anaesthesia can be easily induced using inspired concentrations of 2–4% and maintained with inspired concentrations of 0.5–2.5%. Spontaneous breathing will generally increase the required inspired concentration whereas nitrous oxide, controlled ventilation and opiates will have the opposite effect. Halothane may be administered using a variety of techniques; the open-drop mask, the OMV inhaler in air, the semi-closed circuit and the closed circuit with carbon dioxide absorption. It is advisable to administer halothane through a calibrated temperature/flow-compensated vaporizer.

Halothane tarnishes or corrodes a wide number of metals and alloys including brass, copper, stainless steel, aluminium, bronze and tin. Nickel and titanium are not attacked. The possibility that dichlorohexafluorobutene (DCHFB) might be produced by a reaction between halothane liquid and the metal surface of a copper kettle vaporizer was investigated by Cohen's group (1963). Although they produced some evidence in support of this, other workers disputed their findings (Albin et al 1964). The chemical purity of halothane improved after 1965, and subsequent investigations failed to substantiate Cohen's findings (Nagel et al 1966). The total impurity content is now less than 75 ppm, with any single unsaturated impurity present only in amounts less than 5 ppm (Raventos & Lemon 1965).

Halothane is highly soluble in rubber, and by its uptake and release in rubber anaesthetic circuits can both slow induction and delay recovery.

Cardiovascular system

Halothane causes a fall in arterial blood pressure, the extent of which is proportional to the concentration of inhaled vapour. This is its predominant effect on the circulation. Possible explanations include central sympathetic depression (Price et al 1965), ganglionic blockade (Raventos 1956), myocardial depression (Severinghaus & Cullen 1958, Kaplan et al 1976) and a direct action on vascular smooth muscle (Black & McArdle 1962).

In vitro studies using papillary muscle indicate that halothane has negative inotropic effects on the heart, causing decreased maximal velocity of shortening and decreased maximal isometric force (Sugai et al 1968). In man, Morrow & Morrow (1961) measured the effect of halothane on myocardial contractile force by suturing a Walton–Brodie strain gauge to the ventricle during cardiopulmonary bypass. Halothane (2%) administered through the oxygenator for 10 min decreased contractile force by 30% and mean arterial pressure by 15%. This work has been confirmed by Kaplan et al (1976), who showed by measuring systolic time intervals that contractility was reduced by 30–50% and mean arterial pressure by 11%.

Peripheral blood flow

During halothane anaesthesia the limbs appear warm and peripherally vasodilated. Black & McArdle (1962), using a water-filled plethysmograph, showed that halothane caused substantial increases in limb blood flow. A subsequent study using a mercury-in-rubber strain gauge showed that this is mainly due to an increase in skin flow, and that muscle flow is not increased (Scott et al 1978). However, the means by which halothane produces vasodilatation are multifactorial and include central sympathetic depression, ganglion blockade, interference with baroreceptor activity, as well as α-adrenergic blockade. Recent animal studies indicate that halothane attenuates α_2-, but not α_1-adrenoreceptors (Larach et al 1987).

The addition of nitrous oxide to steady-state halothane–oxygen anaesthesia causes an increase in systemic vascular resistance, and other signs of sympathetic activation (Smith et al 1970).

Coronary blood flow

Domenech and his colleagues (1977) reported marked reductions in coronary vascular resistance in both the intact and isolated heart of the dog during the inhalation of halothane, probably due to direct vasodilatation. In health there is a balance between oxygen supply and demand, and normally this is not compromised by anaesthesia. In the presence of ischaemia, however, increased demand may interrupt supply and the choice of agent used may be crucial. Although halothane reduces myocardial function and oxygen supply it also reduces oxygen demand (Merin et al 1976), and it is a suitable agent for use in the presence of myocardial ischaemia.

Liver blood flow

Halothane, by reducing mean arterial pressure, reduces splanchnic perfusion pressure. Studies in man have shown that hepatic blood flow falls by 25–30% during halothane anaesthesia (Epstein et al 1966, Price et al 1966). Halothane appears to have no significant effect on splanchnic vascular resistance, suggesting that hypotension rather than increased vasomotor tone may be responsible for the reduction in splanchnic blood flow.

Catecholamines

Roizen and colleagues (1974) have shown that in rats the total plasma catecholamine concentration during 1% halothane anaesthesia is only about 12% of that in awake animals, the plasma catecholamine titre continuing to fall proportionally as the concentration of halothane increased. It has since been shown by Sumikawa and co-workers (1982) that halothane has an inhibitory effect on sympathetic preganglionic synapses and thereby inhibits catecholamine release. There is also evidence that halothane inhibits the release of noradrenaline from peripheral venous tissue (Lunn & Rorie 1982).

Effects on heart rate and rhythm

Halothane, in common with other anaesthetics with a hydrocarbon structure, sensitizes the myocardium to the effects of catecholamines (Katz & Katz 1966). The mechanism is not clear, but is probably related to bradycardia and depression of ventricular automaticity (Reynolds et al 1970, Hashimoto & Hashimoto 1972). Halothane frequently causes cardiac slowing which becomes more pronounced as anaesthesia deepens. There may be a shift of pacemaker and nodal rhythm due to unopposed vagal activity, this being more likely when high concentrations of halothane are being inhaled. Both halothane and methoxyflurane produce a dose-dependent increase in the functional refractory period of the AV conducting system (Morrow et al 1972).

Unlike cyclopropane, arrhythmias are not commonly encountered during uncomplicated halothane anaesthesia in man in the presence of normal arterial P_{CO_2} levels (Black 1967). Indeed, correction of a respiratory acidosis will often abolish ventricular irregularities even though the concentration of halothane is unaltered. The indiscriminate use of atropine to correct changes in heart rate or rhythm is fraught with danger and may, by abolishing vagal tone, accentuate their severity and even induce ventricular fibrillation (Black 1965). Hypercarbia is a common cause of tachyarrhythmias during halothane anaesthesia.

Exogenous catecholamines in the form of subcutaneous adrenaline for haemostasis will produce similar undesirable effects in heart rate and rhythm. Johnstone et al (1976) in a study of the arrhythmogenic potentials of enflurane, halothane and isoflurane in man, found that when adrenaline was used, halothane increased the risk of serious arrhythmias. These workers recommend that adrenaline should not be given in a dose exceeding 14 ml of 1:200 000 solution during halothane anaes-

thesia, and not more than 47 ml of 1:200 000 solution during isoflurane anaesthesia. They also suggest that lignocaine 0.5% solution is a useful anti-arrhythmic when used with all three volatile agents.

Oral surgery is associated with a particularly high incidence of cardiac arrhythmias (Alexander & Murtagh 1979). These are accentuated by 'light' anaesthesia and by the use of halothane. In comparative studies in dental patients, Hutchison and colleagues (1989) and other groups of workers found there was a much higher frequency of cardiac arrhythmias with halothane than with either isoflurane or enflurane.

Central nervous system

The electrical activity of the brain as reflected in the electroencephalogram during halothane induction shows a gradual change from a fast low-voltage pattern to a slow high-amplitude waveform. There is no evidence from electroencephalographic studies that halothane has any serious epileptogenic potential (Burchiel et al 1978).

Halothane causes cerebral vasodilatation and increases cerebral blood flow (CBF) provided the systemic blood pressure remains in the normal range (Wollman et al 1964, Smith & Wollman et al 1972). However, it impairs autoregulation (Miletich et al 1976), is associated with increased cerebrospinal fluid pressure (Lassen & Christensen 1976) and appears to increase intracranial pressure to a greater extent than isoflurane (Artu 1983). The cerebral metabolic consumption of oxygen is reduced and oxygen delivery to the brain would appear to be in excess of demand. On account of its tendency to over-perfuse, halothane is not a useful drug for many neurosurgical procedures and it should be avoided in circumstances where there is any possibility of cerebral oedema.

Respiratory system

Halothane is non-irritant to the respiratory tract and can be used to produce rapid, smooth induction of anaesthesia. It does not stimulate salivary or bronchial secretions to any significant extent. At deeper levels it obtunds pharyngeal and laryngeal reflexes and facilitates endotracheal incubation. A further very useful property of halothane is its bronchodilating action, which makes it particularly suitable for patients with chronic bronchitis or asthma.

Halothane alters the control of respiration, and tachypnoea is a feature in patients who have not received opiates. The effect of this is to decrease tidal volume. There may also be a reduction in minute volume and in effective alveolar ventilation. This is particularly likely to happen in children who, as a group, require high concentrations of halothane during induction and whose anatomical dead space is already proportionately larger than that of adults. The cause of the tachypnoea has been attributed to the sensitization of pulmonary stress receptors (Coleridge et al 1968). The effect, however, has been shown to persist following bilateral vagotomy and Berkenbosch and colleagues (1982) claim that tachypnoea is exclusively due to an action of halothane on brainstem structures.

Liver

Careful trials of halothane in animals prior to its release in the early years of its use revealed no hepatotoxicity (Raventos 1956). Nevertheless, its chemical similarity to known hepatotoxins such as chloroform and carbon tetrachloride invited a degree of suspicion which has blighted its otherwise excellent reputation ever since. The first reports of liver damage following halothane were published shortly after the introduction of the drug in 1956 (Burnap et al 1958, Virtue & Payne 1958) and unfortunately were followed by new reports (Brody & Sweet 1963, Bunker & Blumenfeld 1963, Lindenbaum & Leifer 1963).

Difficulties of diagnosis, inconclusive retrospective studies and medicolegal implications have been constant features of the debate that has followed.

The United States National Halothane Study was set up in 1963 to try to resolve some of the uncertainties surrounding the whole question of postoperative liver necrosis. The findings were reported in full in the report of the National Halothane Study (1969), but Mc-Caughey (1972) has outlined the main findings in his summary of the investigation. The overall incidence of massive hepatic necrosis is 82 per 850 000 general anaesthetics regardless of the anaesthetic agents used. In only nine of these patients could the massive hepatic necrosis be attributed to the anaesthetic agent itself, and of these only seven received halothane. Since 250 000 patients in the study received halothane the incidence of hepatic necrosis in those who received the drug is 7 in 250 000, that is, 1 in 35 000 (Carney & Van Dyke 1972). Other findings were that hepatic necrosis did not occur more commonly than with other agents, and that repeated administration of halothane was not associated with a higher mortality rate. The study did not, however, give any insight into factors which might confer an increased risk of damaging hepatitis.

In further retrospective studies Inman & Mushin (1974) reported that there was an increased likelihood of liver dysfunction following repeated exposure to halothane, and that the risk increased as the interval between successive administrations decreased. These findings have been strengthened by the results of three prospective studies in which the activities of certain liver enzymes were raised after repeated exposure to halothane (Trowell et al 1975, Wright et al 1975 Fee et al 1979). However, it is known that, irrespective of the agent used and regardless of whether or not the cause can be explained, there is an increased incidence of jaundice and death after multiple anaesthetics (Strunin & Simpson 1972). Neuberger & Williams (1984) regard the danger interval between administrations as 4 weeks, whereas the Committee on Safety of Medicines (1986) advise against a further exposure within a period of 3 months unless there are over-riding clinical circumstances. Some would argue that there is no safe period and that repeat halothane is best avoided altogether.

Various predisposing factors have been proposed, including obesity (Dundee et al 1981), female gender (Benjamin et al 1985) and genetics (Hoft et al 1981, Gourlay et al 1981). The explanations for these have not been elucidated, although obesity increases halothane biotransformation (Bentley et al 1982) and may also be associated with liver hypoxia, during or after anaesthesia; these patients may also need increased dosage. There is also evidence that halothane may reduce hepatic oxygen supply to a greater extent than other volatile agents (Gelman et al 1987).

Reports of liver damage following halothane in children have been extremely rare, but more cases are being reported (Whitburn & Sumner 1986, Walton 1986). The overall incidence is estimated at 1 in 82 000 halothane anaesthetics.

THE THEORETICAL BASIS OF HALOTHANE HEPATOTOXICITY

In recent years the biotransformation of halothane has gradually been unravelled, and there is now a detailed understanding of many of the biochemical processes involved. There are three aspects of the biotransforming process which, although interdependent, offer clues as to the nature of halothane hepatotoxicity. Much of the current emphasis is on an immunological explanation (Hubbard et al 1988a) but the means by which this might occur remain ill-defined. Broadly, halothane hepatotoxicity may be a consequence, in greater or smaller part, of direct hepatotoxicity, enhanced minor metabolic pathways and immunological reactions. These are not discrete entities and a full explanation of the phenomenon is likely to involve some aspects of each.

Direct toxicity

Most, if not all, the anaesthetic hydrocarbons have been associated with hepatotoxicity to a much greater extent than the ethers (see Chloroform, page 111). Evidence for a direct toxic effect comes both from animal and human studies. Rats exposed to diethyl ether, isoflurane or halothane for long periods had a greater incidence of hepatic damage after halothane despite being given lower concentrations of it than the other agents (Stevens et al 1975a). Several studies of repeat halothane anaesthetics in patients showed that liver enzyme activity increased after multiple halothane exposures but not after enflurane (Fee et al 1979). More recently, Hussey and colleagues (1988) showed that a specific liver enzyme, glutathione S-transferase, was elevated in 50% of those receiving a single administration of halothane, 20% after enflurane, and 11% after isoflurane. In these and other similar studies the elevations in liver enzymes were transient and in none did any patient become jaundiced. The link, if any, between mild liver damage (type I) and jaundice due to massive liver necrosis (type II) is unclear, but may be related to the presence of intermediate metabolites produced by halothane biotransformation.

The hepatotoxicity of both carbon tetrachloride and chloroform is a consequence of their biotransformation. In both, a significant amount of the parent compound is metabolized to substances which are 'reactive' with cellular macromolecules. In the case of carbon tetrachloride, metabolism is mainly a reductive process, whereas chloroform is subject to chemical oxidation.

Thus, while failing to explain halothane hepatitis completely, there is good evidence that halothane is, like other halogenated hydrocarbons, a direct toxin, albeit a mild one.

Enhanced metabolism

The dominant metabolic pathway for volatile anaesthetic agents is an oxidative process mediated by cytochrome P450. In the case of halothane despite the intention to create a stable, non-reactive molecule, up to 45% of the absorbed dose is thought to be oxidatively metabolized (Carpenter et al 1986). The major metabolite is trifluoroacetic acid (TFA), a compound which is of low-level toxicity and which is excreted in the urine with Br^- and Cl^- (see below):

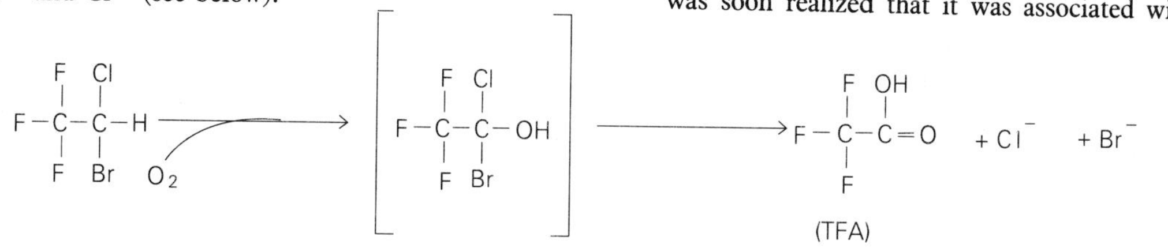

Uniquely among volatile anaesthetic agents, halothane undergoes reductive metabolism. This process also requires cytochrome P450 but under hypoxic conditions there is an increase in plasma inorganic fluoride levels accompanied by the creation of a defluorinated volatile metabolite, 2-chloro-1,1-difluoroethylene (CDF), and a non-defluorinated compound, 2-chloro-1,1,1-trifluoroethane (CTF) (Sharp et al 1979). Thus, both pathways release bromide, but only reductive metabolism releases significant amounts of fluoride. None of the end-products of either metabolic route is likely to cause liver damage, but unstable toxic intermediate compounds are produced by both oxidation and reduction, which are capable of binding to liver macromolecules. This binding may be to hepatic protein or lipids and may result in lipid peroxidation or inhibition of the cytochrome P450 series of enzymes with consequent centrilobular hepatic damage.

Studies in animals showed that when halothane was given under hypoxic conditions and with enzyme inducers, centrilobular liver damage could be induced. The frequent discovery of the two reductive volatile metabolites suggested that in humans under certain conditions, reductive metabolism might predominate and be responsible for hepatic necrosis after halothane. As the sole explanation of halothane hepatitis, this theory has several flaws, particularly in respect of the role of hypoxia. Lunan et al (1985) have now developed an anaesthetic model where hepatotoxicity can be induced without hypoxia. Furthermore, it is rare for halothane hepatitis to occur in circumstances where there is a risk of hypoxaemia — COAD, hypovolaemia, pulmonary aspiration, or indeed in those who have suffered cardiac arrest during or after halothane anaesthesia. Also, the timing of the phenomenon in the clinical situation differs from that produced by halothane/hypoxia in animals.

The importance of metabolic processes may be related to the synthesis of intermediate compounds which can bind to and alter liver cell membranes in such a way as to make them antigenic.

Immunological reactions

It has long been recognized that halothane hepatitis might have an immunological basis, particularly as it was soon realized that it was associated with repeated administrations. Perhaps the most striking evidence for an immunological basis was the occurrence of halothane hepatitis in two anaesthetists following re-exposure to the drug (Belfrage et al 1966, Klatskin & Kimberg 1969). However, the mechanism by which a small molecule, like halothane, could induce an allergic reaction was unclear.

Sensitization to halothane-altered rabbit hepatocytes was shown in some patients who were suffering from halothane hepatitis (Vergani et al 1978) and subsequently antibodies were found in humans which were specific for the trifluoroacetyl (TFA) product of oxidative halothane metabolism (Vergani et al 1980). Trifluoroacetyl chloride binds covalently to cell proteins which, in an altered state, may then act antigenically and stimulate antibody production (Callis et al 1986). Five halothane hepatitis patients out of six were found to produce an antibody which reacted with the protein-bound trifluoroacetyl moiety (Hubbard et al 1988b); the sixth patient was immunosuppressed and failed to generate anti-TFA antibodies, thus raising a doubt as to the precise role of the antibody — was it cause or effect?

A report by Christ and his colleagues (1988) presents evidence that there may be a common hepatotoxic mechanism between volatile anaesthetic agents. The suggestion is that the toxic potential is proportional to the degree of biotransformation, and that using enflurane or isoflurane instead of halothane for a repeat exposure will reduce the incidence of liver damage rather than guarantee its prevention.

Although the above findings provide evidence of an altered immune state in patients with halothane hepatitis, it is difficult to be certain that they represent the 'cause' and not the 'effect'. There have been many reports of halothane-associated hepatitis in patients who had never received the drug before, and who could not therefore have been sensitized to it. Walton and his associates (1976) reported that two patients who had previously developed hepatitis after halothane, and in whom it subsequently recurred following another exposure had, in the intervening period, received halothane without untoward postoperative effects.

Other theories on the aetiology have been advanced by various authorities over the years. Toxic chemical impurities such as dichlorohexafluorobutene (DCHFB) were implicated by Cohen and his colleagues (1965) and the purity of Fluothane was subsequently improved. The question of the role of radiation on the aetiology of the condition has also been raised. Pennington (1968) examined the effect of gamma radiation on samples of halothane and demonstrated that DCHFB was increased in linear fashion as the dose of gamma radiation increased. Gelb & Steen (1973), in confirming this, noted

that thymol reduced the extent of the degradation. These findings prompt questions about the possible effects of radium on body tissues and on drugs or other substances present in the body. The effects of X-ray or other types of radiation on halothane in vaporizers are not known. It is known, however, that routine maintenance of anaesthetic vaporizers is often neglected (Milligan & Rodgers 1983).

It is becoming increasingly apparent that the 'cause' of halothane hepatitis is multifactorial. Mention has already been made of risk factors such as repeat administrations within a short period of time, obesity, hypoxia, enzyme induction and the development of halothane hepatitis in a near relative. In the vast majority of cases this agent causes no problems, its positive advantages greatly outweighing its disadvantages in most situations, particularly when the extent of the risk associated with alternatives is greater, or unknown.

Renal effect

Halothane has been shown to depress renal function (Deutsch et al 1966). Renal blood flow, glomerular filtration rate, urinary sodium excretion and urinary volume are all reduced, whilst the filtration fraction and renal vascular resistance are increased. The mechanisms by which these effects take place are not clear. Halothane can liberate antidiuretic hormone (ADH) by a central autonomic effect (Price et al 1965), or by a fall in circulating blood volume. Other explanations include: the secretion of extrarenal hormones such as aldosterone and catecholamines; reduced cardiac output and peripheral resistance; changes in body temperature and acid–base balance. The clinical importance of the effect of halothane on the kidney remains speculative. Studies in man and animals with chronic renal insufficiency have shown that neither halothane nor enflurane caused further impairment of renal function. Indeed both agents in man were associated with slight improvements in postoperative renal function (Mazze et al 1984). Serum inorganic fluoride levels following halothane have been studied by Cousins and his co-workers (1976), who showed no increase, in contrast to other fluorinated agents. Young and his colleagues (1975) demonstrated a rise in serum inorganic fluoride in obese patients receiving halothane.

Obstetrics

Halothane diminishes the tone of uterine smooth muscle and can safely be used to facilitate external version of the fetus. It also reduces the contractile response of the uterus to ergotamine, syntometrine and oxytocin. In spite of this and its poor analgesic qualities (Dundee & Moore 1960) its use as a supplementary agent in anaesthesia for Caesarean section has much to commend it. Moir (1970) showed that the addition of 0.5% halothane to a standard 50% nitrous oxide/oxygen/tubocurarine technique reduced the incidence of maternal awareness without any increase in maternal blood loss. Furthermore the condition of the newly born was improved compared with the unsupplemented group.

High halothane concentrations in these circumstances are both unnecessary and dangerous, bearing in mind that the MAC for halothane in pregnancy is possibly reduced (Palahniuk et al 1974) and that concentrations of approximately 1% or more may lead to hypotension and the risk of increased uterine blood loss (Moir 1970).

It should be remembered that women of childbearing age are very likely to have had previous anaesthesia (Fee et al 1978) and that repeat exposure to this agent introduces the risk of hepatotoxicity.

VOLATILE ANAESTHETIC AGENTS OF HISTORICAL INTEREST

In the western world, anaesthesia with ether and chloroform may be outdated, but both drugs continue to be manufactured and supplied to less developed countries.

In contrast, a considerable number of volatile agents have become truly obsolete in terms of their use as general anaesthetics world-wide. A few of the more important of these are discussed below.

Ethyl chloride (C_2H_5Cl)

The local anaesthetic properties of this compound were discovered in the mid-nineteenth century about the time of the introduction of chloroform. By nature of its very low boiling point (12°C) ethyl chloride was first used to 'freeze' the skin and mucous membranes prior to incision, its general anaesthetic properties only being recognized around 1900.

The vapour is non-irritant but flammable. Both induction and recovery were rapid using an open-drop method, and for this reason it was popular for use in children. Like other hydrocarbons it causes myocardial depression, sensitizes the myocardium to adrenaline, and occasionally results in liver damage. Its properties have been reviewed by Lawson (1965).

Vinyl ether (divinyl ether, divinyl oxide)

This compound ($CH_2CH)_2O$, was synthesized in the early 1930s in the hope that it might combine the potency of diethyl ether with the low toxicity and speedy induction of ethylene.

Vinyl ether is more volatile than diethyl ether, with a boiling point of 28.3°C, and is flammable. It decomposes readily to formaldehyde, acetaldehyde and formic and acetic acids on exposure to light, air and heat. A stabilizing agent, phenyl alpha naphthylamine (0.01%) was added, together with 3.5% absolute alcohol to reduce volatility. This preparation was known in the United Kingdom as 'Vinesthene'.

Vinyl ether is very potent, and it was used as an induction agent prior to maintenance with ether; induction using an open-drop technique was extremely fast. It was non-irritant and was said not to markedly depress the cardiovascular system. At high concentrations breathing ceased prior to cardiac arrest and this afforded a degree of protection. Vinyl ether appeared not to sensitize the heart to the effects of catecholamines, and although liver damage was reported, this appears to have been much less likely than after chloroform. Recovery was said to be rapid, smooth and free of excitement.

Fluroxene ('Fluoromar')

Fluroxene is a halogenated ether (trifluoroethylvinyl ether) whose structural formula is given in Figure 7.12. It was introduced in 1954 and was the first fluorinated anaesthetic agent for clinical use. Widely used in the USA, fluroxene was never popular in the United Kingdom, probably due to the introduction of halothane in 1956.

Fluroxene is a colourless liquid with a pleasant odour. The vapour is both flammable and explosive, although less so than the non-fluorinated ethers.

In most of its anaesthetic characteristics, fluroxene resembles diethyl ether, although it is not irritant to the respiratory tract and induction was smooth. It was best given by a calibrated vaporizer and could be administered safely in a closed-circuit system. Fluroxene does not sensitize the heart to the catecholamines, and there is no evidence that it caused liver damage. It has a good analgesic effect in sub-anaesthetic doses and was used to provide analgesia during painful nursing procedures such as the dressing of burns.

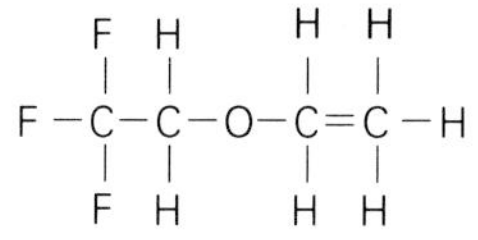

FLUROXENE

Fig. 7.12 Chemical structure of fluroxene.

REFERENCES

Abboud T K, Gangolly J, Mosaad P, Crowell D 1989 Isoflurane in obstetrics. Anesthesia and Analgesia 68: 388–391

Adams R W, Cucchiara R F, Gronert G A, Messick J M, Michenfelder J D 1981 Isoflurane and cerebrospinal fluid pressure in neurosurgical patients. Anesthesiology 54: 97–99

Albin M S, Horrocks L A, Kretchmer H E 1964 Halothane impurities and the Copper Kettle. Anesthesiology 25: 672–675

Alexander J P, Murtagh J G 1979 Arrhythmia during oral surgery: fascicular blocks in the cardiac conducting system. British Journal of Anaesthesia 51: 149–155

Ali H H, Savarese J J 1976 Monitoring of neuromuscular function. Anesthesiology 45: 216–249

Allen P J, Downing J W 1977 A prospective study of hepatocellular function after repeated exposure to halothane or enflurane in women undergoing radium therapy for cervical cancer. British Journal of Anaesthesia 49: 1035–1039

Armstrong-Davison M H 1965 Chloroform. British Journal of Anaesthesia 37: 655–660

Artu A A 1983 Effects of halothane and fentanyl on the rate of CSF production in dogs. Anesthesia and Analgesia 62: 581–584

Azar I, Thiagarajah S 1984 The jury is still out in the case of isoflurane versus halothane in neurosurgical patients. Anesthesiology 61: 786–787

Azar I, Karambelkar D J, Lear E 1984 Neurologic state and psychomotor function following anesthesia for ambulatory surgery. Anesthesiology 60: 347–349

Bastard O G, Carter J G, Moyers J R, Bross B A 1984 Circulatory effects of isoflurane in patients with ischaemic heart disease: a comparison with halothane. Anesthesia and Analgesia 63: 635–639

Belfrage S, Ahlgren I, Axelson S 1966 Halothane hepatitis in an anaesthetist (Letter). Lancet 2: 1466

Benjamin S B, Goodman Z D, Ishak K G, Zimmerman H J, Irey N S 1985 The morphologic spectrum of halothane-induced hepatic injury: analysis of 77 cases. Hepatology 5: 1163–1171

Bentley J B, Vaughan R W, Gandolfi A J, Cork R C 1982 Halothane biotransformation in obese and non-obese patients. Anesthesiology 57: 94–97

Berkenbosch A, de Goede J, Olievier C N, Quanjer Ph H 1982 Sites of action of halothane on respiratory pattern and ventilatory response to CO_2 in cats. Anesthesiology 57: 389–398

Berman M L, Lowe H J, Bochantin J, Hagler K 1973 Uptake and elimination of methoxyflurane as influenced by enzyme induction in the rat. Anesthesiology 38: 352–357

Black G W 1965 A review of the pharmacology of halothane. British Journal of Anaesthesia 37: 688–705

Black G W 1967 A comparison of cardiac rhythm during halothane and methoxyflurane anaesthesia at normal and elevated levels of $Paco_2$. Acta Anaesthesiologica Scandinavica 11: 103–108

Black G W, McArdle L 1962 The effects of halothane on the peripheral circulation in man. British Journal of Anaesthesia 34: 2–10

Black G W, Johnston H M L, Scott M G 1977 Clinical impressions of enflurane. British Journal of Anaesthesia 49: 875–880

Bodley P O, Mirza V, Spears J R, Spilsbury R A 1966 Obstetric analgesia with methoxyflurane. Anaesthesia 21: 457–463

Booth H S, Bixby E M 1932 Fluorine derivatives of chloroform. Industrial Engineering Chemistry 24: 637

Bosnjak Z J, Kampine J P 1983 Effects of halothane, enflurane and isoflurane on the SA node. Anesthesiology 58: 314–321

Bourne W 1936 Anesthetics and liver function. American Journal of Surgery 34: 486–495

Brody G L, Sweet R B 1963 Halothane anesthesia as a possible cause of massive hepatic necrosis. Anesthesiology 24: 29–37

Bunker J P, Blumenfeld C M 1963 Liver necrosis after halothane anesthesia. Cause or coincidence? New England Journal of Medicine 268: 531–534

Burchiel K J, Stockard J J, Calverley R K, Smith N T 1977 Relationship of pre- and post-anesthetic EEG abnormalities to enflurane-induced seizure activity. Anesthesia and Analgesia 56: 509–514

Burchiel K J, Stockard J J, Calverley R K, Smith N T, Scholl, M L, Mazze R I 1978 Electroencephalographic abnormalities following halothane anesthesia. Anesthesia and Analgesia 57: 244–251

Burnap T K, Galla S J, Vandam L D 1958 Anesthetic circulatory and respiratory effects of Fluothane. Anesthesiology 19: 307–320

Callis A H, Brooks S D, Waters S J 1986 Evidence for a role of the immune system in the pathogenesis of halothane hepatitis. In: Roth S H, Miller K W (eds) Molecular and cellular mechanisms of a anaesthetics. Plenum, New York, pp

Calverley R K, Smith N T, Prys-Roberts C, Eger E I (II), Jones C W 1978a Cardiovascular effects of enflurane anesthesia during controlled ventilation in man. Anesthesia and Analgesia 57: 619–628

Calverley R K, Smith N T, Jones C W, Prys-Roberts C, Eger E I (II) 1978b Ventilatory and cardiovascular effects of enflurane anesthesia during spontaneous ventilation in man. Anesthesia and Analgesia 57: 610–618

Carney F M T, Van Dyke R A 1972 Halothane hepatitis: a critical review. Anesthesia and Analgesia 51: 135–160

Carpenter R L, Eger E I (II), Johnson B H, Unadkat J D, Sheiner L B 1986 The extent of metabolism of inhaled anesthetics in humans. Anesthesiology 65: 201–205

Cascorbi H F, Blake D A, Helrich M 1970 Differences in the biotransformation of halothane in man. Anesthesiology 32: 119–123

Cattermole R W, Verghese C, Blair I J, Jones C H J, Flynn P J, Sebel P S 1986 Isoflurane and halothane for outpatient dental anaesthesia in children. British Journal of Anaesthesia 58: 385–389

Chase R E, Holaday D A, Fiserova-Bergerova V, Saidman L J, Mack F E 1971 The biotransformation of Ethrane in man. Anesthesiology 35: 262–267

Christ D D, Kenna J G, Kammerer W, Satoh H, Pohl L R 1988 Enflurane metabolism produces covalently bound liver adducts recognised by antibodies from patients with halothane hepatitis. Anesthesiology 69: 833–838

Churchill-Davidson H C (ed) 1978 Inhalational anaesthetic

agents. In: A practice of anaesthesia, 4th edn. Lloyd-Luke, London, Ch. 6

Cohen E N, Bellville J W, Budzikiewiez H, Williams D H 1963 Impurity in halothane anesthetic. Science 145: 899

Cohen E N, Brewer H W, Bellville J W, Sher R 1965 The chemistry and toxicology of dichlorohexafluorobutene. Anesthesiology 26: 140–153

Coleridge H M, Coleridge J C G, Luck J C, Norman J 1968 The effect of four volatile anaesthetic agents on the impulse activity of two types of pulmonary receptors. British Journal of Anaesthesia 40: 484–492

Committee on Safety of Medicines 1986 Current problems, No. 18. Committee on Safety of Medicines, London

Conway C M 1965 The anaesthetic ethers. British Journal of Anaesthesia 37: 644–654

Cousins M J, Mazze R I 1973 Methoxyflurane nephrotoxicity — a study of dose response in man. Journal of the American Medical Association 225: 1611–1616

Cousins M J, Greenstein L R, Hitt B A, Mazze R I 1976 Metabolism and renal effects of enflurane in man. Anesthesiology 44: 44–53

Crawford J S 1978 Principles and practice of obstetric anaesthesia, 4th edn. Blackwell Scientific Publications, London, pp: 49–58

Cromwell T H, Eger E I (II), Stevens W C, Dolan W M 1971 Forane uptake, excretion and blood solubility in man. Anesthesiology 35: 401–408

Cronnelly R, Salvatierra O Jr, Feduska N J 1984 Renal allograft function following halothane, enflurane or isoflurane anesthesia. Anesthesia and Analgesia 63: 202

Defalque R J 1968 The first delayed chloroform poisoning. Anesthesia and Analgesia 47: 374–375

de Jong R H, Eger E I (II) 1975 MAC expanded. Anesthesiology 42: 384–389

Deutsch S, Goldberg M, Stephen G W, Wein-Hsien W 1966 Effects of halothane anesthesia on renal function in normal man. Anesthesiology 27: 793–804

Dobkin A B, Levy A A 1973 Blood serum fluoride levels with methoxyflurane anaesthesia. Canadian Anaesthetists' Society Journal 20: 81–93

Dobkin A B, Heinrich R G, Israel J S, Levy A A, Neville J F, Ounkasem K 1968 Clinical and laboratory evaluation of a new inhalation agent: compound 347. Anesthesiology 29: 275–287

Dodd R B 1962 Diethyl ether. Springfield, Illinois, C C Thomas

Domenech R J, Macho P, Valdes J, Penna M 1977 Coronary vascular resistance during halothane anesthesia. Anesthesiology 46: 236–240

Drasner K, Bernards C M, Ozanne G M 1988 Intrathecal morphine reduces the minimum alveolar concentration of halothane in humans. Anesthesiology 69: 310–312

Duncum B M 1947 The development of inhalation anaesthesia. Oxford University Press, London

Dundee J W 1953 Tachypnoea during the administration of trichloroethylene. British Journal of Anaesthesia 25: 3–23

Dundee J W, Moore J 1960 Alterations in response to somatic pain associated with anaesthesia. IV: The effect of subanaesthetic concentrations of inhalation agents. British Journal of Anaesthesia 32: 453–459

Dundee J W, Fee J P H, McIlroy P D A, Black G W 1981 Prospective study of liver function following repeat

halothane and enflurane. Journal of the Royal Society of Medicine 74: 286–291

Dykes M H M 1970 Anesthesia and the liver. In: Dykes M H M (ed) International Anesthesiology Clinics Vol 8, No 2. Little, Brown, Boston, pp 189–201

Dykes M H M 1984 Is enflurane hepatotoxic? Anesthesiology 61: 235–237

Eger E I (II) 1974 Anesthetic uptake and action. Williams & Wilkins, Baltimore

Eger E I (II) 1982 Isoflurane, A Compendium and Reference. Anaquest

Eger E I (II) 1984 The pharmacology of isoflurane. British Journal of Anaesthesia 56: 71S–99S

Eger E I 1987 Partition coefficients of I-653 in human blood, saline and olive oil. Anesthesia and Analgesia 66: 971–973

Eger E I, Johnson B H 1987 Rates of awakening from anesthesia with I-653, halothane, isoflurane and sevoflurane. Anesthesia and Analgesia 66: 977–982

Eger E I, Smith N T, Stoelting R K, Cullen D J, Kadis L B, Whitcher C E 1970 Cardiovascular effects of halothane in man. Anesthesiology 32: 396–409

Eger E I (II), Stevens W C, Cromwell T H 1971 The electroencephalogram in man anesthetised with Forane. Anesthesiology 35: 504–508

Epstein R M, Deutsch S, Cooperman L H, Clement A H, Price H L 1966 Splanchnic circulation during halothane anesthesia and hypercapnia in normal man. Anesthesiology 27: 654–661

Fairlie C W, Barss T P, French A B, Jones C M, Beecher H K 1951 Metabolic effects of anesthesia in man. IV: A comparison of the effects of certain anesthetic agents on the normal liver. New England Journal of Medicine 244: 615–622

Fay M L, Holzman R S 1983 Isoflurane for resection of phaeochromocytomas. Anesthesia and Analgesia 62: 955

Fee J P H, McDonald J R, Dundee J W, Clarke R S J 1978 Frequency of previous anaesthesia in an anaesthetic patient population. British Journal of Anaesthesia 50: 917–920

Fee J P H, Black G W, Dundee J W et al 1979 A prospective study of liver enzyme and other changes, following repeat administration of halothane and enflurane. British Journal of Anaesthesia 51: 1133–1141

Fogdall R P, Miller R D 1975 Neuromuscular effects of enflurane, alone and combined with d-tubocurarine, pancuronium and succinylcholine in man. Anesthesiology 42: 173–178

Gelb E J, Steen S N 1973 Effect of gamma radiation on halothane. International Research Communications System (73–4)38–0–2

Gelman S, Dillard E, Bradley E L 1987 Hepatic circulation during surgical stress and anesthesia with halothane, isoflurane or fentanyl. Anesthesia and Analgesia 66: 936–943

Ghaly R G, Flynn R J, Moore J 1988 Isoflurane as an alternative to halothane for Caesarean section. Anaesthesia 43: 5–7

Gion H, Saidman L J 1971 The minimum alveolar concentration of enflurane in man. Anesthesiology 35: 361–364

Gourlay G K, Adams J F, Cousins M J, Hall P 1981 Genetic differences in reductive metabolism and hepatotoxicity in three rat strains. Anesthesiology 55: 96–103

Greene N M 1968 The metabolism of drugs employed in anesthesia. Part II. Anesthesiology 29: 327–360

Griffiths H W C 1964 Effects of chloroform and halothane on liver function in man. Lancet 1: 246–247

Halsey M J 1989 Potency and physical properties of inhalational anaesthetics. In: Nunn J F, Utting J E, Brown B R Jr (eds) General Anaesthesia, 5th edn. Butterworths, London, pp 7–18

Hashimoto K, Hashimoto K 1972 The mechanism of sensitization of the ventricle to epinephrine by halothane. American Heart Journal 83: 652–658

Heiberg J K, Wiberg-Jorgensen F, Skovsted P 1978 Heart rate changes caused by enflurane and halothane anaesthesia in man. Acta Anaesthesiologica Scandinavica 22 (Suppl. 67): 59–62

Heneghan C P H, Bergman N A, Jordan C, Lehane J R, Catley D M 1986 Effect of isoflurane on bronchomotor tone in man. British Journal of Anaesthesia 58: 24–28

Hoft R H, Bunker J P, Goodman H I, Gregory P B 1981 Halothane hepatitis in three pairs of closely related women. New England Journal of Medicine 304: 1023–1024

Holaday D A, Fiserova-Bergerova V, Latto I P, Zumbiel M A 1975 Resistance of isoflurane to biotransformation in man. Anesthesiology 43: 325–332

Holaday D A, Rudofsky S, Treuhaft P S 1970 Metabolic degradation of methoxyflurane in man. Anesthesiology 33: 579–593

Hubbard A K, Gandolfi A J, Brown B R 1988a Immunological basis of anesthetic-induced hepatotoxicity. Anesthesiology 69: 814–817

Hubbard A K, Roth T P, Gandolfi A J, Brown B R, Webster N R, Nunn J F 1988b Halothane hepatitis patients generate an antibody response toward a covalently bound metabolite of halothane. Anesthesiology 68: 791–796

Hussey A J, Aldridge L M, Paul D, Ray D C, Beckett G J, Allan L G 1988 Plasma glutathione S-transferase concentration as a measure of hepatocellular integrity following a single general anaesthetic with halothane, enflurane or isoflurane. British Journal of Anaesthesia 60: 130–135

Hutchison G L, Davies C A, Main G, Gray I G 1989 Incidence of arrhythmias in dental anaesthesia: a cross-over comparison of halothane and isoflurane. British Journal of Anaesthesia 62: 518–521

Inman W H W, Mushin W W 1974 Jaundice after repeated exposure to halothane: an analysis of reports to the Committee on Safety of Medicines. British Medical Journal 1: 5–10

Inman W H W, Mushin W W 1978 Jaundice after repeated exposure to halothane: a further analysis of reports to the Committee on Safety of Medicines. British Medical Journal 2: 1455–1456

Jennett W B, Barker J, Fitch W, McDowall D G 1969 Effect of anaesthesia on intracranial pressure in patients with space-occupying lesions. Lancet 1: 61

Johnstone R R, Eger E I (II), Wilson C 1976 A comparative interaction of epinephrine with enflurane, isoflurane and halothane in man. Anesthesia and Analgesia 55: 709–712

Jones R M 1990 Desflurane and sevoflurane: inhalation anaesthetics for this decade? British Journal of Anaesthesia 65: 527–536

Jones R M, Cashman J N, Mant T G K 1990 Clinical impressions and cardiorespiratory effects of a new fluorinated inhalation anaesthetic, desflurane (I-653), in volunteers. British Journal of Anaesthesia 64: 11–15

Kaplan J A, Miller E D, Bailey D R 1976 A comparative study of enflurane and halothane using systolic time intervals. Anesthesia and Analgesia 55: 263–268

Karis J H, Gissen A J, Nastuk W L 1966 Mode of action of diethyl ether in blocking neuromuscular transmission. Anesthesiology 27: 42–51

Katoh T, Ikeda K 1987 The minimum alveolar concentration (MAC) of sevoflurane in humans. Anesthesiology 66: 301–303

Katz R L 1966 Neuromuscular effects of diethyl ether and its interaction with succinylcholine and d-tubocurarine. Anesthesiology 27: 52–63

Katz R L, Katz G J 1966 Surgical infiltration of pressor drugs and their interaction with volatile anaesthetics. British Journal of Anaesthesia 38: 712–718

Klatskin G, Kimberg D V 1969 Recurrent hepatitis attributable to halothane sensitization in an anesthetist. New England Journal of Medicine 280: 515–522

Kopriva C J, Eltringham R 1974 The use of enflurane during resection of a pheochromocytoma. Anesthesiology 41: 399–400

Korttila K, Tammisto T, Ertama P, Pfaffli P, Blomgren E, Hakkinen S 1977 Recovery, psychomotor skills and simulated driving after brief inhalational anesthesia with halothane or enflurane combined with nitrous oxide and oxygen. Anesthesiology 46: 20–27

Kreul J F, Dauchot P J, Anton A H 1976 Hemodynamic and catecholamine studies during pheochromocytoma resection under enflurane anesthesia. Anesthesiology 44: 265–268

Larach D R, Schuler H G, Derr J A, Larach M G, Hensley F A, Zelis R 1987 Halothane selectively attenuates α_2-adrenoceptor mediated vasoconstriction in vivo and in vitro. Anesthesiology 66: 781–791

Larson C P, Eger E I (II), Muallem M, Buechel D R, Munson E S, Eisele J H 1969 The effects of diethyl ether and methoxyflurane on ventilation. Anesthesiology 30: 174–185

Lassen N A, Christensen M S 1976 Physiology of cerebral blood flow. British Journal of Anaesthesia 48: 719–734

Lawson J I M 1965 Ethyl chloride. British Journal of Anaesthesia 37: 667–670

Lee J A 1953 A synopsis of anaesthesia, 3rd edn, Wright, Bristol, p 79

Lewis J H, Zimmerman H J, Ishak K G, Mullick F G 1983 Enflurane hepatotoxicity: a clinicopathologic study of 24 cases. Annals of Internal Medicine 98: 984–992

Libonati M, Malsch E, Price H L, Cooperman L H, Baum S, Harp J R 1973 Splanchnic circulation during methoxyflurane anesthesia. Anesthesiology 38: 466–472

Lindenbaum J, Leifer E 1963 Hepatic necrosis associated with halothane anesthesia. New England Journal of Medicine 268: 525–530

Lunan C A, Cousins M J, Hall P de la M 1985 Guinea-pig model of halothane-associated hepatotoxicity in the absence of enzyme induction and hypoxia. Journal of Pharmacology and Experimental Therapeutics 232: 802

Lunn J J, Rorie D K 1982 Halothane-induced changes in the release and disposition of norepinephrine at adrenergic nerve endings in dog saphenous vein. Anesthesiology 61: 377–384

McArdle L, Unni V K N, Black G W 1968 The effects of trichloroethylene on limb blood flow in man. British Journal of Anaesthesia 40: 767–772

McCaughey W 1972 A summary of the National Halothane Study. British Journal of Anaesthesia 44: 918

McLeod D D, Ramayya G P, Tunstall M E 1975 Self-administered isoflurane in labour. Anaesthesia 40: 424–426

Major V, Rosen M, Mushin W W 1966 Methoxyflurane as an obstetric analgesic: a comparison with trichloroethylene. British Medical Journal 2: 1554–1561

Mapleson W W 1963 Quantitative prediction of anesthetic concentrations. In: Papper E M, Kitz R J (eds). Uptake and distribution of anaesthetic agents. McGraw-Hill, New York, pp 104–119

Maze M, Birch B, Vickery R G 1987 Clonidine reduces halothane MAC in rats. Anesthesiology 67: 868–869

Maze M, Vickery R G, Merlone S C, Gaba D M 1988 Anesthetic and hemodynamic effects of the alpha$_2$-adrenergic agonist, azepexole, in isoflurane-anesthetized dogs. Anesthesiology 68: 689–694

Mazze R I, Cousins M J, Barr G A 1974 Renal effects and metabolism of isoflurane in man. Anesthesiology 40: 536–542

Mazze R I, Calverley R K, Smith N T 1977 Inorganic fluoride nephrotoxicity. Anesthesiology 46: 265–271

Mazze R I, Sievenpiper T S, Stevenson J 1984 Renal effects of enflurane and halothane in patients with abnormal renal function. Anesthesiology 60: 161–163

Melvin M A, Johnson B H, Quasha A L, Eger E I (II) 1982 Induction of anesthesia with midazolam decreases halothane MAC in humans. Anesthesiology 57: 238–241

Merin R G, Kumazawa T, Luka N L 1976 Enflurane depresses myocardial function, perfusion and metabolism in the dog. Anesthesiology 45: 501–507

Miletich D J, Ivankovich A D, Albrecht R F, Reimann C R, Rosenberg R, McKissic E D 1976 Absence of autoregulation of cerebral blood flow during halothane and enflurane anesthesia. Anesthesia and Analgesia 55: 100–109

Miller R D, Eger E I (II), Way W L, Stevens W C, Dolan W M 1971a Comparative neuromuscular effects of Forane and halothane alone and in combination with d-tubocurarine in man. Anesthesiology 35: 38–42

Miller E D, Greene N M 1990 Waking up to desflurane: the anesthetic for the '90s? (Editorial) Anesthesia and Analgesia 70: 1–2

Miller R D, Way W L, Dolan W M, Stevens W C, Eger E I (II) 1971b Comparative neuromuscular effects of pancuronium, gallamine and succinylcholine during Forane and halothane anesthesia in man. Anesthesiology 35: 509–514

Milligan K, Rodgers R C 1983 Vaporizer failure (Letter). Anaesthesia 38: 997

Moffitt E A, Barker R A, Glenn J J et al 1984 Myocardial metabolism and hemodynamic responses with isoflurane anesthesia for coronary artery surgery. Anesthesia and Analgesia 63: 252

Moir D D 1970 Anaesthesia for Caesarean section. British Journal of Anaesthesia 42: 136–142

Morrow D H, Haley J V, Logic J R 1972 Anesthesia and digitalis. VII: The effect of pentobarbital, halothane and

methoxyflurane on the A-V conduction and inotropic responses to ouabain. Anesthesia and Analgesia 52: 430–438

Morrow D H, Morrow A G 1961 The effects of halothane on myocardial contractile force and vascular resistance. Anesthesiology 22: 537–541

Moss E, Dearden N M, McDowall D G 1983 Effects of 2% enflurane on intracranial pressure and cerebral perfusion pressure. British Journal of Anaesthesia 55: 1083–1088

Munson E S, Embro W J 1977 Enflurane, isoflurane and halothane and isolated human uterine muscle. Anesthesiology 46: 11–14

Munson E S, Eger E I (II), Tham, M K, Embro W J 1978 Increase in anesthetic uptake, excretion and blood solubility in man after eating. Anesthesia and Analgesia 57: 224–231

Murphy F L, Kennell E M, Johnstone R E 1974 The effects of enflurane, isoflurane and halothane on cerebral blood flow and metabolism in man. Anesthesiology 42: 61–2

Murphy M R, Hug C C 1982 The anesthetic potency of fentanyl in terms of its reduction of enflurane MAC. Anesthesiology 57: 485–488

Nagel E L, Moya F, Burg S P, Vestal B, Jalowayski B S 1966 Dichlorohexafluorobutene concentration in clinical vaporizers. Anesthesiology 27: 673–680

National Halothane Study 1969 Bunker J P, Forrest W H, Mosteller F, Vandam L D (eds) A study of the possible association between halothane anesthesia and postoperative hepatic necrosis. US Government Printing Office, Washington

Neigh J L, Garman J K, Harp J R 1971 The electroencephalographic pattern during anesthesia with Ethrane: effects of depth of anesthesia, Pa_{CO_2} and nitrous oxide. Anesthesiology 35: 482–487

Neuberger J, Williams R 1984 Halothane anaesthesia and liver damage. British Medical Journal 289: 1136–1139

Opitz A, Oberwetter W D 1979 Enflurane or halothane anaesthesia for patients with cerebral convulsive disorders? Acta Anaesthesiologica Scandinavica, Suppl 71: 43–47

Palahniuk R J, Shnider S M, Eger E I (II) 1974 Pregnancy decreases the requirements for inhaled anesthetic agents. Anesthesiology 41: 82–83

Parkhouse J 1965 Trichloroethylene. British Journal of Anaesthesia 37: 681–687

Pauca A L, Dripps R D 1973 Clinical experience with isoflurane (Forane). British Journal of Anaesthesia 45: 697–703

Pennington S N 1968 The effects of gamma radiation on halothane. Anesthesiology 29: 153–154

Price H L, Dripps R D 1970 General anesthetics. II: Volatile anesthetics: diethyl ether, divinyl ether, chloroform, halothane, methoxyflurane and other halogenated volatile anesthetics. In: Goodman L S, Gilman A (eds) The pharmacological basis of therapeutics, 4th edn. New York, Macmillan pp 79–92

Price H L, Pauca A L 1969 Effects of anesthesia on the peripheral circulation. Clinical Anesthesia 3: 73–76

Price H L, Price M L, Morse H T 1965 Effects of cyclopropane, halothane and procaine on the vasomotor centre of the dog. Anesthesiology 26: 55–60

Price H L, Deutsch S, Davidson I A, Clement A H, Behar M G, Epstein R M 1966 Can general anesthetics produce splanchnic visceral hypoxia by reducing regional blood flow? Anesthesiology 27: 24–32

Prior F N 1972 Trichloroethylene in air with muscle relaxants. Anaesthesia 27: 66–75

Prior F N 1979 Requiem for trichloroethylene? (Letter). Anaesthesia 34: 904

Quasha A L, Eger E I (II), Tinker J H 1980 Determination and applications of MAC. Anesthesiology 53: 315–334

Rampil I J, Zwass M, Loekhart S, Eger E I (II), Johnson B H 1989 MAC of I-653 in surgical patients. Anesthesiology 71: A269

Raventos J 1956 The action of fluothane — a new volatile anaesthetic. British Journal of Pharmacology 11: 394–410

Raventos J, Lemon P G 1965 The impurities in Fluothane: their biological properties. British Journal of Anaesthesia 37: 716–737

Reisner L S, Lippmann M 1975 Ventricular arrhythmias after epinephrine injection in enflurane and in halothane anesthesia. Anesthesia and Analgesia 54: 468–470

Reiz S, Bålfors E, Sørensen M B, Ariola S Jr, Friedman A, Truedsson H (1983) Isoflurane — a powerful coronary vasodilator in patients with coronary artery disease. Anesthesiology 59: 91–97

Reynolds A K, Chiz J F, Pasquet A F 1970 Halothane and methoxyflurane — a comparison of their effects on cardiac pacemaker fibers. Anesthesiology 33: 602–610

Robertson C E, Sinclair C J, Steedman D, Brown D, Malcolm-Smith N 1985 Use of ether in life-threatening acute severe asthma. Lancet 1: 187–188

Roizen M F, Moss J, Henry D P, Kopin I J 1974 Effects of halothane on plasma catecholamines. Anesthesiology 41: 432–439

Rosen I, Soderberg M 1975 Electroencephalographic activity in children under enflurane anaesthesia. Acta Anaesthesiologica Scandinavica 19: 361–369

Rupp S M, McChristian J W, Miller R D 1985 Neuromuscular effects of atracurium during halothane–nitrous oxide and enflurane–nitrous oxide anesthesia in humans. Anesthesiology 63: 16–19

Rupp S M, Miller R D, Gencarelli P J 1984 Vecuronium-induced neuromuscular blockade during enflurane, isoflurane and halothane anesthesia in humans. Anesthesiology 60: 102–105

Sampaio M M, Crean P M, Keilty S R, Black G W 1989 Changes in oxygen saturation during inhalation induction of anaesthesia in children. British Journal of Anaesthesia 62: 199–201

Saner C A, Foëx P, Roberts J G, Bennett M J 1975 Methoxyflurane and practalol: a dangerous combination. British Journal of Anaesthesia 47: 1025

Scott M G, McArdle L, Black G W 1978 A critical appraisal of venous occlusion plethysmography as a method of assessing limb blood flow during halothane anaesthesia. British Journal of Anaesthesia 50: 630

Segal I S, Vickery R G, Walton J K, Doze V A, Maze M 1988 Dexmedetomidine diminishes halothane anesthetic requirements in rats through a postsynaptic alpha$_2$-adrenergic receptor. Anesthesiology 69: 818–823

Severinghaus J W, Cullen S C 1958 Depression of myocardium and body oxygen consumption with Fluothane in man. Anesthesiology 19: 165–177

Sharp J H, Trudell J R, Cohen E N 1979 Volatile metabolites and decomposition products of halothane in man. Anesthesiology 50: 2–8

Shimosato S 1964 Ventricular function during anesthesia. In: Price H L, Cohen P J (eds) Effects of anesthetics on the circulation. Thomas, Springfield,

Shimosato S, Sugai N, Iwatsuki N, Etsten B E 1969 The effects of Ethrane on cardiac muscle mechanics. Anesthesiology 30: 513–518

Siebecker K L, Bamforth B J, Steinhaus J E, Orth O S 1960 Clinical studies of new and old hydrocarbons. Anesthesia and Analgesia 39: 180–188

Sigurdsson G H, Carlsson C, Lindahl S, Werner O 1983 Cardiac arrhythmias in non-intubated children during adenoidectomy: a comparison between enflurane and halothane anaesthesia. Acta Anaesthesiologica Scandinavica 27: 75–80

Smith A L, Wollman H 1972 Cerebral blood flow and metabolism. Anesthesiology 36: 378–400

Smith N T, Eger E I, Stoelting R K, Whayne T F, Cullen D, Kadis L B 1970 The cardiovascular and sympathomimetic responses to the addition of nitrous oxide to halothane in man. Anesthesiology 32: 410–421

Sørensen M B, Ariola S Jr, Friedman A, Truedsson H 1983 Isoflurane — a powerful coronary vasodilator in patients with coronary artery disease. Anesthesiology 59: 91–97

Special Chloroform Committee 1903 Report of the Special Chloroform Committee of the British Medical Association. British Medical Journal 2 (Suppl cxli)

Steffey E P, Woliner M J, Howland D 1983 Accuracy of isoflurane delivery by halothane-specific vaporizers. American Journal of Veterinary Research 44: 1072

Stevens W C, Cromwell T H, Halsey M J, Eger E I (II), Shakespeare T F, Bahlman S H 1971 The cardiovascular effects of a new inhalation anesthetic, Forane, in human volunteers at constant arterial carbon dioxide tension. Anesthesiology 35: 8–16

Stevens W C, Eger E I (II), Joas T A, Cromwell T H, White A, Dolan W M 1973 Comparative toxicity of isoflurane, halothane, fluroxene and diethyl ether in human volunteers. Canadian Anaesthetists' Society Journal 20: 357–368

Stevens W C, Dolan W M, Gibbons R T, White A, Eger E I, Miller R D, De Jong R H, Elashoff R M 1975b Minimum alveolar concentrations (MAC) of isoflurane with and without nitrous oxide in patients of various ages Anesthesiology 42: 197–200

Stevens W C, Eger E I, White A, Halsey M J, Munger W, Gibbons R D, Dolan W, Sharge R 1975a Comparative toxicities of halothane, isoflurane and diethyl ether at subanesthetic concentrations in laboratory animals. Anesthesiology 42: 408–419

Stoelting R K, Longnecker D E, Eger E I (II) 1970 Minimum alveolar concentrations in man on awakening from methoxyflurane, halothane, ether and fluroxene anesthesia: MAC awake. Anesthesiology 33: 5–9

Strum D P, Eger E I (II) 1987 Partition coefficients for sevoflurane in human blood, saline and olive oil. Anesthesia and Analgesia 66: 654–656

Strunin L, Simpson B R 1972 Halothane in Britain today. British Journal of Anaesthesia 44: 919–924

Stullken E H, Sokoll M D 1975 Anesthesia and subarachnoid intracranial pressure. Anesthesia and Analgesia 54: 494–498

Suckling C W 1957 Some chemical and physical factors in

the development of Fluothane. British Journal of Anaesthesia 29: 466–472

Sugai N, Shimosato S, Etsten B E 1968 Effect of halothane on force–velocity relations and dynamic stiffness of isolated heart muscle. Anesthesiology 29: 267–274

Sumikawa K, Matsumoto T, Ishizaka N, Nagai H, Amenomori Y, Amakata Y 1982 Mechanism of the differential effects of halothane on nicotonic and muscarinic receptor-mediated responses of the dog adrenal medulla. Anesthesiology 57: 444–450

Suzukawa M, Michaels I A L, Ruzbarsky J, Kopriva C J, Kitahata L M 1983 Use of isoflurane during resection of pheochromocytoma. Anesthesia and Analgesia 62: 100–103

Tarnow J, Bruckner J B, Eberlein H J, Hess W, Patschke D 1976 Hemodynamics and myocardial oxygen consumption during isoflurane (Forane) anaesthesia in geriatric patients. British Journal of Anaesthesia 48: 669–675

Tarnow J, Markschies-Hornung A, Schulte-Sasse U 1986 Isoflurane improves the tolerance to pacing-induced myocardial ischemia. Anesthesiology 64: 147–156

Theye R A, Michenfelder J D 1975a Whole-body and organ V_{O_2} changes with enflurane, isoflurane and halothane. British Journal of Anaesthesia 47: 813–817

Theye R A, Michenfelder J D 1975b Individual organ contributions to the decrease in whole body VO_2 with isoflurane. Anesthesiology 42: 35–40

Tinker J H 1988 Anaesthesia for the patient with cardiac disease. Canadian Journal of Anaesthesia 35: 59–513

Trowell J, Peto R, Crampton-Smith A 1975 Controlled trial of repeated halothane anaesthetics in patients with carcinoma of the uterine cervix treated with radium. Lancet 1: 821–824

Unni V K N, McArdle L, Black G W 1970 Sympatho-adrenal, respiratory and metabolic changes during trichloroethylene anaesthesia. British Journal of Anaesthesia 42: 429–433

Vergani D, Tsantoulas D, Eddleston A L W F, Davis M, Williams R 1978 Sensitization to halothane-altered liver components in severe hepatic necrosis after halothane anaesthesia. Lancet 2: 801–803

Vergani D, Mieli-Vergani, G, Alberti A, Neuberger J, Eddleston A L W F, Davis M Williams R 1980 Antibodies to the surface of halothane-altered rabbit hepatocytes in patients with severe halothane-associated hepatitis. New England Journal of Medicine 303: 66–71

Virtue R W, Payne K W 1958 Postoperative death after Fluothane. Anesthesiology 19: 562–563

Wahba W M 1980 Analysis of ventilatory depression by enflurane during clinical anesthesia. Anesthesia and Analgesia 59: 103–109

Wallin R F, Regan B M, Napoli M D, Stern I J 1975 Sevoflurane: a new inhalation anesthetic agent. Anesthesia and Analgesia 54: 758–765

Walton B 1986 Halothane hepatitis in children. Anaesthesia 41: 575–578

Walton B, Simpson B R, Strunin L, Doniach D, Perrin J, Appleyard A J 1976 Unexplained hepatitis following halothane. British Medical Journal 1: 1171–1176

Warren T M, Datta S, Ostheimer G W, Naulty J S, Weiss J B, Morrison J A 1983 Comparison of the maternal and neonatal effects of halothane, enflurane and isoflurane for Cesarean delivery. Anesthesia and Analgesia 62: 516–520

Waters M 1951 Chloroform: a study after 100 years. University of Wisconsin, Madison

Waud B E, Waud D R 1975 The effects of diethyl ether, enflurane and isoflurane at the neuromuscular junction. Anesthesiology 42: 275–280

Weiskopf R B, Holmes M A, Eger E I, Johnson B H, Rampil I J, Brown J G 1988 Cardiovascular effects of I-653 in swine. Anesthesiology 69: 303–309

Whitaker A M, Jones C S 1965 Report of 1500 chloroform anesthetics administered with a precision vaporizer. Anesthesia and Analgesia 44: 60–65

Whitburn R H, Sumner E 1986 Halothane hepatitis in an 11-month-old child. Anaesthesia 41: 611–613

Willatts D G, Harrison A R, Groom J F, Crowther A 1983 Cardiac arrhythmias during outpatient dental anaesthesia: comparison of halothane with enflurane. British Journal of Anaesthesia 55: 399–403

Winter P M, Hornbein T F, Smith G 1972 Hyperbaric nitrous oxide anesthesia in man: determination of anesthetic potency (MAC) and cardiorespiratory effects. Abstracts of Scientific Papers. Annual meeting of American Society of Anesthesiologists 1972

Wollman H, Alexander S C, Cohen P J, Chase P E, Melman E, Behar M G 1964 Cerebral circulation of man during halothane anaesthesia. Anesthesiology 25: 180–184

Wren W S, Allen P, Synnott A, O'Keefe D, O'Griofa P 1987 Effects of halothane, isoflurane and enflurane on ventilation in children. British Journal of Anaesthesia 59: 399–409

Wright R, Chisholm M, Lloyd B et al 1975 Controlled prospective study of the effect on liver function of multiple exposures to halothane. Lancet 1: 817–820

Young S R, Stoelting R K, Peterson C, Madura J A 1975 Anesthetic biotransformation and renal function in obese patients during and after methoxyflurane anesthesia. Anesthesiology 42: 451–457

8. Anaesthetic gases

H. J. L. Craig

The gases nitrous oxide, cyclopropane, ethylene, acetylene and xenon possess anaesthetic properties, but only the first three of these have been used in clinical practice to any great extent. At the present time nitrous oxide is in common usage, cyclopropane is still occasionally administered and ethylene is mainly of historical interest.

These anaesthetic gases have several features in common, all being stored in cylinders compressed to a liquid form at room temperature (below 10°C for ethylene) and moderate pressures and, by definition, having a vapour pressure above ambient pressure at room temperature, can be administered up to a concentration of 100%. They share the property of low blood solubility, thus the induction of general anaesthesia with these agents is rapid, and all are relatively resistant to biotransformation in the body.

NITROUS OXIDE (N_2O)

Nitrous oxide, by far the most commonly used anaesthetic gas, was first prepared by Priestly in 1772 (Priestly 1774), its anaesthetic properties described by Sir Humphry Davy in 1800, and was first used in clinical practice by Colton and Wells in 1844.

Physical properties

Nitrous oxide is a colourless, slightly sweet-smelling, non-irritant gas with a molecular weight of 44.01 and a specific gravity of 1.53 (air = 1). The gas is readily compressible to a clear colourless liquid with a boiling point of −89°C. The oil/water solubility ratio is 3.2 and the blood/gas solubility coefficient 0.47. It is stable in the presence of soda-lime. The gas is neither flammable nor explosive, but it will support combustion of other agents, even in the absence of oxygen, as above 450°C it decomposes into oxygen and nitrogen.

Commercial preparation and storage

Nitrous oxide is prepared commercially by heating ammonium nitrate, impurities being removed by cooling the gas and passing it through water, caustic permanganate and acid scrubbers. The nitrous oxide is dried and stored under pressure in metal cylinders. The critical temperature of the gas is 36.5°C and below that temperature part of the contents of a full cylinder will be in liquid form, the exact proportion and the pressure being dependent on the temperature. At 20°C a full cylinder will have four-fifths of its contents in liquid form at a pressure of 5170 kPa. Latent heat is required for the vaporization of liquid nitrous oxide, and this is obtained from the casing of the cylinder, which rapidly cools and causes freezing of water vapour in the surrounding air. Water must be excluded from inside the cylinder, otherwise it will freeze as the gas passes through the pressure-reducing valve, thus decreasing the rate of gas flow. When the gas is released from a cylinder the pressure at first falls, and is then built up again, as some of the liquid vaporizes. With rapid flows (10 l min^{-1}) there is a sharp linear fall in pressure due to the fall in temperature; however, with low flows (2 l min^{-1}) there is only a small but progressive decrease. Short interruptions in flow allow gas pressure to be built up again as more liquid vaporizes (Jones 1974). A pressure gauge will not indicate the total cylinder contents until all the liquid is exhausted.

Mixtures of nitrous oxide and oxygen can be prepared which will remain gaseous under pressure; the nitrous oxide can be considered as being dissolved in the oxygen. Such premixed cylinders will usually release a gas of constant composition, but the stability decreases as the proportion of nitrous oxide is increased. Equal volumes of nitrous oxide and oxygen are stable unless cooled below −8°C, when the contents separate into liquid nitrous oxide and gaseous oxygen. The cylinder would then deliver a high oxygen mixture at first, but later nearly pure nitrous oxide. If these cylinders are inadvertently chilled they should be stored at room temperature for some hours and then inverted several times to re-establish the original mixture.

Impurities

Impurities created during manufacture of nitrous oxide are ammonia, nitric acid, nitrogen, nitric oxide, nitrogen dioxide, carbon monoxide and water vapour. It is important that these are removed, particularly the higher oxides of nitrogen. Nitrogen dioxide is very toxic and in concentrations greater than 50 parts per million (ppm) causes laryngospasm, reflex inhibition of breathing and cyanosis, due to methaemoglobin formation and altered pulmonary gas exchange. Pulmonary oedema may occur in the acute phase, but characteristically develops after a latent period of a few hours (Greenbaum et al 1967). There is usually a gross impairment of acid–base balance with respiratory acidosis caused by ventilatory failure, and metabolic acidosis from production of nitrous and nitric acids formed from solution of nitrogen dioxide in body fluids. Hypotension may result from the effects of nitrite and nitrate ions on the vascular smooth muscle.

Absorption and fate in the body

When nitrous oxide is inhaled the gas is rapidly absorbed from the alveoli and 100 ml blood will carry 45 ml nitrous oxide in the plasma; it does not combine with haemoglobin. Arterial blood reaches approximately 90% saturation in 10 min, there being a net gas uptake of about 1 l min^{-1} during induction; however, full equilibrium does not occur for several hours. Elimination from the body is rapid, even after prolonged administration, the gas being readily excreted by the lungs with a small amount diffusing through the skin and traces excreted in the urine. While there is no definite evidence of biotransformation there is circumstantial evidence that this may occur. The gas is not biologically inert and metabolism of nitrous oxide by human and rat intestinal contents has been demonstrated (Hong et al 1980).

Transfer of nitrous oxide to closed gas spaces

Nitrous oxide is about 34 times as soluble as nitrogen in the blood, and so will diffuse into any air-containing cavity more rapidly, in proportion to its partial pressure in the blood, than nitrogen molecules will exit. During nitrous oxide anaesthesia any closed gas-filled body cavity will expand and/or gas pressure will increase.

Expansion of a pneumothorax, pneumopericardium or pneumoperitoneum may have serious consequences. Air entering the circulation during nitrous oxide anaesthesia will greatly increase in volume. Spaces enclosed by rigid walls, such as the paranasal sinuses and the middle ear, in which the normal exits are blocked, may undergo rapid increases in pressure during administration of nitrous oxide and barotrauma may occur (Mann et al 1985, Bailie & Restall 1988).

Pharmacology

Central nervous system

Nitrous oxide is a weak anaesthetic with a minimum alveolar concentration value (MAC) of 104% (Hornbein et al 1982). At normal atmospheric pressure it is possible to render some patients unconscious with 80% nitrous oxide in 20% oxygen, but surgical anaesthesia cannot be produced with this agent alone without some degree of hypoxia, as concentrations of 85–90% are necessary. At twice normal atmospheric pressure 50% nitrous oxide with oxygen produces surgical anaesthesia with full oxygenation. The rapid induction of anaesthesia seen when 100% nitrous oxide is inhaled is due more to displacement of oxygen from the brain, rather than to saturation with nitrous oxide to a degree sufficient to cause anaesthesia (Bourne 1954). Consequently, in modern anaesthetic practice, nitrous oxide is never used as the sole agent, but it is widely used in combination with more potent volatile agents where, in concentrations of 60–70%, it reduces by approximately two-thirds the MAC value of the volatile agent. In addition, because of the rapid initial uptake of nitrous oxide, there is a noticeable second gas effect which hastens the uptake of other agents and speeds induction of anaesthesia.

Nitrous oxide alters the sensory thresholds associated with touch, temperature, light and sound (Burns et al 1960). It also alters the sense of time and impairs recent memory (Robson et al 1960). Lower concentrations lead to dissociation from one's environment, whereas higher concentrations produce perseveration, sedation, drowsiness and amnesia (Tomlin et al 1973). The gas also decreases both sensitivity to a stimulus and the ability, or willingness, of a subject to report a perceived stimulus as painful; thus it is a powerful analgesic when used in sub-anaesthetic doses, usually 50% nitrous oxide in oxygen.

Nitrous oxide seems to act primarily by directly depressing spinal transmission of impulses, and inhibitory supraspinal systems may also be activated (Komatsu et al 1981). No consistent changes have been demonstrated in the responsiveness of the thalamic relay nuclei, but a depression of response to nociceptive stimuli by cells in the trigeminal nucleus has been shown during exposure to nitrous oxide (Kitahata et al 1973). There may be a common mechanism of action for opioids and nitrous oxide to explain its analgesic effect. The gas may interact selectively with the opioid receptor–endorphin system, and may stimulate supraspinal centres which in turn activate opioid-releasing spinal cord neurons, which then inhibit the transmission of impulses following painful stimuli. This is supported by the finding that naloxone usually, but not always, partially reverses the analgesic effect of nitrous oxide (Yang et al 1980), but it is probable that other mechanisms of CNS depression also play a part in the analgesic action of the gas.

Investigations into the effects of nitrous oxide on intracranial dynamics give varying results. Sub-anaesthetic doses (50–75%) seem to affect brain metabolism (Fitzpatrick & Gilboe 1982), dilate cerebral blood vessels (Pelligrino et al 1984) and may increase intracranial pressure. However, the deepening of inhalational or intravenous anaesthesia by the addition of nitrous oxide can increase cerebral blood flow and intracranial pressure dramatically (Sakabe et al 1978). Sub-anaesthetic concentrations may also cause large rises in intracranial pressure in patients with a decreased intracranial compliance (Henriksen & Jorgensen 1973).

Cardiovascular system

For many years nitrous oxide was regarded as devoid of cardiovascular side-effects, but recent studies in animals and man show that it has a direct myocardial depressant effect and, possibly due to action on the suprapontine areas of the brain, a sympathomimetic effect (Ebert and Kampine 1989). The latter frequently counters and obscures the former, the end-result being very little overall cardiovascular depression.

It is difficult to measure the effects of nitrous oxide on the circulation because if the gas is used alone in sub-anaesthetic concentrations with adequate oxygenation, psychic factors, such as anxiety and excitement, cause cardiovascular changes, whereas if full anaesthesia is attempted (at normal atmospheric pressure) hypoxia complicates the picture. The addition of other potent anaesthetic agents to maintain anaesthesia will also have an effect on the cardiovascular system. Thus evidence of the effects of nitrous oxide on the circulation must be interpreted with caution.

Price & Helrich (1955) and Motomura and his colleagues (1984) have demonstrated a dose-dependent depression of the dog myocardium in heart/lung preparations, and Eisele et al (1969) found cardiac depressant effects in conscious dogs exposed to 60% nitrous oxide. Inhalation of 40% nitrous oxide results in a 10% reduction in the amplitude of the ballistocardiogram in normal man (Eisele & Smith 1972), with a fall in arterial pressure and a rise in left ventricular end-diastolic pressure in patients suffering from coronary artery disease (Eisele et al 1976). There is substantial evidence of both α- and β-adrenergic effects when nitrous oxide is added during stable halothane (Smith et al 1970) or isoflurane (Dolan et al 1974) anaesthesia, but the sympathomimetic response seems to be less marked in the presence of enflurane anaesthesia (Bennett et al 1977, Smith et al 1978). Hanowell and his colleagues (1982) suggest that in patients with coronary artery disease nitrous oxide is better tolerated during halothane than during enflurane anaesthesia.

Addition of nitrous oxide to high-dose morphine anaesthesia causes an increase in systemic vascular resistance (Stoelting & Gibbs 1973, Lappas et al 1975), an α-adrenergic effect, and a decrease in cardiac output and heart rate, a cardiac depressant effect (McDermott & Stanley 1974). The cardiac depression may be explained by the ability of opioids to block the centrally mediated β-adrenergic stimulation normally associated with nitrous oxide (Flaim et al 1978). Similar depression of myocardial function has been observed when nitrous oxide is added to high-dose fentanyl anaesthesia (Lunn et al 1979, Meretoja et al 1985).

Nitrous oxide usually elevates central venous pressure (Winter et al 1972), and although this may be caused by myocardial depression it is more likely to be due to an increase in venous tone with a consequent decrease in venous compliance (Eisele & Smith 1972). Increased pulmonary vascular resistance also occurs with nitrous oxide, particularly in patients with pre-existing pulmonary hypertension, and this may contribute to an increase in right atrial pressure.

The results of studies of the effects of nitrous oxide on myocardial blood flow are conflicting. Thorburn and colleagues (1979) found no change in coronary blood flow, vascular resistance or myocardial oxygen consumption in dogs exposed to 70% nitrous oxide, while Dottori et al (1976) found an increase in coronary flow and decreased vascular resistance during 80% nitrous oxide. Moffitt et al (1983) found that the addition of 50% nitrous oxide to patients anaesthetized with halothane decreased coronary sinus blood flow by 36%. However Mitchell and colleagues (1989) could find no evidence that nitrous oxide, when used as an adjunct to fentanyl anaesthesia, induced myocardial ischaemia in patients with coronary artery disease.

Nitrous oxide, like all anaesthetics, depresses the baroreceptor reflexes. However, the degree of depression is difficult to estimate because of the limited potency of the gas and the common use of a background anaesthetic.

A leftward shift of the oxyhaemoglobin dissociation curve occurs in blood samples exposed to 50% nitrous oxide (Fournier & Major 1984); this may be important clinically when estimating arterial oxygen tensions from haemoglobin saturation levels.

Respiratory system

Nitrous oxide decreases the tidal volume and increases the respiratory rate and minute ventilation, arterial carbon dioxide tension tending to remain within normal limits (Hornbein et al 1982). However, the normal ventilatory response to increased levels of arterial carbon dioxide is markedly depressed (Winter et al 1972), and the response to hypoxia is also significantly reduced (Knill & Clement 1982).

The greater density of nitrous oxide produces slightly more airway resistance than oxygen or air. Alveolar collapse by absorption of gases in an obstructed lung segment may also be more rapid with nitrous oxide than with nitrogen, due to greater solubility of the former. In addition, nitrous oxide depresses mucociliary flow and neutrophil chemotaxis (Nunn & O'Morain 1982). All these features may predispose to postoperative respiratory complications.

During recovery from nitrous oxide anaesthesia the rapid outpouring of the gas from the lungs will cause dilution of other gases, most importantly oxygen, and this can cause hypoxia (Fink 1955).

Alimentary system

Nitrous oxide is known to cause nausea and vomiting, probably by both a peripheral and a central action (Janhunen & Tammisto 1972; Lonie & Harper 1986). The peripheral effects may be due to distension of the gastrointestinal tract by transfer of nitrous oxide to gas already present in the bowel; this is particularly likely in anxious patients in whom air swallowing results in a high initial gut volume (Eger 1974). Parkhouse and his colleagues (1960) found that the incidence of nausea and vomiting increases when higher concentrations of nitrous oxide are used, and when the duration of administration is prolonged; these are also factors which would favour maximum transfer of nitrous oxide into the gut. It has been suggested that, as nitrous oxide has been shown to interact with the endogenous opioid system, it shares with other opiate and opioid substances substantial central emetic properties (Gillman 1985).

In patients with intestinal obstruction nitrous oxide transfer to gas in the obstructed segment of bowel may make surgical procedures more difficult. However, in the majority of these cases the blood supply to the obstructed segment of gut is much reduced and, as a consequence, gas transfer is slow and may not be of much practical significance.

Muscular system

Nitrous oxide, either by itself or in combination with narcotics, increases skeletal muscle activity and does not seem to have any effect on the neuromuscular blockade produced by non-depolarizing muscle relaxants (Sokoll et al 1972). It is thought that the gas causes increased muscle activity through a supraspinal effect, rather than by an alteration in the stretch reflexes or an increase in reflex excitability of the spinal motor neurons (Freund et al 1973).

Toxic effects

A few hours of exposure to anaesthetic concentrations of nitrous oxide cause almost total inactivation of methylcobalamin (vitamin B_{12}), which is the bound cofactor of the enzyme methionine synthase (Deacon et al 1980, Royston et al 1988). Methionine synthase activity is required for the conversion of homocysteine to methionine, and for the demethylation of methyltetrahydrofolate. The latter is one of the precursors of 5,10-methylene tetrahydrofolate, which is required for the conversion of deoxyuridine to thymidine, a DNA base. Activity of hepatic betaine–homocysteine methyltransferase increases to compensate partially for the decrease in methionine synthase activity (Lumb et al 1983); nevertheless, serum methionine concentrations decrease rapidly to very low levels in patients anaesthetized with nitrous oxide (Koblin et al 1982, Skacel et al 1983). In healthy subjects a measurable effect on DNA synthesis in the bone marrow, as measured by the capacity of the marrow to convert deoxyuridine to thymidine (the deoxyuridine suppression test), does not occur unless exposure continues for 6–12 h (O'Sullivan et al 1981), and the effects appear to be readily reversible on cessation of administration of nitrous oxide. However, in seriously ill patients evidence of depression of DNA synthesis in the bone marrow may be detected following exposure to nitrous oxide for 2 h or less (Amos et al 1982, Nunn et al 1986). This disturbance of DNA synthesis is almost certainly the cause of the megaloblastic changes seen in normal human marrow after 24 h exposure to 50% nitrous oxide (Amess et al 1978); similar changes occurring after much shorter periods of exposure in very ill patients (Nunn et al 1986). Longer exposure to the gas will result in depression of all bone marrow elements and the reticulo-endothelial system, with consequent leucopenia and thrombocytopenia in the peripheral blood, which can be fatal in some cases (Lassen et al 1956).

Hepatic S-adenosylmethionine concentrations also decrease (Lumb et al 1983), and this is thought to be responsible for the neurological changes, resembling those of subacute combined degeneration of the cord, which follow repeated exposure to high concentrations of nitrous oxide, typically seen in chronic abusers of the gas (Layzer et al 1978, Scott & Weir 1981).

Nitrous oxide also has an inhibitory action on methionine synthesis at a concentration very much lower than that at which it exerts any other measurable effect. This provides a mechanism which can explain all of the toxic effects for which exposure to trace concentrations of nitrous oxide have been blamed, except for performance decrement. Methionine synthase inactivation has been clearly demonstrated in rats exposed to concentrations of nitrous oxide of as little as 1000 ppm (Sharer et al 1983). Fetotoxicity in rats has been shown after exposure to 70% nitrous oxide on the 9th day of pregnancy (Lane et al 1980) and following exposure to 1000 ppm (but not 500 ppm or less) of the gas throughout pregnancy (Viera et al 1980). Unscavenged and poorly ventilated operating theatres can accumulate nitrous oxide in concentrations greater than 1000 ppm (Davenport et al 1980, Gray 1989), and dentists and their assistants can be exposed to levels in excess of 5000 ppm (Hillman et al 1981). Therefore there is a real possibility that theatre and dental staff can inhale sufficient amounts of the gas to cause significant inhibition of methionine synthase. A epidemiological study in personnel chronically exposed to trace concentrations of nitrous oxide has found evidence of an increased risk of spontaneous abortion, or damage to the developing fetus, in the early stages of pregnancy, and an increased incidence of liver, kidney and neurological disease (Cohen et al 1980). In contrast, single exposures of less than 6 h to anaesthetic concentrations of nitrous oxide have not been shown to have any adverse effects on the fetus during the first or second trimesters of pregnancy (Crawford & Lewis 1986, Aldridge & Tunstall 1986).

It is suggested that the maximum safe concentration of nitrous oxide is of the order of 100–200 ppm, measured on the basis of a time-weighted sample (Sharer et al 1983), although the American National Institute for Occupational Safety and Health suggest that much lower levels are desirable (25 ppm).

Administration

Equal volumes of nitrous oxide and oxygen are frequently administered to provide analgesia using either a preset intermittent flow machine, such as the Lucy Baldwin, or from premixed cylinders attached to an Entonox demand flow head. For general anaesthesia for minor surgery nitrous oxide can be given using an intermittent-flow machine and supplemented, as necessary, with small concentrations of more powerful volatile agents. For major surgery continuous flows of the gas are used and supplemented with volatile and/or intravenous agents, myoneural blocking drugs providing muscle relaxation if required.

CYCLOPROPANE (C_3H_6)

Cyclopropane was first prepared by Freund in 1882, and in 1929 Lucas and Henderson noted that it possessed good anaesthetic properties, but it was Waters and his colleagues who introduced the gas into clinical anaesthesia in 1933 (Waters & Schmidt 1934).

Physical properties

Cyclopropane is a colourless, sweet-smelling gas which is irritant to the respiratory tract in high concentrations (over 40%). It has a molecular weight of 42.08 and a specific gravity of 1.45 (air = 1). The gas is readily compressible to a liquid with a boiling point of $-33°C$ and a critical temperature of 125°C. The oil/water solubility is 6.8 and the blood/gas solubility coefficient 0.42. It is stable in the presence of soda-lime but it will attack and diffuse through rubber. Cyclopropane is highly flammable and forms explosive mixtures with air (2.4–10.4%), oxygen (2.5–60%) and nitrous oxide (3–30%). The addition of helium, in a concentration of 30% or more, to cyclopropane–oxygen mixtures reduces the risk of explosions.

Commercial preparation and storage

Cyclopropane can be prepared from the natural gas found in the United States, or from trimethylene glycol, which is produced during the fermentation of molasses. Trimethylene glycol is reacted with hydrobromic acid to form trimethylene dibromide, which is then treated with zinc to produce cyclopropane and zinc dibromide.

The gas is stored as a liquid in orange-coloured cylinders at a pressure of 517 kPa at 15°C.

Impurities

Propylene, allene, cyclohexane, carbon dioxide, some halides such as brom- and chlor-propane, and nitrogen are possible impurities. Propylene in concentrations above 3% can be dangerous.

Absorption and fate in the body

Cyclopropane is absorbed from the alveoli and carried in the blood attached principally to the red cells because of their high protein and lipoprotein content. Some is attached to serum protein, but only a small proportion is physically dissolved in the plasma as the water-solubility of the gas is low.

It is unlikely that any significant biotransformation takes place in the body, although Van Dyke and Chenoworth (1965) suggested that cyclopropane could be metabolized into carbon dioxide. The gas is excreted almost entirely by the lungs, although a small quantity diffuses through the skin. Approximately 50% of the gas is eliminated within 10 min of discontinuing the administration.

Pharmacology

Central nervous system

Cyclopropane is a potent anaesthetic agent with a MAC value of 9.2 vol.%. Breathing a 50% mixture of cyclopropane with oxygen produces loss of consciousness within 30 s, which is rapidly followed by central depression of respiration and apnoea. Analgesia can be obtained with 4%, surgical anaesthesia maintained with 9% and deep anaesthesia with 20–30% of the gas.

Cyclopropane increases sympathetic nervous activity by selective depression of certain inhibitory neurons in the medulla, and a possible excitatory action on spinal cord neurons (Price et al 1969).

Low concentrations of cyclopropane reduce cerebral blood flow, whereas high concentrations cause an increased blood flow and a rise in intracranial pressure. Postoperative headache is more common than with other anaesthetics.

Cardiovascular system

Cyclopropane is a direct myocardial depressant; when administered to the heart–lung preparation the depressant effect is directly proportional to the concentration used. In humans this effect is counteracted by the central sympathetic stimulant action so that, under light anaesthesia, there is an increase in cardiac output with a rise in right ventricular stroke volume, stroke work, end-diastolic pressure, total peripheral resistance and arterial blood pressure. Central venous pressure is also raised and skin blood flow is markedly increased (Cullen et al 1969). As depth of anaesthesia is increased cardiac output falls to normal, or below normal, values. Noradrenaline concentration in the myocardium increases proportionately with the cyclopropane concentration, but adrenaline levels are unchanged. Circulating catecholamine levels are also raised and withdrawal of cyclopropane is accompanied by an abrupt fall in these levels. This may be a contributory factor to the hypotension which can follow deep levels of cyclopropane anaesthesia (cyclopropane shock), particularly likely if respiratory acidosis has been allowed to occur.

Cyclopropane may increase vagal activity, though this is usually counteracted by the increased sympathetic action, so that the change in heart rate is negligible in the unpremedicated patient (Price 1961). Following a narcotic premedication cyclopropane usually causes a slowing of the heart rate (Li and Etsten 1957). If the vagal stimulant effect is blocked by i.v. atropine a dramatic increase in heart rate occurs, and this is augmented by the unrestrained sympathetic stimulant effect of the cyclopropane. In this situation there is a high incidence of dysrhythmias with a risk of ventricular fibrillation (Eger 1962). The incidence of dysrhythmias under cyclopropane anaesthesia also increases with increasing depth of anaesthesia, particularly so when arterial carbon dioxide tension is allowed to rise (Lurie et al 1958).

Respiratory system

Cyclopropane is a marked respiratory depressant producing a progressive reduction in alveolar ventilation as anaesthesia deepens. In the unpremedicated patient respiratory rate increases, but not enough to compensate for the reduction in tidal volume. Following a narcotic premedication the respiratory rate may be unchanged, or decreased, as cyclopropane anaesthesia deepens, with profound hypoventilation at an earlier stage. In animal experiments cyclopropane has been shown to cause bronchoconstriction, and in clinical anaesthesia laryngospasm is not uncommon during light anaesthesia.

Muscular system

Depression of skeletal muscle tone is not marked until deep levels of anaesthesia are obtained; plain muscle is unaffected.

Effects on other organs

There is a transient and slight depression of liver and kidney function, and blood flow is reduced in these organs (Price et al 1965). At the same time there is a rise in anti-diuretic hormone and renin plasma levels. Cyclopropane readily crosses the placental barrier to cause respiratory depression in the fetus; uterine contractions are depressed in direct relationship to the concentration used. There is a slight rise in blood sugar during cyclopropane anaesthesia, and post-operative nausea and vomiting are very common.

Toxic effects

There is an adequate margin of safety between anaesthetic and toxic concentrations of cyclopropane, but because of its low blood solubility it is easy to achieve dangerously deep levels of anaesthesia quickly. Cardiac arrhythmias are the principal danger and are most likely with deep levels of anaesthesia combined with inadequate ventilation.

Administration

Cyclopropane is expensive and so the gas, mixed with oxygen, is administered through a closed-circuit anaesthetic system with carbon dioxide absorption. The use of cyclopropane has declined because of its explosive properties and tendency to produce cardiac arrhythmias, though it is still occasionally used for induction of anaesthesia in children.

ETHYLENE (C_2H_4)

There is some doubt as to the exact date of preparation of the hydrocarbon ethylene, perhaps by Becher in 1669, or by Ingenhousz in 1779 (Atkinson et al 1987). Luckhart first observed its anaesthetic and analgesic properties in animals, while in 1923 Luckhart and Carter reported their findings on the use of the gas in human subjects (Luckhart & Carter 1923).

Physical properties

Ethylene is a colourless, non-irritating gas with a slightly sweetish but rather unpleasant odour. It has a molecular weight of 28.03 and a specific gravity of 0.97. Below 9.7°C it is compressible to a liquid with a boiling point of −104°C. The oil/gas coefficient is 1.28 and the blood/gas solubility coefficient 0.14. It is stable in the presence of soda-lime and diffuses through rubber. The gas is highly flammable and forms explosive mixtures with air (3.1–32%) or oxygen (3–80%). The addition of helium or nitrogen reduces the explosive range.

Commercial preparation and storage

Ethylene is prepared commercially by the dehydration of ethyl alcohol with either sulphuric or phosphoric acid.

Impurities

Possible impurities are alcohol, aldehydes, ether, oxides of sulphur or phosphorus, carbon monoxide, carbon dioxide, acetylenes and olefins. These are either contaminants produced during the manufacture or are decomposition products.

Pharmacology

Ethylene is rapidly absorbed from the lungs and in concentrations of 100% will produce unconsciousness slightly more rapidly than nitrous oxide, while 80–90% is required for anaesthesia, and 20–40% for analgesia. Compared to nitrous oxide ethylene produces slightly more muscle relaxation, but has the disadvantages of being a highly explosive gas with an unpleasant smell, and causing a higher incidence of postoperative nausea and vomiting.

Ethylene is rapidly eliminated from the body through the lungs, a small amount diffusing through the skin and a tiny fraction may be broken down in the body to carbon dioxide (Van Dyke & Chenoworth 1965).

XENON

Xenon is manufactured by the fractional distillation of liquid air. This inert gas has similar anaesthetic properties to nitrous oxide with a MAC value of 71% (Cullen et al 1967) it is claimed to be less toxic to the developing fetus (Lane et al 1980), and to produce more stable cardiovascular conditions during surgery with an absence of an increase in plasma adrenaline levels (Boomsa et al 1990). However, its prohibitive cost precludes its widespread clinical use.

REFERENCES

Aldridge L M, Tunstall M E 1986 Nitrous oxide and the fetus. British Journal of Anaesthesia 58: 1348–1356

Amess J A L, Burman J F, Rees G M, Nancekievill D G, Molin D L 1978 Megaloblastic haemopoiesis in patients receiving nitrous oxide. Lancet 2: 339–342

Amos R J, Amess J A L, Hinds C J, Mollin D L 1982 Incidence and pathogenesis of acute megaloblastic bone marrow change in patients receiving intensive care. Lancet 2: 835–838

Atkinson R S, Rushman G B, Lee J A 1987 A synopsis of anaesthesia. Wright, Bristol p 177

Bailie R, Restall J 1988 Otic barotrauma due to nitrous oxide. Anaesthesia 43: 888–889

Bennett G M, Loeser E A, Kawamura R, Stanley T H 1977 Cardiovascular response to nitrous oxide during enflurane and oxygen anesthesia. Anesthesiology 46: 227–229

Boomsma F, Rupreht J, Man in 't Veld A J, de Jong F H, Dzoljic M, Lachmann B 1990 Haemodynamic and neurohumoral effects of xenon anaesthesia. A comparison with nitrous oxide. Anaesthesia 45: 273–278

Bourne J G 1954 General anaesthesia for out-patients with special reference to dental extraction. Proceedings of the Royal Society of Medicine 47: 416–422

Burns B D, Robson J G, Welt P J L 1960 The effects of nitrous oxide upon sensory thresholds. Canadian Anaesthetists' Society Journal 7: 411–422

Cohen E N, Brown B W, Wu M L, Whitcher C E, Brodsky J B, Gift H C, Greenfield W, Jones T W, Driscoll E J, 1980 Occupational disease in dentistry and chronic exposure to trace anesthetic gases. Journal of the American Dental Association 101: 21–31

Crawford J S, Lewis M 1986 Nitrous oxide in early pregnancy. Anaesthesia 41: 900–905

Cullen D J, Eger E I, Gregory G A 1969 The cardiovascular effects of cyclopropane in man. Anesthesiology 31: 398–406

Cullen S C, Eger E I, Gregory P 1967 Use of xenon and xenon-halothane in a study of basic mechanisms of anesthesia in man. Anesthesiology 28: 243–244

Davenport H T, Halsey M J, Wardley-Smith B, Bateman P E 1980 Occupational exposure to anaesthetics in 20 hospitals. Anaesthesia 35: 354–359

Davy H 1800 Researches, Chemical and Philosophical chiefly concerning Nitrous Oxide. London.

Deacon R, Lumb M, Perry J, Chanarin I, Minty B, Halsey M, Nunn J 1980 Inactivation of methionine synthase by nitrous oxide. European Journal of Biochemistry 104: 419–423

Dolan W M, Stevens W C, Eger E I (II), Cromwell T H, Halsey M J, Shakespeare T F, Miller R D 1974 The cardio-vascular and respiratory effects of isoflurane–nitrous oxide anaesthesia. Canadian Anaesthetists' Society Journal 21: 557–568

Dottori O, Haggendal E, Linder E, Nordstrom G, Seeman T 1976 The haemodynamic effects of nitrous oxide on myocardial blood flow in dogs. Acta Anaesthesiologica Scandinavica 20: 421–428

Ebert T J, Kampine J P 1989 Nitrous oxide augments sympathetic outflow: direct evidence from human peroneal nerve endings. Anesthesia and Analgesia 69: 444–449

Eger E I (II) 1962 Atropine, scopolamine, and related compounds. Anesthesiology 23: 365–383

Eger E I (II) 1974 Anesthetic uptake and action. Williams and Wilkins, Baltimore, p. 174

Eisele J H, Trenchard D, Stubbs J, Guz A 1969 The immediate cardiac depression by anaesthetics in conscious dogs. British Journal of Anaesthesia 41: 86–93

Eisele J H, Smith N T 1972 Cardiovascular effects of 40 per cent nitrous oxide in man. Anesthesia and Analgesia 51: 956–963

Eisele J H, Reitan J A, Massumi R A, Zellis R F, Miller R R 1976 Myocardial performance and N_2O analgesia in coronary-artery disease. Anesthesiology 44: 16–20

Fink B R 1955 Diffusion anoxia. Anesthesiology 16: 511–519

Fitzpatrick J H Gilboe D D 1982 Effects of nitrous oxide on cerebrovascular tone, oxygen metabolism and electroencephalogram of the isolated perfused canine brain. Anesthesiology 57: 480–484

Flaim S F, Zelis R Eisele J H 1978 Differential effects of morphine on forearm blood flow: attenuation of sympathetic control of the cutaneous circulation. Clinical Pharmacology and Therapeutics 23: 542–546

Fournier L, Major D 1984 The effect of nitrous oxide on the oxyhaemoglobin dissociation curve. Canadian Anaesthetists' Society Journal 31: 173–177

Freund A 1882 Uber Trimethylene. Monatshefte für Chemie 3: 625

Freund F G, Martin W E, Wond K C, Hornbein T F 1973 Abdominal-muscle rigidity induced by morphine and nitrous oxide. Anesthesiology 38: 358–362

Gillman M A 1985 Nitrous oxide and its opioid emetic properties. Canadian Anaesthetists' Society Journal 32: 315

Gray W M 1989 Occupational exposure to nitrous oxide in four hospitals. Anaesthesia 44: 511–514

Greenbaum R, Bay J, Hargreaves M D, Kain M L, Kelman G R, Nunn J F, Prys-Roberts C, Siebold K 1967 Effects of higher oxides of nitrogen on the anaesthetised dog. British Journal of Anaesthesia 39: 393–403

Hanowell S T, Kim Y D, Jones M, Pierce E, Macnamara T E 1982 N_2O addition to halothane and enflurane: depressant or stimulant in coronary artery disease? Anesthesiology 57: A77

Henriksen H T, Jorgensen P B 1973 The effect of nitrous oxide on intracranial pressure in patients with intracranial disorders. British Journal of Anaesthesia 45: 486–492

Hillman K M, Saloojee Y, Brett I I, Cole P V 1981 Nitrous oxide in the dental surgery. Atmospheric and blood concentrations of personnel. Anaesthesia 36: 257–262

Hong K, Trudell J R, O'Neil J R, Cohen E N 1980 Metabolism of nitrous oxide by human and rat intestinal contents. Anesthesiology 52: 16–19

Hornbein T F, Eger E I (II), Winter P M, Smith G, Wetstone D, Smith K H 1982 The minimum alveolar concentration of nitrous oxide in man. Anesthesia and Analgesia 61: 553–556

Janhunen L, Tammisto T 1972 Postoperative vomiting after different modes of general anaesthesia. Annales Chirurgicae et Gynaecologicae Fennicae 61: 152–159

Jones P L 1974 Some observations on nitrous oxide cylinders during emptying. British Journal of Anaesthesia 46: 534–538

Kitahata L M, McAllister R G, Taub A 1973 Identification of central trigeminal nociceptors and the effects of nitrous oxide. Anesthesiology 38: 12–19

Knill R L, Clement J L 1982 Variable effects of anaesthetics on the ventilatory response to hypoxaemia in man.

Canadian Anaesthetists' Society Journal 29: 93–99

Koblin D D, Waskell L, Watson J E, Stokstad E L R, Eger E I 1982 Nitrous oxide inactivates methionine synthetase in human liver. Anesthesia and Analgesia 61: 75–78

Komatsu T, Shingu K, Tomemori N, Urabe N, Mori K 1981 Nitrous oxide activates the supraspinal pain inhibition system. Acta Anaesthesiologica Scandinavica 25: 519–522

Lane G A, Nahrwold M L, Tait A R, Taylor-Busch M, Cohen P J, Beaudoin A R 1980 Anesthetics as teratogens: nitrous oxide is fetotoxic, xenon is not. Science 210: 899–901

Lappas D G, Buckley M J, Laver M B, Daggett W M, Lowenstein E 1975 Left ventricular performance and pulmonary circulation following addition of nitrous oxide to morphine during coronary artery surgery. Anesthesiology 43: 61–69

Lassen H C A, Henriksen A, Neukirch F, Kristensen H S 1956 Treatment of tetanus. Severe bone marrow depression after prolonged nitrous-oxide anaesthesia. Lancet 1: 527–530

Layzer R B, Fishman R A, Schafer J A 1978 Neuropathy following abuse of nitrous oxide. Neurology 28: 504–506

Li T H, Etsten B 1957 Effect of cyclopropane anesthesia on cardiac output and related hemodynamics in man. Anesthesiology 18: 15–32

Lonie D S, Harper N J N 1986 Nitrous oxide anaesthesia and vomiting. The effect of nitrous oxide anaesthesia on the incidence of vomiting following gynaecological laparoscopy. Anaesthesia 41: 703–707

Lucas G H W, Henderson V E 1929 A new anaesthetic gas: cyclopropane. A preliminary report. Canadian Medical Association Journal 21: 173–175

Luckhart A B, Carter J B 1923 Ethylene as a gas anesthetic; preliminary communication. Clinical experience in 106 surgical operations. Journal of the American Medical Association 80: 1440–1442

Lumb M, Sharer N, Deacon R, Jennings P, Purkiss P, Perry J, Chanarin I 1983 Effects of nitrous-induced inactivation of cobalamin on methionine and S-adenosylmethionine in the rat. Biochimica et Biophysica Acta 756: 354–359

Lunn J K, Stanley T H, Eisele J, Webster L, Woodward A 1979 High dose fentanyl anesthesia for coronary artery surgery: Plasma fentanyl concentrations and influence of nitrous oxide on cardiovascular response. Anesthesia and Analgesia 58: 390–395

Lurie A A, Jones R E, Linde H W, Price M L, Dripps R D, Price H L 1958 Cyclopropane anesthesia. 1. Cardiac rate and rhythm during steady levels of cyclopropane anesthesia at normal and elevated end-expiratory carbon dioxide tensions. Anesthesiology 19: 457–472

McDermott R W, Stanley T H 1974 The cardiovascular effects of low concentrations of nitrous oxide during morphine anesthesia. Anesthesiology 41: 89–91

Mann M S, Woodsford P V, Jones R M 1985 Anaesthetic carrier gases. Their effect on middle ear pressure peri-operatively. Anaesthesia 40: 8–11

Meretoja O A, Takkunen O, Heikkila H, Wegelius U 1985 Haemodynamic response to nitrous oxide during high-dose fentanyl pancuronium anaesthesia. Acta Anaesthesiologica Scandinavica 29: 137–141

Mitchell M M, Prakash O, Rulf E N R, van Daele M E R M, Cahazan M K, Roelandt J R T C 1989 Nitrous

oxide does not induce myocardial ischemia in patients with ischemic heart disease and poor left ventricular function. Anesthesiology 71: 526–534

Moffitt E A, Sethna D H, Gary R J, Raymond M J, Matloff J M, Bussell J A, 1983 Nitrous oxide added to halothane reduces coronary flow and myocardial oxygen consumption in patients with coronary disease. Canadian Anaesthetists' Society Journal 30: 5–9

Motomura S, Kissin I, Aultman D F, Reves J G 1984 Effects of fentanyl and nitrous oxide on contractility of blood-perfused papillary muscle of the dog. Anesthesia and Analgesia 63: 47–50

Nunn J F, O'Morain C 1982 Nitrous oxide decreases motility of human neutrophils in vitro. Anesthesiology 56: 45–48

Nunn J F, Chanarin I, Tanner A G, Owen E R T C 1986 Megaloblastic bone marrow changes after repeated nitrous oxide anaesthesia. British Journal of Anaesthesia 58: 1469–1470

O'Sullivan H, Jennings F, Ward K, McCann S, Scott J M, Weir D G 1981 Human bone marrow biochemical function and megaloblastic hematopoiesis after nitrous oxide anesthesia. Anesthesiology 55: 645–649

Parkhouse J, Henrie J R, Duncan G M, Rome H P 1960 Nitrous oxide analgesia in relation to mental performance. Journal of Pharmacology and Experimental Therapeutics 128: 44–54

Pelligrino D A, Miletich D J, Hoffman W E, Albrecht R F 1984 Nitrous oxide markedly increases cerebral cortical metabolic rate and blood flow in the goat. Anesthesiology 60: 405–412

Price H L 1961 Circulatory actions of general anesthetic agents and the homeostatic roles of epinephrine and norepinephrine. Clinical Pharmacology and Therapeutics 2: 163–176

Price H L, Helrich M 1955 The effects of cyclopropane, diethyl ether, nitrous oxide, thiopentone and hydrogen ion concentration on the myocardial function of the dog heart–lung preparation. Journal of Pharmacology and Experimental Therapeutics 115: 206–216

Price H L, Deutsch S, Cooperman L H, Clement A J, Epstein R M 1965 Splanchnic circulation during cyclopropane anesthesia in normal man. Anesthesiology 26: 312–319

Price H L, Warden J C, Cooperman L H, Millar R A 1969 Central sympathetic excitation caused by cyclopropane. Anesthesiology 30: 426–438

Priestly J 1774 Experiments and observations on different kinds of Air. London

Robson J G, Burns B D, Welt P J L 1960 The effect of inhaling dilute nitrous oxide upon recent memory and time estimation. Canadian Anaesthetists' Society Journal 7: 399–410

Royston B D, Nunn J F, Weinbren H F, Royston D, Cormack R S 1988 Rate of inactivation of human and rodent hepatic methionine synthase by nitrous oxide. Anesthesiology 68: 213–216

Sakabe T, Kuramoto T, Inoue S, Takeshita H 1978 Cerebral effects of nitrous oxide in the dog. Anesthesiology 48: 195–200

Scott J M, Weir D G 1981 The methyl folate trap. Lancet 2: 337–340

Sharer N M, Nunn J F, Royston J P, Chanarin I 1983 Effects of chronic exposure to nitrous oxide on methionine synthase activity. British Journal of Anaesthesia 55: 693–701

Skacel P O, Hewlett A M, Lewis J D, Lumb M, Nunn J F, Chanarin I 1983 Studies on the haemopoietic toxicity of nitrous oxide in man. British Journal of Anaesthesia 53: 189–200

Smith N T, Eger E I (II), Stoelting R K, Whayne T F, Cullen D, Kadis L B 1970 The cardiovascular and sympathomimetic responses to the addition of nitrous oxide to halothane in man. Anesthesiology 32: 410–421

Smith N T, Calverley R K, Prys-Roberts C, Eger E I (II), Jones C W 1978 Impact of nitrous oxide on the circulation during enflurane anesthesia in man. Anesthesiology 48: 345–349

Sokoll M D, Hoyt J L, Gergis S D 1972 Studies in muscle rigidity, nitrous oxide and narcotic analgesic agents. Anesthesia and Analgesia 51: 16–20

Stoelting R K, Gibbs P S 1973 Hemodynamic effects of morphine and morphine-nitrous oxide in valvular heart disease and coronary-artery disease. Anesthesiology 38: 45–52

Thorburn J, Smith G, Vance J P, Brown D M 1979 Effects of nitrous oxide on the cardiovascular system and coronary circulation of the dog. British Journal of Anaesthesia 51: 937–942

Tomlin P J, Jones B C, Edwards R, Robin P E 1973 Subjective and objective responses to inhalation of nitrous oxide and methoxyflurane. British Journal of Anaesthesia 45: 719–724

Van Dyke R A, Chenoworth M B 1965 Metabolism of volatile anesthetics. Anesthesiology 26: 343–357

Viera E, Cleaton-Jones P, Austin J C, Moyes D G, Shaw R 1980 Effects of low concentrations of nitrous oxide on rat fetuses. Anesthesia and Analgesia 59: 175–177

Waters R M, Schmidt E R 1934 Cyclopropane anesthesia. Journal of the American Medical Association 103: 975–983

Winter P M, Hornbein T F, Smith G, Sullivan D, Smith K H 1972 Hyperbaric nitrous oxide anesthesia in man: Determination of anesthetic potency (MAC) and cardiorespiratory effects. Abstracts of American Society of Anesthesiologists Annual Meeting, Boston, October 1972, pp. 103–104

Yang J C, Crawford Clark W, Ngai S H 1980 Antagonism of nitrous oxide by nalaxone in man. Anesthesiology 52: 414–417

9. Barbiturates

J. W. Dundee

The barbiturates are compounds prepared from the combination of malonic acid and urea. They were once widely used as sedative–hypnotic drugs, but the dangers of dependence and tolerance and a very organized anti-barbiturate lobby (CURB – Campaign for the Use and Restriction of Barbiturates, 1976–1977) aimed at reducing over-prescribing, led to their almost complete replacement by the safer benzodiazepines. Their main use is now as anti-epileptics or intravenous anaesthetics, and this chapter concentrates mainly on the latter. The term 'barbiturate' is used here also to include the thiobarbiturates.

HISTORY

Barbituric acid, alternatively known as malonyl urea, was first prepared in 1864 by Adolf von Baeyer, who achieved fame in 1905 by receiving the award of the Nobel Prize for chemistry for work unconnected with the barbiturates. The word *Barbiturate* is a combination of the name *Barbara* with urea. It has been suggested that Barbara was either his mother or a girlfriend — his wife's name was not Barbara and he was not married until several years later. An alternative story suggests that von Baeyer celebrated the discovery of the drug by visiting a nearby tavern frequented by artillery officers on St Barbara's Day, Barbara being the patron saint of artillery officers, and in the ensuing festivities Barbara was amalgamated with urea to give the new compound its name. Barbituric acid was devoid of hypnotic activity and in 1903 Fischer and von Mering synthesized barbitone (the sodium salt of di-ethyl barbituric acid) which was given the trade name of 'Veronal', derived from Verona where Fischer had recently spent a holiday. Later in 1921 they introduced Somnifen, a combination of the diethyl amines of diethyl barbituric acid and diallyl barbituric acid, which achieved some popularity in continental Europe. There are few clinical data on its use and the lack of scientific interest in this field is shown by the formulation of the drug being changed from a diallyl to allypropyl side chain without any record of it in the literature. The early 1930s saw a profusion of new barbiturates, some of which were, for a time, adapted for intravenous anaesthesia. These included amylobarbitone and pentobarbitone.

Intravenous anaesthesia came of age in 1932 with the report by Weese and Scharpff on hexobarbitone (Evipal or Evipan) the first rapidly acting intravenous barbiturate, and its acceptance was widespread and enthusiastic. It was estimated that within the first 12 years some 10 million administrations of the drug had taken place. In contrast to previous barbiturates, adequate doses of hexobarbitone would induce anaesthesia in one arm–brain circulation time, allowing a flexibility of dosage comparable with the inhalational agents.

Meanwhile research had been progressing with a new group of hypnotically active thiobarbiturates (Tabern & Volwiler 1935) and in 1934 John S. Lundy from the Mayo Clinic, and Ralph M. Waters from Madison, Wisconsin, started clinical trials of thiopentone; these men worked simultaneously and although Lundy published the first report (Lundy & Tovell 1934) Waters had the distinction of giving the first clinical administration of thiopentone (Pratt et al 1936).

The acceptance of intravenous barbiturates varied from country to country. The early popularity of this form of induction was greater in the United States than elsewhere, but showed a distinct falling off in the 1942–1943 period following the tragic results from its indiscriminate use at Pearl Harbor. By contrast, induction of anaesthesia by intravenous agents in Britain was limited up to 1944–1945, after which it grew rapidly, and by 1955 it was used in about 90% of all anaesthetics.

The first demonstration of the synergistic action of thiopentone with nitrous oxide and oxygen was by Organe & Broad from the Westminster Hospital, London, in 1938, and is an almost forgotten landmark in the development of its clinical use. It is the forerunner of our present-day 'balanced techniques', and played a major part in the universal acceptance of thiopentone as an induction agent. Despite some competition from other barbiturates, thiopentone has remained essentially unchallenged among the intravenous anaesthetics. *Thiamylal*, an equally good agent, was passed over for another 15 years (Dornette 1954) and today remains a comparatively little-used but very acceptable substitute for thiopentone.

The next advance came in 1957 with the synthesis of methohexitone, known originally as Lilly 25 398 (Stoelting 1957). It is the only member of the barbiturate series which offers any real competition to thiopentone, although now in a rather different and limited field, such as outpatient operations, dental procedures and electroconvulsive therapy. Its more rapid recovery, as compared with thiopentone, has been convincingly confirmed.

Two other thiobarbiturates, buthalitone and methitural, were later introduced into anaesthesia but abandoned after a time because of the high incidence of induction complications. Thialbarbitone is another satisfactory thiobarbiturate, which for a time enjoyed a limited popularity, but is now withdrawn from clinical use.

CLINICAL GROUPING

The classical grouping of the barbiturates, based on the expected duration of action of normal therapeutic doses, includes drugs given by mouth and those injected intravenously.

Long: Oral (or intramuscular) preparations used mostly as hypnotics.
Medium and short: Usually employed as oral (or intramuscular) sedatives or hypnotics, but can be given intravenously.
Ultra-short: Drugs normally given by intravenous injection for induction of anaesthesia.

This terminology is illogical; the intravenous barbiturates are not ultra-short-acting, their clinical effect is related to dosage and, even after return of consciousness, mental clouding may persist for some time. Even the 'short-acting' compounds can, in suitable doses, cause drowsiness for many hours, the duration and intensity of action depending partly on the route of administration. Furthermore, it is not always possible to distinguish between the clinical effects of the long- and short-acting groups. The most useful classification for the drugs in current use is:

Short-acting: Oral hypnotics which can also be given parenterally, but where there is some delay in onset of action after intravenous injection.

Rapidly acting: Intravenous anaesthetics with no delay in onset of action and dose-related duration.

The almost universal acceptance of hexobarbitone and thiopentone as intravenous anaesthetics, in preference to pentobarbitone or amylobarbitone was undoubtedly due to the ability of effective doses to cause sleep in one arm–brain circulation time. Where an excessive response to the barbiturate can be anticipated — such as hypotension in poor-risk patients — the slow injection of small doses is desirable, but this can only be done safely with 'rapidly acting' drugs. As will be seen, there is a fairly clear relationship between this suggested clinical classification and the chemical structure of the groups of drugs.

Phenobarbitone, amylobarbitone, butobarbitone, pentobarbitone and quinalbarbitone are the only barbiturates in common use outside anaesthetic practice. All can be given by mouth and the first two are available in solution for i.m. or i.v. use. The injectable preparations have a limited use in anaesthetic practice, pentobarbitone and amylobarbitone having been used as induction agents prior to the discovery of hexobarbitone and thiopentone but abandoned because of the slow onset of action and delayed recovery. They could still be used to produce light sleep during operations under local analgesia or in psychiatric practice, but in general they have been replaced by the benzodiazepines. Oral pentobarbitone is still used as pre-anaesthetic medication.

CHEMISTRY

The drugs used in anaesthetic practice are the water-soluble sodium salts prepared by the combination of urea (or thiourea) with malonic (propanedioc) acid.

Although it is more correct to regard barbituric acid as a pyrimidine derivative it is usually depicted as the cyclical ureide of malonic acid (Fig. 9.1). The acidity is due to the hydrogen ion which migrates from the nitrogen (keto form) in the 1 position (enol form). In aqueous solution it dissociates into hydrogen ion and barbiturate ion.

Barbituric acid has no hypnotic action but substitution of the 5-hydrogens by organic radicals endows the resultant drugs with the ability to depress consciousness. Many side chains can be used in the 5 and 5' positions, but these are concerned with potency and have less effect on the basic action of the drugs than changes in the 1 and 2 positions (Tables 9.1 and 2). A sulphur atom in position 2 results in a rapidly acting drug. A methyl (CH_3) group in position 1 results in a more rapid onset of action, but also produces a high incidence of dose-related excitatory phenomena. The net

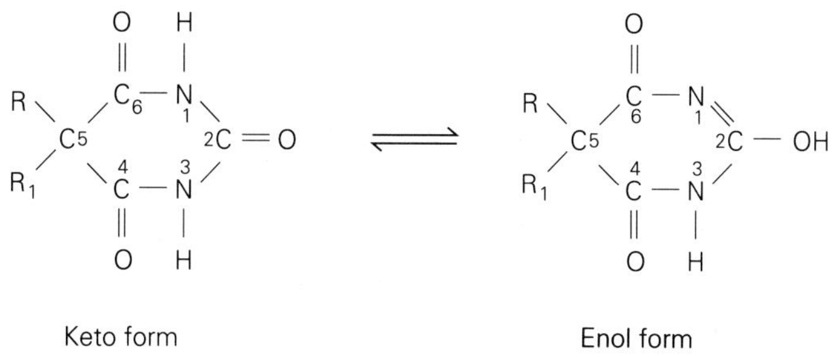

Fig. 9.1 Differing forms of representation of barbituric acid.

Table 9.1 Relationship of chemical grouping to clinical action of barbiturates

	Substituents		
Group	Position 1	Position 2	Group characteristics when given intravenously
(Oxy) barbiturates	H	O	Delay in onset of action, degree depending on 5 and 5' side chains. Useful as basal hypnotics. Prolonged action.
Methylated barbiturates	CH_3	O	Rapidly acting, usually with rapid recovery. High incidence of excitatory phenomena.
Thiobarbiturates	H	S	Rapidly acting, usually smooth onset of sleep and fairly prompt recovery.
Methylated thiobarbiturates	CH_3	S	Rapid onset of action and very rapid recovery but with so high an incidence of excitatory phenomena as to preclude use in clinical practice.

Table 9.2 Changes in potency of barbiturates and thiobarbiturates with changes in 5 and 5' side chains (Dundee 1974)

	Positions on barbiturate molecule					
5	5'	2				Relative potency
$CH_3\text{—}CH_2\text{—}$	$CH_3\text{—}CH_2\text{—}CH_2\text{—}CH\text{—}$ with CH_3	O S	Pentobarbitone THIOPENTONE	(Nembutal) (Pentothal)	1.0	 1.0
$CH_2\text{=}CH\text{—}CH_2\text{—}$	$CH_3\text{—}CH_2\text{—}CH_2\text{—}CH$ with CH_3	O S	Quinalbarbitone THIAMYLAL	(Seconal) (Surital)	1.1	 1.1
$CH_3\text{—}CH_2\text{—}$	$CH_3\text{—}CH\text{—}CH_2\text{—}CH_2\text{—}$ with CH_3	O S	Amylobarbitone THIOETHAMYL	(Amytal) (Venesetic)	0.5	 0.5
$CH_3\text{—}CH_2\text{—}$	$CH_3\text{—}CH_2\text{—}CH\text{—}$ with CH_3	O S	Butobarbitone THIOBUTOBARBITONE	(Soneryl) (Inactin)	0.7	 0.7

effect of substitutions at four possible sites can be predicted with a reasonable degree of certainty, and this is illustrated in Figure 9.2. This shows a barbiturate (pentobarbitone) with a slow onset of action when injected i.v. and its rapidly acting thio-analogue (thiopentone). Removal of one CH_2 linkage produces thiobutobarbitone, which is less potent than thiopentone and has a similar incidence of side-effects; methylation

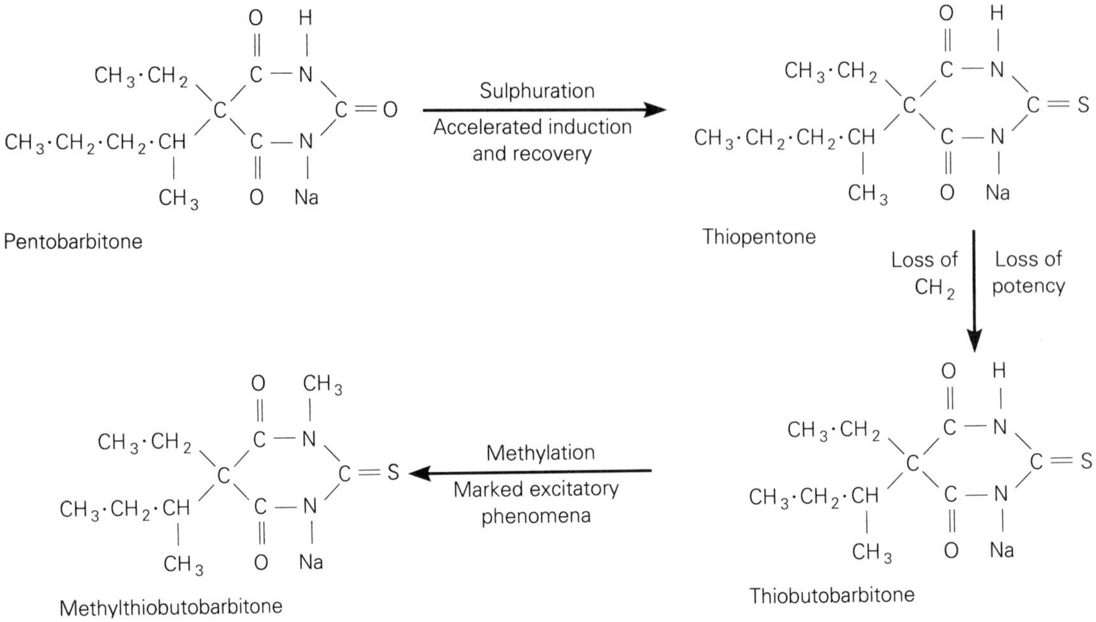

Fig. 9.2 Chemical relationship between four compounds and the effects produced by various structural alterations.

of thiobutobarbitone results in a most unsatisfactory drug which produces an excessively high incidence of excitatory effects.

MODE OF ACTION

Barbiturates reversibly depress activity of all excitable tissues. The central nervous system (CNS) is particularly sensitive to their action, and therapeutic doses have remarkably little effect on skeletal, cardiac or even smooth muscle.

The exact mode of action of the barbiturates is not known, but a likely mechanism is a direct effect on the specialized portions of the neural membrane, modifying synaptic transmission. The ability of a number of agents to depress Na-dependent excitatory synaptic transmission can be correlated with hydrophobicity which, in turn, is strongly correlated with anaesthetic potency in vivo. Available evidence suggests that excitatory synaptic transmission is mainly depressed by barbiturates, while inhibitory synaptic transmission is usually unaffected or enhanced. The site of action appears to be at a component of the ion channel control mechanism rather than on the associated receptor.

The effects of barbiturates on the various pathways and subsystems of the CNS represent the total effect of these complex and diverse actions of the drugs on many millions of individual neurons. For obvious reasons, pathways subserving the maintenance of consciousness

and centripetal transfer of sensory information have been the main objects of study in investigations of barbiturate action. The spinal cord dorsal horn has an important modulatory role in the onward transfer of sensory information. Monosynaptic spinal reflexes are depressed by barbiturates, as are spontaneous and evoked activity in dorsal horn cells. Thus, action at spinal cord level contributes to the overall picture of barbiturate anaesthesia. In contrast, the classical sensory pathways of the spinal cord and brainstem, which contain only two or three synapses, appear to be relatively resistant to the effects of barbiturates.

However, information also travels to the cortex in the multisynaptic reticular formation. The demonstration (Moruzzi and Magoun 1949) that stimulation of the reticular formation causes electroencephalographic (EEG) and behavioural arousal, suggests that the formation might have a role in the production of the anaesthetic state. Pentobarbitone blocks sensory and auditory cortical evoked response by a direct action on the reticular formation (French et al 1953), while EEG arousal in response to direct reticular stimulation is also blocked by barbiturates (Arduini & Arduini 1954). Analysis of the effects of thiopentone on the human sensory evoked response shows that the late component of the response, which is believed to be due to reticular stimulation, is blocked by anaesthetic doses of the drug, while the early, specific component remains intact (Abrahamian et al 1963). These results suggest that reticular formation blockade is an essential component of the mechanism of barbiturate action on the brain. King et al (1957) have attributed depression by barbiturates of transmission through the ventrobasal thalamus to an effect on reticular tone.

Functional denervation of the cortex, through increased inhibitory and decreased facilitatory reticular stimulation of the ventrobasal thalamus, might be a general mechanism of anaesthesia. However, there is no simple relationship between the concentration of a drug which produces anaesthesia and that which blocks cortical evoked responses (Clarke & Rosner 1973). Furthermore the complex effects of barbiturates and other anaesthetics on synaptic transmission in isolated slices of cortex provides evidence of the probable importance of direct cortical effects, as well as on ascending systems, in the mechanism of barbituate anaesthesia.

ORAL HYPNOTICS AND SEDATIVES

Phenobarbitone

Chemical name: ethyl phenyl barbiturate.

Phenobarbitone is used as an anti-convulsant and this is the only drug in this series to have a specific clinical indication. The anti-epileptic action of phenobarbitone is attributed to the presence of the phenyl ring in the side chain, but even with this drug it is not possible to achieve the desired effect without producing some general depression of the CNS.

Phenobarbitone is a long-acting drug with an elimination half-life in the region of 80–120 h. Despite this it is recommended in small (15–30 mg) doses as a daytime sedative and a night-time hypnotic (100 mg). One feature of its use is stimulation of liver enzymes (enzyme induction), and in view of the wide implications of this it should be reserved for specific use in epileptics.

Pentobarbitone

Chemical name: sodium 5 ethyl 5-(1 methyl) butyl barbiturate

Pentobarbitone is the oxygen analogue of thiopentone (Table 9.2) but differs from the thiobarbiturates in having a lower (0.05 cf 3.30) heptane-water partition coefficient of the non-ionized form. It was at one time a very popular night-time hypnotic with a duration of action of 6–8 hours, the elimination half life being 2–3 times that of thiopentone.

An injectable preparation is available, either freshly prepared from dry powder in a glycerol-containing aqueous solution which is mainly used in veterinary practice. Historically it was used as an induction agent before thiopentone, but there was a 20–30 s delay in onset of action which made practical administration difficult. It is still used, in subhypnotic doses, for 'cover' for local anaesthesia but is gradually being replaced by the injectable benzodiazepines.

Rectal (suppositories) preparations of pentobarbitone are available and have some popularity in paediatric practice.

Other oral barbiturates

Amylobarbitone

Chemical name: sodium 5-ethyl-5-isopentyl barbiturate

Butobarbitone

Chemical name: sodium 5n-Butyl-5-ethyl barbiturate.

Cyclobarbitone

Chemical name: sodium 5-ethyl-5 cyclohex-1'(enyl) barbiturate.

Quinalbarbitone

Chemical name: sodium-allyl-5(1-methylbutyl) barbiturate.

Apart from differences in potency (Table 9.2) and duration of action, the effects of these drugs are very similar. Butobarbitone is intermediate in potency between pentobarbitone and amylobarbitone. In effective doses all cause drowsiness in 15–20 min after oral administration, with peak effect occurring in 40–60 min. Duration of action varies between 4 and 8 h, with quinalbarbitone being the shortest-acting and butobarbitone the longest.

All of these drugs have a high addiction potential and their long-term use leads to tolerance with the need for higher doses to produce the desired effect. Frequent use can lead to confusional states. Symptoms of dependence include confusion, impaired judgement and loss of emotional control. Symptoms which follow a prompt withdrawal after prolonged use include delirium and even convulsions, and in less severe cases insomnia and general irritability.

Their hypnotic use should be limited to a few nights when other drugs are not readily available, but they should be avoided in patients in whom enzyme induction could be a problem. These include those on warfarin preparations, oral contraceptives and anti-diabetic drugs. All barbiturates are absolutely contra-indicated in patients with known or suspected porphyria.

INTRAVENOUS ANAESTHETICS

Thiopentone and methohexitone are the only two drugs in widespread use for this purpose. Thiamylal is so similar to thiopentone that it is not discussed separately. It is proposed to discuss the pharmacology of thiopentone in detail and only refer to methohexitone when its action differs from that of the thiobarbiturate. The formulae for thiopentone and methohexitone are shown in Figure 9.3.

The barbiturates used for induction of anaesthesia are sodium salts, freely soluble in water, forming aqueous solutions of limited stability. Their important physical properties are shown in Table 9.3. Commercial preparations contain a mixture of 6 parts anhydrous sodium carbonate and 100 parts w/w of the barbiturate. This additive prevents precipitation of the insoluble free acid by atmospheric carbon dioxide and results in an alkaline solution (pH 10.5–11.0).

Thiopentone (Fig. 9.3) is a thiobarbiturate. It is the sulphur analogue of pentobarbitone (Table 9.2) and its formula can be remembered from the proprietary name Nembutal, Na Ethyl Methyl BUTyl barbitAL, *al* being the American ending for all barbiturates.

Methohexitone (Fig. 9.3) is a racemic mixture of alpha-*d* and alpha-*l* isomers (that is, the optically active isomers are present in such proportions as to render the mixture optically inactive). It was found that the beta-

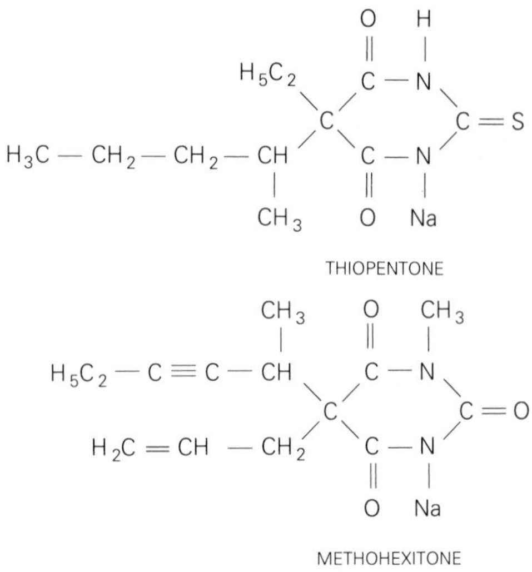

Fig. 9.3   Formulae of thiopentone and methohexitone.

isomer produced excessive motor activity. The most desirable configuration proved to be alpha-*dl*, which is available in the commercial compounds 'Brietal' and 'Brevital Sodium'.

Pharmacokinetics

Until about 1948 it was believed that the duration of action of thiobarbiturates was determined by the rate of their metabolic transformation. It is now appreciated that brevity of action is related to redistribution rather than to metabolism, and patients regain consciousness with a large amount of undetoxicated drug in the body. Blood and tissue levels are changing continuously, and since many factors might be affecting them at the same time, often in different directions, it is not always possible to predict what will happen in any given set of circumstances. Furthermore there is no good correlation between the clinical depth of anaesthesia and blood thiopentone levels, and it is often difficult to correlate changes in tissue levels with clinical effects.

The three most important drug factors affecting the distribution and fate of barbiturates are *lipid solubility* (partition coefficient), *protein binding* and the degree of *ionization*. In addition to their more rapid onset of action (and brevity of effect), the highly lipid-soluble agents tend to be more rapidly degraded metabolically with minimal renal excretion.

Protein binding

Immediately on injection a large proportion of the barbiturate is rendered pharmacologically inactive by being bound to the non-diffusible constituents of plasma.

Table 9.3   Comparative properties of thiopentone and methohexitone

	Thiopentone	Methohexitone
Chemical group	Thiobarbiturate	Methylated oxybarbiturate
Powder	Pale yellow	White
Solution	Pale yellow	Clear
Molecular weight	264.3	284.3
Melting point	158–159°C	93°C
Iso-osmotic concentration of aqueous solution	3.1%	3.7%
Concentration for clinical use	2–2.5%	1–2%
Relative potency	1	2.5–3
pKa (clinically used solution)	7.6	8.1

Thiobarbiturates are bound to a greater extent than their oxygen analogues, the figure for thiopentone being 60–85%. The degree of binding varies with the pH: with increasing barbiturate concentration the percentage of bound drug diminishes, although the total amount activated by this means increases and at low concentrations practically all the drug is bound to the plasma protein, especially albumin. Enhancement of the action of thiopentone from changes in binding, if it occurs at all, would seem to be limited to the immediate effects of very large doses. However, pretreatment with oral probenecid or intravenous acetylsalicylic acid, drugs which have a high affinity for albumin binding sites, reduces the induction doses of thiopentone, presumably due to the effect on plasma binding of the barbiturate (McMurray et al 1984, Dundee et al 1986).

The binding of drugs such as the barbiturates to plasma albumin is an unstable bonding readily reversible with changes in concentration, and can be considered as a means of barbiturate transport in the blood stream, somewhat analogous to oxygen transport by haemoglobin except that the oxygen in haemoglobin exists as a chemical compound whereas albumin and barbiturate form a loose structural complex held together by forces of physical attraction acting at their surfaces. Unbound, undissociated barbiturate molecules pass blood–brain and other blood–tissue barriers at speeds related to their lipid solubilities, and these determine the speed of transit of the barbiturates across the blood–brain barrier. Thiopentone enters but is not extensively carried in red cells.

Uptake

The rate at which barbiturates penetrate the CNS can be correlated with the lipid solubility of the unionized molecules or the partition coefficient between lipid solvents and aqueous buffer. The slower onset of hypnotic action with intravenous pentobarbitone compared with thiopentone is due to the higher ($\times$ 60) partition coefficient of the latter. Thiopentone is largely non-ionic at plasma pH and has a very high partition coefficient.

Thus, to summarize, the rapid onset of sleep following the intravenous injection of adequate doses of thiopentone, thiamylal and methohexitone is due to their high lipid solubility and lack of ionization, leading to immediate penetration of the blood–brain barrier.

Barbiturates are weak acids and, at a pH near 1 in the stomach, they are practically unionized. Absorption from the stomach varies with their lipid solubility and oral administration of large doses (10 mg kg^{-1}) of thiopentone produces rapid intense sedation of short duration.

Following a single injection of thiopentone, the high cerebral blood flow results in a rapid increase in brain barbiturate content; the effects on the electroencephalogram can be detected in 8–15 s and consciousness is usually lost after one deep inspiration. The temporal relationship of this respiratory effect to the onset of anaesthesia suggests that it is mediated by the chemoreceptors in the carotid body. The brain continues to take up thiopentone for a further 30–60 s and thereafter the concentration of the drug in the efferent venous blood slightly exceeds the afferent arterial level; the brain concentration then falls as the drug is removed from the brain. Thus, the maximum depressant action of thiopentone on the nervous system does not occur until $\frac{1}{2}$ min or so after its initial effect.

The immediate uptake of thiopentone by the brain is accompanied by a similar rapid uptake in other important non-nervous tissues such as the liver and kidneys (vital organs), and the plasma level falls quickly. The concentration of drug reaching the brain is thus lowered, brain content falls and anaesthesia lightens. The initial peak concentration of drug in the liver exceeds that in the plasma, and thereafter they decline at a similar rate. The cerebrospinal fluid concentration reaches a level almost as high as that of the unbound drug in the plasma, and thereafter it declines as in other tissues.

Redistribution

With the exception of muscle and fat, the maximum tissue concentration of thiopentone is reached within 1 min of a single intravenous injection. It is the rapid redistribution which is responsible for the short action of small doses. Equilibrium with the muscles is not attained until about $\frac{1}{4}$ h after injection, and thereafter its concentration declines at a rate parallel to the plasma level. Despite the affinity of thiopentone for fat, because of the poor blood supply, uptake of the drug in adipose tissues is relatively slow. By 1 h the concentration in fat exceeds that of other tissues. Maximum deposition of thiopentone in fat does not occur until 1 h or so after uptake by muscle has ceased, about one-third of the injected dose being located there within 30 min and half of the drug is in fat depots by 90 min.

Price (1960) presented a mathematical analysis of the kinetics of thiopentone distribution, validating his conclusions by direct measurements of drug concentrations in tissues (Price et al 1960). Following a bolus injection, the course of anaesthesia depends passively upon a competition between nervous and non-nervous tissues for thiopentone. His concept was of injection into a central 'pool' of blood with the rapid onset of anaesthesia resulting from the high blood supply and affinity of the

CNS for thiopentone. Within 1 min the blood has given up 90% of the injected dose to the highly perfused tissues, principally CNS, heart and liver. During the subsequent $\frac{1}{2}$ h they were depleted as a result of further redistribution, with about 80% of the thiopentone given up by these highly perfused viscera to other aqueous 'lean' tissues in the body, while the remainder entered fat.

Figure 9.4 differs from Price's concept by allowing for early metabolism of thiopentone. Saidman & Eger (1966) showed that, although the uptake in muscle plays a dominant role in the early fall of arterial concentration, this is equalled by the additive effects of metabolism and uptake in fat. Earlier studies by Brodie et al (1950), and Brodie (1952) showed that 10–15% of thiopentone is broken down per hour.

Since virtually no thiopentone is eliminated unchanged in the urine, the positive role of the liver in the metabolism of thiopentone is now recognized. The range of thiopentone hepatic extraction ratio varies from 0.08 to 0.20 with a total body clearance of the drug ranging from 1.6 to 4.3 mg kg^{-1} min^{-1} (Morgan et al 1981a, b, Stanski & Watkins 1982, Burch & Stanski 1983). These values are lower than the 0.3 ratio used by Saidman in calculating Figure 9.4, and suggest a less important, but not insignificant, role of drug metabolism. Animal experiments and observations in humans have shown that prolongation of the action of thiopentone in the presence of hepatic dysfunction only occurs after very large doses. The low hepatic extraction shows that thiopentone has capacity-limited binding-sensitive elimination. Thus changes in protein binding and in hepatic enzyme activity will affect the clearance of the drug.

Due to differences in dosage there are some major differences in the reported pharmacokinetic data for thiopentone and methohexitone. In some patients the plasma decay follows a bi-exponential pattern, while in others (as in Fig. 9.5) these correlate well with a tri-exponential equation. The only comparison of strictly equivalent doses of thiopentone and methohexitone is that of Hudson et al (1983a), who compared the pharmacokinetics of equivalent doses in two groups of nine subjects (Table 9.4). The volumes of distribution, both central compartment (V_c) and steady state (Vd_{ss}), were similar for drugs, and the clearance of methohexitone was similar to that described by Breimer (1976). The hepatic extraction ratio of methohexitone was approximately 0.5, indicating that the liver metabolized about half the amount of methohexitone passing through it during any given interval, and this is higher than the comparable figure for thiopentone. The clearance of a drug with such a high hepatic extraction is dependent largely on the magnitude of hepatic blood flow. Although the distribution half-life and Vd_{ss} were similar there were major differences between methohexitone and thiopentone disposition. Methohexitone was cleared three times more rapidly than thiopentone, and thus the elimination half-life of methohexitone was one-third that of thiopentone. Using complicated pharmacokinetic calculations Burch & Stanski (1983) have calculated the

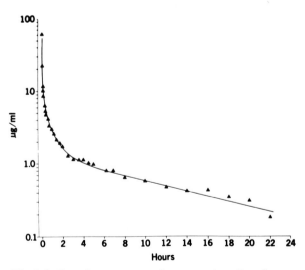

Fig. 9.5 Log plasma concentration versus time. Data from a patient given 6.4 mg kg^{-1} thiopentone as an intravenous bolus. The solid line represents the tri-exponential equation determined by non-linear regression. The triangles represent the measured thiopentone plasma concentrations (Stanski and Watkins 1982).

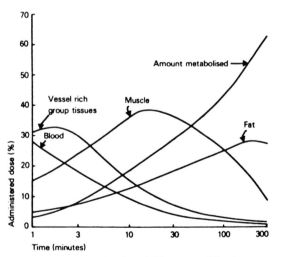

Fig. 9.4 Tissue distribution of thiopentone following intravenous injection (according to Saidman and Eger 1966).

Table 9.4 Pharmacokinetic parameters of thiopentone and methohexitone (Mean ± SD)

	Methohexitone	Thiopentone
Dose (mg kg^{-1})	2.4 ± 0.4[‡]	6.7 ± 0.7[‡]
Distribution half-lives (min)		
Rapid	5.6 ± 2.7	8.5 ± 6.1
Slow*	58.3 ± 24.6	62.7 ± 30.4
Elimination half-life (h)	3.9 ± 2.11[†]	11.6 ± 6.0[†]
Clearance (ml kg^{-1} min^{-1})	10.9 ± 3.0[‡]	3.4 ± 0.5[‡]
Vc (ℓ kg^{-1})	0.35 ± 0.10	0.38 ± 0.09
Vd$_{ss}$ (ℓ kg^{-1})	2.2 ± 0.7	2.5 ± 10

*Slow distribution phase for the three patients given methohexitone and the eight patients given thiopentone exhibiting tri-exponential kinetics.
[†] $P < 0.005$.
[‡] $P < 0.001$.
From Hudson et al 1983a.

fraction of thiopentone lost from the central compartment which they could attribute to metabolism. Applying these principles, Hudson et al (1983a) estimated that at 30 min the ratio of metabolic loss to total loss is 0.38 for methohexitone and 0.22 for thiopentone.

Prolonged administration

As more drug is administered, the concentration in some tissues approaches equilibrium with the thiopentone in blood. Since the CNS equilibrates rapidly with blood, and thus ceases to take up the drug, continuous administration will result in an increasing proportion of the total dose administered being located in non-nervous tissues. Thus the body gradually loses its ability to remove the thiopentone from the brain, and theoretically there should be a grave risk of overdosage and very prolonged narcosis. Studies in patients given the very large infusion doses of thiopentone used in cerebral resuscitation have shown a change in elimination from the expected first-order (rate of elimination and elimination half-life constant, irrespective of plasma concentration) to non-linear or Michaelis–Menten elimination, in which the rate of elimination varies with the plasma concentration (Stanski et al 1980). This results in a decrease in the rate of elimination and an increase in the apparent elimination half-life as the plasma concentration increases. With the highest doses (477–600 mg kg^{-1}) the calculated $t\frac{1}{2}\beta$ values were in the range of 16–30 h, compared with the accepted 6–10 h after smaller doses. This is presumably due to progressively increasing

saturation of the hepatic enzyme systems that oxidize thiopentone. With doses of this order desulphuration occurs to an appreciable degree, and at the end of the infusions plasma pentobarbitone concentrations were approximately 10% of thiopentone levels. Similar findings have been reported in two patients given very large doses of thiopentone as treatment for uncontrollable seizures.

Placental transfer

The placenta offers no barrier to the passage of barbiturates to the fetus (Morgan et al 1981b). These workers found an extremely high correlation between umbilical venous and arterial plasma concentrations at delivery, and also between maternal and umbilical venous thiopentone levels at delivery. This is expected from the passage of highly lipoid-soluble agents across a barrier like the placenta.

pH effect

Thiopentone has a pK value of 7.6 and the degree of ionization can change considerably with physiological variations in blood pH. The effect can be understood by regarding thiopentone as being distributed *in vitro* between two immiscible phases; one (mainly water) consists of blood and parenchymatous tissues, and the other (organic phase) is fat. The concentration of undissociated acid relative to that ionized largely determines the distribution of a weak organic acid, such as barbituric acid, between an aqueous buffer and an immiscible organic solvent. The lower the pH, the more drug will be in the organic phase, while at a higher pH the opposite is true. Brodie and his colleagues (1950) found that decreasing the pH of plasma of dogs to 6.8 by the inhalation of 10% carbon dioxide, reduced the concentration of thiopentone in the plasma by about 40%. On stopping the inhalation the blood pH returned to near the control level, and the plasma level of the drug rose rapidly. However, the brain content would rise with acidosis, which would enhance the effect of the drug.

Renal excretion

The degree of ionization governs the renal excretion of the unionized drug which appears in the glomerular filtrate, diffusing back into the circulation through the renal tubules. This will be less if the drug is ionized and with weak organic acids ionization will be maximal at a high (alkaline) pH. Only very minimal amounts of thiopentone or methohexitone are excreted unchanged in the urine. Alkalinization of urine will not facilitate excretion.

Metabolism

Site of metabolic transformation. The liver is the primary site of ion inactivation the barbiturates.

Thiopentone and similar drugs are broken down by non-synthetic (phase 1) reactions, mainly oxidation, the resulting polar compound having no hypnotic activity and being excreted by the kidney.

The main route of metabolism of thiopentone is ω-oxidation to the pharmacologically inactive thiopentone carboxylic acid.

$$-CH-CH_2-CH_2-CH_3 \rightarrow CH-CH_2-CH_2-COOH$$
$$\;\;\;|\qquad\qquad\qquad\qquad\quad |$$
$$\;\;CH_3\qquad\qquad\qquad\qquad CH_3$$

The role of desulphuration to pentobarbitone is only important following the administration of very large doses, and possibly might contribute to delayed recovery in appropriate circumstances.

The metabolic fate of methohexitone has not been studied to the same extent as that of thiopentone. Less than 1% of the administered dose can be found in bile and urine (Sunshine et al 1966). The major pathway is ω-1-oxidation of the triple bond side chain, resulting in hydroxymethohexitone (Murphy 1974).

$$-CH \equiv C-CH_2CH_3 \rightarrow CH \equiv C-C-CH_3$$
$$\;\;\;|\qquad\qquad\qquad\qquad |\quad\;\; |$$
$$\;\;CH_3\qquad\qquad\qquad CH_3\quad OH$$

Factors influencing pharmacokinetics

Pregnancy

A secondary peak in plasma concentration has been noted around the time of delivery in patients anaesthetized for Caesarean section (Morgan et al 1981b). Otherwise the pharmacokinetics are very similar to those in non-pregnant subjects. There are wide variations in elimination half-life of thiopentone in pregnant patients ranging from 6 to 46 h (mean 26.1 h). The clearance of thiopentone is greater in pregnant patients, and Morgan and colleagues attributed the longer elimination half-life to a larger volume of distribution of the drug. The higher clearance of thiopentone, which is a low clearance drug, is most likely due to induction of the hepatic drug-metabolizing enzymes, particularly near term.

The widely recognized phenomenon of an alert infant being born to a mother anaesthetized with thiopentone can be explained on a pharmacokinetic basis. Suggestions include a preferential uptake of thiopentone by the fetal liver (Finster et al 1966, 1972), the higher water content of the brain (Flowers & Hill 1959) and a fall in carbon dioxide tension at delivery. There is also more redistribution of drug into maternal tissues, causing a rapid reduction in maternal to fetal concentration gradient in addition to the dilution in the fetal circulation. A combination of these factors might prevent thiopentone from achieving sufficiently high concentration in the fetal brain to depress the infant at birth. The studies of Morgan et al (1981b) suggest that the rapid redistribution of thiopentone in the maternal tissues during the period between induction and delivery is the major factor responsible for the discrepancy in the states of consciousness of the mother and neonate at delivery. Venous plasma concentrations of thiopentone in the umbilical cord, which should be similar to those entering the fetal brain, were well below the arterial plasma concentrations required to produce anaesthesia in adults.

Renal disease

In chronic renal failure the dose of thiopentone necessary to induce anaesthesia is reduced to about one-half. The plasma protein binding of the drug is markedly reduced in patients with chronic renal failure (Ghoneim & Pandya 1975), resulting in an increased free fraction of drug and thus the need for decreased dosage. Burch & Stanski (1981) estimated that the increased free drug concentration in chronic renal failure resulted in a larger total drug clearance because elimination is proportional to the amount of free drug available. Vd_{ss} (ml kg^{-1}) was increased due to the increased free fraction in plasma available for tissue distribution. Since changes in clearance and volume of distribution were equal, the terminal elimination half-life was unaffected. Clearance was estimated as 4.5 mg kg^{-1} min^{-1} compared with 3.2 in normal subjects, and elimination half-life was 9.7 h compared with 10.2 h in a corresponding control series. Thus it would seem that the pharmacokinetic changes are due solely to alterations in binding of thiopentone to plasma; clinically it is necessary to reduce the induction dose but recovery should not be prolonged.

Liver disease

It is only with very large doses of thiopentone that one can detect a prolongation of action in patients with liver dysfunction. In the clinical dose range Ghoneim & Pandya (1975) found an increase in the free thiopentone fraction, and the pharmacokinetic basis of an exaggerated response to thiopentone in patients with hepatic dysfunction is probably similar to that described earlier for chronic renal failure patients.

Hepatic cirrhosis indicates a severe derangement of liver function and in such patients Pandela and colleagues (1983) have demonstrated an increase in free thiopentone fraction similar to that mentioned above. Although patients with very severe liver dysfunction might have a decreased capacity to metabolize thiopentone, a prolonged effect is unlikely in cirrhotic patients provided small doses are given: the other toxic effects of the drug should also be no more marked provided the injections are not given too rapidly.

Age

The induction dose of thiopentone in elderly patients is significantly lower than in the young (Christensen & Andreasen 1978, Christensen et al 1982, Dundee et al 1982). Christensen and his colleagues (1981, 1982), however, did not find the venous and arterial blood concentrations on induction of anaesthesia to be different in the 60–80 year age range as compared with a younger age group. Using a three-compartment open model to describe the disappearance of thiopentone from venous blood they found a significant increase in $t_{\frac{1}{2}}\beta$ from 8 to 13 h in the elderly, but this would not explain the lower induction dose. A significantly decreased early redistribution rate constant ($K_{1.2}$) which is found in the early stage could be responsible. It is the initial redistribution rate constant rather than the size of Vd_{ss} that is the important factor in determining the induction dose of this drug. Cardiac output is a major determinant in this redistribution, and in young subjects Christensen et al (1980) have demonstrated a significant positive relationship between the cardiac output before induction and the dose that was necessary for induction. The recognized depressant effect of thiopentone on cardiac function is normally compensated for by an increase in heart rate so that cardiac output is maintained; however, this compensation might be impaired in the elderly in whom the cardiovascular effects of the drug are more marked. This explanation can also apply to other patients classified as 'poor-risk', and in whom clinical experience has shown that the induction dose is less than normal, and in whom the response of the cardiovascular system to a normal dose is exaggerated.

Sorbo et al (1984) examined the pharmacokinetics of thiopentone in 16 healthy children, with an average age of 6 years (5 months–13 years) and showed that distribution kinetics did not differ from those of adults (Table 9.5), but the elimination half-life was about one-half of the adult value. In addition, clearance of thiopentone was twice as great in infants and children as in adults. The ratio of $t_{\frac{1}{2}}\beta$ to age did not reach statistical signifi-

Table 9.5 Pharmacokinetic data for paediatric (5 months–13 years) and adult patients given 4 mg kg^{-1} thiopentone.

Parameter	Paediatric patients	Adult patients
Distribution $t_{\frac{1}{2}}$ (min)		
Rapid	6.3 ± 6.6	3.7 ± 1.1
Slow	43.0 ± 16.0	61.0 ± 34.0
Elimination $t_{\frac{1}{2}}$(h)	$6.1 \pm 3.3^{\star}$	12.0 ± 6.0
Clearance (ml kg^{-1} min^{-1})	$6.6 \pm 2.2\dagger$	3.1 ± 0.5
Vd_{ss} (ℓ kg^{-1})	2.1 ± 0.71	2.2 ± 0.11
V_c (ℓ kg^{-1})	0.4 ± 0.19	0.28 ± 0.11
Free thiopentone (percentage unbound)	$13,2 \pm 1.5$	13.6 ± 1.3

$^{\star}P < 0.0005$ significant difference.
$^{\dagger}P < 0.001$.
From Sorbo et al 1984.

cance, but clearance significantly decreased with age. Plasma binding was similar in adults and children.

The need for a higher induction dose of thiopentone in children, as compared with adults, is difficult to explain purely on a pharmacokinetic basis (decrease in free drug and increased binding or more rapid early distribution), and may be due to decreased sensitivity of the brain to thiopentone as compared with adults.

Poor-risk patients

This ill-defined group includes patients with cardiovascular and other diseases which most affect the pharmacokinetic mechanisms influencing the induction dose of thiopentone. The most important factor is probably the altered pharmacokinetics in patients with cardiac failure and hypervolaemia affecting the initial redistribution phase (Christensen et al 1985). Many of these patients will also have alterations in plasma proteins, the effects of which have already been mentioned. There might also be acid–base disturbances and, while these have to be marked to alter the amount of free drug, severe acidosis will decrease the plasma concentration of thiopentone due to an increased unionized fraction, thus increasing penetration into the brain and enhancing its depressant effect. This includes the effect on the vasomotor and respiratory centres as well as those responsible for consciousness.

Obesity

In clinical practice thiopentone is given on an approximate bodyweight basis, but if adhered to in the case of patients with morbid obesity it would result in very large doses being given. Vd$_{ss}$ is significantly larger in obese as compared with age-matched lean patients (Jung et al 1982). Total drug clearance, adjusted for body weight, does not differ significantly between obese and lean patients. The elimination half-life was found to be significantly longer in obese (27.8 h) than in lean patients (6.3 h), this difference being primarily due to the larger apparent volume of distribution of thiopentone in the obese.

Sex

Edwards & Ellis (1978) and Dundee et al (1982) found a significantly lower induction dose requirement in women compared with men, irrespective of the age of the patients. Christensen et al (1981) found a higher venous concentration at the moment of sleep in elderly men (34.3 μg ml^{-1}) as compared with women of the same age group (19.2 μg ml^{-1}). The early distribution thus differs between men and women with a relatively large apparent initial volume of distribution in women. In practice the sex differences are less important than the influence of age or pathological factors.

Pharmacodynamics

The effects of thiopentone on the body have been studied in more detail than those of methohexitone. The former will be described with appropriate reference to the oxybarbiturate where they differ from thiopentone and when the data are available.

In effective doses both thiopentone (4–5 mg kg^{-1} and methohexitone (1.2–1.6 mg kg^{-1}) will induce anaesthesia in one arm–brain circulation time, and maximum depression of vital centres occurs within 1 min of administration. The loss of consciousness is usually smooth with thiopentone, although occasionally accompanied by slight spontaneous muscle movement, particularly in unpremedicated subjects. The plasma thiopentone level necessary for anaesthesia in fit patients is around 40 μg ml^{-1} with the free drug concentration for surgical anaesthesia in the region of 6 μg mg^{-1} (Becker 1978).

Central nervous system

Thiopentone has no analgesic action and small doses may increase sensitivity to somatic pain. This hyperalgesic (antanalgesic) action limits its use as sole anaesthetic, and it has also been demonstrated in the postoperative period following large doses (Dundee 1960, 1964).

The EEG changes induced by thiopentone follow a constant pattern (Kiersey et al 1951) and can be correlated with the clinical depth of anaesthesia, although it is difficult to relate them to plasma drug concentration in different patients. Initially there is high-amplitude, fast spiky activity of mixed frequency (10–30 Hz). Amplitudes vary greatly; short runs of two or three waves with amplitude of 25–80 μV are interspersed with runs of lower amplitude. This is followed by a complex pattern of mixed frequency characterized by the presence of predominantly short wave forms of irregular contour and random occurrence, and with much variation in voltage. As anaesthesia deepens, the EEG is characterized by a progressive suppression of cortical activity and increasing periods of relative quiescence separating groups of waves, which appear abruptly and consist of a short series of high-voltage waves, with a frequency of 10 Hz, for about 1 s followed immediately by two or more short waves (2 Hz) tailing off into the next suppression phase. In surgical anaesthesia the duration of cortical quiescence varies from 3 to 10 s, and there is a reduction in the amplitude of the components which might fall below 25 μv.

Thiopentone causes a reduction in cerebral metabolic rate, especially in areas of high activity. This is accompanied by a corresponding reduction in cerebral blood flow, resulting in cerebral vasoconstriction and reduction in intracranial pressure. Doses sufficient to produce light general anaesthesia will reduce cerebral blood flow by one-third, with a 50% fall in deep anaesthesia. However, the main effects of barbiturates are secondary to those of blood pressure, and cerebral blood flow showed a proportionate fall in acute hypotension. To maintain blood flow in the presence of a falling blood pressure the cerebral arterioles relax and thus lower cerebrovascular resistance.

Induction doses of thiopentone also have a marked anticonvulsant action, although methohexitone is not recommended for this purpose.

With the barbiturates, more so than any other drugs used in anaesthesia, the clinical level of anaesthesia is related to the intensity of the surgical stimulus as well as to the degree of cerebral depression. After thiopentone an undisturbed patient with depressed respiration, and abdominal and masseter relaxation, might give a picture of moderately deep surgical anaesthesia, but on application of a surgical stimulus the respiration is stimulated, relaxation lost and reflex movement of a limb may occur. If given sufficient thiopentone to produce surgical anaesthesia in the presence of strong stimulation, a dangerous degree of respiratory depression might occur when the stimulation ceases. Pretreatment with opioids will reduce the dose of thiopentone required to produce surgical anaesthesia, but they also depress respiration and might be long-acting, and a similar state of affairs can be produced at the end of the operation. With the use of nitrous oxide–oxygen to supplement thiopentone it is possible to produce a pattern of anaesthesia somewhat similar to that observed with other drugs without excessive dosage, and without causing dangerous and prolonged periods of depression of vital functions.

Acute tolerance is one aspect of the cerebral action of thiopentone which cannot be explained readily. With single doses, return of consciousness will occur at a higher plasma concentration than following smaller doses. A large induction dose usually needs to be followed by larger increments to maintain a constant level of anaesthesia than after smaller induction doses. Equally baffling is the finding that with continuous administration the plasma levels at which certain signs occur increase with time. Subjects have been known to converse seemingly rationally with plasma levels in excess of those at which they were anaesthetized 6 h or so previously (Dundee et al 1956). A pharmacokinetic explanation for this has been suggested, but is far from proven (Hudson et al 1983b).

Induction of anaesthesia with methohexitone is less smooth than with thiopentone. Excitatory effects (tremor, spontaneous muscle movement and hypertonus) and cough and/or hiccough, occur in about one-fifth of unpremedicated patients. Their frequency and severity increase with large doses, and with a fast rate of injection. The excitatory effects of methohexitone are reduced markedly by opioids (premedication or immediate pretreatment) while atropine and hyoscine will reduce the respiratory side-effects.

Cardiovascular system

Heart rate is increased slightly on induction of anaesthesia, and systolic blood pressure and cardiac output fall to a significant degree when surgical anaesthesia is achieved. Immediately on administration of thiopentone one sees marked vasodilatation, and measurements of intrathoracic blood volume suggest that blood has been shunted from the central pool to the periphery, resulting in a decreased venous return which in turn reduces cardiac output and arterial pressure. In normal doses, thiopentone causes minimal depression of the heart but marked depression occurs with large doses (Chamberlain et al 1977). On repeat or prolonged administration there is a delay in recovery of arterial pressure, suggesting that direct myocardial depression is playing an important role. The degree of cardiovascular depression is related to both the rate of administration (more marked with

rapid administration) and the total dose given. Even large doses given as an infusion may cause less hypotension than a small rapid injection. The response varies with the condition of the patient, particularly with regard to blood volume, acid–base balance and cardiovascular disease and hypertension: these relate mainly to the ability to compensate for the effects of peripheral vasodilatation. Concurrent or previous administration of drugs, which themselves cause vasodilatation or reduce comparative tachycardia, will also enhance the hypotensive effect of thiopentone. Thiopentone abolishes the compensatory vasoconstriction produced by an increase in intrathoracic pressure, and persistent hypotension can accompany hyperventilation. In the absence of hypercarbia, arrhythmias are uncommon after thiopentone.

The hypotensive effect of methohexitone is less than that of equivalent doses of thiopentone; this is due to its tendency to cause tachycardia, which can be very marked on occasions.

Hypotension will be more marked in the undisturbed patient and surgical stimulation or laryngoscopy and tracheal intubation will usually result in a rise in pressure — in many instances a marked overshoot occurs. Lightening of anaesthesia does not necessarily reverse the hypotension which may persist into the postoperative period, and if accompanied by respiratory depression will lead to hypoxia.

Respiratory system

Thiopentone is a powerful central depressant of respiration and transient apnoea (up to $\frac{1}{2}$ min) usually occurs. In normal doses in fit patients this is not a clinical problem except after 'heavy' opioid premedication. As with most anaesthetics, the sensitivity of the respiratory centre to carbon dioxide is depressed proportionately to the depth of anaesthesia. In deep anaesthesia the action of hypoxia on the carotid sinus plays an important part in the maintenance of respiration, but the shift of control of respiration from carbon dioxide to hypoxia is accompanied by a decrease in minute volume. Carbon dioxide retention may be particularly difficult to detect since the thiopentone may also obtund the usual rise in pressure which it causes.

Cough and hiccough are uncommon during induction with thiopentone, but there is some heightening of laryngeal reflexes, particularly in light anaesthesia and a tendency to laryngospasm which will be induced by minor stimuli. Bronchospasm is a rare, but not unknown, complication with this drug, particularly in asthmatic subjects in whom its use may be better avoided. In many cases the term 'bronchospasm' is used to describe a complex situation involving spasm of intercostal and other muscles, which can be reversed by the use of muscle relaxants. The respiratory effects of methohexitone include a high incidence of cough and hiccough, particularly after the rapid administration of high doses to unpremedicated subjects. These often persist during the intermittent administration of the drug, and are of such severity as to make methohexitone an unsuitable drug for continuous infusion (McMurray et al 1986).

Hepatic and renal function

Although hepatic dysfunction has been described following the use of large doses of thiopentone in animals, there are no clinical data to suggest that normal induction doses have a hepatotoxic effect, even in patients with an already damaged liver. It is, however, possible to demonstrate transient impairment of liver function tests following large doses and after infusions (Kawar et al 1982).

In common with other anaesthetics, oliguria occurs during barbiturate anaesthesia — partly as the result of reduction in renal blood flow and partly from an increase in circulating anti diuretic hormone. This is of no clinical importance.

Other systems

In therapeutic doses neither drug affects the tone of the gravid uterus, but tone is reduced in deep anaesthesia. There is no obvious interaction between the barbiturates and any of the commonly used myoneural blocking drugs.

A mild hypoglycaemia occurs during anaesthesia, during which patients' ability to handle a glucose load is impaired. Hyperglycaemia may, however, be the normal response to stress rather than an effect of the drug on glucose metabolism.

The most serious toxic action of the barbiturates is their ability to induce an acute attack in patients with latent porphyria. This is brought about by stimulation of ALA synthetase, the enzyme which catalyses the rate-limiting reaction for haem production. Not every type of porphyria is adversely affected by thiopentone (Leading Article 1985) but the outcome is so serious following an acute attack that any suspicion of porphyria should be an absolute contra-indication to their use.

Local effects

Pain on injection is uncommon with 2.5% thiopentone, even when small veins are used, but occurs in 25–30%

of patients with 1% methohexitone. Venous thrombosis is also a rare occurrence with either drug.

Thiopentone can cause tissue damage if injected subcutaneously, particularly with large volumes and in elderly patients with a poor peripheral circulation or sparseness of subcutaneous tissue. Arterial injection can cause serious sequelae and care must be taken to avoid this problem. The degree of damage varies with the concentration of solution used (Table 9.6). Intense pain, radiating into the fingers often, but not invariably, follows an intra-arterial injection. Pain usually disappears after a few minutes but with large amounts of drug it can persist for several hours. The radial pulse will usually disappear and there may be blanching of the limb. If the circulation is quickly re-established this may be followed by reactive hyperaemia. Oedema of the limb will occur when the muscles have been invaded by thiopentone. Depending on the degree of spasm of blood vessels and anatomical distribution of blood from affected vessels, sequelae can vary from transient hyperaesthesia of the affected area to loss of a digit or even a limb, but the latter has not been reported with a 2.5% solution.

Damage results from unrelieved vascular spasm being followed by thrombosis. Spasm is related to the production of crystals of insoluble thiopentone acid in a bloodstream of decreasing capacity: direct blockage is unlikely but release of ATP from damaged blood cells or platelets and an area of intimal damage at the puncture site could initiate the intravascular thrombosis.

Table 9.6 A survey of cases showing the sequelae of intra-arterial thiopentone related to the strength of solution used

Percentage solution	n	Nature	Permanent n	Permanent %	Nil n	Nil %
10	11	Amputation required	5	45	2	18
		Gangrene of fingers	3	28		
		Skin slough	1	9		
5	16	Amputation	3	19	11	69
		Skin slough	1	6		
		Area of hypo-aesthesia	1	6		
2.5–5.0	5				5	100
2.5 or less	33	Slight hypo-aesthesia	1	3	32	97

From Dundee & Wyant 1988

The effects of extravenous injection of methohexitone are less than those of thiopentone. This cannot be fully explained on the basis of using a less concentrated solution, and there is a lesser tendency for the oxybarbiturate to form intravascular crystals.

Hypersensitivity reactions

Transient erythema is a common occurrence after administration of thiopentone: this appears to be more frequent in women and occurs in the 'blushing' area.

More serious reactions are rare with thiopentone, although the incidence appears to be increasing in recent years. It is often difficult to distinguish between relative overdose ('normal' dose given to an unfit patient) and true hypersensitivity to thiopentone. The latter resembles the effects of histamine liberation and might involve this as an intermediary. A small number of thiopentone reactions occur in patients with previous exposure (type 1) and involve the production of IgE antibodies. However, the majority are not antibody-mediated, occurring in patients with a history of atopy (hay fever or eczema or other sensitivity), involving non-immune mechanisms such as the direct release of histamine (Dundee et al 1978, Fee et al 1978).

The clinical picture is one of sudden onset of pallor, cardiovascular collapse (tachycardia and hypotension) and bronchospasm. The latter is most difficult to treat, but the hypotension, due to sudden expansion of the cardiovascular tree, usually responds quickly to rapid colloid infusion and vasopressors. There is also usually a slight delay in onset of action of the anaesthetic.

The majority of reactions have oedema of the eyelids as a feature and some have massive wheals. A 1 mm layer of subcutaneous fluid throughout the body can produce a circulatory loss of 1.5 litres. This is usually exceeded when visible oedema is present. Bronchospasm may in part be due to oedema. However, the most serious form is oedema of the glottis, and when this occurs one must administer intravenous adrenaline.

It is estimated that hypersensitivity reactions to thiopentone occur in between 1 in 23 000 (Shaw 1974) and 1 in 36 000 (Beamish & Brown 1981) administrations. This may seem a negligible risk, but even with aggressive treatment it causes a 50% mortality which is higher than with other intravenous anaesthetics. This may be because the drug remains in the body for a long time, but there is the additional factor of the greater toxic effects of thiopentone on the cardiovascular system than methohexitone or etomidate.

Clinical aspects

Table 9.7 summarizes the important clinical differences between thiopentone and methohexitone which are of clinical importance. These have all been referred to in the text.

Dosage

The induction dose varies with:

1. age of the patient,
2. fitness of the patient,
3. premedication,
4. pretreatment with opioids immediately prior to induction.

Taking the normal induction dose of thiopentone as $4-5$ mg kg^{-1} this can be as high as $6-8$ mg kg^{-1} in children, and as low as $2-2.5$ mg kg^{-1} in the elderly. There is a marked reduction in requirements over the age of 60, irrespective of physical fitness, and this appears to be mainly a true pharmacodynamic (rather than pharmacokinetic) effect. Any degree of 'unfitness' will reduce dosage requirements.

Subjects with an acquired tolerance to sedatives, hypnotics, opioids or even alcohol, have increased requirements of thiopentone, and this may occur in patients with a degree of cardiovascular or other disease which would engender sensitivity to the toxic effects of such doses. This situation is best dealt with by prior

Table 9.7 Clinical relevance of differences (and some similarities) of thiopentone and methohexitone.

Both rapidly acting	
Induction	Smoother with thiopentone
	Excitatory effects troublesome with methohexitone in unpremedicated subjects: greater with rapid injection and large doses
	Cough and hiccough often troublesome with methohexitone
Cardiovascular effects	Slightly less with methohexitone, which frequently causes tachycardia
Recovery	More rapid with methohexitone
	Methohexitone is pharmacokinetically more suitable for infusions but needs opioid supplementation because of excitatory effects
	Extravenous thiopentone does more damage than extravenous methohexitone
	Both absolutely contra-indicated in porphyria

administration of a suitable dose of fentanyl or alfentanil.

With the exception of acquired tolerance decreased dosage requirements occur in any patient who is classed as unfit. This is particularly marked in patients with a raised blood urea (Dundee & Hassard 1983) and in those with cardiac disease (Christensen et al 1985).

Prevention and treatment of cerebral ischaemia

Since Michenfelder (1974) has shown that doses of barbiturates which render the EEG isoelectric reduce the cerebral metabolic rate by about half, with no further effects from larger doses, the value of continuous infusions of thiopentone in minimizing the sequelae from hypoxic episodes has been investigated. A recent study of the randomized application of prophylactic barbiturate coma in the treatment of severe head injury failed to demonstrate any beneficial effect from the therapy; rather in some patients there was a deleterious effect

from its hypotensive action (Ward et al 1985). Earlier claims for a therapeutic effect were probably due to the intensive therapy to which their patients were subjected. Thiopentone can, however, be of value in patients with post-hypoxic convulsions. These seizures increase cerebral metabolic rate at a time when compensatory increases in cerebral blood may be limited.

The value of thiopentone in reducing the size of the brain in neurosurgical operations is not questioned, but similar effects can be produced by moderate hyperventilation. A second dose given immediately prior to tracheal intubation will prevent the increase in blood pressure and cerebrospinal pressure which often accompany this event (Unni et al 1984). Another similar indication for a supplementary dose of thiopentone is during carotid endarterectomy; 4–5 mg kg^{-1} given just before internal carotid artery occlusion will result in around 5 min ECG burst suppression, which, although less than the total period of arterial occlusion, will be followed by local metabolic depression in the poorly perfused brain areas (Bendsten et al 1984).

REFERENCES

Abrahamian H A, Allison T, Goff W R, Rosner B S 1963 Effects of thiopental on human cerebral evoked responses. Anesthesiology 24: 650–657

Arduini A, Arduini M G 1954 Effect of drugs and metabolic alterations on brain-stem arousal mechanism. Journal of Pharmacology and Experimental Therapeutics 110: 76–85

Beamish D, Brown D T 1981 Adverse responses to i.v. anaesthetics. British Journal of Anaesthesia 53: 55–58

Becker K E 1978 Plasma levels of thiopental necessary for anesthesia. Anesthesiology 49: 192–196

Bendsten A O, Cold G E, Astrup J, Rosenorn J 1984 Thiopental loading during controlled hypotension for intracranial aneurysm surgery. Acta Anaesthesiologica Scandinavica 28: 473–477

Breimer D D 1976 Pharmacokinetics of methohexitone following intravenous infusion in humans. British Journal of Anaesthesia 48: 643–649

Brodie B B 1952 Physiological disposition and chemical fate of thiobarbiturates in the body. Federation Proceedings 11: 632–639

Brodie B B, Mark L C, Papper E M, Lief P A, Bernstein E, Rovenstine E A 1950 Fate of thiopental in man and method for its estimation in biological material. Journal of Pharmacology and Experimental Therapeutics 98: 85–96

Burch P G, Stanski D R 1983 Thiopental pharmacokinetics in renal failure. Anesthesiology 55: A176

Chamberlain J H, Sede R G F L, Chung D C W 1977 Effect of thiopentone on myocardial function. British Journal of Anaesthesia 49: 865–870

Christensen J H, Andreasen F 1978 Individual variation in response to thiopental. Acta Anaesthesiologica Scandinavica 22: 303–313

Christensen J H, Andreasen F, Jansen J A 1980 Pharmacokinetics of thiopentone in a group of young women and a group of young men. British Journal of Anaesthesia 52: 913–917

Christensen J H, Andreasen F, Janssen J A 1981 Influence of age and sex on the pharmacokinetics of thiopentone. British Journal of Anaesthesia 53: 1189-1195

Christensen J H, Andreasen F, Janssen J A 1982 Pharmacokinetics and pharmacodynamics of thiopentone: a comparison between young and elderly patients. Anaesthesia 37: 398–404

Christensen J H, Andreasen F, Janssen J A 1985 Increased thiopental sensitivity in cardiac patients. Acta Anaesthesiologica Scandinavica 29: 702–705

Clarke D L, Rosner B S 1973 Neurophysiologic effects of general anesthetics. I: The electroencephalogram and sensory evoked responses in man. Anesthesiology 38: 564–582

Dornette W H L 1954 From ampule to beaker. Current Researches in Anesthesia 33: 38

Dundee J W 1960 Alterations in response to somatic pain. II: The effect of thiopentone and pentobarbitone. British Journal of Anaesthesia 32: 407–414

Dundee J W 1964 Alterations in response to somatic pain associated with anaesthesia. XVI: Methohexitone. British Journal of Anaesthesia 36: 798–800

Dundee J W 1974 Molecular structure–activity relationships of barbiturates: In: Halsey M J, Millar R A, Sutton J A (eds) Molecular mechanisms in general anaesthesia. Churchill Livingstone, Edinburgh, p 22

Dundee J W, Hassard T H 1983 The influence of haemoglobin and plasma urea levels on the induction dose of thiopentone. Anaesthesia 38: 26–28

Dundee J W, Wyant G M 1988 Intravenous anaesthesia.

2nd ed. Churchill Livingstone, Edinburgh

Dundee J W, Price H L, Dripps R S 1956 Acute tolerance to thiopentone in man. British Journal of Anaesthesia 28: 344–352

Dundee J W, Fee J P H, McDonald J R, Clarke R S J 1978 Frequency of atopy and allergy in an anaesthetic patient population. British Journal of Anaesthesia 50: 793–798

Dundee J W, Hassard T H, McGowan W A W, Henshaw J 1982 The 'induction' dose of thiopentone. A method of study and preliminary illustrative results. Anaesthesia 37: 1176–1184

Dundee J W, Halliday N J, McMurray T J, Harper K W 1986 Pretreatment with opioids. The effect on thiopentone induction requirements and on the onset of action of midazolam. Anaesthesia 41: 159–161

Edwards R, Ellis F R 1978 Clinical significance of thiopentone binding to haemoglobin and plasma protein. British Journal of Anaesthesia 45: 891–893

Fee J P H, McDonald J R, Dundee J W, Clarke R S J 1978 Frequency of previous anaesthesia in an anaesthetic patient population. British Journal of Anaesthesia 50: 917–920

Finster M, Mark L C, Morishima H O, Moya F, Perel J M, James L S, Dayton P G 1966. Plasma thiopental concentration in the newborn following delivery under thiopental–nitrous oxide anesthesia. American Journal of Obstetrics and Gynecology, 95: 621–629

Finster M, Morishima H O, Mark L C, Perel J M, Dayton P G, James L S 1972 Tissue thiopental concentration in the fetus and newborn. Anesthesiology, 36: 155–158

Fischer E, von Mering J 1903 Ueber eine neue Klasse von Schlafmitteln. Therapie der Gegenwart 5: 97–101

Flowers C E, Hill C 1959 The placental transmission of barbiturates and thiobarbiturates and their pharmacological action on the mother and infant. American Journal of Obstetrics and Gynecology, 78: 730–740

French J D, Verzeano M, Magoun H W 1953 An extralemniscal sensory system in the brain. Archives of Neurology and Psychiatry 69: 505–518

Ghoneim M M, Pandya H 1975 Plasma protein binding of thiopental in patients with impaired renal or hepatic function. Anesthesiology 42: 545–549

Hudson R J, Stanski D R, Burch P G 1983a Pharmacokinetics of methohexital and thiopental in surgical patients. Anesthesiology 59: 215–219

Hudson R J, Stanski D R, Saidman L F, Meathe E 1983b A model for studying depth of anesthesia and acute tolerance to thiopental. Anesthesiology 59: 301–308

Jung T, Mayersohn M, Perrier D, Calkins J, Saunders R 1982 Thiopental disposition in lean and obese patients undergoing surgery. Anesthesiology 56: 269–274

Kawar P, Briggs L P, Bahar M, McIlroy P D A, Dundee J W, Merrett J D, Nesbitt G S 1982 Liver enzyme studies with disoprofol (ICI 35868) and midazolam. Anaesthesia 37: 305–308

Kiersey D K, Bickford R G, Faulconer A 1951 EEG patterns produced by thiopental sodium during surgical operations: description and classification. British Journal of Anaesthesia 23: 141–152

King E E, Naquet R, Magoun H W 1957 Alterations in somatic afferent transmission through thalamus by central

mechanisms and barbiturates. Journal of Pharmacology and Experimental Therapeutics 119: 48–63

Leading Article 1985 Latent acute hepatic porphyria. Lancet 1: 197–198

Lundy J S, Tovell R M 1934 Some of the newer local and general anaesthetic agents. Methods of their administration. Northwest Medicine (Seattle) 33: 308–311

McMurray T J, Dundee J W, Henshaw J S 1984 The influence of probenecid on the induction dose of thiopentone. British Journal of Clinical Pharmacology 17: 224P

McMurray T J, Robinson F P, Dundee J W, Riddell J G, McClean E 1986 A method for producing constant plasma concentrations of drug: application to methohexitone. British Journal of Anaesthesia 58: 1085–1090

Michenfelder J D 1974 The interdependency of cerebral functional and metabolic effects following massive doses of thiopental in the dog. Anesthesiology 41: 231–236

Morgan P J, Blackman G L, Paull J D and Wolff L J 1981a Pharmacokinetics and plasma binding of thiopental. I: Studies in surgical patients. Anesthesiology 54: 468–473

Morgan P J, Blackman G L, Paull J D and Wolff L J 1981b Pharmacokinetics and plasma binding of thiopental. II: Studies in Caesarean section. Anesthesiology 54: 474–480

Moruzzi G, Magoun H W 1949 Brain stem reticular formation and activation of the EEG. Electroencephalography and Clinical Neurophysiology 1: 455–473

Murphy P J 1974 Biotransformation of methohexital. International Anesthesiology Clinics 12 (2): 139–143

Organe G S W, Broad R J B 1938 Pentothal with nitrous oxide and oxygen. Lancet 2: 1170–1172.

Pandela G, Chaux F, Salvadori C, Farinotti M, Duvaldestin P 1983 Thiopentone pharmacokinetics in patients with cirrhosis. Anesthesiology 59: 123–126

Pratt T W, Tatum A L, Hathaway H R, Waters R M 1936 Sodium ethyl (1-methylbutyl) thiobarbiturate: preliminary experimental and clinical study. American Journal of Surgery 31: 464

Price H L (1960) A dynamic concept of the distribution of thiopental in the human body. Anesthesiology 21: 40–45

Price H L, Kovnat P J, Safer J N, Conner E H, Price M L 1960 The uptake of thiopental by body tissues and its relation to the duration of narcosis. Clinical Pharmacology and Therapeutics 1: 16–22

Saidman L J, Eger E I 1966 The effect of thiopental metabolism on the duration of anesthesia. Anesthesiology 27: 118–126

Shaw H 1974 Anaesthetic complications. New Zealand Society of Anaesthetists Newsletter 21: 144

Sorbo S, Hudson R J, Loomis J C 1984 The pharmacokinetics of thiopental in pediatric surgical patients. Anesthesiology 61: 666–670

Stanski D R, Mihm F G, Rosenthal M H, Kalman S M 1980 Pharmacokinetics of high-dose thiopental used in cerebral resuscitation. Anesthesiology 53: 169–171

Stanski D R, Watkins D W 1982 Drug disposition in anesthesia. Grune & Stratton, New York.

Stoelting V K 1957 Use of a new intravenous oxygen barbiturate 25 398 for intravenous anesthesia. Anesthesia and Analgesia, Current Researches 36: 49–51

Sunshine I, Whitwam, J G, Fike W W, Finkle B, LeBeau J

1966 Distribution and excretion of methohexitone in man. A study using gas and thin layer chromatography. British Journal of Anaesthesia 38: 23–28

Tabern D L, Volwiler E H 1935 Sulfur-containing barbiturate hypnotics. Journal of the American Chemical Society 57: 1961–1963

Unni V K N, Johnston R A, Young H S A, McBride R J 1984 Prevention of intracranial hypertension during laryngoscopy and endotracheal intubation: use of a second dose of thiopentone. British Journal of Anaesthesia 56: 1219–1223

Ward J D, Becker D P, Miller J D, Choi S C, Marmarou A, Wood C, Newlon P G, Keenan R 1985 Failure of prophylactic barbiturate coma in the treatment of severe head injury. Journal of Neurosurgery 62: 383–388

Weese H, Scharpff W 1932 Evipan, ein neuartiges einschlafmittel. Deutsche medizinische Wochenschrift 58: 1205–1207

10. Non-barbiturate intravenous anaesthetics

J. W. Dundee   R. S. J. Clarke

To put these drugs into perspective it is helpful to look at a classification of intravenous anaesthetics based on their speed of onset. Table 10.1 includes some drugs which are no longer in clinical use: these will be referred to briefly in so far as their removal leaves a vacuum in the armamentarium of the anaesthetist. The benzodiazepines used for induction of anaesthesia or sedation are only listed in the table as they are discussed in chapter 11. This chapter therefore mainly deals with etomidate, propofol and ketamine.

Table 10.1 Classification of intravenous anaesthetics

Rapidly acting agents: induction of anaesthesia
1. Thiobarbiturates: thiopentone, thiamylal
   Barbiturates: methohexitone
2. Imidazole compounds: etomidate
3. Sterically hindered alkyl phenols: propofol
4. Steroids: Althesin†, minaxolone†
5. Eugenols: propanidid†

Slower-acting agents: basal hypnotics
6. Ketamine
7. Benzodiazepines: diazepam, midazolam, flunitrazepam
8. Large-dose opioids: fentanyl, alfentanil, sufentanil
9. Neurolept combinations: opioid + neuroleptic

†Withdrawn from clinical use.

Solutions

The sodium salts of the barbiturates are freely soluble in water, as is ketamine. Because of lack of stability of the aqueous solution, etomidate, which is freely soluble in water, is marketed in an organic solvent. This leads to problems of injection pain and thrombosis. Cremophor EL was used as a solubilizing agent for propanidid and Althesin, neither of which is now available, because of the high incidence of hypersensitivity reactions mainly attributable to this solvent (Chapter 34). Propofol was first used clinically in a cremophor solvent, but this was abandoned for the same reason. It is now prepared in a freely flowing emulsion which does not have this hazard. However, there is a clinical impression that this formulation is less potent than the previous cremophor form. A similar situation applied when the organic solvent form of diazepam was replaced by an emulsion, and this view is supported by data on bioavailability. These emulsion preparations cause a very low incidence of venous thrombosis.

Etomidate

Chemical name: R-(+)-ethyl-1-(1-methyl benzyl)
                 -1H-imidazole-5-carboxylate
                 sulphate.

This is a white crystalline powder with a molecular weight of 342.4. Only the *dextro* isomer is active as a hypnotic. The salt is soluble in water, but unstable in aqueous solution. The base is soluble in propylene glycol and ethanol, freely soluble in polyethylene glycol and chloroform, sparingly soluble in acetone and water, and practically insoluble in ether and *n*-hexane. The drug is commercially available as an induction agent in a 35% propylene glycol solvent containing 2 mg ml^{-1} (0.2% solution) and is stable at room temperature for 2 years. The pH at 37°C is around 4.25.

Pharmacology

Central nervous system.   In effective doses etomidate is a rapidly acting drug with onset times similar to those of thiopentone and methohexitone (Kay 1976).

155

The minimum anaesthetic dose in fit unpremedicated adults is around 0.25 mg kg^{-1} and 0.3 mg kg^{-1} is recommended for clinical use. On a w/w basis etomidate is approximately 12 times more potent than thiopentone and 4–5 times more potent than methohexitone.

The duration of an induction dose of 0.3 mg kg^{-1} is such as to allow for uptake of a volatile agent, or for tracheal intubation with suxamethonium or with a non-depolarizing relaxant. It is a reliable induction agent with variations in the induction doses similar to thiopentone.

The EEG pattern of anaesthesia is similar to that with the barbiturates and propanidid (Doenicke 1974). The onset of sleep is accompanied by a high incidence of excitatory effects similar in frequency and severity to those with equivalent doses of methohexitone (Boralessa & Holdcroft 1980). These can be troublesome if induction is followed by a non-relaxant sequence, or with intermittent use of etomidate.

The excitatory effects can be reduced by opioid premedication or an opioid given intravenously 2–3 min before induction (Carlos & Innerarity 1979; Zacharias et al 1979b). Fentanyl or alfentanil would appear to be the drugs of choice for this purpose, and many anaesthetists feel that etomidate is only clinically acceptable after such pre-treatment. With small doses (50 μg fentanyl or 150 μg fentanyl) it is possible to sustain spontaneous breathing.

Recovery.   Recovery from etomidate is dose-related within the range 0.1–1.0 mg kg^{-1} (Fig. 10.1) in which respect it differs from the barbiturates but resembles propanidid (Clarke & Dundee 1966). There is a general consensus of clinical opinion that recovery from etomidate is slightly faster than from equivalent doses of methohexitone and markedly shorter than that from thiopentone.

Cardiovascular system.   One of the outstanding features of etomidate is its relative lack of cardiovascular toxicity, as compared with thiopentone. This was shown in the first reported animal studies and later in clinical studies. Therapeutic doses have no depressant effect on atrial muscle function or conduction, and the drug has no effect on dp/dt_{max}, mean aortic pressure or on coronary blood flow in man.

Clinical studies in general have confirmed this low cardiovascular toxicity (Zindler 1975). In fit patients Bruckner and colleagues (1974) found that 0.3 mg kg^{-1} produced a slight increase in cardiac index, accompanied by a slight fall in heart rate, a slight fall in arterial pressure (14%) and peripheral resistance (17%); dp/dt_{max} rose (9%) with maximum effects occurring about 3 min after injection. These changes are small in comparison with

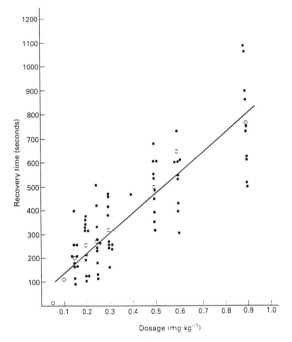

Fig. 10.1   Duration of sleep (time from end of injection until opening of eyes on command) related to the dosage of etomidate. ● = individual patients; ○ = average of groups of 10 (Dundee & Zacharias 1979).

the effects of other intravenous anaesthetics. Clinical doses of etomidate reduce peripheral vascular resistance and arterial blood pressure, an action which may be potentiated by other drugs (Dubois-Primo et al 1976, Kettler & Sonntag 1974, Zacharias et al 1979b).

Kettler & Sonntag (1974) also investigated coronary blood flow and myocardial oxygen consumption (MVO$_2$) in healthy patients. Increases in heart rate are in the main responsible for the increases in MVO$_2$ which were found with ketamine (+ 78%), thiopentone (+ 55%) and methohexitone (+ 44%). In contrast, etomidate did not produce significant changes in MVO$_2$. Coronary arteriovenous difference was not significantly altered by any of the agents, and etomidate alone seemed to have a true but weak coronary vasodilator effect. In another study they gave an induction dose of 0.3 mg kg^{-1} etomidate followed by an infusion of 0.12 mg kg^{-1}, min^{-1}, and found that coronary blood flow was increased by 19% and coronary resistance decreased 19%, leaving a constant coronary perfusion pressure.

Reports which deal mostly with infusions of etomidate (Lees 1983, Cohn et al 1983, Edbrooke et al 1983) or its use in poor-risk patients (Oduro et al 1983), confirm this comparative lack of cardiovascular toxicity. As suggested above, it is established practice to give etomidate with fentanyl or alfentanil: these opioids have minimal effects on the cardiovascular system and pretreatment with them will reduce the induction dose of etomidate. This might play some part in the reported low cardiovascular toxicity of etomidate; nevertheless it remains the drug of choice for many anaesthetists in dealing with poor-risk patients (Gooding et al 1979, Lindeburg et al 1982).

Etomidate causes a reduction in cerebral blood flow and intracranial pressure similar to thiopentone. It has been used therapeutically for patients with head injuries (Dearden & McDowall 1985) and also for neurosurgical anaesthesia, but in view of the adverse effects of prolonged infusions on adrenocortical function the justification for this application is in doubt.

Venous irritation. Pain on injection occurs in about one-quarter of patients given a direct intravenous injection of the propylene glycol preparation; the incidence is higher when small veins are used, particularly on the back of the hand or at the wrist. Slow injection is a major factor influencing the occurrence of pain; presumably the time the drug is in contact with the vein wall is the important factor. Opioid premedication reduces the incidence of injection pain and the common practice of preceding etomidate with fentanyl also minimizes the problem. Pain is reduced when the drug is given into a rapidly running infusion (Thomas et al 1976) but attempts by Kay (1976) to reduce injection pain by combining etomidate with lignocaine were not very successful.

A 2–3-day follow-up has shown a high incidence of venous thrombosis after direct intravenous injection of etomidate. In one study this occurred in about 25% of patients with the commercially available preparation (Zacharias et al 1979a). The incidence was related to the dose of drug injected, increasing from 13% with 0.3 mg kg^{-1} to 37% with doses in excess of 0.9 mg kg^{-1}. In a similar study carried out on patients undergoing major operations Olesen et al (1984) found a 24% incidence of thrombophlebitis up to the 14th postoperative day with etomidate, compared with 4% after thiopentone. There was no correlation between pain on injection and the subsequent thrombophlebitis.

Respiratory system. Cough and hiccough are uncommon with etomidate. If they occur they are of short duration and do not interfere with the course of anaesthesia, their frequency and severity being reduced by premedication with an opioid or diazepam.

Equipotent doses of etomidate $(0.3$ mg kg$^{-1})$ and methohexitone $(1.5$ mg kg$^{-1})$ cause a similar shift in the CO_2 response curve (Choi et al 1985), indicating a similar depression of the medullary centres that modify the ventilatory drive in response to changing CO_2 tensions. However, at any given CO_2 tension ventilation is greater after etomidate than after the barbiturate. This may suggest a CO_2-independent stimulation of ventilation. It would thus have advantages as an induction agent where maintenance of spontaneous ventilation is desirable.

Interactions with relaxants. Etomidate is a noncompetitive, as well as a competitive, inhibitor of pseudocholinesterase (Calvo et al 1979). Because of an early clinical impression that suxamethonium was less effective when given with etomidate than with thiopentone, Dundee & Zacharias (1979) measured the average duration of respiratory depression and apnoea following 50 mg suxamethonium. Although they found little difference in the duration of apnoea with the two induction agents, respiratory depression lasted significantly longer in those patients induced with thiopentone. The difference may not be of great clinical significance but it can be important if etomidate–suxamethonium is used for bronchoscopy with the apnoeic-ventilation technique or for electroconvulsive therapy.

There is a possibility of a prolonged action when suxamethonium is given after etomidate in patients with low plasma pseudocholinesterase activity (Booij 1984). Etomidate also potentiates the non-depolarizing relaxants (Booij & Crul 1979).

Histamine release. Unlike other intravenous anaesthetics, etomidate does not release significant amounts of histamine, but there are reports of rashes occurring in varying parts of the body — mainly head, neck and upper trunk — following its use (Holdcroft et al 1976) but this incidence is low (approx. $1:500$). Watkins (1983) considers etomidate to be an 'immunologically safe' anaesthetic agent but the possibility of a genuine immune response occurs, on repeated exposure to any drug, in addition to the normal risk of an anaphylactoid response. Those reactions which are reported appear to be free from severe cardiovascular effects and etomidate is recommended in high-risk patients such as those who previously have had a severe anaphylactoid response. The situation has, however, become less clear with two case reports in the German literature. Krumholz and colleagues (1984) observed generalized erythema, severe urticaria and hypotension when 4 mg etomidate was given near the end of an anaesthetic in a patient who had already received a number of drugs. The second patient (Sold & Rothhammer 1985) was given five drugs at induction, including 4 mg etomidate, and developed a severe tachycardia and hypotension which, on the basis of subsequent skin tests, was likely to be due to etomidate. Although Doenicke and his co-workers

(1973) found no evidence for direct histamine liberation with etomidate they were able to demonstrate an effect when it was used in conjunction with suxamethonium, alcuronium, pancuronium or lormetazepam (Doenicke et al 1980), i.e. synergistic histamine release. Sold & Rothhammer may have reported the first genuine anaphylactic reaction involving etomidate but Watkins (1985) considered that, since several million people have been anaesthetized with the drug, the risk is very small and 'the combination fentanyl–etomidate–pancuronium must still be the safest option open for the anaesthetist for the induction of anaesthesia'.

Liver and kidney function. Dundee & Zacharias (1979) found no changes in five liver function tests on the 3rd–4th and 13th–15th postoperative days in 20 patients given an average of 1.2 mg kg^{-1} etomidate for minor operations lasting about 10–12 min. The influence of etomidate on renal function has not been studied in detail. Contrary to the effects of volatile and some other intravenous anaesthetics, it does not decrease renal perfusion (Tarnow et al 1974).

Postoperative emetic effects. When used as the main agent for minor operations or for dental procedures etomidate has a higher incidence of emesis than other induction agents (Dundee & Zacharias 1979, Boralessa & Holdcroft 1980). This is a problem when etomidate is given as an infusion particularly when combined with an opioid.

Use in porphyria. The uneventful use of etomidate in a known porphyric who had developed acute abdominal pain and lower motor neuron paralysis following injection of a barbiturate suggested that the drug might be safe for induction of anaesthesia in such patients (Famewo 1985). However, Harrison et al (1985) have carried out experiments on a DDC-primed rat model of latent variegate porphyria which show potential porphyrogenicity of etomidate but not of ketamine when administered as a continuous infusion. Etomidate resulted in a change from control in 5-aminolaevulinate synthesase (ALAS) activity which increased by 47% with a corresponding 85% increase in corproporphyrin and a 40% increase in photoporphyrin content. On these grounds the drug must be regarded as potentially porphyrogenic.

Adrenocortical function. The pharmacokinetic profile of etomidate made it an ideal drug for long-term infusions, and its use was recommended for sedation in the intensive care unit to reduce intracranial pressure or during and following neurosurgical operations, or as a controllable method of achieving general anaesthesia in combination with an opioid and neuromuscular blocking drugs.
The safety of long-term use of etomidate was first challenged by Ledingham & Watt in 1983. During the years 1981–1982 they noted a significant increase in mortality in patients surviving more than 5 days from the time of injury, and whose lungs were mechanically ventilated. There was no difference in the severity of injury or in the degree of sepsis when compared with a lower mortality group who, apart from the sedation, were treated in a similar manner during 1979–1980. The more recent group were sedated with etomidate, in comparison with morphine and benzodiazepines in the previous group. They suggested that the causative mechanism might be suppression of adrenocortical function by etomidate by a direct effect on steroid synthesis in the adrenal cortex. This resulted in a more detailed look at adrenal function during etomidate infusions.

The actual cause of death in the Glasgow patients was usually related to infection, with adrenocortical suppression by etomidate as a possible contributory factor.

Ledingham & Watt's hypothesis was supported by in vitro animal experiments in which Preziosi and Vacca (1982) and Preziosi (1983) showed that 20 μmol kg^{-1} d-etomidate inhibited stress and drug-induced corticosteroid production in the adrenal gland as well as inhibiting the ACTH-mediated response. Etomidate also appeared to inhibit the rises in prolactin which normally follow surgical or other forms of stress, the findings being similar to those of another in vitro study (Lambert et al 1983), which found etomidate to be an even more potent inhibitor of steroid synthesis than metyrapone. Subsequent studies by Sear and his colleagues (1983) confirmed the suppressant effects of etomidate on adrenal function. They compared the response to induction followed by infusion of etomidate to that in similar patients anaesthetized with thiopentone, nitrous oxide and halothane. In response to a similar stimulus plasma cortisol increased significantly with the latter technique, whereas a slight decrease was seen in the etomidate group. Fragen et al (1983) found similar changes in comparing the responses to etomidate and thiopentone. In the etomidate group plasma cortisol concentrations decreased to less than the control concentrations, compared with an increase following thiopentone. In a subsequent publication Fragen et al (1984) reported that in patients who had been given thiopentone both cortisol and aldosterone concentrations were greater than the control level in the 2nd to 4th hours after induction, while with etomidate both levels were below baseline values in the 1st and 2nd hour after induction, and significantly lower than in those who had received thiopentone. Because aldosterone was also suppressed they suggest that etomidate exerts its effect by inhibiting the early stages of steroidogenesis in the adrenal cortex.

Sebel et al (1983) compared plasma cortisol concentrations following induction of anaesthesia with etomidate and with thiopentone. They found no significant differences in the two groups, in both of which cortisol had increased by the end of the operation. A subsequent, more detailed study by Wagner & White (1984) compared induction (bolus) and maintenance (infusion) with thiopentone and etomidate and a third group of patients induced with etomidate and maintained with thiopentone. They showed no difference in noradrenaline levels between the series, but a very marked decrease in plasma cortisol in those given etomidate. The suppression occurred even when the use of etomidate was limited to induction of anaesthesia. The authors point out that steroid supplementation might be required if patients given etomidate are exposed to an unexpected stress during the operation. These views are compatible with the results of the in vitro studies of Kenyon et al (1985).

In a more recent study Wanscher et al (1985) studied the adrenocortical response to a short tetracosactrin (Synacthen) test in patients having major gynaecological operations. Etomidate completely blocked the adrenocortical response to corticotropin stimulation for at least 24 h after operation, but no suppression was found in patients given thiopentone infusion. They conclude that etomidate cannot be recommended for routine induction and maintenance of anaesthesia.

Pharmacokinetics

This aspect of the action of etomidate has not been studied in detail, and there is some disagreement in findings by different workers. During transport in the blood about 76% of etomidate is bound to plasma proteins. The distribution of the two optical isomers [R(+)] and [S(−)] does not differ substantially in the blood, brain or liver but S(−) has considerably less hypnotic activity, suggesting stereospecificity of the 'receptor' area of the brain.

The first reported pharmacokinetic data showed a rapid fall in plasma concentration of unchanged etomidate in a biphasic manner, with an elimination half-life of 75 min. Plasma concentrations of metabolites increase over the first 30 min after administration then decrease with $t_{\frac{1}{2}}\beta$ of 160 min. Van Hamme et al (1978) followed plasma concentrations after an induction dose of 0.3 mg kg^{-1} etomidate in patients in whom anaesthesia was maintained with 1.5–2% enflurane in nitrous oxide–oxygen. These results are consistent with the drug following a three-compartment model distribution, the individual half-lives being 2.6, 29 and 275 min respectively. Subsequent studies by Shuttler et al (1980) in patients given 20 mg etomidate, who, like those of van

Hamme and colleagues also received enflurane, gave plasma levels which were best fitted to a two-compartment model with an elimination half-life of 68 min. Van Hamme et al (1978) found the apparent volume of distribution to be 4.5 l kg^{-1} and the systemic or plasma clearance rate was 11.7 ml kg^{-1} min^{-1}, the corresponding figures for the Shuttler study being 2.2 l kg^{-1} and 23.8 ml kg^{-1} min^{-1}. The differences between these two studies are not readily accountable.

Later work from Shuttler and his colleagues (1982) has shown that, in the presence of a steady-state concentration of fentanyl (10 ng ml^{-1}) the clearance of etomidate was reduced from about 1600 to 400 ml min^{-1}, with little alteration of the elimination half-life.

However V_1 decreased from 21 l to 5 l and Vd from 160 l to about 40 l. The exact kinetic drug interactions are not known: they might involve saturation of the enzymes responsible for the metabolism of etomidate. If substantiated by subsequent studies, the clinical implications of this opioid–etomidate reaction are important, as they suggest prolonged recovery after fentanyl–etomidate anaesthesia.

Etomidate is metabolized mainly in the liver by ester hydrolysis to pharmacologically inactive metabolites, the main metabolite in man being the corresponding carboxylic acid. About three-quarters of the administered dose is excreted in the urine in that form, with only about 2% being excreted unchanged.

Propofol

Chemical name: di-isopropyl phenol.
Propofol is a hindered phenol which is chemically dissimilar to any other compounds used in anaesthesia. It is insoluble in water and was originally solubilized in Cremophor EL. The currently available preparation is a 1% w/v aqueous emulsion containing 10% w/v soya bean oil, 1.2% w/v egg phosphatide and 2.25% w/v glycerol. The pH is 6–8.5 and the pKa of the drug in water is 11.

The emulsion formulation, which contains 10 mg ml^{-1} is free-flowing and is as easy to inject as an aqueous solution. it is made isotonic with glycerol and is sealed under nitrogen. The precautions which apply to intravenous fat emulsions must be taken with propofol; that is it should be stored below 25°C but must not be frozen and the ampoules should be shaken before use. Filters should not be used during administration of the emulsion, which should not be mixed before administration with other therapeutic agents or infusion fluids.

Pharmacology

Central nervous system.   Intravenous propofol rapidly and reliably induces anaesthesia, and side-effects are comparable with those of other induction agents. It has less anticonvulsant and central anticholinergic action than comparable doses of thiopentone. Propofol is a 'rapidly acting' induction agent and doses of 2.0–2.5 mg kg^{-1} injected at the height of forearm reactive hyperaemia will induce anaesthesia in unpremedicated adults in around 11 s (Robinson et al 1985). This is similar to the times with equivalent doses of thiopentone.

In contrast to thiopentone (Dundee 1960) sub-

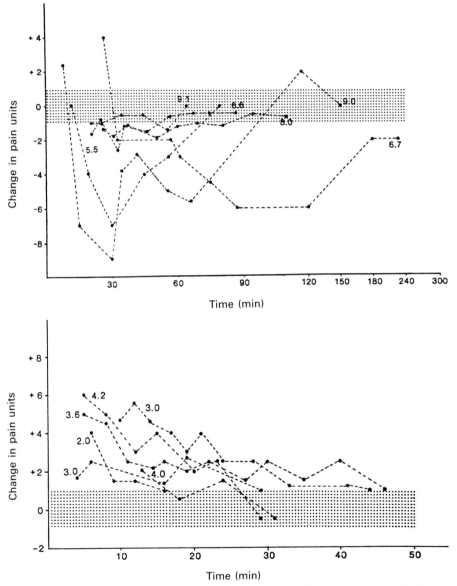

Fig. 10.2   Changes in postoperative pain readings from pre-operative controls following large doses of thiopentone (upper) and propofol (lower). Dotted line shows range of expected normal variations in readings (Briggs et al 1982).

Table 10.2 Frequency (percentage) of adequate induction of anaesthesia, hypotension and apnoea with varying single bolus doses of propofol in two age groups ($n = 30$, except $\star n = 20$)

Dose (mg kg^{-1})	Anaesthesia induced	Under 60 years: systolic BP fall (mmHg)		Apnoea (s)		Anaesthesia induced	Over 60 years: systolic BP fall (mmHg)		Apnoea (s)	
		21–40	41+	+ 31–60	61+		21–40	41+	31–60	61+
1.25						$\star$100 (30)	35	15	10	15
1.50	53 (13)	20	3	17	3	97 (3)	27	13	23	7
1.75	83 (17)	40	0	30	7	100 (0)	50	13	40	7
2.00	87 (10)	23	0	20	10	97 (0)	40	20	53	20
2.25	97 (0)	50	0	30	13	$\star$100 (0)	35	45	30	25
2.50	100 (3)	33	13	64	13					
2.75	100 (0)	40	3	20	40					
3.00	100 (0)	33	10	23	43					

Figures in parentheses indicate rapid lightening of anaesthesia (Dundee et al 1986).

hypnotic doses of propofol in cremophor do not cause an increase in sensitivity to experimentally induced somatic pain (Briggs et al 1982). Of more clinical importance are the postoperative findings when the drugs are used as sole agent for minor operations (Fig. 10.2). Thiopentone was consistently followed by hyperalgesia, which lasted for up to 4 h, while propofol caused a short period of analgesia. Clinical experience confirms the absence of antanalgesia (Briggs & White 1985, Lees et al 1985, Grounds et al 1985).

Propofol exhibits a very marked relationship between the age of the subject and the induction dose (see Ch. 4, p. 57, and Fig. 4.6). The reduction in dosage with increasing age becomes clinically obvious at 60 years. In subjects studied by Dundee et al (1986) the induction dose for those under 60 years averaged 2 mg kg^{-1}, while that for patients older than 60 years was 1.6 mg kg^{-1}. This is further illustrated by another study in which bolus doses ranging from 1.5 to 3.0 mg kg^{-1} were given over 20 s to fit patients under or over 60 years (Table 10.2). In these unpremedicated patients 2.25 mg kg^{-1} was adequate for the younger age group, whereas in the elderly patients a dose of 1.75 mg kg^{-1} sufficed. There was also increasing cardiorespiratory depression with dosage in both of these series.

The preoperative administration of 100 μg fentanyl with 5 mg droperidol reduced the induction dose of propofol to as low as 1.5 mg kg^{-1} (Rolly and Versichelen 1985, Rolly et al 1985). McCollum et al (1986), who studied the effect of a number of premedicants, found no potentiating effect from diazepam 10 mg or pethidine 50–75 mg, but papavaretum 20 mg with hyoscine 0.4 mg, made 1.75 mg kg^{-1} an effective induction dose in young subjects.

Recovery. Using reaction times and subjective assessment of coordination Herbert et al (1985) showed a faster return to baseline reaction times after 2.5 mg kg^{-1} propofol as compared with 5 mg kg^{-1} thiopentone, and performance after the latter remained significantly impaired until the morning of the second postoperative day.

Figure 10.3 compares changes in critical reaction time after equivalent doses of thiopentone, methohexitone and propofol. It also shows changes in a comparable group of patients who had no anaesthesia, showing some improvement due to learning. In the doses used, early recovery from propofol was clearly superior to that after the other two intravenous anaesthetics. By 40 min there was little to choose between propofol and methohexitone, but thiopentone recovery was still delayed at the end of 1 h.

In clinical studies, although Noble & Ogg (1985) found no difference between recovery from methohexitone (average 2.8 mg kg^{-1}) and propofol (3.3 mg kg^{-1}), most other workers have demonstrated an earlier recovery from propofol. The difference was most marked in the immediate postoperative period, and patients were ready to eat earlier after propofol than after methohexitone. This has made it the drug of choice for many anaesthetists for outpatient surgery (Mirakhur 1990)

Cardiovascular effects. Most workers have commented adversely on the cardiovascular effects of propofol, and many have considered these to be worse

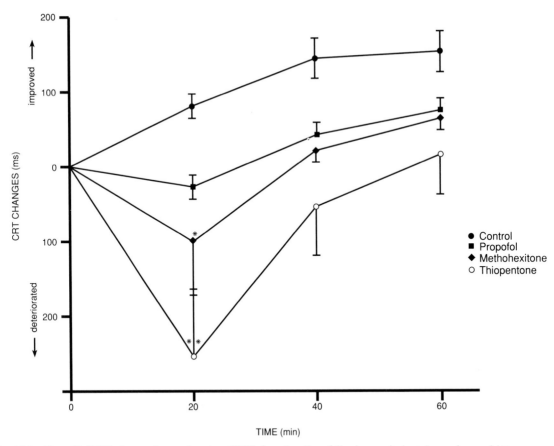

Fig. 10.3 Mean (± SEM) changes in reaction time (CRT) from baseline, following equivalent doses of propofol ■, methohexitone ♦, and thiopentone ○, and in patients having no anaesthetic. *Significant difference from propofol (Milligan et al 1987).

than those of equivalent doses of thiopentone (Prys-Roberts et al 1983, Youngberg et al 1985, Mouton et al 1985). Changes in the heart rate are less than with thiopentone and, together with decreased systemic vascular resistance, this could account for the relatively greater hypotensive effect of the propofol. Fahmy et al (1985) found that propofol caused a greater reduction in systemic vascular resistance than equivalent doses of thiopentone. In an in-depth study, Patrick et al (1985) compared the cardiovascular effects of propofol 1.5 mg kg^{-1} and thiopentone 2 mg kg^{-1} for induction of anaesthesia in patients scheduled for elective coronary artery operations. Anaesthesia with propofol was accompanied by a reduction in arterial pressure which was largely due to a decrease in systemic vascular resistance, and while thiopentone resulted in a small decrease in arterial pressure there was a greater rise in arterial pressure following tracheal intubation after the barbiturate.

The hypotensive effect of propofol as compared with thiopentone is more marked when the drug is given by intermittent administration even for short procedures. However, Robinson (1985), who gave large doses up to 16 mg kg^{-1} over a period of 40–60 min, found that the maximum fall in blood pressure occurred within the first few minutes of administration of the bolus induction dose; thereafter systolic and diastolic blood pressures remained virtually unchanged for the duration of the procedure. She also found a stable heart rate with intermittent administration of propofol.

Age affects not only the induction dose of propofol but also the cardiovascular response to the drug (Dundee et al 1986). In studies carried out on patients in ASA status 1 or 2 who were unlikely to have severe undetected cardiac disease, Table 10.2 shows a greater degree of hypotension indicating the need for caution in the administration of propofol in the elderly. The importance of speed of injection is shown when one compares the degree of hypotension in the initial dose-finding study reported by the same workers, where the drug was administered slowly over a period which could have been as long as 60–90 s compared with the effect of a bolus administration (over 20 s). Even in the elderly patients hypotension was not a problem with the slow injection, whereas Table 10.2 shows a high incidence with more rapid administration. These elderly subjects could probably benefit from preparation with a small dose of fentanyl or alfentanil, which should reduce the induction dose and minimize the cardiovascular effects, albeit at the risk of causing respiratory depression. Slow injection in the elderly is probably the most important prophylactic measure in reducing adverse cardiovascular effects of propofol.

Comparing the acute cardiovascular effects of 2.5 mg kg^{-1} propofol and 4 mg kg^{-1} thiopentone in patients without cardiovascular disease Grounds et al (1985) found significant differences between the drugs. There was a slight fall from baseline in cardiac output with both drugs, this reaching statistical significance only at 2 min after propofol and 8 min after thiopentone. Heart rate did not change significantly with either drug, although there was a tendency to tachycardia after thiopentone. Significant falls in mean arterial blood pressure occurred following both drugs, and these were always greater after propofol.

Arrhythmias do not appear to be a feature of propofol in humans. Animal experiments showed that induction and maintenance by propofol increased the threshold to adrenaline arrhythmias as compared with either propofol–halothane or thiopentone–halothane (Glen and his colleagues, 1985) The same workers found that propofol does not possess any significant ganglion-blocking or β-adrenoreceptor antagonist properties.

Venous irritation. Pain on injection has been reported since the first studies of propofol (Kay & Rolly 1977). There is a marked association between the site of injection and the incidence and severity of pain — 39% when injected into a vein at the back of the hand, compared with 3% when veins at the forearm or antecubital fossa were used. While pain is less with the emulsion, the relationship to the site of injection still applies (Briggs & White 1985). Venous thrombosis is not a clinical problem with the currently available formulation (Mattila & Koski 1985).

Of the various remedies tried to minimise the injection pain, premixing with 20–40 mg lignocaine immediately before administration, or prior injection of 40 mg lignocaine followed by venous occlusion for 20 s appear to be the most successful (Helbo-Hansen et al

1988, Scott et al 1988, Johnson et al 1990). The rate of injection does not appear to influence this complication, but administration of a solution at 4°C reduces pain (McCrirrick and Hunter 1990).

Respiration. There is an initial reduction in tidal volume following a normal induction dose of propofol, often amounting to a period of apnoea varying from 30 to 60 s. This is not a problem for the clinical anaesthetist, and patients easily tolerate artificial ventilation. However, there might be some difficulty in uptake of volatile agents if respiration is not assisted. There seems to be some degree of tachypnoea which Goodman et al (1985) found usually preceded the reduction in tidal volume and was also apparent on the return of respiration after a period of apnoea. Cough and hiccough are uncommon.

The intravenous injection of 2.5 mg kg^{-1} propofol had no effect on resting bronchomotor tone in the anaesthetized guinea pig (Glen et al 1985). In contrast to thiopentone, propofol depresses laryngeal reflexes, an oropharyngeal airway is tolerated in light anaesthesia and laryngospasm is uncommon after its use. In agreement with this de Grood et al (1985) found a greater degree of relaxation of the vocal cords after topical lignocaine in patients anaesthetized with propofol as compared with thiopentone.

Adrenocortical function. In vitro studies reported by Robertson et al (1985), Lambert et al (1985) and Kenyon et al (1985) showed that thiopentone, propofol and etomidate all inhibited ACTH-stimulated cortisol secretion in a dose-related manner. Similar inhibition of LH-stimulated testosterone secretion in a dose-related manner was found with thiopentone and propofol but not with etomidate, a finding in keeping with the known inhibitory site of action of the latter drug. The relevance of the findings is not clear, but on the basis of the relationship of inhibition to effective concentrations Robertson and colleagues (1985) suggest that it seems unlikely that either thiopentone or propofol will have any deleterious effect in vivo on adrenal or testicular steroidogenesis, while Kenyon et al conclude that, on the basis of its effects on in vitro cortisol synthesis, 'the clinical use of propofol should not be accompanied by the sort of steroidogenic problems seen with etomidate'. This view is supported by the animal experiments of Blackburn et al (1985), who found a reduced corticosteroid response to ACTH in rats anaesthetized with etomidate, but not with methohexitone or propofol.

Others

Liver function. Two reported studies of the influence of propofol on liver function tests (Kawar et al 1982, Robinson & Patterson 1985) showed no significant changes in liver enzymes (aspartate transaminase and alanine transaminase) or in serum alkaline phosphatase in either series.

Histamine release. The emulsion formulation caused no untoward effects in rats whereas the cremophor formulation produced a marked increase in plasma histamine concentration (Glen & Hunter 1984). Likewise there were no adverse effects following repeat administration of the emulsion preparation to the minipig, whereas the cremophor formulation had produced anaphylactic responses when a second injection was given 1 week after an uneventful first exposure (Glen & Hunter 1984). In a randomized study in healthy volunteers, Doenicke et al (1985) found no changes in immunoglobulin levels, complement C_3 or plasma histamine concentration consistent with a propensity to produce anaphylactoid reactions.

Coagulation. The drug has no significant effect on blood coagulation or fibrinolytic activity (Sear et al 1985). These workers found a significant fall in haematocrit value and haemoglobin concentration following its use, with a slight rise in blood sugar, but their significance is not known (Stark et al 1985).

Renal function. Apart from causing a slight reduction in excretion of sodium ions there is no evidence that propofol impairs renal function. By contrast thiopentone causes a marked reduction in sodium excretion and a decrease in the elimination of chloride.

Intra-ocular pressure. Propofol causes a reduction in intra-ocular pressure similar to that produced by comparable doses of thiopentone (Mirakhur & Shepherd 1985). These studies were carried out in elderly patients and the authors commented unfavourably on the significant fall in arterial pressure that occurred with propofol.

Pharmacokinetics

A highly lipophilic drug such as propofol would be expected to distribute rapidly but extensively from blood to tissues with a high estimated volume of the central compartment and a very high Vd_{ss} (Cockshott 1985). Studies with single 2 mg kg^{-1} doses of the cremophor preparation showed a decline in blood levels which could be described by a two-compartment open model with a mean α-phase half-life of 2.5 min and a mean β-phase half-life of 54 min (Adam et al 1983). The plasma levels were similar, irrespective of whether the drug was injected as a fast bolus or over 20–40 s. Patients opened their eyes at an average of 4.4 min after this dose, and by 5.2 min they were able to give date of

birth on request. This would suggest that with the intermittent injection technique supplementary doses would be required every 4–5 min.

Two studies indicate that the pharmacokinetics of the emulsion preparation of propofol can be described by a three-compartment open model (Kay et al 1985, Briggs et al 1985). In both there was a very rapid initial distribution of the drug from blood, a rapid intermediate phase and a slower final elimination. In the post-distributive phase propofol concentration declined biphasically with a mean $t_{\frac{1}{2}}\beta$ in the range 35–45 min — thought to reflect metabolic clearance of propofol from the blood. A slower final phase was observed in all patients giving a terminal half-life of 200–300 mins; it is likely that this phase represents slower return of propofol to blood from a poorly perfused compartment, probably fat. Both studies confirm the high clearance of the drug, the rate being in excess of the estimates of hepatic blood flow during anaesthesia, suggesting some possible extrahepatic metabolism of propofol. In patients who did not receive fentanyl or halothane clearance has been estimated as 1.8–1.9 l min^{-1}, and the volume of distribution 722–755 l.

Both fentanyl and halothane modify these figures (Briggs et al 1985). Fentanyl, but not halothane, significantly reduced the clearance from an average of 1.9 to 1.3 l min^{-1}. This was probably because propofol levels were higher in patients pretreated with fentanyl than in a comparable control group, reflecting a reduced degree of propofol distribution in the former.

A similar pharmacokinetic profile was noted when propofol was administered for induction and maintenance of anaesthesia by repeat bolus doses in patients having subarachnoid anaesthetic blocks. The blood concentration declined rapidly between 2 and 6 min after injection, indicating rapid distribution of propofol from blood into tissues (Knell & McKean 1985).

Secondary peaks have been observed in the blood decay concentrations in many patients following propofol. These might reflect local or systemic changes occurring on recovery, such as drug coming from muscle when exercised, or other alterations in regional blood flow; these appear to have no clinical or dynamic sequelae.

Most (88%) of the radioactivity detected following administration of labelled propofol can be accounted for in the urine in the form of glucuronides of propofol and the corresponding quinol, with approximately 2% in faeces (Cockshott 1985). Animal studies have shown that the drug is completely and rapidly metabolized to the sulphate and glucuronide conjugates of 2,6-diisopropyl-1,4-quinol and other related compounds which are eliminated mainly via the kidneys.

In vitro binding of propofol has been investigated using equilibrium dialysis techniques. Over the concentration range 0.1–20 μl ml^{-1} the drug was 98% bound to proteins in humans; data for animals were similar.

These pharmacokinetic data suggest that propofol would be very suitable for administration by intermittent injection or by continuous infusion. Gepts et al (1985) found that infusion rates of 9 mg kg^{-1} h^{-1} did not consistently maintain the desired hypnotic effect, and they suggested that an analgesic premedication followed by an average of 6 mg kg^{-1} h^{-1} might be a simple and convenient method of achieving good operating conditions. Robinson (1985) suggests that, given with nitrous oxide, 11.25 mg kg^{-1} h^{-1} would be an adequate dose for maintenance of anaesthesia.

Preliminary studies suggest that the pharmacokinetics of propofol are generally similar in patients with impaired renal function to those in normal patients (Morcos & Payne 1985). Interim results in the study of the effect of liver cirrhosis on the pharmacokinetics of propofol indicate that even in patients with a reduced capacity for metabolism by liver the clearance of propofol from blood is similar to that in hepatically normal patients (Cockshott 1985). This confirms the high capacity of the liver to metabolize propofol.

There are recent reviews by Dundee & Clarke (1989) and by Sebel & Lowdon (1989).

Ketamine

Chemical name: *dl* 2-(O-chlorophenyl)-2-(methylamino) cyclohexanone hydrochloride.

Ketamine is chemically related to phencyclidine and cyclohexamine (CI–400). It is an acidic solution (pH 3.5–5.5) available in 10, 50 and 100 mg ml^{-1} strengths, and is suitable for intravenous or intramuscular injection. It contains 1:10 000 benzethonium chloride as a preservative, but this is not included in the dilute solutions marketed in Britain. The 10 mg ml^{-1} has been made isotonic with sodium chloride.

Pharmacology

Central nervous system. Ketamine produces a condition known as dissociative anaesthesia, which is quite different from conventional anaesthesia. It is characterized by catalepsy, light sedation, amnesia and marked analgesia. This state has been described as 'a dissociation of the limbic from the thalamo-neocortical systems' (Corssen & Domino 1966).

Ketamine is described as a compound with a cataleptic, analgesic action but without hypnotic properties. Catalepsy may be defined as a characteristic akinetic state with a loss of orthostatic reflexes but without impairment of consciousness, in which the extremities appear to be paralysed by motor and sensory failure. Early animal studies showed the therapeutic index of ketamine to be higher than that of the barbiturates. There has been much speculation about its mode of action: it may exert its anaesthetic effect by a pharmacologically specific interaction with the NMDA (N-methyl-d-aspartate) receptor (Yamamura et al 1990).

Analgesia. The effects of ketamine on the central nervous system are intimately related to the profound analgesia it induces, and to its ability to produce dreams and emergence hallucinations. It blocks afferent signals associated with pain perception in the spinoreticular tracts without impairing spinothalamic conduction. It depresses nociceptic cells in the medial medullary reticular formation and the medial thalamic nuclei. Thus the analgesic effect of ketamine appears to be largely related to the blockage of the affective–emotional, rather than the somatic, components of pain perception. There is some evidence that ketamine binds to opioid receptors, an observation which, however, was not corroborated by all workers. The analgesia produced by ketamine, which can be produced even by sub-anaesthetic doses, extends well into the post-anaesthetic period.

Failure to obtain anaesthesia occurs occasionally, and may be associated with the absence of appropriate cerebral development; intact cortical function is necessary for the production of analgesia. However failure to obtain anaesthesia with ketamine, even in the presence of a normal central nervous system, has been reported. Self-induced enzyme induction must be remembered as a cause of resistance on repeat administration.

Electroencephalographic changes. In anaesthetic doses in humans, ketamine depresses the alpha rhythm and produces fairly continuous theta waves and rarely delta wave bursts (Domino et al 1965, Virtue et al 1967). This onset of theta activity coincides with the loss of consciousness, but some theta wave activity persists into the recovery period, even after analgesia has passed off. Ketamine also causes depression of late portions of the auditory evoked response. Detailed studies of the electroencephalogram show a function dissociation between the thalamo-neocortical and limbic systems, the former being depressed before there is a significant ob-tunding of the reticular activating and the limbic systems (Corssen et al 1968). The site of action of minimal anaesthetic doses of ketamine thus appears to be the non-specific thalamo-neocortical system.

Ketamine is excitatory to the thalamus and limbic system, where it provokes a seizure pattern limited to these particular structures but not extending to the cerebral cortex (Kayama & Iwama 1972, Ferrer-Allado et al 1973, Corssen et al 1974). Ketamine has been used in patients with seizure disorders (Sybert & Kyff 1983) and anticonvulsant properties have been attributed to the drug (Fisher 1974).

Anaesthesia with ketamine. The rate of onset is much slower than after the barbiturates. Figure 10.4 shows a comparison of times until patients stopped counting when varying doses of ketamine were injected during the period of reactive hyperaemia which follows arterial occlusion. They are compared with average figures obtained for methohexitone. In contrast to the barbiturates, it may be difficult to get a clear endpoint indicative of onset of sleep, particularly after slow injection, as patients appear to gaze sightlessly into space and may not close their eyes for several minutes. The eyelash, corneal and laryngeal reflexes remain unimpaired, and there is usually increased muscle tone accompanied by grimacing or involuntary muscle movement, but there is no response to auditory stimuli. While the usual adult induction dose is 2 mg kg^{-1} most patients will fall asleep with doses as low as 1 mg kg^{-1}.

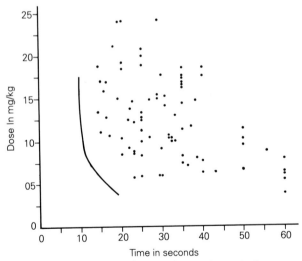

Fig. 10.4 Plotting points: time to onset of anaesthetic action of varying doses of ketamine, judged by time from end of rapid injection until patient stops counting, compared with average time (solid line) for methohexitone (Bovill et al 1971c).

With intramuscular injection the induction dose is 5–10 mg kg^{-1} and consciousness is usually lost in 2–4 min, but the onset may be delayed for 6–8 min.

Tremor and spontaneous involuntary muscle movements are not uncommon during induction with ketamine, and may be accompanied by hypertonus. In contrast to the barbiturates the incidence of excitatory phenomena is not influenced by premedication. Occasionally purposeless and tonic–clonic movements of the extremities occur during the course of anaesthesia. These might be taken to indicate a light plane of anaesthesia and the need for an additional dose, and unless this possibility is recognized one can readily give an overdose.

Memory of events occurring after apparent recovery is often impaired, amnesia increasing with the total dose of ketamine given. A much higher incidence is found when ketamine is given after heavy premedication, but no greater than that encountered when barbiturates are given after the same premedicants.

Cerebral blood flow, metabolism and intracranial pressure. In contrast to the action of the barbiturates, ketamine increases both cerebral blood flow (CBF) and oxygen consumption (CMRO$_2$). In dogs anaesthetized with nitrous oxide–halothane and paralysed with suxamethonium Dawson et al (1971) found that 2 mg kg^{-1} ketamine increased CBF by 80% and CMRO$_2$ by 16%. CBF returned to normal in 30 min and CMRO$_2$ in 20 min. Cerebrospinal fluid pressure changes closely followed changes in CBF. These rises occurred with repeated doses of ketamine. In their study the rise in mean arterial blood pressure was not very marked, presumably due to the concomitant use of halothane. The effects of ketamine on CBF, CMRO$_2$ and cerebrospinal fluid pressure were blocked by the prior injection of thiopentone. The rise in cerebrospinal fluid pressure after ketamine has been confirmed in its clinical use for pneumoencephalography (Tjaden et al 1969); it may be dangerous in patients with intracranial pathology in whom it is more marked. The rise in blood flow, cerebrospinal fluid pressure and intracranial pressure can be abolished by the hypocarbia produced by controlled ventilation.

Recovery. Consciousness returns in about 10–15 min after the normal dose of 2 mg kg^{-1} ketamine but, like the onset of anaesthesia, it is difficult to determine the exact moment when this occurs. Muscle tone reverts to normal first, after which there may be a period when the patient seems 'distant' and unaware of their surroundings. The final apparent return of full contact with the environment may be sudden, and the time varies from a few minutes to over an hour after first evidence of awakening. Diplopia and other visual disturbances are frequently present on return of consciousness, and can be both persistent and distressing. Some patients think they are blind at this stage, and this can be the cause of severe emergence delirium, particularly when accompanied by difficulty in speaking.

Emergence sequelae.   Manifestations vary in severity from pleasant dream-like states, a floating feeling, vivid imagery to hallucinations and emergence delirium. These may be accompanied by irrational behaviour, and may or may not be remembered. There are three related aspects of this problem which will be discussed together: (a) emergence reactions, (b) dreams and hallucinations and (c) longer-term psychotomimetic effects.

It is difficult to improve on the description of emergence sequelae by Domino et al (1965) in the first detailed report of the use of ketamine in man:

> During the recovery period the subjects showed considerable variation in psychic reaction. Some were completely orientated in time and space and showed no significant changes. Others showed marked alteration in mood and affect, some becoming apprehensive and aggressive and others markedly withdrawn. Almost all subjects felt entirely numb, and in extreme instances stated that they had no arms or legs or that they were dead. Other reactions noted included feelings of estrangement or isolation, negativism, hostility, apathy, drowsiness, inebriation, hypnogenic states and repetitive motor behaviour.

Because of the number of factors which can influence emergence disturbances it is difficult to get reliable figures as to their incidence when other agents were not used. The figures in Table 10.3 apply to the use of ketamine as the main anaesthetic in women undergoing minor gynaecological operations lasting for 5–10 min.

Table 10.3 shows a relationship in severity of symptoms (as judged by the need for medication) with dosage. This is a much higher incidence than the 2.8% incidence of 'confusion, with or without vocalization, excitement or irrational behaviour' of early reports. The symptoms may occur if patients are aroused early in the recovery phase, but this is not a universal finding. The incidence of disturbing emergence upset is much less after body surface operations (30–40 min) and even less after abdominal operations (60–80 min), although the duration of anaesthesia per se is not an important factor. Symptoms are less common in men than women, and the incidence is reduced markedly by opioid, opioid–hyoscine or opioid–droperidol premedication. Intravenous droperidol 5 mg, either immediately before or during recovery, will almost abolish emergence upset after ketamine. It can often be controlled by talking to the patient or, if this is ineffective, a small intravenous dose of 2.5–5.0 mg diazepam will exert a rapid calming

Table 10.3.   Percentage incidence of severity and nature of emergence sequelae in unpremedicated women undergoing minor gynaecological operations under ketamine–nitrous oxide–oxygen

	< 2 mg kg^{-1}	2–3 mg kg^{-1}	3+ mg kg^{-1}
Severity			
Mild	13	27	9
Severe	19	12	27
Requiring medication	4	6	24
Visual disturbances			
Nystagmus	4	8	20
Focusing problems	10	6	8
Diplopia	0	6	8
Colours	4	12	8
Dreams			
Pleasant	19	13	18
Unpleasant	23	33	38

From Knox et al 1970.

effect. Larger doses may reinduce anaesthesia and cause respiratory depression. A small dose of thiopentone will promptly terminate a severe reaction. Few patients have any memory of emergence delirium, particularly if diazepam is given, and it is more distressing to the attendants than to the patient. Lorazepam 2–4 mg is probably the most effective benzodiazepine premedicant for reducing ketamine sequelae (Lilburn et al 1978).

In contrast, dreams can be very upsetting to the patient. These have been described as dreams, hallucinations, psychological responses or altered affect. Again, to quote from the original description of Domino et al (1965)

> At times some of the subjects had vivid dreamlike experiences or frank hallucinations. Some of these involved the recall of television programmes or motion pictures seen a few days before, or they were at home with their relatives or even in outer space. Some of these phenomena were so real that the subject could not be certain they had not actually occurred.

When ketamine is used as an analgesic with nitrous oxide–oxygen following thiopentone induction, sequelae are rare and consist only of slight confusion. If sub-hypnotic doses of ketamine are given as analgesics for minor procedures without other cerebral depressants unpleasant reactions do occur occasionally, but are often minor.

It is of some importance to note that both emergence delirium and dreaming are virtually absent following the administration of ketamine in obstetrics (Moore et al

1971). This cannot be explained entirely by the other drugs given during labour. Perhaps the altered psychological state of the mother with her new baby may be all-important.

It is probable that neither emergence upset nor unpleasant dreams occur in very young children after ketamine (Ginsberg & Gerber 1969, Spoerel & Kandel 1971). While it is difficult to determine the incidence of hallucinations in small children, Roberts (1967) did not detect any personality disturbance with multiple ketamine anaesthetics, and only a 1:20 incidence of possible psychotomimetic effects. Wilson et al (1969) found that about 1 in 20 children reacted unfavourably to the repeated administration of the drug, but its 'acceptance' by the remainder improved with successive anaesthetics. None had problems with auditory or visual hallucinations. Although the incidence and severity of sequelae is greatly reduced in geriatric patients, the sequelae are not completely eliminated.

In burned adults subjected to daily administrations it is noted that disturbing emergence sequelae following the first administration are less after the second and do not occur at all thereafter. Reference has already been made to ketamine causing induction of the enzyme which is responsible for its own metabolism, and perhaps one particular breakdown product may have a psychotomimetic action and metabolism to this compound could be reduced by repeat administration. Domino et al (1984) have looked at a similar explanation for the reduction of sequelae by the prior administration of diazepam. This benzodiazepine reduces ketamine clearance to a significant degree, but there is no evidence that this may have psychomimetic metabolites. Alternatively they suggest that diazepam may enhance aminobutyric acid-mediated transmission which may be altered by ketamine. It is more likely that diazepam reduces delirium by use of its sedative and/or amnesic properties. This latter would fit in with this protective effect of thiopentone.

Any suggestion that the sequelae are not due to ketamine itself is dispelled by the work of Moretti et al (1984): in a double-blind comparison in female volunteers 2.5 mg kg^{-1} ketamine caused a significantly greater incidence of 'abnormalities of mental status' than 5.0 mg kg^{-1} thiopentone. The changes were short-lived and not evident on the following day, and there were no long-term sequelae.

Cardiovascular effects. In contrast to almost all other anaesthetic induction agents, ketamine tends to maintain the integrity of the cardiovascular system under most clinical circumstances by causing a dose-related rise in the rate–pressure product without significant changes in the stroke index (Tweed et al 1972, Idvall et al 1979). Tokics and co-workers (1983) have found a relationship between oxygen uptake and cardiac output similar to that seen with some other general anaesthetics, but they have not been able to establish a relationship between plasma catecholamine concentrations and central haemodynamics. However, significant cardiovascular depression can occur when ketamine is used with halothane or enflurane (Bidwai et al 1975, Stanley 1973) or in critically ill patients or those who have been subjected to acute trauma (Waxman et al 1980).

In the absence of depressant premedication the rise in systolic pressure in adults receiving clinical doses of ketamine is in the region of 20–40 mmHg, with a slightly lower rise in diastolic pressure. In the majority of patients the blood pressure rises steadily over the 3–5 min following injection and then declines to normal limits over the next 10–20 min. There is often a slight delay in the rise in diastolic pressure, which may still be rising when the systolic has begun to drop. This is a highly individual reaction and on occasions the pressure may be alarmingly high (Corssen & Domino 1966). The heart rate almost invariably increases following intravenous ketamine in humans.

The cardiovascular stimulating effects of ketamine are almost certainly due to primary direct stimulation of the central nervous system. In the absence of autonomic control it is a direct myocardial depressant (Traber et al 1968); the apparent paradoxical response in critically ill patients is likely to be due to an inability of ketamine and its sympathomimetic effect to counterbalance the direct myocardial depression and vasodilation, a direct effect on smooth muscle removed from normal autonomic influence (Liao et al 1979). The cardiovascular stimulation from ketamine can be blocked with thiopentone, diazepam (Jackson et al 1978) or flunitrazepam. On the other hand pressure rises and tachycardia, when ketamine is given with pancuronium, are greater than when tubocurarine or alcuronium are used, in keeping with the cardiovascular stimulant action of pancuronium. Cardiac arrhythmias are very uncommon following ketamine, and a number of workers have shown that it has an anti-arrhythmic action.

There are no differences in response to ketamine between patients found to have cardiac disease and those with normal hearts. Tweed et al (1972) found that the drug had both cardiac and peripheral effects, causing an increase in blood pressure, cardiac index (29%) and heart rate (33%) and pulmonary arterial pressure (44%) with a constant stroke volume index. In paced patients a 26% increase in cardiac index occurred with a corresponding increase in stroke volume index, thus indicating that ketamine enhances myocardial contractility. This is accompanied by a rise in oxygen consumption, and on this basis one would not recommend the use of ketamine in patients with severe coronary disease.

With doses in excess of 1 mg kg^{-1} there is very little variation in the hypertensive action of ketamine which has been noted even with sub-hypnotic doses (Domino et al 1965, Knox et al 1970). As shown in Figure 10.5, when a dose of 2 mg kg^{-1} was injected over 20 s or at 20 mg min^{-1} the peak rise was significantly greater at the slow rate as compared with the standard rate of injection (Bovill et al 1971a). This difference may have resulted from slight agitation during the slower onset of sleep.

In adults an intramuscular dose of 8 mg kg^{-1} is followed by a similar pressure as 2 mg kg^{-1} intravenously, although pressure rises do not occur until 4–6 min after injection, reaching a peak in 8–10 min. This effect lasts longer than that following intravenous injection. Premedication has little effect on the hypertensive action of ketamine. There is no clear relationship between the age of the patient and the hypertensive response to ketamine. The initial blood pressure does not affect the degree of hypertension produced by ketamine.

Relatively little is known of the effect of ketamine on the pulmonary circulation in man. Ketamine causes marked elevation of pulmonary pressure and right ventricular stroke work due to increase in pulmonary vascular resistance. Gooding and colleagues (1977) have shown that there is a 40% increase in pulmonary vascular resistance in individuals free of cardiovascular disease.

Respiratory effects. Respiratory depression is minimal and transient after clinical doses of ketamine when given in the absence of depressant premedication, and some have even found evidence of respiratory stimulation. The peak depressant effect occurs about 2 min after intravenous injection. Significant respiratory depression with reduction of PaO_2 occurs only after the rapid single-dose injection of 2 mg kg^{-1} in spontaneously breathing patients on room air (Zsigmond et al 1976). Respiratory depression, and even apnoea, have been noted when ketamine is given after opiate premedication, especially after rapid injection or when it is given intramuscularly to small children. There is a slight increase in respiratory rate in most patients. Cough, hiccough or laryngospasm are more frequent in children than in adults.

Ketamine dilates the bronchial tree and antagonizes the broncho-constrictive effect of histamine, acetylcholine and 5-hydroxytryptamine (5-HT) on both the trachea and bronchi, and ketamine has proved to be a most satisfactory agent for the asthmatic (Corssen et al 1972).

Salivary and tracheo-bronchial secretions are enhanced by the administration of ketamine and prophylactic administration of a drying agent is recommended, particularly in children.

Laryngeal reflexes are not markedly depressed with normal adult doses, but the extent to which the protective reflexes remain intact is not as great as was originally thought (Taylor & Towey 1971). Studies where 20 ml of a radio-opaque contrast medium were injected over the back of the tongue 1 min after loss of consciousness show a low incidence of inhalation of dye after 1 mg kg^{-1} ketamine, but there is less effective protection with 2 mg kg^{-1} and the lungs invariably contained the contrast when any premedication was given prior to the ketamine (Carson et al 1973).

Others. Intra-ocular pressure. There is a slightly increased intra-ocular pressure following the intravenous administration of ketamine (Corssen et al 1968) which has been attributed to a possible imbalance in the tone of the extra-ocular muscles.

Uterus. Uterine tone is not depressed with clinical doses of ketamine (Moore et al 1971), the tendency being towards increased tone. Galloon (1973) has shown that ketamine increases the pressure in the pregnant uterus for 5–15 min after injection, and during this same period increases the intensity and frequency of contractions. Marx et al (1979), investigating the effects of ketamine in doses ranging from 5 to 100 mg using in-

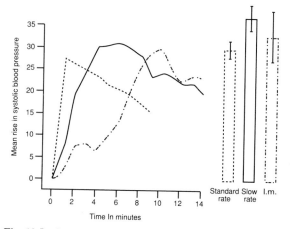

Fig. 10.5 Average rise in systolic blood pressure (mmHg) after ketamine. Columns on right show mean peak rise (drawn from data of Bovill et al 1971a).

ternal tocography of the term-pregnant uterus immediately following delivery, concluded that 100 mg or less has no unphysiological effect on the pregnant uterus at term under normal conditions. However, during situations in which increased uterine activity may be harmful — such as tetanic contraction, abruptio placenta or cord prolapse — the dose of ketamine should not exceed 25 mg. Idvall and co-workers (1983) have established that ketamine increases the basal tone and intensity of contractions of the non-pregnant uterus, and that these effects coincide with the phase of haemodynamic stimulation and peak plasma ketamine levels. Moore and his colleagues found some evidence of increased muscle tone in infants when ketamine was given to the mothers.

Blood sugar.   Ketamine causes a slight rise in blood sugar but this effect is quite variable. It does not exacerbate the metabolic response to surgical trauma (Lacoumenta et al 1984).

Porphyria.   There is no evidence that ketamine can precipitate an attack of porphyria in susceptible subjects.

Histamine liberation.   An erythematous rash is seen in about one-fifth of the patients given ketamine, but this is transient and of no particular significance.

Salivation.   This may be profuse after either route of administration of ketamine.

Pharmacokinetics

Because of its high lipid solubility the pattern of distribution of ketamine in the body is similar to that of the rapidly acting barbiturates, with short duration of anaesthesia due to both rapid breakdown and redistribution to peripheral tissues (Wieber et al 1975). Peak plasma levels occur within 1 min of intravenous and within 5 min of intramuscular injection. Initially ketamine is distributed to highly perfused tissues, including the brain, then to less well-perfused organs. Ketamine relies to some extent on biliary excretion, and significant prolongation of sleeping time and increase in its plasma concentration is seen after ligation of the common bile duct in rats (Ireland & Livingston 1980). The tissue concentrations follow the pattern of a two-compartment open-model system (Clements & Nimmo 1981, Zsigmond & Domino 1980). The initial distribution time is around 10 min, and the elimination half-life is in the region of 2–3 h following single-dose administration.

Ketamine is metabolized extensively by liver enzymes. *N*-desmethylation via cytochrome P450 is a major metabolic pathway forming nor-ketamine which

can then be hydroxylated at one or more positions in the cyclohexanone ring to form hydroxy-nor-ketamine compounds; these in time can be conjugated to the more water-soluble glycuronide derivatives. Ketamine can also undergo ring hydroxylation, but this pathway is of minor importance. Less than 4% of ketamine can be recovered from the urine as either unchanged drug or nor-ketamine, and only 16% as hydroxylated derivatives. Faecal excretion accounts for less than 5% of injected ketamine. Diazepam decreases the clearance of ketamine, resulting in higher plasma levels (Domino et al 1984)

The main metabolite of ketamine, like that of diazepam, has hypnotic properties, and nor-ketamine is about one-third to one-fifth as potent as ketamine as an anaesthetic. This might explain the prolonged residual drowsiness sometimes seen after return of consciousness. More interesting is the suggestion by White et al (1982) that the other metabolites might contribute to the cardiovascular or central nervous system effects of ketamine — the time-pattern could well explain the unpleasant psycho-sequelae, which were discussed earlier. As with the barbiturates, at the termination of ketamine anaesthesia the body will contain a large amount of unchanged drug, and this might have significance with regard to a cumulative effect and drug interactions.

Resistance often builds up to repeated administrations of ketamine: this could be explained by its effect on hepatic drug-metabolising enzymes by a process of self-induction. Marietta et al (1977) suggest that by increasing the levels of P450, NADPH reductance and metabolism of Type I substance ketamine behaves like the well-established enzyme-inducing drug, pentobarbitone.

Ketamine isomers

Ketamine enantiomers have been tested in animals, and have been subjected to clinical studies by White and associates (1980). Both quantitative and qualitative differences have been demonstrated between the isomers on one hand and the racemic compound on the other. It has been shown that there are unique pharmacodynamic and pharmacokinetic differences between these three substances. While no differences in duration of anaesthesia could be demonstrated for equipotent doses, there was a definite difference in potency, the ratio being 3.4:1 for the (+) ketamine as compared to (−) ketamine. (+) Ketamine seems to produce more effective anaesthesia than either the racemic or (−) ketamine preparation, with significantly more psychic emergence reactions. Postoperative pain was more prominent with the racemic and (−) ketamine than with the (+) ketamine variety, while the instance of dreaming was identical for the three groups. In a more general sense patients found the (+) ketamine more acceptable than either of the other two. Since the plasma decay curves and the patterns of appearance in excretion of the ketamine metabolites are parallel in all three groups, the difference can only be explained as being due to pharmacodynamic factors.

Despite the apparent superiority of (+) ketamine over the other two preparations the substance has not been marketed.

Clinical applications

Ketamine is one of the most interesting intravenous anaesthetics to have been introduced into clinical practice. It has properties both desirable and undesirable which are unique in the realm of pharmacology, and because of these its exact role is still undecided and even controversial after 25 years of use (Domino 1990, Dundee 1990). Because of the excellent tissue tolerance and its consequent suitability for intramuscular administration, and because of the profound analgesia obtained, it is a most desirable agent in instances when there is difficulty finding a suitable vein, or where venepuncture is poorly tolerated, particularly in young children and patients with extensive burns. Ketamine is also a very suitable single anaesthetic for minor diagnostic procedures, such as examination under anaesthesia, probing of tear ducts, certain neurological investigations in the absence of intracranial hypertension, paediatric dentistry and radiotherapy. Even the oral route has been found effective in children (Hain 1983, Morgan & Dutkiewicz 1983) while Maltby & Watkins (1983) have found the rectal route as acceptable as the intramuscular one for repeat anaesthesia in children, despite the low bioavailability of rectal ketamine (Idvall et al 1983).

Other non-barbiturate anaesthetics

Steroids

Hydroxydione was the first widely accepted non-barbiturate induction agent. It was freely soluble in water but had a delayed onset of action and a prolonged effect. Continuing research in this field pioneered the mixture of two steroids known commercially as Althesin or Al-

fathesin (no BP name). The main constituent of this was alphaxalone, and while alphadolone acetate had some hypnotic action its main property was to increase solubility. The contents of Althesin are:

Alphaxalone	0.90 g
Alphadolone acetate	0.30 g
Polyoxyethylated castor oil	20.00 g
Sodium chloride	0.25 g
Water for injection	to 100 ml

This was a rapidly acting drug which, in effective doses, induced sleep in one arm–brain circulation time. Anaesthesia was smooth and side-effects were few. The mixture had a very good dose–response curve as far as side-effects were concerned, and it was widely used for poor-risk patients. Recovery was rapid and the pharmacokinetic profile made it a very suitable drug for use as an infusion.

As shown above, this preparation is solubilized in cremophor, and an increasing number of anaphylactic reactions, and evidence to attribute these to the solvent, led to its withdrawal from clinical use. Unlike propofol, attempts at other formulations were unsuccessful.

Minaxolone, a water-soluble steroid, overcame the seeming impasse between water-solubility (slow onset) and insolubility (rapidly acting). It proved unsuitable for clinical use, despite its water-solubility, as it was accompanied by a high incidence of muscle movements and had a prolonged recovery time.

Propanidid

This is one of three eugenols (derivatives of oil of cloves) which have been studied as intravenous anaesthetics and the only one marketed in Britain (Clarke & Dundee 1966). Like Althesin, it was solubilized in cremophor.

Propanidid differed from all other intravenous anaesthesia in being an ultra-short-acting drug. Recovery, while partly due to redistribution from nervous to non-nervous tissues, was mainly due to rapid and complete inactivation by plasma cholinesterase to hypnotically inactive compounds. This breakdown process was dependent on the same enzyme as suxamethonium, and the duration of action of the latter was prolonged during propanidid anaesthesia. Unlike thiopentone it caused stimulation of respiration, followed by some depression or apnoea.

REFERENCES

Adam H K, Briggs L P, Bahar M, Douglas E J, Dundee J W 1983 Pharmacokinetic evaluation of ICI 35 868 in man. British Journal of Anaesthesia 55: 97–102

Bidwai A V, Stanley T H, Graves C L, Kawamura R, Sentker C R 1975 The effect of ketamine on cardiovascular dynamics during halothane and enflurane anesthesia. Anesthesia and Analgesia, Current Researches 54: 588–592

Blackburn T P, Glen J B, Hunter S C, Wood P 1985 Adrenocortical function in rats during anaesthesia with etomidate, methohexitone or propofol. British Journal of Pharmacology 86: 497P

Booij L H D J 1984 Benzodiazepine and non-barbiturate hypnotic drugs. In: Sear J W (ed), Clinics in Anaesthesia: Intravenous Anesthesiology, vol 2, W B Saunders Company, London pp 65–87

Booij L H D J, Crul J F 1979 The comparative influence of gamma-hydroxy butyric acid, Althesin and etomidate on a neuromuscular blocking potency of pancuronium in man. Acta Anaesthesiologica Belgica 30: 219–223

Boralessa H, Holdcroft A 1980 Methohexitone or etomidate for induction of dental anaesthesia. Canadian Anaesthetists' Society Journal 27: 578–583

Boulton T B (ed) 1985 Anaesthesia beyond the major medical centre. Current techniques with ketamine. Blackwell, Oxford.

Bovill J G, Clarke R S J, Davis E A, Dundee J W 1971a Some cardiovascular effects of ketamine. British Journal of Pharmacology 41: 411

Bovill J G, Clarke R S J, Dundee J W, Pandit S K, Moore J 1971b Clinical studies of induction agents. XXXVIII: Effect of premedicants and supplements on ketamine anaesthesia. British Journal of Anaesthesia 43: 600–608

Bovill J G, Coppel D L, Dundee J W, Moore J 1971c Current status of ketamine anaesthesia. Lancet i: 1285–1288

Briggs L P, White M 1985 The effects of premedication on anaesthesia with propofol (Diprivan). Postgraduate Medical Journal 61 (Suppl 3): 35–37

Briggs L P, Dundee J W, Bahar M, Clarke R S J 1982 Comparison of the effect of diisopropylphenol (ICI 35 868) and thiopentone on response to somatic pain. British Journal of Anaesthesia 54: 307–311

Briggs L P, White M, Cockshott I D, Douglas E J 1985 The pharmacokinetics of propofol (Diprivan) in female patients. Postgraduate Medical Journal 61 (Suppl 3): 58–59 (Suppl 3): 58–59

Bruckner J B, Gethmann J W, Patschke D, Tarnow J, Weymar A 1974 Untersuchungen zur Wirkung von Etomidate auf den Kreislauf des Menschen. Anaesthesist 23: 322–340

Calvo R, Carlos R, Erill S 1979 Etomidate and plasma esterase activity in man and experimental animals. Pharmacology 18: 294–298

Carlos R, Innerarity S 1979 Effect of premedication on etomidate anaesthesia. British Journal of Anaesthesia 51: 1159–1162

Carson I W, Moore J, Balmer J P, Dundee J W, McNabb G 1973 Laryngeal competence with ketamine and other drugs. Anesthesiology 38: 128–133

Choi S D, Spaulding B C, Gross J B, Apfelbaum J L 1985 Comparison of the ventilatory effects of etomidate and methohexital. Anesthesiology 62: 442–447

Clarke R S J, Dundee J W 1966 Survey of experimental and clinical pharmacology of propanidid. Current Researches in Anesthesia and Analgesia 45: 250–262.

Clements J A, Nimmo W S 1981 Pharmacokinetics and analgesic effect of ketamine in man. British Journal of Anaesthesia 53: 27–30

Cockshott I D 1985 Propofol (Diprivan) pharmacokinetics and metabolism — an overview. Postgraduate Medical Journal 61 (Suppl 3): 45–50

Cohn B F, Rejger V, Hagenouw-Taal J C W, Voormolen J H C 1983 Results of a feasibility trial to achieve total immobilisation of patients in a neuro-surgical intensive care unit with etomidate. Anaesthesia 38 Suppl: 47–50

Corssen G, Domino E F 1966 Dissociative anesthesia; further pharmacologic studies and first clinical experience with the phencyclidine derivative CI-581. Anesthesia and Analgesia, Current Researches 45: 29

Corssen G, Gutierrez J, Reves J G, Huber F C Jr 1972 Ketamine in anesthetic management of asthmatic patients. Anesthesia and Analgesia, Current Researches 51: 588–596

Corssen G, Little S, Tavakoli M 1974 Ketamine and epilepsy. Anesthesia and Analgesia, Current Researches 53: 319–335

Corssen G, Miyasaka M, Domino E F 1968 Changing concepts in pain control during surgery: dissociative anesthesia with CI-581: a progress report. Anesthesia and Analgesia, Current Researches 47: 746–759

Dawson B, Michenfelder J D, Theye R A 1971 Effects of ketamine on canine cerebral blood flow and metabolism: modification by prior administration of thiopental. Anesthesia and Analgesia, Current Researches 50: 443–447

Dearden N M, McDowall D G 1985 Comparison of etomidate and Althesin in the reduction of increased intracranial pressure after head injury. British Journal of Anaesthesia 57: 361–368

de Grood P M R M, van Egmond J, van de Watering M, van Beem H B, Booij L H D J, Crul J F 1985 Lack of effects of emulsified propofol (Diprivan) on vecuronium pharmacodynamics — preliminary results in man. Postgraduate Medical Journal 61 (Suppl 3): 28–30

Doenicke A 1974 Etomidate, a new intravenous hypnotic. Acta Anaesthesiologica Belgica 25: 307–315

Doenicke A, Lorenz W, Beigl R, Bezecny H, Uhlig G, Kalmar L, Praetorius B, Mann G 1973 Histamine release after intravenous application of short-acting hypnotics. A comparison of etomidate, Althesin CT 1341 and propanidid. British Journal of Anaesthesia 45: 1097–1104

Doenicke A, Lorenz W, Dittman J, Hug P 1980 Histaminfreisetzung nach Diazepam/ Lormetazepam in Kombination mit Etomidat. In: Doenicke A, Ott H (eds) Lormetazepam. Springer, Berlin, pp 11–15

Doenicke A, Lorenz W, Stanworth D, Duka Th, Glen J B 1985 Effects of propofol (Diprivan) on histamine release, immunoglobulin levels and activation of complement in healthy volunteers. Postgraduate Medical Journal 61 (Suppl 3): 15–20

Domino E F (Ed) 1990 Status of ketamine in anesthesiology. NPP Books, Ann Arbor.

Domino E F, Chodoff P, Corssen G 1965 Pharmacologic effects of CI-581, a new dissociative anesthetic in man. Clinical Pharmacology and Therapeutics 6: 279–290

Domino E F, Domino F E, Smith R E, Domino L E, Goulet J R, Domino K E, Zsigmond E K 1984 Ketamine kinetics in unpremedicated and diazepam-premedicated subjects. Clinical Pharmacology and Therapeutics 36: 645–653

Dubois-Primo J, Bastenier-Geens J, Genicot C, Rucquoi M 1976 A comparative study of etomidate and methohexital, as induction agents for analgesic anesthesia. Proceedings of the Belgian Congress of Anesthesiology II, Brussels, 10–13 September 1975. Acta Anaesthesiologica Belgica 27: 187–195

Dundee J W 1960 Alterations in response to somatic pain associated with anaesthesia. II: The effect of thiopentone and pentobarbitone. British Journal of Anaesthesia 32: 407–414

Dundee J W 1990 Twentyfive years of ketamine. Anaesthesia 45: 159–160

Dundee J W, Clarke R S J 1989 Propofol. European Journal of Anesthesiology 6: 5–22

Dundee J W, Robinson F P, McCollum J S C, Patterson C C 1986 Sensitivity to propofol in the elderly. Anaesthesia 41: 482–485

Dundee J W, Zacharias M 1979. Etomidate. In: Dundee J W (ed) Current topics in anaesthesia series. 1: Intravenous anaesthetic agents. Arnold, London, ch 6, pp 46–66

Edbrooke D L, Newby T.M, Mather S J 1983 Use of etomidate in an intensive care unit. Anaesthesia 38 Suppl: 44–46

Fahmy N R, Alkhouli H M, Sunder N, Smith D, Kelley M M 1985 Diprivan: a new intravenous induction agent. A comparison with thiopental. Anesthesiology 63: A363

Famewo C E 1985 Induction of anaesthesia with etomidate in a patient with acute intermittent porphyria. Canadian Anaesthetists' Society Journal 32: 171–173

Ferrer-Allado T, Brechner V L, Dymond A, Cozen H, Crandall P 1973 Ketamine-induced electroconvulsive phenomena in the human limbic and thalamic region. Anesthesiology 38: 333–334

Fisher M McD 1974 Use of ketamine hydrochloride in the treatment of convulsions. Anaesthesia and Intensive Care 2: 266–268

Fragen R J, Shanks C A, Molpeni A 1983 Etomidate. Lancet 2: 265

Fragen R J, Shanks C A, Molpeni A, Avram M J 1984 Effects of etomidate hormonal responses to surgical stress. Anesthesiology 61: 652–656

Galloon S 1973 Ketamine and the pregnant uterus. Canadian Anaesthetists' Society Journal 20: 141–145

Gepts E, Claeys A M, Camu F 1985 Pharmacokinetics of propofol (Diprivan) administered by continuous intravenous infusion in man. A preliminary report. Postgraduate Medical Journal 61 (Suppl 3): 51–52

Ginsberg H, Gerber J A 1969 Ketamine hydrochloride: a clinical investigation in 60 children. South African Medical Journal 43: 627–628

Glen J B, Hunter S C 1984 Pharmacology of an emulsion formulation of ICI 35 868. British Journal of Anaesthesia 56: 617–625

Glen J B, Hunter S C, Blackburn T P, Wood P 1985 Interaction studies and other investigations of the pharmacology of propofol (Diprivan). Postgraduate Medical Journal 61 (Suppl 3): 7–14

Gooding J M, Dimick A R, Tavakoli M 1977 A physiologic analysis of cardio-pulmonary responses to ketamine anesthesia in non-cardiac patients. Anesthesia and Analgesia, Current Researches 56: 813–816

Gooding J M, Wang J T, Smith R, Beringer J T, Kirby R R 1979 Cardiovascular and pulmonary response following etomidate induction of anaesthesia in patients with demonstrated cardiac disease. Anesthesia and Analgesia 58: 40–41

Goodman N W, Carter J A, Black A M S 1985 Some ventilatory effects of propofol (Diprivan) as a sole anaesthetic agent. Preliminary studies. Postgraduate Medical Journal 61 (Suppl 3): 21–22

Grounds R M, Morgan M, Lumley J 1985 Some studies on the properties of the intravenous anaesthetic propofol. (Diprivan) — a review. Postgraduate Medical Journal 61 (Suppl 3): 90–95

Hain W R 1983 Oral ketamine. Anaesthesia 38: 810–811

Harrison P G, Moore M R, Meissner T M 1985 Porphyrinogenicity of etomidate and ketamine as continuous infusions: screening in the DDC-primed rat model. British Journal of Anaesthesia 57: 420–423

Helbo-Hansen S, Westergaard V, Krogh B L and Svendsen H P 1988 The reduction of pain on injection of propofol: the effect of addition of lignocaine. Acta Anaesthesiologica Scandinavica 32: 502–504

Herbert M, Makin S W, Bourke J B, Hart E A 1985 Recovery of mental abilities following general anaesthesia induced by propofol (Diprivan) or thiopentone. Postgraduate Medical Journal 61 (Suppl 3): 132

Holdcroft A, Morgan M, Whitwam J G, Lumley J 1976 Effect of dose and premedication on induction complications with etomidate. British Journal of Anaesthesia 48: 199–204

Idvall J, Ahlgren L, Aronsen K F, Stenberg P 1979 Ketamine infusions: Pharmacokinetics and clinical effects. British Journal of Anaesthesia 51: 1167–1173

Idvall J, Holaset J, Stenberg P 1983 Rectal ketamine for induction of anaesthesia in children. Anaesthesia 38: 60–64

Ireland S J, Livingstone A 1980 Effect of biliary excretion on ketamine anaesthesia in the rat. British Journal of Anaesthesia 52: 23–28

Jackson A P F, Omadahale P C, Callaghan M L, Alser S 1978 Haemodynamic studies during induction of anaesthesia for open heart surgery using diazepam and ketamine. British Journal of Anaesthesia 50: 375–378

Johnson R A, Harper N J N, Chadwick S, Vohra A 1990 Pain on injection of propofol. Anaesthesia 45: 439–442

Kawar P, Briggs L P, Bahar M, McIlroy P D A, Dundee J W, Merrett J D, Nesbitt G S 1982 Liver enzyme studies with disoprofol (ICI 35 868) and midazolam. Anaesthesia 37: 305–308

Kay B 1976 A clinical assessment of the use of etomidate in children. British Journal of Anaesthesia 48: 207–211

Kay B, Rolly G 1977 ICI 35 868 — the effect of a change of formulation on the incidence of pain after intravenous injection. Acta Anaesthesiologica Belgica 28: 317–322

Kay N H, Uppington J, Sear J W, Douglas E J, Cockshott I D 1985 Pharmacokinetics of propofol (Diprivan) as an induction agent. Postgraduate Medical Journal 61 (Suppl 3): 55–57

Kayama Y, Iwama K 1972 The EEG evoked potentials and

single unit activity during ketamine anesthesia in cats. Anesthesiology 36: 316–328

Kenyon C J, McNeil L M, Fraser R 1985 Comparison of the effects of etomidate, thiopentone and propofol on cortisol synthesis. British Journal of Anaesthesia 57: 509–511

Kettler D, Sonntag H 1974 Intravenous anesthetics: coronary blood flow and myocardial oxygen consumption (with special reference to Althesine). Acta Anaesthesiologica Belgica 25: 384–399

Knell P J W, McKean J F 1985 An investigation of the pharmacokinetic profile of propofol (Diprivan) after administration for induction and maintenance of anaesthesia by repeat bolus doses in patients having spinal anaesthetic block. Postgraduate Medical Journal 61 (Suppl 3): 60–61

Knox J W D, Bovill J G, Clarke R S J, Dundee J W 1970 Clinical studies of induction agents. XXXVI: Ketamine. British Journal of Anaesthesia 42: 875–885

Krumholz W, Muller H, Gerlach H, Russ W, Hempelmann G 1984 Ein Fall von anaphylaktoider Reaktion nach Gabe von Etomidat. Anaesthesist 33: 161–162

Lacoumenta S, Walsh E S, Waterman A E, Ward I, Paterson J L, Hall G M 1984 Effects of ketamine anaesthesia on the metabolic response to pelvic surgery. British Journal of Anaesthesia 56: 493–497

Lambert A, Mitchell R, Frost J, Ratcliffe J G, Robertson W R 1983 Direct in vitro inhibition of adrenal steroidogenesis by etomidate. Lancet 2: 1085

Lambert A, Mitchell R, Roberston W R 1985 Effect of propofol, thiopentone and etomidate on adrenal steroidogenesis in vitro. British Journal of Anaesthesia 57: 505–508

Ledingham I McK, Watt I 1983 Influence of sedation on mortality in critically ill multiple trauma patients. Lancet 1: 1270

Lees N W 1983 Experience with etomidate as part of a total intravenous technique. Anaesthesia 38 Suppl: 70–73

Lees N W, McCulloch M, Mair W B 1985 Propofol (Diprivan) for induction and maintenance of anaesthesia. Postgraduate Medical Journal 61 (Suppl 3): 88–89

Liao J C, Koehntop D E, Buckley J J 1979 Dual effect of ketamine on the peripheral vasculature. Anesthesiology 51: S116

Lilburn J K, Dundee J W, Nair S G, Fee J P H, Johnston H M L 1978 Ketamine sequelae — evaluation of the ability of various premedicants to attenuate its psychic actions. Anaesthesia 33: 307–311

Lindeburg T, Spotoff H, Pregard-Sorensen M, Skopsted T 1982 Cardiovascular effects of etomidate used for induction and in combination with fentanyl–pancuronium for maintenance of anaesthesia in patients with valvular heart disease. Acta Anaesthesiologica Scandinavica 26: 205–208

McCollum J S C, Dundee J W, Carlisle R J T 1986 Premedication — effect on induction of anaesthesia with propofol. British Journal of Anaesthesia 58: 1330P

McCrirrick A, Hunter S 1990 Pain on injection of propofol: the effect of injectate temperature. Anaesthesia 45: 443–444

McLennan F M 1982 Ketamine tolerance and hallucinations in children. Anaesthesia 37: 1214–1215

Maltby J R, Watkins D M 1983 Repeat ketamine anaesthesia of a child for radiotherapy in the prone position. Canadian Anaesthetists' Society Journal 30: 526–530

Marietta M P, Way W L, Castagnoli N 1977 On the pharmacology of ketamine enantimorphs in the rat. Journal of Pharmacology and Therapeutics 202: 157–165

Marx G F, Hwang H S, Chandra P 1979 Postpartum uterine pressures with different doses of ketamine. Anesthesiology 50: 163–166

Mattila M A K, Koski E M J 1985 Venous sequelae after intravenous propofol (Diprivan) — a comparison with methohexitone in short anaesthesia. Postgraduate Medical Journal 61 (Suppl 3): 162–164

Milligan K R, O'Toole D P, Cooper J C, Dundee J W 1987 Recovery from outpatient anaesthesia: a comparison of propofol, methohexitone and thiopental. Anesthesia and Analgesia 66: s118

Mirakhur R K 1990 Drugs used by anaesthetists. Anaesthesia 45: 500–501

Mirakhur R K, Shepherd W F I 1985 Intraocular pressure changes with propofol (Diprivan): comparison with thiopentone. Postgraduate Medical Journal 61 (Suppl 3) : 41–44

Moore J, McNabb T G, Dundee J W 1971 Preliminary report on ketamine in obstetrics. British Journal of Anaesthesia 43: 779–782

Morcos W E, Payne J P 1985 The induction of anaesthesia with propofol (Diprivan) compared in normal and renal failure patients. Postgraduate Medical Journal 61 (Suppl 3): 62–63

Moretti R J, Hallan S Z, Goodman L I, Meltzer H Y 1984 Comparison of ketamine and thiopental in healthy volunteers: effects on mental status, mood and personality. Anesthesia and Analgesia 63: 1087–1096

Morgan A J, Dutkiewicz T W 1983 Oral ketamine. Anaesthesia 38: 293

Mouton S M, Bullington J, Davis L, Fisher K, Ramsey S, Wood M 1985 A comparison of Diprivan and thiopental for the induction of anesthesia. Anesthesiology 63: A364

Noble J, Ogg T W 1985 The effect of propofol (Diprivan) and methohexitone on memory after day case anaesthesia. Postgraduate Medical Journal 61 (Suppl 3): 103–104

Oduro A, Tomlinson A A, Voice A, Davies G K 1983 The use of etomidate infusions during anaesthesia for cardiopulmonary bypass. Anaesthesia 38 Suppl: 66–69

Olesen A S, Huttel M S, Hole P 1984 Venous sequelae following the injection of etomidate or thiopentone intravenously. British Journal of Anaesthesia 56: 171–173

Patrick M R, Blair I J, Feneck R O, Sebel P S 1985 A comparison of the haemodynamic effects of propofol (Diprivan) and thiopentone in patients with coronary artery disease. Postgraduate Medical Journal 61 (Suppl 3): 23–27

Preziosi V 1983 Etomidate, sedative and neuroendocrine changes. Lancet 2: 276

Preziosi V, Vacca M 1982 Etomidate and the corticotrophic axis. Archives of International Pharmacodynamic and Therapy 256: 308–310

Prys-Roberts C, Davies J R, Calverley R K, Goodman N W 1983 Haemodynamic effects of infusions of diisopropyl phenol (ICI 35 868) during nitrous oxide in anaesthesia in man. British Journal of Anaesthesia 55: 105–111

Roberts F W 1967 A new intramuscular anaesthetic for small children. Anaesthesia 22: 23–28

Robertson W R, Reader S C J, Davison B, Frost J, Mitchell R, Kayte R, Lambert A 1985 On the biopotency and site of action of drugs affecting endocrine tissues with special reference to the antisteroidogenic effect of anaesthetic agents. Postgraduate Medical Journal 61 (Suppl 3): 145–151

Robinson F P 1985 Propofol ('Diprivan') by intermittent bolus with nitrous oxide in oxygen for body surface operations. Postgraduate Medical Journal 61 (Suppl 3): 116–119

Robinson F P, Patterson C C 1985 Changes in liver function tests after propofol (Diprivan). Postgraduate Medical Journal 61 (Suppl 3): 160–161

Robinson F P, Dundee J W, Halliday N J 1985 Age affects the induction dose of propofol (Diprivan). Postgraduate Medical Journal 61 (Suppl 3): 157–159

Rolly G, Versichelen L 1985 Comparison of propofol and thiopentone for induction of anaesthesia in premedicated patients. Anaesthesia 40: 945–948

Rolly G, Versichelen L, Herregods L 1985 Cumulative experience with propofol (Diprivan) as an agent for the induction and maintenance of anaesthesia. Postgraduate Medical Journal 61 (Suppl 3): 96–100

Scott R P F Saunders D A, Norman J 1988 Propofol: clinical strategies for preventing the pain of injection. Anaesthesia 43: 492–494

Sear J W, Allen M C, Gales M, McQuay H J, Kay N H, McKenzie P J, Moore R A 1983 Suppression by etomidate of normal cortisol response to anaesthesia and surgery. Lancet 2: 1028

Sear J W, Uppington J, Kay N H 1985 Haematological and biochemical changes during anaesthesia with propofol (Diprivan). Postgraduate Medical Journal 61 (Suppl 3): 165–168

Sebel P S, Lowdon J P 1989 Propofol: a new intravenous anesthetic. Anesthesiology 71: 260–277

Sebel P S, Verghese C, Macken H L J 1983 Effect on plasma cortisol concentrations of single induction dose of etomidate or thiopentone. Lancet 2: 625

Shuttler J, Wilms M, Lauven P M, Stoeckel H, Koenig A 1980 Pharmakokinetische untersuchungen uber etomidat beim menschen. Anaesthesist 29: 658–661

Shuttler J, Lauven P M, Schwilden H, Stoeckel H 1982 Alterations of the pharmacokinetics of etomidate caused by fentanyl. Anaesthesia, Volume of summaries, Sixth European Congress of Anaesthesiology, London, 1982. Abstract 700, p 368

Sold M J, Rothhammer A 1985 Lebensbedrohliche anaphylaktoide Reaktion nach Etomidat. Anaesthesist 34: 208–210

Spoerel W E, Kandel P F 1971 CI-581 in anaesthesia for tonsillectomy in children. Canadian Anaesthetists' Society Journal 17: 37–51

Stanley T H 1973 Blood pressure and pulse rate responses to ketamine during general anesthesia. Anesthesiology 39: 648–649

Stark R D, Binks S M, Dutka V N, O'Connor K M, Arnstein M J A, Glen J B 1985 A review of the safety and tolerance of propofol (Diprivan). Postgraduate Medical Journal 61 (Suppl 3): 152–156

Sybert J W, Kyff J V 1983 Ketamine treatment of status epilepticus. Anesthesiology 58: 203

Tarnow J, Passian J, Patschke D, Weymar A, Bruckner J B 1974 Nierendurchblutunt unter Etomidate. Anaesthesist 23: 421–422

Taylor P A, Towey R M 1971 Depression of laryngeal reflexes during ketamine anaesthesia. British Medical Journal 2: 688–689

Thomas B, Meirlaen L, Rolly G, Weyne L 1976 Clinical use of etomidate. Proceedings of the Belgian Congress of Anesthesiology II, Brussels, 10–13 September 1975. Acta Anaesthesiologica Belgica 27: 167–174

Tjaden R J, Ethier R, Gilbert R G B, Straja A 1969 The use of CI-581 (Ketalar) for paediatric pneumoencephalography. Journal of the Canadian Association of Radiologists 20: 155–156

Tokics L, Brismar B, Hedenstierna G, Lundh R 1983 Oxygen uptake and central circulation during ketamine anaesthesia. Acta Anaesthesiologica Scandinavica 27: 318–322

Traber D L, Wilson R D, Priano L L 1968 Differentiation of the cardiovascular effects of CI-581. Anesthesia and Analgesia, Current Researches 47: 769–778

Tweed W A, Minuck M, Mymin D 1972 Circulatory response to ketamine anesthesia. Anesthesiology 37: 613–619

van Hamme M J, Ghoneim M M, Ambre J J 1978 Pharmacokinetics of etomidate, a new intravenous anaesthetic. Anesthesiology 49: 274

Virtue R W, Alanis J M, Mari M, Lafargue R T, Vogel J H K, Metcalf D R 1967 An anesthetic agent: 2-orthochlorophenyl, 2-methylamino cyclohexanone HCl (CI-582). Anesthesiology 28: 823–833

Wagner R L, White P F 1984 Etomidate inhibits adrenocortical function in surgical patients. Anesthesiology 61: 647–651

Wanscher M, Tonnesen E, Huttel M, Larsen K 1985 Etomidate infusion and adrenocortical function. A study in elective surgery. Acta Anaesthesiologica Scandinavica 29: 483–485

Watkins J 1983 Etomidate: 'immunologically safe' anaesthetic agent. Anaesthesia 38 Suppl: 34–38

Watkins J 1985 Letter: Etomidate: an 'immunologically safe' anaesthetic agent? Anaesthesia 40: 145

Waxman K, Shoemaker W C, Lippmann M 1980 Cardiovascular effects of anesthetic induction with ketamine. Anesthesia and Analgesia, Current Researches 59: 355–358

White P F, Ham J, Way W L, Trevor A J 1980 Pharmacology of ketamine isomers in surgical patients. Anesthesiology 52: 231–239

White P F, Way W L, Trevor A J 1982 Ketamine — its pharmacology and therapeutic uses. Anesthesiology 56: 119–136

Wieber J, Gugler R, Hengstmann J K Dengler H J 1975 Pharmacokinetics of ketamine in man. Der Anaesthetist 24: 260–263

Wilson R D, Traber D L, Evans B L 1969 Correlation of psychologic and physiologic observations from children undergoing repeated ketamine anesthesia. Anesthesia and Analgesia, Current Researches 48: 995–1001

Yamamura T, Karado K, Okamuro A, Kemmotsu O 1990 Is the site of action of ketamine anesthesia the n-methyl-d-aspartate receptor? Anesthesiology 72: 704–710

Yoshikawi K, Murai Y 1971 The effect of ketamine on

intraocular pressure in children. Anesthesia and Analgesia, Current Researches 50: 199–202

Youngberg J A, Grogono A W, Sehon C K, White J, Texidor M 1985 Comparative evaluation of diprivan, thiopental and thiamylal for induction of anesthesia. Anesthesiology 63: A365

Zacharias M, Clarke R S J, Dundee J W, Johnston S B 1979a Venous sequelae following etomidate. British Journal of Anaesthesia 51: 779

Zacharias M, Dundee J W, Clarke R S J, Hegarty J E 1979b Effect of preanaesthetic medication on etomidate. British Journal of Anaesthesia 51: 127–133

Zindler M 1975 In: Arias A, Llaurado R, Nalda M A, Lunn J N (eds) Recent progress in anaesthesiology and resuscitation, Proceedings of the IV European Congress of Anaesthesiology, Madrid 5–11 September 1974. Excerpta Medica, Amsterdam; American Elsevier, New York, p 118–121

Zsigmond E K, Domino E F 1980 Ketamine — clinical pharmacology, pharmacokinetics, and current clinical uses. Anesthesiology Review 7: 13–33

Zsigmond E K, Matsuki A, Kothary S P, Jallad M 1976 Arterial hypoxemia caused by intravenous ketamine. Anesthesia and Analgesia, Current Researches 55: 311–314

11. Benzodiazepines

J. W. Dundee J. N. Halliday

The benzodiazepines are part of the recent 'drug explosion' which has affected all branches of medicine. In the 1950s the phenothiazines were introduced into anaesthetic practice and were the first drugs which could be truly called multipurpose. The most popular of these, chlorpromazine, had the British trade name of Largactil, indicating its large number of actions: it was used as pre-anaesthetic medication, with narcotics to induce anaesthesia, to facilitate the production of hypothermia, to 'potentiate' anaesthetic agents, as an anti-emetic and to augment the action of analgesic drugs. The benzodiazepines are the second of this multipurpose group and the most popular of these, diazepam, has been used for most of the above indications. Like chlorpromazine it is available in oral and injectable forms. At one time it was estimated that between 30 and 40 phenothiazines had been used clinically, and today the situation is very similar with respect to the benzodiazepines. This chapter, while discussing their pharmacology in general, will deal in detail only with those drugs which are of immediate interest to the anaesthetist (Table 11.1). Emphasis will placed on diazepam and midazolam.

MODE OF ACTION

The benzodiazepine group of drugs all possess the same range of actions on the central nervous system. They act on specific receptor sites throughout the brain and spinal cord, though radio-isotopic binding studies have shown these to be most dense in the cerebral cortex, the hippocampus and the cerebellum (Mohler & Okada 1977).

Their effect is produced by the potentiation of certain inhibitory interneurons which utilize the neurotransmitter gamma-aminobutyric acid (GABA). Upon release of GABA into the synapse an increase in the flow of Cl^- ions into the target neuron occurs, resulting in hyperpolarization. The nerve cell is thus made more refractory to any excitatory impulse (Haefely et al 1975).

The benzodiazepine receptors form part of a larger structure: the GABA receptor–chloride channel complex (Fig. 11.1). Like other ion channels, this is composed of a number of protein subunits arranged around the channel. In this case there are two types of protein; the benzodiazepine receptor exists on the alpha subunit, while the GABA receptor is on the beta (Mohler and Richards 1988). GABA receptor agonists act on the GABA receptor to cause opening of the chloride channel. The benzodiazepine receptor is a modulating unit, so that substances acting on it modify the GABA-mediated chloride channel gating process, either enhancing or reducing it. The benzodiazepines act as agonists at the benzodiazepine receptors and enhance a submaximal response to GABA (they cannot increase a maximal effect, which may explain the high therapeutic index of these drugs) and produce the classical benzodiazepine effects — sedative, anticonvulsant and anti-anxiety. There are two other classes of ligand at the

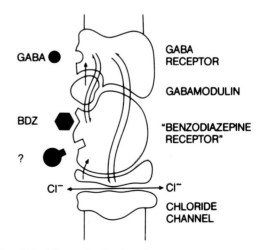

Fig. 11.1 The mode of action of benzodiazepines and their antagonists on their receptors.

benzodiazepine receptor. Competitive antagonists, including flumazenil, bind to the receptor and inhibit benzodiazepine effects. The third group of drugs bind to the receptors, but inhibit GABA-mediated chloride channel opening and so cause opposite effects to the benzodiazepines. These have been termed 'inverse agonists' (Nutt et al 1981). Chemically, they are mainly beta-carbolines.

Similarity of clinical action

There is growing evidence that all of the benzodiazepines have a similar pharmacological profile, and that the therapeutic use is related more to the form of pharmaceutical preparation rather than to any inherent drug differences. The currently available benzodiazepines range from those which are marketed as 'daytime sedatives' to longer-acting drugs which are used as hypnotics. Certain preparations are recommended for control of epileptic convulsions and a small number for induction of anaesthesia.

The benzodiazepines can be regarded as drugs which cause a dose-related cerebral depression. A hypothetical representation of this is shown on Figure 11.2. In increasing doses all of these drugs will cause mild sedation, drowsiness, sleep and even anaesthesia, but it is only possible to produce this wide spectrum of actions with a small number which are available as oral, intravenous and intramuscular preparations. Certain pharmacokinetic differences determine the time of onset of intravenous benzodiazepines but in anaesthetic practice these are less important than their metabolism, particularly their breakdown to hypnotically active

metabolites and the duration of action of both the parent compound and the metabolite.

The variability of action of the benzodiazepines is quite different from that of other drugs used in anaesthesia. With an increasing degree of cerebral depression there is an increasing variability of dose required to produce the desired therapeutic effect. As will be shown later, this difference is more marked in younger patients and is one of the factors limiting their more widespread acceptance as induction agents.

While anaesthetists will generally agree with the views expressed in Figure 11.2 it is interesting to note that recently the Committee on Review of Medicines (1980) made a similar comment with regard to the similarity of the anxiolytic and sedative properties of different benzodiazepines. They based their classification of the different drugs on their pharmacokinetic properties and their clinical classification (similar to Table 11.1) divides them according to their elimination half-life ($t_{\frac{1}{2}}\beta$). This will be discussed later.

In addition to the common pharmacological actions shown in Figure 11.2, all benzodiazepines have anticonvulsant activity, and the injectable ones are useful as anticonvulsants although their potency is limited in comparison with intravenous thiobarbiturates or neuromuscular blocking drugs.

PHARMACOKINETICS

As already mentioned, the benzodiazepines have a number of similar pharmacodynamic actions but vary in their metabolism and elimination. They may be classified according to their elimination half-life (Table 11.1) and this bears a close relationship to their clinical action. In this table chlordiazepoxide and flurazepam are included in the long-acting group because of their metabolites. There are certain exceptions to this (McKenzie 1983), e.g. the clinical effects of lorazepam do not conform to this classification. This drug has a longer clinical action than one expect from its elimination half-life; this is because of its extensive distribution in the central nervous system.

Absorption and administration

The rate and extent of absorption of the benzodiazepines following oral and intramuscular injection varies greatly, and is dependent upon the physicochemical and pharmaceutical properties of the individual preparations. Unlike most other drugs, in man diazepam is more reliably absorbed following oral administration than when given by the intramuscular route (Hillstead et al 1974, Gamble et al 1975, Assaf et al 1974, 1975). With

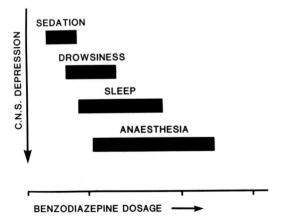

Fig. 11.2 Dose-effect response to an injectable benzodiazepine showing increasing dose requirements and variability in response.

Table 11.1 Classification of the duration of action of some benzodiazepines based on their elimination half-lives (h) in healthy subjects

Ultra-short	Short	Intermediate	Long
Midazolam (1.5–5)★	Oxazepam (5–15)	Flunitrazepam (15–35)★	Diazepam (20–70)★
[Triazolam (2–5)]	Temazepam (7–20)	Nitrazepam (20–40)	[Chlordiazepoxide (5–30)]
		Lorazepam (10–20)★	[Flurazepam (2–3)]
		[Clonazepam (20–40)★]	

★Indicates a commercially available injectable form.
Those in brackets are of little interest to anaesthetists.

oral diazepam, peak plasma levels occur within 1 h following administration. These studies were carried out with the organic solvent preparation, Valium, from which the delayed and incomplete absorption of the drug may be due to precipitation in muscle. Lower plasma levels follow intramuscular injection of Diazemuls as compared with Valium (Dundee & Kawar 1982). As Diazemuls is very painful on intramuscular injection, this point is of purely theoretical interest.

Midazolam is rapidly and completely absorbed when given by mouth, with peak levels attained by 45 min. However as two-thirds of the drug is cleared following its first passage through the liver it is not ideal for oral administration: at the time of writing it is only commercially available in an injectable form. When given intramuscularly midazolam is rapidly and consistently absorbed (Hildebrand et al 1983).

By contrast with the above, both flunitrazepam and lorazepam are absorbed less rapidly than diazepam when given by mouth, taking up to 2 h to attain peak plasma levels. Intramuscular uptake of both drugs from injection sites is similar to that following oral administration, and is more reliable than diazepam. Temazepam, which is not available in an injectable form, varies in its uptake depending on the pharmaceutical formulation used. The soft gelatine capsule available in Britain is rapidly absorbed, while the hard capsule used in North America leads to slow absorption (Fucella et al 1977, 1979, Divoll et al 1981). This is an important point which may on occasions be ignored.

Factors influencing absorption

Several other factors alter the absorption of the benzodiazepines. In the case of intramuscular injection, exercise is probably the most important (Gamble 1975, Hildebrand et al 1983). These latter workers also showed a more rapid uptake when midazolam was injected with hyaluronidase. Oral absorption is most readily speeded up by the simultaneous administration of metoclopramide, which hastens passage of the drug into the upper small intestine from which the bulk of absorption takes place. In social concentrations (10% v/v) alcohol will decrease the rate of absorption of diazepam; however, concentrations of 50% and greater will increase uptake from the stomach (Greenblatt et al 1978a). It has a variable effect on absorption of other benzodiazepines.

Effect of gastric acidity and emptying

The histamine-2 antagonists, cimetidine (McGowan and Dundee 1982) and ranitidine (Elwood et al 1983) have been shown to increase the absorption of orally administered diazepam, lorazepam and midazolam.

The resultant increase in gastric pH leads to a greater concentration of unionized benzodiazepine in the stomach, and hence more will be absorbed. When midazolam absorption is enhanced by ranitidine (Elwood et al 1983), there is a clinically significant increase in the soporific effects associated with higher plasma levels of the benzodiazepines.

Benzodiazepines are better absorbed if the stomach is empty, as following the administration of intravenous metoclopramide. The presence of food or an aluminium-containing antacid will delay gastric emptying and absorption (Greenblatt et al 1978b). This effect of delaying gastric emptying by antacid administration outweighs the influence of pH changes upon absorption. This delayed gastric emptying associated with slower absorption is also a feature with concurrent morphine, pethidine and atropine administration (Gamble et al 1975, 1976b).

Protein binding

The benzodiazepines are all highly bound to plasma albumin, ranging from 80% in the case of flunitrazepam to 98% with diazepam (Greenblatt et al 1982). The rank order for binding of other preparations is shown in

Table 11.2. Small changes in this protein binding will produce large alterations to concentrations of available free drug, and will markedly affect the clinical action of the benzodiazepine. This has been demonstrated to be important in clinical practice in the case of midazolam (Dundee et al 1984). Patients with liver or renal disease and in states of malnutrition with resulting hypo-albuminaemia, have an enhanced response to benzo-diazepines as compared with normal subjects (Vinik et al 1982), and this may be attributable to their plasma binding.

Distribution and metabolism

The disappearance of benzodiazepines from the plasma is in the biphasic manner of a two-compartment model, although there is great inter-individual variability in the pharmacokinetics of these drugs. As an example, the elimination half-life of diazepam can range from 20 to 70 h. Pharmacokinetic parameters do not vary with the dose of drug given, or with the duration of therapy, and as a rule the benzodiazepines follow first order kinetics. There is no evidence to suggest that with prolonged ad-ministration these drugs induce hepatic enzymatic activity and hasten their own metabolism.

Following administration of a benzodiazepine there is the usual initial distribution phase to vessel-rich tissues including the central nervous system, kidneys, liver and heart, from where it is distributed to muscle and later to body fat. The elimination phase is then depen-dent on hepatic biotransformation. Some degree of 'enterohepatic recirculation' occurs with diazepam: fol-lowing biliary excretion of the drug into the gastrointestinal tract there is reabsorption by the intes-tinal mucosa which results in a second peak effect as illustrated in Figure 11.3. This usually occurs within about 4–6 h after the initial administration, and may be accompanied by a period of re-sedation. Figure 11.3 shows an additional peak in the 10–12 h period: this can only be detected when very large doses are given, such

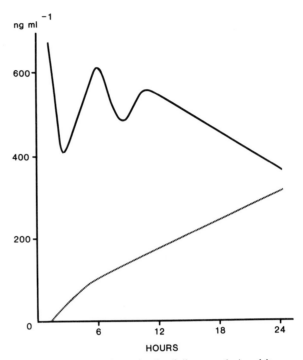

Fig. 11.3 Average plasma levels of diazepam (—) and its metabolite, N-desmethyl diazepam (.....), up to 24 hours following 1 mg kg^{-1} intravenously. Free hand drawing of average readings in 10 patients: calculated from unpublished data.

as the 1 mg kg^{-1} in these patients. There are alternative theories for the cause of this 'second peak' effect, but these are less important than appreciating that this is not an uncommon finding. The elimination of the benzodiazepines follows one of the patterns shown in Table 11.3. Oxidation occurs in the liver; drugs can be considered to have a low extraction ratio when the he-patic clearance is lower than hepatic blood flow. Available evidence suggests that benzodiazepine oxida-tion is a 'susceptible' metabolic pathway and it may be impaired in subjects with liver disease and in some elderly patients. Furthermore it is impaired by the ad-ministration of drugs which are known to inhibit the activity of microsomal oxidising enzymes such as cimetidine, isoniazid and certain oestrogens which are contained in oral contraceptives. In these circumstances the clearance of the benzodiazepine may be delayed. With the high extraction drugs, liver blood flow is an important factor in determining alterations in the rate of their metabolism. Oxidation may occur to a compound which itself has some hypnotic activity, such as desmethyldiazepam in the case of diazepam and a simi-lar related compound in the case of flurazepam. Both of

Table 11.2 Rank order of certain properties which influence the pharmacokinetics of the bezodiazephines

Lipid solubility	MDZ < FNZ < TMZ < LZ < DZ
Plasma protein binding	LZ <FNZ < MDZ < TMZ <DZ
Volume of distribution	LZ < FNZ < MDZ < TMZ < DZ
Elimination half-life	MDZ < TMZ = LZ < FNZ < DZ
Plasma clearance	LZ = FNZ < DZ < TMZ <MDZ

DZ = diazepam; MDZ = midazolam; LZ = Lorazepam; FNZ = flunitrazepam; TMZ = temazepam

Table 11.3 Classification of benzodiazepines according to their route of metabolism and extraction ratios

	Low extraction	High extraction
Oxidation	Diazepam Chlordiazepoxide Flunitrazepam	Triazolam Midazolam
Conjugation	Oxazepam Lorazepam Temazepam	
Nitroreduction	Nitrazepam Clonazepam	

Modified from Greenblatt et al 1982.

these metabolites have a longer elimination half-life than the parent compound, and this can be of great clinical importance following their repeated use and even more important following their long-term use at short intervals. Gamble et al (1976b) have demonstrated a very marked buildup of *N*-desmethyl diazepam in patients who received the parent compound at 4-hourly intervals for periods of 10–17 days (Fig. 11.4). This slowly eliminated metabolite resulted in a very long recovery period.

Figure 11.5 illustrates the biotransformation pathways of some of the benzodiazepines, showing that a number have desmethyl diazepam (nordiazepam) as a common metabolite.

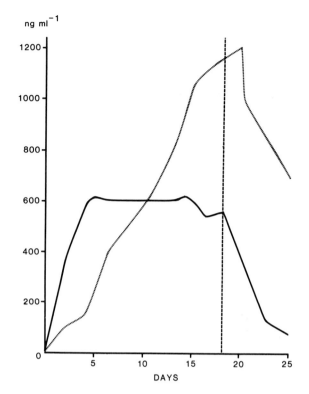

Fig. 11.4 Plasma levels of diazepam (—) and N-desmethyl diazepam (-----) following administration of 10 mg diazepam 4-hourly for 17 days (Gamble, Dundee and Gray, 1976).

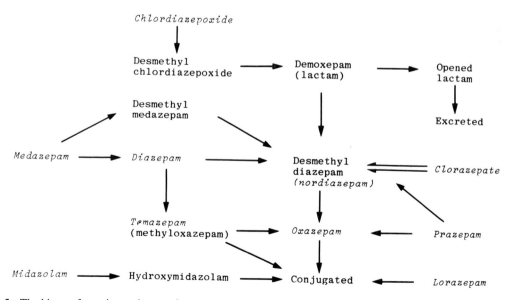

Fig. 11.5 The biotransformation pathways of some commonly used benzodiazepines.

The wide range of elimination half-lives quoted for the benzodiazepines is partly due to the fact that this is increased in elderly patients. With their intravenous use, Harper and his colleagues (1984) have shown that, when given before minor operations, the elimination half-life of midazolam is in the region of 2.5 h but is increased to 5–6 h following major surgery. This possibly reflects alterations in hepatic blood flow.

Placental transfer

Being very lipophilic it is not surprising that the benzodiazepines cross the placental barrier rapidly. This has been shown by a number of workers for diazepam, and the most important finding with this drug is that diazepam levels in infants were higher than those in mothers following a single premedicant dose (Erkkola et al 1974, Gamble et al 1977). The placental transfer of lorazepam is less marked than that of diazepam (McBride et al 1979). Evidence from animal studies suggests that the fetal/maternal ratio following a single dose of midazolam is much lower than with the other drugs (Vree et al 1984). Kanto et al (1983) studied the placental transfer and maternal kinetics of a single 15 mg oral dose of midazolam on the night before Caesarean section. The findings are complicated by individual variations in gastrointestinal absorption in full-term pregnant women, but results suggest that placental transfer takes place more slowly than with diazepam.

Following delivery the plasma diazepam levels fall less rapidly in the fetus than in the mother. In one reported study the fetal/maternal ratio was 1.46 at birth and 1.64 after 24 h (Gamble et al 1977). This can be attributed to the inability of the neonate to metabolize diazepam as readily as does the mother. Of the two pathways of metabolism of diazepam — demethylation and hydroxylation — the former is less efficient in the neonate (Morselli 1983).

PHARMACODYNAMICS

As pointed out previously all the benzodiazepines have similar multiple pharmacological actions. These will now be reviewed in general and later the properties of individual drugs which make them of specific value in different clinical settings will be reviewed.

Central nervous system

As a group the benzodiazepines cause a dose-related depression of the central nervous system (Fig. 11.2).

Their effects range from mild daytime sedation to full general anaesthesia, depending on the dosage used and the preparation employed.

Animal experiments have demonstrated an anti-conflict action for most of the benzodiazepines with doses which produce little sedation. This is the basis for their anxiolytic action in humans, which is one of the main clinical indications for their use. In larger doses their hypnotic properties predominate and pharmacokinetic differences determine which drug is best suited for this usage. In still larger doses, given intravenously, some drugs will induce anaesthesia. These include diazepam, flunitrazepam and midazolam which may induce sleep in periods ranging from 2 to 5 min. There is a wide individual variation in this response, and this will be discussed later. Their onset of action does not occur in one arm–brain circulation time as with thiopentone. Although they may not produce any marked hypnotic effect, small doses of diazepam (0.2 mg kg^{-1}) have been shown to reduce the MAC for halothane (Perisho et al 1971).

Amnesia

The ability to produce amnesia with low doses is one of the desirable effects of the injectable benzodiazepines. It has not been reported with oral medication except with lorazepam (McKay & Dundee 1980). Figure 11.6 summarizes experimental amnesic studies with intravenous doses of diazepam, midazolam and lorazepam given in equivalent doses. Subjects who did not lose consciousness were shown objects at varying times following administration and their ability to recall these was tested 6 and 24 h later. With diazepam and midazolam there was a brief but very intense period of amnesia but this effect had mainly passed off by 20–30 min. In contrast, the onset of amnesic action of lorazepam was very slow, had not reached a peak until about 60 min, and was still present in the majority of subjects by 90 min (Dundee & Pandit 1972, George & Dundee 1977, Dundee & Wilson 1980). Flunitrazepam behaves similarly to diazepam in this respect. Retrograde amnesia was not reported in any patient. A reliable amnesic effect of these benzodiazepines has only been demonstrated following their intravenous use, and this effect is variable when given by intramuscular injection or by mouth (Dundee et al 1970, McKay & Dundee, 1980).

Anti-convulsant action

All the benzodiazepines possess anti-convulsant proper-

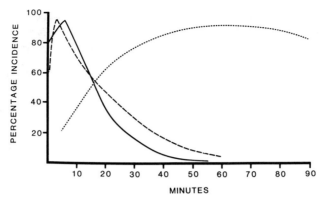

Fig. 11.6 Percentage incidence of patients who could not recall being shown objects at various times following intravenous administration of diazepam 10 mg (—), midazolam 5 mg (--) and lorazepam 4 mg (. . .) (from George & Dundee, 1977; Dundee & Wilson, 1980).

ties but not all are used for this purpose. Their action of enhancing the inhibitory neurons in the central nervous system enables them to suppress generalised abnormal activity rather than a primary epileptic focus. Although strictly defined as 'muscle relaxants' this action on the internuncial neurons of the spinal cord is different from that of the neuromuscular blocking drugs, and the action of these is not potentiated to any important degree. Unlike these, the benzodiazepines do not reduce either the fasciculations or the incidence of myalgia following the use of suxamethonium in ambulant patients (Chestnutt et al 1984).

Anti-hallucinatory effects

This is the basis for the use of certain benzodiazepines in minimizing alcohol withdrawal states. If one considers the action of the central nervous system as a balance between inhibition and excitation in normal subjects, and that chronic alcoholic intoxication suppresses the normal inhibitory action, then drugs like diazepam may act by increasing or producing inhibitory actions on the neuronal populations of the mesencephalic reticular formation and the limbic system (Kaim 1973). There may be some relationship between this widely used clinical application and the ability of diazepam, flunitrazepam and lorazepam to minimize the emergence sequelae following the use of moderately large doses of ketamine, particularly in unpremedicated patients undergoing minor operations (Coppel et al 1973). Those benzodiazepines which have been studied in this respect also have the ability to reduce unpleasant dreams following ketamine.

Hypnotic effect

One of the main long-term clinical uses of the benzodiazepines is as a night-time hypnotic. Effective doses of these drugs reduce the amount of REM sleep and the amount of time spent in slow-wave sleep. These alterations in sleep patterns are not fully understood. Normal subjects spend 20–25% of their time in the REM-dreaming state of sleep, but this does not appear to affect the 'restful' effect. There may, however, be a period of rebound wakefulness following the use of the very short-acting benzodiazepines as hypnotics, particularly when they are prescribed for patients who have problems with onset of sleep.

Tolerance occurs after the long-term use of the benzodiazepines, particularly for night-time sedation, but it is not as marked as with the barbiturates when used for the same purpose.

Analgesia

In clinical doses the benzodiazepines have no analgesic action. More importantly, when used for induction of anaesthesia small doses do not have the antanalgesic action of the barbiturates.

As a group, the benzodiazepines are frequently used in the management of chronic pain. This, however, is related not to any analgesic action, but to a reduction in the anxiety which often accompanies chronic pain.

There have been a few reports of patients complaining of "sexual trespass" by their attendant when under the influence of sedative doses of intravenous diazepam or midazolam (Dundee 1990). In many instances this appears to be a misinterpretation of a stimulus, but such are the medicolegal implications of such cases that endoscopists, dentists and anaesthetists should not give these drugs in the absence of a third person.

Cardiovascular system

Even in large doses given by injection, the benzodiazepines tend not to depress the cardiovascular system, the effects being much smaller than those of other intravenous anaesthetics. Combined with high doses of opioid analgesics, diazepam (Knapp & Dubow 1970) and midazolam (Kawar et al 1983) have proved very safe in the management of poor-risk patients undergoing major cardiac operations.

Midazolam causes a fall in systemic vascular resistance rather than the rise seen with thiopentone (Al-Khudhairi et al 1982). The effects of this are evident when vascular resistance is raised, as in hypertensive patients and in the stressful period immediately prior to operation (Muller et al 1981). Venous pooling and the fall in the systemic vascular resistance induced by midazolam can be helpful in reducing pre-load and after-load performance in the failing heart, but this effect will be more marked in hypovolaemic patients (Muller et al 1981, Schulte-Sasse et al 1982). In contrast with results in intact humans, in patients on cardiopulmonary bypass diazepam causes more pronounced arterial and venous dilatation than midazolam (Samuelson et al 1980).

Some of the early claims by anaesthetists for lesser cardiovascular effects of the benzodiazepines as compared with orthodox induction agents may have been due to their slower onset of action (Clarke & Lyons 1977). If sufficient time is allowed before tracheal intubation the fall in arterial pressure with equivalent doses of diazepam and thiopentone was similar, but in clinical practice intubation is usually carried out before the maximum depressant effect of the benzodiazepines occurs. Notwithstanding, as a group the injectable benzodiazepines in clinical doses cause less depression of the cardiovascular system than do orthodox induction agents, and this beneficial effect is more marked when they are combined with large doses of an appropriate opioid.

With marked sedation or loss of consciousness there is the usual peripheral vasodilatation and a slight drop in cardiac output and peripheral resistance, but this is of no clinical significance and in anaesthesia these effects are reversed by surgical stimulation.

Sedative doses of the benzodiazepines are sometimes given to patients in the upright or semi-upright position, as in dental surgery, or where there is already a marked vasodilatation, as following spinal or epidural anaes-

thesia. There have been occasional reports of collapse in the former situation, and in the latter their use should be followed carefully and adequate fluid therapy given. When used for cardioversion the benzodiazepines are associated with fewer ventricular extrasystoles than the barbiturates (Muenster et al 1967) and this, combined with their minimal cardiovascular depression, has made them the drugs of choice for cardioversion. Tachycardia following these drugs is probably a manifestation of vasodilatation and relative hypovolaemia, and is of little clinical importance.

Organ blood flow

The benzodiazepines cause minimal changes in coronary or cerebral blood flow or in myocardial or cerebral oxygen consumption in anaesthetized, ventilated dogs (Hilfiber et al 1980). Cerebral perfusion pressure is slightly decreased due to a fall in mean aortic pressure. Like other anaesthetics, the benzodiazepines depress renal blood flow and renal function (Lebowitz et al 1982). Midazolam has a more profound effect on renal blood flow than do equivalent doses of thiopentone, although this does not appear to apply to renal vascular resistance. Benzodiazepines reduce liver blood flow in parallel with the small decreases in cardiac output (Gelman et al 1983).

Respiration

Here one must distinguish between the oral uses of these drugs as anxiolytics or hypnotics and their intravenous use for sedation or induction of anaesthesia. There is nothing to suggest that, in the normal therapeutic doses, the oral administration of any of the benzodiazepines is followed by respiratory depression. Their use is not accompanied by bronchoconstriction and they can be safely given to asthmatic subjects.

With intravenous injection one has to consider the dose used, the rate of administration, the concomitant use of opioids and the physical status of the patient. As consciousness is lost so is sensitivity to carbon dioxide, and under different circumstances the response to a normal induction dose can vary from no detectable effect to apnoea. The normal effect would be a slight decrease in tidal volume, but this may be compensated for by an increase in respiratory rate. The dose–response curve is different from that of the opioid: while both shift the CO_2 response curve to the right (Forster et al 1980), midazolam and diazepam flatten the slopes, indicating a less profound dose-response effect (Zsigmond & Shiveley 1966). Nevertheless, in patients with chronic obstructive airway disease the respiratory depressant effect of benzodiazepines may be greater than in normal subjects (Catchlove & Hefer 1971, Gross & Smith 1981) and as consciousness is lost, so is sensitivity to carbon dioxide.

The liability to produce respiratory obstruction is the most important effect of hypnotic doses of intravenous diazepam (Healey et al 1970, Dixon et al 1973). It is respiratory obstruction rather than depression which is more likely to result in the cyanosis which has been noted by a number of workers.

Parenchymatous organs

Alterations in liver or kidney function have not been reported after the benzodiazepines (Kawar et al 1982) and any changes associated with their use are the result of the accompanying cardiovascular effects.

Local effects

Apart from midazolam, the injectable benzodiazepines use either an organic solvent or an emulsion and the former, particularly, cause pain on injection, and venous thrombosis. However, many early reports do not mention thromboses with the Valium brand of diazepam since, in many incidents, this does not appear until the 7th or 10th day after administration (Hegarty & Dundee 1977). Both injection pain and venous thrombosis are more likely to occur with the use of small veins on the dorsum of the hand. In practice the Diazemuls brand of diazepam, and the aqueous solution of midazolam, are to be preferred for injection because of their minimal irritant effects.

Other effects

Even after long-term use the benzodiazepines do not cause enzyme induction to the same degree as the barbiturates. Even after the long-term administration of clonazepam in epileptics there does not appear to be any evidence of stimulation of hepatic microsomal activity (Browne 1982).

Despite some early reports to the contrary, pretreatment with diazepam or midazolam does not reduce the myalgia which follows $1 \, mg \, kg^{-1}$ suxamethonium in ambulant patients (Chestnutt et al 1984). Neither do they affect the onset and offset time of the relaxant.

Abuse

Being the most widely currently prescribed medicines, it is not surprising that there have been many reports of abuse of the benzodiazepines. It is claimed that about 6% of Americans felt they needed benzodiazepines on a regular basis, while 15% needed them from time to time: the comparable figures for Britain were 8 and 14%. Women are more frequent users than men, presumably because of their greater frequency of anxiety. It is well established that the main improvement in anxiety will occur within 1 week of starting benzodiazepine therapy, and patients do not derive further benefit after 16 weeks of treatment. However, a number may continue on the drugs in the hope of improvement. The dangers of long-term benzodiazepine therapy vary from cerebral damage, as demonstrated on the CT scanner, to withdrawal symptoms. The latter have been reported with diazepam (Priest 1980) and are least likely to occur with the long-acting drugs such as flurazepam and quazepam, but even with these their occurrence is related to the duration of therapy. It has been estimated that the risk of benzodiazepine dependence is about one case in 50 million patient-months, and that all patients with withdrawal symptoms had increased their dosage beyond the normal therapeutic range. However, as with morphine, specific withdrawal symptoms have been demonstrated following normal therapeutic doses, although as with the opioid these would not have been detected clinically (Dundee 1983).

Overdosage

Benzodiazepine overdosage, either accidental in the case of children or premeditated in adults, is not uncommon. Because of the relative lack of cardiovascular depression with these drugs compared with the barbiturates, recovery should occur provided ventilation is maintained and vital functions supported. In many cases patients are very sleepy, but respiration is not so depressed as to require assistance. However, the warning regarding the occurrence of respiratory obstruction with the benzodiazepines should be noted and, in some instances, tracheal intubation and assisted respiration may be the treatment of choice, even though this may necessitate the use of a neuromuscular blocking drug. Physostigmine is a non-specific antidote to benzodiazepine depression (see below) but there are no reports of its use in cases of marked overdosage. The antagonist flumazenil will be discussed later.

Physostigmine reversal

Physostigmine, being a tertiary amine, crosses the blood-brain barrier and increases brain acetylcholine concentration by inhibition of cholinesterase. It has been used successfully in ameliorating the 'central cholinergic syndrome' which may be induced by atropine, hyoscine, tricyclic antidepressants and anti-parkinsonian drugs (Holzgrafe et al 1973). There is increasing clinical evidence that it can reverse central depression induced by benzodiazepine tranquillizers.

Little is known about the specificity of this action, but there are several reports which show that physostigmine may act as an antidote to an occasional marked depressant effect of diazepam (Larson et al 1977). It has also proved effective in overdose in a child (DiLiberti et al 1975). As mentioned above, untoward effects of diazepam, such as respiratory arrest, are uncommon and are best treated with ventilation. Delirium following lorazepam has also been treated successfully with physostigmine (Blitt & Petty 1975).

THE INDUCTION OF ANAESTHESIA

This section will be limited to diazepam and midazolam. The physico-chemical and pharmacokinetic properties of these two drugs relevant to the induction of anaesthesia are summarized in Table 11.4. Although there is a wide scatter of the induction times with both of these drugs, in no reported incident has this been in the range of the rapidly acting thiobarbiturates. Figure 11.7 shows the onset time following an injection of 0.3 mg kg^{-1} of midazolam given over a 20 s period in 166 patients. This also shows that younger patients appear to have more resistance to the drug, and that in most of the elderly patients the onset time is in the region of 20–40 s. An appreciable number of younger patients do not lose consciousness within 3 min of administration of what is generally considered to be an adequate induction dose. Halliday et al (1984) have demonstrated a direct negative relationship between the age of the patient and induction time. Although similar studies have not been carried out with diazepam a very wide range of doses is required to induce sleep. These can vary from 0.2 to 2 mg kg^{-1} (Brown & Dundee 1968).

Benzodiazepines are highly bound drugs and small changes in plasma binding will lead to a wide variation in the amount of free drug. Halliday and his colleagues (1984) have demonstrated a correlation between plasma albumin and the onset time following 0.3 mg kg^{-1} midazolam. Clinical reports would suggest that this also applies to diazepam.

The onset time of the benzodiazepines can be reduced by drugs which will affect plasma binding, such as probenecid by mouth or aspirin i.v. (Halliday et al 1984). A small dose of fentanyl (50–100 μg) will increase the number of patients anaesthetized with 0.3 mg kg^{-1} mid-

Table 11.4 Physicochemical and pharmacokinetic properties of diazepam and midazolam

	Diazepam	Midazolam
Physicochemical		
Solubility	Insoluble in water. Available in organic solution or lipid emulsion	Solubility in water because hydrophilic imidazole group
Form of i.v. presentation	Organic solvent. Emulsion	Aqueous solution
pKa	3.4	6.2
Lipophilicity		
Octanol : buffer partition ratio	309	34
Pharmacokinetics		
Plasma protein binding	97–99%	94–98%
Volume of distribution (Vd(1kg^{-1})	0.7–1.6	0.8–1.6
Elimination half-life (h) ($t_{\frac{1}{2}}\beta$)	20–70	1.5–5
Clearance		
Total body (ml min^{-1}kg^{-1})	0.24–0.53	6.4–11.1
Plasma (ml min^{-1})	20–47	268–630
Metabolism	To desmethyldiazepam and oxazepam. Both hypnotically active	Active metabolite α-hydroxymidazolam which is very rapidly conjugated to inactive form ($t_{\frac{1}{2}}\beta$ 1 h)
Second peak	Present at 6–8 h due to enterohepatic recirculation and is of clinical significance	If present, is very small and not clinically significant

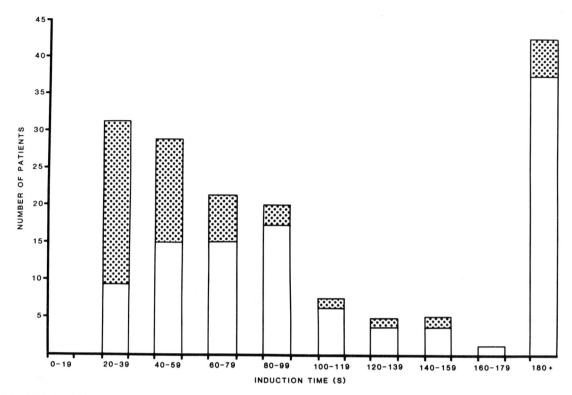

Fig. 11.7 Variability in the time to the onset of sleep following the injection of midazolam 0.3 mg kg^{-1} to 166 unpremedicated patients of varying ages (from Dundee et al, 1984). Patients over 50 years are indicated by hatched area.

azolam and also reduces the induction time in the young resistant patients. Given by the intravenous route, midazolam is one and a half times to twice as potent as diazepam (w/w).

It is interesting to note that on clinical grounds the onset of action of intravenous diazepam and midazolam appears to be similar despite the greater fat solubility of the former. This is probably compensated for by the lower plasma binding of midazolam, thus leaving more pharmacologically active drug.

In clinical practice recovery from equivalent doses of midazolam occurs much more rapidly than following diazepam. The effects of the latter are prolonged both by enterohepatic recirculation and also by the presence of the hypnotically active metabolite nordiazepam, which has a particularly long elimination half-life. On theoretical grounds one would not expect the action of diazepam, which has a relatively slow clearance, to be prolonged in the presence of liver damage, but this could occur with midazolam. The action of midazolam will, however, be markedly affected by alterations in hepatic blood flow.

There is no suggestion that induction with the benzodiazepines is not compatible with standard techniques for balanced anaesthesia, but there has been some difference of opinion as to the relative value of midazolam and thiopentone as routine induction agents (Reves et al 1979, 1982, Dundee & Kawar 1982). In the case of thiopentone the advantages are reliability and rapid onset of action. The reliability of midazolam is certainly better in the elderly patients and in those given narcotic premedication. When used for day-case surgery, in combination with fentanyl, recovery was quicker in patients given thiopentone but this was more than compensated for by the lower incidence of nausea in those given midazolam (Crawford et al 1984). At the time of writing the relative situation of these two drugs as induction agents is still not clear. Thiopentone is a well-tried drug with marked toxic effects on the cardiovascular and respiratory systems. Midazolam is less well tried but in certain circumstances the slow onset of action and the unreliability (which can be overcome with the judicious use of narcotics) may be more than compensated for by cardiovascular stability.

The inter-patient variation shown by two induction doses of midazolam and diazepam is less important when these drugs are used for sedation. Although some variation does occur, it does not interfere with their usefulness as sedatives or hypnotics.

Workers in continental Europe have used flunitrazepam as an induction agent in similar ways to diazepam and midazolam, but lorazepam is not acceptable for this purpose because of the very great delay in onset of action.

INDIVIDUAL DRUGS

As a group the benzodiazepines are insoluble in water and all the commercially available preparations are available in tablet or capsule, and in some cases syrup, form. The first four drugs described below are those of most interest to anaesthetists. Midazolam is the newest member of this group and is a water-soluble imidazole benzodiazepine derivative.

Diazepam

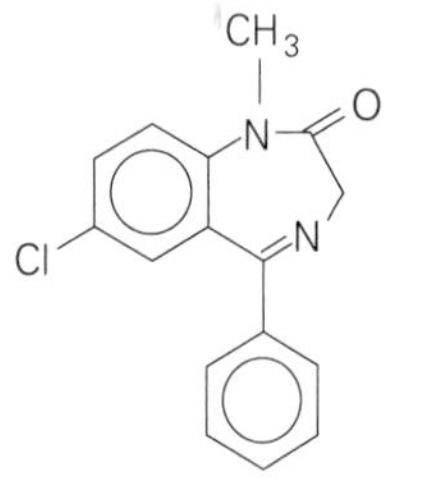

Chemical name: 7-chloro-1,3-dihydro-
1-methyl-5-phenyl-2H-1,
4-benzodiazepin-2-one.

Diazepam is a colourless crystalline base, insoluble in water with a molecular weight of 285. It is available both in oral and injectable forms. There are two preparations of the latter.

The established preparation (Valium) contains 5 mg ml^{-1} in an aqueous vehicle composed of organic solvents consisting mainly of propylene glycol, ethyl alcohol and sodium benzoate in benzoic acid. This is a slightly viscid solution with a pH in the range 6.4 to 6.9, and it requires a large-bore needle for rapid intravenous injection.

An emulsion preparation (Diazemuls) contains 5 mg ml^{-1} in a lipid emulsion made from soya bean oil similar to the fat emulsion used for parenteral nutrition (Intralipid). The solution, which has a pH of 6.0, is easy to inject but the opacity may cause slight difficulties with venepuncture.

There was a preparation of diazepam solubilized in Cremophor EL, but this is no longer commercially available because of the high incidence of hypersensitivity reactions. The trade name of this preparation, Stesolid, is now used for one brand of diazepam BP solubilized with propylene glycol.

Diazepam is also available in tablet and capsule form (2, 5 and 10 mg), a syrup (2 mg in 5 ml), in 5 and 10 mg suppositories and in a form suitable for rectal administration.

Midazolam

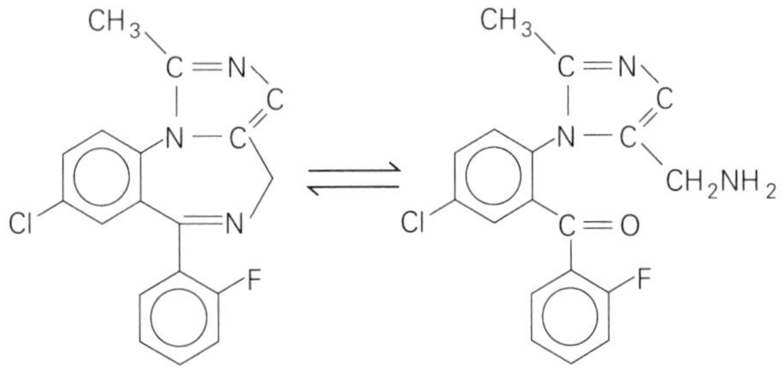

Chemical name: (8-chloro-6
(2-fluorophenol)-l-methyl-4H
imidazo (1,S-a) (1,4))
benzodiazepine.

Midazolam is an imidazo benzodiazepine derivative. The nitrogen in the imidazole ring, which is attached to positions 1 and 2 in the diazepine ring, imparts to the molecule a higher basicity and hence water-solubility, as well as a shorter duration of action than other injectable drugs. It can be prepared as a water-soluble salt with hydrochloric, malic or lactic acid, and is commercially available in a stable aqueous solution as in the hydrochloride salt.

Although midazolam is stable in an aqueous solution and freely water-soluble, the latter is pH-dependent. As shown in the diagram, the ring opens reversibly at pH values below 4, imparting water-solubility. At the pH of plasma the ring closes and the lipid-solubility is enhanced, this closing process having a half-life of about 10 min. Care should be taken to ensure that midazolam is not mixed with acidic solutions.

Flunitrazepam

Chemical name: 5-(2 fluorophenyl)-1,3 dihydro-
7-nitro-1-methyl-(2H-1,4-
benzodiazepin-1-one.

Flunitrazepam is marketed widely as a hypnotic and in some countries in an injectable form (2 mg ml^{-1}) for induction of anaesthesia and sedation. Like diazepam the solution is made up in an organic solvent with pH around 6.0 and pKa of 1.8, which causes less pain on injection and fewer sequelae than Valium (Hegarty & Dundee 1977).

Lorazepam

Chemical name: 7-chloro-5-(O-chlorophenyl)-
                  1,3-dihydro-3 hydroxy-2H-
                  1,4-benzodiazepam-2-one.

Lorazepam is available in tablet form (differing strengths in different countries) and as a solution (organic solvent), with pH around 6.4 and pKa of 1.3, containing 4 mg ml^{-1}. Like flunitrazepam, lorazepam causes less pain on injection and fewer venous sequelae than the comparable solution of diazepam.

OTHER BENZODIAZEPINES

Chlordiazepoxide

This was the first clinically used benzodiazepine (Randall 1960), being introduced as methaminodiazepoxide. It is used in the treatment of acute and chronic anxiety states, but is an example of a relatively short-acting drug with a long-acting metabolite. A solution for intramuscular injection (drug ampoules containing 100 mg mixed with 2 ml of organic solvent supplied) can be prepared but should not be injected intravenously.

Clonazepam

Clonazepam is available in oral and injectable forms and is insoluble in aqueous solution. It is rapidly absorbed when given by mouth, reaching peak plasma concentrations 1–3 h following administration. The drug has an elimination half-life ranging from 20 to 40 h, being metabolized by nitro reduction to inactive metabolites.

Clonazepam acts, as do other benzodiazepines, by increasing the convulsive threshold of the cerebrum, preventing the spread of electrical activity from an epileptic focus. It is best used in the prophylaxis of infantile spasms or petit mal and myoclonic seizures (Browne 1978). However one-third of patients on long-term clonazepam will develop tolerance to its anti-convulsant action. A starting dose of 1 mg before bedtime is given, increasing up to a daily maintenance dose of 8 mg.

As with other drugs used in the control of seizures, withdrawal from clonazepam should be gradual because of the possibility of inducing convulsions. Intravenous clonazepam is used in the control of status epilepticus, up to 1 mg being given initially by slow injection.

Flurazepam

Flurazepam, with a short elimination half-life, can be looked on as a pro-drug for its hypnotically active, long-lasting ($t_{\frac{1}{2}}\beta$ 40–100 h) metabolite, N-desalkyl flurazepam. It is used as a night-time hypnotic in doses of 15–30 mg. While there must be an accumulation of active metabolite on repeated use, this reduces the likelihood of withdrawal symptoms when medication is stopped.

Nitrazepam

This is mainly used in the short-term treatment of insomnia (dosage 2.5–5 mg), although it has been used as pre-anaesthetic medication. With a $t_{\frac{1}{2}}\beta$ of around 24 h there is little danger of 'early-morning' insomnia or of rebound insomnia and anxiety when the drug is stopped, although it has not an hypnotically active metabolite. Clinically it is a useful drug for 'night before operation' sedation.

Oxazepam

This is more slowly absorbed than diazepam following oral administration, and is preferable for the treatment of anxiety than as night sedation. It has a short plasma half-life of 5–15 h and is transformed directly to an inactive gluconamide by the liver (Fig. 11.5). Hence the kinetics of oxazepam are independent of patient age and liver function. The dosage is 15–30 mg three times daily.

Temazepam

Temazepam (4-hydroxydiazepam) is a minor metabolite of diazepam. It has a relatively short half-life of about 5–11 h, being longer in some subjects and in the elderly. It has no active metabolites of any clinical significance and is considered more suitable for use as a night-time hypnotic than longer-acting drugs such as diazepam, nitrazepam or flurazepam, where residual effects on the next day are undesirable. Although morning performance is usually normal after temazepam, there is some evidence of impairment of psychomotor and cognitive function at the upper end (30 mg) of the recommended dose.

Temazepam is available commercially as a hard gelatine capsule and as a solution in polyethylene glycol within a soft gelatine capsule. The two dose forms have different absorption characteristics, peak plasma concentrations occurring more rapidly with the soft capsule form (Fucella et al 1977, Fucella, 1979). The differences (45 and 86 min with 20 mg dose) are of clinical importance when the drug is used as pre-anaesthetic medication, but probably less important when used as a night-time hypnotic (Heel et al 1981).

The hypnotic dose of temazepam varies from 10 to 30 mg, the adult premedicant dose is 20 mg. Greenwood & Bradshaw (1983) have found this dose to be satisfactory when given 1 h before day-case surgery. It can be prescribed for patients on cimetidine or ranitidine therapy without fear of over-sedation; the reduction of liver blood flow by these two H_2 receptor blockers would not affect the bioavailability or subsequent hepatic clearance by a drug with a low hepatic ratio such as temazepam (Elliott et al 1984a).

Triazolam

Triazolam as with midazolam, has a high hepatic extraction ratio and displays an ultrashort plasma half-life of 1.5–5 h. It is favoured as a night sedative in the elderly as this short half-life would ensure minimal morning drowsiness. However, other drugs are preferred for insomniacs with early-morning wakening. There is a loss of sleep-inducing efficacy at the end of 2 weeks of triazolam therapy; furthermore withdrawal may lead to rebound insomnia (Kales et al 1976).

BENZODIAZEPINE ANTAGONISTS

Flumazenil

The imidazobenzodiazepine flumazenil, one of a series initially investigated by Hunkeler and colleagues (1981) appears to act as a competitive antagonist at the benzodiazepine receptor. It antagonizes the effects of benzodiazepines in humans, without altering bioavailability or blood levels (Darragh et al 1981, O'Boyle et al 1983). The specific activity at the benzodiazepine receptor complex is confirmed by its inability to inhibit the central effects of drugs such as meprobamate or phenytoin (Bonetti et al 1982), and other similar studies. However, flumazenil has been found to hasten recovery from halothane anaesthesia (Geller et al 1988). The mechanism of this is not known. There is evidence from animal studies, with some confirmation in humans, that flumazenil does have a slight partial agonist profile, seen at higher doses, and may also at lower doses show 'inverse agonist' activity, but such actions appear to be weak, and in general flumazenil given alone in recommended doses is largely devoid of intrinsic activity.

Pharmacokinetics

Flumazenil is insoluble in water, and is currently available as a 'micelles' preparation for parenteral use. Intramuscular injection may be painful. Flumazenil is rapidly absorbed after oral administration, but undergoes extensive first-pass metabolism, so that bioavailability is only about 16%. It is rapidly distributed, with maximal brain levels being achieved 5–8 min after intravenous injection (Persson et al 1985). A plasma level around $20 \ \mu l^{-1}$ seems to be effective in reversing benzodiazepine effects. Protein binding is low, at around 40%. Elimination is rapid, with a plasma half-life of generally under 1 h, and a high clearance of around 700 ml min^{-1} (Roncari & Ziegler 1986, Klotz & Kanto 1988).

Clinical use

Flumazenil may have a place in several areas, and is

undergoing investigation in accelerating recovery from general anaesthesia, or sedative techniques, in facilitating weaning from ventilation in intensive-care patients sedated with benzodiazepines, and in management of benzodiazepine overdosage.

Dosage and administration

Flumazenil may be given by injection as a bolus, or as an infusion. The dose required for reversal of midazolam sedation is generally in the range $0.005-0.01$ mg kg^{-1} which should be titrated carefully in increments of $0.1-0.2$ mg. Resedation is unlikely but not unknown in this situation, as the half-lives of midazolam and flumazenil are reasonably 'matched' if flumazenil is given as midazolam effect is waning. If flumazenil is used to antagonize the action of benzodiazepine overdose, or after prolonged use, or use

of a longer-acting drug, then an infusion may be appropriate, at a dose range of $100-400$ μg h^{-1}.

Side-effects

These are mainly slight. There is a small incidence of nausea, and some patients may experience a degree of agitation on reversal of benzodiazepine activity. However, an increase in intracranial pressure has been reported in some patients with head injury on reversal of sedation, and this may be clinically significant. In general, cardiovascular stability is maintained during flumazenil reversal of benzodiazepines, but caution has been advised in mixed-drug overdose or where the patient's state of benzodiazepine dependency is not known, as ventricular arrhythmias have been seen (Short et al 1988).

REFERENCES

Al-Khudhairi D, Whitwam J G, Chakrabarti M K, Askitopoulou H, Grundy E M Powrie S 1982 Haemodynamic effects of midazolam and thiopentone during induction of anaesthesia for coronary artery surgery. British Journal of Anaesthesia 54: 831–835

Assaf R A E, Dundee J W, Gamble J A S 1974 Factors influencing plasma diazepam levels following a single administration. British Journal of Clinical Pharmacology 1: 343P–344P

Assaf R A E, Dundee J W, Gamble J A S 1975 The influence of the route of administration on the clinical action of diazepam. Anaesthesia 30: 152–158

Blitt C O, Petty W C 1975 Reversal of lorazepam delirium by physostigmine. Anesthesia and Analgesia, Current Researches 54: 607–608

Bonetti E P, Pieri L, Cumin R, Schaffner M, Pieri M et al 1982 Benzodiazepine antagonist Ro 15–1788: neurological and behavioural effects. Psychopharmacology 78: 8

Braestrup C; Nielsen M 1982 Neurotransmitters and CNS disease. Lancet 2: 1030–1034

Brown S S, Dundee J W 1968 Clinical studies of induction agents. XXV: Diazepam. British Journal of Anaesthesia 40: 108–112

Browne T R 1978 Clonazepam. New England Journal of Medicine 299: 812–816

Browne T R 1982 Enzyme induction and drug interaction. In: Usdin E, Skolnick P, Tallman Jr J F, Greenblatt D, Paul S M (eds) Pharmacology of benzodiazepines. Macmillan, London, p 330

Catchlove R F H, Hefer E R 1971 The effects of diazepam on respiration in patients with obstructive pulmonary disease. Anesthesiology 34: 14–18

Chestnutt W N, Lowry K G, Elliott P, Mirakhur R K, Pandit S K, Dundee J W 1984 A comparison of the efficacy of benzodiazepines with tubocurarine in prevention of suxamethonium-induced muscle pain. British Journal of Clinical Pharmacology 17: 222P

Clarke R S J, Lyons S M 1977 Diazepam and flunitrazepam as induction agents for cardiac surgical operations. Acta Anaesthesiologica Scandinavica 21: 282–292

Committee on the Review of Medicine 1980 Systematic review of benzodiazepines. British Medical Journal 280: 910–912

Coppel D L, Bovill J G, Dundee L W 1973 The taming of ketamine. Anaesthesia 28: 293–296

Crawford M E, Carl P, Andersen R S, Mikkelsen B O 1984 Comparison between midazolam and thiopentone-based balanced anaesthesia for day-case surgery. British Journal of Anaesthesia 56: 165–169

Darragh A, Lambe R, Brick I, Downie W W 1981 Reversal of benzodiazepine-induced sedation by intravenous Ro 15–1788. Lancet 2: 1042

Di Liberti J, O'Brien M L, Turner T 1975 The use of physostigmine as an antidote in accidental diazepam intoxication. Journal of Pediatrics 86: 106–107

Divoll M, Greenblatt D J, Harmatz J S, Shader R I 1981 Effect of age and gender on disposition of temazepam. Journal of Pharmaceutical Science 70: 1104–1107

Dixon R A, Day C D, Eccersley P S, Thornton J A 1973 Intravenous diazepam in dentistry monitoring results from a controlled clinical trial. British Journal of Anaesthesia 45: 202–206

Dundee J W 1983 Editorial: Abuse of benzodiazepines. British Journal of Anaesthesia 55: 1–2

Dundee J W 1990 Fantasies during sedation with intravenous midazolam or diazepam. Medical Legal Journal 58: 29–34

Dundee J W, Kawar P 1982 Benzodiazepines in anaesthesia. In: Usdin E, Skolnick P, Tallman Jr J F, Greenblatt D, Paul S M (eds) Pharmacology of benzodiazepines. Macmillan, London, pp 314–316

Dundee J W, Pandit S K 1972 Anterograde amnesic effects of pethidine, hyoscine and diazepam in adults. British Journal of Pharmacology 44: 140–144

Dundee J W, Wilson D B 1980 Amnesic action of midazolam. Anaesthesia 35: 459–461

Dundee J W, Haslett W H K, Keilty S R, Pandit S K 1970 Studies of drugs given before anaesthesia. XX: Diazepam-containing mixtures. British Journal of Anaesthesia 42: 143–150

Dundee J W, Halliday N J, Loughran P G 1984 Variation in response to midazolam. British Journal of Clinical Pharmacology 17: 645P–646P

Elliott P, Dundee J W, Collier P S, McClean E 1984a The influence of two H₂-receptor antagonists, cimetidine and ranitidine, on the systemic availability of temazepam. British Journal of Anaesthesia 56: 800–801

Elwood R J, Hildebrand P J, Dundee J W 1983 Influence of ranitidine on uptake of oral midazolam. British Journal of Anaesthesia 55: 241P

Erkkola R, Kanto J, Sellman R 1974 Diazepam in early human pregnancy. Acta Obstetrica et Gynecologica Scandinavica 53: 135–138

Forster A, Gardaz J-P, Suter P M, Gemperle M 1980 Respiratory depression by midazolam and diazepam. Anesthesiology 53: 494–497

Fucella L M 1979 Bioavailability of temazepam in soft gelatin capsules. British Journal of Clinical Pharmacology 8: 31–35

Fucella L M, Bolcioni G, Tamassia V, Ferrario L, Tognoni G 1977 Human pharmacokinetics and bioavailability of temazepam administered in soft gelatin capsules. European Journal of Clinical Pharmacology 12: 383–386

Gale G D, Galloon S, Porter W R 1983 Sublingual lorazepam: a better premedication? British Journal of Anaesthesia 55: 761–765

Gamble J A S 1975 Some factors influencing the absorption of diazepam. Proceedings of the Royal Society of Medicine 68: 772

Gamble J A S, Dundee J W, Assaf R A E 1975 Plasma diazepam levels after single dose oral and intramuscular administration. Anaesthesia 30: 164–169

Gamble J A S, Dundee J W, Gray R C 1976a Plasma diazepam concentrations following prolonged administration. British Journal of Anaesthesia 48: 1087–1090

Gamble J A S, Gaston J H, Nair S G, Dundee J W 1976b Some pharmacological factors influencing the absorption of diazepam following oral administration. British Journal of Anaesthesia 48: 1181–1185

Gamble J A S, Moore J, Lamki H, Howard P J 1977 A study of plasma diazepam levels in mother and infant. British Journal of Obstetrics and Gynaecology 84: 588–591

Geller E, Weinbrum A, Schiff B et al 1988 The effects of flumazenil on the process of recovery from halothane anaesthesia. European Journal of Anaesthesia Suppl 2: 151–153

Gelman S, Reves J G, Harris D 1983 Circulatory responses to midazolam anaesthesia: emphasis on canine splanchnic circulation. Anesthesia and Analgesia 62: 135–139

George K A, Dundee J W 1977 Relative amnesic actions of diazepam, flunitrazepam and lorazepam in man. British Journal of Clinical Pharmacology 4: 45–50

Greenblatt D J, Shader R I, Weinberger D R, Allen M D, MacLaughlin D S 1978a Effect of a cocktail on diazepam absorption. Psychopharmacology 57: 199

Greenblatt D J, Allen M D, MacLaughlin D S 1978b Diazepam absorption: effects of antacids and food. Clinical Pharmacology and Therapeutics 24: 600–609

Greenblatt D J, Shader R I, Abernethy D R, Ochs H R, Divoll M and Sellers E M 1982 Benzodiazepines and the challenge of pharmacokinetic taxonomy. In: Usdin E, Skolnick P, Tallman Jr J F, Greenblatt D, Paul S M (eds) Pharmacology of benzodiazepines. Macmillan, London, pp 257–269

Greenwood B K, Bradshaw E G 1983 Preoperative medication for day-case surgery. British Journal of Anaesthesia 55: 933–937

Gross J B, Smith T C 1981 Ventilation after midazolam and thiopental in subjects with COPD. Anesthesiology 55: A384

Gross J B, Zebrowski M E, Carel W D, Gardner S, Smith T C 1983 Time course of ventilatory depression after thiopental and midazolam in normal subjects and in patients with chronic obstructive pulmonary disease. Anesthesiology 58: 540–544

Haefely W, Kulcsar A, Mohler H, Pieri L, Polc P, Schaffner R 1975 Possible involvement of GABA in the central actions of benzodiazepines. Advances in Biochemistry and Psychopharmacology 14: 131

Halliday N J, Dundee J W, Loughran P G, Harper K W 1984 Age and plasma proteins influence the action of midazolam. Anesthesiology 61: A357

Harper K W, Lowry K G, Elliott P, Collier P S, Halliday N J, Dundee J W 1984 Age and nature of operation influence the pharmacokinetics of midazolam. British Journal of Anaesthesia 56: 1288P–1289P

Healey T E J, Robinson J S, Vickers M D 1970 Physiological responses to intravenous diazepam as a sedative for conservative dentistry. British Medical Journal 3: 10–13

Heel R C, Brogden R N, Speight T M, Avery G S 1981 Temazepam: a review of its pharmacological properties and therapeutic efficacy as an hypnotic. Drugs 21: 321–340

Hegarty J E, Dundee J W 1977 Sequelae after the intravenous injection of three benzodiazepines — diazepam, lorazepam and flunitrazepam. British Medical Journal 2: 1384–1385

Hildebrand P J, Elwood R J, McClean E, Dundee J W 1983 Intramuscular and oral midazolam. Some factors influencing uptake. Anaesthesia 38: 1220–1221

Hilfiber O, Larsen R, Stafforst D, Kettler D 1980 Midazolam: Wirkung auf allgemeine, coronare und cerebrale Hamodynamik. Anaesthesist 29: 337–338

Hillstead L, Hansen T, Melsom H 1974 Diazepam metabolism in normal man. I: Serum concentrations and clinical effects after intravenous, intramuscular and oral administration. Clinical Pharmacology and Therapeutics 16: 479–484

Holzgrafe K E, Vandroll J J, Mintz S M 1973 Reversal of postoperative reactions to scopolamine with physostigmine. Anesthesia and Analgesia, Current Researches 52: 921–925

Hunkeler W, Mohler H, Pieri L, Polc P, Bonetti E P, Cumin R, Schaffner R, Haefely W 1981 Selective antagonists of benzodiazepines. Nature 290: 514–516

Kaim S C 1973 Benzodiazepines in treatment of alcohol withdrawal states. In: Garattini S, Mussini E, Randall L O (eds) The benzodiazepines. Raven Press, New York, pp 571–574

Kales A, Kales J D, Bixler E O, Scharf M B, Russek E 1976 Hypnotic efficacy of triazolam: sleep laboratory evaluation of intermediate-term effectiveness. Journal of Clinical Pharmacology 16: 399–406

Kanto J, Sjovall S, Enkola R, Himberg J–J, Kangas L 1983 Placental transfer and midazolam kinetics. Clinical Pharmacology and Therapeutics 33: 786

Kawar P, Briggs L P, Bahar M, McIlroy P D A, Dundee J W, Merrett J D, Nesbitt C J 1982 Liver enzyme studies with disoprofol (ICI 35 868) and midazolam. Anaesthesia 37: 305–308

Kawar P, Carson I W, Lyons S M, Clarke R S J, Dundee J W 1983 Comparative study of haemodynamic changes during induction of anaesthesia with midazolam and diazepam in patients undergoing coronary artery bypass surgery. Irish Journal of Medical Science 152: 215

Klotz U, Kanto J 1988 Pharmacokinetics and clinical use of flumazenil (Ro 15–1788) Clinical Pharmacokinetics 14: 1–14.

Knapp R B, Dubow H 1970 Comparison of diazepam with thiopental as an induction agent in cardiopulmonary disease. Anesthesia and Analgesia 49: 722

Larson G F, Hurlbert B J, Wingard D W 1977 Physostigmine reversal of diazepam-induced depression. Anesthesia and Analgesia, Current Researches 56: 348–451

Lebowitz P W, Cote M E, Daniels A L, Bonventre J 1982 Comparative renal effects of midazolam and thiopental. Anesthesiology 57: A35

McBride R J, Dundee J W, Moore J, Toner W, Howard P J 1979 A study of the plasma concentrations of lorazepam in mother and neonate. British Journal of Anaesthesia 51: 971–978

McGowan W A W, Dundee J W 1982 The effect of intravenous cimetidine on the absorption of orally administered diazepam and lorazepam. British Journal of Clinical Pharmacology 14: 207–211

McKay A C, Dundee J W 1980 Effect of oral benzodiazepines on memory. British Journal of Anaesthesia 52: 1247–1257

McKenzie S G 1983 Introduction to the pharmacokinetics and pharmacodynamics of benzodiazepines. Progress in Neuro-Psychopharmacology and Biological Psychiatry 7: 623–627

Mohler H, Okada T 1977 Benzodiazepine receptors: demonstration in the central nervous system. Science 198: 849–851

Mohler H, Richards J G 1988 The benzodiazepine receptor: a pharmacological control element of brain function. European Journal of Anaesthesia Suppl 2: 15–24

Morselli P L 1983 Clinical pharmacokinetics in neonates. In: Gibaldi M and Prescott L (eds) Handbook of clinical pharmacokinetics. ADIS, Auckland, pp 79–97

Muenster J J, Rosenberg M S, Carleton R A, Graettinger J S 1967 Comparison between diazepam and sodium pentothal during direct current countershock. Journal of the American Medical Association 199: 758

Muller von H, Schleussner E, Stoganov M, Kling D, Hempelmann G 1981 Hamodynamische Wirkungen und Charakteristika der Narkoseeinleitung mit Midazolam. Arzneimittel-Forschung/Drug Research 31: 2227–2232

Nutt D J, Cowen P J, Little H J 1981 Unusual interactions of benzodiazepine receptor antagonists. Nature 295: 436

O'Boyle C, Lambe R, Darragh A, Taffe W, Brick I, Kenny M 1983 Ro 15–1788 antagonizes the effects of diazepam in man without affecting its bioavailability. British Journal of Anaesthesia 55: 349–456

Perisho J A, Buechel D R, Miller R D 1971 The effect of diazepam (Valium) on minimum alveolar anaesthetic requirement (MAC) in man. Canadian Anaesthetists' Society Journal 18: 536

Persson A, Ehrin E, Eriksson L, Farde L, Hedstrom C–G et al 1985 Imaging of [^{11}C]-labelled Ro 15–1788 binding to benzodiazepine receptors in the human brain by positron emission tomography. Journal of Psychiatric Research 19: 609–622

Power S J, Morgan M, Chakrabarti M K 1983 Carbon dioxide response curves following midazolam and diazepam. British Journal of Anaesthesia 55: 837–841

Priest R G 1980 The benzodiazepines: a clinical review. In: Priest R G, Vianna Filho U, Amtein R, Skreta M (eds) Benzodiazepines Today and Tomorrow. MTP Press Lancaster, pp 77–83.

Randall L O 1960 Pharmacology of methaminodiazepoxide. Disease of the Nervous System 21: 7–10

Reves J C, Vinik R, Hirschfield A M, Holcomb C, Strong S 1979 Midazolam compared with thiopentone as a hypnotic component in balanced anaesthesia. A randomized, double-blind study. Canadian Anaesthetists' Society Journal 26: 42–49

Reves J C, Samuelson P N, Vinik H R 1982 Consistency of action of midazolam. Anesthesia and Analgesia 61: 545–546

Roncari G, Ziegler W H 1986 Pharmacokinetics of a new benzodiazepine antagonist Ro 15-1788 in man following intravenous and oral administration. British Journal of Clinical Pharmacology 22: 421–428

Samuelson P N, Reves J G, Smith L R, Kouchoukos N T 1980 Midazolam versus diazepam: different effects on systemic vascular resistance. Arzneimittel Forschung/Drug Research 31: 2268

Schulte-Sasse U, Hess W, Tarnow J 1982 Haemodynamic responses to induction of anaesthesia using midazolam in cardiac surgical patients. British Journal of Anaesthesia 54: 1053–1058

Short T G, Maling T, Galletly D C 1988 Ventricular arrhythmia precipitated by flumazenil. British Medical Journal 296: 1070–1071

Vinik H R, Reves J G, Greenblatt D J, Nixon D C, Whelchel J D, Luke R, Wright D, McFarland L 1982 Pharmacokinetics of midazolam in renal failure patients. Anesthesiology 57: A366

Vree T B, Reeken-Ketting J J, Fragen R J, Arts T H M 1984 Placental transfer of midazolam and its metabolite 1-hydroxymethylmidazolam in the pregnant ewe. Anesthesia and Analgesia 63: 31–34

Zsigmond E K, Shiveley J C 1966 Spirometric and blood gas studies on the respiratory effects of hydroxyzine hydrochloride in the human volunteer. Journal of New Drugs 6: 128

12. Other sedatives and hypnotics

J. A. S. Gamble

PHENOTHIAZINES

The phenothiazines are a group of drugs widely used in many fields of medicine. They are primarily employed for the treatment of patients with serious psychiatric illness, but are also used in the treatment of nausea and vomiting, for the production of peripheral vasodilatation and as antihistamines and sedatives. In anaesthetic practice they are generally used either in premedication in combination with other drugs, or to control postoperative emetic symptoms. A large number of phenothiazines are now available, but apart from having a common nucleus their actions differ widely. The phenothiazine nucleus has no antihistaminic effect and little or no CNS depressant effect, but these effects are present in the aminated derivatives.

Figure 12.1 shows the general structural formula of the aminated phenothiazine derivatives. In this formula X is either a two- or three-carbon chain, sometimes with an additional methyl substitution at the second carbon atom, and R_1 and R_2 are alkyl groups or may form part of a heterocyclic ring. At Y the hydrogen atom may be substituted by a halogen, methyl or methoxy group.

In the late 1930s a derivative of phenothiazine, promethazine, was prepared and was found to have antihistamine properties and a strong sedative effect. It was also found to cause a marked prolongation of barbiturate sleeping time. A decade later chlorpromazine was synthesized, and Laborit et al (1952) described how it potentiated anaesthetics. They noted that by itself chlorpromazine did not cause loss of consciousness but produced a tendency to sleep and a lack of interest in the surroundings. These central actions became known as ataractic or neuroleptic. Phenothiazines were thus used initially as adjuvants to anaesthesia, and their application to psychiatry followed later. Cholestatic jaundice, blood dyscrasias and extrapyramidal side-effects may follow their use. While hundreds of phenothiazine derivatives have been studied, those which have been useful in anaesthetic practice include chlorpromazine, promethazine, trimeprazine, promazine and prochlorperazine.

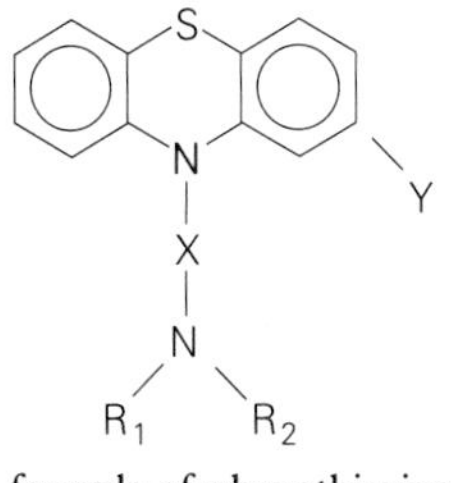

Chlorpromazine is the most widely studied drug of the phenothiazines and has become the standard by which the other members are judged.

Chlorpromazine hydrochloride

Chemical name: 2-chloro-10-(3-dimethyl-
aminopropyl) phenothiazine
hydrochloride.

Pharmacology

Central nervous system. Chlorpromazine has an inhibitory effect on all cellular activity. It is a central depressant with a marked effect on the reticular formation, the basal ganglia and the hypothalamus. It produces drowsiness and relieves anxiety. Sleep is induced, but the subject is usually easily aroused although consciousness may be lost if large doses are given. EEG changes are similar to those produced by normal sleep. It potentiates the action of anaesthetics, sedatives and analgesics, and antagonizes the stimulant effect of the analeptics. It has a marked anti-emetic effect due to depression of the chemoreceptor trigger zone. Large doses depress the vomiting centre. These effects are due to action at dopamine (D_2), muscarinic and histamine (H_1)

Fig. 12.1 General formula of phenothiazines.

195

receptors (Peroutka & Snyder 1982). The anti-emetic effects of the phenothiazines are discussed in more detail in Chapter 15.

Chlorpromazine can also induce a parkinsonism-like syndrome similar to that found following the use of nearly all the anti-psychotic drugs. Parkinson's disease is associated with a deficiency of dopamine in the basal ganglia. It would thus appear that interference with the transmitter function of dopamine in the mammalian forebrain might contribute to the neurological and anti-psychotic effects of these drugs. This is supported by the findings that neuroleptic drugs increase the concentrations of the metabolites of dopamine but have variable effects on the metabolism of other neurotransmitters (Carlsson & Lindqvist 1963, Carlsson 1978). The increase in the turnover of dopamine suggests a secondary or compensatory response to dopamine receptor blockade.

Autonomic nervous system. Chlorpromazine has marked α-adrenergic antagonist activity, and can either block or reverse the pressor effects of adrenaline. It also produces a mild anticholinergic action.

Cardiovascular system. The actions of chlorpromazine on the cardiovascular system are complex because the drug produces direct effects on the heart and blood vessels, and also indirect ones through its effects on the CNS and autonomic reflexes. However, its main cardiovascular effects are due to its adrenergic blocking action.

Intravenous administration of chlorpromazine produces hypotension which may be profound, especially in the upright position — orthostatic hypotension — and a reflex tachycardia. Oral therapy produces mild hypotension, the fall in systolic pressure being more pronounced than the fall in diastolic pressure. Tolerance develops to the hypotensive effects although orthostatic hypotension may persist. Chlorpromazine has a direct depressant action on the heart. Vasodilation following its use is due both to its α-blocking effect and a direct action on blood vessels. Vasodilation reduces peripheral resistance and cardiac output may increase. ECG changes include tachycardia and an increase in the conduction time.

Respiratory system. There is little effect on the pulmonary ventilation if given in moderate doses. Large doses, however, may cause respiratory depression. It has an antagonistic effect to respiratory depression caused by pethidine. Bronchial and laryngeal reflexes may be depressed. A decrease in bronchial secretions may result in dryness of the mucosa of the respiratory tract.

Temperature regulation. A reduction in body temperature may follow due to:

(a) peripheral vasodilation,

(b) depression of temperature-regulating centre,
(c) reduction in muscle tone,
(d) inhibition of shivering.

Gastrointestinal tract. Chlorpromazine causes a reduction in salivary and gastric secretions. A reduction in intestinal motility may result in constipation.

Liver. Jaundice has frequently been reported following its use, even in small doses. Patients with alcoholic liver disease are particularly at risk. The jaundice is due to cholestasis and usually clears after discontinuation of the drug for a few days. Prolonged periods of jaundice leading to biliary cirrhosis have been reported.

Antihistaminic action. Chlorpromazine has only a mild antihistamine effect.

Miscellaneous effects. Chlorpromazine increases the effects of both non-depolarizing and depolarizing muscle relaxants; it also had a local analgesic action. Chlorpromazine causes skeletal muscle relaxation in some types of spastic conditions. Since it has little effect at spinal levels, and does not produce blockade at the neuromuscular junction, its effect on motor activity must be mediated at a higher level.

Absorption, metabolism and excretion

While chlorpromazine is well absorbed following oral and intramuscular administration its effects following the oral route are very variable. This may be because the drug is metabolized in the gut wall and in the liver, and the rate of metabolism is dependent upon the individual. Parenteral administration bypasses this 'first-pass effect'. Chlorpromazine is highly protein-bound (98%). Following intramuscular administration it has a volume of distribution (V_d) of 21 l kg^{-1} and a plasma half-life ($t_{\frac{1}{2}}$) of 30 h. Chlorpromazine, like the other phenothiazines, is metabolized by two main pathways: (a) ring hydroxylation and subsequent conjugation, and (b) sulphoxide formation. The large number of metabolites, these being mainly inactive, are excreted in the urine and faeces.

Toxicity

Large doses may cause extrapyramidal side-effects. These disappear on stopping the drug, or may be controlled by concurrent administration of anti-parkinsonian drugs. Leucopenia and rarely agranulocytosis may occur. Skin rashes have occurred in personnel handling the drug, and urticaria and other allergic effects have been observed in patients.

Clinical uses

Chlorpromazine is used in premedication and to allay anxiety for minor surgical procedures and investigations. It is a useful anti-emetic, especially in the treatment of drug-induced or radiation-induced emetic symptoms. While it has no analgesic properties it is useful in combination with analgesic drugs in the treatment of intractable pain. It may be used in the treatment of hiccough. Its main use is in psychiatry, in the symptomatic control of most types of severe psychomotor excitement.

Dosage and administration

Chlorpromazine can be given by the oral, intramuscular or intravenous route. When given intravenously the solution should be diluted in water and given very slowly, as severe falls in blood pressure frequently occur following intravenous administration. Elderly patients are likely to be more sensitive to both therapeutic and toxic effects of neuroleptic drugs, as a result of age-related alterations in pharmacodynamic drug sensitivity, as well as pharmacokinetic drug disposition (Salzman 1987).

The oral dose ranges from 50 to 100 mg, and the intramuscular and intravenous doses are generally 25–50 mg. However, much larger doses are frequently employed in psychiatry in the treatment of severely disturbed patients. A mixture of chlorpromazine 50–100 mg, promethazine 50–100 mg and pethidine 50–100 mg in 500 ml of dextrose, the so-called 'lytic cocktail', may be given by slow intravenous infusion until the desired level of sedation is produced.

Promethazine

Chemical name: 10-(2-dimethylaminopropyl) phenothiazine hydrochloride.

Pharmacology

Nervous system. The effect on the CNS is similar to that of chlorpromazine. However, it is a more potent sedative and sleep is more readily induced.

Cardiovascular system. Its effect on the cardiovascular system is much less than that caused by chlorpromazine, as it has only a slight anti-adrenaline effect. However, a small fall in blood pressure may follow its use.

Respiratory system. It has an atropine-like action on the respiratory system in that secretions are reduced and bronchial musculature is relaxed.

Anti-histamine action. It has a marked anti-histamine effect and so is useful in the treatment of allergic phenomena.

Clinical uses

It is used in premedication for its sedative and anti-emetic properties. It is used in the management of allergic reactions, and is useful in the control of travel sickness. However, drivers of vehicles should avoid its use as its strong sedative effect may impair their driving ability.

Dosage and administration

It may be given by the oral, intramuscular or intravenous route. It has a plasma half-life $(t_{\frac{1}{2}})$ of 12 h and a volume of distribution (Vd) of 13 l kg^{-1}. For premedication the usual dose is 25 mg intramuscularly combined with 100 mg pethidine, while 25–50 mg by mouth is used to prevent travel sickness and in the treatment of allergic conditions. This dose may be repeated 4-hourly if necessary.

Prochlorperazine

Chemical name: 2-chloro-{10-3-[4-methyl piperazin-l-yl] propyl} phenothiazine.

Prochlorperazine has similar pharmacological effects to those of chlorpromazine. It has, however, a more powerful anti-emetic effect and its use in anaesthetics is as an anti-emetic agent. It may be given either preoperatively or postoperatively. The usual adult dose is 12.5 mg intramuscularly. When repeat doses are given the dose should be reduced to prevent the occurrence of extrapyramidal side-effects.

Trimeprazine

Chemical name: 10-(3-dimethylamino-2-methylpropyl) phenothiazine tartrate.

Trimeprazine has similar central effects to those of chlorpromazine and an antihistamine effect more powerful than that of promethazine. Its use in anaesthetics is a premedication, usually in children, where it is given orally in a dose of 3–4.5 mg/kg.

Miscellaneous phenothiazines

These include fluphenazine, methotrimeprazine, promazine, propiomazine, trifluoperazine and many other minor drugs.

BUTYROPHENONES

The butyrophenones, along with several of the pheno-thiazines, belong to a class of drug named neuroleptics. Neurolepsis is described as a drug-induced behavioural syndrome. Neuroleptic compounds produce a quiescent state of reduced motor activity, which may be sufficiently marked to be described as cataleptic immobility, together with reduced anxiety and mental detachment, in which the patient is mildly sedated and indifferent to his/her surroundings. Sleep is not necessarily induced and patients are easily aroused and responsive to commands. They are capable of giving appropriate answers to direct questions and seem to have their intellectual functions intact.

It is believed that neuroleptics block dopamine receptors at postsynaptic membranes in the brain and thus decrease transmission. Their main effects are thus in areas of the brain which are rich in dopaminergic receptors, namely the chemoreceptor trigger zone and basal ganglia. They thus exert a powerful anti-emetic effect and may produce a parkinsonian state if large doses are administered.

Neuroleptanalgesia is a term which describes the state of a patient following the administration of a sedative of the butyrophenone series, e.g. droperidol, together with a potent analgesic, e.g. phenoperidine or fentanyl. Major surgery can be carried out using this technique provided ventilation is controlled if large doses of analgesics are required.

The two main butyrophenones used in clinical practice are droperidol and haloperidol.

Droperidol

Chemical name: 1-1-[3-(4-fluorobenzoyl)propyl]-1,2,3,6-tetrahydro-4-pyridyl benzimidazolin-2-one.

Pharmacology

Droperidol produces a state of mental detachment but has little hypnotic effect. Voluntary movement is inhibited. It has a specific inhibitory effect on the chemoreceptor trigger zone, controlling nausea and vomiting. It has a weak α-adrenergic receptor blocking action and hypotension may follow intravenous administration. Its α-blocking effect gives some protection against catecholamine-induced arrhythmias during anaesthesia.

It acts within 5–10 min following intravenous injection and has a duration of action of up to 12 h. It is metabolized in the liver.

Toxicity

Extrapyramidal side-effects may occur if large doses are given.

Uses

Droperidol may either be used alone or in combination with a potent analgesic.

In psychiatry it may be used for tranquillization and for the emergency control of psychiatric states, e.g. mania and in behavioural disturbances.

In anaesthesia it is used as a premedicant, or an anti-emetic, and when given intravenously in conjunction with a potent analgesic to produce neuroleptanalgesia. In premedication 5–10 mg may be given intramuscularly 1 h preoperatively, either alone or in combination with an analgesic. As an anti-emetic 2.5–5 mg may be given intramuscularly or intravenously postoperatively. Its anti-emetic use is discussed in more detail in Chapter 15. As droperidol increases the central nervous depression produced by other CNS-depressant drugs, including hypnotics, sedatives and analgesics, the dose of these may have to be reduced for up to 12 h following droperidol.

Neuroleptanalgesia

Neuroleptanalgesia is a useful anaesthetic technique when the patient's conscious co-operation is required during surgery. It may also be used for unpleasant diagnostic procedures, e.g. aortography or angiocardiography. In addition it may be used as a supplement to thiopentone, relaxant, gas-oxygen anaesthesia where the use of a volatile agent is contra-indicated. During surgical procedures under local anaesthetic it may be used to produce varying degrees of sedation.

Haloperidol

Chemical name: 4-[4-(4-chlorophenyl-4-hydroxypiperidino]-4-fluorobutyrophenone.

Pharmacology

Haloperidol is similar in action to droperidol producing a cataleptic state with little hypnosis. It is a powerful anti-emetic. It has virtually no α- adrenergic blocking activity and thus produces no hypotension even following intravenous administration. Its action is longer than that of droperidol, lasting 24 h.

Uses

1. Its main use is in psychiatry in the treatment of schizophrenia and related psychoses, and tranquillization and emergency control in behavioural disturbances.
2. Premedication: 5 mg intramuscularly.
3. Neuroleptanalgesia: 2.5–5 mg intravenously followed by an analgesic, usually phenoperidine or fentanyl.

Miscellaneous drugs

Chlormethiazole edisylate

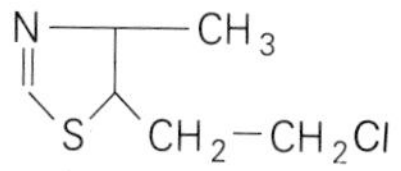

Chemical name: 5-(2-chloroethyl)-4-methylthiazole ethane-1,2 disulphonate.

Chlormethiazole is both a hypnotic and an anticonvulsant, and also has anti-emetic properties. Available evidence suggests that chlormethiazole enhances GABA-ergic transmission in the brain, by a mechanism which partly differs from that of the barbiturates and the benzodiazepines (Ogren 1986). Chlormethiazole appears to act on an allosteric site of the GABA receptor complex, which is closely related to chloride channel function. It also enhances glycine-mediated inhibition. At higher doses chlormethiazole also affects more general functions of GABA which underlie the hypnotic effects of the drug and its action on other transmitter systems.

It has little effect on the cardiovascular system other than causing tachycardia (Sinclair et al 1985), but in large doses some hypotension may occur. It is also respiratory-depressant at higher doses.

Pharmacokinetics

Chlormethiazole is well absorbed but undergoes exten-

sive first-pass hepatic metabolism, with a systemic bioavailability of about 15% after oral administration. This effect is markedly reduced in patients with advanced cirrhosis, in whom doses may consequently have to be reduced. After intravenous administration there is rapid redistribution with a biphasic fall in plasma concentration, with half-lives of 0.54 and 4.05 h (Moore et al 1975). Following prolonged infusion the fall in plasma level is slower, as it is dependent on metabolism, and half-lives of 7.9–17 h have been found (Scott et al 1980, Robson et al 1984)

Clinical usage

It is used as a night-time sedative, especially in the elderly where its rapid elimination and lack of hangover may be advantageous. Intravenous infusion of 0.8% solution may be used for sedation in the intensive care unit, or during regional anaesthetic procedures (Seow et al 1985, Sinclair et al 1985), and this route is also used in treatment of alcoholic withdrawal states, eclampsia (Campbell 1986) and of other convulsive disorders. It may be effective in treatment of status epilepticus resistant to benzodiazepines and barbiturates. A rapid infusion (30–50 ml 0.8% solution) is given at a rate of about 4 ml min^{-1} until drowsy, and the rate is then reduced. Because of its short half-life, treatment may have to be continued by infusion or orally for some time.

Adverse effects include an incidence of thrombophlebitis, and haemolysis can occur if concentrations greater than 0.8% are used. Chlormethiazole inhibits the hepatic mono-oxygenase system — it is 10 times more effective than cimetidine in doing this (Hoensch 1986).

Chloral derivatives

Chloral, chemical name 2,2,2-trichloroacetaldehyde, is an unstable compound, and its derivatives are used as

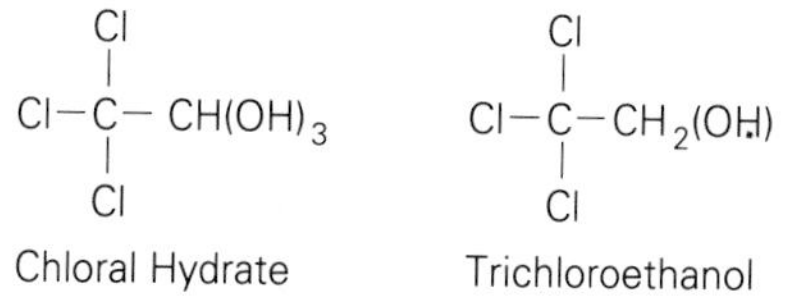

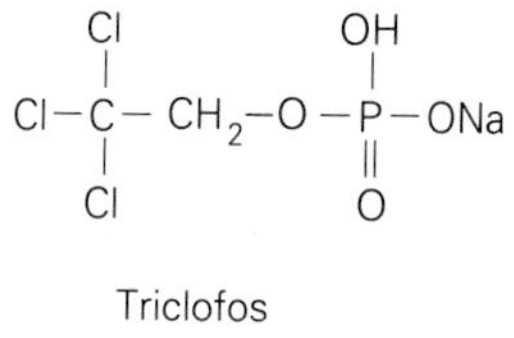

Chloral Hydrate

Trichloroethanol

Triclofos

medicines. These include chloral hydrate, dichloralphenazone and triclofos.

The main effects of chloral hydrate are due to trichloroethanol, to which it is very rapidly reduced in the body. Triclofos is rapidly metabolized to chloral hydrate and trichloroethanol. The drugs have a depressant effect on the central nervous system, causing sedation, but like barbiturates there is little or no analgesic activity. They have some anticonvulsant activity, but are less effective than the benzodiazepines in this respect. They are stated to have relatively little effect on REM sleep.

In normal doses there is little depression of respiration or blood pressure, but in overdose (see Chapter 35) there may be severe respiratory and cardiovascular depression.

All these compounds are well absorbed after oral administration. Distribution of chloral hydrate is rapid as it is lipid-soluble. Triclofos is more hydrophilic but is rapidly metabolized as described above, and distributes rapidly.

Chloral hydrate is metabolized to trichloroethanol in erythrocytes, liver and other tissues, mainly by alcohol dehydrogenase. Some chloral hydrate and trichloroethanol are oxidized to trichloroacetic acid, but the main pathway for excretion is conjugation of trichloroethanol with glucuronic acid and excretion mainly in the urine, with a plasma half-life of 4–12 h. Trichloroacetic acid is excreted more slowly with a half-life of around 67 h (Sellers et al 1973).

Clinical usage and dosage

Chloral derivatives are considered to be relatively non-toxic hypnotic drugs, and are often recommended for sedation of paediatric and geriatric patients; the usual adult doses are: chloral hydrate 0.5–2 g, triclofos sodium 1–2 g dichloralphenazone 1.3–2 g orally, and the hydrate is recommended to be taken with milk because of its gastric irritant effect.

Adverse effects

Apart from gastric irritation, the main effects worth noting at normal doses are the occurrence of enzyme induction, and the displacement of other drugs from protein-binding sites, mainly by trichloroethanol. Thus there may be interaction with other drugs — e.g. oral anticoagulants. Enzyme inhibition may also occur. Chronic intake of chloral may lead to tolerance, dependence and addiction, similar to alcohol dependence. In toxic doses there is depression of myocardial contractility, and both ventricular and supraventricular

tachyarrhythmias may also occur. Supraventricular tachycardias have also been reported with normal doses of chloral hydrate given to children following cardiac surgery (Hirsch and Zauder 1986). Arrhythmias may in part be due to sensitization of the heart to the effects of catecholamines, by the halogenated hydrocarbon metabolite, trichloroethanol (Marshall 1977).

Meprobamate

$$CH_2-O-\overset{\displaystyle O}{\overset{\displaystyle \|}{C}}-NH_2$$
$$C_3H_7-\overset{\displaystyle |}{\underset{\displaystyle |}{C}}-CH_3$$
$$CH_2-O-\overset{\displaystyle O}{\overset{\displaystyle \|}{C}}-NH_2$$

Chemical name: 2-methyl-2-propyl trimethylene dicarbamate.

Meprobamate belongs to the carbamate group of tranquillizers, and as well as causing anxiolysis it has some anticonvulsant and muscle relaxant properties. Its central effects may be due to a generalized depression of neuronal excitability. Meprobamate is a potent inhibitor of adenosine uptake, and may exert its effects by potentiating the effects of endogenously released adenosine by reducing uptake of this inhibitory neurotransmitter (De Long et al 1985).

Pharmacokinetics

Meprobamate is rapidly absorbed from the gastrointestinal tract, with peak concentrations occurring in 1–2 h, and is widely distributed. Ninety per cent is excreted in the urine, mainly as a hydroxylated metabolite and its glucuronide conjugate; less than 10% is found in the faeces. The elimination half-life is 6–16 h, but is prolonged in patients with renal or hepatic insufficiency.

Clinical usage

Meprobamate is used mainly as a tranquillizer, in an oral dosage of 400 mg three times daily to a maximum of 2.4 g per day. Its efficacy as a tranquillizer has been questioned.

Adverse effects

These are mostly minor. Hypersensitivity reactions occur occasionally, and agranulocytosis rarely. Hepatic enzyme induction occurs, and so it is contra-indicated in acute intermittent porphyria.

Paraldehyde

Paraldehyde is a cyclic polymer of acetaldehyde. It is a colourless or pale yellow liquid (if darker, toxic degradation compounds should be suspected), with a powerful and unpleasant smell.

Paraldehyde is a rapidly acting hypnotic, usually causing sleep in 10–15 min after oral administration. In normal clinical dosage it has little effect on respiration or blood pressure, but in large doses or in overdosage, hypotension and respiratory depression occur. In poisoning, respiration is commonly rapid and laboured. Damage occurs to various organs including the lungs; the lethal dose is probably about 50 g, but is variable. A common feature of paraldehyde toxicity is the occurrence of acidosis, presumably associated with its route of metabolism.

Pharmacokinetics

Paraldehyde is rapidly absorbed, and crosses the placenta. Metabolism in the liver, where it is depolymerized to acetaldehyde and then oxidized to acetic acid, accounts for 70–80% of the drug. The remainder is excreted unchanged, mainly from the lungs together with a small amount in the urine. Elimination is slowed, and the excretion from the lungs becomes more important in hepatic insufficiency.

Clinical usage

Paraldehyde is largely of historic interest. It has been used in treatment of convulsive conditions including tetanus, eclampsia, status epilepticus, etc., and in management of alcohol withdrawal, and still has a limited use for some of these.

The drug is irritant whether given orally, intramuscularly or intravenously, and nerve injury or other tissue necrosis may occur. The adult dose is 5–10 ml by deep intramuscular injection (not more than 5 ml at one site); or 4–5 ml, diluted by several volumes of normal saline, given intravenously, or the same dose rectally as a 10% enema diluted in normal saline.

ALCOHOLS

Several alcohols have been used for their sedative actions, but none is in popular use now — except for ethyl alcohol in its traditional medicinal and social roles.

Ethyl alcohol, ethanol

Chemical formula: C_2H_5OH

The general properties of alcohol are well known. It acts on the central nervous system in much the same way as other general anaesthetics, inhibiting the higher centres and functions first. There is little effect on the respiratory centre at moderate doses, but respiratory depression occurs at higher blood levels (400 mg $100\ ml^{-1}$ and above), and can be lethal. Again, although alcohol is a vasodilator, there is little overall effect on cardiovascular dynamics at moderate doses. At higher doses the effects on the heart in patients with coronary artery disease are deleterious, and although there is no overall cerebral vasodilatation, there may be areas of localized ischaemia.

In the digestive tract, alcohol stimulates gastric acid production by several pathways. It may thus be associated with peptic ulcer disease, and there is also an association between alcohol intake and the occurrence of pancreatitis. There is little acute effect on liver function, but chronic excessive intake leads to cirrhosis (some of the effects of this on drug handling are described in Chapter 4).

Alcohol as an anaesthetic

Before the discovery of modern anaesthesia in 1844, alcohol was, with opium, one of the few drugs capable of producing some degree of relief from the pain of surgical procedures. Perhaps surprisingly, it has received attention in more recent times. Marin, a Mexican army surgeon, attempted to use it as a 30% intravenous solution in 1929, but side-effects were unacceptable. More scientific study of its properties show that in a 10% v/v (8% w/v) solution it is capable of inducing anaesthesia, and that it is characterized by good cardiovascular and respiratory stability (Dundee and Isaac 1969). However, awakening is accompanied by a high incidence of emergence delirium, more troublesome to staff and other patients than to the subject, and this makes alcohol unacceptable as an anaesthetic in comparison to other available drugs.

Absorption of alcohol is rapid from the stomach, small intestine and colon. In the stomach the initial rapid uptake soon slows to a very low rate; food may delay emptying and complete absorption may then take 2–6 h. Absorption from the intestine remains rapid irrespective of food in stomach or intestine. After absorption it is distributed widely throughout the body.

Alcohol is metabolized to acetaldehyde in the liver, a small amount — 2–10% being excreted unchanged in urine and breath. Metabolism is mainly by alcohol dehydrogenase, but also to a small extent by the mixed-function oxidases. The enzyme systems are saturated at most blood levels, and so metabolism is by zero-order kinetics.

Drug interaction

The commonest effect is an additive action with other CNS depressant drugs such as tranquillizers, antihistamines, etc. The inebriated patient has a reduced requirement for general anaesthetic drugs, but tolerance develops with chronic alcohol intake, so that the chronic imbiber who is not drunk will show resistance. However, this tolerance does not extend to the cardiovascular system, so care must be taken that increased doses of anaesthetic do not cause cardiovascular depression. Hepatic enzyme systems may be acutely depressed but chronically induced. This may lead to unpredictable interaction with, for example, oral hypoglycaemic and anticoagulant drugs.

REFERENCES

Campbell D M 1986 Clinical experience and a review of chlormethiazole in the management of pre-eclampsia and eclampsia. Acta Psychologica Scandinavica Suppl 329: 175–181

Carlsson A 1978 Mechanism of action of neuroleptic drugs. In: Lipton M A, DiMascir A, Killam K F (eds) Psychopharmacology: a generation of progress. Raven Press, New York, pp 1057–1070

Carlsson A, Lindqvist M 1963 Effect of chlorpromazine and haloperidol on formation of 3-methoxytyramine and normetanephrine in mouse brain. Acta Pharmacologica et Toxicologica (Kbh) 20: 140–144

De Long R E, Phillips J W, Barraco R A 1985 A possible role of endogenous adenosine in the sedative action of meprobamate. European Journal of Pharmacology 118: 359–362

Dundee J W, Isaac M 1969 Clinical trials of induction agents. XXIX: Ethanol. British Journal of Anaesthesia 41: 1063–1069

Hirsch I A, Zauder H L 1986 Chloral hydrate — a potential cause of arrhythmias. Anesthesia and Analgesia 65: 691–692

Hoensch H P 1986 Effect of chlormethiazole on the hepatic monooxygenase system. Acta Psychologica Scandinavica Suppl 329: 66–68

Laborit H, Huguenard P, Alluaume R 1952 Un noveau stabilisateur vegetatif, le 4560 RP. Presse Medicale 60: 206–208

Marshall A J 1977 Cardiac arrhythmias causes by chloral hydrate. British Medical Journal 2: 294

Moore R G, Tripp E J, Shanks C A, Thomas J 1975 Pharmacokinetics of chlormethiazole in humans. European Journal of Clinical Pharmacology 8: 353–357

Ogren S O 1986 Chlormethiazole — mode of action. Acta Psychologica Scandinavica Suppl 329: 13–27

Peroutka S T, Snyder S H 1982 Antiemetics: neurotransmitter receptor binding predicts therapeutic action. Lancet 1: 658–659

Robson D J, Blow C, Gaines P, Flanagan R J, Henry J A 1984 Accumulation of chlormethiazole during intravenous infusion. Intensive Care Medicine 10: 315–316

Salzman C 1987 Treatment of agitation in the elderly. In: Meltzer H Y (ed) Psychopharmacology: The third generation of progress. Raven Press New York pp 1167–1176

Scott D B, Beamish D, Hudson I N, Joskell K-G 1980 Prolonged infusion of chlormethiazole in intensive care. British Journal of Anaesthesia 52: 541–545

Sellers E M, Lang M L, Koch Weser J, Cooper S D 1973 Chloral hydrate and triclofos metabolism. Clinical Pharmacology and Therapeutics 14: 147

Seow L T, Mathers L E, Cousins M J 1985 Comparison of the efficacy of chlormethiazole and diazepam as IV sedatives for supplementation of extradural anaesthesia. British Journal of Anaesthesia 57: 747–752

Sinclair C J, Fagan D, Scott D B 1985 Cardiovascular effects of a chlormethiazole infusion in combination with extradural anaesthesia. British Journal of Anaesthesia 57: 587–590

13. Opioids

J. G. Bovill

The pharmacological effects of opium, derived from the juice of the unripe seed heads of the poppy plant, *Papaver somniferum*, have been recognized for more than 2000 years. Raw opium contains at least 25 active alkaloids of which only three — morphine, codeine and papaverine — remain in clinical use. Opium smoking, however, remains a common form of addiction in middle and far eastern countries.

The opium alkaloids, together with a large number of synthetic or semi-synthetic compounds, form a group of drugs which produce analgesia by an agonist action at one or more specific receptors in the nervous system, either centrally or in the spinal cord. Various terms are used to describe these compounds. In Britain they are commonly referred to as opiates, i.e. opium-like drugs. However, many of the newer synthetic compounds, although having pharmacological properties similar to that of the opium alkaloids, have chemical structures which bear little resemblance to them. For this reason the term 'opioid' is preferable to describe this class of drugs and will be used throughout this chapter. An 'opioid' has been defined as any substance, whether derived from opium, or of synthetic origin, or produced within the body, having morphine-like actions that are potently and competitively blocked by naloxone.

The terms 'narcotic or narcotic analgesic' are prevalent in North America. The word narcotic is derived from the Greek word for stupor or sleep, and was at one the used to describe any drug which induced sleep. Although in sufficient doses all opioids induce sleep, or even anaesthesia, so do countless other substances, e.g. thiopentone, halothane, which are never referred to as 'narcotics'. Today the term narcotic is increasingly used in a legal context to refer to any drug which can cause physical dependence. It should be abandoned in medical nomenclature.

OPIOID RECEPTORS

The concept that the several pharmacologically distinct actions of the opioids might be due to an interaction with specific receptors was first proposed in 1965 (Portoghese 1965). Several factors suggested the existence of such receptors, both within the central nervous system and elsewhere.

1. All opioids are stereospecific, with activity usually exhibited only by the laevorotatory isomer.
2. Some opioids are extremely potent — etorphine, for example, is 10 000 times more potent than morphine. Only a selective receptor with high affinity could account for such potency.
3. The existence of drugs such as naloxone which have pure antagonist activity, i.e. they antagonize almost all the effects of opioids but have virtually no pharmacological activity themselves, favours specific receptors.
4. Many opioids exhibit structural specificity in that small alterations in their chemical structure can alter their pharmacological profile. A good example is the change caused by forming the *N*-allyl derivative of most opioids, e.g. Oxymorphone is a pure agonist yet its *N*-allyl derivative (naloxone) is a pure antagonist.

The existence of specific opioid binding sites in the central nervous system of vertebrates has been confirmed using ligands of high specificity. These sites combine stereospecifically with all known opioid agonists and antagonists. Their pharmacological significance is suggested by a high correlation between the affinity which a wide range of opioid-like compounds have for these sites and their pharmacological potency.

Most of the original knowledge about opioid receptors derives from the work of Martin and his colleagues, who studied behavioural effects on non-dependent chronic spinal dogs (Martin et al 1976, Gilbert and Martin 1976). They found that morphine and allied opioids produced three distinct syndromes which they attributed to separate receptors. They named these receptors after the prototype agonist producing the distinct physiological effect: μ (mu) for morphine, κ (kappa) for ketocyclazocine and σ (sigma) for SKF-10 047 (*N*-allylnormetazocine).

It has been hypothesized that μ-receptors mediate analgesia, κ-receptors mediate sedation and σ-receptors mediate mania and other psychomimetic effects of opioid drugs. This is, however, an oversimplification as a variety of responses are observed from stimulation of a specific receptor, although one response may predominate. The possible role of the various receptors in mediating physiological responses is summarized in Table 13.1.

More recently other receptors have been identified. A receptor with high affinity for leucine-enkephalin which is preponderant in the mouse vas deferens (δ-receptor), has been described (Lord et al 1977). An ϵ-receptor has also been identified in rat vas deferens (Schultz et al 1981) which is thought to be more specific for β-endorphin.

The μ-receptor

This subspecies of the opioid receptors is the one most widely studied. This is due mainly to the existence of a variety of μ-selective agonists, which can be used as pharmacological probes. Morphine is the prototype μ-agonist but many other drugs in this class — e.g. heroin, codeine, pethidine and fentanyl — are μ-agonists as defined by their animal and human pharmacology and their ability to substitute for morphine in dependent subjects.

There is a high correlation between the analgesic potency of opioid agonist drugs and their binding affinity for μ-receptors. Only a small proportion of μ-receptors need to be occupied to produce analgesia, and deep surgical anaesthesia is produced in rats when only 25% of the available CNS receptors are occupied. It has been postulated, from studies using naloxazone, a long-acting possibly irreversible opioid antagonist, that subpopulations of the μ-receptor exist: A high-affinity receptor (μ_1) responsible for analgesia and a low-affinity μ_2 receptor that appears to be involved in the produc-

tion of respiratory depression (Pasternak 1988). The central effects of opioids on gastrointestinal function may also be mediated solely by the μ_2 receptor. This obviously raises the possibility of the development of μ-selective drugs which could provide analgesia without respiratory side-effects.

The μ-receptors are also involved in opioid addiction, a phenomenon characterized by tolerance, physical dependence and compulsive drug abuse. Tolerance is the decreasing effect produced by a drug after repeated administration of the same dose. Physical dependence has been defined as the altered physiological state produced by the repeated administration of a drug which necessitates its continued use to prevent the appearance of a recognizable withdrawal syndrome (Jaffe 1985). There is evidence that the μ_2 receptor, but possibly not the μ_1 receptor is involved in physical dependence (Ling et al 1984). The neuronal mechanism of drug addiction is not fully known, but it probably reflects the adaptation of nerve cells to an altered environment caused by the continuous presence of the drug. Collier (1968) postulated that post-synaptically located receptors became supersensitive on prolonged opioid-induced inhibition of a presynaptically released excitatory neurotransmitter, probably adenylate cyclase. This concept closely resembles the phenomenon of denervation- or disuse-supersensitivity. Tolerance and physical dependence to enkephalin and β-endorphin can be produced in animals.

The functioning of enkephalin neurons themselves may play a part in addiction to opiates. A simple model can explain how alterations in the firing rate of enkephalin neurons could account at least in part for the behavioral manifestations of tolerance and physical dependence. Under resting conditions opiate receptors are exposed to a certain basal level of enkephalin. On treatment with morphine, cells with opiate receptors find themselves 'overloaded' with opiate-like material, and by some hypothetical neuronal feedback loop, they convey a message to the enkephalin neurons, 'Please turn off the enkephalin machine!' Whereupon, the enkephalin neurons cease firing and stop releasing enkephalin. At this point the postsynaptic cells are exposed c 'v to morphine so that they can 'tolerate' more of it to make up for the enkephalin they are no longer receiving. When morphine administration is terminated, the opiate receptors find themselves with neither morphine nor enkephalin, and hence are abstinent, which initiates a sequence of events resulting in withdrawal symptoms (Snyder 1977)

Chronic treatment of rats with morphine or an opioid antagonist results in an increase in brain μ-opioid binding sites, i.e. receptor up-regulation (Rothman et al 1989). It has been suggested that there is a relationship between μ receptor regulation and the development of tolerance, although no direct evidence exists at present

Table 13.1 Agonist responses of the opiate receptors

Mu (μ)	Kappa (κ)	Sigma (σ)
Supraspinal analgesia	Spinal analgesia	Dysphoria
Respiratory depression	Respiratory depression	Vasomotor stimulation
Euphoria	Sedation	Hallucinations
Dependance	Miosis	Mydriasis
Miosis		

to support this hypothesis. Rothman et al (1989) postulated that chronic morphine administration releases 'anti-opioids' into the CSF, leading to receptor up regulation, thereby producing tolerance and dependence. Among possible candidates for these 'anti-opioids' are cholecystokinin-8 (CCK) and some β-endorphin fractions. CCK is a gastrointestinal octapeptide hormone that is also found in the CNS where it is thought to function as a neurotransmitter or neuromodulator. It acts as an opioid antagonist following systemic or central administration in animals (O'Neill et al 1989). CCK may be an endogenous opioid antagonist acting through a negative feedback mechanism to return the organism to its basal level of sensitivity to pain after a nociceptive insult (Han et al 1985). The possible role of receptor regulation in opioid tolerance and dependence has been the subject of a recent review (Loh et al 1988).

In animals high concentrations of μ-receptors occur in lamina IV of the cerebral cortex and in the thalamus, amygdala, mesolimbic areas and periaqueductal grey matter of the brainstem. In the spinal cord, dense collections of μ-receptors are found in the substantia gelatinosa. Direct application of morphine to this site causes intense analgesia. Outside the nervous system opioid receptors are found mainly in the gastrointestinal tract — perhaps because both systems arise from a common embryological structure. High concentrations of μ-receptors are found in guinea-pig ileum and this tissue has proved extremely useful for in vitro μ-receptor studies. μ-Receptors have been isolated and purified from both bovine and rat brain (Gioannini et al 1985; Cho et al 1986). The receptor is a protein with a molecular weight between 58 000 and 65 000 Daltons.

The κ-receptors

Due to the lack of a highly selective ligand, until recently less was known about these receptors than about the μ-receptor. However, the isolation of dynorphin, a 17 amino acid peptide with potent opioid properties, from porcine pituitary and ileum, has allowed the distribution and pharmacology of κ-receptors to be studied. Dynorphin is a highly selective κ-receptor agonist. Immunohistochemical studies using this peptide have demonstrated the presence of κ-receptors in rat brain and spinal cord. It is possible that spinal analgesia is mediated in part by κ-agonists.

With the development of highly selective ligands for the κ-receptor, it has become increasingly apparent that there are subtypes of this receptor, just as for the μ-receptor (Traynor 1989). The physiological significance of these subtypes remains undetermined.

The human placenta contains opioid receptors, whose physiological function is unknown, but they may be involved in the analgesia of pregnancy, an elevation in pain thresholds during the terminal stages of pregnancy. Recently a glycoprotein, with a molecular weight of 63 000 Daltons, was purified from human placental villus membranes (Ahmed et al 1989). This glycoprotein bound κ ligands with high affinity and the binding was saturable and specific, indicating that it was a κ-receptor. This is the first report on the purification of an active κ receptor from human or any other tissue.

Several drugs used clinically are κ-receptor agonists. Many of these belong to the mixed agonist–antagonist subclass of opioids, i.e. those which show agonist and antagonist action at different receptor subtypes. Nalorphine is the prototype for this group of drugs and shows agonist activity at κ-receptors and antagonist activity at μ-receptors. Others include pentazocine, buprenorphine, butorphanol and nalbuphine. Bremazocine, a benzomorphan derivative, which has been widely studied in animals but not yet in humans, appears to be an almost pure κ-agonist. It is twice as potent an analgesic as morphine, and appears to be devoid of respiratory depression effects (Freye et al 1983). Another promising κ-agonist it spiradoline, which even in high doses has little cardiovascular or respiratory effects (Althaus et al 1988).

Physical dependence for κ-receptor agonists occurs, although the risk is much less than with morphine-like drugs. The type of dependence and the withdrawal symptoms are also distinct from that seen with the classical opioids.

The σ-receptor

The σ-receptor is thought to mediate the psychomimetic and mania-producing effects of opioids. SKF-10 047, the prototype drug for this class of receptor, is a μ-receptor antagonist which produces delirium and autonomic stimulation in the dog and delusional and hallucinatory effects in humans. Similar effects are seen with some of the mixed agonist–antagonist drugs, e.g. nalorphine, pentazocine, which are thought to be partial σ-receptor agonists. Naloxone, a μ-receptor antagonist, has extremely low affinity for σ-receptors. σ-Receptors have been demonstrated in the guinea-pig ileum and brain where highest levels were found in the brainstem, midbrain and cerebellum. This is in contrast to μ-receptors, which are only sparsely present, or absent, in the cerebellum. σ-Receptors have also been demonstrated in human post-mortem brains (Weissman et al 1988). The densities of the σ receptors was highest in the cerebellum, nucleus accumbens and cerebral cortex.

Similarities between the effects of SKF-10 047 and phencyclidine, a potent psychomimetic agent related to ketamine, have been demonstrated in binding assays. Based on this and other evidence, it is now considered that the σ-receptor is not a true opioid receptor but one which can coincidentally be activated by benzomorphans (Zukin & Zukin 1981). It is still uncertain what the role is of σ receptors but the identification of a putative endogenous σ ligand ('sigmaphin') in guinea pig brains suggest a functional σ system (Contreras et al 1987; Su et al 1986). This may be involved in human behaviour and some psychological disorders.

The δ-receptor

Lord et al (1977) reported an opioid receptor in the mouse vas deferens having a high affinity for leucine-enkephalin, which they designated as a δ-receptor. δ-Receptors are distributed diffusely in the central nervous system with highest densities found in the limbic system of bovine brain and in the frontal cortex of human brain. They are also present in the periaqueductal grey and spinal cord. δ-Receptor agonists are antinociceptive at the spinal cord level, but their role in mediation of supraspinal analgesia is controversial. Traditionally supraspinal antinociception was considered to be due solely to activation of μ receptors. There is however, a growing body of evidence which suggests that δ-receptors also may be involved (Heyman et al 1988), especially for thermal nociceptive stimuli. δ-Receptor activation may also initiate and modulate some forms of μ mediated supraspinal analgesia (Heyman et al 1989). Some supraspinal μ and δ receptors exist in an opioid receptor complex. The δ receptor was the first of the opioid receptors to be purified. It is a glycoprotein with a molecular weight of 58 000 Daltons (Simonds 1988).

Molecular biology of opioid receptors

The opioid system has widespread physiological functions in addition to the modulation of nociception. It is involved in the control of pituitary and adrenal medullary hormone release and activity, and in regulation of cardiovascular and respiratory function. Evidence for a possible role of opioids in regulation of the immune system has been comprehensively reviewed by Sibinga and Goldstein (1988). The endogenous opioid system also is involved in the regulation of cell proliferation, both in the brain of the fetus and neonate (Zagon & McLaughlin 1987) and in human and animal neoplasias (Zagon & McLaughlin 1986). In the gastrointestinal tract, the opioid system has an important function not only in regulating peristalsis but also of water and electrolyte regulation in the gut (Kromer 1988). All of these activities occur as the result of interactions between endogenous opioid peptides and one or more of the opioid receptors. These receptors, in the membranes of nerve and other tissue cells, are the key elements in a regulatory system which allows opioids to modify intracellular events and alter cell function (Simonds 1988). Several mechanisms are involved in this signal transmission at cellular level. As with many hormone and receptor-mediated systems, opioid receptor activation involves inhibition of adenylyl cyclase. This inhibition is mediated via receptor-effector coupling involving guanine nucleotide regulatory protein (G protein), particularly G_I (I for inhibitory). Electrophysiological evidence suggests that μ and δ receptors couple to a G-protein which activates potassium channels to cause an increase in transmembrane conductance and hence membrane depolarization. This is similar to muscarinic potassium channel activation in the heart. κ-Receptors are coupled to inhibition of voltage-dependent calcium channels.

ENDOGENOUS OPIOID PEPTIDES

The discovery of opioid receptors intensified the search for endogenous morphine-like substances which would interact with these receptors. That such substances existed was supported by experimental evidence, e.g. electrical stimulation of certain midbrain centres in animals produced analgesia which was reversed by naloxone. Early attempts to isolate an endogenous ligand for the opioid receptors were unsuccessful, since it was assumed that it would be chemically similar to morphine. However, in 1975, Hughes and his colleagues reported the identification of two similar pentapeptides in aqueous extracts of pig brain which produced morphine-like depression of motor activity of the mouse vas deferens and guinea-pig ileum, reversible by naloxone. Hughes and his group identified the two pentapeptides as methionine-enkephalin (H-tyrosine-glycine-glycine-phenylalanine-methionine-OH) and leucine-enkephalin (H-tyrosine-glycine-glycine-phenyl-alanine-leucine-OH). The amino acid sequence of methionine-enkephalin is identical to the sequence between residues 61 and 65 of β-lipoprotein, a 91 amino acid peptide found in the pituitary. Various fragments of β-lipoprotein possessing opioid activity have been isolated. Residue 61–91, called β-endorphin (*endogenous morphine*) or C-fragment, has the greatest activity and has been shown to interact with opioid receptors. α-endorphin (residue 61–76) and γ-endorphin (residue 61–77) have also been isolated from the pituitary.

At present it is possible to identify three main groups of endogenous opioid peptides, all of which by definition contain an enkephalin pentapeptide (either met5- or leu5-enkephalin). These three groups are distinct in their anatomical localization, as well as being synthesized differently in the body.

1. Endorphin. The large peptide pro-opiomelanocortin in the hypothalamic–pituitary region is the precursor of β-endorphin (and of α- and γ-endophins which are not opioid agonists) as well as of corticotrophin and of the MSH hormones. β-Endorphin includes the sequence of met-enkephalin.
2. The enkephalins are derived from a larger pro-enkephalin molecule, which contains met- and leu-enkephalin sequences in the ratio 6 : 1, separated by basic dipeptide cleavage markers.
3. The third important group, which includes dynorphin, are peptides based on the leu-enkephalin sequence, extended by two or more amino acids.

Although the final physiological role of the enkephalins has yet to be determined, the weight of evidence at present suggests that they have an important function as inhibitory neurotransmitters or neuromodulators within the central and peripheral nervous system. With a fast onset of action and rapid enzymatic termination of activity they are well suited for this role. These peptides constitute a major proportion of the opioid-like activity found in the brain and spinal cord with approximately ten times more enkephalin than β-endorphin. The enkephalins are widely but unevenly distributed throughout the central nervous system. Their concentration is low in the cortex and, in most species, absent from the cerebellum. Highest concentrations are found in the limbic structures (particularly the medial hypothalamus and amygdala) and in those regions of the paleospinothalamic tract which conduct dull diffuse pain. These latter include the medial part of the thalamus, laminae I and II and the periventricular and periaqueductal areas of the upper medulla and midbrain. The limbic system is involved with the perception and expression of emotion and with homeostatic responses. This regional CNS distribution is very similar to that of the opioid receptors. Within the spinal cord, enkephalin-containing neurons are localized in a dense band in the substantia gelatinosa, where initial integration of incoming sensory information takes place. Enkephalin and opioid receptors are also found in the gastrointestinal tract. There is a high association between regions with rich enkephalin innervation and those with high densities of opioid receptors. The chromaffin cells of the adrenal medulla contain enkephalins and catecholamines, both of which are released into the circulation on stimulation of the splanchnic nerve. The role of circulating enkephalins is not known.

Enkephalin, and possibly also endorphin, has a role in the regulation of pain perception. Modulation of pain is likely to occur at both supraspinal and spinal cord sites. In the spinal cord there is a close relationship between enkephalin and substance P (Fig. 13.1), a polypeptide believed to be involved in excitatory spinal processes specifically associated with nociception. There is evidence that whereas both β-endorphin and enkephalins participate in analgesic mechanisms centrally, only enkephalins act in the spinal cord. The analgesia produced by morphine-like drugs is thought to occur at both spinal and supraspinal levels.

The question arises, however, as to the normal physiological role of enkephalin/endorphin analgesic activity. Naloxone is an almost pure antagonist and yet has little pharmacological effect on its own, in contrast to other pure antagonists, e.g. atropine and d-tubocurarine. In human volunteers large doses of intravenous naloxone, up to 10 mg, are without effect on subjective pain ratings, whereas less than 1 mg will reverse profound opioid-induced analgesia. It seems likely that the analgesic role of the enkephalin/endorphin system is not tonically active, except in pathological states. This is supported by the report of a case of congenital insensitivity to pain in which 1.2 mg i.v. naloxone temporarily brought the greatly elevated pain threshold into the normal range (Dehen et al 1977). Intense activity of this system can also explain the almost complete absence of pain sensation in subjects who have suffered severe wounds at times of intense psychological tension, e.g. during battle.

Because the naturally occurring enkephalins are rapidly inactivated by peptidases they have little analgesic activity, even when injected into the cerebral ventricles. Enzyme-resistant analogues such as D-Ala^2-methionine enkephalin are, however, potent antinociceptive peptides. β-Endorphin is more resistant to enzymatic degradation and is a potent analgesic (it is as potent as morphine) when injected into the cerebral ventricle. Although β-endorphin produces analgesia in the whole body, others produce analgesia in specific body areas, i.e. α-endorphin produces analgesia only in the head and neck regions.

Endorphin is present in high concentration in the hypothalamic–pituitary axis, where it is thought to mediate control of endocrine function, particularly that of prolactin and growth hormone.

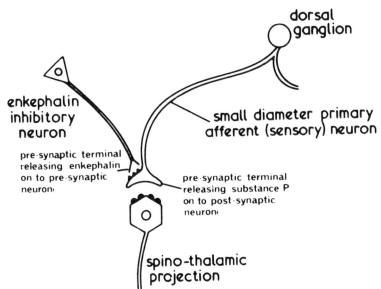

Fig. 13.1   Postulated interaction of enkephalin inhibitory neuron and substance P releasing primary afferent neuron in the dorsal horn of the spinal cord. (Reproduced with permission from Krug and Pycock 1979.)

OPIOID PHARMACOLOGY

Definition of terms

Opioid drugs produce a pharmacological effect through an interaction with receptors, discrete regions of post-synaptic membranes which can selectively bind molecules of a specific structure. Whether the process is initiated by the initial occupation of the receptor or by the whole process of binding to, and detachment from, the receptor is unknown.

The terminology used to describe the possible combinations of drug and receptor of a drug is described in Chapter 2. Although the terms antagonist or partial antagonist are often used to describe those opioids which have a low or intermediate intrinsic activity at the receptor, the term mixed agonist–antagonist is probably more meaningful, since these drugs can have different actions at different receptors. For example nalorphine is a competitive μ-antagonist, a partial κ-agonist, and a σ-agonist; pentazocine is a weak μ-antagonist, a strong κ-agonist and a σ-agonist.

A useful in vitro test as to whether an opioid drug is an agonist or an antagonist is the sodium index. The binding of antagonist drugs is enhanced in the presence of sodium ions, whereas agonist binding is inhibited (Chapman & Way 1980). The sodium index is defined as the ratio of IC_{50} value determined in the presence and absence of sodium ions. For agonists the index is high, and for antagonists it is low. This phenomenon also occurs with lithium but not other positive monovalent ions

such as potassium. The sodium effect is particularly marked with μ-receptors. Guanosine triphosphate has a similar effect on δ-receptors where the sodium influence is much weaker.

AGONISTS

Morphine

Morphine is the most important alkaloid of opium and constitutes about 10% by weight of raw opium. Chemically morphine is a phenanthrene with the structure shown in Figure 13.2. It was first isolated by Serturner in 1803 who named it after the Greek god of dreams, Morpheus. Its synthesis in the laboratory is extremely difficult and has only recently been achieved, although many semisynthetic derivatives, e.g. heroin (diacetylmorphine), can be readily prepared. Morphine is an almost pure μ-receptor agonist and is the yardstick against which all other agonist opioids are measured. Morphine is usually available as the sulphate salt; a hydrochloride salt is also available.

Morphine is especially effective in relieving continuous dull pain, e.g. that arising from hollow viscera, although sharp intermittent pain is also obtunded. A major factor in morphine's pain-relieving ability is the alteration which it produces in the subject's awareness of pain — it is still perceived but fails to elicit the former unpleasant response. Morphine is effective orally and parenterally. The usual adult intramuscular dose is 10–15 mg, which will produce analgesia reaching a peak

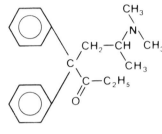
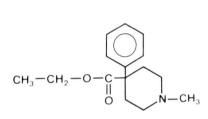

Fig. 13.2 Chemical structure of morphine and allied drugs.

in about 30 min and lasting from 4 to 5 h. With larger doses the incidence of side-effects increases out of proportion to the increase in analgesia.

For severe pain, for example postoperatively, it is preferable to titrate small doses, e.g. 2 mg intravenously until adequate analgesia is achieved, rather than rely on a fixed p.r.n. dose intramuscularly. Morphine is well absorbed from the gastrointestinal tract although significant presystemic metabolism occurs and larger doses are required. The effect is also more variable than with parenteral administration but the oral route can be useful in the management of patient with chronic cancer pain. Recently the administration of morphine intrathecally or epidurally has received widespread attention for providing analgesia of long duration. This application is discussed below.

Respiratory system. Morphine produces a direct, dose-related, depressant effect on the medullary respiratory centre. The primary effect is a reduction in the sensitivity of the respiratory centre to carbon dioxide so that initially respiratory rate is affected more than tidal volume, which may even increase. With increasing doses respiratory rhythmicity and reflexes are also disturbed, resulting in the irregular, gasping breathing characteristic of opioid overdose. This has been described as 'pharmacological decerebration'. Administration of oxygen to a patient whose respiration is depressed by morphine may produce apnoea by decreasing hypoxic stimulation of chemoreceptors. Patients who have been given large doses of morphine will often breathe on command, but when left unstimulated are indifferent to respiration and become apnoeic. Other stimuli, especially pain, are also effective in counteracting morphine-induced depression. Elderly patients are more sensitive to the respiratory depressant effects of morphine than younger patients, and the dose used needs to be adjusted accordingly. It is also important to remember that other central nervous system depressants such as barbiturates, alcohol and inhalational anaesthetics will potentiate the respiratory effects of morphine. Morphine-induced respiratory depression is reversed by naloxone and the mixed agonist–antagonist drugs, e.g. nalorphine. The latter may be preferable in the immediate postoperative period since they cause a less abrupt and complete reversal of analgesia.

Opioid-induced respiratory depression may be related to inhibition of acetylcholine release from neurons in the central nervous system. Physostigmine, an anticholinesterase, increases the level of acetylcholine in the brain and can antagonize morphine-induced respiratory depression in animals without antagonizing analgesic activity. Studies in humans have clearly demonstrated that physostigmine, 13–33 μg/kg intravenously, can rapidly reverse the somnolent effect of morphine and restore ventilation to pre-drug values without altering analgesia. The effect lasts approximately 35–45 min. The use of physostigmine may be accompanied by an increased incidence of nausea and vomiting.

Cardiovascular system.   Clinical doses of morphine produce minimal effect on the cardiovascular system of normal subjects in the supine position. Morphine does, however, decrease vascular resistance and this can lead to venous pooling and postural hypotension in semi-supine or erect subjects. Hypotension may be severe in hypovolaemic patients in whom morphine, if required, should be titrated slowly intravenously, restricting the dose to the mininum required to achieve pain relief. The intramuscular administration of morphine is potentially dangerous in shocked patients since absorption can be slow and unpredictable due to low muscle blood flow. Subsequent resuscitation and improvement in muscle blood flow may then result in a sudden increase in plasma morphine concentration.

Morphine has both a local and a central action on the peripheral circulation. Particularly with higher concentrations it can cause a direct inhibition of the contractile response of veins to noradrenaline. Morphine, and other opioids, also interact with specific pulmonary opioid receptors, initiating a pulmonary chemoreceptor reflex via vagal afferents.

Morphine-induced depression of the medullary vasomotor centre is also responsible for its observed cardiovascular effect. The onset of this effect is slower, however, than the peripheral effect due to slow uptake of morphine into the central nervous system. It is mediated via opioid receptors and can be reversed by naloxone.

Morphine causes release of histamine in humans, and this may also be responsible for decreased systemic vas-

cular resistance and hypotension. Prior administration of H_1 and H_2 receptor antagonists block morphine-induced histamine release and the accompanying vasodilation.

Morphine produces a negative inotropic effect on isolated cardiac muscle and isolated heart experiments. However, in intact animals morphine has a positive inotropic effect unaffected by carotid sinus denervation or vagotomy.

In patients without cardiovascular disease morphine 1 mg/kg produces minimal alteration in haemodynamics. The same dose given to patients with severe aortic valve disease about to undergo cardiac surgery, resulted in improvement in cardiac function (Lowenstein et al 1969). This observation laid the groundwork for the subsequent widespread use of high doses of morphine to produce anaesthesia for cardiac surgery.

Although it has long been recognized that morphine can decrease heart rate, in clinical practice this response is unpredictable. Therapeutic doses given to healthy supine subjects produce an increase in heart rate, and the initial tachycardia in response to abrupt tilting is greater after morphine than before (Drew et al 1946). Morphine in clinically effective doses has little effect on the sinoatrial node, and bradycardia, when it occurs, is thought to be vagal in origin. Morphine-induced central vagal activation may be valuable in reducing the vulnerability of the heart to ventricular fibrillation.

Morphine is a valuable drug in the management of patients with acute left ventricular failure. Part of this beneficial effect is due to the sedation and alleviation of fear which it produces. More important, however, may be its peripheral vascular effects. Reduction in systemic vascular resistance, and particularly the increase in venous capacitance, by reducing both preload and afterload, will allow the left ventricle to function more efficiently.

Gastrointestinal tract.   Outside the central nervous system the gastrointestinal tract is the only system with significant concentrations of opioid receptors. These, together with regions showing enkephalin-like immunoreactivity, are found throughout the gut, with highest concentration in the upper small intestine and stomach antrum. Morphine and allied drugs delay gastric emptying and the passage of food through the duodenum may be delayed for up to 12 h after morphine administration. This has important clinical implications for the anaesthetist dealing with patients presenting for emergency surgery. Where such patients have received morphine for either pain relief or premedication it must always be assumed that they have a full stomach, and appropriate steps taken to prevent regurgitation during induction of anaesthesia. Morphine also delays transit time through the ileum and colon by increasing resting tone and diminishing propulsive activity. This latter effect accounts for a major part of the constipating effect of morphine-like drugs, which are frequently used in the treatment of diarrhoea. In patients with ulcerative colitis, however, morphine is potentially dangerous. The gastrointestinal action of morphine-like drugs is partly mediated via a central mechanism which can be blocked by vagotomy. Morphine also has an effect on the biliary system, increasing common bile duct pressure and decreasing bile production and flow, primarily as a result of spasm of the choledochoduodenal sphincter (sphincter of Oddi) but also due to increased tone in the bile duct itself. Morphine should be avoided in patients with biliary colic and in those undergoing radiographical investigations of the biliary system.

Central nervous system. The therapeutically useful effects of morphine are almost all mediated via central nervous system activity. By far the most important of these is analgesia which results from a μ-agonist action both supraspinally in the brain and via opioid receptors in the spinal cord. In the brain morphine acts at two levels. Firstly it interferes with the transmission, integration and interpretation of pain impulses arriving via pain pathways. The most important sites for this action are the periaqueductal grey matter and medullary and thalamic nuclei, such as the raphe magnus and ventral caudalis. This component of morphine's analgesic effect can be demonstrated by an increase in the threshold for experimentally induced pain. Secondly morphine acts on the significance of pain by altering the subject's attitude to the pain process. This component is perhaps the most important, and is part of the overall effect of morphine on mood, thought to be mediated by an action on the limbic system which has high concentrations of opioid receptors. Euphoria, an unrealistic sense of well-being, is another manifestation of a limbic system effect and these mood changes are largely responsible for the abuse potential of morphine-like drugs. When given in the absence of pain morphine may sometimes produce dysphoria — an unpleasant sensation of fear and anxiety.

Central nervous system depression is the usual effect of morphine, and sedation and drowsiness are frequently observed with therapeutic doses. Morphine reduces the frequency content of the electroencephalogram and with doses sufficient to produce anaesthesia (1–3 mg/kg) δ-rhythm is the predominant feature of the EEG. Respiratory depression is another manifestation of morphine's depressive activity. Some animals, however, react to morphine not by central nervous depression but by excitation leading to convulsion. These include cats, pigs, cows and horses. Excitatory effects are rare in humans given even large doses of morphine, but are seen with pethidine. The most important stimulatory effects

of morphine in man are emesis and miosis. The former results from stimulation of the chemoreceptor trigger zone, although stimulation of the vestibular nerve may be important in producing nausea, especially in ambulatory patients. Miosis occurs with all morphine-like drugs and is due to stimulation of the Edinger–Westphal nucleus of the third nerve. The combination of pin point pupils, coma and respiratory depression are classical signs of morphine overdosage. Stimulation of the solitary nuclei may also be responsible for depression of the cough reflex (anti-tussive effect).

Epidural and subarachnoid morphine. The demonstration of opioid receptors and enkephalin-containing neurons in the spinal cord, and the realization that these played a major role in the production of analgesia by opioids, has led to a widespread interest in the administration of morphine into both the epidural and subarachnoid space to produce analgesia of long duration. In contrast to local analgesic drugs, opioid-induced spinal or epidural analgesia is accompanied by minimal sympathetic efferent and motor blockade. The principle behind this application of opioids has recently been extensively reviewed (Yaksh 1987).

Intrathecal morphine has been given in a wide range of doses, from 0.5 to 20 mg, although the optimal dose appears to be 0.5 to 1 mg. The intrathecal route has the advantage of minimal systemic uptake compared to epidural administration. This reduces both the total dose required (about one-tenth of the epidural dose) and the time to maximum effect. Nonetheless the onset of analgesia is slow compared to local analgesic drugs. The limiting factor in determining speed of penetration from the water phase of the CSF to the lipid phase of the neural tissue is the relative aqueous and lipid solubility of the drug. Morphine, being a highly hydrophilic compound which is poorly lipid-soluble, tends to remain in the CSF, and this is responsible for the slow onset of action. In rabbits given intraventricular injections of radioactive morphine it took 20 min for the drug to penetrate to a depth of 1.2 mm (Teschemacher et al 1973). The substantia gelatinosa of the spinal cord, which is the presumed site of action of spinal opioids, lies at an average depth of 1–2 mm. The duration of the analgesia produced by intrathecal administration of opioids is, in contrast, inversely related to lipid solubility. Drugs such as morphine cross lipid barriers with difficulty — i.e. they take a long time to enter neural cells but once they have arrived also have difficulty in leaving.

Morphine administered via the epidural space has an extra barrier to cross before it reaches the CSF. In addition there may be considerable systemic uptake of morphine via the epidural venous plexus, so that larger doses are required than with intrathecal administration. Commonly used doses are 2.5 to 10 mg, diluted in 10 ml normal saline. The latency of onset of analgesia is longer than with intrathecal administration, averaging about 35–45 min. Systemic uptake can result in blood morphine concentrations similar to those seen with intramuscular injections of the same dose (Sjöström et al 1987). In obstetric patients blood levels may reach that capable of fetal depression.

The intensity of analgesia is satisfactory for postoperative pain relief but insufficient to allow surgery. Epidural morphine therefore is often combined with a local analgesic which provides blockade for the surgical procedure, the morphine being given either simultaneously or at the end of surgery via an epidural catheter. The success rate with epidural morphine (about 40%) is lower than with intrathecal morphine (about 80%) and also much lower than with other opioids, e.g. pethidine or fentanyl.

The side-effects and complications are similar with both routes of administration. By far the most troublesome side-effect is pruritus, the incidence of which is much higher with morphine than with other opioids, and is higher with intrathecal (70%) than with epidural (40%) administration. Pruritus can be very severe and extremely distressing for patients. The mechanism is unknown but possible causes have been reviewed (Ballantyne et al 1988). It most commonly affects the head and trunk region initially, but may spread to all areas of the body and begins about 3 h after injection. It may be related to cephalad spread of morphine within the CSF. Naloxone will relieve the pruritus but may also reverse the analgesia. Surprisingly, pethidine has been found useful in alleviating the symptoms.

Rostral spread is also largely responsible for emetic symptoms and respiratory depression. Nausea and vomiting has a reported incidence of up to 75% and again is worse with intrathecal than epidural morphine. The incidence of respiratory depression is low (0.25–0.5%) but is potentially the most serious complication with these routes and is frequently delayed until several hours after drug administration. It can be profound and long-lasting. The respiratory depressant effects and pharmacokinetics of spinal opioids have been reviewed by Etches et al (1989). The other important side-effect is urinary retention with an overall incidence of about 40%. It can develop insidiously and since bladder sensation is partially or wholly lost may not be reported by the patient until gross overdistension of the bladder has occurred. Although administration of parasympathetic agents (e.g. bethanechol) has been recommended as the first line of treatment for urinary retention there is a high failure rate. Naloxone, 0.4 mg intravenously, will immediately restore normal micturition.

Endocrine and metabolic effects. The highest concentrations of the endogenous opioid peptide, β-endorphin, are found in the pituitary and medial hypothalamus, and enkephalin-containing cells are present in significant numbers in various hypothalamic nuclei. These are regions which have a direct effect on endocrine and metabolic function so it is not surprising that exogenous opioids, e.g. morphine, can also influence these functions. Morphine, even in small doses, will inhibit ACTH release and block the pituitary-adrenal response to surgery. Larger doses (1–4 mg/kg) will also block hormonal and metabolic responses to major abdominal and cardiac surgery. Many textbooks continue to state that morphine causes an increase in ADH secretion. While morphine is known to stimulate ADH secretion in dogs and rats, it does not do so in humans. The changes in urine production seen in some patients who have received morphine, i.e. decrease in volume without alteration in specific gravity or chloride composition, are inconsistent with an ADH mechanism. They may be due to alterations in glomerular filtration rate and renal plasma flow, possibly related to morphine-induced increases in circulating cathecolamines.

Pharmacokinetics and metabolism. One of the problems in the investigation of morphine kinetics has been, until recently, the lack of a sensitive and specific assay. Many of the older methods could not distinguish between morphine and its major metabolites, particularly morphine-3-glucuronide. The development in recent years of radioimmunoassays which are sensitive and specific has done much to alleviate this problem.

Morphine is rapidly and completely absorbed after subcutaneous and intramuscular injection with peak plasma concentrations reached after about 15 min (Stanski et al 1978). The rate of absorption when the deltoid muscle is used may be greater than with other muscles, e.g. gluteus maximus, since the deltoid has a significantly higher muscle blood flow. The terminal elimination half-life of morphine is relatively short (2–4 h) in comparison to fentanyl or pethidine. Also, unlike fentanyl or pethidine, plasma morphine concentrations are poorly correlated with pharmacological response, due to the very low lipid solubility of morphine. The drug distribution coefficient, i.e. the partition coefficient between lipid and water adjusted for the fact that only unionized drug distributes in the lipid phase, is 1.4 for morphine and 39 for pethidine. The hydrophilicity of morphine is related to the presence of hydrophilic hydroxyl groups on the molecule. Low lipid solubility restricts drug movement across lipid-rich cell membranes (see discussion of epidural and intrathecal morphine, above).

About one-third of morphine present in plasma is bound to protein, mainly albumin. The protein binding is pH-dependent and increases by 3% for each 0.2 unit increase in pH. Protein binding is also concentration-dependent.

The physiochemical property of the morphine molecule responsible for hydrophilicity also results in a low dissociation constant (pKa) so that at a plasma pH of 7.4 about 80% of the morphine in plasma is in the ionized state. Only the non-ionized moiety can readily cross the blood–brain barrier. There are two sites on the morphine molecule where ionization occurs — the phenolic group ($pKa = 9.36$ at 37°C) and the tertiary nitrogen ($pKa = 7.93$ at 37°C). For this reason the pKa value is often quoted as 7.93/9.36, although ionization at the phenolic group is of minimal consequence at physiological pH.

Morphine undergoes extensive hepatic biotransformation and less than 10% of a parenterally administered dose is excreted unchanged in the urine. Because of the high hepatic 'first-pass' effect the dose of oral morphine required to produce a therapeutic effect is much larger than with parenteral administration. The principal metabolite, morphine-3-glucuronide (M-3-G), accounts for about 80% of an administered dose 1 h after i.v. administration, with morphine-6-glucuronide (M-6-G) representing 5–10%. M-3-G is biologically inactive but M-6-G is pharmacologically active. It is a respiratory depressant with a potency substantially in excess of that of free morphine (Pelligrino et al 1989). Even allowing for its slower penetration into the brain, it may be that 50 percent or more of the respiratory depression observed by 1 h after systemic administration of morphine is due to this metabolite, and this contribution will increase with time. M-6-G makes a significant contribution to morphine intoxication in patients with renal failure (Osborne et al 1986).

Papaveretum

Papaveretum (Omnopon) is a mixture of the water-soluble alkaloids of opium standardized to contain 50% anhydrous morphine. Available preparations of morphine contain the alkaloid in salt form, usually as the sulphate combined with five molecules of water of crystallization. Since, in papaveretum, morphine is in the anhydrous form, it contains more than 50% effective alkaloid. Papaveretum 20 mg contains morphine alkaloid equivalent to that contained in 13.3 mg morphine sulphate. Papaveretum is claimed to be more sedative than morphine, possibly due to the non-morphine alkaloids

which it contains. It is popular as a premedicant drug, often given in combination with scopolamine. The side-effects are similar to those with morphine. Papaveretum is well absorbed after oral administration.

Levorphanol

Levorphanol (Dromoran) is a synthetic opioid of the morphinan series (Fig. 13.2), containing the *l*-isomer of the original synthetic product. The *d*-isomer (dextrorphan) is devoid of analgesic activity but is used as an anti-tussive. Levorphanol is a potent analgesic which is effective both parenterally and orally. Levorphanol 2 mg is equipotent with 10 mg morphine. Sedation is considerably less than with equivalent doses of morphine and the incidence of nausea and vomiting is also lower. Other side-effects are similar to those seen with morphine. Levorphanol is a valuable analgesic for post-operative use, and in one large comparative study of 14 drugs emerged as the most effective agent.

Codeine phosphate

Codeine is one of the principal alkaloids of opium. Its chemical structure is shown in Figure 13.2. Its analgesic efficacy is much lower than other opioids, possibly due to an extremely low affinity for opioid receptors. It has a low abuse potential and does not fall under the Control of Drugs Act. In contrast to other opioids, with the exception of oxycodone, codeine is relatively more effective when administered orally than parenterally. This is due to methylation at the C-3 site which may protect it from conjugating enzymes. It is used in the management of mild to moderate pain, often in combination with non-opioid analgesics such as aspirin or paracetamol. It is valuable as an anti-tussive and for the treatment of diarrhoea. Side-effects are uncommon and respiratory depression, even with large doses, is seldom a problem.

Potency. Codeine is approximately one-sixth as potent as morphine and 5–10 times as potent as aspirin. An oral dose of 30–60 mg produces a good pharmacological effect. Doses above 60 mg do not improve analgesic activity but may increase the incidence of side-effects.

Pharmacokinetics and metabolism. Codeine is metabolized in the liver mainly to inactive conjugates of glucuronic acid. About 10% undergoes demethylation to norcodeine and morphine — the morphine possibly contributing to the analgesic activity of codeine. About 10% of an oral dose appears as unchanged drug in the urine. The elimination half-life of codeine in plasma is 2.5–3 h (Findlay et al 1978).

RELATED COMPOUNDS

Dihydrocodeine

This is a semisynthetic derivative of codeine. It is more potent than the parent compound, 30 mg being approximately equianalgesic with 10 mg of morphine. It is effective both orally and parenterally, and is useful in the management of mild to moderate pain. It is available commercially as DF118, as tablets containing 30 mg dihydrocodeine tartrate and as ampoules for injection containing dihydrocodeine tartrate 50 mg per ml. Constipation is the commonest side-effect but in some patients nausea and vomiting occur. Overdosage causes respiratory depression.

Diamorphine

Diamorphine (diacetylmorphine, heroin) is a semisynthetic derivative of morphine. Its chemical structure is shown in Figure 13.2. Diamorphine is a potent analgesic with a high potential for addiction and its manufacture and use, even for medical purposes, is illegal in many countries including the United States of America. Although it is claimed that diamorphine produces more sedation and less nausea and vomiting than morphine, it is likely that the incidence of side-effects with equianalgesic doses is similar to other opioids.

Potency. A dose of 5 mg diamorphine is equipotent with 10 mg morphine, but the duration of action is shorter, about 2 h. Because diamorphine in solution rapidly undergoes deacetylation, injections should always be freshly prepared.

Pharmacokinetics and metabolism. Diamorphine undergoes rapid deacetylation in the plasma and tissues to monoacetylmorphine (MAM) and then to morphine. This liberated morphine may account for a major part of heroin's activity. Both diamorphine and MAM are more lipid-soluble than morphine and may act as carriers to facilitate the entry of morphine into the central nervous system.

Methadone

Methadone is a synthetic opioid with the chemical structure shown in Figure 13.2. Although the two-dimensional structure does not resemble that of other opioids, in three dimensions the molecule has an opioid-like pseudopiperidine configuration. Methadone is commercially available as a racemic mixture but almost all of the activity resides in the *l*-isomer which is up to 50 times more potent than the *d*-isomer. The pharmacological properties of methadone are qualitatively similar to those of morphine. It produces less sedation and euphoria but in other respects the side-effects are the same. It is well absorbed following both intramuscular and oral administration. The latter makes it useful in the management of severe chronic pain, e.g. due to cancer. It is widely used in the treatment of withdrawal symptoms in opioid addicts. Methadone is also commonly used in anaesthesia as a premedicant, and for the relief of postoperative pain.

Potency. Although it is often quoted that intramuscular methadone is equipotent with morphine in terms of analgesic effect, evidence (Gourlay et al 1982) suggests that, at least intravenously, methadone is less potent than morphine and that a dose of 20 mg gives optimal postoperative pain relief. The oral dose is 5–15 mg depending on the severity of the pain. In addicts, 1 mg methadone is equivalent to 1 mg heroin or 3 mg morphine.

Pharmacokinetics and metabolism. Methadone is rapidly absorbed after oral administration, and the biological availability is high, resulting in plasma concentrations comparable to those with intramuscular injection. About 85% in the plasma is protein-bound. It is also highly bound to tissue protein and this, together with a high lipid solubility, accounts for its very large volume of distribution (6 l kg^{-1}). The terminal half-life is very long with a mean value of 35 h (Gourlay et al 1982) and therefore with repeated doses it is easy for cumulation to lead to development of symptoms of overdosage. Analgesia is well correlated with plasma concentration. Methadone undergoes hepatic biotransformation by *N*-demethylation to form pyrrolidines.

Related compounds. Dextromoramide (Palfium) and Dipanone are analogues of methadone with similar pharmacological properties and potencies. It is claimed that they produce less constipation than methadone. Both are effective orally and are useful in the management of chronic cancer pain. The adult dose of dextromoramide is 5 mg intramuscularly or orally. Dipanone is available as a tablet containing 10 mg dipanone and 30 mg cyclizine, an anti-emetic (Diconal). The initial recommended dose is one tablet repeated if necessary every 6 h.

Dextropropoxyphene is structurally very similar to methadone. It is less potent than codeine, 90–120 mg dextropropoxyphene orally producing similar analgesia to 60 mg codeine. The hydrochloride salt is water-soluble and is well absorbed orally and parenterally. The napsylate salt is less soluble. It is available as Doloxene capsules, containing dextropropoxyphene hydrochloride 32.5 mg and paracetamol 325 mg. Although widely prescribed, dextropropoxyphene is not without risk, and overdosage will result in respiratory depression and later paracetamol hepatotoxicity. Prolonged use can lead to physical dependence.

Etorphine

Etorphine (Immobilon) is a semisynthetic opioid derived from thebaine, a benzylisoquinoline alkaloid of opium. The affinity of etorphine for the opioid receptor is 83 times greater than morphine but it is 2210 times as potent as morphine in the tail withdrawal reflex in the rat (Stahl et al 1977). Etorphine is about 400 times as potent as morphine in humans. It has a short duration of action and has rarely been used clinically. It is, however, a useful tool in laboratory studies of opioid binding, and because of its extreme potency is used in veterinary medicine, especially for the immobilization of large animals. Its effects can be rapidly reversed by naloxone.

Pethidine

Pethidine (meperidine) was the first totally synthetic opioid to be introduced. It is chemically related to atropine and was synthesized by Eisleb and Schaumann in 1939 for its possible smooth muscle relaxant properties. However, when given to mice it produced a Straub phenomenon (erection of the tail due to anal sphincter spasm), a characteristic of morphine-like drugs, and this attracted attention to its analgesic properties. The chemical structure of pethidine is shown in Figure 13.2. It is an effective analgesic widely used for the treatment of severe pain, as a premedicant and as analgesic component of balanced anaesthesia.

Potency. Pethidine is less potent than morphine, 75 mg pethidine being approximately equivalent to 10 mg morphine. It is well absorbed from the gastrointestinal tract, with peak plasma concentrations reached within 2–3 h of administration. It is less potent by the oral route than by injection. The duration of analgesia after parenteral administration is shorter than with equivalent doses of morphine.

Respiratory system. Like other opioids pethidine causes a dose-related respiratory depression. Small doses decrease respiratory rate but cause insignificant changes in tidal volume. With larger doses tidal volume is also decreased. Because of its atropine-like activity pethidine may be preferable to other opioids in patients who are liable to bronchospasm.

Cardiovascular system. Although doses of pethidine in the range 0.5–1 mg/kg cause minimal cardiovascular disturbances, with higher doses hypotension is more likely to occur than after equipotent doses of morphine. This is in part due to decreases in systemic vascular resistance, but is also related to pethidine's negative inotropic effect. In the isolated cat papillary muscle, pethidine produces 100–200 times more depression than morphine. In contrast to other opioids, pethidine administration often results in tachycardia. This may be related to the atropine-like structure of pethidine.

Pethidine may have a quinidine-like action which reduces myocardial irritability and can prevent or control ventricular arrhythmias after myocardial infarction. Like morphine, it can cause histamine release.

Central nervous system. The incidence of sedation and euphoria is similar to that observed after equianalgesic doses of morphine. Pethidine differs from morphine, however, in that with increasing doses signs of CNS excitation — tremors, muscle twitching and eventually convulsions — predominate over CNS depression. Norpethidine, a major metabolite of pethidine, may be the principal mediator of those CNS excitatory effects.

CNS toxicity is most likely to occur in patients taking pethidine for long periods, in patients with renal failure and where the oral route is used. This latter is due to the significant (50%) presystemic metabolism, which results in rapid accumulation of norpethidine. Toxic CNS symptoms should be treated by withdrawal of pethidine (substituting another analgesic if required), supporting respiration and controlling convulsions. It may take several days for normal neurological functions to return. It is important to realize that naloxone may exacerbate rather than antagonize the convulsions caused by toxic doses of pethidine.

Gastrointestinal tract. Pethidine causes less constipation than morphine, although the effect on gastric emptying and upper small intestine propulsive activity is similar. The incidence of nausea and vomiting is similar to that seen with morphine.

It has often been assumed that pethidine, perhaps due to its atropine-like activity, produces less biliary spasm than other opioids, and could therefore be safely used in patients with biliary colic or undergoing biliary surgery involving cholangiography. The weight of evidence suggests, however, that pethidine causes changes in biliary mechanics similar to that produced by other opioids.

Interaction with MAOI drugs. Pethidine should be avoided in patients taking monoamine oxidase inhibitory drugs, since the combination can cause serious adverse reactions (see Chapter 34).

Pharmacokinetics and metabolism. Absorption after intramuscular administration is almost complete with peak plasma levels within 5–15 min. The measured plasma terminal half-life of pethidine in many studies has averaged about 4 h. However, a study (Verbeeck et al 1981) in which blood sampling was continued for up to 24 h, instead of the more usual 6–8 h, found a terminal half-life of 6–8 h, a value more in keeping with pethidine's large volume of distribution of about $4 \, l \, kg^{-1}$. Plasma protein-binding is about 65%. Pethidine undergoes extensive hepatic metabolism by N-demethylation and hydrolysis. A number of metabolites have been identified, the most important being norpethidine, pethidinic acid and norpethidinic acid.

Norpethidine is the only metabolite found in the plasma, and is thought to be responsible for most of the excitatory effects of pethidine overdosage. Norpethidine's binding affinity for opioid receptors is similar to that of pethidine. It has a long plasma half-life in normal patients (14–21 h) and even longer in those with diminished renal function. This results in accumulation of norpethidine with prolonged use of the parent drug. Both pethidine and norpethidine readily cross the placental barrier and can accumulate in the fetus. Both compounds are weak bases (the pKa of pethidine is 8.5 and that of norpethidine higher) and ion-trapping in the fetal plasma occurs. The elimination of pethidine in neonates is also longer than in adults with half-lives prolonged up to 6 days.

The hepatic extraction ratio of pethidine is high so that significant amounts of an orally administred dose undergo hepatic 'first-pass' metabolism, and only about 60% of the dose reaches the systemic circulation. About 7% of an administered dose appears in the urine as unchanged drug. This proportion increases to 20% if the urine is made alkaline.

Related compounds. *Loperamide* is a piperidine derivative which is poorly absorbed from the gastro-intestinal tract. It inhibits peristalsis by an effect on the intestinal smooth muscle. This is partly due to an inter-action with opioid receptors and partly to a non-opioid cholinergic mechanism. It is effective in the control of diarrhoea and is available as capsules containing 2 mg loperamide hydrochloride (Imodium). The usual dose is 4–8 mg per day.

Diphenoxylate is another pethidine analogue which is used in the treatment of diarrhoea. It is insoluble in aqueous solutions and thus cannot be administered par-enterally. It is available as the commercial preparation Lomotil, as tablets containing diphenoxylate hydro-chloride 2.5 mg with 25 μg atropine sulphate. A liquid formulation contains the same quantities per 5 ml. Al-though safe in adults, caution should be observed with young children, in whom overdosage may result in symptoms of both opioid and atropine poisoning.

Piritramide

Piritramide was the first of the four aminopiperidine derivatives to be introduced into medical practice. It is an effective analgesic which has been mainly used for the treatment of postoperative pain. In adults 20 mg piritramide is equivalent to 15 mg morphine. It has a greater hypnotic effect than morphine and is more car-dio-depressant, but the incidence of other side-effects, particularly nausea and vomiting, is less. Piritramide is usually given intramuscularly when the maximum anal-gesia is reached within 5–15 min and lasts for 3–4 h.

Phenoperidine

Phenoperidine is an N-phenylpropyl derivative of norpethidine. It was introduced in 1957, 3 years before fentanyl, to which it is chemically closely related. The chemical structure of phenoperidine is shown in Figure 13.3. The use of phenoperidine has been almost totally restricted to use as a supplement to inhalational anaes-thesia (often in combination with droperidol) and in the management of patients requiring prolonged mechanical ventilation.

Potency. Phenoperidine is approximately 50 times as potent as pethidine. As a supplement during anaes-thesia the usual dose is 0.5–1 mg intravenously in spontaneously breathing patients, and up to 5 mg in those where IPPV is used. For postoperative pain relief 2 mg phenoperidine is equipotent with 10 mg mor-phine. Phenoperidine 2 mg will provide adequate analgesia for approximately 1 h.

Side-effects. Phenoperidine in the recommended doses has minimal effect on the cardiovascular system. Respiratory depression occurs as with all opioids.

Metabolism. About 50% of phenoperidine is ex-creted in the urine. The remainder undergoes hepatic biotransformation, with pethidine, norpethidine and pethidinic acid as the most important metabolites.

Fentanyl

Fentanyl is a phenylpiperidine of the 4-anilopiperidine series which is structurally related to, but not derived from, pethidine. Its chemical structure is shown in Fig-ure 13.3. Fentanyl is commercially available as the citrate salt in an aqueous solution containing 50 μg fen-tanyl base per ml. For many years after its introduction in 1959 the main use of fentanyl was as a component of neuroleptanalgesia in combination with droperidol. In recent years, however, it has become extremely popular as a supplement during balanced anaesthesia and as a total anaesthetic for cardiac surgery.

Potency. On a milligram basis fentanyl is between 60 and 80 times as potent as morphine. When the in-trinsic potencies of these two drugs at the opioid receptor are examined, however, morphine is only slightly less potent than fentanyl (Stahl et al 1977).

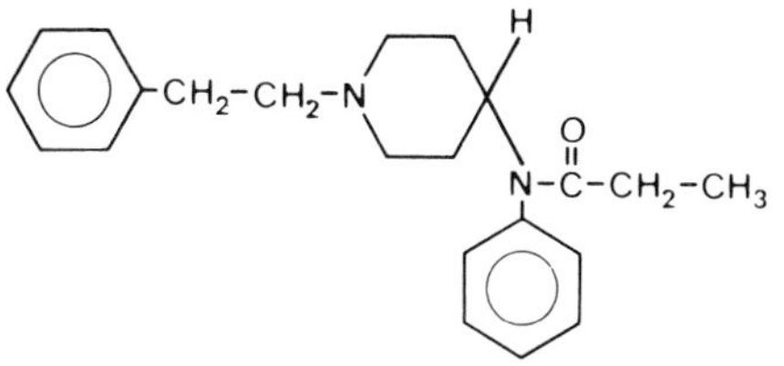

FENTANYL

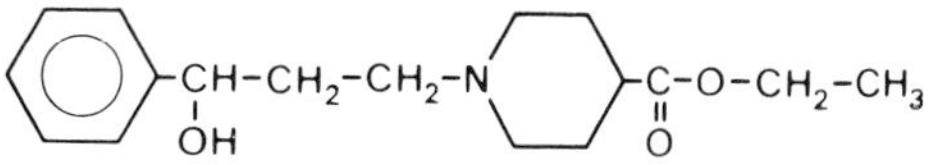

PHENOPERIDINE

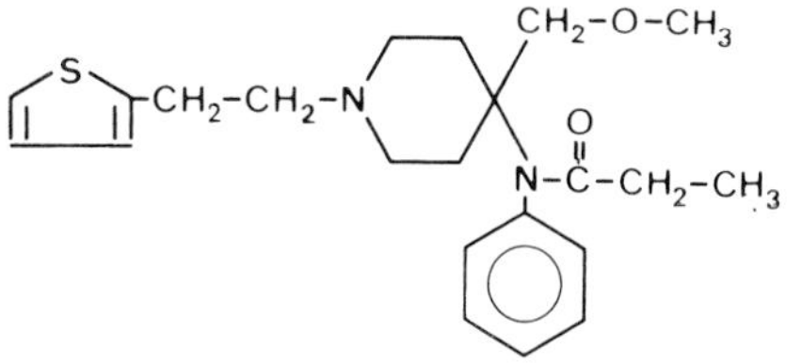

SUFENTANIL

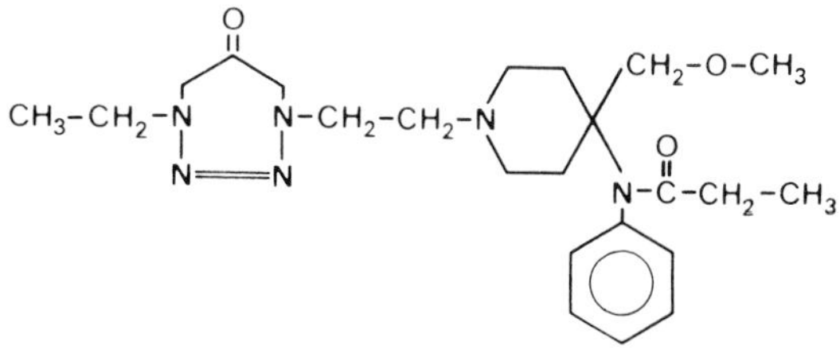

ALFENTANIL

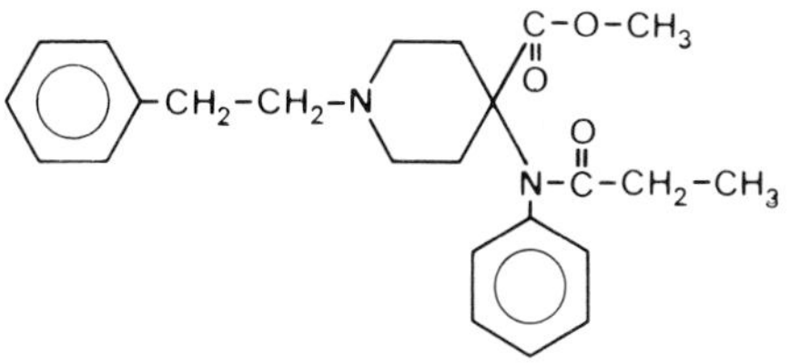

CARFENTANIL

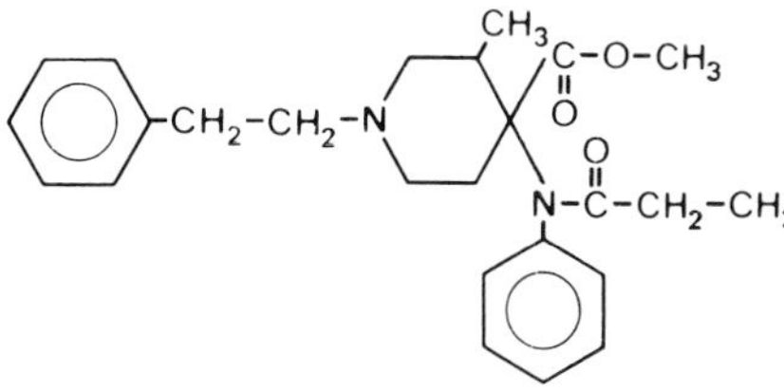

LOFENTANIL

Fig. 13.3 Chemical structure of fentanyl and allied drugs.

Respiratory system. Like all opioid agonists, fentanyl causes a dose-related depression of respiration. With small doses (2 $\mu g\ kg^{-1}$) respiratory rate decreases and there is a compensatory rise in tidal volume. With higher doses tidal volume also decreases, leading to irregular periodic respiration and finally apnoea. The central response to carbon dioxide is also affected, with the ventilation response curve shifted to the right. A plasma fentanyl concentration of about 3 $ng\ ml^{-1}$ causes a 50% depression of the CO_2 response curve, results in a resting $Paco_2$ of about 46 mmHg, and provides adequate analgesia in most patients.

Delayed respiratory depression in the postoperative period has been reported after small intravenous doses of fentanyl given during anaesthesia. This biphasic respiratory depression is probably related to secondary peaks in the plasma fentanyl concentration during the elimination phase. There is enterohepatic recirculation of fentanyl, with sequestration of fentanyl in the stomach and subsequent reabsorption from small intestine. This is unlikely, however, to account for the secondary peaks, since fentanyl undergoes almost complete presystemic metabolism and little or none of the absorbed drug would reach the systemic circulation. A more likely explanation is release of fentanyl from body stores, especially muscle, as a result of increased patient activity in the postoperative period.

Cardiovascular system. The effect of fentanyl on the cardiovascular system has been extensively investigated in isolated muscle preparations, isolated hearts and in intact animals. Many of the laboratory results are conflicting, due to differences in experimental design and species used, and it is difficult to assess their relevance for the clinical situation. The concentrations used were often at least 100 times those anticipated clinically.

Fentanyl appears to exert a protective effect on the heart during periods of ischaemia, by decreasing myocardial energy demand mainly as a result of its negative chronotropic effect. In doses up to 150 $\mu g\ kg^{-1}$ it is popular as an anaesthetic for patients undergoing cardiac surgery. Even with these high doses there is good cardiovascular stability.

Fentanyl, like all opioid agonists with the exception of pethidine, will induce bradycardia. This is more marked in the anaesthetised subject, although the severity is less when nitrous oxide is used. This may be due to the stimulating effect of nitrous oxide on the sympathetic system. Atropine is usually effective in treating fentanyl-induced bradycardia, although on occasion even doses of 2 mg are ineffective. Bradycardia can be especially severe in patients taking β adrenergic blocking agents. The severity of the bradycardia can be reduced by giving fentanyl slowly. The mechanism of fentanyl-induced bradycardia is incompletely understood, but is probably similar to that responsible for the phenomenon with morphine.

Fentanyl causes some peripheral vasodilatation but much less than is seen with morphine. This may partly be due to the absence of histamine release by fentanyl.

In patients with intracranial space-occupying lesions ventilated to normocapnia fentanyl reduces CSF and intracranial pressure. Cerebral perfusion pressure is only moderately decreased in the presence of hypocarbia but can become dangerously low in the presence of hypotension.

Muscle rigidity.   Muscle rigidity associated with the use of opioids is a particular problem with the more lipophilic drugs such as fentanyl. The phenomenon is characterized by increased muscle tone progressing to severe stiffness, particularly in the abdominal and thoracic muscles although limb muscles are also affected. Rigidity of the thoracic muscles, so-called 'wooden chest', can cause severe difficulties with ventilation in non-paralysed patients. The severity of rigidity is increased by rapid injection and by concomitant use of nitrous oxide. Fentanyl-induced muscle rigidity is not due to a direct action on muscle fibres since it can be blocked by neuromuscular blocking drugs, and is not associated with increases in creatinine phosphokinase. Opioids do not have significant effects on nerve conduction and cause only minimal depression of the monosynaptic spinal reflexes associated with muscle stretch receptors. The muscle rigidity is probably a manifestation of the catatonic state, a basic pharmacological property of all opioids, which may be related to enhancement of dopamine biosynthesis in the caudate nucleus.

Central nervous system.   Fentanyl produces less sedation than equianalgesic doses of morphine, although EEG changes can be observed with doses as low as 2 μg kg^{-1} in human volunteers. Nonetheless large doses of fentanyl will cause unconsciousness in ventilated subjects, and doses greater than 75 μg kg^{-1} are regularly used

to provide anaesthesia for cardiac surgery. With doses of this magnitude very striking EEG changes are produced, characterized by large increases in the amplitude of the very low frequencies in the delta band (0.5–3.5 Hz) and virtual disappearance of frequencies above about 6 Hz. In occasional patients isolated sharp waves can be seen in the EEG, although epileptic activity has never been proven to occur with the doses used clinically in humans. Convulsions are seen in dogs given extremely large doses (4 mg kg^{-1}) of fentanyl. This is some 20 times the highest dose given to humans.

Low doses of fentanyl, 5 μg kg^{-1}, are effective in blocking the hypertensive circulatory responses to endotracheal intubation. This may be simply an analgesic effect, but may also be due to a more specific blockade of afferent nerve impulses from the pharynx and larynx. There are high concentrations of opioid receptors in the solitary nucleus and the nuclei of the 9th and 10th cranial nerves. These nuclei are associated with visceral afferent fibres originating in the pharynx and larynx.

Fentanyl, when given into the epidural space, produces a more consistent and intensive analgesia than morphine. The incidence of side-effects is also less than with morphine or pethidine, although nausea, sedation and itching occur. When 100 μg fentanyl is given into the epidural space the duration of analgesia varies from 2–7 h. This short duration of action and the low incidence of side-effects is probably related to the high lipid-solubility of fentanyl, which results in rapid uptake by epidural blood vessels and nervous tissue.

Metabolic and endocrine effect.   Fentanyl 50 μg kg^{-1} as a supplement to nitrous oxide anaesthesia abolishes the hyperglycaemic response and reduces the cortisol and growth hormone responses to abdominal surgery. High-dose fentanyl (75 μg kg^{-1}) anaesthesia also prevents increases in catecholamines, non-esterified free fatty acids and vasopressin during the pre-bypass period of cardiac surgery, but not the response to bypass itself. The continued administration of fentanyl postoperatively fails to prevent postoperative endocrine and metabolic responses. The significance of these changes for the ultimate well-being of the patient remains to be determined.

Gastrointestinal tract.   Fentanyl in the low to moderate doses often used during balanced anaesthesia causes a varying incidence of nausea and vomiting. This is reduced if droperidol is given concurrently. These emetic effects have a central and peripheral mechanism. The central one is via stimulation of the chemoreceptor trigger zone located in the area postrema in the floor of the fourth ventricle in close proximity to the respiratory centre. Fentanyl, like other opioids, also reduces gastrointestinal motility. The volume but not the pH of gastric secretions is reduced by fentanyl. Larger doses of fentanyl have an anti-emetic effect thought to be due to central depression of the vomiting centre. Possibly for this reason emetic symptoms are uncommon in patients anaesthetized with high-dose fentanyl for cardiac surgery.

Fentanyl causes an increase in common bile duct pressure, due to both direct stimulation of biliary smooth muscle and spasm of the choledochoduodenal sphincter. This can be reversed by glucagon or naloxone but not by atropine. Tachyphylaxis to biliary pressure changes caused by fentanyl may occur.

Pharmacokinetics and metabolism. Fentanyl is a highly lipophilic substance which is rapidly distributed to the tissues after intravenous injection. Large amounts of an administered dose are distributed initially to tissues which are highly perfused such as muscle and lung. There is also rapid uptake into the brain. Fentanyl elimination is almost totally hepatic with only 4–7% of the drug excreted unchanged in the urine. The primary metabolic pathway in man is N-dealkylation, which converts fentanyl to norfentanyl. Several hydroxylation products can also be detected in the urine using gas chromatographic–mass spectrometric techniques. Inhibition of fentanyl metabolism by halothane and enflurane has been demonstrated in man.

The plasma terminal half-life of fentanyl is approximately 200 min, but this is prolonged in elderly patients, due to decreased clearance and in patients using cimetidine. Fentanyl is moderately bound to plasma protein (84%). The degree of binding is pH-sensitive and the free fraction decreases to 10% at a pH of 7.6. Thus changes in plasma pH caused by, e.g. hyperventilation could alter the pharmacodynamics of fentanyl.

Alfentanil

Alfentanil is a short-acting opioid chemically related to fentanyl. Its chemical structure is shown in Figure 13.3. Alfentanil is commercially available, as the hydrochloride, in a saline solution containing 500 μg base per ml. In animal studies it is between 30 and 70 times more potent than morphine. Acute toxicity studies in dogs have shown it to have a safety index intermediate between that of fentanyl and morphine. In animals and in humans it has a very rapid onset of action and has been used as an induction agent for general anaesthesia, as a supplement to balanced anaesthesia and in high doses as the sole anaesthetic for cardiac surgery.

Potency. Clinical experience suggests that alfentanil is one-third to one-fifth as potent as fentanyl.

Respiratory system. Like all opioids, alfentanil causes depression of respiration. In human volunteer studies using doses between 1.6 and 6.4 μg kg^{-1} alfentanil intravenously, Kay & Pleuvry (1980) found a dose- related shift to the right in the respiratory CO_2 response curve with maximum depression 3–5 min after injection. Respiratory depression with these doses lasted less than 30 min. With higher doses respiratory depression will of course last longer. As with fentanyl, there have been several occurrences of delayed, life threatening respiratory depression following the intraoperative use of alfentanil. In these cases alfentanil was given by continuous infusion during surgery. In addition to possible causes for delayed depression discussed above for fentanyl, it is likely that a contributing factor in the cases involving alfentanil was the administration by continuous intravenous infusion. When a drug is given in this way then the decline in plasma concentration when the infusion is stopped is less rapid than from a comparable concentration following a single bolus injection. This is because redistribution, the major cause of the initial decrease in concentration, following a prolonged infusion is less marked because the tissues are already partially saturated. Indeed if the infusion were to be continued until a true steady state was reached between plasma and all tissue compartments, then there would be no distribution phase and plasma concentration would decline only as a result of the much slower metabolic elimination of the drug. When administering alfentanil by infusion it is important, therefore, to terminate the infusion in good time before the end of surgery to allow for this effect.

Cardiovascular system. In ventilated dogs cardiovascular stability is well maintained with doses up to 5 mg kg^{-1}. There have been several reports of its use as the sole anaesthetic agent during cardiac surgery. A typical dose regimen for this application is induction of anaesthesia with alfentanil 125 μg kg^{-1} followed by a maintenance intravenous infusion at a rate between 4 and 8 μg kg^{-1} min^{-1}. Stable haemodynamics are obtained for both coronary artery and valve replacement surgery.

Pharmacokinetics and metabolism. The findings from animal experiments and initial clinical experience that alfentanil has a short duration of action has been confirmed by several kinetic studies (Bovill et al 1982b, Bower & Hull 1982). After bolus intravenous administration alfentanil is very rapidly distributed from the plasma to the tissues. The terminal half-life is about 1.5 h. The short half-life — the shortest of all the opioids — is the result of a low volume of distribution (approximately 0.9 l kg^{-1}) and a moderate plasma clearance. Alfentanil has a much lower lipid solubility than fentanyl or sufentanil but is highly protein-bound, mainly to the 'acute-phase' protein alpha$_1$-acid glyco-protein. Alfentanil differs from other opioids in having a pKa value below physiological pH (pKa = 6.8). Thus at a physiological pH of 7.4, 85% of alfentanil will be present in plasma in the unionized form, in comparison to fentanyl where only 9% is present in the unionized form. Since only the unionized form of a drug can readily cross cell membranes this may explain why, despite a low lipid solubility, alfentanil has such a rapid onset of effect. In humans, as in rats and dogs, alfentanil is metabolized very rapidly into a large number of metabolites. As with fentanyl, oxidative N-dealkylation at the piperidine nitrogen is the major metabolic pathway, to noralfentanil. Thirty-one per cent of a dose is excreted in the urine as noralfentanil. Oxidative O-demethylation accounts for only about 5% of the metabolism of alfentanil in humans, but is more important in dogs and rats.

Total hepatic clearance of alfentanil in humans is lower than with fentanyl or sufentanil, with a hepatic extraction ratio of approximately 0.5. The 'first-pass' effect will therefore be less important than with the other drug, and oral administration of alfentanil could result in analgesic plasma concentrations.

Sufentanil citrate

Sufentanil is a thienyl derivative of the 4-anilino-piperidine series chemically related to fentanyl. Its chemical structure is shown in Figure 13.3. In animal experiments it is very potent with an extremely high safety index. In the tail withdrawal reflex test in rats it is 4500 times as potent as morphine with an LD_{50}/ED_{50} ratio of 25 000 (morphine = 67 and fentanyl = 277).

Potency. Sufentanil is 5 to 10 times as potent as fentanyl in humans. It is currently available in ampoules containing either 5 μg or 50 μg sufentanil base per ml for intravenous administration.

Respiratory system. Similar degrees of respiratory depression occur clinically as with fentanyl or other opioids. One study, however, suggested that intraoperative sufentanil resulted in less profound respiratory depression and greater analgesia in the immediate postoperative period than fentanyl (Clark et al 1987). Like other opioids sufentanil can produce muscle rigidity which, by reducing chestwall compliance, can interfere with ventilation.

Cardiovascular system. In animals, sufentanil has minimal effects on myocardial function or haemodynamics. In humans, sufentanil in very high doses, up to 20 μg kg^{-1}, is used to provide anaesthesia for cardiac surgery with good haemodynamic stability (Sebel &

Bovill, 1987). High dose sufentanil anaesthesia is also effective for cardiac surgery in infants. In particular, the modification of the pathological stress responses to surgery is considered a significant advantage in neonates. Sufentanil is also popular in neuroanaesthesia, partly because of its favourable haemodynamic profile and the possibility that postoperative respiratory depression may be less than with fentanyl.

Central nervous system. At low doses sufentanil may produce more drowsiness than fentanyl. Higher doses produce surgical anaesthesia, with electroencephalographic changes similar to those seen with fentanyl and morphine, i.e. marked increase in slow-wave (delta) activity (Bovill et al 1982a). Recently, epidural sufentanil has been widely used for the treatment of postoperative pain. The onset of analgesia is rapid and lasts 4–6 h. Respiratory depression can occur within the first 30 min after epidural injection and may be related to systemic vascular uptake. Combination of sufentanil and low concentrations of bupivacaine (0.125% or 0.0625%) have proven valuable in obstetric analgesia.

Pharmacokinetics and metabolism. Sufentanil is extremely lipid-soluble with an octanol–water partition coefficient double that of fentanyl. It is also highly bound to plasma protein (93%), with the 'acute-phase' protein, alpha$_1$-acid glycoprotein, being an important binding component. Sufentanil is rapidly distributed after intravenous administration with a terminal half-life of 165 min (Bovill et al 1984). It is metabolized almost exclusively in the liver, principally by N-dealkylation. Oxidative O-demethylation is a minor metabolic pathway, but may be of clinical significance since its end-product, desmethyl sufentanil, is pharmacologically active with a potency about one-tenth that of sufentanil, i.e. equivalent to that of fentanyl. The hepatic intrinsic clearance is more than 4 times normal liver blood flow. This means that the 'first-pass' effect will be almost total, and that almost none of an oral dose of sufentanil would reach the systemic circulation.

Carfentanil citrate

Carfentanil is a novel ultra-potent member of the group of chemical compounds which include fentanyl. Its chemical structure is shown in Figure 13.3. Carfentanil has not been used in humans, but its extreme potency has led to its use as an immobilizer of wild animals. It is one of the most potent opioids in existence — about 32 times as potent as fentanyl or 18 000 times as potent as pethidine. A dose of less than 1 mg/ton is sufficient to immobilize a 6000 kg elephant (de Vos 1978). The potency of carfentanil has been emphasized by a recent report showing that surgical anaesthesia could be attained in dogs allowed to breathe nebulized carfentanil (Port et al 1983).

Lofentanil

Lofentanil is an ultra-potent opioid chemically similar to carfentanil, with a methyl group substituted in the 3-position of the piperidine ring. Its chemical structure is shown in Figure 13.3. Lofentanil is 10 000 times as potent as pethidine and is extremely long-acting. In rats the duration of action of lofentanil at two times its lowest analgesic dose is more than 10 h. Respiratory depression lasting longer than 48 h has been reported after a dose of 0.7 μg kg^{-1} in humans. This extremely long duration of action is probably related to long-lasting receptor occupancy. The half-life of dissociation of the lofentanil–opioid receptor complex in binding assays is 208 min at 37°C. This makes lofentanil a particularly valuable tool for in vitro studies of opioid receptors. Lofentanil has been used epidurally in patients but the initial experiences have been disappointing.

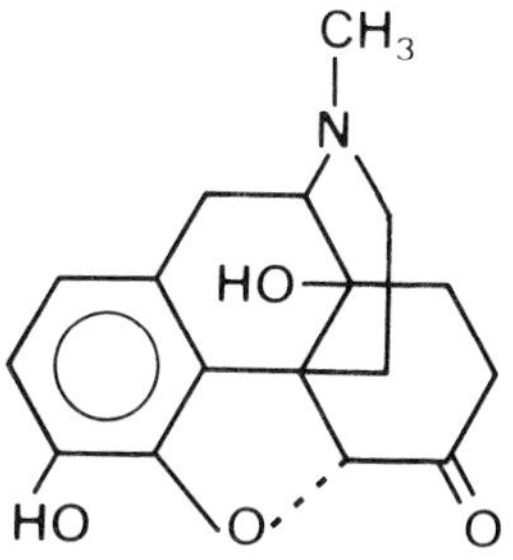

PURE ANTAGONISTS

Naloxone

Naloxone (Narcan) is the N-allyl derivative of oxymorphone (Fig. 13.4). In contrast to oxymorphone, which is a pure agonist, naloxone is a pure opioid antagonist. Naloxone, unlike the mixed agonist–antagonists nalorphine and levalorphan, is by itself virtually devoid of pharmacological activity in the intact animal. It will precipitate withdrawal symptoms in opioid addicts and has been used for the detection of addiction.

Naloxone is widely used to reverse the depressant effects of overdosage with opioid drugs. While there is no doubt that naloxone is the drug of choice in the emergency treatment of cases of overdose with morphine-like drugs, or where the diagnosis is in doubt, the author has grave doubts concerning the routine use of naloxone in the immediate postoperative period and prefers to use nalorphine. Bennett & Adams (1983) consider naloxone 'a wholly inappropriate drug to use postoperatively'. It must be remembered that naloxone will reverse not only the respiratory depression produced by intraoperative (or preoperative) opioids but also all other opioid effects including analgesia. There have been reports of intense pressor responses, tachycardia and severe pulmonary oedema occurring when naloxone has been used to reverse the effects of opioids. In one instance two patients died

OXYMORPHONE

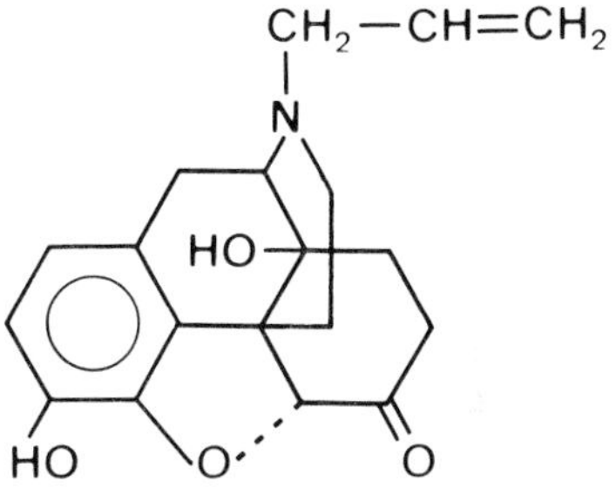

NALOXONE

Fig. 13.4 Chemical structure of oxymorphone, a μ-agonist and naloxone, the N-allyl derivative of oxymorphone. Naloxone is a pure μ-antagonist.

immediately after receiving naloxone (Andree 1980). These responses are probably due to release of catecholamines and sympathetic overactivity resulting from acute reversal of analgesia. Naloxone administered to subjects who have not been given opioids has no influence on blood pressure or plasma catecholamine levels. Another explanation for the pressor response after naloxone administration in patients given opioids may be alteration of baroreceptor reflexes so that an exaggerated haemodynamic response occurs to subsequent stimulation. Naloxone may also have an analeptic action unrelated to opioid receptor antagonism.

Recently attention has been given to the therapeutic use of naloxone in patients with hypovolaemic endotoxic shock. There is considerable animal evidence to support this therapeutic approach, which is thought to work by antagonizing the high-levels of circulating β-endorphin produced by endotoxins. The results of naloxone treatment of shock in patients remains controversial.

Dose. In reversing opioid-induced respiratory depression a dose of 0.2–0.4 mg is effective. However, it should be realized that the plasma half-life of naloxone (1.0–1.5 h) is considerably shorter than most opioids. An intravenous dose of naloxone 0.4 mg will antagonize the effects of morphine for only 30–45 min and one must therefore be prepared if necessary to give repeated doses or use a continuous intravenous infusion.

Naltrexone

Naltrexone is an analogue of naloxone created from oxymorphone by the substitution of a cyclopropylmethyl group on the nitrogen atom. It has similar pharmacological properties to naloxone but with a duration of action twice as long. It is used mainly in the management of addicts.

MIXED AGONIST-ANTAGONISTS

The history of the mixed agonist–antagonist drugs dates from 1914 when Pohl, in an attempt to improve the analgesic properties of codeine, synthesized N-allylcodeine, which he found could antagonise respiratory depression produced by morphine (Pohl 1915). This discovery remained almost unnoticed by the medical fraternity until Weijland and Erickson (1942) synthesized N-allylmorphine (nalorphine). Nalorphine is an example

of how minor structural changes to an existing opioid can give compounds with very different pharmacological properties. Morphine is the prototype μ-receptor agonist while nalorphine is a μ-receptor antagonist and a κ-receptor agonist. Alkylation of the piperidine nitrogen in an agonist molecule with a three-carbon side-chain, usually propyl, allyl or methylallyl, results in a compound with mixed agonist–antagonist activity. Changing the side-chain back to an amyl group restores agonist activity.

Nalorphine is equipotent with morphine as an analgesic and in causing respiratory depression. Unfortunately nalorphine's severe psychotomimetic activity, including unpleasant visual hallucinations, precludes its clinical use as an analgesic. Until the discovery of naloxone it was widely used for its antagonist properties in the treatment of opioid overdose. The recommended dose is 5–10 mg intravenously.

Levallorphan, the N-allyl derivative of levorphanol, is another mixed agonist–antagonist which has been used mainly for its antagonist properties. It produces fewer psychotomimetic side-effects, and possibly also less respiratory depression, than nalorphine. It was not as popular as nalorphine in Europe, although it had a longer duration of action and was also active orally. Levallorphan is five times as potent as nalorphine, the usual

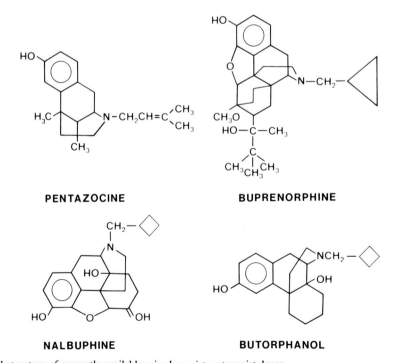

PENTAZOCINE

BUPRENORPHINE

NALBUPHINE

BUTORPHANOL

Fig. 13.5 Chemical structure of currently available mixed agonist–antagonist drugs.

dose being 1–2 mg. Levallorphan was also used in combination with pure opioid agonists, e.g. Pethilorfan, (pethidine 100 mg and levallorphan 1.25 mg). The rationale for the use of these mixtures was that such a combination would reduce the side-effects of the agonist drug, especially respiratory depression, without antagonizing the analgesia. They were particularly popular in obstetric practice, where it was claimed that the risk of neonatal depression was decreased while adequate maternal analgesia was maintained. However, accurate clinical investigation failed to corroborate these claims.

Pentazocine

Pentazocine, the N-dimethylallyl derivative of phenazocine (Fig. 13.5), was the first member of the mixed agonist–antagonist opioids to prove clinically successful. Its analgesic potency is approximately one-third to one-fifth that of morphine. Pentazocine is available for oral and parenteral administration. Peak blood concentrations after oral administration are reached by 1–3 h and between 15 and 45 min after intramuscular administration. Blood levels correlate well with analgesic effect.

Respiratory system. In equianalgesic doses pentazocine causes the same degree of respiratory depression as morphine. However, as with other drugs in this class both the response curves for respiratory depression and analgesia are plateau-shaped, with the plateau being reached at a dose of approximately 60 mg for the average adult. Pentazocine-induced respiratory depression can be reversed by naloxone, but not by other mixed agonist–antagonists such as nalorphine.

Pentazocine itself has been used at the end of anaesthesia to reverse the respiratory depression induced by fentanyl, so-called sequential anaesthesia. The philosophy of this technique was that the respiratory depression but not analgesia would be reversed. This is probably not so.

Cardiovascular system. Unlike morphine, pentazocine causes an increase in blood pressure, heart rate and plasma catecolamines. This is associated with increased systemic vascular resistance, pulmonary artery pressure and myocardial workload and decreased myocardial contractility. Pentazocine is contra-indicated in the treatment of patients with acute myocardial infarction.

Central nervous system. Psychotomimetic side-effects such as hallucinations, bizarre dreams and sensations of depersonalization occur in about 6–10% of patients. They are more common in elderly patients, in those who are ambulatory and when doses above 60 mg are given. Nausea occurs in approximately 5% of patients although vomiting is less common. Other

commonly reported side-effect are dizziness and drowsiness. Euphoria is less common than with pure agonist drugs, which may account in part for the lower risk of physical dependence and 'drug-seeking' behaviour. However, despite earlier suggestions to the contrary, repeated use of pentazocine will result in physical dependence. A popular form of abuse in the United States has been the combination of pentazocine and the anti-histamine pyribenzamine intravenously. Withdrawal symptoms in pentazocine addicts are usually milder than with morphine addicts. Where it is necessary that they should be alleviated, this should be done by a gradual reduction of pentazocine rather than substitution with another drug.

Pharmacokinetics and metabolism. Most of an administered dose of pentazocine undergoes hepatic biotransformation, mainly to glucuronide conjugates. There is considerable inter-individual variation in pentazocine metabolism, which may account for the variability of its analgesic response. There is a large hepatic 'first-pass' effect and less than 20% of an oral dose may reach the systemic circulation. Pentazocine is highly lipophilic with a brain/plasma ratio of 3.6 compared to 0.046 for morphine.

Butorphanol tartrate

Butorphanol is a fully synthetic morphinan dervative. Its chemical structure is shown in Figure 13.5. One milligram of tartrate salt is equivalent to 0.68 mg base. Butorphanol is a strong κ-receptor agonist and weak μ-receptor competitive antagonist. The relatively low incidence of psychotomimetic effects in humans compared to pentazocine suggests a lack of significant σ-receptor action.

Potency. Butorphanol is 3.5–5 times as potent an analgesic as morphine. The recommended doses are 1–4 mg intramuscularly every 3–4 h or 0.5–2 mg intravenously. The onset of analgesia occurs within 10 min after i.m. administration and peak analgesic activity is reached within 30–45 min. Given intravenously peak analgesia is reached in less than 30 min.

Respiratory system. Respiratory depression produced by butorphanol 2 mg i.v. is similar to that of 10 mg morphine. However, unlike morphine, a ceiling effect for respiratory depression is seen with increasing doses of butorphanol. Clinically, near-maximum depression occurs after 4 mg in normal adults. The respiratory depression is reversible by naloxone.

Cardiovascular system. In healthy volunteers, butorphanol 0.03–0.06 mg kg^{-1} produces no significant cardiovascular changes. However, in patients with cardiac disease progressive increases in cardiac index and pulmonary artery pressure occur. These changes are similar to those produced by pentazocine, and butorphanol is therefore best avoided in patients with recent myocardial infarction.

Central nervous system. Butorphanol produces more drowsiness than equianalgesic doses of pentazocine, a property which makes it useful as a premedicant. Other side-effects include dysphoria and hallucinations, although these are claimed to be less than with pentazocine. Butorphanol will antagonize the analgesia produced by pure agonist drugs, e.g. morphine, and will precipitate withdrawal symptoms in patients who are physically dependent an morphine-like drugs. As with all opioids there is risk of physical dependence developing with prolonged use, although the liability for abuse is less than with the pure agonists.

Pharmacokinetics and metabolism. Butorphanol is metabolized mainly in the liver to inactive metabolites, hydroxy and norbutorphanol, which are excreted principally in the urine, although some biliary excretion occurs. The terminal half-life is 2.5–3.5 h. Butorphanol crosses the placenta, and plasma levels in the neonate may exceed maternal levels.

Nalbuphine hydrochloride

Nalbuphine hydrochloride is structurally related to oxymorphone and naloxone (Fig. 13.5). Nalbuphine produces analgesia by a κ-receptor agonist interaction and has low μ-receptor intrinsic activity. It can, however, precipitate withdrawal signs in morphine-dependent monkeys. Acute toxicity in animals is low, even with high doses. One unusual side-effect that occurs in rats and dogs after chronic subcutaneous administration is reversible hair loss. This side-effect has not been reported in humans.

Potency. Nalbuphine is approximately equipotent with morphine. The onset of analgesia is within 2–3 min of intravenous administration and 15 min after intramuscular injection, and lasts 3–6 h with an adult dose of 10 mg.

Respiratory system. With equianalgesic doses, similar degrees of respiratory depression to that of morphine occur up to a dose of approximately 0.45 mg/kg. Beyond that dose a 'ceiling effect' is seen in the CO_2 response curve (Fig. 13.6). This 'ceiling effect' is paralleled by the dose–response curve for analgesia. Adequate postoperative ventilation is maintained after intraopera-

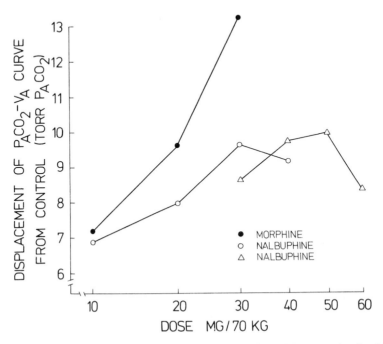

Fig. 13.6 Dose–effect curve for respiratory depression by cumulative doses of morphine (●) and nalbuphine (○) in eight subjects. Data of larger doses of nalbuphine (△) were obtained from an additional 10 subjects who did not receive morphine. Abcissa is log scale. (Reproduced with permission from Romagnoli and Keats 1980.)

tive doses up to 3 mg/kg. If respiratory depression occurs it can be reversed with naloxone.

Cardiovascular system. Intravenous nalbuphine causes minimal haemodynamic changes in patients with cardiac disease. In contrast to pentazocine and butorphanol, nalbuphine does not increase cardiac workload or pulmonary artery pressure, and is thus safe in the management of patients after acute myocardial infarction. Unlike morphine, nalbuphine does not cause histamine release.

Central nervous system. Sedation occurs in one-third of subjects given doses of 10–20 mg. The incidence of psychotominetic side-effects is lower than with pentazocine. A 5% incidence of dizziness and vertigo has been reported. Chronic administration can result in physical dependence which resembles that seen with pentazocine rather than morphine, although the abuse potential would seem to be low. Nalbuphine causes withdrawal symptoms in opioid-dependent subjects. Nalbuphine in doses of up to 0.2 mg/kg is an effective antagonist of opioid-induced respiratory depression (Jaffe et al 1988). Its use is sometimes associated with a number of side effects, including nausea, hypertension, tachycardia and confusion. Larger doses also tend to antagonize analgesia. However, by careful titration of small incremental doses, it is possible to achieve satisfactory reversal of respiratory depression without precipitating pain and haemodynamic side effects. Nalbuphine can in many situations be a good alternative to naloxone, not least because of its much longer duration of action.

Pharmacokinetics and metabolism. Nalbuphine is metabolized in the liver to inactive metabolites which are excreted mainly in the bile. About 7% of administered nalbuphine is excreted in the urine as unchanged drug or conjugates. The plasma terminal half-life is approximately 5 h in humans.

Buprenorphine

Buprenorphine is a semisynthetic derivative of thebaine, one of the most chemically reactive of the opium alkaloids. Its chemical structure is shown in Figure 13.5. Unlike other mixed agonist–antagonists buprenorphine has significant μ-receptor agonist activity, although its intrinsic activity is low. Buprenorphine binds to and dissociates from the μ-receptor very slowly, which may account for its low potential for physical abuse. This stable interaction with the μ-receptor is also likely to be the explanation for the difficulty with which naloxone will reverse the agonist effects of buprenorphine once these have

been established, although the agonist effects can be blocked by naloxone given prior to buprenorphine.

Potency. Buprenorphine is approximately 30 times as potent as morphine as an analgesic. A dose of 0.3 mg intramuscularly has a duration of analgesic action of 6–18 h. Buprenorphine is also effective sublingually, absorption from the buccal mucosa being rapid. The onset of action is rather slow (5–15 min) after both intramuscular and intravenous administration, possibly due to slow receptor association. However, this slow receptor dissociation also allows excellent analgesia with low plasma concentrations — $0.4–0.6$ ng ml^{-1} (Bullingham et al 1982).

Respiratory system. In animals there is a bell-shaped response curve for respiratory depression with buprenorphine, rather than the typical flattened dose-response curve of the partial antagonists. This is presumably due to increasing antagonist activity at higher doses. There is some evidence for a similar effect in humans, with the response curve peaking at doses between 0.3 and 0.6 mg intramuscularly. In one study large intravenous doses, up to 7 mg, given to patients after Caesarean section, did not produce respiratory depression (Budd 1981). However, buprenorphine may have a synergistic respiratory depressant effect with fentanyl and other opioids. When respiratory depression occurs, it is important to realize that no satisfactory antagonist exists: naloxone even with doses as large as 14–16 mg may only partially reverse this side-effect. Doxapram may in some situations prove a useful alternative.

Cardiovascular system. Buprenorphine has minimal effect an the cardiovascular system in normal patients and in those with cardiac disease, including recent myocardial infarction.

Central nervous system. Drowsiness and dizziness are the most common CNS side-effects, although they rarely constitute a major problem. In comparison with other opioids buprenorphine appears to have a very low abuse potential. This may be due to the lack of euphoria and the nature of the drug interaction with the opioid receptor. Symptoms after withdrawal of long-term opioid therapy are thought to be related to the rate of dissociation of drug from receptor and consequent loss of homeostatic control. Since buprenorphine dissociates very slowly from the receptor this allows for homeostatic adaptation when the drug is withdrawn. When addiction occurs withdrawal results in a slowly emerging abstinence syndrome with maximum symptoms occurring only several days after stopping the drug.

Pharmacokinetics and metabolism. Buprenorphine is almost completely metabolized by hepatic activity.

The hepatic extraction is close to unity, so that systemic availability after oral administration is low due to the large first-pass effect. Systemic availability when given intramuscularly is greater than 90% with peak plasma concentrations reached between 2 and 5 min. Within 10 min the concentration after intramuscular administration is the same as that achieved by giving the same dose intravenously. The terminal half-life is approximately 3 h. Because of slow receptor binding there is no direct relationship between plasma concentration and clinical effect. Buprenorphine is highly bound (96%) to plasma proteins.

MISCELLANEOUS DRUGS

Meptazinol

Meptazinol is a centrally acting analgesic first introduced into clinical trials in 1975. It is a hexahydroazepine derivative (Fig. 13.7) currently available only for parenteral use. Some of its pharmacological properties suggested that it belonged to the mixed agonist–antagonist group of opioids. Meptazinol-induced analgesia can be almost completely reversed by naloxone, although higher doses are needed than for pure opioid agonists. Meptazinol will also reverse the signs of acute morphine overdosage and precipitate withdrawal symptoms in morphine-dependent animals. However, in isolated tissue experiments using guinea-pig ileum, a tissue with a rich supply of opioid receptors, meptazinol behaved very differently from opioids. Opioids, whether pure agonist or mixed agonist–antagonists, produce a characteristic depression of the twitch response of the ileum to electrical stimulation, which is restored by adding naloxone to the bath. Low concentrations of meptazinol, in contrast, cause an increase in the electrically induced twitch and with higher concentrations the ileum goes into spasm which can only be relaxed by washing out the meptazinol or adding atropine (Bill et al 1983). This effect is probably due to inhibition of cholinesterase (Hetherington et al 1987). Experimental evidence in conscious animals has also shown

that a component of meptazinol's analgesic activity is mediated by an effect at central cholinergic synapses, a mode of action different from all other conventional analgesics (Green 1983). Unlike opioids, each of the isomers of meptazinol possesses equal analgesic potency (Bill et al 1983), although its cholinergic mediated analgesia is stereospecific.

Potency.   Meptazinol is rapidly absorbed following intramuscular administration, peak analgesic effect occurring within 15–30 min. It is approximately equipotent with pethidine.

Respiratory system.   Meptazinol in clinically effective analgesic doses appears to be almost devoid of respiratory side-effects. However, when given intraoperatively to patients anaesthetized with halothane, meptazinol produces a dose-related fall in respiratory rate and elevation in end-tidal CO_2 concentration, reversible with naloxone (Slattery et al 1982).

Cardiovascular system.   Meptazinol has minimal effect on haemodynamics after intramuscular administration. It may have mild positive inotropic activity and increases in blood pressure and heart rate lasting up to 20 min have been reported after meptazinol 1.6 mg kg^{-1} intravenously. Administration of meptazinol to animals with haemorrhagic shock causes rapid and sustained restoration of blood pressure (Chance et al 1981). This effect is similar to that produced by naloxone in the same animal model; and may be due to an antagonism of the cardiodepressant actions of endorphins released during shock.

Pharmacokinetics and metabolism.   Meptazinol is a basic lipophilic drug with a low (23%) protein binding over the therapeutic range of plasma concentrations (25–250 ng/ml). It is rapidly conjugated in the liver to the glucuronide, less than 5% of the unchanged drug being excreted in the urine. None of the metabolites has biological activity. The terminal half-life in adults is approximately 2 h. When meptazinol is given to women in labour, the neonatal/maternal plasma ratio is 0.6. The neonate eliminates the drug with a half-life of about 3 h. However, bilirubin and meptazinol share a common metabolic pathway, conjugation with glucuronic acid, and this pathway may be impaired in the neonate. In one double-blind study a higher incidence of jaundice was reported in neonates whose mother received meptazinol than in those in which pethidine was used (Birks & Nicholas 1982).

APPENDIX

Pharmacokinetic properties of some of the drugs discussed in this chapter.

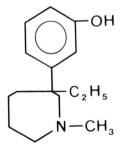

Fig. 13.7   Chemical structure of meptazinol.

Morphine

Salt	sulphate or hydrochloride
pKa	7.93/9.3; the morphine molecule has two sites of ionization — the phenolic group with a pKa of 9.36 and the tertiary nitrogen group with a pKa of 7.93; the latter is the only important one at physiological pH
Lipid solubility	very low
Protein binding	23–36%, mainly to albumin
Volume of distribution	3–5 l kg^{-1}
Clearance	12–15 ml kg^{-1} min^{-1}
Terminal half-life	3–4.5 h
Minimal effective blood level	40–80 ng ml^{-1}

References: Mazoit et al 1987

Codeine

pKa	8.1
Volume of distribution	3–6 l kg^{-1}
Clearance	0.6–0.75 ml kg^{-1} min^{-1}
Terminal half-life	2.5–3 h

References: Findlay et al 1978 Rogers et al 1982.

Methadone

Salt	hydrochloride
pKa	8.62
Lipid solubility	high
Protein binding	85%
Volume of distribution	6 l kg^{-1}
Clearance	2.7 ml kg^{-1} min^{-1}
Terminal half-life	35 h
Minimal effective blood level	30–40 ng ml^{-1}

References: Gourlay et al 1982.

Pethidine

pKa	8.5
Lipid solubility	moderate; the n-octanol water partition coefficient is 11.5
Protein binding	65–82%; alpha$_1$-acid glycoprotein is an important binding protein
Volume of distribution	2.8–4.2 l kg^{-1}
Clearance	10–17 ml kg^{-1} min^{-1}
Terminal half-life	3–4 h
Minimal effective blood level	0.4 μg ml^{-1}

References: Mather & Meffin 1978, Stambaugh et al 1976.

Fentanyl

Salt	citrate
pKa	8.43
Lipid solubility	very high; the n-octanol/water partition coefficient is 816
Protein binding	84%, of which 46% is bound to albumin, alpha$_1$-acid glycoprotein is also an important binding site
Volume of distribution	3.7 l kg^{-1}
Clearance	11–13 ml kg^{-1} min^{-1}
Terminal half-life	3–4 h
Minimal effective blood level	0.6–1 ng ml^{-1}

References: Bower & Hull 1982, McClain and Hug 1980, Meuldermans et al 1982

Alfentanil

Salt	hydrochloride
pKa	6.5
Lipid solubility	low; the n-octanol/water partition coefficient is 129
Protein binding	92%, mainly to alpha$_1$-acid glycoprotein
Volume of distribution	0.5–1 l kg^{-1}
Clearance	6 ml kg^{-1} min^{-1}
Terminal half life	$1\frac{1}{2}$ h
Minimal effective blood level	100–200 ng ml^{-1}

References: Bovill et al 1982b, Bower & Hull 1982; Meuldermans et al 1982.

Sufentanil

Salt	citrate
pKa	8.0
Lipid solubility	very high; the n-octanol/water partition coefficient is 1757

Protein binding	92.5%,
Volume of distribution	$1.7 \, \text{l kg}^{-1}$
Clearance	$12.7 \, \text{ml kg}^{-1} \, \text{min}^{-1}$
Terminal half-life	3 h
Minimal effective blood level	approximately $0.2 \, \text{ng ml}^{-1}$

References: Bovill et al 1984, Meuldermans et al 1982.

Pentazocine

Lipid solubility	high, brain/plasma ratio 3.57
Protein binding	50–75%
Elimination half-life	2–3 h

References: Ehrnebo et al 1974, Pittman & Portmann 1974.

Butorphanol

Salt	tartrate
Protein binding	80%
Volume of distribution	$5 \, \text{l kg}^{-1}$

Clearance	$3.8 \, \text{l kg}^{-1} \, \text{min}^{-1}$
Terminal half-life	2.7 h

References: Smith et al 1979.

Buprenorphine

Lipid solubility	high
Protein binding	96%
Volume of distribution	$1.5–2.8 \, \text{l kg}^{-1}$
Clearance	$13–19 \, \text{ml kg}^{-1} \, \text{min}^{-1}$
Terminal half-life	1.5–2.8 h
Minimal effective blood level	$0.4–6.6 \, \text{ng ml}^{-1}$

References: Bullingham et al 1980, 1982.

Naloxone

Lipid solubility	high
Volume of distribution	$1.81 \, \text{l kg}^{-1}$
Clearance	$14–30 \, \text{ml kg}^{-1} \text{min}^{-1}$
Terminal half-life	1–1.5 h

References: Fishman et al 1973, Ngai et al 1976.

REFERENCES

Ahmed M S, Zhou D H, Cavinato A G, Maulik D 1989 Opioid binding properties of the purified kappa receptor from human placenta. Life Sciences 44: 861–871

Althaus J S, DiFazio C A, Moscicki J C, von Voigtlander P F 1988 Enhancement of anesthetic effect of halothane by spiradoline. A selective κ-agonist. Anesthesia and Analgesia 67: 823–827

Andree R A 1980 Sudden death following naloxone administration. Anesthesia and Analgesia 59: 782–784

Ballantyne J C, Loach A B, Carr D B 1988 Itching after epidural and spinal opiates. Pain 33: 149–160

Bennett M R D, Adams A P 1983 Postoperative respiratory complications of opiates. In: Bullingham R E S (ed) Opiate analgesia. Clinics in anaesthesiology, vol 1. W B. Saunders, London, ch. 3, p 50

Bill D J, Hartley J E, Stephens R J, Thompson A M 1983 The antinociceptive effect of meptazinol depends on both opiate and cholinergic mechanisms. British Journal of Pharmacology 79: 191–199

Birks R J, Nicholas A D G 1982 Meptazinol in labour. A preliminary report. Anaesthesia 37: 373

Bloom F E, 1983 The endorphins: a growing family of pharmacologically pertinent peptides. Annual Review of Pharmacology and Toxicology 23: 151–170

Bovill J G, Sebel P S, Wauquier A, Rog P 1982a Electroencephalographic effects of sufentanil anaesthesia in man. British Journal of Anaesthesia 54: 45–52

Bovill J G, Sebel P S, Blackburn C L, Heykants J 1982b The pharmacokinetics of alfentanil (R 39209): a new opioid analgesic. Anesthesiology 57: 439–443

Bovill J G, Sebel P S, Blackburn C L et al 1984 The pharmacokinetics of sufentanil in surgical patients. Anesthesiology 61: 502–506

Bower S, Hull C J 1982 Comparative pharmacokinetics of fentanyl and alfentanil. British Journal of Anaesthesia 54: 871–877

Budd K 1981 High dose buprenorphine for postoperative analgesia. Anaesthesia 36: 900–903

Bullingham R E S, McQuay H J, Moore R A, Bennett M R D 1980 Buprenorphine kinetics. Clinical Pharmacology and Therapeutics 28: 667–672

Bullingham R E S, McQuay H J, Porter E J B et al 1982 Sublingual buprenorphine used postoperatively: ten hour plasma drug concentration analysis. British Journal of Clinical Pharmacology 12: 117–122

Chance E, Todd M H, Waterfall J F 1981 A comparison of the cardiovascular effects of meptazinol, morphine and naloxone in haemorrhagic shock in rats. British Journal of Pharmacology 74: 930

Chapman D B, Way E L 1980 Metal ion interactions with opiates. Annual Review of Pharmacology and Toxicology 20: 533–579

Cho T M, Hasegawa J I, Ge B L, Low H H 1986 Purification to apparent homogeneity of a mu-type opioid receptor from rat brain. Proceedings of the National Academy of Sciences, USA 83: 4138–4142

Clark N J, Meuleman T, Liu W-S, Zwanikken P, Pace N L, Stanley T H 1987 Comparison of sufentanil-N_2O and fentanyl-N_2O in patients without cardiac disease undergoing general surgery. Anesthesiology 66: 130–135

Collier H O J 1968 Supersensitivity and dependence. Nature 220: 228–231

Contreras P C, DiMaggio D A, O'Donoghue T L 1987 An

endogenous ligand for the sigma opioid binding site. Synapse 1: 57–61

Dehen H, Willer J C, Boureau F, Cambier J 1977 Congenital insensitivity to pain and endogenous morphine-like substances. Lancet 2: 293–294

Drew J H, Dripps R D, Comroe J H 1946 Clinical studies on morphine II. The effect of morphine upon the circulation of man and upon the circulatory and respiratory responses to tilting. Anesthesiology 7: 44–61

Ehrnebo M. Agwrell S, Boréus L O et al 1974 Pentazocine binding to blood cells and plasma protein. Clinical Pharmacology and Therapeutics 16: 424–429

Etches R C, Sandler A N, Daley M D 1989 Respiratory depression and spinal opioids. Canadian Journal of Anaesthesia 36: 165–185

Findlay J W A, Jones E C, Butz R F, Welch P M 1978 Plasma codeine and morphine concentrations after therapeutic oral doses of codeine-containing compounds. Clinical Pharmacology and Therapeutics 24: 60–68

Fishman J, Roffwarg H, Hellman L 1973 Disposition of naloxone-7,8-[^{3}H] in normal and narcotic dependent men. Journal of Pharmacology and Experimental Therapeutics 187: 575–580

Freye E, Hartung E, Schenk G K 1983 Bremazocine: an opiate that induces sedation and analgesia without respiratory depression. Anesthesia and Analgesia 62: 483–488

Gilbert P E, Martin W R 1976 The effects of morphine- and nalorphine-like drugs in the nondependent, morphine-dependent and cyclazocine-dependent chronic spinal dog. Journal of Pharmacology and Experimental Therapeutics 198: 66–82

Gioannini T L, Howard A D, Hiller J M, Simon E J 1985 Purification of an active opioid-binding protein from bovine striatum. Journal of Biochemical Chemistry 260: 15117–15121

Gourlay G K, Wilson P R, Glynn C J 1982 Pharmacodynamics and pharmacokinetics of methadone during the perioperative period. Anesthesiology 57: 458–467

Green D 1983 Current concepts concerning the mode of action of meptazinol as an analgesic. Postgraduate Medical Journal 59 (Suppl 1): 9–12

Han J S, Ding X Z, Fan S G 1985 Is cholecystokinin octapeptide (CCK-8) a candidate for endogenous antiopioid substrates? Neuropeptides 5: 399–402

Hetherington M S, Hughes I E, Lees A 1987 An investigation of the mechanism involved in the cholinergic actions of meptazinol. Journal of Pharmacy and Pharmacology 39: 185–189

Heyman J S, Vaught J L, Raffa R B, Porreca F 1988 Can supraspinal δ-opioid receptors mediate antinociception? Trends in Pharmacological Science 9: 134–138

Heyman J S, Vaught J L, Mosberg H I, Haaseth R C, Porreca F 1989 Modulation of μ-mediated antinociception by δ agonists in the mouse: Selective potentiation of morphine and normorphine by [D-Pen^2, D-Pen^5] enkephalin. European Journal of Pharmacology 165: 1–10

Hughes J, Smith T W, Kosterlitz H W et al 1975 Identification of two related pentapeptides from the brain with potent opiate agonist activity. Nature 258: 577–579

Jaffe R S, Moldenhauer C C, Hug C C jr, Finlayson D C, Tobia V, Kopel M E 1988 Nalbuphine antagonism of fentanyl-induced ventilatory depression: A randomized trial. Anesthesiology 68: 254–260

Jaffe J H 1985 Drug addiction and drug abuse. In: Gilman A G, Goodman L S, Rall T W, Murad F (eds). The pharmacological basis of therapeutics, 7th edition Macmillan, New York, pp 532–581

Kay B, Pleuvry B 1980 Human volunteer studies of alfentanil (R39209), a new short-acting narcotic analgesic. Anaesthesia 35: 952–956

Kromer W 1988 Endogenous and exogenous opioids in the control of gastrointestinal motility and secretion. Pharmacological Reviews 40: 121–162

Krug Z L, Pycock C J 1979 Neurotransmitters and drugs. Croom Helm Biology in Medicine Series. Croom Helm, London, ch 8, p 139

Ling G S F, MacLeod J M, Lee S, Lockhart S H, Pasternak G W 1984 Separation of morphine analgesia from physical dependence. Science 226: 462–464

Loh H H, Dwoskin L P, Zahniser N R 1988 Role of receptor regulation in opioid tolerance mechanisms. Synapse 2: 457–462

Lord J A H, Waterfield A A, Hughes J, Kosterlitz H W 1977 Endogenous opioid peptides: multiple agonists and receptors. Nature 267: 495–499

Lowenstein E, Hallowell P, Levine F N et al 1969 Cardiovascular response to large doses of intravenous morphine in man. New England Journal of Medicine 281: 1389–1393

Martin W R, Eades C G, Thompson J A, Hoppler R E, Gilbert P E 1976 The effects of morphine- and nalorphin-like drugs in the nondependent and morphine-dependent chronic spinal dog. Journal of Pharmacology and Experimental Therapeutics 197: 517–532

Mather L E, Meffin P J 1978 Clinical pharmacokinetics of pethidine. Clinical Pharmacokinetics 3: 352–368

Mazoit J-X, Sandouk P, Zetlaoui P, Scherrmann J-M 1987 Pharmacokinetics of unchanged morphine in normal and cirrhotic subjects. Anesthesia and Analgesia 66: 293–298

Meuldermans W E G, Hurkmans R M A, Heykants J J P 1982 Plasma protein binding and distribution of fentanyl, sufentanil, alfentanil and lofentanil in blood. Archives Internationales de Pharmacodynamie et de Thérapie 257: 4–19

McClain D A, Hug C C 1980 Intravenous fentanyl kinetics. Clinical Pharmacology and Therapeutics 28: 106–114

Napolitano L, Chernow B 1988 Endorphins in circulatory shock (editorial). Critical Care Medicine 16: 566–567

Ngai S H, Berkowitz B A, Yang J C et al 1976 Pharmacokinetics of naloxone in rats and in man. Anesthesiology 44: 398–401

Niemegeers C J E 1971 The apomorphine antagonism test in dogs. Pharmacology 6: 353–364

O'Neill M F, Dourish C T, Iversen S D 1989 Morphine-induced analgesia in the rat paw pressure test in blocked by CCK and enhanced by the CCK antagonist MK-329. Neuropharmacology 28: 243–247

Osborne R J, Joel S P, Slevin M P 1986 Morphine intoxication in renal failure: The role of morphine-6-glucuronide. British Medical Journal 292: 1548–1549

Pasternak G W 1988 Multiple morphine and enkephalin receptors and the relief of pain. Journal of the American Medical Association 259: 1362–1367

Pelligrino D A, Riegler F X, Albrecht R F 1989 Ventilatory effects of fourth cerebroventricular infusion of morphine-6-glucuronide in the awake dog. Anesthesiology 71: 936–940

Pittman K A, Portmann G A 1974 Pharmacokinetics of pentazocine in the rhesus monkey. Journal of Pharmaceutical Science 63: 84–88

Pohl J 1915 Uber das N-allylnorcodeine, einen Antagonisten des Morphins. Journal of Experimental Pathology and Therapeutics 17: 370–378

Port J D, Stanley T H, McJames S 1983 Topical narcotic anesthesia. Anesthesiology 59: A325

Portoghese P S 1965 A new concept of the mode of interaction of narcotic analgesics with receptors. Journal of Medicinal Chemistry 8: 609–616

Rogers J F, Findlay J W A, Hull J H et al 1982 Codeine disposition in smokers and non smokers. Clinical Pharmacology and Therapeutics 32: 218–227

Romagnoli A, Keats A S 1980 Ceiling effect for respiratory depression by nalbuphine. Clinical Pharmacology and Therapeutics 27: 478–485

Rothman R B, Bykov V, Long J B, Brady L S, Jacobson A E, Rice K C, Holaday J W 1989 Chronic administration of morphine and naltrexone up-regulate μ-opioid during binding sites labeled by [^{3}H] [D-Ala^2, MePhe^4, Gly-ol^5] enkephalin: Further evidence for two μ-binding sites. European Journal of Pharmacology 160: 71–82

Schultz R, Wuster M, Herz A 1981 Pharmacological characterisation of the epsilon receptor. Journal of Pharmacology and Experimental Therapeutics 216: 604–606

Sebel P S, Bovill J G 1987 Opioid analgesia in cardiac anesthesia. In: Kaplan J A (ed) Cardiac Anesthesia, 2nd ed, Grune & Stratton, Orlando, pp 67–123

Sibinga N E S, Goldstein A 1988 Opioid peptides and opioid receptors in cells of the immune system. Annual Review of Immunology 18: 219–249

Simonds W F 1988 The molecular basis of opioid receptor function. Endocrine Reviews 9: 200–212

Sjöström S, Hartvig P, Persson M D, Tamsen A 1987 Pharmacokinetics of epidural morphine and meperidine in humans. Anesthesiology 67: 877–888

Slattery P J, Harmer M, Rosen M, Vickers M D 1982 Naloxone reversal of meptazinol-induced respiratory depression. Anaesthesia 37: 1163–1166

Smith R D, Pittman K A, Gaver R C 1979 Human pharmacokinetics and metabolism of butorphanol. Clinical Pharmacology and Therapeutics 25: 250–257

Snyder S H 1977 Opiate receptors in the brain. New England Journal of Medicine 296: 266–271

Stahl K D, van Bever W, Janssen P, Simon E J 1977 Receptor affinity and pharmacological potency of a series of narcotic analgesics, anti-diarrheal and neuroleptic drugs. European Journal of Pharmacology 46: 199–205

Stambaugh J E, Wainer I W, Sanstead J K et al 1976 The clinical pharmacology of meperidine; comparison of routes of administration. Journal of Clinical Pharmacology 16: 245–256

Stanski D R, Greenblatt D J, Lowenstein E 1978 Kinetics of intravenous and intramuscular morphine. Clinical Pharmacology and Therapeutics 24: 52–59

Su T P, Weissman A D, Yeh S Y 1986 Endogenous ligands for sigma receptors in the brain ('sigmaphin'): Evidence from binding assays. Life Science 38: 2199–2210

Teschemacher H J, Schubert P, Herz A 1973 Autoradiographic studies concerning the supraspinal site of the antinociceptive action of morphine when inhibiting the hindleg flexor reflex in rabbits. Neuropharmacology 12: 123–131

Traynor J 1989 Subtypes of the κ-opioid receptor: Fact or fiction? Trends in Pharmacological Science 10: 52–53

Verbeeck R K, Branch R A, Wilkinson G R 1981 Meperidine disposition in man: influence of urinary pH and route of administration. Clinical Pharmacology and Therapeutics 30: 619–628

de Vos V 1978 Immobilization of free-ranging wild animals using a new drug. Veterinary Record 103: 64–68

Wang R I H, Robinson N 1981 Doxpicomine in postoperative pain. Clinical Pharmacology and Therapeutics 29: 771–775

Weijland J, Erickson A E 1942 N-allylnormorphine. Journal of the American Chemical Society 64: 869–870

Weissman A D, Su T-P, Hedreen J C, London E D 1988 Sigma receptors in post-mortem human brains. The Journal of Pharmacology and Experimental Therapeutics 247: 29–33

Yaksh T L 1987 Spinal opiates: A review of their effect on spinal function with emphasis on pain processing. Acta Anaesthesiologica Scandinavica 31 (Suppl 85): 25–37

Zagon I S, McLaughlin P J 1987 Endogenous opioid systems regulate cell proliferation in the developing rat brain. Brain Research 412: 68–72

Zagon I S, McLaughlin P J, 1986 Endogenous opioid systems, stress and cancer. In: Plotnikoff N P, Murgo A J, Faith R E, Good R A (eds) Enkephalins–Endorphins: Stress and the immune system. Plenum, New York, pp 81–100

Zukin R S and Zukin S R 1981 Multiple opiate receptors: emerging concepts. Life Science 29: 2681–2690

14. Non-steroidal anti-inflammatory analgesics

J. G. Bovill

This is a group of drugs which produce analgesia by a peripheral action, unlike the opioids which have a predominantly central action. The primary mechanism of action of these drugs is inhibition of prostaglandin synthesis, which also explains their anti-inflammatory and antipyretic properties. Although all produce analgesia, many have a high toxicity which restricts their routine use to the treatment of chronic inflammatory conditions such as rheumatoid arthritis. Structurally they form a heterogeneous group, although most can be broadly classified according to chemical class (Table 14.1).

Aspirin

Aspirin (acetylsalicylic acid) is a derivative of salicylic acid. The latter was first obtained from the glycoside salicin, the bitter principle of the willow bark, which was first introduced in 1875 as an antiseptic, antipyretic and antirheumatic. Acetylsalicylic acid was first synthesized in 1859 but was not used in medical practice until 1899. Although in the intervening years many other antipyretic/anti-inflammatory compounds have been produced, aspirin is still the most widely available

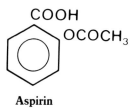

Aspirin

and most commonly used drug in this class, and remains the one against which all others are judged. It has been estimated that in the United States alone over 10 000 tons of the drug are consumed annually.

Unlike the opioids, which produce analgesia by a central mechanism, the analgesia produced by aspirin and similar drugs has been convincingly demonstrated to have a peripheral site of action. Topically applied aspirin suppresses the electrical activity recorded from stimulation of the dentine in cats' teeth, whereas application at sites proximal to the termination of the sensory fibres has no effect. Aspirin thus affects the site at which pain is generated, i.e. the sensory nerve terminals, by interfering with the metabolic activities involved. There is now overwhelming evidence that the analgesic and anti-inflammatory properties of aspirin and other non-steroidal anti-inflammatory drugs results from their inhibition of prostaglandin synthesis and release (Ferreira & Vane 1974). These drugs cause inhibition of the enzyme cyclo-oxygenase which converts arachidonic acid to the cyclic endoperoxides PGG_2, and PGH_2, critical prostaglandin precursors. Prostaglandins are synthesized in all mammalian cells (with the possible exception of the erythrocyte) and are released by a variety of inflammatory stimuli. Prostaglandin release occurs due to activation of phospholipase A, which converts membrane phospholipids to arachidonic acid which, when exposed to the enzyme cyclo-oxygenase, is rapidly converted to prostaglandin. Prostaglandins are not stored within cells and are rapidly removed if they reach

Table 14.1 Classification of non-steroidal anti-inflammatory analgesics according to chemical structure

Salicylate	Aspirin
Para-amino phenol	Paracetamol
Arylpropionic acids	Ibuprofen, Indoprofen, Naproxen
Indol-pyrrol acetic acids	Indomethacin, Zomepirac
Pyrazolon	Phenylbutazone
Phenylanthranilic acid	Mefenamic acid

the systemic circulation during passage through the lungs. Intramuscular injection of prostaglandin PGE_2, and PGF_2, given to pregnant women to induce abortion, caused intense local pain (Karim 1971). In contrast, however, low concentrations of prostaglandin PGE_1, similar to those present in inflammatory exudate, cause long-lasting hyperalgesia, i.e. a state where pain can be induced by mechanical or chemical stimuli which would normally be painless. Aspirin does not affect this hyperalgesia, suggesting that its activity is at the stage of prostaglandin synthesis and release. Therapeutic doses of aspirin and indomethacin induce almost maximum inhibition of prostaglandin turnover in females after 1 day of treatment (Hamberg 1972).

Since their first introduction to medicine the salicylates have been used in the treatment of conditions where pyrexia occurs. The causes of pyrexia are multifactorial, e.g. infection, tissue damage, etc. Temperature regulation, which requires a delicate balance between heat production and heat loss, is controlled by the hypothalamus, which sets the point at which body temperature is maintained. In fever this is adjusted upwards, possibly under the influence of substances released from the inflammatory process, including pyrogens and prostaglandins. Considerable rises in prostaglandin E_1 concentration in the brain and CSF occur during pyrexia. The antipyretic activity of aspirin-like drugs is therefore, in part, explainable by their influence on prostaglandin synthesis. Aspirin also prevents the release of endogenous pyrogens from white cells.

Aspirin has no effect on temperature regulation in normal doses in subjects with normal body temperature. However, toxic doses produce hyperpyrexia as a result of intracellular uncoupling of oxidative phosphorylation, which inhibits a number of ATP-dependent reactions. The increased energy released by this abnormal cellular respiration is dissipated as heat instead of being used to convert inorganic phosphate and ADP to ATP. There is a concomitant rise in oxygen consumption and carbon dioxide production. These effects can be measured with the large doses used in the treatment of rheumatoid arthritis.

Therapeutic uses. Aspirin is indicated for the relief of mild to moderate pain, particularly of inflammatory origin. It is also frequently used in the management of febrile states. The usual dose for mild pain is 300–600 mg orally. In the treatment of rheumatic diseases larger doses, 5–8 g daily, are often required.

Because of gastrointestinal irritation oral aspirin is seldom used for the early treatment of postoperative pain. A soluble salt, lysine acetylsalicylic acid (LAS), having similar pharmacological properties to aspirin, is available for parenteral administration. LAS, 1.8 g, intramuscularly or intravenously, has been reported to give analgesia similar to that with morphine 10 mg or oxycodone 6 mg after abdominal surgery (Kweekel-de Vries et al 1974). Other workers, however, have not found this compound valuable postoperatively (McAteer and Dundee 1981). The analgesia lasts for approximately 2 h and causes fewer side-effects than opioids.

Platelet function. As well as inhibiting prostaglandin synthesis at sites of inflammation and tissue damage, aspirin also exerts this effect in platelets by an irreversible inactivation of cyclo-oxygenase. Platelets occupy a primary role in haemostasis, maintaining vascular integrity and contributing to the complex process of coagulation. They have also been implicated in the promotion of arteriosclerotic lesions. Two substances play a major role in platelet function. Thromboxane A_2, a prostaglandin-like compound, is a potent stimulator of platelet aggregation and a powerful vasoconstrictor. Prostaglandin I_2, officially known as epoprostenol and also as prostacyclin, is generated in vessel walls and is the most potent inhibitor of platelet aggregation currently known. PGI_2 causes an increase in platelet cyclic AMP, which prevents them from aggregating but not from adhering to the endothelium, thus allowing minor endothelial injury healing. In health there is a balance between PGI and thromboxane A_2.

Aspirin inhibits production of both platelet thromboxane and vessel wall PGI_2. The predominant effect of aspirin therapy is, however, inhibition of platelet aggregation. Since platelets are unable to synthesise new proteins, and thus cannot regenerate cyclo-oxygenase, small doses of aspirin have effect on platelet function for 8–11 days — the life of a platelet. Eskimos, who have a diet rich in eicosapentanoic acid, a precursor of PGI_3 (which has properties similar to PGI_2), have low platelet aggregability and a very low incidence of heart disease.

Aspirin reduces the incidence of myocardial infarction and cardiac mortality in patients with unstable angina (Lewis et al 1983; Cairns et al 1985). These patients often have evidence of platelet activation with increased urinary prostanoid excretion (Hamm et al 1987). Aspirin, either alone or more commonly combined with dipyridamole is widely used to prevent graft occlusion after coronary artery surgery.

Gastrointestinal tract. Aspirin and the other nonsteroidal anti-inflammatory drugs, with the exception of paracetamol, cause gastric irritation, ulceration and haemorrhage. In patients who are regular users of aspirin the faecal blood loss can amount to 8 ml daily, and result in iron-deficiency anaemia. Occasionally massive haemorrhage occurs, requiring admission to hospital. The incidence of gastric irritation can be reduced by using buffered preparations of aspirin, and it has been suggested that the gastric side-effects are related to the pH of gastric juice. A link between aspirin-induced inhibition of prostaglandin synthesis and gastric irritation has also been proposed (Ferreira and Vane 1974). Reduction in prothrombin and fibrinogen levels caused by aspirin may also contribute to gastric bleeding.

Respiratory system. As mentioned above, aspirin causes uncoupling of oxidative phosphorylation, primarily in skeletal muscle. After full therapeutic doses this effect causes an increase in oxygen consumption and carbon dioxide production. The latter stimulates ventilation, essentially by increasing the depth of alveolar ventilation, and $PaCO_2$ does not change. Should other respiratory depressant drugs, e.g. opioids which lower the respiratory response to carbon dioxide, be given concomitantly, large increases in $PaCO_2$ can occur. With higher plasma concentrations, such as occur with overdose, salicylates directly stimulate the respiratory centre, resulting in marked hyperventilation with increases in both rate and depth. In humans these effects are seen with plasma salicylate concentrations over 350 μg ml^{-1}. The respiratory changes induced by aspirin are accompanied by changes in acid–base and electrolyte balance. Most commonly observed with full therapeutic doses is a compensated respiratory alkalosis. However, when toxic doses are ingested, particularly by infants and children, metabolic acidosis occurs, due to accumulation of acids caused by salicylic acid derivatives, circulatory collapse and renal impairment. Respiratory acidosis will also occur if plasma salicylate concentration become high enough to cause medullary depression of respiration. This stage of intoxication is accompanied by dehydration, hypernatraemia and hypokalaemia.

Cardiovascular system. Normal doses of aspirin have no significant effect on haemodynamics. Toxic doses cause circulatory and central vasomotor depression.

Aspirin intolerance. Aspirin is the non-steroidal anti-inflammatory analgesic most commonly involved in adverse hypersensitivity reactions. With the exception of indomethacin, cross-sensitivity to other drugs in this class is uncommon. Because these reactions have no proven immunological mechanism, the term 'aspirin intolerance' is used instead of the old term 'aspirin allergy'. Aspirin intolerance is strictly defined as the presence of acute urticaria, angioneurotic oedema, bronchospasm, severe rhinitis or shock occurring within 3 h of aspirin ingestion (Settipane 1981). The first case of aspirin intolerance, acute angioneurotic oedema, was reported in the literature only 3 years after the drug was introduced (Hirschberg 1902). In the normal population the incidence is between 0.3 and 0.9%, and in asthmatic

patients 4%. However patients suffering from chronic urticaria have an incidence of 23% (Settipane 1981). In this latter group intolerance is mostly manifested by urticarial-type reactions while in asthmatic patients bronchospastic symptoms predominate. These two types of manifestation seem to be mediated by different mechanisms. Aspirin inhibits PGE (a bronchodilator) more than PGF (a bronchconstrictor), disturbing the normal ratio of prostaglandins, and $PGF_{2\alpha}$ produces acute bronchospasm in patients with aspirin intolerance. Unfortunately there is no safe clinical test at present which can distinguish patients at risk from aspirin intolerance.

Pharmacokinetics and metabolism. Aspirin and other salicylates are rapidly absorbed from the stomach due to a low pKa value (3.5). The presence of food, by raising pH, will delay gastric absorption. Considerable absorption also occurs from the upper intestine and this site, because of its large absorbing surface, may be more important than the stomach. About one-third of an oral dose is hydrolysed to salicylic acid during absorption. The absorption half-life of orally ingested unbuffered aspirin is 30 min and somewhat shorter for buffered preparations. Peak plasma levels are reached within 2–3 h although appreciable concentrations are found within 30 min. Rectal absorption is slower and peak plasma concentrations reached are lower than with the same dose given orally, the relative bioavailability being 76% of the oral dose. Aspirin is rapidly hydrolysed in the plasma, liver and erythrocytes to salicylic acid. The latter is responsible for some, but not all, of the analgesic activity. Salicylic acid is too irritating to be used systemically. Salicylates undergo extensive biotransformation to glucuronides and conjugation, mainly in the liver, but also in many other tissues. Both the unchanged drug and its metabolites are excreted in the urine — in normal circumstances 10% appears as free salicylic acid and 75% as salicyluric acid. Excretion is facilitated by alkalinization of the urine, when up to 85% of the ingested drug is eliminated as salicylate. In acidic urine this proportion may be as low as 5%. Metabolism in normally very rapid and aspirin has a plasma half-life of only 2–3 h. However, liver enzymes that form salicyluric acid and phenolic glucuronide are easily saturated (Levy et al 1972) and after multiple doses the terminal half-life may increase to 10 h.

Paracetamol

Paracetamol (Acetaminophen) is the major active metabolite of phenacetin, an analgesic which has been withdrawn from the UK market because of renal toxicity. The structural formula of paracetamol is shown in

$$O = C - CH_3$$

$$NH$$

(benzene ring)

$$OH$$

Paracetamol

the diagram. Its analgesic and antipyretic effects are similar to those of aspirin, but is has negligible anti-inflammatory activity. Like aspirin it is a potent prostaglandin inhibitor.

Paracetamol is widely used in the treatment of mild to moderate pain, and is incorporated as an ingredient of many proprietary compounds together with aspirin, codeine or other mild analgesics. It is well absorbed from the gastrointestinal tract and does not cause the gastric irritation or blood loss seen with aspirin. Indeed, side-effects with paracetamol are uncommon with normal doses. Occasional haemolytic anaemia has been reported in patients with glucose-6-phosphate dehydrogenase deficiency in the erythrocytes.

In contrast to the lack of toxicity with therapeutic doses, overdosage with paracetamol is extremely dangerous and potentially fatal, due to liver damage. This hepatotoxicity is due to the N-hydroxyl metabolite, which binds covalently to essential macromolecules in hepatic cells, particularly those with sulphydryl (—SH) groups. With normal doses this toxic metabolite is excreted as the harmless conjugates of sulphur-containing amino acids such as glutathione or methionine. However, after ingestion of toxic doses this process becomes swamped, resulting in free metabolite in the plasma which causes cellular damage. Liver damage has been reported after a single dose of 5 g paracetamol, and deaths have occurred after 15 g (30 tablets). Since the hepatic damage is caused by a metabolite, signs of liver damage may not become apparent for many hours after an overdose has been taken. The treatment of paracetamol poisoning is dealt with in Chapter 35.

Dose. The adult dose of paracetamol is 0.5–1 g orally.

Ibuprofen

Ibuprofen is a propionic acid derivative with analgesic properties similar to aspirin. It is better tolerated than aspirin, mainly due to less severe gastrointestinal disturbances, which occur in about 10–15% of patients. Nevertheless it should not be used by patients with a history of peptic ulcers. Other reported side-effects have included skin rashes, thrombocytopenia, blurred vision and dizziness. There have been a few reported cases of toxic amblyopia, and any patient developing ocular symptoms should discontinue ibuprofen treatment immediately.

Ibuprofen is very highly bound (99%) to plasma albumin, but does not displace warfarin or oral hypoglycaemic drugs, probably because ibuprofen itself occupies only a small fraction of the available binding sites when given in conventional doses. It is rapidly absorbed after oral administration with peak analgesia being reached within 1–2 h. Absorption is more rapid when taken on an empty stomach. The usual dose for mild to moderate pain is 400 mg every 4–6 h. It is useful in the management of arthritic and musculoskeletal conditions.

Indoprofen

Indoprofen is an iso-indoline propionic acid derivative which is rapidly absorbed after oral administration. It is a weak acid so that most of the drug present in the blood is in the ionized form and little passes the blood–brain barrier.

Pharmacologically it is similar to ibuprofen and is an effective and relatively safe analgesic with fewer side-effects than aspirin. It has low antipyretic activity, possibly due to poor penetration of the CNS, but is anti-inflammatory and is useful in the symptomatic treatment of arthritic conditions. The dose is 50–200 mg every 4–6 h.

Naproxen

Naproxen is available both as the free acid and as the sodium salt, although therapeutically there is no distinction between them since naproxen has a pKa of 4.2 and is almost completely dissociated in blood. Absorption from the gastrointentinal tract is, however, more rapid with the sodium salt. Like other drugs in this class it is highly bound to albumin, and caution should be observed in patients simultaneously receiving anticoagulants or oral hypoglycaemic agents, although the risk of interaction is minimal. Naproxen can cause dyspeptic symptoms, although the incidence is less than with aspirin. It is indicated in the treatment of arthritic conditions, musculoskeletal disorders and dysmenorrhoea. Naproxen and other non-steroidal anti-inflammatory drugs suppress menstrual prostaglandin release. Inhibition of uterine prostaglandin synthesis reduces uterine contractility and improves uterine perfusion so that both spasmodic and ischaemic pain are relieved. The dose of naproxen is 500–1000 mg per day in divided doses. Naproxen has a terminal half-life of approximately 13 h so that in most patients twice-daily administration is satisfactory.

Indomethacin

Indomethacin is a methylated indole derivative with the chemical structure shown in the diagram. It is a potent anti-inflammatory drug but less effective as an analgesic for pain of non-inflammatory origin than aspirin. Like aspirin, its analgesic and anti-inflammatory properties are in the main due to inhibition of prostaglandin synthesis by inactivation of the enzyme cyclo-oxygenase. It is also an inhibitor of leucocyte motility.

Indomethacin is rapidly and almost completely absorbed from the gastrointestinal tract after oral administration. The recommended dosage is initially 25 mg three times daily, gradually increasing to about 100 mg per day. To diminish gastrointestinal disturbances it should be taken with food. It is also well absorbed from the rectum and a suppository containing 100 mg indomethacin is available. Due to the high incidence of side-effects indomethacin is not routinely used as an analgesic or antipyretic, and is reserved for the treatment of rheumatoid and osteoarthritis and ankylosing spondylitis. It is also useful in the management of acute attacks of gout, and can be of value in relieving the pain and inflammation of uveitis after ophthalmic surgery. Indomethacin in low doses is often combined with steroid therapy. Troublesome side-effects occur in approximately 30–35% of patients, and in 20% are severe enough to require reduction of dosage or complete withdrawal of the drug. The most common complaints are headache and gastrointestinal disturbances. The incidence of side-effects is dose-related.

Gastrointestinal tract, Dyspepsia, abdominal cramps, nausea and loss of appetite are common. Silent giant peptic ulcers similar to those seen during corticosteroid therapy can occur, and perforation and haemorrhage have been reported. Diarrhoea sometimes associated with bowel ulceration also occurs.

Central nervous system. Dizziness, vertigo and mental confusion, and blurred vision are frequent. More worrying is the occurrence of severe depressive symptoms and psychoses, which have led to suicide.

Cardiovascular system. Indomethacin causes salt and water retention and will inhibit the action of antihypertensive drugs. In particular indomethacin has been shown to antagonize the hypotensive effect of β-adrenergic blocking agents. The mechanism of this appears to be related to its effect on prostaglandin synthesis. Indomethacin also antagonizes the diuretic effect of frusemide, and this may contribute to fluid retention in patients treated with this diuretic. An interesting application of indomethacin has been in the treatment of cardiac failure in neonates caused by a patent ductus arteriosus (Heymann et al 1976). The rationale behind this application is the prostaglandin inhibitory activity of indomethacin. Prostaglandin E causes dilatation of the ductus arteriosus and inhibition by indomethacin may allow the ductus to close, thereby reducing the load on the heart.

Haematopoietic system. Evidence of marrow depression such as neutropenia, thrombocytopenia and occasionally aplastic anaemia has been reported. Indomethacin and other non-steroidal anti-inflammatory acidic drugs are highly bound to site 1 on serum albumin and, in vitro, can displace warfarin from this site. Although there is no evidence that these drugs interfere with the therapeutic effects of warfarin it is recommended that patients receiving anticoagulant therapy should be carefully monitored if indomethacin is added to their drug regimen.

Occular effect. Infrequently orbital and peri-orbital pain and blurred vision occur. Corneal deposits and retinal disturbances have been reported and patients on long-term indomethacin therapy should undergo routine ophthalmic examination.

Pharmacokinetics and metabolism. Indomethacin is rapidly absorbed and peak plasma concentrations are reached within 3 h. In patients taking probenecid concurrently with indomethacin, plasma levels of the latter will be higher than normal due to diminished renal excretion of unchanged drug. This may allow a lower dose of indomethacin to be used. Indomethacin undergoes hepatic biotransformation, the most important metabolites being ortho-demethylation products (50%) and glucuronic acid conjugates (10%). Between 10 and 20% of an oral dose is excreted in the urine. The metabolites are excreted mainly via the bile and urine, and enterohepatic recycling of the conjugates has been described (Duggan et al 1972).

Phenylbutazone

Phenylbutazone is a pyrazolon derivative with the chemical structure shown in the diagram. It is an effective anti-inflammatory analgesic which, because of its significant toxicity, is used only in the management of patients with arthritis and acute gout. It can be administered orally, rectally or intramuscularly. The recommended initial oral dose is 400–600 mg daily in divided doses with meals. This should be reduced to 200–300 mg daily for long-term use. A rectal dose of 250–500 mg daily will give the equivalent effect. Peak plasma levels are reached within 2–3 h by both routes. Injections should be given deeply intramuscularly to avoid deposition in fat. Because phenylbutazone becomes fixed to muscle, there is a considerable delay of 6–10 h in attaining peak plasma concentrations with this route. The intramuscular dose is 600 mg every 2–3 days.

Side-effects. These are similar to those described above for indomethacin. Sodium and water retention is more marked with phenylbutazone, and it is estimated that about 10% of patients taking this drug will develop oedema. Phenylbutazone is contra-indicated in a patients at risk of cardiac failure. Isolated occurrences of an 'acute pulmonary syndrome' – characterized by fever, dyspnoea and radiographic changes, have been reported.

Pharmacokinetics and metabolism. Phenylbutazone is rapidly absorbed after oral administration with a biological availability of about 90%. It is very highly bound to the same site on albumin as indomethacin and warfarin. Unlike indomethacin, phenylbutazone increases the hypoprothrombinaemic effect of warfarin, due to inhibition of warfarin metabolism rather than to displacement of warfarin from its protein-binding sites. Phenylbutazone can displace thyroid hormone from protein-binding sites and this may interfere with tests of thyroid function.

Phenylbutazone undergoes extensive hepatic metabolism, particularly by glucuronidation and hydroxylation. An important metabolite, oxyphenbutazone, has similar pharmacological properties to phenylbutazone and may contribute significantly to the parent drug's activity.

Oxyphenbutazone is also available as an independent drug. Metabolism of phenylbutazone is slow and the terminal half-life is extremely long — up to 100 h. Significant concentrations may persist in synovial fluid for up to 3 weeks after the drug is stopped.

Mefenamic acid

Mefenamic acid is an *N*-substituted derivative of phenylanthranilic acid. Its chemical structure is shown in the diagram. It has an analgesic spectrum similar to aspirin but although it is also anti-inflammatory it has mainly been used as an analgesic and antipyretic. The recommended dose is 250–500 mg orally, and it is best taken with food. It is well absorbed and peak plasma concentrations are reached by 2 h after ingestion.

Side effects. Gastrointestinal side-effects can occur in up to one-quarter of patients and include nausea, bleeding and ulceration. Diarrhoea may occur with ordinary doses and can be severe and associated with inflammation of the bowel. Other side-effects include skin rashes, temporary disturbances of hepatic and renal function and haematological problems such as agranulocytoses, pancytopenia, thrombocytopenic purpura and haemolytic anaemia of the autoimmune type. Blood studies should therefore be carried out in patients on long-term therapy.

Mefenamic acid and its metabolites in urine can give false positive results with certain tests for bile.

Diclofenac

Diclofenac is a derivative of phenylacetic acid, with anti-inflammatory and analgesic activity, and is a potent inhibitor of prostaglandin synthesis. Its anti-inflammatory activity is similar to indomethacin and greater than aspirin.

Analgesic activity. Several studies have shown that diclofenac given peri-operatively has a good analgesic activity. For example Hodsman and colleagues (1987) showed a reduction in morphine requirement of around 20 mg following abdominal surgery. Although it is a prostaglandin inhibitor, increase in β-endorphin levels in the hypothalamic region may contribute to its analgesic effect (Sacerdote et al 1985).

Gastrointestinal. With most anti-inflammatory drugs the ability to cause peptic ulceration is related to the degree of reduction in gastric prostaglandin. However, diclofenac is an exception in that it has a higher therapeutic ratio than most while having high potency for prostaglandin inhibition (Todd and Sorkin 1988). Nevertheless, gastric irritation and occult blood loss is a feature of diclofenac also.

Platelet function. There is inhibition of induced platelet aggregation, but little change in platelet count or in various indices of coagulation, although some studies have found slightly increased bleeding time following diclofenac.

Pharmacokinetics. Diclofenac administered orally is almost completely absorbed, with peak plasma concentrations reached in 10–30 min. These occur at 1.5–2.5 h with enteric-coated preparations, but these times may be greatly prolonged when there is food in the stomach.

The drug is subject to first-pass metabolism, about 60% reaching the systemic circulation unchanged. Diclofenac is highly protein-bound, 99.5% or over, binding mainly to two specific sites on serum albumin. These are a high-affinity site, which is probably the benzodiazepine site; and a low affinity site, probably the warfarin site (Chamouard et al 1985). It crosses the placenta.

Metabolism is mainly in the liver, and its metabolites have low or no activity. The elimination of the drug is rapid with a terminal half-life of around 1.1–1.8 h. Diclofenac is administered orally or intramuscularly in a dose of 75–150 mg.

Drug interactions. There are few. Despite high protein binding it does not appear to interact with oral anticoagulants or hypoglycaemics. It does reduce lithium clearance and has been found to increase digoxin concentrations.

MISCELLANEOUS DRUGS

Nefopam

Nefopam hydrochloride is a potent analgesic which cannot be classified as an opioid or a non-steroidal anti-inflammatory drug, since apart from its ability to relieve pain it shares no pharmacological properties with either group. Unlike aspirin it has no anti-inflammatory or anti-pyretic properties, and is not a CNS-depressant like the opioids. Chemically it is related to diphenhydramine. It blocks the re-uptake of noradrenaline and can produce atropine-like side-effects, e.g. dry mouth, blurred vision and tachycardia. It does not produce the gastrointestinal and other side-effects seen with aspirin, and has been successfully used to treat postoperative and musculoskeletal pain. It is available in tablet and injection form as Acupan, the usual dose being one or two tablets (20 mg) three times daily or 20 mg intramuscularly or intravenously repeated 6-hourly is necessary.

Carbamazepine

Carbamazepine (Tegretol) is chemically related to the tricyclic antidepressants. It is an anticonvulsant which is particularly indicated in the treatment of temporal lobe epilepsy. It has no analgesic properties but is included here because of its efficacy in controlling attacks of pain due to trigeminal neuralgia, for which it is the drug of choice.

However, only about 70% of patients achieve continuing relief with carbamazepine, and in up to 20% it must be discontinued because of adverse side-effects. Drowsiness, nausea and vomiting, and dyspepsia are common but may disappear on continued use. Skin rashes occur in about 3% of patients. More serious problems are blood dyscrasias, including aplastic anaemia, and renal and hepatic damage. Patients taking carbamazepine should have renal, hepatic and bone-marrow function regularly monitored. Cardiovascular effects also occur, e.g. hypertension and left ventricular failure, and carbamazepine should not be used in patients with atrioventricular conduction abnormalities because of depression of A-V conduction.

Carbamazepine is rapidly absorbed after oral administration. It induces hepatic enzymes so that the dose of concurrently administered drugs which undergo hepatic metabolism may have to be increased, e.g. anticoagulants. Enzyme induction also effects the metabolism of carbamazepine itself so that tolerance to the drug may occur due to altered pharmacokinetics. Carbamazepine reduces the activity of hormones contained in the combined oral contraceptive pill, and an oral contraceptive containing at least 50 μg oestrogen is recommended to avoid breakthrough bleeding. It should not be administered with, or within 2 weeks of cessation of monoamime oxidase inhibitor therapy. The dose required in controlling trigeminal neuralgia pain is very variable and a gradually increasing dosage is advised starting with 100–200 mg daily. Some patients may need up to 1600 mg per day to achieve effective control.

APPENDIX

Aspirin

pKa	3.5
Protein binding	80–90%, mainly albumin
Volume of distribution	0.15 l kg^{-1}
Terminal half-life	for aspirin itself only 15 min, but for salicylates 2–3 h; elimination is dose-dependent and with high doses the half-life of salicylates may exceed 15 h.
Minimal effective blood level	20 μg ml^{-1}

References: Davison 1971, Levy et al 1972.

Paracetamol

Protein binding	20–50%
Terminal half-life	1–4 h

Indomethacin

Protein binding	90%
Terminal half-life	2–3 h
Minimal effective blood level	0.5–1 μg kg^{-1}

Reference: Alvan et al 1975.

Phenylbutazone

pKa	4.5
Protein binding	98%
Terminal half-life	50–100 h

REFERENCES

Alvan G, Orme M, Bertilsson L, Ekstrand R, Palmer L 1975 Phamacokinetics of indomethacin. Clinical Pharmacology and Therapeutics 18: 364–373

Cairns J A, Gent M, Singer J, et al 1985 Aspirin, sulphin-pyrazone or both in unstable angina. New England Journal of Medicine 313: 1369–1375

Chamouard J-M, Barre J, Urien S, Houin G, Tillement J-P 1985 Diclofenac binding to albumin and lipoprotein in human serum. Biochemical Pharmocology 34: 1695–1700

Davison C 1971 Salicylate metabolism in man. Annals of the New York Academy of Sciences 179: 249–268

Duggan D E, Hogans A F, Kwam K C, McMahon F G 1972 The metabolism of indomethacin in man. Journal of Pharmacology and Experimental Therapeutics 201: 8–13

Dunn M J, Zambraski E J 1980 Renal effects of drugs that inhibit prostaglandin synthesis. Kidney International 18: 609–622

Ferreira S H, Vane J R 1974 New aspects of the mode of action of nonsteroid anti-inflammatory drugs. Annual Review of Pharmacology 14: 57–73

Hamberg M 1972 Inhibition of prostaglandin synthesis in man. Biochemical and Biophysical Research Communications 49: 720–726

Hamm C W, Lorenz R L, Bleifeld W, Kupper W, Wober W, Weber P C 1987 Biochemical evidence of platelet activation in patients with persistent unstable angina. Journal of the American College of Cardiology 10: 998–1004

Heymann M A, Rudolph A M, Silverman N H 1976 Closure of the ductus arteriosus in premature infants by inhibition of prostaglandin synthesis. New England Journal of Medicine 295: 530–533

Hirschberg S R 1902 Mitterlung über einen Fall von Nebenwirkung des Aspirin. Deutsche Medizinische Wochenschrift 28

Hodsman N B A, Burns J, Blyth A, Kenny G N C, McArdle C S, Rotman H 1987 The morphine sparing effects of diclofenac sodium following abdominal surgery. Anaesthesia 42: 1005–1007

Karim S M M 1971 Action of prostaglandin in the pregnant woman. Annals of the New York Academy of Sciences 180: 483–398

Kweekel-de Vries W J, Spierdijk J, Mattie H, Hermans J M H 1974 A new soluble acetysalicylic acid derivative in the treatment of postoperative pain. British Journal of Anaesthesia 46: 133–135

Levy G, Tsuchiya T, Amstel L P 1972 Limited capacity for salicyl phenolic glucuronide formation and its effect on the kinetics of salicylate elimination in man. Clinical Pharmacology and Therapeutics 13: 258–268

Lewis H D, Davis J W, Archibald D G et al 1983 Protective effects of aspirin against acute myocardial infarction and death in men with unstable angina. New England Journal of Medicine 309: 396–403

McAteer E, Dundee J W 1981 Injectable aspirin as a postoperative analgesic. British Journal of Anaesthesia 53: 1069–1071

Sacerdote P, Monza G, Mantegazza P, Panerai A E 1985 Dicofenac and pirprofen modify pituitary and hypothalamic beta-endorphin concentrations. Pharmacological Research Communications 17: 679–684

Settipane G A 1981 Adverse reactions to aspirin and related drugs. Archives of Internal Medicine 41: 328–332

Todd P A, Sorkin E M 1988 Diclofenac: a reappraisal of its pharmacodynamic and pharmacokinetic properties and therapeutic efficacy. Drugs 35: 244–285

15. Anti-emetics and antihistamines

J. W. Dundee

Anti-emetic drugs are used for the symptomatic control of nausea and vomiting, and it is desirable first to look at the causes of these and the occasions where such drugs might be used. It need hardly be mentioned that anti-emetics should be used only when the cause of vomiting cannot readily be removed. The problems of passive regurgitation in the patient with a full stomach will not be discussed here.

CLINICAL CAUSES OF NAUSEA, VOMITING AND RETCHING

1. Morphine, pethidine and similar drugs are among the most potent emetic compounds in clinical use, although there is a great individual variation in response to these. This is less important in the postoperative period and in patients suffering from pain, but does apply to their pre and intraoperative use and may extend into the postoperative period after short operations. Within certain limits the frequency and severity of emetic sequelae increase with dosage and there is some variation in the emetic potential of different potent analgesics. Unfortunately in some instances the emetic effect of the opioid outlasts its analgesic action. It is well established that movement increases the likelihood of the opioid causing sickness. Fortunately, for long-term use, some patients become tolerant to the emetic stimulant effects of the opioids.

2. Some inhalational anaesthetics are more prone to cause nausea and vomiting than others, e.g. ether, chloroform, cyclopropane and trichloroethylene, and this may be very prolonged with the latter. In contrast, halothane has a slight anti-emetic effect (Dundee et al 1965a).

3. Certain emesis-inducing metabolic disturbances or intoxications, e.g. hyperemesis gravidarum, radiation therapy, hyperglycaemia or hypoglycaemia, may be present in patients scheduled for operation.

4. Psychogenic stimuli, including fear and anxiety and offensive sights, smells or tastes, can induce sickness in the preoperative or postoperative period.

5. Patients with vestibular disturbances may be scheduled for operations, and here the tendency to sickness is great.

6. Vomiting can be caused by the peripheral reflex reaction to disease, inflammation, injury or irritation of various abdominal organs.

7. The local irritant effect of drugs on the gastrointestinal tract can cause vomiting, particularly in cases of poisoning, and under this cause one can include changes in intra-luminal pressure due to tumours, infection, ulcers, etc.

8. Drugs given in the routine preoperative preparation of the surgical patient may lead to vomiting, particularly in relative overdose (e.g. digitalis) and their importance as a differential diagnosis of unexplained vomiting must be remembered. This also applies to certain antibiotics.

9. Vomiting can be caused by a rise in intracranial pressure, and this is likely to occur in certain neurological conditions. The physical movement associated with the act of vomiting can upset the beneficial effects of some plastic operations. It can also lead to a loss of vitreous humour in ophthalmic operations and routine action to prevent it is essential in certain cases. Also important is the rise in cerebrospinal fluid pressure that accompanies vomiting, since this can accentuate an already raised intracranial tension to a dangerous degree, even leading to apnoea.

10. Other factors influencing the incidence of emetic symptoms:

a. Sex: women are more prone to nausea and vomiting than men, especially in the third and fourth weeks of the menstrual cycle.

b. Age: emesis decreases with age — children are more prone, and the elderly less prone, than adults.

c. Site of operation: intra-abdominal and intra-oral operations have a higher risk of emetic symptoms, and in minor gynaecological procedures, dilatation of the cervix markedly increases emetic sequelae (Morrison et al 1968).

d. Duration of anaesthesia: this is an important factor after both major and minor surgery, there being a consistent increase in the incidence of vomiting as duration of anaesthesia increases (Bodman et al 1960, Morrison et al 1968).

e. Gastric tubes: a number of workers have noted that decompression of the stomach by a gastric tube causes a substantial reduction in postoperative nausea and vomiting.

These factors must be considered when planning routines of anti-emetics, and because of the lack of standardization many published papers on this subject are worthless.

PHYSIOLOGY

The following descriptive definitions are taken from the reviews of Borison & Wang (1953), Borison and McCarthy (1983), Wang and Borison (1952) and Editorial (1987).

Vomiting

Vomiting, or emesis, is a primitive protective function in which substances detrimental to the well-being of the organism are actively evacuated from the gastrointestinal tract. However, in a variety of situations, such as in motion sickness, vomiting may play no useful purpose and in certain circumstances, e.g. hyperemesis gravidarum, it may be harmful to the body. It is usually accompanied by a rise in arterial blood pressure, intracranial pressure and intra-ocular pressure and, as mentioned above, these can be deleterious in certain conditions.

Nausea

Nausea, a purely subjective feeling, often precedes or accompanies vomiting and is frequently associated with hypersalivation, but both vomiting and nausea can occur independently.

Retching

Retching is the laboured rhythmic activity of the respiratory musculature which usually precedes or accompanies vomiting. Vomiting is neither synonymous with retching nor an invariable consequence of it.

The classical concept first postulated by Gianuzzi in 1865, and later confirmed by Thumas in 1891, is of a vomiting centre — a bilateral structure — deep in the medulla. The vomiting centre is anatomically located in the dorsal portion of the lateral reticular formation in the midst of other sites concerned with various motor activities which are affected during the act of vomiting. These include the centres for inspiration and expiration, salivation, vasomotor control, postural tone control as well as the vestibular nuclei. Their proximity explains many of the features of vomiting such as the typical posture, the excess salivation, breath-holding or deep breathing, the occurrence of bradycardia during retching or tachycardia during nausea and the tendency to cardiac arrhythmias.

More important is the functional nature of the vomiting centre in the integration of the act of vomiting and of stimuli from both central and peripheral receptor sites (Fig. 15.1). These may be from higher centres (including psychogenic stimuli), vestibular apparatus, the local irritant action of drugs on the gastrointestinal tract or from the chemoreceptor trigger zone (CTZ).

The CTZ lies superficially in the medulla on the floor of the fourth ventricle. In animals this is sensitive to certain emetic chemicals but not to electrical stimulation. In carefully designed studies, Wang & Borison (1952) demonstrated that apomorphine is a centrally acting emetic agent which has no peripheral activity (via the afferent nervous pathways from the gut), its site of action being on the CTZ and not the vomiting centre; this may apply to all the opioids. Experiments with copper sulphate emesis have shown that CTZ is not an integral part of the vomiting centre.

Although different stimuli appear to cause vomiting by different mechanisms, there is often a summation of effects, e.g. opiates (CTZ) are more likely to cause sickness in the ambulant patient (labyrinthine upset) and sickness is more likely to follow an emetic stimulus if the patient can see and hear another patient who is actually vomiting.

Because emesis involves activity at several discrete locations in the body, it is more difficult to ascribe anti-emetic activity of drugs to action at one particular type of receptor. In fact it has been suggested that three separate receptor types are involved (Peroutka & Snyder

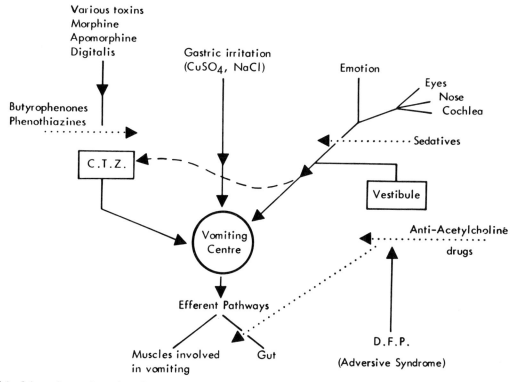

Fig. 15.1 Schematic representation of the vomiting mechanism, causes of vomiting and some therapeutic approaches to its control. Modified from Borison and Wang (1949), Wang and Borison (1950). CTZ: Chemoreceptor trigger zone; DFP: diflurophosphate.

1982). These are muscarinic cholinergic, histamine H_1 and dopamine D_2 (different from the vascular dopamine receptor). Dopamine D_2 receptors are found in high concentrations in the area postrema, which contains the chemoreceptor trigger zone. Histamine H_1 receptors are concentrated in the nucleus tractus solitarius, which processes sensory information relating to emesis, and in the dorsal motor nucleus of the vagus. This nucleus and the nucleus ambiguus also contain muscarinic cholinergic receptors, and these initiate the motor components of vomiting (Stefanini & Clement-Cormier 1981, Palacios et al 1981, Wamsley et al 1981). The relative potencies of some representative drugs are shown in Table 15.1. Thus a single drug will usually act mainly at one receptor type, but a suitably chosen combination of drugs might, by acting at several receptor types, be more effective than any of its constituents at their optimal dosage.

In addition to these receptors, it has been suggested that enkephalins are involved in some parts of this process. Harris (1982) hypothesizes that enkephalins, or

opioids, cause release of dopamine in the CTZ, with stimulation of dopaminergic receptors; and that cytotoxic drugs, by inhibiting the enzymes which break down enkephalins, may allow them to build up, thus causing nausea.

In contrast there may be an enkephalin-mediated anti-emetic 'tone'. The anti-emetic effect of opioid drugs is expressed at the vomiting centre, not the CTZ (Costello & Borison 1977), and is probably an effect on synaptic transmission here. Costello & Borison found in cats that systemic naloxone blocked the anti-emetic effects of opioids (at the emetic centre), but that higher naloxone levels achieved by intraventricular injection were needed to block emetic effects (at the CTZ). These differential sensitivities of the two regions might be explained by their containing μ and δ receptors respectively (Harris 1982).

Acupuncture, which is known to influence enkephalin concentrations has been shown to have an anti-emetic action (Dundee et al 1986, 1989c).

5-HT or serotonin may also be a possible neurotrans-

Table 15.1 Anti-emetic drug potencies at neurotransmitter receptor sites (modified with permission from Peroutka and Snyder 1982)

Drug group	Receptor type		
	Dopamine D_2	Muscarinic cholinergic	Histamine H_1
Anticholinergic			
Scopolamine	−	+ + + +	−
H_1 Antihistamine			
Diphenhydramine	−	+	+ +
Promethazine	+	+ +	+ + +
Neuroleptic			
Chlorpromazine	+ +	+	+ +
Metoclopramide	+	−	−
Droperidol	+ + +	−	−
Tricyclic			
Amitriptylene	+	+ +	+ + +

K_1 (nanomolar): + + + +, very high (<1); + + +, High (1–10); + +, moderate (10–100); +, low (100–1000); −, very low (>1000).

mitter involved in emesis, as antagonists to the 5-HT M (5-HT$_3$) receptor have be found to be effective in cisplatin-induced vomiting (Miner & Sanger 1986, Leading Article 1987). Metoclopramide in high doses may also act through this pathway rather than as a dopamine antagonist.

DRUGS

The drugs which are therapeutically useful for the control of vomiting and/or nausea can be grouped as follows:

1. parasympatholytic agents (belladonna alkaloids)
2. phenothiazines
3. butyrophenones
4. antihistamines
5. metoclopramide; domperidone
6. general sedatives and tranquillizers
7. Miscellaneous.

Parasympatholytic (vagolytic) drugs — the belladonna alkaloids

Hyoscine (scopolamine), atropine

The most common examples of the use of these are the preoperative use of atropine with pethidine and the time-honoured papaveretum–hyoscine (omnopon and scopolamine), the regular use of atropine with morphine dating back to 1907 (Stewart 1963). The general pharmacology of these is described Chapter 19, and only the data relevant to their anti-emetic action are described here.

Hyoscine is a well-proven remedy for motion sickness. It is given in the form of the hydrobromide (scopolamine), 1 mg of which contains 0.7 mg of laevo-hyoscine base. Initially doses in the region of 1 mg were recommended and these caused troublesome side-effects, but studies by Brand and Perry (1966) show that a good anti-emetic action can be obtained with doses as small as 0.1 mg of base. Commercially available seasickness tablets usually contain 0.3 mg and two are recommended as a single dose for protection for short journeys. Side-effects (drowsiness, blurred vision and dry mouth) preclude the long-term use of hyoscine for travel sickness. It is surprising that atropine does not appear to have been used for this purpose, since its lack of soporific action may offer advantages over hyoscine.

The ability of clinically used premedicant doses of atropine (0.6 mg) and hyoscine (0.4 mg) to suppress the emetic effects of 100 mg pethidine and 10 mg morphine is shown in Table 15.2. These studies were carried out in women having minor gynaecological operations with a standard anaesthetic. The emetic effects of intramuscular pethidine occurred mostly in the 90 min before operation and the incidence of vomiting, but not nausea, was significantly reduced by both atropine and hyoscine. If it were not for the widespread use of these antisialogogues it is doubtful if pethidine would be clinically acceptable as a premedicant. This does not apply to morphine, when most of the sickness occurs at a later period. Although both vagolytic agents give good protection in the early postoperative period, it is obvious that the emetic action of 10 mg morphine lasts longer than the anti-emetic action of either atropine or hyoscine. Table 15.2 shows that 0.4 mg hyoscine is a better

Table 15.2 Percentage incidence of vomiting (including retching) and nausea when pethidine 100 mg or morphine 10 mg was given as pre-anaesthetic medication, with or without an antisialogogue

	Opioid					
	Pethidine 100 mg			Morphine 10 mg		
Cholinergic drug	—	Atropine 0.6 mg	Hyoscine 0.4 mg	—	Atropine 0.6 mg	Hyoscine 0.4 mg
Preoperative 0–90 min						
Vomiting	12	3	4	3	2	1
Nausea	34	24	22	7	9	1
Pre- and postoperative						
Vomiting	34	30	20	45	35	28
Nausea	21	19	20	15	17	13
Nil	45	51	60	40	48	59

Figures are percentage incidence of emetic sequelae, and format of study is outlined in the text (Clarke et al 1965; Dundee et al 1964).

anti-emetic than 0.6 mg atropine, but neither has any notable effect on the incidence of nausea. Both of these drugs have very limited anti-emetic activity in tolerated doses and will have little beneficial effect on the sequelae following larger doses of opioids. A transdermal delivery system has been used to deliver hyoscine continuously for up to three days. The initial results from this approach are encouraging (Bailey et al 1990).

In a comprehensive evaluation of anti-motion sickness drugs Wood and Graybiel (1968) found best results when hyoscine was combined with dextroamphetamine. The summative effects of the two provided greater protection than any single drug, and although they are not combined in a commercially available preparation, the administration of a sympathomimetic and parasympatholytic drug may be beneficial in intractable travel sickness.

Muscarinic receptors occur centrally in the nucleus tractus solitarius and the nucleus ambiguus. Hyoscine, which penetrates the blood–brain barrier, may act here, and its action and that of atropine may also be in part attributable to their antimuscarinic (antispasmodic) action on the gastrointestinal tract. Salivary secretion is reduced, gastric secretion is reduced in volume and possibly in acidity, motor activity is reduced both as regards tone and frequency of contractions, and relaxation of sphincters is inhibited. Excessive motility and hypertonus induced by morphine are partly antagonized by atropine, which also antagonizes most of the stimulant effects of the opioid on the large intestine (Adler et al 1942, Atkinson et al 1943). Brand & Perry (1966) suggest that the anti-emetic action of hyoscine does not depend solely on peripheral anti-acetylcholine activity, but that its effect on the vestibular mechanism plays a major role in its efficacy in motion sickness.

Phenothiazines

The general pharmacology of these drugs appears in Chapter 12 and this section is limited to their anti-emetic action. As a generalization it seems that those with a piperazine amino propyl side chain (see below) are more effective as anti-emetics than those with dimethyl amino propyl side chains (such as chlorpromazine). Chemical structures are shown in Figure 15.2.

(a) Diethyl aminophenothiazines

Chlorpromazine

Chlorpromazine, then known as 4560 RP, was one of the first drugs to be used specifically for the symptomatic control of vomiting and nausea. In animal experiments it appeared to be particularly effective against drugs which act on the CTZ (Courvoisier et al 1953), while larger doses may also depress the vomiting centre (Glaviano & Wang 1954). Early clinical results supported these claims, and although chlorpromazine is now seldom used primarily as an anti-emetic, other phenothiazines are justifiably popular in this field.

Promethazine

Promethazine, one of the older phenothiazines, is available as the hydrochloride (Phenergan) or theoclate (Avomine). It is a long-acting antihistmaine with anti-emetic properties, which is used mainly for its antihistaminic and soporific action rather than primarily in the control of sickness. It may cause motor restlessness if taken alone, and the risk of postural hypotension which occurs with all the phenothiazines is always present. It is too soporific to recommend for ambulant

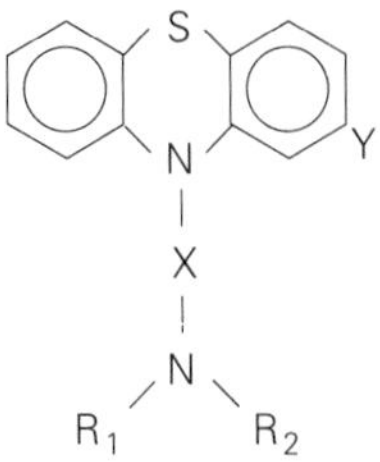

	Y	X	R₁	R₂
Chlorpromazine	Cl	$-(CH_2)_3-$	CH_3	CH_3
Promethazine	H	$-CH_2-CH^-$ CH_3	CH_3	CH_3
Fluphenazine	CF_3	$-(CH_2)_3-$	N N $-CH_2-CH_2-OH$	
Prochlorperazine	Cl	$-(CH_2)_3-$	N N $-CH_3$	
Perphenazine	Cl	$-(CH_2)_3-$	N N $-CH_2-CH_2-OH$	
Trifluperazine	CF_3	$-(CH_2)_3-$	N N $-CH_3$	

Fig. 15.2 Structures of phenothiazines.

patients. It is available as 10 and 25 mg tablets and in a 2.5% solution, and in some countries in suppositories containing 25 or 50 mg promethazine hydrochloride. Injections should be given deep intramuscularly rather than subcutaneously. Where a rapid effect is desired the drug can be given intravenously, preferably in a more dilute solution.

In their review of drugs used in motion sickness Brand & Perry (1966) noted that 25–35 mg doses of promethazine were not as effective as 50 mg cyclizine or meclozine. Neither drug is a particularly effective anti-emetic when given with an opioid prior to minor operations, even in doses of 50 mg. This may be due to early postoperative restlessness. Its antanalgesic action may adversely affect the course of anaesthesia, particularly with methohexitone (Dundee & Moore 1961, Moore & Dundee 1961).

Promethazine is used as a sedative and tranquilliser in obstetrics, and in these circumstances its anti-emetic action is more useful, particularly since it is usually given with pethidine. Here the antanalgesic action,

which applies to somatic pain, does not occur; rather there is an enhancement of the degree of patient relief.

Promethazine chlorotheophyllinate or theoclate (Avomine) has an action similar to the hydrochloride but may be less soporific. It is available only in 25 mg tablet form, and is recommended for travel sickness and hyperemesis gravidarum.

Therapeutic doses of both preparations of promethazine appear to be effective for about 4 h, but their soporific action may be more prolonged.

(b) Phenothiazines with a piperazine ring

Perphenazine

Perphenazine was at one time the most widely used antiemetic phenothiazine. Considering both efficacy and toxicity this popularity appears to be justified (Moore et al 1958, Dobkin 1959, Bellville et al 1960, Lind & Breivik 1970). Dundee et al (1975a) have studied the efficacy of 2.5 and 5.0 mg against the emetic action of

100 mg pethidine and 10 and 15 mg morphine (see Table 15.4) and found that perphenazine has a rapid onset of action, but its anti-emetic activity does not last as long as the emetic effect of morphine. The 5 mg dose may be needed to effectively control the emetic sequelae from morphine or pethidine, but the less toxic 2.5 mg dose has an appreciable anti-emetic activity. Oral doses of 2–4 mg are useful for prophylaxis in patients having radiation or chemotherapy, but they may have to be repeated in 4–6 h. It should not be forgotten that perphenazine is a potent tranquillizer, being useful in severe anxiety and tension states, particularly where agitation is present. It may also enhance the soporific action of opiates or other sedatives. When given alone the intramuscular injection of 5 mg perphenazine is accompanied by an unacceptably high incidence of restlessnes and dyskinesia, and Robbie (1959) has reported this complication following its repeated use. It can occur following 4 mg by mouth.

Prochlorperazine

Although less potent (w/w) than perphenazine, the anti-emetic and other effects of these two drugs are very similar but prochlorperazine has not been as widely studied as perphenazine and is promoted mainly for the treatment of vertigo due to Ménière's syndrome or other labyrinthine disturbances, and for the sickness which accompanies migraine. It appears to be particularly effective where an attack is accompanied by severe emotional upset. It can also be taken in low doses (about 15–20 mg daily) for the prevention of migraine. Like perphenazine it carries the risk of dyskinesia and oculogyric crises, but in 100 patients the author and colleagues (1965b) did not see dystonic reactions following the single intramuscular injection of 12.5 mg of the maleate (Stemetil), although they occurred in 2% of patients following 5 mg perphenazine and 3% of those having 2 mg trifluperazine.

Prochlorperazine may have a slightly less soporific action than the effective anti-emetic doses of other drugs in this group, but the difference is negligible. It is available in a 1.25% solution, in 5 and 25 mg tablets and in 5 mg suppositories as well as in a 3 mg buccal preparation. The latter two may be useful in patients having radiotherapy but as yet there is no controlled study on their efficacy in this field. In addition to the above, prochlorperazine is available in sustained-release capsules (as the maleate) containing 10 and 15 mg (Vertigon). Peikes (1957) found a bedtime dose to be effective in controlling nausea and vomiting of pregnancy. Its prolonged action has also been utilized in the control of seasickness (Wheeler et al 1959) and radiation sickness (Stoll 1962). No appreciable toxicity was reported in any of these studies.

Thiethylperazine

This is a good anti-emetic in doses of 10 mg. Like prochlorperazine it is claimed to be less soporific than equivalent doses of perphenazine, and while this concurs with clinical impressions it is by no means proven. Neither is there support for the claims of its greater anti-emetic activity because it acts on both the CTZ and the vomiting centre (Lovelace et al 1963). Its main clinical use is in the relief of vertigo associated with labyrinthine disturbances of surgery. It carries the same risk of extrapyramidal effects as related compounds. Thiethylperazine is available in tablets, ampoules and suppositories containing 10 mg of the maleate.

Trifluoperazine

The main use of this drug, which is a potent anti-emetic, is in psychiatric practice and anxiety states, possibly senile agitation and confusion. It appears to have all the advantages and disadvantages of the other related compounds. A sustained-release capsule — Stelazine spansule — consisting of a hard gelatine capsule with a clear, colourless, body and an opaque yellow cap containing an attractive mixture of blue and white spherical pellets, is available containing 2, 10 and 15 mg of the hydrochloride. This can cause severe and persistent extrapyramidal effects with repeated use and the long-acting preparation is not recommended as an anti-emetic.

Conclusion

There are four useful phenothiazine anti-emetics which vary only in their w/w potency. Their action is mainly on the CTZ and there they are most effective against opiate-induced emesis and least effective against opiate-induced emesis and least effective in the prevention of travel sickness. Each carries the risk of extrapyramidal side-effects, particularly after repeated use or when given in the absence of an opioid. Perphenazine is probably the most investigated of these, but the less soporific prochlorperazine or thiethylperazine may be preferred on occasions.

Butyrophenones

Droperidol

Droperidol is the most widely used member of this

group and its pharmacology has been discussed in Chapter 12. Although primarily used in neurolept anaesthesia or analgesia for its 'dissociative' action, it is a powerful anti-emetic in clinical doses (Janssen et al 1963, Patton et al 1974, Wheeler & Campman 1971). The work of Van den Driessché and Eben-Moussi (1971) suggests that its action is on the CTZ. Haloperidol has also been shown to have a powerful anti-emetic action (Stoll 1962) but is not principally used for this purpose.

The anti-emetic dose of droperidol has been taken as 2.5–10 mg for adults, given intravenously or intramuscularly. However, Morrison (1970) found a disturbing incidence of motor restlessness and anxiety when 5 or 10 mg were given alone, and its anti-emetic use in this way should be limited to patients who have been given opioids. It should be remembered that droperidol will enhance the soporific effects of these. Motor restlessness and drowsiness may last longer than its anti-emetic action. Both droperidol and haloperidol can cause oculogyric crises, and this precludes their repeated parenteral administration in anti-emetic doses. Unpublished reports suggest that standard doses of droperidol should not be combined with agonist — antagonist opioids.

Droperidol has more recently been found to be an effective anti-emetic given in 'ultra-low' dosage, 0.005 mg kg^{-1} (Rita et al 1981) or 0.25 mg as an adult dose (Shelley & Brown 1978). The ultra-low dose may actually be more effective than higher doses (O'Donovan & Shaw 1984), and avoids most of the adverse extrapyramidal effects and prolonged sedation associated with these.

Antihistamines

A number of seemingly chemically unrelated compounds — most of which contain an ethylamine chain — have been shown to possess useful anti-emetic properties. They appear to be most effective in suppression of motion sickness. This action which was first discovered in dimenhydrate (Dramamine) followed by diphenhydramine (Benadryl), is not a general property of antihistamines. Drugs active in this respect may also relieve the emetic complications of labyrinthine disturbances and are of value in controlling vomiting from other causes.

Although most antihistamines possess a local anaesthetic action their anti-emetic action is central in origin. Since motion sickness is more affected than apomorphine-induced, vomiting the action is not likely to be solely on the vomiting centre or CTZ (Brand & Perry

1966). Many of these compounds have a powerful soporific action which may play a minor role in their anti-emetic action, but which can be used with advantage in therapy. The antihistamines with proven anti-emetic activity fall into the following chemical groups:

Ethanolamines: Diphenhydramine hydrochloride
                 Dimenhydrinate theoclate
Piperazines: Cyclizine hydrochloride or lactate
                 Buclizine
                 Cinnarizine
Phenothiazines: Promethazine.

The latter has already been discussed under the phenothiazines.

Ethanolamines

Both diphenhydramine and dimenhydrinate are potent and effective antihistamines. In clinical doses they possess significant atropine-like activity and have a marked soporific effect, both of which may contribute to their anti-emetic action. Both drugs are relatively insoluble in water. Discussion is here limited to the latter preparation. Although its site of action is not fully understood it appears to have a primary inhibitory action on the overstimulated labyrinth and also to depress transmission of neural stimuli between the labyrinth and vomiting centre.

Dimenhydrinate

Chemical name: β-dimethyl amino ethyl benzohydrl
                 ether theoclate.

This was initially used in the control of vertigo associated with Ménière's disease and as a prophylaxis following surgery of the middle ear. It has also been recommended for controlling vertigo and sickness due to labyrinthitis, and has been given intravenously with most gratifying results to control the dizziness and sickness of acute migraine (Vaisberg 1954).

In two studies on postoperative vomiting Moore and his colleagues (1952, 1955) found that the parenteral administration of 50 mg was most effective in reducing sickness. They established the 'dramamine routine' of giving 50 mg intramuscularly as the patient left his or her room for the operation, 50 mg on return from surgery and the same dose at 4-hourly intervals for four doses. This results in a very drowsy patient, but no ill-effects are reported following these large doses. Kerman (1951) has used dimenhydrinate in the prevention and treatment of nausea and vomiting following electro-convulsant therapy.

Other reports on the efficacy of dimenhydrinate as an anti-emetic refer to its use in controlling the nausea and vomiting of early pregnancy. There is no evidence to suggest that it has any teratogenic effects. Radiation sickness is another field in which it has been proved useful.

Cyclizine

$$CH_3\ N \diagup\!\!\!\diagdown N\ CH(C_6H_5)_2\ H\ Cl$$

Chemical name: 1-methyl-4-α-phenyl-benzpiperazin hydrochloride.

Cyclizine is a competitive antihistamine which is primarily used for its anti-emetic rather than antihistamine effects. It is available in tablet form as the hydrochloride and in injectable form as the lactate. Cyclizine is well tolerated by both intramuscular and intravenous injection, and it may be diluted and given slowly by the latter route. It is rapidly absorbed from the gastrointestinal tract and its effects start within 15–30 min of administration, persisting for about 3–6 h. Kuntzman et al (1967) found that cyclizine is mainly demethylated to the corresponding 'nor' compound, although some is metabolized to the oxide.

It is justifiably popular as an anti-emetic for prevention and treatment of travel sickness (Chinn et al 1956) although there are no recent scientific data to confirm early reports on its efficacy. Many workers have studied the use of cyclizine — usually in 50 mg adult doses — in postoperative vomiting (Dent et al 1955, Moore et al. 1956, Davies & Gallagher 1957). In a comprehensive study Dundee et al (1975a, 1976) found that 50 mg reduced vomiting and nausea associated with morphine and pethidine premedication to approximately the same extent as 5 mg perphenazine. It was noticable that its efficacy against pethidine sickness was maximal in the first 90 min after administration, pointing to its short action.

As one of the most widely used anti-emetics there have been remarkably few side-effects reported following cyclizine in humans; the main one being drowsiness. When given simultaneously with an opioid it also enhances the soporific effect of both pethidine and morphine. This complication was not specifically commented on in studies in which the cyclizine was given

in the postoperative period. Drowsiness has been noted when cyclizine is given by mouth, and this is a major drawback to its use in seasickness. When taken concurrently with potent analgesics its soporific action becomes noticeable only when large doses of opioids are given. Its possible teratogenic effect will be discussed later, with that of meclozine.

Cyclizine also has an atropine-like action and produces dryness of the mouth in clinical doses. This may be troublesome if it is combined with large doses of opioids. Tachycardia may become a problem when it is given by rapid intravenous injection, when it also causes a slight rise in blood pressure. Although oculogyric crises have not been reported following cyclizine, patients may become restless and agitated after high or repeated doses.

Stoll (1957) has found the drug to be effective in controlling sickness for radiotherapy. Dundee & Jones (1968) combined a number of potent oral analgesics with 50 mg cyclizine and compared the incidence of nausea and vomiting following these with that after the opioid alone. Their study, carried out in ambulant patients suffering from intractable pain, showed a reduced incidence of vomiting with all analgesics, but cyclizine was less effective in suppressing nausea. This led to the formulation of Cyclimorph (morphine 10 and 15 mg with cyclizine 50 mg) and Diconal (dipipanone 10 mg with cyclizine 30 mg).

Meclozine

$$Cl\text{—}\bigcirc\text{—}CH\text{—}N\diagup\!\!\!\diagdown N\text{—}CH_3\text{—}\bigcirc\text{—}CH_3 \quad 2HCl$$

Chemical name: 1(4-Chloro phenylbenzyl)-4-(3-methylbenzyl) piperazine dihydrochloride.

This is an antihistamine with three bencyclic rings in addition to piperazine. It is available only in tablet form. In the USA, but not in Britain, these tablets are chewable, but this seems pointless with a drug which is poorly soluble in water but fairly soluble in dilute acid.

The early pharmacological studies of P'an et al (1954) showed that the onset of action of meclozine and of the related compound buclizine was relatively slow, and that its action was prolonged. Both compounds are potent antihistamines and are relatively non-toxic.

In their extensive evaluation of sea sickness remedies in 16 920 soldiers and airmen crossing the Atlantic, the US army, navy and air force motion sickness team found that 50 mg meclozine taken one to three times daily gave good protection, and was as effective as the same dosage of cyclizine (Chinn et al. 1956). In other studies, Wood & Graybiel (1968) found the best protection using dextro-amphetamine and hyoscine, but meclozine was reasonably effective, although probably not as good as cyclizine. The effectiveness of meclozine in treating vertigo of vestibular origin has also been demonstrated. Sickness following irradiation is another field in which meclozine has proved beneficial, but in the reported studies it was given in combination with pyridoxine (vitamin B_6).

In two reported studies of prophylaxis of postoperative nausea and vomiting, meclozine (25 mg) was given in combination with pyridoxine (50 mg) as preanaesthetic medication. In one of these, Bentley (1959) gave it before ocular surgery, while Albertson et al (1956) used it in unselected cases. Neither of these studies involved a number of anti-emetics, and although the therapy significantly reduced the incidence of sickness below the 'control level', one would have liked a more critical evaluation of the mixture.

Teratogenicity of cyclizine or meclozine. The suggestion that cyclizine may be teratogenic in humans came from the work of Tuchmann-Duplessis and Mercier-Parot (1963) in rats, mice and rabbits. Morphogenetic lesions were seen in groups receiving 50–75 mg, as compared with the recommended clinical dose of about 1 mg/kg three times daily. King (1963) and King et al (1965a,b) later made similar observations in the rat with meclozine.

An extensive survey of congenital abnormalities in children born in the Women's Hospital in Sydney between 1951 and 1962 was carried out by McBride (1963), one of the two people who first detected the teratogenic effect of thalidomide. In the latter years of his survey about 100 patients per month had been given cyclizine for morning sickness, yet this widespread use revealed no suggestion of a teratogenic action (Stalsberg 1965). The months of December 1962 and January 1963 saw 14 publications in the *British Medical Journal* or *Lancet* on fetal abnormalities, mostly associated with meclozine (Sadusk & Palmisano 1965). However, in a later survey Midwinter (1971) pointed out that five large epidemiological series, each with over 200 patients on meclozine or cyclizine, have shown that 'although it can-

not be ruled out, they can give a reasonable assurance that these drugs are not teratogenic'.

Buclizine

Chemical name: [1-(4 tert-butylbenzyl)-4-
                 (4-chloro-α-phenylbenzyl)
                 piperazine].

Buclizine is a long-acting antihistamine. When it was available on its own it was used mainly in the treatment of allergic conditions, vomiting of pregnancy and travel sickness. At present it is available only in combination with other drugs for the treatment of migraine.

Cinnarizine

Chemical name: (trans-1-cinnamy 1-4-(diphenyl
                 methyl) piperazine.

Cinnarizine is an antihistamine which is virtually insoluble in water. It is available in tablet form and although promoted for the control of labyrinthine disorders — including vertigo, tinnitus and the nausea and vomiting of Ménière's disease — there is good experimental and clinical evidence for its anti-emetic action. This applies particularly to its use in motion sickness.

Metoclopramide

Chemical name: *N*-(diethylaminoethyl)-2-methoxy-
                 4-amino-5 chlorbenzamide
                 monohydrochloride.

Chemically this is related to the procaine derivative, orthoclopramide. It is a white crystalline substance, freely soluble in water and stable in aqueous solution. Its pharmacology has been described fully by Robinson (1973). Among its actions in animals is its ability to inhibit emesis due to locally acting emetics such as copper sulphate and to apomorphine which acts on the CTZ (Justin-Besancon & Laville 1964). Metoclopramide has no antihistaminic effects, but has a moderately high potency at dopaminergic (D_1) receptor sites (Peroutka & Snyder 1982, Table 15.1).

Metoclopramide hastens emptying of the stomach and aids propulsion through the upper gastrointestinal tract (Margieson et al 1966), as well as abolishing irregular peristaltic activity (Johnson 1973). Thus it is not surprising that it has been used in radiology of the gastrointestinal tract (Kreel 1973), to aid emptying of the stomach prior to operation in obstetrical (Howard & Sharp 1973) and surgical emergencies (Howells et al 1971) and as an anti-emetic (Clark & Storr 1969, Tornetta 1969, McGarry 1971).

Metoclopramide in intramuscular doses of 10–20 mg is a poor sedative; in one study these doses caused restlessness in 12 and 26% of patients respectively (Dundee et al 1974). This complication occurs more frequently after its intravenous use in radiology; otherwise it appears to be a very safe drug in single doses but extrapyramidal symptoms, including oculogyric crises, have occurred after its prolonged use. The author has seen a 14-year-old patient who was admitted to hospital with suspected tetanus following the administration of 40 mg metoclopramide daily for 2 days. His symptoms, which included marked stiffness of the jaw, subsided almost immediately following the intravenous injection of 25 mg promethazine.

Despite its widespread popularity there is considerable doubt as to the anti-emetic efficacy of metoclopramide, particularly in relation to postoperative sickness. Handley (1967) and Lind & Breivik (1970) have shown the effectiveness of 10 and 20 mg doses when given at the end of minor gynaecological procedures, but Dundee & Clarke (1973) found that it did not significantly reduce the incidence of postoperative sickness below that which occurred in patients premedicated with 0.4 mg atropine. McGarry (1971) found the incidence of vomiting to be decreased in women in normal labour who had received 100 mg pethidine, while Dundee & Clarke (1973) and Assaf et al (1974) found it markedly reduced the incidence of sickness which follows 100 mg pethidine. In contrast, Ellis & Spence (1970) and Shah & Wilson (1972) failed to demonstrate any anti-emetic effect of either 10 or 20 mg metoclopramide in patients premedicated with either morphine or papaveretum. Its limited efficacy against morphine was confirmed by Assaf and his colleagues (1974), who have shown that this is due, at least in part, to its brevity of action (Table 15.3).

While metoclopramide (Maxolon) is actively promoted for its anti-emetic action in doses of 10 mg three times daily by mouth or by intramuscular injection, its limitations should be appreciated. It may be of value in nausea and vomiting due to gastrointestinal disorders but a longer-acting drug may be preferred in drug intolerance, malignant disease, or after radiation therapy. A single dose may be recommended postoperatively but if ineffective another anti-emetic should be used.

The other clinical use of metoclopramide is with cytotoxic drugs, and here best results were obtained with high doses (Gralla et al 1981). It was studies in this field which led to the postulation of an anti-$5HT_3$ action from high doses, and the ultimate study of more specific antagonists such as ondansetron.

Table 15.3 Percentage incidence of vomiting (V) and nausea (N) during the first 6 h after a minor gynaecological operation carried out in women under methohexitone–N_2O–O_2 anaesthesia

Metoclopramide		Morphine 10 mg			Pethidine 100 mg		
Preoperative	End of Operations	V	N	Nil	V	N	Nil
—	—	44	17	39	31	18	51
10 mg	—	12	25	63	10	21	69
20 mg	—	20	17	63	12	20	68
10 mg	10 mg	30	10	60	5	5	90
10 ng	20 mg	20	15	65	0	15	85

Patients were premedicated with 10 mg morphine or 100 mg pethidine and metoclopramide given as shown (Assaf et al. 1974).

The gastrointestinal actions of metoclopramide are antagonized by atropine.

Domperidone

Domperidone is a benzimidazole derivative, chemically unrelated to the phenothiazines or butyrophenones. Experimental work showed that it inhibited the CTZ and increased gastric emptying. An increase in the tone of the lower oesophageal sphincter may also contribute to its anti-emetic effect (Brock-Utne et al 1980). Clinically 4–10 mg has been shown to be more effective than placebo in treating postoperative vomiting (Fragen and Caldwell 1978). However the drug has a short duration of action (2–4 h), and Wilson and Dundee (1979) found that it was not effective as a prophylactic against pethidine- or morphine-induced emesis when given in a 10 or 15 mg dose with the opioid. Similar results have been reported by Waldmann et al (1985).

Sedatives and tranquillizers

As expected these drugs may reduce emetic symptoms when there is a large psychogenic element in their causation. They also reduce postoperative sickness by reducing the mobility of the patient, but adequate analgesia and avoidance of hypoxia are also essential to avoid restlessness. It is difficult to be sure whether some sedatives have a specific anti-emetic action, but this may apply to diazepam. In a series of patients given pethidine, or pethidine and diazepam, there was no obvious delay in recovery in the patients receiving pethidine and diazepam, yet the reduction in nausea and vomiting in the first 6 h after operation was highly significant compared with patients premedicated with pethidine alone.

Others

Pyridoxine — vitamin B6

This is included in several of the commercially available anti-emetics (Diggory & Tomkinson 1962). In two very early studies of a postoperative vomiting, Kernis & Stodsky (1950) and Hill (1951) failed to demonstrate any therapeutic benefit from doses of 100 mg given intravenously before and also 1 h after operation, and there has been no subsequent evidence to contradict this finding.

The earliest use of pyridoxine as an anti-emetic was in radiation sickness or pregnancy. Its efficacy in the latter is in doubt, but Contractor & Shane (1970) have produced evidence that a deficiency of this vitamin often occurs in pregnancy, even in the absence of vomiting. Correction of this would appear to be its main use. Its use in combination with meclozine has already been discussed.

Benzquinamide

This is a non-amine-depleting benzquinoline derivative, chemically unrelated to other anti-emetics. It is not available for clinical use in Europe, but has been introduced in North America. It is available in ampoules containing 25 mg/ml for intravenous or intramuscular administration. Absorption following both oral and rectal administration is rapid and reliable.

Initial reports of its anti-emetic activity are encouraging, and 50 mg benzquinamide has been found to be as effective as 10 mg perphenazine (Larrauri 1969) and more effective than 10 mg thiethylperazine (Lutz & Immich 1972) or 10 mg prochlorperazine (Klein et al 1970).

One promising aspect of this drug is its apparent lack of toxicity. No extrapyramidal side-effects have been reported, and in contrast to the phenothiazines it may have some pressor activity (Burstein 1963) and also has been shown to antagonise morphine-induced respiratory depression (Steen & Yates 1972, Mull & Smith 1974).

Betahistine hydrochloride

Chemical name: (2-2′-methyl-amino-ethyl-pyridine dihydrochloride.

This histamine analogue qualitatively resembles histamine in some of its actions, particularly on the microcirculation of the inner ear (Hicks et al 1967). Although classed among the antinauseant and anti-emetic drugs in some of the literature, it is used only for the treatment of Ménière's disease. Here is it useful for controlling vertigo and nausea (Elia 1970) and improving vestibular function (Wilmot 1971).

Stimulation of P6 Acupuncture Point

Over a period of 6 years researchers attached to the Belfast Medical School have investigated the anti-emetic effects of stimulation of the Neiguan point on the acupuncture (ACP) pericardial meridian (P6). (Dundee 1990, Dundee et al 1986, 1989a, 1989b, 1990: Ghaly et al 1987). As far as possible this 'complimentary' technique was studied with the same scientific approach (patient selection, elimination of variables, randomisation etc) as one would use in the investigation of a new drug. Premedication (nalbuphine 10 mg IM), anaesthesia (methohexitone-nitrous oxide-oxygen) and observations (double blind assessment) were standardised. On the basis of over 500 observations the following conclusions can be drawn.

1. When given with the premedication, 5 minutes of invasive ACP (manual rotation of needle or electrical stimulation 10 Hz DC) is a very effective anti-emetic, reducing the incidence of nausea and vomiting for up to 8 hours.
2. This action cannot be explained on a psychological basis
   (a) patients did not know what to expect from ACP
   (b) stimulation of a 'dummy' point near the elbow had no therapeutic effect.
3. Blocking the site of insertion of the ACP needle abolishes the anti-emetic action: infiltration with saline does not impair anti-emesis.
4. The anti-emetic action is mainly prophylactic. ACP given before the opioid is much more effective than when applied immediately before or during operation. (This applies to most orthodox anti-emetics).
5. Non-invasive stimulation of the P6 point, by pressure (sea bands) or transcutaneous electrical stimulation (via a conducing stud) is intially as effective as the use of invasive techniques, but the anti-emetic action does not last as long.
6. Under the conditions of these studies both invasive and non-invasive ACP were as effective anti-emetics as IM cyclizine 50 mg or metoclopramide 10 mg and lacked the toxicity of droperidol 2.5 mg.

These findings have been confirmed in general by Fry (1986), Barsoum et al (1990) and by Ho and colleagues (1990). As yet their role in anaesthesia is not clear, and it is possible that their main use may be in the field of cancer chemotherapy. Here their action is synergistic with that of standard anti-emetics (Dundee et al 1989c, Dundee and Yang, 1990).

Ondansetron

As described above and in chapter 5, there are several receptors for serotonin (5HT) — $5HT_1$ and subtypes, $5HT_2$ and $5HT_3$ which has subtypes in different species. Some of the anti-emetic effect of metoclopramide, at high doses, is due to $5HT_3$ antagonism, but at the expense of side-effects from profound antagonism of the dopamine D_2 receptors.

Ondansetron is a specific antagonist at the $5HT_3$ receptor. These receptors are situated in the visceral afferent vagus and/or the area postrema, as well as the gut (Blackwell and Harding 1989). Ondansetron has been shown to be effective in antagonising the nausea and vomiting associated with cytotoxic therapy and radiation (Tyers et al 1989), and is marketed for this purpose. It is ineffective against motion sickness (Stott et al 1989), and its action as an anti-emetic in other situations is under investigation at present.

Ondansetron is well absorbed after oral administration. After oral or intravenous use it is eliminated mainly by hepatic metabolism with a plasma half life of about 3.5 h; about 10% is excreted unchanged (Blackwell and Harding 1989).

The dosage usually recommended in cisplatin therapy is 8 mg IV followed by 1 mg h^{-1} infusion for 8–24 hours. Oral therapy may also be effective.

Side effects are few and generally mild.

Comparative studies of anti-emetics

Despite their widespread use there have been remarkably few comparative studies involving more than two or three anti-emetic drugs.

The largest reported long-term study has been carried out by the Belfast Department of Anaesthetics. The results are summarised in Table 15.4. Under the conditions of these studies 5 mg perphenazine or 50 mg cyclizine appear to be the most satisfactory anti-emetics.

Table 15.4 Percentage incidence of emetic sequelae found during the first 6 h after minor gynaecological operations in groups of not less than 100 patients receiving the premedicants, shown

	mg	Vomiting	Nausea	Nil	P
Saline		11	7	82	
Cyclizine	50	10	14	76	
Diazepam	10	16	9	75	
Metoclopramide	10	8	8	84	
Metoclopramide	20	6	8	86	
Trimethobenzamide	100	10	11	79	
Chlorpromazine	25	11	0	89	
Perphenazine	5	7	0	93	0.05
Prochlorperazine	12.5	9	3	88	
Promazine	100	9	9	82	
Thiethylperazine	10	9	9	82	
Trifluperazine	2	9	8	83	
Triflupromazine	20	11	3	86	
Morphine	10	44	17	39	
With atropine	0.6	35	17	48	
With hyoscine	0.4	28	13	59	0.05
With cyclizine	50	9	14	77	0.001
With metoclopramide	10	12	25	63	0.001
With metoclopramide	20	20	17	63	0.001
With perphenazine	5	16	4	80	0.01
With perphenazine	2.5	34	13	53	0.05
Pethidine	100	31	18	51	
With atropine	0.6	30	19	51	
With hyoscine	0.4	20	20	60	
With cyclizine	50	13	12	75	0.001
With diazepam	10	16	9	75	0.001
With metroclopramide	10	10	21	69	0.01
With metroclopramide	20	12	20	68	0.01
With trimethobenzamide	100	17	23	60	
With perphenazine	5	7	9	84	0.001
With perphenazine	2.5	8	11	81	0.001
With promaizne	25	22	30	48	
With promethazine	25	10	22	68	0.01
With promethazine	50	15	15	70	0.01
With promethazine	20	16	15	69	0.01
With thiethylperazine	10	12	13	75	0.001
With trifluperazine	10	21	10	69	0.01
Morphine	15	65	15	20	
With cyclizine	50	37	16	47	0.0005
With perphenazine	5	34	18	48	0.0005
With perphenazine	2.5	38	17	45	0.0005

P = significance of difference in incidence (combined vomiting and nausea) compared with control drug shown in italics in the same group.

Taking the risk of side-effects into consideration, cyclizine is preferred to perphenazine. Even including travel sickness these two drugs can probably meet the demands of all clinical situations, except gastrointestinal disturbances when metoclopramide may be more effective.

Other aspects

Route and details of administration.   Not all anti-emetics are available in forms suitable for oral, intramuscular and intravenous administration, and the form of pharmaceutic presentation may, on occasions, affect the choice of drug. There are two important aspects to be considered.

1. For patients already nauseated, or actually vomiting, a parenteral preparation is obviously desired. Quite a few anti-emetic drugs can be given intravenously but some of these, such as the phenothiazines, carry a distinct risk if injected too rapidly. Intramuscular injection should be deep into the buttock or outer aspect of the thigh, to ensure good absorption.
2. Oral preparations are desirable for long-term use, particularly when taken outside hospital, and are naturally the drugs of choice for motion sickness. It must be appreciated that many drugs can cumulate in the body with repeated administration, and side-effects occurring 4–5 days after starting treatment may not be readily associated with the anti-emetic.

For effective self-medication patients must be made aware that prophylaxis is often easier than cure, and that the appropriate drugs should be taken well in advance of the emetic stimulus. This applies not only to travel sickness, but to opioid administration, cancer therapy or radiotherapy. In these circumstances it should be appreciated that the duration of the emetic stimulus may outlast the effective period of action of the anti-emetic which should be repeated towards the end of the period of its excepted duration of action.

Nausea.   Generally speaking, it is easier to control vomiting than nausea, and in some circumstances these two manifestations of the problem may occur independently. Persistent nausea is very unpleasant, and is associated with dizziness, anorexia and listlessness and often with a 'drugged' feeling. Where possible bed rest may be the most appropriate therapy for this distressing symptom. Again prophylaxis may be easier than cure, and repeated doses of medication may be required.

Side-effects.   The relative merits of anti-emetic drugs cannot be divorced from their side-effects. If the patient is required to be mobile and ambulant (as in air crew or sea crew, or travellers suffering from motion sickness) a drug with a soporific action, or one which will produce postural hypotension, is unacceptable. In contrast some bedridden patients may benefit when sickness results from radiotherapy or chemotherapy. Patients quickly become tolerant to the soporific effect of anti-emetics and this is a not a problem in long-term therapy.

Akathisia (motor restlessness) and other extrapyramidal side-effects are undesirable and generally unacceptable complications of anti-emetic therapy. Akathisia, which literally means 'the inability to sit down', is aptly termed 'the jitters' by patients, who feel a compulsion to move about and may be very apprehensive. Drug-induced dystonic extrapyramidal side-effects may not occur until 6–24 h after administration, and the relationship of these to the anti-emetic may be missed (Ayd 1961, Dundee et al 1965b). Acute dystonia is characterized by painless spasmodic contractions of one or more muscle groups (Forrest 1974). Trismus, torticollis and opisthotonos indicate muscular spasms of the jaw, neck and spine respectively. The best-known dystonic condition is the oculogyric crisis, during which the eyes, after being fixed in a stare, later move to one side, while the head tilts uncomfortably and alarmingly backwards and towards the same side (Dundee et al 1975b).

Oculogyric crises or often severe dystonic reactions can be quickly controlled by the intravenous injection of 10–25 mg promethazine. Because of its anti-emetic properties this is preferred to anti-parkinsonism drugs such as benztropine (Cogentin), biperiden (Akineton) or procyclidine (Kemadrin). A similar dose of promethazine should be given subcutaneously or intramuscularly, since the extrapyramidal dyskinesia may last longer than the action of a single intravenous dose.

The oral administration of 50 mg diphenhydramine (Benadryl) also can be of benefit in preventing the recurrence of dyskinesia because of its prolonged action. The risk of extrapyramidal side-effects precludes the prophylactic use of 'depot' preparations of anti-emetics which can cause this side-effect (Ayd 1974).

Use in early pregnancy.   Since early morning sickness occurs in between 50 and 80% of pregnancies, mostly between the 6th and 14th weeks of gestation (Midwinter 1971) and about 40% of patients are still vomiting, albeit less persistently, at 14 weeks (Diggory & Tomkinson 1962), this aspect of the use of anti-emetics is very important.

The teratogenic effect of most anti-emetic drugs is not known, but by virtue of their long-term extensive use most are considered to be safe. In a large study of drug consumption in 458 mothers who gave birth to infants with congential abnormalities, out of a total of 1369 Nelson & Forfar (1971) found only 48 who had taken anti-emetics during the first trimester.

Where such data are available the teratogenic effects of anti-emetics have been discussed with the individual drugs. Woolham (1965) has given a most exhaustive list of drugs capable of producing embryopathy in laboratory animals. This writer states that 'the contemplation of this list [of over 100 drugs] makes one wonder whether there is any effective medicine which, if it were tested with sufficient thoroughness, would not appear on the list'. This is an extreme view which is shared to some extent by many subsequent workers. A leading article in the *British Medical Journal* (1964) says:

there may be a real danger that valuable drugs which are in reality innocuous to the fetus, but which have come into disrepute as a result of laboratory tests will be withdrawn . . . while other drugs of less therapeutic value and more danger to the fetus remain available, because they have passed less rigorous tests or because they have yet to be tested.

The compromise view of Wade & Dundee (1969) is probably good advice:

It is now considered undesirable to give any drug during the first trimester of pregnancy for fear of causing fetal abnormality, but occasionally a pregnant woman is so nauseated and anorexic that it is considered justifiable to use anti-emetics such as cyclizine, meclozine or promethazine.

This supported by the view of an obstetrician. In her review of 'Vomiting in pregnancy', Midwinter (1971) lists the available anti-emetics and comments, 'All these have been used widely for many years in early pregnancy in large series of patients . . . suggesting with reasonable assurance that they are not teratogenic.'

Choice of anti-emetic

It is obvious that there is a large number of safe and effective anti-emetics available for clinical use. In deciding which drug to use in a particular situation one should consider the cause of the symptoms and, where possible, use these as the basis for the choice of type of drug. Figure 15.3 enlarged from the review of Stewart (1963), is a useful basis to work on.

Table 15.5 Rationale for the use of various anti-emetics modified from Stewart (1963).

Psychogenic stimuli: fear	Diazepam: sedative
Motion sickness	Hyoscine, cyclizine
CTZ stimulation	Perphenazine, prochlorperazine, thiethylperazine, trifluperazine
Gastrointestinal upset	Metoclopramide

While Table 15.5 does not include all available anti-emetics, it is recommended as a useful working hypothesis for the rational use of these drugs. Within each group one can choose the drug which is not only most effective, but which produces the lowest incidence of side-effects in the particular patient.

REFERENCES

Adler H F, Atkinson, A J, Ivy A C 1942 Effect of morphine and Dilaudid on the ileum and of morphine, Dilaudid and atropine on the colon of man. Archives of Internal Medicine 69: 974–985

Albertson H A, Trout H H Jr, Daily F W 1956 Prophylaxis of postoperative nausea and vomiting. American Journal of Surgery 92: 423–427

Assaf R A E, Clarke R S J, Dundee J W, Samuel I O 1974 Studies of drugs given before anaesthesia. XXIV: Metoclopramide with morphine and pethidine. British Journal of Anaesthesia 46: 514–519

Atkinson A J, Adler H F, Ivy A C 1943 Motility of the human colon. The normal pattern, dyskinesia and the effect of drugs. Journal of the American Medical Association 9: 646–652

Ayd F J Jr 1961 A survey of drug-induced extrapyramidal reactions. Journal of the American Medical Association 175: 1054–1060

Ayd F J Jr 1974 Side effects of depot fluphenazines. In: Phenothiazines and structurally related drugs, vol 9. New York, Raven Press, pp 301–309

Bailey P L, Streisland J B, Pace N L, Bubbers S J M, East K A, Mulder S, Stanley T H 1990 Transdermal scopolamine reduces nausea and vomiting after outpatient laparoscopy. Anesthesiology 72: 977–980

Barsoum G, Perry E P and Fraser I A 1990 Postoperative nausea is relieved by acupressure. Journal of the Royal Society of Medicine 83: 86–89

Bellville J W, Bross I D J, Howland W S 1960 Postoperative nausea and vomiting. V: Anti-emetic efficacy of trimethobenzamide and perphenazine. Clinical Pharmacology and Therapeutics 1: 590–596

Bentley M D 1959. Adjunctive use of meclizine-pyridoxine (Bonadoxin) in the prevention of preoperative and postoperative nausea and emesis. Michigan Medical Society 58: 1483–1484

Blackwell C P and Harding S M 1989 The clinical pharmacology of ondansetron. European Journal of Cancer and Clinical Oncology 25 Suppl.1, s21–s24

Bodman R I, Morton H T V, Thomas E T 1960 Vomiting by out-patients after nitrous oxide anaesthesia. British Medical Journal 1: 1327–1329

Borison H L, Wang S C 1953 Physiology and pharmacology of vomiting. Pharmacological Review 5: 193

Borison H L, McCarthy L E 1983 Neuropharmacology of chemotherapy induced emesis. Drugs 28: 8–17

Brand J J, Perry W L M 1966 Drugs used in motion sickness. Pharmacological Reviews 18: 895–924

Brock-Utne J G, Downing J W, Dimopoulos G E, Rubin J, Moshal M G 1980 Effect of domperidone on lower oesophageal sphincter tone in later pregnancy. Anesthesiology 52: 321–323

Burstein C L 1963 Respiratory effects of benzquinamide during anesthesia. Anesthesia and Analgesia. Current Researches 42: 435–437

Chinn H I, Bayne-Jones S, Gersoni C S et al 1956 Evaluation of drugs for protection against motion sickness aboard transport ships. Journal of the American Medical Association 160: 755–760

Clark M M, Storr J A 1969 The prevention of postoperative vomiting after abortion. British Journal of Anaesthesia 41: 890–892

Clarke R S J, Dundee J W, Love W J 1965 Studies of drugs given before anaesthesia VIII: Morphine 10 mg alone and with atropine or hyoscine. British Journal of Anaesthesia 39: 772–779

Contractor S F, Shane B 1970 Blood and urine levels of vitamin B6 in the mother and fetus before and after loading of the mother with vitamin B6. American Journal of Obstetrics and Gynecology 107: 635–640

Costello D J, Borison H L 1977 Naloxone antagonises narcotic self blockade of emesis in the cat. Journal of Pharmacology and Experimental Therapeutics 203: 222–230

Courvoisier S, Fournel J, Ducrot R, Kolsky M, Koetschet P 1953 Proprietes pharmacodynamiques de chlorhydrate de chloro-3 (dimethyl amino-3 propyl) — 10 phenothiazine (4560 R P). Etudes experimentale d'un nouvel corps utilise dans l'anesthesie potentialisee et dans l'hibernation artificelle. Archives Internationales de Pharmacodynamie et de Therapie 92: 305

Davies R, Gallagher E 1957 Post anaesthetic vomiting: a trial of cyclizine tartrate. Journal of the Irish Medical Association 40: 84

Dent S J, Ramachandra V, Stephen C R 1955 Postoperative vomiting: incidence, analysis and therapeutic measures in 3000 patients. Anesthesiology 16: 564–572

Diggory P L, Tomkinson J S 1962 Nausea and vomiting in pregnancy, a trial of meclozine dihydrochloride with and without pyridoxine. Lancet 2: 370–372

Dobkin A B 1959 Perphenazine in clinical anaesthesia. Canadian Anaesthetists' Society Journal 6: 341–346

Dundee J W 1990 Belfast experience with acupuncture anti-emesis. Ulster Medical Journal 59: 63–70

Dundee J W, Assaf R A E, Loan W B, Morrison J D 1975a A comparison of the efficacy of cyclizine and perphenazine in reducing the emetic effects of morphine and pethidine. British Journal of Clinical Pharmacology 2: 81–85

Dundee J W, Clarke R S J 1973 The premedicant and anti-emetic action of metoclopramide. Postgraduate Medical Journal 48 (Suppl 4): 34–38

Dundee J W, Fitzpatrick K T J, Ghaly R G and Patterson C C 1988 Does dextrability or sinistrability affect the outcome of P6 acupuncture anti-emesis? British Journal of Clinical Pharmacology 25: 679–680

Dundee J W, Ghaly R G and McKinney M S 1989a. P6 Acupuncture anti-emesis comparison of various techniques. Anesthesiology 71 A130

Dundee J W, Ghaly R G, Bill K M, Chestnutt W N, Fitzpatrick K T J, Lynas A G A 1989b Effect of stimulation of the P6 antiemetic point in postoperative nausea and vomiting. British Journal of Anaesthesia 63: 612–618

Dundee J W, Ghaly R G, Fitzpatrick K T J, Abram W P, Lynch G A 1989c Acupuncture prophylaxis of cancer chemotherapy-induced sickness. Journal of Royal Society of Medicine 82: 268–271

Dundee J W, Jones P O 1968 The prevention of analgesic-induced nausea and vomiting by cyclizine. British Journal of Clinical Practice 22: 379–382

Dundee J W, Moore J 1961. The effects of premedication with phenothiazine derivatives on the course of methohexitone anaesthesia. British Journal of Anaesthesia 33: 382

Dundee J W, Moore J, Clarke R S J 1964 Studies of drugs given before anaesthesia V Pethidine 100 mg alone and with atropine or hyoscine. British Journal of Anaesthesia 36: 703–710

Dundee J W, Kirwan M J, Clarke R S J 1965a Anaesthesia and premedication as factors in postoperative vomiting. Acta Anaesthesiologica Scandinavica 9: 223–231

Dundee J W, Moore J, Love W J, Nicholl R M, Clarke R S J 1965b Studies of drugs given before anaesthesia. VI: The phenothiazine derivatives. British Journal of Anaesthesia 37: 332–353

Dundee J W, Halliday F, Nicholl R M, Moore J 1966 Studies of drugs give before anaesthesia. X: Two non-phenothiazine anti-emetics — cyclizine and trimethobenzamide. British Journal of Anaesthesia 38: 50–57

Dundee J W, Clarke R S J, Howard P J 1974. Studies of drugs given before anaesthesia. XXIII: Metoclopramide. British Journal of Anaesthesia 46: 509–513

Dundee J W, Clarke R S J, Carruthers S G 1975b Drug-induced extrapyramidal disorders. Prescribers' Journal 15: 26–31

Dundee J W, Chestnutt W N, Ghaly R G, Lynas A G A 1986. Traditional Chinese acupuncture: a potentially useful anti-emetic? British Medical Journal 293: 583–584

Dundee J W and Yang J 1990 Prolongation of the anti-emetic action of P6 acupuncture by acupressure in patients having cancer chemotherapy. Journal of the Royal Society of Medicine 83: 360–362

Editorial 1987 The Chemoreceptor Trigger Zone revisited. Lancet i: 144

Elia J C 1970 Long term treatment of Ménière's disease. International Surgery 53: 24–27

Ellis F R, Spence A A 1970 Clinical trials of metoclopramide (Maxolon) as an anti-emetic in anaesthesia. Anaesthesia 25: 460

Forrest F M 1974 In Phenothiazines and structurally related drugs. Advances in Biochemical Psychopharmacology, vol. 9 Raven Press, New York, pp 255–268

Fragen R J, Caldwell N 1978 A new benzimidazole anti-emetic, domperidone for the treatment of postoperative nausea and vomiting. Anesthesiology 1: 289–290

Fry E N S 1986 Acupressure and postoperative vomiting. Anaesthesia 41: 661–662

Ghaly R C, Fitzpatrick K T J and Dundee J W 1987 Antiemetic studies with traditional chinese acupuncture: A comparison of manual needling with electrical stimulation and commonly used anti-emetics. Anaesthesia 42: 1108–1110

Giannuzi C 1865 Untersuchungen uber die Organe, welche an dem Brechact theilnehmen, und uber die physiologische Wirkung des Tartarus stibiatus. Zentralblatt fur die medizinischen Wissenschaften 3: 1

Glaviano V V, Wang S G 1954 Dual mechanism of anti-emetic action of chlorpromazine. Federation Proceedings 13: 358

Gralla R G, Itri L M, Pisko S C 1981 Antiemetic efficacy of high doses of metoclopramide in patients with chemotherapy-induced nausea and vomiting. New England Journal of Medicine 305: 905–909

Handley A J 1967 Metoclopramide in the prevention of postoperative nausea and vomiting. British Journal of Clinical Practice 21: 460

Harris A L 1982 Cytotoxic-therapy-induced vomiting is mediated via enkephalin pathways (Hypothesis). Lancet 1: 714–716

Hicks J J, Hicks J N, Cooley H N 1967 Ménière's disease. Archives of Otolaryngology 86: 610–613

Hill F W 1951 Pyridoxine in the treatment of postanaesthetic nausea and vomiting. Anaesthesia 6: 52–53

Ho R T, Jawan B, Fury S T, Cheung H K, Lee J H 1990 Electro-acupuncture and postoperative emesis. Anaesthesia 45: 327–329

Howard F A, Sharp D S 1973 Effects of metoclopramide on gastric emptying during labour. British Medical Journal 1: 446

Howells T H, Khanam T, Kreel L, Seymour C, Oliver B, Davies J A H 1971 Pharmacological emptying of the stomach with metoclopramide. British Medical Journal 2: 558

Janssen P A J, Niemeegers C J E, Schellekens K H I, Verbruggen F J, Van Nueten J M 1963 The pharmacology of dehydrobenzperidol, new potent and short acting neuroleptic agent chemically related to haloperidol. Arzneimittel-Forschung 13: 205–211

Johnson A G 1973 Gastroduodenal motility and synchronisation. Postgraduate Medical Journal 48 (Suppl 4): 29

Justin-Besancon L, Laville C 1964 Anti-emetic action of metoclopramide against apomorphine and hydergine. Compte Rendu des Seances de la Societé de Biologie de Paris 158: 723

Kerman E F 1951 Dramamine in the prevention and treatment of nausea and vomiting following electroshock therapy. Diseases of the Nervous System 12: 83

Kernis L, Stodsky B 1950 Failure of pyridoxine in postanesthetic nausea and vomiting. Anesthesiology 11: 212–214

King C T G 1963 Teratogenic effects of meclozine hydrochloride on the rat. Science 141: 353–355

King C T G, Weaver S A, Derr J E 1965a Benhydrylpiperazine antihistamines, hydraminos and congenital malformations in the rat. American Journal of Obstetrics and Gynecology 93: 563–565

King C T G, Weaver S A, Narrod S A 1965b Antihistamines and teratogenicity in the rat. Journal of Pharmacology and Experimental Therapeutics 147: 391–398

Klein R L, Graves Constance L, Yong I K, Blatnick R 1970 Inhibition of apomorphine-induced vomiting by benzquinamide. Clinical Pharmacology and Therapeutics 11: 530–537

Kreel L 1973 The use of metoclopramide in radiology. Postgraduate Medical Journal 48 (Suppl 2): 42

Kuntzman R, Philips A, Tsai I, Klutch A, Burns J J 1967 N-oxide formation: a new route for inactivation of the antihistaminic chlorcyclizine. Journal of Pharmacology and Experimental Therapeutics 155: 337–344

Larrauri R M 1969 Benzquinamide parenteral for the treatment of postoperative nausea and vomiting. Current Therapeutic Research 11: 118–120

Leading Article 1964 Drugs and the embryo. British Medical Journal 1: 195

Leading Article 1987 5-HT$_3$ receptor antagonists: a new class of anti-emetics. Lancet 1: 1470–1471

Lind B, Breivik H 1970 Metoclopramide and perphenazine in the prevention of postoperative nausea and vomiting. British Journal of Anaesthesia 42: 614–617

Lovelace F R, Poe M F, Dornette W H L 1963 A clinical evaluation of the anti-emetic properties, thiethylperazine maleate. Anaesthesia and Analgesia 42: 653–657

Lutz H, Immich H 1972 Anti-emetic effect of benzquinamide in postoperative vomiting. Current Therapeutic Research 14: 178–184

McBride W 1963 Cyclizine and congenital abnormalities. British Medical Journal 1: 1157–1158

McGarry J M 1971 A double-blind comparison of the anti-emetic effects during labour of metoclopramide and perphenazine. British Journal of Anaesthesia 43: 613

Margieson G R, Sorby W A, Williams H B L 1966 The action of metoclopramide on gastric emptying: a radiological assessment. Medical Journal of Australia 2: 1272–1274

Midwinter A 1971 Vomiting in pregnancy. Practitioner 206: 743–750

Miner W D, Sanger G J 1986 Inhibition of cisplatin-induced vomiting by selective 5-hydroxytryptamine M-receptor antagonism. British Journal of Pharmacology 88: 497–499

Moore D C, Anderson L, Wheeler G, Scheidt J 1952 The use of parenteral dramamine to control postoperative vomiting: a report of 1192 cases. Anesthesiology 13: 354–360

Moore D C, Bridenbaugh L D, Green J C, Piccioni V F, Adams P A, Linstrom C A 1955 Intramuscular use of dimenhydrinate (Dramamine) to control postoperative vomiting. Journal of the American Medical Association I59: 1342–1345

Moore D C, Bridenbaugh L D, Piccioni V F, Adams P A, Lindstrom C A 1956 Control of postoperative vomiting with Merazine: a double blind study. Anesthesiology 17: 690–695

Moore D C, Bridenbaugh L D, van Acheren E G, Cole F V 1958 Control of postoperative vomiting with perphenazine (Trilafon): a double blind study. Anesthesiology 19: 72–74

Moore J, Dundee J W 1961 Alterations in response to somatic pain associated with anaesthesia. V: The effect of promethazine. British Journal of Anesthesia 33: 3

Morrison J D 1970 Studies of drugs given before anaesthesia. XXII: Phenoperidine and fentanyl, alone and in combination with droperidol. British Journal of Anaesthesia 42: 1119–1126

Morrison J D, Hill G B, Dundee J W 1968 Studies of drugs given before anaesthesia. XV: Evaluation of the method of study after 10,000 observations. British Journal of Anaesthesia 40: 890–900

Mull T D, Smith T C 1974 Comparison of the ventilatory

effects of two anti-emetics, benzquinamide and prochlorperazine. Anesthesiology 40: 581–587

Nelson M M, Forfar J O 1971 Associations between drugs administered during pregnancy and congenital abnormalities of the fetus. British Medical Journal 1: 523–527

O'Donovan N, Shaw J 1984 Nausea and vomiting in day-care dental anaesthesia. The use of low-dose droperidol. Anaesthesia 39: 1172-1176

Palacios J M, Wamsley J K, Kuhar M J 1981 The distribution of Histamine H1 receptors in the rat brain: an autoradiographic study. Neuroscience 6: 15–17

P'an S Y, Gardocki J F, Reilly J C 1954 Pharmacological properties of two new antihistaminics of prolonged action. Journal of the American Pharmaceutical Association 43: 653–656

Patton C M, Moon M R, Dannemiller F J 1974 The prophylactic anti-emetic effect of droperidol. Anesthesia and Analgesia, Current Researches 53: 361–364

Peikes I L 1957 Nausea and vomiting of pregnancy treated with a sustained release form of prochlorperazine. Clinical Medicine 4: 1385–1387

Peroutka S J, Snyder S H 1982 Anti-emetics: Neurotransmitter receptor binding predicts therapeutic actions. Lancet 1982 (i): 658–659

Rita L, Goodarzi M, Seleny F 1981 Effect of low dose droperidol on postoperative vomiting in children. Canadian Anaesthetists' Society Journal 259–262

Robbie D S 1959 Post anaesthetic vomiting and anti-emetic drugs. Anaesthesia 14: 349–354

Robinson O P W 1973 Metoclopramide — a new pharmacological approach? Postgraduate Medical Journal 49 (Suppl 4): 9–13

Sadusk J F Jr, Palmisano P A 1965 Teratogenic effect of meclozine, cyclizine and chlorcyclizine. Journal of the American Medical Association 194: 987–989

Schallek W, Heise G A, Keith E F, Bagdon R E 1959 Anti-emetic activity of 4-(2-dimethyl amino-ethoxy) N-(3,4,5-trimethoxybenzoyl) benzylamine hydrochloride. Journal of Pharmacology and Experimental Therapeutics 126: 270

Shah Z P, Wilson J 1972 An evaluation of metoclopramide Maxolon) as an anti-emetic in minor gynaecological survey. British Journal of Anaesthesia 44: 865

Shelley G S, Brown H A 1978 Anti-emetic effect of ultra-low dose droperidol. American Society of Anesthesiologists Annual Meeting Abstracts 633–634

Stalsberg H 1965 Anti-emetics and congenital deformities — meclozine, cyclizine and chlorcyclizine. Norwegian Medical Journal 85: 1840–1841

Steen S N, Yates M 1972 The effects of benzquinamide and prochlorperazine, separately and combined, on the human respiratory center. Anesthesiology 36: 519–520

Stefanini E, Clement-Cormier Y 1981 Detection of dopamine receptors in the area postrema. European Journal of Pharmacology 74: 257–260

Stewart H C 1963 The pharmacology of anti-emetic drugs. British Journal of Anaesthesia 35: 174–179

Stoll B A 1957 New drugs for irradiation sickness. Radiology 68: 380–385

Stoll B A 1962 Radiation sickness: an analysis of over 1000

controlled drug trials. British Medical Journal 2: 507–510

Stott J R R, Barnes G R, Wright R J and Ruddock C J S 1989 The effect on motion sickness and oculomotor function of GR 38032F, a 5HT$_3$-receptor antagonist with anti-emetic properties. British Journal of Clinical Pharmacology 27: 247–257

Thumas L J 1891 Ueber das Brechcentrum und uber die Wirkung einiger pharmakologischer Mittel auf dasselbe. Virchows Archiv fur pathologische Anatomie and Physiologie and fur klinische Medizin 123: 44

Tornetta F J 1969 Clinical studies with the new anti-emetic metoclopramide. Anesthesia and Analgesia, Current Researches 48: 198

Tuchmann-Duplessis H, Mercier-Parot L 1963 Action du chlorhydrate de cyclizine sur la gestation et la developpement embryonaire du rat, de la souris et du lapin. Comptes Rendus Hebdomadaires des Seances de l'Academie des Science 256: 3359–3362

Tyers M B, Bunce K T, Humphrey P P A 1989 Pharmacological and antiemetic properties of ondansetron. European Journal of Cancer and Clinical Oncology 25 Suppl.1 s15–s19

Vaisberg M 1954 Dramamine (injectable) in migraine. Annals of Allergy 12: 180

Van den Driessché J, Eben-Moussi E 1971 Essais de prevention des vomissements provoques chez le chien par la L-dopa. Pathologie et Biologie 19: 797–800

Wade O L, Dundee J W 1969 Anti-emetic drugs. Prescribers' Journal 9: 69–74

Waldmann C S, Verghese C, Short D R, Goldhill D R and Evans S J W 1985 The evaluation of domperidone and metoclopramide as anti-emetics in day case abortion patients. British Journal of Clinical Pharmacology 19: 307–310

Wamsley J K, Lewis M S, Young W S III, Kuhar M J 1981 Autoradiographic localisation of muscarinic cholinergic receptors in rat brainstem. Journal of Neuroscience 1: 176–191

Wang S C, Borison H L 1952 A new concept of organisation of the central emetic mechanism. Gastroenterology 22: 1

Wheeler M W, Campman K L 1971 A comparative study of droperidol v. hydroxyzine hydrochloride as premedication. Journal of the American Association of Nurse Anesthetists 401–404

Wheeler W L, Howland J M Smith W, Corso J E 1959 The use of prochlorperazine in seasickness. Industrial Medicine and Surgery 28: 405–406

Wilmot T J 1971 An objective study of the effect of betahistine hydrochloride on hearing and vestibular function tests in patients with Meniere's disease. Journal of Laryngology and Otology 85: 369–373

Wilson D B, Dundee J W 1979 Evaluation of the anti-emetic action of domperidone. Anaesthesia 34: 765–767

Wood C D, Graybiel A 1968 Evaluation of sixteen anti-motion sickness drugs under controlled laboratory conditions. Aerospace Medicine 39: 1341–1344

Woolham D H M 1965 Principles of teratogenesis: mode of action of thalidomide. Proceedings of the Royal Society of Medicine 58: 497–501

Drugs acting peripherally on the nervous system

16. Autonomic and peripheral nerves; cholinergic and adrenergic transmission

J. R. Carpenter

Role of the autonomic nervous system

The autonomic nervous system is responsible for the regulation (rather than the initiation) of processes in the body which are not under voluntary control, and provides a control system which is able to produce more rapid responses than can be achieved through the endocrine system. All control systems are composed of both an afferent limb and an efferent limb, and although afferent fibres travel in major autonomic nerve trunks, the autonomic nervous system *per se* is composed only of efferent fibres. The rest of this chapter will be devoted to these efferent nerves. The functions controlled by the autonomic nervous system do not need either the rapid reactions or the precision of the somatic system, which accounts for the major differences between the two efferent nervous systems.

Structure and organization

Autonomic nerves leave the central nervous sytem in three anatomically distinct groups. These outflows can be most simply described as cranial, thoracolumbar and sacral. In the mid-eighteenth century the term 'sympathetic' began to be applied to the chain of paravertebral ganglia which have since been shown to be connected to the thoracolumbar outflow. The descriptions of the autonomic nervous system were formalized by Langley (1921), who was responsible for the term 'autonomic'. He preserved the by then classical term 'sympathetic' for the nerves arising from the thoracolumbar outflow, and introduced the term 'parasympathetic' for the nerves leaving the CNS in the cranial and sacral nerves. This terminology, although not without its problems, has proved to be remarkably useful and even prophetic, as it anticipated the discovery of the chemical differences between the two divisions, and is now used universally.

Control centres in the central nervous system

The primitive origins of the autonomic nervous system are reflected in the location of the control centres in the brainstem. Most autonomic functions appear to be controlled from the hypothalamus, sympathetic outflow originating primarily in the posterior and lateral hypothalamic nuclei, whereas the anterior nuclei and midline nuclei close to the tuber cinereum control the parasympathetic outflow, although influences from higher levels, including conscious cerebral inputs, can have important effects upon autonomic function. Descending fibres from the sympathetic centres run in the anterolateral bundles of white matter in the cord, innervating cell bodies in the lateral horns of the thoracic and lumbar segments from which outflow occurs. There are also connections to higher and lower segments within the cord through segmental and intersegmental interneurons, the cell bodies of which have been traced to the medial nucleus of grey matter in the cord.

Peripheral distribution

In both divisions the peripheral autonomic innervation comprises two neurons in series, and although it is only in the sympathetic system and the cranial nerves III, VI and IX that the nerve–nerve synapses occur in anatomically discrete ganglia, it is usual to describe the two neurons as being preganglionic and postganglionic, whether the synapse occurs in a real ganglion or not. (The swelling on the vagus just below the skull, known as the nodose ganglion, is in fact composed of the cell bodies of afferent nerves running in the vagus, approximately 75% of vagal fibres at this point being afferent fibres.)

The peripheral nerves of both divisions are small, the preganglionic neurons being myelinated B-fibres (1–3 μm in diameter) whereas the postganglionic fibres are unmyelinated C-fibres (<1μm in diameter). Conduction velocity in these unmyelinated C-fibres is no more than about 5 m s^{-1}, which dictates that the impulse frequency is kept low. It has been shown, for example, that impulse frequency in sympathetic vasomotor neurons seldom, if ever, exceeds 10 Hz.

Another reflection of the functional differences between the somatic and autonomic nervous systems is to be found in the arrangement of terminal branches and the sites of transmitter release. Terminal somatic neurons branch profusely, and each branch ends in a single, specialized region for transmitter storage and release, the terminal knob or button. There is a very narrow synaptic cleft (approx. 50 nm) separating the nerve ending from an equally highly specialized region on the muscle cell, the muscle endplate, which is richly endowed with cholinoceptors, has specialized electrical properties and is densely supplied with acetylcholinesterase. (A rather similar arrangement has been described for the innervation of ganglion cells.)

Autonomic neurons, however, do not show this 'focal' system of innervation. Instead the fine C-fibres begin to branch and rebranch as soon as they enter the innervated organ, to form a diffuse reticulum. Fluorescence microscopy shows the fine terminal branches of noradrenergic neurons to bear 'beads' or 'varicosities' periodically along the fine fibres. These varicosities show a much higher intensity of fluorescence than the axons themselves, indicating that they contain very high concentrations of noradrenaline. Similar structural arrangements have been described for cholinergically innervated tissues. Confirmation that the varicosities represent the sites of transmitter storage and release comes from electron microscopy, which shows varicosities to be packed with transmitter storage vesicles. (In osmium-stained preparations these vesicles are electron-translucent in cholinergic neurons and electron-opaque in noradrenergic neurons.) Transmission between autonomic nerves and effector organs, then, shows several differences from transmission at skeletal neuromuscular junctions and ganglia. These differences may be summarized as follows: firstly the synaptic gap is not only much wider in autonomically innervated tissues, but is very variable (up to 2000 nm). Secondly, transmitter release sites (varicosities) are arranged in series rather than in parallel, an arrangement known as 'en passage' transmission. Finally, there are no specialized regions on the effector organs analogous to skeletal muscle endplates. Instead receptors are distributed over the whole surface of the cells of the effector organ.

SYMPATHETIC DIVISION

The sympathetic nervous system is summarized in dia-grammatic form in Figure 16.1. The preganglionic neurons of most sympathetic nerves have their cell bodies in the lateral horns of spinal segments T1 to L3, and leave the cord in the ventral roots along with somatic motor fibres which merge with afferent fibres entering the dorsal root to become the segmental mixed spinal nerves. The preganglionic sympathetic neurons leave the mixed spinal nerves almost immediately and travel in short, discrete trunks known as the white communicating rami to enter the paravertebral ganglia, where they synapse. Postganglionic sympathetic fibres supplying viscera and blood vessels associated with that segment leave the paravertebral ganglia in the postganglionic trunks and travel to their respective effector organs, often in association with blood vessels. Many preganglionic sympathetic neurons, however, travel up or down the chain of paravertebral ganglia before they synapse and leave in segments some distance from their original outflow from the cord. This applies particularly to neurons supplying the head and neck above the highest segment in which sympathetic outflow from the cord occurs (T1), and to those supplying organs in the lower abdomen, the pelvis and legs (the lowest spinal segment from which sympathetic outflow occurs being L3). Thus sympathetic nerves to the head and parts of the neck travel up the chain of cervical paravertebral ganglia before leaving either as postganglionic trunks or in the mixed spinal nerves. In the latter case the fibres reach the mixed spinal nerves in the grey communicating rami. In the sacral extensions of the paravertebral chain, postganglionic sympathetic fibres reach the lower parts of the body mainly via the grey rami and the mixed spinal nerves. Some preganglionic, sympathetic fibres do not synapse in the paravertebral ganglia, but after entering the paravertebral chain in the white rami, pass straight through to synapse in the prevertebral ganglia. These are many and unpaired, forming a diffuse plexus ventral to the great vessels in the abdominal cavity. However, there are several sites at which considerable numbers of preganglionic fibres converge and synapse, giving rise to identifiable, named structures — viz. the coeliac, superior mesenteric, aorticorenal and inferior mesenteric ganglia.

The final component of the sympathetic nervous system is the adrenal medulla, which arises from the same part of the embryonic neural ectoderm that gives rise to postganglionic sympathetic neurons. Each adrenal medulla can be considered to be a modified extension of the coeliac ganglion; the medulla of each adrenal gland receives a preganglionic supply of fibres which have passed straight through the coeliac ganglion without synapsing. These fibres are essentially identical to any other preganglionic sympathetic fibres in terms both of their anatomy (lumbar outflow) and chemical transmit-

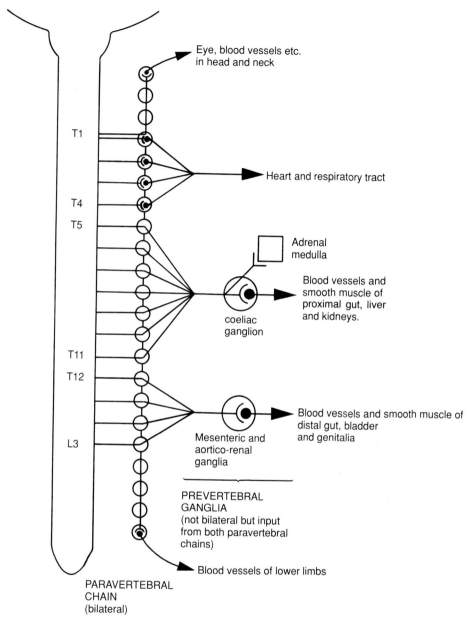

Fig. 16.1 The sympathetic nervous system.

ter (cholinergic). The chromaffin cells of the medulla, instead of acquiring long, conducting axons, become compact, cuboidal cells, specialized for secretion by being packed with transmitter storage vesicles. These chromaffin cells bear nicotinic cholinoceptors but have rather lower resting membrane potentials than ganglion cells (25 mV as opposed to 70 mV), and respond to stimulation by neurotransmitter with only a very small depolarization. In addition the transmitter released from

the adrenal medulla is adrenaline rather than noradrenaline (see below), and as it is released almost directly into the inferior vena cava, it is rapidly distributed throughout the body and can therefore exert an effect upon effector cells that have no sympathetic innervation.

Sympathetic innervation of organs

The distribution of postganglionic sympathetic neurons

Table 16.1 Responses to activity in sympathetic nerves

Organ	Adrenoceptor type	Effect
Cardiovascular system		
Heart		
SA node	β_1	(a) slope of prepotential increased
		(b) rate of rise of and amplitude of AP increased
AV node and His–Purkinje system	β_1	(a) slope of prepotential increased (can become dominant pacemaker)
		(b) conduction velocity increased
		(c) refractory period reduced
Atria	β_1	(a) force of contraction and rate of rise of tension increased
		(b) conduction velocity increased
Ventricles	β_1	(a) force of contraction and rate of rise of tension increased
		(b) 'oxygen wasting' (i.e. though force increased disproportionate rise in O_2 uptake)
		(c) conduction velocity increased
		(d) development of spontaneous depolarisation (especially papillary muscle)
Arterioles		
Skin, mucosae, viscera, skeletal muscle	α, β_2	(a) under physiological conditions these beds constrict as though only α-adrenoceptors present
		(b) circulating adrenaline from adrenal medulla causes dilation (bulk of fall in BP due to skeletal muscle vessels as high proportion of body mass)
Salivary glands	α	constriction
Coronary	α, β_2	under physiological conditions dilation via β-adrenoceptors
Veins (systemic)	α	constriction
Gastrointestinal system		
Propulsive muscle of gut	α, β_2	inhibition
Parasympathetic ganglia in Auerbach's plexus	α	impaired transmission
Sphincters	α	contraction
Biliary tract	α, β_2	relaxation
Pancreas		
acini	α	inhibition
B-cells of islets	α	insulin secretion inhibited (note that β-adrenoceptors on B-cells activated by circulating adrenaline increase insulin secretion)
Genito-urinary system		
Bladder		
detrusor	β_2	relaxation[*]
trigone and sphincter	α	contraction[*]
Vas deferens and seminal vesicles	α	contraction (component of ejaculation)

Table 16.1   Contd

Organ	Adrenoceptor type	Effect
Erectile tissue	α	vasoconstriction (detumescence)
Eye		
Smooth muscle of eyelid	α	contraction — widening of palpebral fissure
Radial muscle of iris	α	contraction (mydriasis)
Ciliary muscle	β?	relaxation — functional significance unproven
Respiratory tract		
Bronchial smooth	α	contraction†
muscle	β₂	relaxation†
Skin		
Pilomotor muscles	α	contraction ('goose-flesh')
Sweat glands (palms of hands and some parts of face only)	α	sweating (most sweat glands receive anatomically sympathetic but cholinergic innervation)

*More important in preventing entry of urine into urethra and sperm into bladder during ejaculation than in control of micturition.

†Functional significance of noradrenergic nerves minimal in health. In asthmatics compensatory bronchodilation achieved via sympathetic nerves and adrent medulla.

to the various organs throughout the body is summarised in Table 16.1, which also indicates the type of response induced by sympathetic neuronal activity to each organ listed, as well as the adrenoceptor type involved in the transmission. (Classification of adrenoceptors is dealt with later in this chapter.) In addition to being mediated through noradrenergic innervations, some important responses are brought about by blood-borne adrenaline acting upon adrenoceptors in parts of the body devoid of sympathetic innervations. These are listed in Table 16.2.

The nerves to most eccrine sweat glands, the sympathetic dilator fibres to blood vessels in skeletal muscle and to certain areas of skin are cholinergic, although they are anatomically sympathetic. The cholinoceptors at these sites are muscarinic. However, whereas sweating is normally mediated through cholinergic sympathetic fibres, the cholinergic supply to blood vessels in skeletal muscle is unimportant in the normal, physiological control of blood flow, although it probably plays a part in the vasodilation associated with the fainting reflex.

Table 16.2   Adrenoceptor mediated responses in systems without noradrenergic innervations

Organ	Adrenoceptor type	Response
Liver	β₂	glycogenolysis
	β₂	gluconeogenesis
	β₁	calorigenesis
	α	K^+ release
Fat cells	β₁	lipolysis (generation of free fatty acids)
Skeletal muscle	β₂	tremor
	β₂	glycogenolysis
Myometrium (near term)	β₂	inhibition

Synthesis and storage of noradrenaline

Synthesis

Although the concept of humoral transmission from what we now know as endocrine glands was established by the end of the nineteenth century, and although chemical transmission at nerve endings was proposed as early as 1904, it was not until 1921 that this concept began to find general acceptance. Shortly after the discovery in 1938 of an enzyme capable of decarboxylating L-DOPA to dopamine a theoretical series of reactions was proposed by which adrenaline could be synthesized from the amino acid tyrosine. (It was only in 1945 that it was demonstrated that the sympathetic transmitter was actually noradrenaline rather than adrenaline.) This scheme proved to be remarkably accurate, and was eventually confirmed for sympathetic neurons in 1958 by experiments with radioactively labelled tyrosine. The sequence is shown in Figure 16.2.

Tyrosine hydroxylase. This can be considered as the first enzyme unique to the noradrenaline synthesis pathway as L-tyrosine is produced in abundance from the essential dietary amino acid L-phenylalanine by the enzyme phenylalanine hydroxylase as part of normal cellular metabolism. (In phenylketonuria there is a congenital absence of phenylalanine hydroxylase, which accounts for the gross neurological abnormalities which develop if this disease is not treated by dietary management.) Tyrosine hydroxylase is concentrated in the endoplasmic reticulum of noradrenergic neurons, and catalyses the hydroxylation of the phenol tyrosine to the catechol dihydroxyphenylalanine (DOPA). Tyrosine hydroxylase is perhaps the most important enzyme in the noradrenaline synthesis pathway because it is both the rate-limiting enzyme and also displays the characteristic of end-product inhibition, in which high intra-neuronal concentrations of noradrenaline (the end product) inhibit the enzyme. This is the mechanism by which the synthetic pathway is regulated; the enzyme, and as it is the rate-limiting step, the whole rate of noradrenaline synthesis, is activated when intra-neuronal noradrenaline levels are low, and conversely is inhibited when stores are replete. This homeostatic mechanism is complemented by the ability of noradrenergic cell bodies to increase the rate at which tyrosine hydroxylase is synthesized *de novo* when neuronal activity is maintained at a high level.

Tyrosine hydroxylase is inhibited by metirosine, a close structural analogue of the natural substrate, tyrosine. By reducing the rate of synthesis of noradrenaline (and therefore also of adrenaline), metirosine is useful

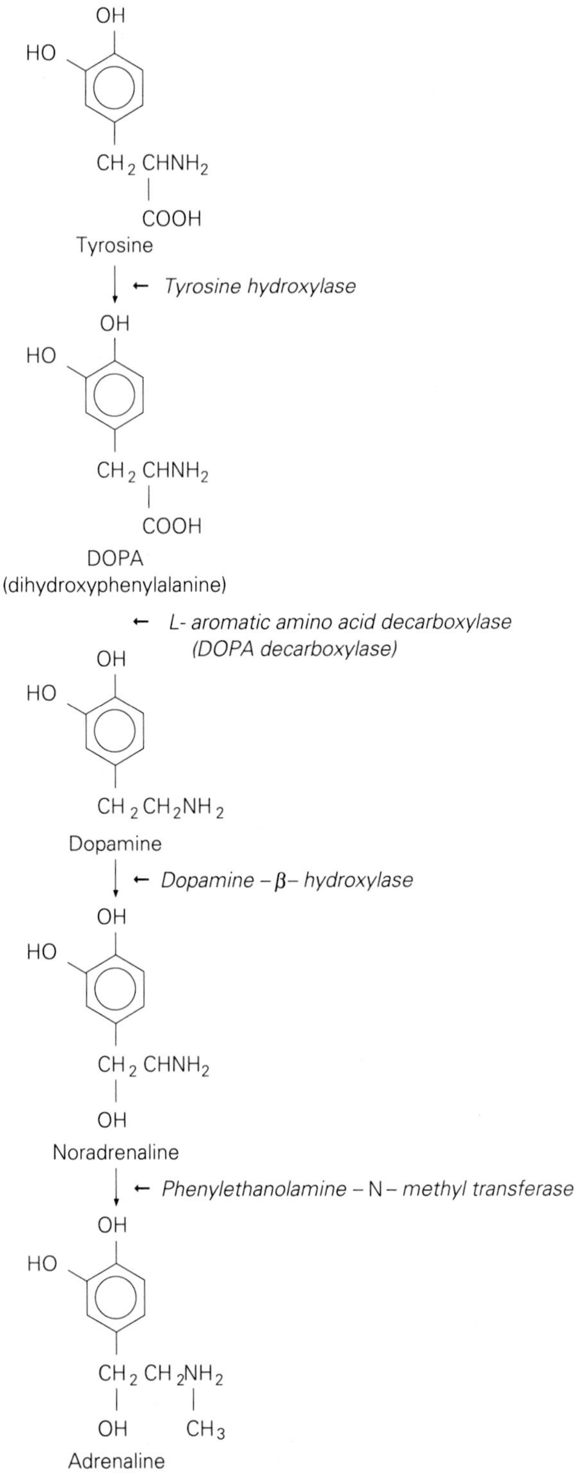

Fig. 16.2 Synthesis of adrenaline.

in the management of phaeochromocytoma, both in preparation for surgery and as a longer-term treatment in patients for whom surgery is inappropriate.

L-*aromatic amino acid decarboxylase* (DOPA decarboxylase). This enzyme is in free solution in the cytoplasm of noradrenergic nerves and requires pyridoxal phosphate as a coenzyme. It catalyses the conversion of the amino acid DOPA to the catecholamine, dopamine, but again is of relatively low specificity as it will decarboxylate many aromatic L-amino acids. In dopaminergic neurons this is the final enzyme in the synthetic pathway. Aromatic L-amino acid decarboxylase is susceptible to inhibition by analogues of DOPA, therapeutically important compounds being benserazide and carbidopa which are useful adjuncts to levodopa (L-DOPA) in the treatment of Parkinson's disease. These two inhibitors are highly polar, and therefore do not penetrate the blood–brain barrier. Consequently, relatively selective peripheral inhibition of decarboxylation can be achieved, thereby preserving peripherally circulating L-DOPA for conversion into dopamine in the CNS. This both reduces the necessary levodopa dose levels and decreases the incidence of adverse effects. (see Chapter 34 and page 562).

Dopamine-beta-hydroxylase. The conversion of dopamine to noradrenaline by the addition of a hydroxyl group to the beta-carbon atom is achieved by the enzyme dopamine-beta-hydroxylase, an enzyme which requires ascorbate or fumarate as a cofactor and which contains a Cu^{2+} prosthetic group. This enzyme is located exclusively within the noradrenaline storage vesicles so that noradrenaline is synthesized at the location at which it is stored. To allow this to occur, the vesicle membrane is equipped with an active accumulation mechanism which pumps dopamine from the cytoplasm to the inside of the vesicle (see under Storage). The copper prosthetic group can be removed by chelating agents, notable among which is diethyldithiocarbamate, one of the metabolic products of disulfiram. Consequently there is a risk of impairing noradrenergic neuron function in alcoholics given long-term aversion therapy with disulfiram. This is most commonly manifested as postural hypotension.

Phenylethanolamine-N-methyltransferase. In chromaffin cells of the adrenal medulla, the final synthetic step from noradrenaline to adrenaline is achieved by the addition of a methyl group to the terminal nitrogen, catalysed by phenylethanolamine-*N*-methyltransferase using adenosyl-methionine as the methyl donor. The level of this enzyme is controlled in part by the level of adrenocortical hormones which facilitate production of the enzyme.

Storage

For chemical transmission to be efficient it is necessary that high concentrations of transmitter are produced rapidly in the vicinity of the receptors. To achieve this, high concentrations of pre-formed transmitter are stored, these stores having been built up slowly over a period of time by the synthetic process and preserved by mechanisms which render the transmitter less susceptible to diffusion. The most important of these diffusion barriers is the membrane of the storage vesicle. This membrane is similar to the lipid bilayer of the plasma membrane of cells, and is therefore relatively impermeable to highly polar molecules such as noradrenaline. The second mechanism that contributes to the maintenance of the high intravesicular concentrations of noradrenaline is an active pump in the vesicle membrane which can transport noradrenaline (and its immediate precursor, dopamine) against a concentration gradient into the core of the vesicle. This active process utilises energy from ATP and requires Mg^{2+}. Thus although noradrenaline synthesized in the vesicle will slowly leak through the vesicle membrane into the cell cytoplasm, it will be pumped back into the vesicle by the uptake pump. The diffusion barrier offered by the vesicle membrane is supplemented by the effects of other vesicular components. Noradrenaline storage vesicles have a remarkably high content of ATP. In chromaffin cells of the adrenal medulla there is one molecule of ATP for every four molecules of adrenaline, in which proportions a weak chemical complex can be shown to form in vitro. This 1:4 stoichiometry, however, does not appear to exist in vesicles from noradrenergic neurons, although noradrenaline, like adrenaline, will form a complex with ATP. Noradrenaline storage vesicles also contain a family of related proteins which are acidic and water-soluble, to which the name 'chromogranins' has been given. The principal component, chromogranin A, is a highly acidic protein with a molecule composed of two similar subunits. The function of these chromogranins is presumably to reduce the diffusibility of the noradrenaline (or noradrenaline–ATP complex) further, but it has not proved possible to demonstrate the formation of a chemical complex between any of the chromogranins and noradrenaline in vitro, with or without ATP. However, the primary structure of chromogranin A suggests that the molecule exists in the form of a random coil, and that the noradrenaline is rendered less diffusible by being trapped within the coils of the protein when this latter is in a gel form. The diffusibility of the transmitter could conceivably be increased by a contraction of the gel matrix induced by the change in ionic environment occasioned by exocytosis (i.e. an extracellular environment as opposed to that within vesicles). In addition to ATP and the chromogranins, noradrenaline storage vesicles contain a sulphomucopolysaccharide in the form of a protein complex. This sulphomucopolysaccharide is similar to chondroitin sulphate, and has also been detected in acetylcholine storage vesicles, the histamine storage vesicles of mast cells and the 5-HT containing vesicles of platelets, suggesting that it plays an important role in the sequestration of transmitters and mediators in general.

Drugs that modify noradrenaline storage. Drugs which are substrates for uptake at both the neuron membrane (see below) and at storage vesicle membranes produce a net efflux of noradrenaline from vesicles by competing for the uptake pump and for sequestration. Extravesicular noradrenaline is then either broken down by cytoplasmic monoamine oxidase (see below) or diffuses out into the extracellular space, where it may activate adrenoceptors. Drugs which are themselves devoid of activity at adrenoceptors, but which can release noradrenaline from vesicular stores, are known as indirect sympathomimetics. Examples are ephedrine, amphetamine and tyramine. The latter, the amine formed by decarboxylating the amino acid tyrosine, is of interest because it is present in high concentrations in a variety of foodstuffs, the preparation of which involves fermentation with micro-organisms (e.g. cheeses, autolysed yeast products, pickled fish and some alcoholic beverages) and is responsible for the serious interaction that can occur between these foodstuffs and monoamine oxidase inhibitors. Reserpine and its congeners cause depletion of noradrenaline stores in a way that involves at least two mechanisms. At low concentrations, reserpine inhibits the vesicular uptake pump so that noradrenaline that has been released during normal nerve activity cannot be resequestered in storage vesicles. Additionally, de novo synthesis of noradrenaline is prevented as the uptake of dopamine is also blocked. Consequently transmission fails first in those noradrenergic nerves with the highest impulse traffic, usually those to the heart and peripheral resistance vessels. This action of reserpine is reversible and inhibited vesicles resume normal pumping once the reserpine has been eliminated from the body. At higher concentrations reserpine causes irreversible damage to the vesicle membrane and disrupts the storage complex, so that transmitter stores are rapidly lost and transmission fails in all noradrenergic nerves, whether active or inactive. Repletion and consequent restoration of transmission depends upon synthesis of new vesicles in the cell body and their subsequent transport down the axon to the varicosities. Some of the effects of reserpine can be duplicated by large doses of guanethidine, although at normal therapeutic doses, guanethidine impairs transmission by blocking the propagation of action potentials and leaves transmitter stores intact. Tetrabenazine has a reserpine-like mechanism of action, but is highly selective for dopaminergic neurons. It therefore depletes dopamine stores in the CNS without impairing peripheral sympathetic nerve function. It is useful in controlling the involuntary movements in Huntingdon's chorea.

Release of noradrenaline

The mechanisms involved in the release of transmitter from autonomic nerves have proved to be rather less amenable to experimental investigation than those at skeletal neuromuscular junctions. This is because of the diffuse nature of autonomic innervation, the system of 'en passage' transmission, the electrical linking between effector cells and the fact that transmitter released from a single varicosity diffuses outwards in an expanding sphere, becoming progressively diluted and stimulating many effector cells as it goes. However, it is likely that the overall process of transmitter release is similar from all nerves, irrespective of the nature of the nerve or the transmitter. The precise way in which exocytosis is triggered by the nerve impulse is equally obscure, except that Ca^{2+} influx is an absolute requirement for transmitter release from all nerves studied to date. The two most likely explanations are either that the Ca^{2+} influx triggers a mass migration of vesicles to the membrane, perhaps involving microtubules, or simply that the presence of high Ca^{2+} concentrations near the membrane allows more of the random collisions between vesicles and the membrane to result in fusions and subsequent release of vesicular contents. Following release of transmitter the vesicles are pinched off and move (or are moved) back into the cytoplasm ready for re-use.

Classification of adrenoceptors

As long ago as 1906 it was shown that only some of the effects of adrenaline could be prevented by ergot extracts, although it was not until 1948 that a satisfactory explanation was provided for this and a variety of other problems associated with the actions of the sympathomimetics. The current view that there are two types of adrenoceptors (designated α and β) is based up on experiments in which the potencies of a number of sympathomimetics were measured on several test systems. When these sympathomimetics are arranged in their rank order of potency for each system, only two rank orders are found, which is most simply explained by proposing the existence of two types of adrenoceptor, each having different structural requirements for stimulation. Although a number of antagonists were available in 1948 (e.g. ergotamine, dibenamine, tolazoline), there were none that were selective for β-adrenoceptors until 1958 when dichloroisoprenaline was found to be an antagonist at β-adrenoceptors. The therapeutic potential offered by selective antagonists at β-adrenoceptors was recognized, and this led to the production of the first potent, selective and safe antagonist at β-adrenoceptors, namely propranolol. The α/β-adrenoceptor classification has been strengthened over the years as new drugs have appeared all fitting easily into these original categories. However, a number of minor inconsistencies have arisen concerning the classification of agonists selective for β-adrenoceptors. For example, although noradrenaline is very potent at cardiac β-adrenoceptors, it is much less potent at β-adrenoceptors on blood vessels, whereas adrenaline has similar potency at both. Another example is that noradrenaline is more potent than adrenaline at the β-adrenoceptors of the gut when, in the original study, the characteristic rank order of potency of agonists at β-adrenoceptors has adrenaline more potent than noradrenaline. Experimental comparisons of potencies of a variety of agonists has led to the proposed existence of two subclasses of β-adrenoceptors, referred to as β_1 and β_2. Further credence was given to this classification by the discovery of agonists at β-adrenoceptors that

showed bronchoselectivity; that is they could produce useful bronchodilation at doses that produced minimal cardiac stimulation (e.g. salbutamol). Similarly, a class of cardioselective antagonists was discovered (e.g. practolol). However, it should be noted that the selectivity ratios of these drugs (i.e. the ratios between doses causing effects on tissues bearing β_1- or β_2-adrenoceptors), are unimpressive when compared with the selectivities of drugs such as methoxamine and propranolol (practolol has a cardioselectivity of less than 100-fold, whereas selectivities of 10 000 or more are not uncommon in drugs that differentiate between α and the major classes of β-adrenoceptors). Further difficulties with the β_1, β_2 subclassification have arisen when rigorous numerical analyses are used. These problems are particularly acute when dispositional mechanisms (uptake and metabolism) are taken into account and in such studies $\beta_1-\beta_2$ selectivities are often greatly reduced, particularly for agonists. However, strong support for the existence of these two subclasses has come from radioligand binding studies, which although not showing persuasive differences in the binding affinities of agonists, do show clear differences between the antagonists. Genetic engineering techniques have led to the identification of at least three distinct β-adrenoceptor sub-types. The complete amino acid sequences of two of these have been established. Consequently, although the explanation for the undoubted organ selectivity of certain agonists at β-adrenoceptors may include other factors, it is clear that at least two subpopulations of β-adrenoceptors exist and thus the $\beta_1- \beta_2-$ -adrenoceptor classification is in practice a very useful way of summarising the pharmacology of drugs acting at β-adrenoceptors. A summary of this subclassification is given in Table 16.3. The classification of α-adrenoceptors into α_1 and α_2 subtypes is described later in this chapter.

Table 16.3 Subclassification of β-adrenoceptors

	β_1 Heart, gut, fat cells liver (glycogenolysis, gluconeogenesis)	β_2 Arterioles, bronchioles, uterus (term), skeletal muscle (tremor)
Agonist	NORADRENALINE adrenaline ISOPRENALINE salbutamol	noradrenaline ADRENALINE ISOPRENALINE SALBUTAMOL
Antagonists	PROPRANOLOL [PRACTOLOL] BUTOXAMINE ATENOLOL	PROPRANOLOL PRACTOLOL BUTOXAMINE atenolol

The selectivities of drugs are indicated by the relative sizes of the typefaces.

Termination of the effects of noradrenaline

The enzyme monoamine oxidase (MAO) was first isolated in 1928, although it was not until 1937 that it was shown to inactivate adrenaline. Until the development of selective inhibitors of MAO in the 1950s, this enzyme was assumed to be responsible for terminating the effects of the transmitter released from sympathetic neurons. However, inhibitors of MAO were soon shown to have little effect on tissue responses to either sympathetic nerve stimulation or exogenous noradrenaline. A second enzyme capable of inactivating noradrenaline was soon discovered, namely catechol-O-methyl transferase, but experiments with selective inhibitors were as unimpressive as those with MAO inhibitors. The observation that cocaine greatly augmented the effects of sympathetic nerve stimulation, known since 1910, was eventually explained when radioactively-labelled noradrenaline of high specific activity became available. It was found that sympathetically innervated tissues take up noradrenaline avidly, and that this process is potently inhibited by cocaine. The characteristics of this uptake system were studied in great detail and can be summarized as follows. There exist two uptake processes for noradrenaline, one of high affinity located in the membrane of noradrenergic neurones, named uptake$_1$, and a second process of lower affinity located in non-neuronal cell membranes called uptake$_2$.

Uptake$_1$

Uptake$_1$ shows a reasonable degree of specificity, transporting L-isomers better than D-isomers and noradrenaline better than adrenaline. The process has the characteristics of a carrier-mediated active transport system — it is saturable, requires metabolic energy derived either from aerobic or anaerobic sources and can pump against a concentration gradient, although it seldom if ever does, as noradrenaline pumped into the cytoplasm is rapidly removed by the vesicular uptake system described earlier or is oxidized by cytoplasmic MAO. Uptake$_1$ also requires Na$^+$ ions and is inhibited by high concentrations of K$^+$ ions. A variety of structures related to noradrenaline are substrates for uptake$_1$, providing certain structural requirements are met. The presence of large substituents on the terminal nitrogen atom reduces affinity for uptake$_1$ — adrenaline has about half the affinity of noradrenaline whereas isoprenaline is not transported at all. The presence of ring hydroxyl groups favours the process, compounds devoid of these being poor substrates whereas those with 3,4-dihydroxy substitution in the ring (catechols) have higher affinities than either their monohydroxy or 3-

methoxy, 4-hydroxy counterparts. The indirect sympathomimetics ephedrine and amphetamine appear to be poorly transported, so it must be concluded that their ability to cause noradrenaline release from vesicles within intact noradrenergic neurons depends upon their being able to penetrate the axon membrane readily by simple diffusion. This hypothesis is consistent both with their structures which show them to be considerably less polar than noradrenaline, and with the ease with which amphetamine and ephedrine are known to cross the blood–brain barrier.

The neuronal uptake mechanism, uptake$_1$, serves not only to terminate the action of released noradrenaline, a prerequisite for efficient chemical transmission, but also to increase the efficiency of the overall transmission process by minimizing the extent of de novo synthesis of noradrenaline. It has been estimated that at least 70% of the noradrenaline released during normal transmission is taken back into noradrenergic neurons (uptake$_1$), sequestered in storage vesicles and subsequently made available for release again.

Interference with uptake$_1$. The classical inhibitor of uptake$_1$ is cocaine, which exhibits this property at concentrations at least an order of magnitude lower than those necessary for local anaesthesia. Other local anaesthetics do not share this property of cocaine. Inhibitors of uptake$_1$ abolish responses to tyramine but augment the effects of both exogenous noradrenaline and those due to activity in sympathetic nerves. The effects of other drugs that depend upon uptake$_1$ for their action are also impaired (e.g. the noradrenergic neuron blocking agents, with the exception of reserpine). At sites where noradrenergic neurons are tonically active, uptake$_1$ inhibitors will cause an overt response. This may explain the central action of drugs such as the tricyclic antidepressants and methylphenidate. Inhibitors of uptake$_1$ can be classified as being either substrates themselves, in which case the inhibition is usually competitive, or as non-transported inhibitors (which may or may not be competitive). Substrates that inhibit neuronal uptake of noradrenaline include sympathomimetics (e.g. tyramine) and noradrenergic neuron blocking agents (e.g. guanethidine, but not reserpine). Non-transported inhibitors include cocaine, the tricyclic antidepressants (e.g. imipramine), CNS stimulants (e.g. methylphenidate), many of the phenothiazines (e.g. chlorpromazine — note that some of the effects are likely to be offset because phenothiazines are often antagonists at α-adrenoceptors as well), haloalkylamines (e.g. phenoxybenzamine), and Na$^+$/K$^+$-ATPase inhibitors (e.g. digoxin). Low concentrations of Li$^+$ actually enhance neuronal uptake of noradrenaline, resulting in a lowering of the concentration of transmitter in the region of adrenoceptors. This may contribute to the beneficial effects of long-term therapy with lithium in manic depression.

Uptake₂

Uptake₂

Like uptake₁, the noradrenaline pumping system designated uptake₂ displays saturation kinetics, although it has a much lower affinity for substrates than does uptake₁ (i.e. it saturates at much higher concentrations). Thus at the concentrations of noradrenaline used experimentally to induce responses, uptake₁ and metabolic degradation mask the small contribution of uptake₂ to the overall inactivation of noradrenaline. In general the structural requirements for uptake₂ are less rigorous than for neuronal uptake, although clear rules appear to apply. In contrast to uptake₁, *N*-substitution and ring *O*-methylation favour uptake₂. Thus both isoprenaline and normetadrenaline (the *O*-methylated derivative of noradrenaline) are substrates for uptake₂ but not for uptake₁.

Another important difference between the two processes is their location. Uptake₁ is located exclusively at the membrane of noradrenergic neurons, whereas uptake₂, although probably present at the same site, is primarily located at the membrane of smooth muscle cells. Classical uptake₂ into smooth muscle cells is characteristically followed rapidly by enzymic degradation, largely by catechol-*O*-methylation, a phenomenon which is particularly noticeable at low concentrations. In addition to terminating the action of that small portion

of noradrenaline released from neurons but not recaptured by them, it is possible that uptake₂ is responsible, in part at least, for the inactivation of catecholamines released into the circulation from the adrenal medulla. This would be of even greater significance in terminating the effects of adrenaline on effector organs devoid of a noradrenergic innervation.

Drugs that interfere with uptake₂. Inhibitors of uptake₁, such as cocaine and imipramine, do not in general inhibit uptake₂. An exception, however, is phenoxybenzamine, which has similar inhibitory potency on both systems. Studies with other 2-haloalkylamines have shown inhibition of uptake to be independent of affinity for α-adrenoceptors. Treatment with phenoxybenzamine will therefore potentiate agents which act at β-adrenoceptors and are substrates for either uptake₁ or uptake₂ (or both).

Other drugs that inhibit uptake₂ include certain steroids, notably hydrocortisone and oestradiol, which partly explains the finding that treatment with hydrocortisone can augment responses to subsequently administered sympathomimetics.

Enzymic degradation

Enzymic degradation

Although uptake is responsible for the removal of noradrenaline from the region of the adrenoceptors, there exist a variety of enzymic processes capable of transforming phenylethylamines into inactive metabolites. These are summarized in Figure 16.3

Monoamine oxidase (MAO). This enzyme is lo-

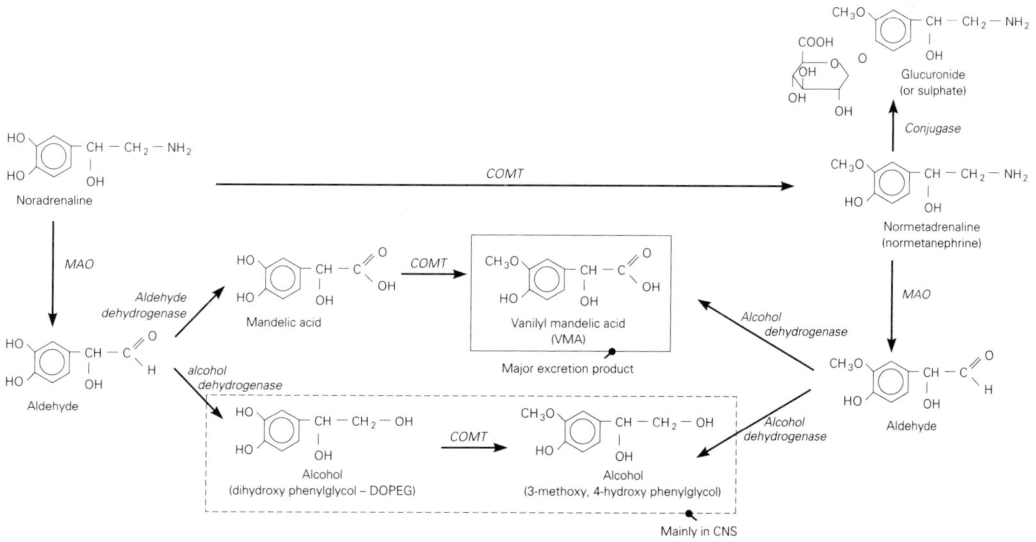

Fig. 16.3 Summary of enzymic processes capable of transforming phenylethylamines into active metabolites.

cated in the membranes of the mitochondria which are so abundant in the varicosities of noradrenergic nerves and chromaffin cells. MAO is also found in the mitochondria of liver and intestinal mucosa. The enzyme uses FAD (flavine adenine dinucleotide) as a prosthetic group and requires a heavy metal ion as cofactor. The basic structural requirement of substrates for MAO is that they should possess an ethylamine chain attached to an aromatic ring. Ring substituents, e.g. catechol or 3-methoxy-4-hydroxy-groups on a phenyl ring, make little or no difference to the affinity, whereas substitutions in the side chain tend to reduce affinity, this effect being more marked the bigger the substituent and the nearer it is to the terminal nitrogen. Thus noradrenaline (with a hydroxyl group on the β-carbon atom of the side chain) has lower affinity than dopamine; adrenaline (N-methyl) has lower affinity than noradrenaline whereas isoprenaline (N-isopropyl) is totally resistant. Substitution on the α-carbon atom abolishes susceptibility, e.g. ephedrine, methoxamine, metaraminol, phenylpropanolamine. The enzyme catalyses the conversion of the amine to the aldehyde, which may then be further oxidized to the acid by virtue of aldehyde dehydrogenase, or the aldehyde may be reduced to the alcohol by alcohol dehydrogenase. MAO appears to subserve two functions, that in noradrenergic nerves and chromaffin cells being concerned with removing surplus transmitter from the cytoplasm. This is important to cell economy as high cytoplasmic noradrenaline concentrations inhibit tyrosine hydroxylase, thereby reducing the overall rate of noradrenaline synthesis. The MAO in the liver and intestinal mucosa seems to have a role in protecting the body from ingested amines or amines generated by bacterial action in the gut.

MAO in fact comprises several isozymes, which are generally classified into two major types referred to as MAO-A and MAO-B. Although most nerves contain both isozymes, the liver and intestinal mucosa contain mainly the A type, whereas certain parts of the brain, particularly the striatum, contain predominantly MAO-B.

Originally, inhibitors of MAO were non-selective, e.g. phenelzine and tranylcypromine, and although they found a place in the therapy of depressive illness, and at one time as hypotensive agents, their usefulness is compromised by a serious interaction with several medicaments and dietary components, notably indirect sympathomimetics in cough and cold remedies and tyramine-containing foodstuffs. In the case of indirect sympathomimetics, though they themselves may not be substrates for MAO, a proportion of the noradrenaline they displace from the storage vesicles is normally oxidized before diffusing out of the neurons.

More recently it has proved possible to synthesize inhibitors selective for MAO-B. The first of these available for use in man was selegiline (deprenyl), which although having a short plasma half-life, has a prolonged action as it is itself a substrate and forms an irreversible complex with the enzyme once activated by MAO — an example of 'suicide inhibition'. Selegiline does not cause the 'cheese reaction' in response to dietary tyramine, as the intestinal and hepatic MAO-A is uninhibited and noradrenergic nerves are therefore protected from ingested tyramine. While selegiline does benefit depressed patients, its primary use is in Parkinson's disease as an adjunct to levodopa treatment, allowing the daily dose of levodopa to be reduced by as much as 30% with a concomitant reduction in the incidence and severity of adverse reactions. There have been some reports that selegiline actually slows down the development of Parkinson's disease. This is under investigation, but could result from reduced formation of neurotoxic intermediates.

Catechol-O-methyl transferase (COMT). There are high concentrations of COMT in the liver as well as in cells receiving a noradrenergic innervation, especially smooth muscle and cardiac cells (see pp. 264–5). Although there is probably COMT in noradrenergic neurons, its physiological significance here is uncertain (see below). The enzyme exists in solution in the cytoplasm, requires Mg^{2+} ions and acts upon catechols to produce the methoxy-derivative. All the catecholamines are therefore substrates, whereas drugs such as ephedrine, metaraminol, methoxamine, phenylephrine, salbutamol, tyramine and tyrosine are not. The function of COMT in the liver seems to be similar to that of MAO, i.e. to protect the body from potentially harmful catechol-containing agents in the diet. COMT in muscle cells of noradrenergically innervated tissues probably has a role in inactivating noradrenaline and adrenaline when the local concentration is high enough to saturate the neuronal uptake system (see above). It is also likely to play a part in terminating the actions of adrenaline (from the adrenal medulla) in tissues without a noradrenergic innervation. Although a number of inhibitors of COMT are used in experimental pharmacology, e.g. pyrogallol and β-thujaplicin, none has any place in therapeutics.

PARASYMPATHETIC DIVISION

Innervation of organs and effects mediated

The parasympathetic nervous system is shown diagrammatically in Figure 16.4 and effects mediated through the parasympathetic system are summarized in Table 16.4

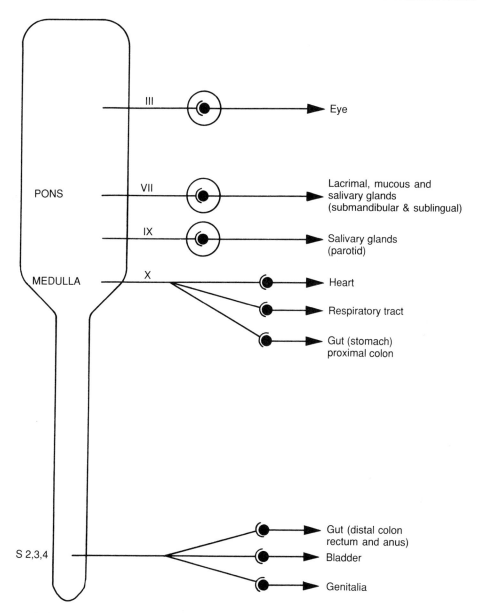

III → Eye

PONS

VII → Lacrimal, mucous and salivary glands (submandibular & sublingual)

IX → Salivary glands (parotid)

MEDULLA

X → Heart

→ Respiratory tract

→ Gut (stomach) proximal colon

S 2,3,4

→ Gut (distal colon rectum and anus)

→ Bladder

→ Genitalia

Fig. 16.4 Parasympathetic nervous system.

The preganglionic neurons of the parasympathetic system leave the CNS in cranial nerves III (occulomotor), VII (facial), IX (glossopharyngeal) and X (vagus) and also in the ventral roots of segments S–2 to S–4 of the spinal cord. The effects of activity in parasympathetic nerves to the various organs are summarized in Table 16.4. The parasympathetic fibres in cranial nerve III arise from Edinger–Westphal nucleus and run with the nerve trunk into the orbit where they synapse in the ciliary ganglion which lies in the fat pad behind the eyeball. Postganglionic fibres from the ciliary ganglion radiate around the back of the eyeball and penetrate to supply the ciliary muscle and the circular muscles of the iris (constrictor pupillae). Parasympathetic fibres in cranial nerve VII leave the main nerve and travel in one of two small branches, either the greater superficial petrosal nerve, in which case they synapse in the sphenopalatine ganglion lying in the upper part of the pterygopalatine fossa from which postganglionic fibres supply the mucous glands of the

Table 16.4   Responses to activity in parasympathetic nerves

Organ	Effect
Cardiovascular system	
Heart	
SA node	(a) membrane hyperpolarised (hence longer to reach threshold and slope of prepotential decreased)
	(b) AP duration reduced
	(c) refractory period reduced
	(d) conduction velocity reduced
AV node	(a) refractory period increased
	(b) conduction velocity reduced
Atria	(a) membrane hyperpolarized
	(b) conduction velocity reduced
	(c) refractory period reduced
	(d) force of contraction reduced (partly direct effect, partly due to reduced rate)
Ventricles	no parasympathetic innervation; hence reduced force of contraction seen on vagal stimulation indirect and caused by bradycardia
Arterioles	
Salivary glands	dilated
Resistance vessels	*Note:* Most resistance vessels bear muscarinic cholinoceptors despite not having parasympathetic innervation; stimulation by circulating agonists causes vasodilation
Gastrointestinal system	
Propulsive muscle	activity increased
Sphincters	relaxed
Biliary tract	constricted
Digestive glands (Salivary, acini of pancreas, gastric, intestinal)	increased secretion
Genito-urinary system	
Bladder	
detrusor	contraction
trigone and sphincter	relaxation
Erectile tissue	vasodilation (engorgement and erection)
Eye	
Radial muscle of iris	contraction (miosis)
Ciliary muscle	contraction (accommodation for near vision)
Lachrymal glands	increased secretion
Respiratory tract	
Bronchial smooth muscle	contraction
Mucous glands	increased secretion

nasopharynx and the lachrymal glands, or in the chorda tympani, which joins with the lingual nerve in the pharynx. Preganglionic parasympathetic fibres then leave the lingual nerve near the root of the tongue to synapse in the submandibular and sublingual ganglia lying on the surfaces of the submandibular and sublingual salivary glands respectively, to which their postganglionic fibres are distributed. Parasympathetic fibres from cranial nerve IX leave the nerve trunk and synapse in the otic ganglion, which lies at the base of the skull immediately below the foramen ovale. Postganglionic fibres from the otic ganglion innervate the parotid salivary glands. (The otic ganglion may also receive some preganglionic parasympathetic fibres from the facial nerve via the lesser petrosal nerve.) Parasympathetic fibres in cranial nerve X (the vagus — from the Latin meaning 'the wanderer') innervate organs outside the head and neck. The cell bodies of the postsynaptic fibres are not located in discrete ganglia but are distributed diffusely throughout the innervated organs so that postganglionic fibres are very short. Fibres from the vagus innervate the heart (SA node, atria and AV node only), the respiratory tract and the propulsive muscle and secretory cells of the gut down to the proximal colon. Beyond this level the gut receives its parasympathetic supply from the sacral outflow, which also supplies the bladder and genitalia. In the gut the cell bodies of the postganglionic fibres are found mostly in the two nerve plexi, namely Auerbach's plexus and Meissner's plexus.

In all cases cholinoceptors on effector organs are of the muscarinic type, having high affinity for the choline esters methacholine and carbachol as well as for the alkaloid pilocarpine. The effects shown in Table 16.4 can be reduced or abolished by antagonists at muscarinic cholinoceptors such as atropine, glycopyrronium and hyoscine.

Synthesis and storage of acetylcholine

Acetylcholine is an ester formed from two chemicals that are both widely distributed in the body and relatively abundant — namely choline, which is a vital component of the lecithins and consequently of many lipid structures within the body, and acetate in the form of acetyl coenzyme A (acetyl-CoA), an essential part of normal energy metabolism. The formation of acetylcholine is catalysed by the enzyme choline acetyltransferase, which is located in free solution in the cytoplasm of cholinergic neurons and also in association with cholinergic storage vesicles. Choline, although freely available in the plasma, does not penetrate membranes easily as it is highly polar. However, presumably because choline is an essential ingredient for normal cellular function, there exists an energy-dependent pump system capable of transporting choline into cholinergic neurons at a rate high enough to maintain adequate acetylcholine synthesis, even during prolonged periods of maximal nervous activity. This system, which probably comprises at least two distinct pumps, also serves to remove that choline from the synaptic cleft which has been produced by acetylcholinesterase from the acetylcholine released in response to action potentials. Acetyl-CoA, which is synthesized in mitochondria, like choline, is unable to penetrate membranes easily and hence is unavailable to the synthetic process in the cytoplasm. It is believed that the acetyl-CoA is converted in the mito-

chondria to citrate by the agency of the enzyme citrate synthetase. The citrate diffuses out into the cytoplasm where it once more becomes acetyl-CoA under the influence of ATP-citrate lyase.

The precise mechanisms by which the acetylcholine synthesized in the cytoplasm enters the storage vesicles and is there sequestered are unknown, but it is likely that there is a transport pump in the vesicle responsible for the movement of at least part of the acetylcholine stored in the vesicles. Like noradrenergic vesicles, vesicles in cholinergic nerves are rich in ATP and also contain a sulphomucopolysaccharide and a soluble protein which are believed to play a role in the storage of the acetylcholine. This protein has been named 'vesiculin', and has a molecular weight in excess of 10 000, although it has not yet been fully characterized or sequenced. A diagrammatic summary of acetylcholine synthesis is given in Figure 16.5.

A number of drugs that interfere with acetylcholine synthesis have been discovered, but they are of no therapeutic significance. Hemicholinium-3 (HC–3) inhibits the choline uptake pump so that, as acetylcholine is released from vesicular stores, the neuron gradually becomes depleted as there is insufficient raw material for transmitter synthesis. Triethylcholine produces a similar failure of transmission by a different mechanism. This agent is accumulated by neurons in place of choline and acetylated to inactive acetyltriethylcholine. Substances such as acetyltriethylcholine, formed from analogues of natural transmitter precursors but lacking normal activity, are known as 'false transmitters'. Triethylcholine is also believed to inhibit choline acetyltransferase to some extent, which causes further interference with transmission.

Release of acetylcholine

Like the release of noradrenaline and other transmitters, the release of acetylcholine in response to the depolarization of the axon membrane is dependent upon extracellular Ca^{2+} ions. The massive release of acetylcholine is the result of synchronous discharge of the contents of many storage vesicles (exocytosis). This parallels the release of noradrenaline almost exactly — depolarization causes an influx of Ca^{2+} ions which in some way stimulate the storage vesicles to fuse with the axon membrane. The fusion sites then break down so that the contents of the vesicles are expelled into the extracellular space, whereupon the vesicles pinch off again from the membrane, are recycled and refilled with transmitter.

Acetylcholine release can be inhibited by reducing the

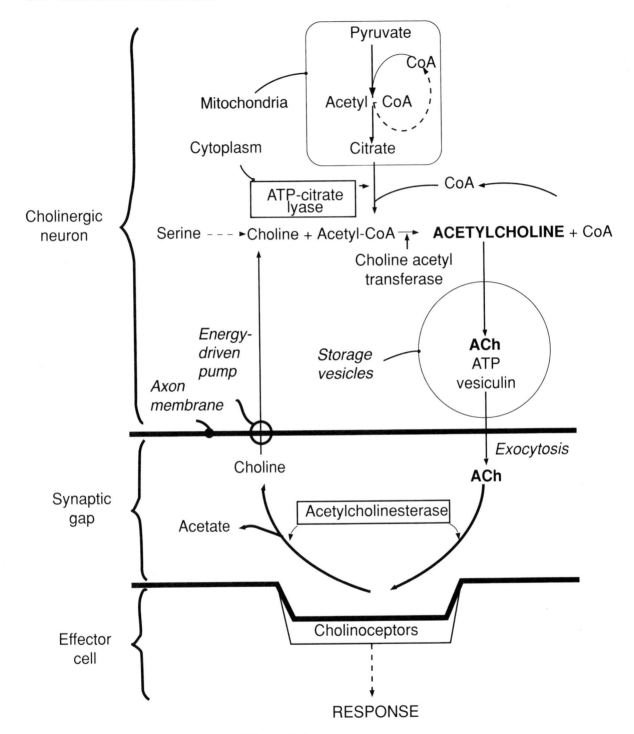

Fig. 16.5 Diagrammatic summary of acetylcholine synthesis.

extracellular Ca^{2+} ion concentration or by raising the extracellular Mg^{2+} ion concentration. Perhaps of more therapeutic importance is the inhibition of acetylcholine release caused by botulinus toxin. Food poisoning by *Clostridium botulinum* results from the production by the bacillus of the toxin known as botulinus toxin, one of the most potent toxins known; fortunately poisoning with this toxin is rare in developed countries. The toxin does not interfere with action potential development or transmission but selectively and persistently disrupts the acetylcholine release mechanism by binding irreversibly to some component of the nerve membrane, probably a ganglioside. Although prevention of acetylcholine release from autonomic nerves is not in itself life-threatening, botulism is potentially fatal because failure of transmission at somatic neuromuscular junctions causes respiratory paralysis which may be of several months duration.

Other toxins that inhibit release of acetylcholine include β–bungarotoxin, a component of a cobra venom (*Bungarus multicinctus*), and the venom of two closely related species of spiders, the American black widow (*Latrodectus mactans tredicimguttatus*) and the Australian red back (*L. mactans hasseltii*). While β-bungarotoxin appears to be selective for cholinergic somatic motor nerves and preganglionic cholinergic nerves in the autonomic system, the spider toxins also disrupt release from noradrenergic neurons. Death from the venoms of these spiders is also due to respiratory paralysis. Fatal poisoning resulting from the bite of *Bungarus* is more complex, as the venom contains other components, one of which is curare-like and another of which causes haemolysis.

Termination of the action of acetylcholine

Once acetylcholine has been released from nerves, the majority is rapidly inactivated by a cholinesterase enzyme, which hydrolyses the transmitter, thereby producing choline and acetate ions. In fact there are many related cholinesterases, the spectrum of activity of which varies somewhat but allows classification into two major types.

Acetylcholinesterase

Acetylcholinesterase (also referred to as true or specific cholinesterase) is located at cholinergic nerve endings and at skeletal muscle endplates, at both sites being responsible for the primary inactivation of transmitter acetylcholine. Curiously, this form of cholinesterase is also found in erythrocytes and in association with certain non-cholinergic nerves, the significance of this distribution being unknown. Apart from acetylcholine, methacholine is a good substrate for acetylcholinesterase, whereas suxamethonium and benzoyl-choline are resistant (see Chapter 19).

Butyrylcholinesterase

Butyrylcholinesterase (also known simply as cholinesterase or pseudocholinesterase) is found in the liver and in solution in the plasma, with a limited distribution to certain glial cells within the CNS. This form of the enzyme is not found in association with cholinergic nerves or skeletal muscle endplates. In addition to acetylcholine, butyrylcholinesterase will hydrolyse suxamethonium, butyrylcholine and benzoylcholine but not methacholine. The function of butyrylcholinesterase is unknown.

Both types of the enzyme are susceptible to inhibition by physostigmine, whereas butyrylcholinesterase is in general more susceptible to inhibition by the organophosphorus anticholinesterases (see Chapter 20). Carbachol is totally resistant to both forms of the enzyme.

Prejunctional receptors

In 1957 it was found that phenoxybenzamine increased the overflow of noradrenaline when the nerve supply to the perfused cat spleen was stimulated. At first it was proposed that this phenomenon was due to inhibition of noradrenaline uptake. However, more selective uptake inhibitors such as cocaine and imipramine were shown not to increase transmitter overflow. Later, when it was shown that other antagonists at α-adrenoceptors had the same effect as phenoxybenzamine, it was proposed that the α-adrenoceptors on the postjunctional membrane had some sort of influence on the function of prejunctional nerve terminals. This theory was abandoned when it was shown that antagonists at α-adrenoceptors also augmented the release of noradrenaline from nerves supplying organs with only β-adrenoceptors — e.g. sympathetic nerves to the heart. It is now accepted that the phenomenon is due to disinhibition, i.e. interference with the feedback inhibition of noradrenaline release, mediated through prejunctional (sometimes called presynaptic) α-adrenoceptors.

Pharmacological studies have revealed that in general there are different structural requirements for binding to prejunctional and postjunctional α-adrenoceptors. This gives further validity to the subclassification of α-adrenoceptors into α_1 and α_2, which was originally made on the basis of location — α_1-adrenoceptors being the classical postjunctional receptors whereas α_2-adrenoceptors are those located on noradrenergic nerve terminals. The selectivities of agonists and antagonists for the two types of adrenoceptors are shown in Table 16.5.

Table 16.5 Subclassification of α-adrenoceptors

	α_1 (postjunctional)	α_2 (prejunctional)
Agonists	cirazoline methoxamine phenylephrine adrenaline noradrenaline	guanabenz clonidine a-CH$_3$-noradrenaline adrenaline noradrenaline
Antagonists	prazosin labetalol phentolamine phenoxybenzamine	rauwolscine yohimbine phentolamine phenoxybenzamine

In addition to α_2-adrenoceptors, noradrenergic neurons are now believed to bear a variety of other types of prejunctional receptors, some of which inhibit noradrenaline release and some of which facilitate release. These are listed in Table 16.6.

Table 16.6 Prejunctional receptors on noradrenergic neurons

Receptors mediating inhibition

α_2-adrenoceptors	prostanoid receptors (E series)
dopamine receptors	adenosine receptors
muscarinic cholinoceptors	tryptamine receptors
opioid receptors	histamine receptors

Receptors mediating facilitation
β-adrenoceptors (possibly β_2)
nicotinic cholinoceptors
GABA receptors
angiotensin receptors

It is now the view that many, if not all, types of nerves bear prejunctional receptors, both for their own transmitter, in which case they are referred to as *autoreceptors*, and which are usually inhibitory, or for other mediators, which may be either inhibitory or facilitatory. (Some workers refer to this latter type of prejunctional receptor as *heteroreceptors*). Nerve types known to bear inhibitory autoreceptors include noradrenergic, adrenergic, dopaminergic, cholinergic, tryptaminergic and GABA-containing neurons.

The functional significance of prejunctional receptors is unclear. It is likely that many of the prejunctional receptors are evolutionary freaks or remnants which no

longer have any physiological significance, but which have not been selected out as they have no adverse effect upon survival. However, a rational proposal for a role for inhibitory autoreceptors can easily be made, the central theme of which is again conservation of transmitter. If neuronal activity is so high that the junctional concentration of transmitter rises above that necessary to produce a near-maximal response (say $> EC_{90}$), then it seems entirely reasonable that a mechanism should exist whereby this high junctional transmitter concentration should inhibit the release of further transmitter through an action on autoreceptors on the nerve membrane. The process by which this feedback inhibition is actually achieved, however, is not fully understood, although it appears that activation of inhibitory prejunctional receptors reduces an availability of Ca^{2+} to the exocytotic mechanism. In the case of facilitatory β-adrenoceptors on noradrenergic neurons, it has been suggested that they play a role in promoting efficient transmission by augmenting noradrenaline release when low rates of nerve activity pertain, so that the junctional noradrenaline concentration is kept above threshold for stimulation of the postjunctional adrenoceptors. In addition prejunctional β-adrenoceptors may serve to augment noradrenaline output from nerves in response to high circulating levels of adrenaline from the adrenal medulla. It is less simple to find a rational role for prejunctional receptors sensitive to substances which are not that neuron's transmitter. However, it is possible that these prejunctional receptors exist to modify nerve function in response to circulating factors such as angiotensin.

Therapeutic significance

It has long been appreciated that classical antagonists at α-adrenoceptors, such as phenoxybenzamine and phentolamine, are of limited value in the treatment of essential hypertension. This is in part because they cause a marked degree of reflex tachycardia, presumably initiated by the baroreceptors in response to the drug-induced fall in blood pressure. An additional cause of this tachycardia is now recognized to be the removal by the antagonist of the feedback inhibition of noradrenaline release mediated by prejunctional α_2-adrenoceptors on the sympathetic nerves to the heart. Prazosin, however, has found a useful place in the armamentarium as it appears not to cause this excessive reflex tachycardia, despite being an antagonist at α-adrenoceptors with a potency no less than phentolamine. This is probably due to its relative selectivity for α_1-adrenoceptors, which are located only on effector organs (e.g. smooth muscle of blood vessels). Hence the release of noradrenaline from sympathetic nerves to the heart is still subject to feedback autoinhibition through prejunctional α_2-adrenoceptors.

It has also been proposed that part of the hypotensive action of angiotensin converting enzyme inhibitors (e.g. captopril) results from a reduction in circulating angiotensin II and a consequent reduction in the release of noradrenaline due to the reduced facilitatory effect of the peptide. The centrally acting drugs clonidine and α-methyl-noradrenaline (formed from the pro-drug methyldopa) may also be exerting their hypotensive action by selective stimulation of prejunctional α-adrenoceptors (i.e. α_2) on central adrenergic or noradrenergic neurons in those pathways concerned with maintenance of normal blood pressure.

Axonal conduction

Although an analogy is often drawn between axons and telephone wires, this is rather misleading, as conduction of impulses in nerve fibres is a very much more active process than the passive conduction of electricity down a copper wire. This results from the relatively poor conductance of even the best biological conductors (e.g. axoplasm) in comparison with that of metals such as copper. Consequently efficient, rapid conduction in nerves can occur without unacceptable attenuation of the signal only if energy is expended and the signal continuously amplified. A better analogy is to view the nerve cell as a cross between a telephone wire and an electrical accumulator, using its stored electrical energy to send a signal in the form of a self-propagating change in the insulating properties of the outer case (axon membrane). To understand this better it is necessary to examine the origin of the resting membrane potential.

Resting membrane potential

The potential difference across a typical neuron membrane is about 70 mV with the inside negative relative to the outside. This potential difference arises because the membrane is permeable to K^+ ions but relatively impermeable to Na^+ ions and totally impermeable to most intracellular anions — mainly proteins and organic phosphates. The intracellular K^+ concentration is high (ca. 140 mM inside as opposed to only 5 mM outside) whereas the intracellular Na^+ concentration is low (10 mM inside, 140 mM outside). As the membrane is relatively permeable to K^+, intracellular K^+ ions tend to diffuse outwards, down their concentration gradient. Electrical neutrality would be maintained if there were

either an efflux of intracellular anions or an influx of extracellular cations. However, as the membrane is totally impermeable to the major intracellular anions and almost totally impermeable to the main extracellular cation, Na^+, the result is a net efflux of positive charge, leaving the inside of the neuron negative respect to the extracellular fluid. This diffusion of K^+ ions down their concentration gradient continues until the inwardly directed electrical gradient this generates (negative inside tending to pull K^+ ions into the neuron) equals the outwardly directed concentration gradient. The potential at which these two opposing forces are equal is known as the *equilibrium potential* for K^+, and can be calculated from the Nernst equation:-

$$E = \left(\frac{RT}{F}\right) \times \log_e \left(\frac{[K^+]_{out}}{[K^+]_{in}}\right)$$

where R is the thermodynamic gas constant,
T is the thermodynamic temperature,
F is the Faraday constant.

If this expression is evaluated using the values for K^+ concentration given above, the equilibrium potential is found to be 88 mV, which is some 15–20 mV higher than that obtained by direct measurement with microelectrodes. The discrepancy cannot be explained by a Cl^- potential as the evidence indicates that Cl^- ions simply equilibrate across the membrane in response to the potential difference generated by the difference in K^+ ion concentrations. The residual potential is in fact due to the small, but nevertheless important, permeability to Na^+ ions, so that the outward movement of positive charge carried by K^+ ions is partly offset by a much smaller inward movement of positive charge carried by Na^+ ions. A modification to the Nernst equation was proposed by Hodgkin and Horowicz (1959) which gives a theoretical value for the resting membrane potential very close to that found experimentally:-

$$E = \left(\frac{RT}{F}\right) \times \log_e \left(\frac{[K^+]_{out} + a[Na]_{out}}{[K^+]_{in} + a[Na]_{in}}\right)$$

where a is the *permeability ratio*, P_{Na}/P_K, and is usually of the order of 0.01.

This small permeability to Na^+ would result in the gradual exchange of Na^+ for K^+ and the disappearence of the K^+ concentration gradient and hence of the membrane potential. This run-down is prevented by the presence in the nerve membrane of an energy-requiring ionic pump that extrudes Na^+ ions in exchange for K^+ ions. This pump utilizes ATP and is often referred to as Na^+/K^+ ATPase. In the final analysis it is the continuous expenditure of chemical energy by this pump that allows the charge separation to occur, and this in its turn provides the electrical energy for the propagation of the action potential.

The origin of the action potential

Although the nerve membrane at rest is relatively impermeable to Na^+ ions, a dramatic change in permeability occurs if the membrane potential changes. If the inside of the cell becomes less negative relative to the outside (either because positive charges are injected artificially, e.g. through a microelectrode, or because of an action potential), when the potential is reduced to about 15 mV, there is a sudden increase in the permeability to Na^+ ions. This critical potential is known as the *threshold*. The sudden influx of Na^+ ions is sufficient to bring the potential across the membrane close to the equilibrium potential for Na^+ predicted by the Nernst equation (56 mV, inside positive). This Na^+ influx is believed to be due to the simultaneous opening of numerous specific channels or pores in the membrane, each being sufficiently large to accommodate a hydrated Na^+ ion. These Na^+ channels open only briefly, and appear to close in response to the increase in positive charge inside the membrane, a process known as *inactivation*. Depolarization also causes a small but sustained increase in the permeability of the membrane to K^+ ions which does not inactivate, so that as the Na^+ channels are inactivated, an increased efflux of positive charge (K^+ ions) persists, and this hastens repolarization. In addition, the Na^+/K^+ ATPase is stimulated and the excess Na^+ ions are extruded in exchange for K^+ ions.

In reality the total number of ions moving across the membrane during each action potential is very small in comparison with the total ion content of the nerve. However, the localized changes in concentration close to the membrane are large. This explains why repolarization can in fact occur without ionic pumping by Na^+/K^+ ATPase. If the enzyme is inhibited then the surplus Na^+ ions near the membrane at the end of the action potential are rapidly distributed by passive diffusion into the axoplasm, so that the concentration of Na^+ in the region of the inner surface of the membrane returns rapidly to near the resting level. A typical neuron can conduct many thousands of action potentials once the Na^+/K^+ ATPase has been inhibited before action potential generation fails due to the ionic gradients becoming insufficient to support a resting potential greater (i.e. more negative) than the threshold.

Propagation of action potentials

For non-myelinated neurons action potential propagation is a relatively simple process in which a wave of activity passes along the nerve. As one patch of the membrane becomes active, its potential briefly reverses (i.e. it becomes positive inside) relative to the adjacent patch of resting membrane. This results in current flowing in a local 'short-circuit' which progressively reduces the potential across the patch of resting membrane. In response, the permeability of the resting membrane to Na^+ gradually increases, allowing further depolarization until the threshold is reached and the massive increase in Na^+ influx of the action potential is triggered. The previously resting patch of membrane is now active and itself short-circuits the next patch of resting membrane, while the recently active patch, now behind the wave front, repolarizes as the Na^+ channels are inactivated. In this way the region of activity moves continually forward down the nerve in a process that has been likened to the spread of fire down a lighted fuse.

Under normal physiological circumstances the impulse will always be initiated at the same end of the axon, so that propagation is always unidirectional. However, an artificial stimulus or injury to the other end of the axon will cause an impulse to be propagated just as easily in the reverse direction. Normal propagation is known as *orthodromic*, whereas propagation in the reverse direction is known as *antidromic*. Parenthetically it should be pointed out that an impulse applied to the middle of a fibre will cause two impulses to be propagated at equal velocities away from the stimulus.

In myelinated neurons, impulse propagation is more complex but more efficient. The insulating sheath of myelin prevents the active patch of the membrane from short-circuiting the adjacent resting membrane. However, depolarization at a node of Ranvier, where the membrane has no sheath, causes a potential difference to develop between the active node and the nearest resting node. This induces a flow of current as the resting node is in electrical continuity with the active node, through both the extracellular fluid and the axoplasm. Consequently the resting node begins to depolarize until it too crosses the threshold and fires an action potential which in turn activates the next node along the nerve. This kind of propagation, in which activity jumps from node to node, is known as *saltatory conduction*, and is much more rapid than that in unmyelinated fibres of a similar diameter. An additional benefit is that because only a few discrete patches of membrane become active, relatively few Na^+ and K^+ ions cross the membrane so that relatively little metabolic energy is expended in maintaining the necessary ionic gradients.

REFERENCES AND FURTHER READING

This list contains both works of general interest as well as those cited in the chapter.

Alquist R P 1948 A study of adrenotropic receptors. American Journal of Physiology 153: 586–600

Bowman W C, Rand M J 1980 Textbook of Pharmacology. Blackwell, Oxford

Day M D 1979 Autonomic pharmacology. Churchill Livingstone, Edinburgh

Gilman A G, Goodman L S, Gilman A 1985 Goodman and Gilman's The Pharmacological basis of therapeutics, 7th edn. Macmillan, New York

Hodgkin A L, Horowicz 1959 Movement of Na and K in single muscle fibres. Journal of Physiology 145: 405–432

Iversen L L 1973 Catecholamine uptake processes. British Medical in 29: 130–135

Kandel E R (Ed) 1977 Neurophysiology. Handbook of physiology, Section 1, Volume 1. American Physiological Society, Bethesda, Maryland

Langley J N 1921 The autonomic nervous system, 4th edn. W. Heffer, Cambridge

Lands A M, Luduena F P, Buzzo H J 1967 Differentiation of receptors responsive to isoproterenol. Life Sciences 6: 2241–2249

Starke K 1981 Presynaptic receptors. Annual Review of Pharmacology and Toxicology 21: 7–30

17. Local anaesthetic drugs; neurolytic drugs

J. Moore

LOCAL ANAESTHETICS

Drugs classified as local anaesthetics produce a reversible block of impulse transmission in a nerve. Many other agents impede the conduction process in isolated or intact nerves, but because this action is irreversible they are of limited clinical value. The term 'local' may lead the unwary administrator to underestimate the systemic effects produced by uptake of the drug, but with high dosage these are of considerable importance. The pharmacology of the local anaesthetics therefore is considered in two parts: (1) their effect on the formation and transmission of the nerve impulse; and (2) the systemic actions following their absorption from the injection site or their intravenous administration.

Chemical structure

The molecular structure of a local anaesthetic contains three subgroups: an aromatic lipophilic portion, a linkage group of length 6–8 Å and a terminal hydrophilic tertiary (occasionally secondary) amine group (Fig. 17.1) The linkage group is connected to the aromatic portion of the molecule by either an ester or an amide bond, and it is this bond which determines the pathway of the drug's metabolism.

The amine group acts as a weak base, being in equilibrium with hydrogen ions (Fig. 17.2).

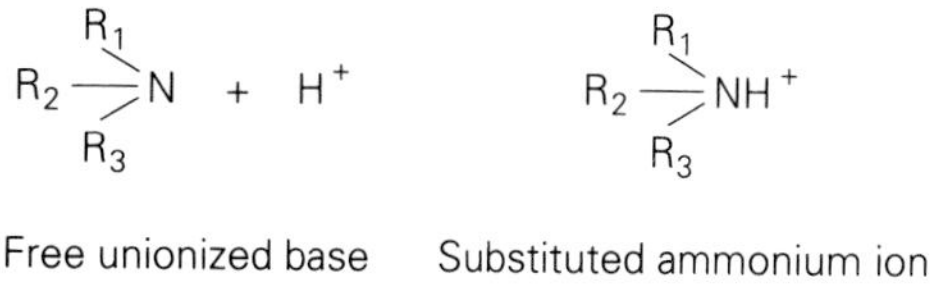

$$R_2 \overset{R_1}{\underset{R_3}{\rlap{\diagup}{\diagdown}}}N \; + \; H^+ \qquad R_2 \overset{R_1}{\underset{R_3}{\rlap{\diagup}{\diagdown}}}NH^+$$

Free unionized base   Substituted ammonium ion

Fig. 17.2

The proportion of the two forms of the drug present depends on the pKa of the molecule and the pH of the environment. The ionic form is highly soluble and stable in aqueous solution (the drugs are normally marketed in the form of their salts — usually the hydrochloride). The unionized form of the molecule is lipid-soluble and can penetrate tissue barriers to reach its site of action.

Variations in any of the three molecular subdivisions produce differences in the physical and chemical properties and are mainly responsible for differences in toxicity, potency and duration of effect. The chemical structures of the ester and amide local anaesthetics are shown in Table 17.1.

The aromatic portion of the procaine molecule is para-amino benzoic acid. Substitution of a butyl group for one of the hydrogen atoms in the amino side chains occurs in tetracaine. The introduction of a chlorine molecule at the 2-position in the benzene ring gives chloroprocaine. The remainder of the molecule of these

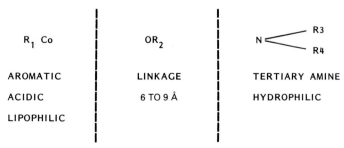

Fig. 17.1 General characteristics of local anaesthetic molecule.

Table 17.1 Chemical Structure of Ester and Amide local anaesthetics

Drug	Structure	Chemical name
Cocaine		2β - CARBOMETHOXY-3β - BENZOXYTROPANE
Procaine		p- AMINO - [2 - (DIETHYL AMINO) ETHYL] - BENZOATE
Chloroprocaine		p - AMINO - O- CHLORO [2 - (DIETHYL AMINO) ETHYL] - BENZOATE
Tetracaine		p n - BUTYLAMINO - [2 - (DIETHYL AMINO) ETHYL] - BENZOATE
Procainamide		p - AMINO - N - [2 - (DIETHYL AMINO) ETHYL] - BENZAMIDE
Cinchocaine		2 - n - BUTOXY -N - 12 - (DIETHYL (AMINO) ETHYL) - CINCHOMINAMIDE
Lignocaine		2 - (DIETHYLAMINO) - 2',6' - ACETOXYLIDIDE
Prilocaine		2 - (PROPYLAMINO) - 2 - PROPIO - O - TOLUIDINE
Mepivacaine		1 - METHYL - 2',6' - PIPECOLOXYLIDIDE
Bupivacaine		1, BUTYL - 2',6' - PIPECOLOXLIDIDE
Etidocaine		2N - ETHYL PROPYLAMINO - 2', 6' - BUTYROXYLIDIDE

three ester compounds is diethylamino ethanol. Other ester local anaesthetics have been produced by re-positioning of the amino group, substitution of the hydrogens of the amino group or by introduction of side chains to the benzene ring, but none has shown clinical advantage over the above three drugs. Replacement of the ester link by the amide in procaine gives procainamide, which has a much longer duration of effect due to its slow breakdown and excretion by liver and kidney. The effect of increasing the complexity of the aromatic portion and replacing the ester by amide link group is best shown by cinchocaine, whose potency, toxicity and duration of action are much greater than those of procaine. Cocaine, derived from *Erythroxolon coca*, is the only naturally occurring local anaesthetic still used in clinical practice. Rarely administered by injection and now mainly used as a surface anaesthetic, cocaine is hydrolysed to the base ecgonine, benzoic acid and methyl alcohol.

Lignocaine, prilocaine, mepivacaine, bupivacaine and etidocaine belong to the amino amide group. All are 2–6-dimethyl xylidide derivatives, except prilocaine in which the aromatic portion is derived from *o*-toluidine. All are tertiary amines except prilocaine, which is a secondary amine with a branched linkage group. Despite the marked structural similarity of bupivacaine and mepivacaine, the former is 3 to 4 times more potent and longer-acting than the latter.

Commonly used local anaesthetics are available in a modified isotonic Ringer's solution as water-soluble hydrochloride salts. These solutions have a pH range of 4–5 and may contain an antioxidant, a preservative and a fungicide.

Carbonated forms of local anaesthetics are now available, but despite claims of shorter latent period and more intense blockade (Bromage et al 1967) have still not attained widespread use. The solutions are bottled at a Pco_2 of 700 mmHg and remain stable at sea level and ambient temperature of 35°C for more than 2 years. The Pco_2 of an open but undisturbed ampoule falls to 500–600 mmHg in 30 min but no precipitate of base occurs for many hours. Heat or agitation speeds release of carbon dioxide. Carbon dioxide may also be added to hydrochloride solutions, the pH being slightly reduced by the process.

Effects of local anaesthetics on nerves

In the untreated nerve a 'resting' electrical potential exists across the nerve membrane, the interior being negative relative to the exterior by some 50–70 mV. This is due to differing ionic concentrations on either side of the membrane as detailed in the preceding chapter. The external concentration of the sodium ion is many times greater than that in the interior of the fibre, while the reverse is true for potassium. Ionic migration across the membrane takes place at pores, and different channels for potassium and sodium have been described. In the 'resting' state the sodium channel has a diameter of 2 nm, thus barring transmembrane movement of this ion whose diameter is 3.4 nm. During depolarization this channel enlarges and allows free inward passage of the sodium ion from the extracellular fluid while potassium migrates outward. The transmembrane potential changes, the interior becoming electropositive relative to the exterior during the final stage of depolarization. During repolarization potassium re-enters the pore and sodium is actively extruded until the resting ionic distribution is re-established. No impulse propagation takes place unless a critical or threshold level of depolarization is achieved. Agents which impede potassium movement such as tetraethyl ammonium do not possess local anaesthetic activity. All drugs which reversibly impair impulse formation and transmission block sodium movement across the nerve membrane. Some compounds can penetrate into and through the membrane easily, whereas others are only effective as blocking agents when applied to one side of the membrane, suggesting different receptors along the sodium channel. The commonly used local anaesthetics are considered to act on a receptor at the axoplasmic side of the membrane and through a physicochemical mechanism (Ritchie 1975). Since the local anaesthetic molecule is too bulky to traverse the slender sodium channel it must first diffuse through the lipid framework of the membrane to reach this site. The lipid-soluble neutral base can do this, but it is the cationic form which plugs the channel (Strichartz 1976, de Jong 1976).

Extracellular calcium concentration affects the stability of the nerve membrane and it may have a regulatory role in the movement of sodium. Calcium is bound to phospholipids in the cell membrane and its displacement may be the initial step in the alteration in membrane permeability leading to depolarization. Local anaesthetics may occupy the calcium binding site and prevent subsequent ionic migrations. Blaustein and Goldman (1966) have postulated a possible relationship between the calcium displacement effect and local anaesthetic potency.

When applied to the nerve membrane, local anaesthetics do not alter the size of the resting membrane potential or the threshold potential for impulse propagation. Measurement of the rate of rise (depolarization phase) and rate of fall (repolarization phase) of the action potential before and after exposure to these drugs reveals a marked decrease in the rate of depolarization, whereas the rate of repolarization is minimally affected. Local anaesthetics slow the rate of rise and decrease the size of the depolarization potential so that it does not reach the critical threshold level for propagation of the nerve impulse.

Other theories for the mechanism of action of local anaesthetics have been reviewed by Ritchie (1975). The acetylcholine hypothesis, based on the chemical resemblance of this compound to some of these agents, is unlikely because of the lack of cogent evidence that this substance is involved in conduction of the nerve impulse. The surface charge theory postulated that the local anaesthetic molecule is bound to the nerve membrane by its lipophilic aromatic end with its cationic head remaining in solution. As a result the fixed negative charges in the membrane are partly or wholly neutralized, so that although the resting potential remains constant, the potential across the membrane increases considerably. If the increase in the transmembrane potential is sufficiently great, the action currents from neighbouring unanaesthetized nerve membrane may be insufficient to reduce the membrane potential to its threshold level, and conduction block will occur. In the membrane expansion theory the nerve membrane is regarded as being essentially impermeable to cations except at its special regions where pores or channels exist. Local anaesthetics are postulated to increase the freedom of movement of the lipid molecules with the result that some part of the membrane critical for conduction is in an expanded state. Either the change in proteins intimately associated with the lipid or the resultant membrane expansion restricts and finally totally impedes cationic transfer across the membrane.

Depolarization and impulse transmission occur in a similar manner in all nerves irrespective of size, type or function, yet variations in these characteristics produce differing sensitivity to the blocking effect of local anaesthetics. The large myelinated motor fibres in which depolarization occurs at the nodes of Ranvier are most resistant. The saltatory spread of the impulse in these nerves may allow transmission even though two or three such sites are affected by the local anaesthetic. A certain length of fibre must be reached to completely block impulse conduction. Differing sensitivities may also be explained by the presence or absence of the myelin sheath as the latter attracts the drugs.

The non-myelinated nerves are very sensitive to the actions of local anaesthetics. However, β fibres, myelinated preganglionic autonomic axons, despite being larger than unmyelinated C fibres, are blocked more readily than the latter (Heavner and de Jong 1974). This could be due to differing physicochemical properties of the local anaesthetics or the presence of fewer sodium channels in B as compared to C type fibres. The most accepted explanation is that, unlike B and A fibres, individual C axons lack separate myelin sheaths; instead several are enclosed in a single Schwann cell sheath. The smallest A and C fibres are of particular importance because they carry pain and temperature impulses. Block of B fibres causes hypotension in spinal and extradural anaesthesia.

Successful nerve block is dependent upon placement of the local anaesthetic in close association with the nerve. The latent period between the time of injection and onset of sensory loss is many times shorter for infiltration techniques than for those requiring conduction block in a mixed nerve. The thicker the nerve coverings the longer the period of latency will be, hence the slow onset of extradural anaesthesia is due to slow penetration by the local anaesthetic of the dense dural sheath enveloping the nerves. In a mixed nerve, axons at the periphery are blocked before those centrally placed. Recovery takes place in a similar direction.

The conduction block produced by local anaesthetics is related to their dissociation constant, lipid solubility, protein binding affinity and the pH of the tissue into which they are administered. Values of some of these parameters are shown in Table 17.2. A lower pKa and higher lipid-solubility are associated with a more rapid onset, while a higher protein binding capacity is related to a longer duration of effect.

Following injection of the water-soluble hydrochloride salt into body tissues free base is liberated and is present in ionized and unionized form, depending upon the dissociation constant and the hydrogen ion concentration of the surrounding medium. As the pKa for the commonly used drugs ranges between 7.5 and 9.0, appreciable quantities of base and cation co-exist at body pH. The uncharged molecule being highly lipid-soluble traverses tissue barriers easily, hence a reduction of hydrogen ion concentration will facilitate penetration to the receptor site on the nerve membrane (Ritchie et al 1965, Ritchie 1975). Once there, however, it is the ionized form which forms the attachment. Local anaesthetics are much less effective if injected into infected tissues, probably because there acidity favours ionization and limits the quantity of free base for diffusion to the nerve membrane. It should be remembered however that n-butanol, a compound with considerable local anaesthetic properties, exists only in the uncharged form and presumably must act by

Table 17.2

Drug	Dissociation Constant	Percentage Protein-bound	Lipid Solubility	Molecular Weight
Procaine	8.9	6	<1	236
Chloroprocaine	8.7	—	>1	271
Tetracaine (Amethocaine)	8.5	76	80	264
Cocaine	8.8	—	>1	—
Cinchocaine (Nupercaine)	8.5			380
Lignocaine	7.9	64	3	234
Prilocaine	7.9	55	2	220
Mepivacaine	7.6	77	2	246
Bupivacaine	8.1	95	28	288
Etidocaine	7.8	94	141	276

dissolving in the nerve membrane and so altering the diameter of the sodium channels.

More rapid onset and greater spread of analgesia are the main advantages attributed to the carbonated solutions of local anaesthetics. Using the bicarbonate form the conversion to the undissociated base is rapid and the partial pressure falls to that of the tissue. Although the pH of the carbonated solution is practically the same as that of the equivalent hydrochloride solution, the rapid diffusion of carbon dioxide across cell membranes causes a fall of intracellular pH in the immediate neighbourhood and the resulting electrochemical gradient favours a greater uptake of local anaesthetic base.

Repetitive doses of local anaesthetics are used to give continuous subarachnoid and extradural anaesthesia. After a period of time the repeat dose produces a less effective and shorter-lasting blockade. This tachyphylaxis is most obvious with the shorter-acting drugs such as chloroprocaine. The aqueous solutions of the hydrochloride form of local anaesthetics are acid. Thus tissue acidosis, relative to the body pH, will occur at the site of injection, favouring formation of ionized base which cannot penetrate the various tissue barriers to reach the nerve membranes. In tissues with poor buffering capacity such as cerebrospinal fluid, tachyphylaxis will occur rapidly.

Uptake and distribution

The chief factors influencing the uptake of local anaesthetics from tissue to blood are: (1) the site of injection; (2) the drug used and (3) the associated use of a vasoconstrictor agent. Variations in uptake are related to varying vascularity of the injection sites: the greater this

is the more rapidly higher plasma levels occur. The addition of adrenaline or other vasoconstrictor drug slows the rate of uptake and limits the peak plasma concentration. Adrenaline has a vasodilator effect in muscle, and it will not reduce uptake of local anaesthetics if used in such tissue. Plasma lignocaine levels following intercostal, extradural, subcutaneous, vaginal and abdominal field blocks were reported to be highest following intercostal nerve block (Scott et al 1972). Rapid uptake is associated with topical application of local anaesthetics to mucous membranes. Total dosage, droplet size, coughing, presence or absence of secretions, spontaneous or positive pressure ventilation all affect uptake from the respiratory tract.

Plasma levels following administration of similar doses and concentrations of different drugs show marked variation. Such differences are related to their differing physicochemical and vasodilator properties. The effectiveness of adrenaline in limiting plasma levels varies with the agent with which it is given, because of varying vasodilator effect. Unlike increase in dosage, increasing the concentration does not increase the maximum blood level. The rate of injection is only significant if the intravenous route is used. Plasma levels are not directly related to the weight of the patient and dosage on a mg kg^{-1} basis can be dangerous. In the young and elderly, uptake, distribution and excretion may differ from the common pattern and plasma levels may reach toxic proportions with dosage which would be acceptable in young adults. Techniques involving repetitive doses of drugs which are slowly detoxicated and excreted can also lead to dangerous blood levels.

Following absorption there is a rapid distribution to all body tissues, but differences in relative distribution exist between specific agents. Tissue blood flow and physicochemical properties of the drug are important determinants. Etidocaine, the most lipid-soluble, has a volume of distribution of 666 ± 493, as compared to 212 ± 53 litres for lignocaine (Tucker & Mather 1975). A local anaesthetic is distributed according to a two-compartment model, the drug initially rapidly entering highly vascular tissues which achieve rapid equilibration, and from where a redistribution takes place to other tissues which reach equilibration more slowly (Boyes et al 1971). Prilocaine is initially present in higher concentrations in lung and brain than lignocaine, while mepivacaine, like the latter, accumulates rapidly in liver, kidney, salivary glands and brain. Simultaneous measurements of drug levels in arterial and peripheral venous blood provide some indication of skeletal muscle uptake. While this tissue does not show particular affinity for local anaesthetics, prilocaine concentrations in muscle are greater than those for lignocaine.

Concentrations of local anaesthetics are measured either in whole blood or plasma. The distribution between the plasma and the red blood cells is determined by the protein-binding properties of the drug, those having a low binding index being distributed evenly between the cell and plasma. Whole blood concentrations of bupivacaine or etidocaine, which are highly protein-bound, are lower than plasma levels.

Metabolism and excretion

The ester local anaesthetics are broken down by the plasma pseudocholinesterase, procaine being metabolized to para-aminobenzoic acid and diethylamino ethanol. Chlorprocaine has many times the affinity of procaine for pseudocholinesterase and its rapid destruction accounts for its brevity of action and low toxicity. Other drugs used in anaesthesia, such as propanidid and succinylcholine, are broken down by this enzyme and their concurrent administration with ester-type local anaesthetics leads to competition for metabolism. Atypical pseudocholinesterases may be unable to metabolize this group of local anaesthetics and their administration in such circumstances can give rise to unexpected toxicity (Davies et al 1960).

The liver plays an important role in the breakdown of the amide-type agents, only small amounts being excreted by the kidney. Caution with dosage is needed where liver function is impaired. The hepatic breakdown varies in rate and type for individual drugs, oxidative and conjugative processes together with hydrolysis being involved (Greene 1968). The metabolites are excreted via the biliary tract into the intestine, where complete reabsorption occurs. These, together with others absorbed directly from the liver into the bloodstream, are then removed via the kidneys. Descriptions of the individual metabolic processes have been detailed by Covino (1972). Prilocaine, less resistant to hydrolysis and more rapidly broken down than other members of the amide group, is also metabolized to some extent by the kidney. Their renal excretion can be enhanced by acidification of the urine.

Certain aromatic amines and their derivatives can cause methaemoglobinaemia in humans and other animals. Both prilocaine and lignocaine are aromatic amines but the former is a much more potent inducer of methaemoglobin formation (Hjelm and Holmdahl 1965). Prilocaine does not form methaemoglobin in vitro, suggesting that a product of metabolism is the causal factor. Hydrolysis of its amide link produces o-toluidine and the further metabolism of this compound by N-hydroxylation gives an N-hydroxy derivative which is a potent inducer of methaemoglobin. The severity of the methaemoglobinaemia is dose-related and is insignificant if 500 mg or less of prilocaine has been given. Its repetitive use as in continuous extradural block is therefore contra-indicated.

Systemic actions

Central nervous system

The prodromal warnings of overdosage accompanying the intravenous administration or rapid uptake of local anaesthetics include sleepiness, sensation of cold, tremor, shivering, numbness of lips and tongue, tinnitus and speech difficulty. If unheeded these give way to a convulsive seizure of a grand-mal type with tonic and clonic muscular movement. Unconsciousness and postictal amnesia follow, with complete recovery at about 1 h later (Usubiaga et al 1966).

Electroencephalographic records taken immediately pre-seizure show predominant delta–theta activity. Convulsions are associated with generalized rapid, high-voltage spike activity which occurs in bursts lasting 3–5 s with electrically silent periods between. Following this period of CNS excitation a flattening of brain wave pattern coincides with the clinical depression. While these ECG changes are broadly similar for different local anaesthetics, onset time varies for individual agents. Marked electrical changes occur early and for a longer time with lignocaine as compared to bupivacaine, which causes no changes until shortly before convulsions (Englesson & Matoussek 1975).

Local anaesthetics have a depressant effect on excitable membranes and their high lipid-solubility facilitates access to the central nervous system. The initial clinical signs and symptoms suggest a stimulating effect on the brain and spinal cord. Nevertheless intravenous lignocaine has been used in the treatment of status epilepticus (Bernhard et al 1955). Cerebral cortical activity is modified by facilitatory and inhibitory neurons and selective depression of the latter in the initial phase of local anaesthetic effect gives rise to the apparent stimulatory clinical action. Increasing doses leads to depression of both regulating systems giving a generalized state of central nervous depression. Wagman, et al (1967) studied the effects of progressively increasing doses of lignocaine on brain electrical activity and found the amygdaloid nuclear complex to be particularly involved.

Respiratory and metabolic acidosis lower the convulsive threshold to local anaesthetics. An elevated Pco_2 may enhance cerebral blood flow so that more drug reaches the brain, or it may exert an excitatory CNS effect which augments their convulsive action. The acidosis may lower intracellular pH, which in turn will cause an increase in the intraneuronal level of the active cationic form of the local anaesthetic.

Anticonvulsant drugs such as barbiturates or benzodiazepines have been used as premedicants to raise the convulsive threshold to local anaesthetics. Thiopentone sodium or diazepam can be given intravenously in the management of established convulsions. While such treatment is effective it is usually the associated hypoxaemia which either kills or causes permanent neurological deficit. Oxygen treatment must be given immediately prodromal signs of CNS toxicity occur. It may be necessary to use a short-acting muscle relaxant to allow adequate ventilatory support to be applied. The post-seizure depression is associated with respiratory arrest, so apparatus for artificial ventilation must always be to hand where local anaesthesia is practised.

Cardiovascular effects

The haemodynamic effects of local anaesthetics are dependent upon the drug used, the total dose given, the rate and site of administration, the associated use of a vasoconstrictor and the physical status of the patient. Massive doses produce cardiovascular collapse due to a reduction in cardiac output and peripheral vasodilatation. Smaller amounts act: (1) by direct action on cardiac and vascular smooth muscle (2) by direct action in the innervating autonomic nerves (3) by evoked reflexes and (4) indirectly via the central nervous system.

Cardiac effects

Non-toxic doses of local anaesthetics do not reduce cardiac output. Lignocaine consistently increases cardiac output and heart rate while the stroke volume effect varies (Blair 1975). Myocardial depression due to barbiturates, halothane, ganglion blocking drugs and hypoxaemia is augmented by local anaesthetics. On increasing dosage to toxic levels those agents do exert a negative inotropic action, the severity of which shows reasonable correlation with their local anaesthetic potency. The mechanism of the initial increase in heart rate and cardiac output may be a central nervous system effect evoked through the sympathetic nervous system.

Lignocaine is commonly used in the treatment of ventricular arrhythmias. For successful treatment venous blood levels in excess of 2 μg ml^{-1} are required and levels up to 10 μg ml^{-1} may be needed. The Purkinje fibre system is selectively affected at low concentrations, the slow depolarization phase being altered or abolished in diastole together with a shortening of the duration of the action potential and the effective refractory period. At the junction between ventricular muscle and Purkinje fibres conduction is enhanced, whereas it is minimally altered in the Purkinje system itself. Intra-atrial, intraventricular and atrioventricular conduction rates are little affected by therapeutic doses, but overtreatment prolongs conduction time and increases the diastolic threshold (Bigger & Mandel 1970).

Local anaesthetics have different actions on the resistance and capacitance vessels. They exert a biphasic effect on smooth muscle causing either stimulation or inhibition which is dependent upon the concentration of the agent used and the resting state of tone of the vascular bed. More increase in tone is shown by the capacitance vessels. The variable response of blood vessels may be due to alterations in calcium concentration within their cellular cytoplasm caused by the local anaesthetic (Blair 1975). High plasma concentrations of local anaesthetics cause vasodilation by inhibiting myogenic activity in the vessel wall. Cocaine inhibits the uptake of catecholamines, particularly noradrenaline, at tissue binding sites and the increased availability leads to arteriolar constriction.

The cardiovascular actions of local anaesthetics are greatly modified by the type of regional nerve block for which they are used. Subarachnoid and extradural anaesthesia, by blocking the thoracic sympathetic outflow, cause hypotension. The addition of a vasoconstrictor drug will also modify the cardiovascular response. Plasma levels sufficient to cause convulsions, if associated with hypoxaemia, cause severe depression.

Respiratory system

Local anaesthetics applied directly to the mucosa of the respiratory tract impair the sensitivity of the laryngeal and cough reflexes. Their use introduces the risk of retention of secretions or pulmonary soiling from aspiration of pharyngeal contents. Cocaine, tetracaine, lignocaine and prilocaine have been employed for this purpose. While the two ester drugs have a longer duration of action, their use is associated with a higher incidence of toxic reactions.

Subconvulsant doses of local anaesthetics do not cause central respiratory depression but a seizure will be followed by a period of transient respiratory arrest. They augment the respiratory depressant effect of general anaesthetics and opioid analgesics. Procaine and lignocaine have been used as bronchodilators in the treatment of asthma, this effect being attributed to their smooth muscle-depressant properties.

Neuromuscular transmission

Local anaesthetics impair neuromuscular transmission: (1) by decreasing the amount of acetylcholine released at the nerve terminals (Katz & Gissen 1969) and (2) by attachment to the receptor endplate where they block the ion channel which opens as a result of the combination of acetylcholine with the receptor. They also have a direct depressant action on the muscle fibre itself. Partial neuromuscular block due either to depolarizing or non-depolarizing relaxants is enhanced by local anaesthetics. Ester agents are hydrolysed by the plasma cholinesterase, an enzyme for which they have a marked affinity. Succinylcholine hydrolysis is also dependent upon the same enzyme and prolongation of its neuromuscular block will occur if it is given concurrently.

Uterine contractility

The administration of local anaesthetics during labour for either extradural or pudendal block is associated with a temporary reduction in intensity and frequency of uterine contractions. Adrenaline added to the local anaesthetic solution produces a further decrease in uterine activity because of β-adrenergic stimulation. Reduction in uterine contractility attributed to local anaesthetics may be partly due to diminished blood supply resulting from occlusion of the inferior vena cava in the supine position.

Hypersensitivity and allergic reactions

Some fatalities due to injudicious dosage of local anaes-

thetics have been wrongly attributed to an allergic or anaphylactoid response (Moore & Bridenbaugh 1960). Nevertheless the symptoms and signs of true systemic anaphylaxis may be indistinguishable from the cardiovascular collapse associated with high blood levels of these drugs. Hypersensitivity responses are more common with ester-type local anaesthetics (Aldrete & Johnson 1970). Reactions to the vasoconstrictor agent or preservative added to the solution must be excluded before the drug is implicated as the causal agent.

Placental transfer

Local anaesthetics, because of their molecular size and high lipid-solubility, readily reach the fetus by passive diffusion. There is a marked variation in the umbilical venous (UV) to maternal venous (MV) blood ratio for individual drugs. Differences in protein binding characteristics for different agents may explain the transfer variations. The rank order of binding in human plasma for a series of amide local anaesthetics is bupivacaine > mepivacaine > lignocaine, and of these bupivacaine has the lowest UV/MV ratio. Plasma binding is inversely related to the total drug concentration so that high plasma levels will make more free drug available for transfer. Prilocaine is readily transferred and can cause methaemoglobinaemia in the infant.

Skin application of local anaesthetics

A eutectic mixture is one in which the constituents show maximum fusibility. EMLA, a eutectic mixture of local anaesthetics, incorporating lignocaine and 2.5% prilocaine, provides approximately 80% active local anaesthetic in each droplet compared with only 20% if lignocaine alone is emulsified. Layered on the skin and covered with a protective dressing the mixture produces dermal analgesia in about $\frac{1}{2}$–1 h. Detectable plasma levels of both local anaesthetics occur, and have been demonstrated up to 8 h after its application. A cream containing 4% amethocaine applied to the skin provides more rapid and longer-lasting analgesia than the lignocaine/prilocaine combination. However, the amide preparation may be preferable in view of the greater risk of toxicity with the ester agent and their frequent use in small children.

INDIVIDUAL AGENTS

Cocaine

Cocaine, introduced in 1884 by Koller as a local anaesthetic for topical use, is an ester of benzoic acid and a nitrogen-containing base. It has proved to be too toxic for other forms of regional anaesthesia. Cocaine is the only local anaesthetic with addicting properties. The initial central nervous system stimulation causes a sense of well-being and euphoria, and with small amounts motor activity is well co-ordinated. With increasing dosage generalized tremors and ultimately clonic–tonic convulsions occur. The vasomotor and vomiting centre are also stimulated, causing hypertension and emetic effects. The postconvulsant depression involves both the vasomotor and respiratory centres, and death results from respiratory failure. Cocaine interferes with the uptake of noradrenaline by the adrenergic nerve terminals and this probably explains its mydriatic and vasoconstrictive effects. The increasing heart rate produced by cocaine is probably of similar origin.

Solutions used clinically for surface anaesthesia vary from 1.0 to 10.0%, the local vasoconstrictive property being of particular value in decreasing vascularity of the nasal cavities. In view of the dangerous potentiation interaction between cocaine and catecholamines, the addition of adrenaline is to be condemned.

Procaine

Procaine, synthesized in 1905, was the first reliable injectable local anaesthetic, being relatively stable in solution and non-irritant to tissues. Used in concentrations from 0.5 to 2%, depending on the regional nerve block required, procaine provided about 1 h of analgesia which could be prolonged by the addition of adrenaline. It is hydrolysed by plasma cholinesterase to para-amino benzoic acid and diethylamino ethanol. Para-amino benzoic acid inhibits the action of sulphonamides. Long-acting preparations of procaine containing benzyl alcohol have a destructive action on nerves, and should be used only in intractable pain situations where permanent sequelae of nerve block treatment are justifiable.

Chloroprocaine

Chloroprocaine is a halogenated derivative of procaine. It is twice as potent as procaine and is less toxic; the lesser toxicity is due to the rapid metabolism by plasma cholinesterase, for which its affinity is many times greater than procaine. The rapid breakdown makes it a short-acting local anaesthetic, and for prolonged procedures and epidural block a catheter technique is required. Even with this method of administration, tachyphylaxis to chloroprocaine develops rapidly, and it is unsatisfactory for procedures lasting several hours.

The 3% solution is very suitable for extradural blockade for Caesarean section, its rapid onset and negligible transfer to the infant being of particular advantage. Inadvertent administration of large volumes of the 3% solution into the cerebrospinal fluid have been associated with persisting neurological deficit. Extensive investigation of the neurotoxic effects of this local anaesthetic have been carried out (Gissen 1986). The amide local anaesthetic derivatives, especially bupivacaine and etidocaine, inhibit the rapid detoxification of chloroprocaine in blood. Reporting four cases of chloroprocaine neurotoxicity, two of whom had both amide- and ester-type drugs administered, Moore et al (1982) suggest that this practice should be avoided. Solutions of chloroprocaine contain the preservatives sodium bisulphite and methylparaben, and these are a possible cause of the neuropathies (Wang et al 1984). In animal experiments sodium bisulphite produces long-lasting hind limb paralysis, and this effect appears to be related to the dose and duration of contact.

Chloroprocaine competes with other ester compounds for plasma cholinesterase and will prolong their duration of effect. In patients with atypical plasma cholinesterase this local anaesthetic has produced prolonged neural blockade (Kuhnert et al (1982).

Amethocaine

Amethocaine, or tetracaine, is a derivative of para-amino benzoic acid and is approximately 4 times more potent and 10 times more toxic than procaine. It is now used mainly for spinal anaesthesia, the hyperbaric solution being 0.1% amethocaine in 6% dextrose. Doses of 0.5–2 ml injected into the CSF provide anaesthesia of $2\frac{1}{2}$–3 h duration. Amethocaine 0.25–0.5% aqueous solutions provide excellent topical anaesthesia in the eye and mucous membranes. Great care with dosage is necessary when it is applied to the respiratory tract as absorption is rapid. The maximum dose should not exceed 40 mg. Availability of less toxic agents makes the continued use of this local anaesthetic questionable.

Cinchocaine

Cinchocaine (dibucaine hydrochloride) is a quinoline derivative and is one of the most potent, most toxic and longest-acting of the local anaesthetic agents. It is approximately 15 times as potent and as toxic as procaine, and the anaesthetic action lasts about 3 times as long. Cinchocaine is now only used for spinal anaesthesia. It is administered as a hyperbaric 1:200 solution in 6% dextrose, 0.5–2 ml being injected according to the level of analgesia required. The duration of the resultant block is approximately 2–2½ h.

Lignocaine (Lidocaine)

The synthesis of lignocaine in 1943 by Lofgren was a major breakthrough in the chemistry of local anaesthetics. It represented such a significant pharmacological advance over procaine that it soon replaced the latter as the standard local anaesthetic drug. Solutions (0.5%) of procaine and lignocaine are equitoxic, but the latter is 1½ times more toxic in 2% concentrations. Lignocaine can be used for any type of local anaesthetic procedure and aqueous solutions of the hydrochloride salt are non-irritating and highly stable. Lignocaine is metabolized in the liver to monoethylglycine xylidide and further hydrolysed by liver amidases to 2, 6-xylidine and 4-hydroxy-2, 6-xylidine. Only 10% is excreted in the urine unchanged. The rate of metabolism is decreased in severe liver disease or by impairment of hepatic blood supply, and is increased by induction of liver enzyme activity by barbiturates.

Lignocaine has a duration of action of 60–90 min, which can be prolonged by the addition of adrenaline. It is impossible to state a maximum safe dose as this will vary with such factors as the general condition of the patient, the site of the injection and whether or not a vasoconstrictor drug has been added to the solution. If large amounts of the more concentrated solutions are required in a vascular site, then the addition of adrenaline will reduce the risk of toxic reaction. For infiltration analgesia a 0.5% solution is employed while nerve blocks and extradural anaesthesia require concentrations of 1–2%. In healthy patients a dose of 300 mg has been administered for such techniques without untoward effect. Lignocaine is an excellent surface analgesic, 2% solution being used in ophthalmic work and up to 4% for topical anaesthesia of the mouth and air passages. Other preparations include a 2% jelly lozenge containing 250 mg, and a 5% ointment.

Lignocaine is used in the management of cardiac arrhythmias. When given intravenously the plasma level declines in two distinct phases. The first phase lasts approximately 30 min and exhibits a half-life of approximately 10 min. This decline primarily reflects a redistribution of the drug into various body tissues, including the heart. The rapid uptake into the heart is responsible for the immediate onset of anti-arrhythmic effect and the rapid fall in blood levels is probably responsible for the short duration of its cardiac action following a single bolus injection. To obtain and maintain therapeutic blood levels it is therefore necessary to follow the loading bolus dose by a continuous infusion. The initial intravenous treatment should be 50–100 mg given slowly, and this should be followed by a continuous infusion at a rate of 2.4 mg min^{-1} usually by way of an 0.2% solution.

Prilocaine

Prilocaine is an amide-type local anaesthetic which in clinical use resembles lignocaine. It is used in similar concentration and dosage. Prilocaine differs chemically from lignocaine in that it is a toluidine derivative and secondary amine, whereas lignocaine is a xylidine derivative and tertiary amine. It undergoes more rapid metabolism and tissue distribution and with similar doses the plasma levels are lower with prilocaine. Being regarded as slightly less toxic than lignocaine, it is a better choice for intravenous regional anaesthesia. Large doses or repetitive treatments give rise to methaemoglobinaemia and this, together with its ease of placental transfer, limit its usefulness in obstetrics.

Mepivacaine

Mepivacaine is an amide local anaesthetic whose potency is similar to lignocaine but with a duration of nerve blocking effect twice as long. Adrenaline added to mepivacaine solutions has little effect on uptake or duration of local anaesthesia. This local anaesthetic has no vasodilator action and in animal experiments vasoconstriction has been demonstrated.

Fetal bradycardia and acidosis have often been associated with the administration of amide local anaesthetics for paracervical block. Mepivacaine is probably the most frequently implicated and fetal/maternal blood concentration ratios in excess of unity have occurred. In the adult, mepivacaine undergoes dealkylation and hydroxylation, ring hydroxylation occurring as the primary reaction. The metabolites are conjugated and then excreted in the urine. In the newborn, the metabolism of mepivacaine is markedly slower than in the adult, as it is unable to produce significant quantities of the ring hydroxylated metabolites of mepivacaine. The infant has to rely on renal excretion as the primary route of elimination. Therefore mepivacaine has a half-life in the newborn some 5 times that of the adult. Adverse effects in the fetus may also be due to the vasoconstricting effects of mepivacaine on the uterine and placental blood supply.

Mepivacaine is used infrequently in the United Kingdom, except perhaps as a hyperbaric solution for spinal anaesthesia. This latter is a 4% solution of mepivacaine in 6% dextrose with a specific gravity of 1.035–1.040 at 20°C. Aqueous solutions of the soluble hydrochloride form are also available in concentrations from 0.5 to 3%.

Bupivacaine

Bupivacaine is about 4 times more potent and more toxic than lignocaine, with a duration of nerve blocking effect some 3–4 times longer. For nerve blocks the maximum recommended dose in any 4 h period is 2 mg kg^{-1}, representing 25–30 ml of 0.5% solution for an adult weighing 65–70 kg. Overdosage symptoms and signs with bupivacaine follow the general pattern outlined for all local anaesthetics. However, it has been suggested that this drug and etidocaine are more cardiotoxic (Albright 1979) than other members of the amide group. Important factors are: (1) inadvertent intravenous administration of the more concentrated solution; (2) concurrent acidosis or hyperkalaemia (Gould & Aldrete 1983) and (3) hypoxaemia. Signs of bupivacaine cardiotoxicity include depressed cardiac conduction and cardiac arrhythmias leading to cardiovascular collapse. Animal studies support the hypothesis that bupivacaine is more cardiotoxic than lignocaine irrespective of the presence of acidosis, hyperkalaemia or hypoxaemia (Kotalko et al 1984).

Despite having a close chemical likeness to mepivacaine, bupivacaine has become the local anaesthetic of choice for extradural analgesia in obstetrics, its long duration of effect, absence of tachyphylaxis and limited transfer to the fetus being of particular advantage. Serious infant effects do not occur providing maternal hypotension is avoided. Although bupivacaine is highly protein-bound and fetal/maternal ratios are low, free drug concentrations may be expected to be similar in mother and baby once equilibrium is established.

Aqueous solutions of bupivacaine hydrochloride are available in varying concentrations from 0.125 to 0.5%. The hyperbaric spinal anaesthetic solution containing bupivacaine 5 mg ml^{-1} and glucose 80 mg ml^{-1} provides 2–3 h anaesthesia for lower limb surgery, but for intra-abdominal procedures only 1 h can be expected.

Etidocaine

Etidocaine, the most recent of the amide local anaesthetics, is the most lipid-soluble of this group and is 94–97% bound to plasma proteins. These properties account in part for its short latent period and long duration of effect. It is about 2–3 times more potent than lignocaine and is used mainly as a 0.5 or 1.0% solution providing analgesia or anaesthesia of similar duration to bupivacaine. Given for extradural blockade the resultant anaesthesia is characterized by greater loss of motor function than that produced by equivalent amounts of other agents. This may be of advantage in abdominal surgery, greater muscle relaxation being provided. In obstetrics the high protein-binding limits transfer to the infant, but the greater maternal weakness is disadvantageous.

NEUROLYTIC AGENTS

Intractable pain can be treated by intrathecal sensory blockade. Alcohol, phenol and chlorocresol (Maher 1957, 1963) have been used mainly as palliative therapy for malignant conditions. The objective is to selectively destroy the pain fibres leaving the motor and other sensory fibres intact. Injected into the cerebrospinal fluid the target site is the posterior nerve root and ganglia. Accurate placement of these substances is essential, otherwise unwanted neurological deficit will occur. They should not be used by the inexperienced and where radiological control of the procedure is not available. Intrathecal blocks are used occasionally for benign conditions, but they are best reserved for pain associated with terminal cancer (Ball et al 1969).

Absolute alcohol provides adequate destruction of pain fibres. It is hypobaric relative to the cerebrospinal fluid and requires careful attention to posture if unpredicted spread is to be prevented. Such spread is augmented by its quick dispersal throughout the cerebrospinal fluid. Positioning must be maintained for 1 h after its intrathecal administration. Volumes up to 1.0 ml are used. Neuritis and sloughing of tissues are two serious complications associated with the injection of absolute alcohol.

The spread of hyperbaric solutions within the cerebrospinal fluid is more controllable, and Maher (1957) introduced their use with neurolytic agents. Phenol added to either glycerine or iophendylate in varying concentrations is the most common. Both of these solutions have a much greater specific gravity than cerebrospinal fluid. The solvents not only act as carriers but also determine to some extent the rate of liberation of the phenol. Phenol (5%) in glycerine is approximately equal to 10% phenol in iophendylate. Use of high concentrations increases the likelihood of motor loss. The glycerine solution needs to be warmed beforehand to reduce viscosity and to facilitate injection. Iophendylate is less viscous and more easily administered with the further advantage of being radio-opaque.

REFERENCES

Albright J A 1979 Cardiac arrest following regional anesthesia with etidocaine or bupivacaine. Anesthesiology 51: 285–287

Aldrete J A, Johnson D A 1970 Evaluation of intracutaneous testing for investigation of allergy to local anesthetic agents. Anesthesia and Analgesia, Current Researches 49: 172–178

Ball H C J, Pearce D J, Davies J A H 1969 Anaesthesia: experiences with therapeutic nerve blocks. Technic XV: 10–14

Bernhard C G, Bohm E, Hojeberg S 1955 A new treatment of status epilepticus. Intravenous injections of a local anesthetic (lidocaine). Archives of Neurology and Psychiatry 74: 208–214

Bigger J T, Mandel W J 1970 Effect of lidocaine on conduction in canine Purkinje fibers and at the ventricular muscle–Purkinje fiber junction. Journal of Pharmacology and Experimental Therapeutics 172: 239–254

Blair M R 1975 Cardiovascular pharmacology of local anaesthetics. British Journal of Anaesthesia 47: 247–252

Blaustein M P, Goldman D E 1966 Competitive action of calcium and procaine on lobster axon: a study of the mechanism of action of certain local anaesthetics. Journal of General Physiology 49: 1043–1063

Boyes R N, Scott D B, Jebson P J R, Godman M J, Jowan D C 1971 Pharmacokinetics of lidocaine in man. Clinical Pharmacology and Therapeutics 12: 105–116

Bromage P R, Burfoot M E, Crowell D E, Truant A P 1967 Quality of epidural blockade. III: Carbonated local anaesthetic solutions. British Journal of Anaesthesia 39: 197

Covino B C 1972 Local anaesthesia. New England Journal of Medicine 286; 975–983; 1035–1041

Davies R O, Martin A U, Kalow W 1960 The action of normal and atypical cholinesterase of human serum upon a series of esters of choline. Canadian Journal of Biochemistry 38: 545–551

De Jong R H 1976 Molecular basis of neural blockade. Anesthesiology 45: 375–376

Englesson S, Matoussek M 1975 Central nervous system effects of local anaesthetic agents. British Journal of Anaesthesia 47: 241–246

Gissen A J 1986 Toxicity of local anesthetics in obstetrics. II: Chloroprocaine research and clinical aspects. Clinics in Anesthesiology Obstetric analgesia and anesthesia 4: 101–111. W B Saunders, London

Gould D B, Aldrete J A 1983 Bupivacaine cardiotoxicity in a patient with renal failure. Acta Anaesthesiologica Scandinavica 27: 18–21

Greene N M 1968 The metabolism of drugs employed in anesthesia. Anesthesiology 29: Part 1, 127–144; Part 2, 327–360

Heavner J E, De Jong R H 1974 Lidocaine block concentrations for B and C nerve fibers. Anesthesiology 40: 228–233

Hjelm M, Holmdahl M H 1965 Biochemical effects of aromatic amines. II: Cyanosis, methaemoglobinaemia and Heinz-body formation induced by a local anaesthetic agent (Prilocaine). Acta Anaesthesiologica Scandinavica 9: 99–120

Katz R L, Gissen A J 1969 Effects of intravenous and intra-arterial procaine and lidocaine on neuromuscular transmission in man. Acta Anaesthesiologica Scandinavica, Suppl 36: 103–113

Kotalko D M, Shnider S M, Dailey P A, Brizgys R V, Levinson G, Shapiro W A, Koike M, Rosen M A 1984 Bupivacaine-induced cardiac arrhythmias in sheep. Anesthesiology 60: 10–18

Kuhnert B R, Philipson E H, Pimental R, Kuhnert P M 1982 A prolonged chloroprocaine epidural block in post partum patients with abnormal pseudocholinesterase. Anesthesiology 56: 477–478

Maher R M 1957 Neurone selection in relief of pain. Further experiences with intrathecal injections. Lancet i: 16–19

Maher R M 1963 Intrathecal chlorocresol in the treatment of pain in cancer. Lancet i: 965–967

Moore D C, Bridenbaugh L D 1960 Oxygen: the antidote for systemic toxic reactions from local anesthetic drugs. Journal of the American Medical Association 174; 842–847

Moore D C, Spierdijk J, Van Kleef J D, Coleman R L, Love G F 1982 Chloroprocaine neurotoxicity: four additional cases (note a fifth case is included as an addendum). Anesthesia and Analgesia 61: 155–159

Ritchie J M 1975 Mechanism of action of local anaesthetic agents and biotoxins. British Journal of Anaesthesia 47: 191–198

Ritchie J M, Ritchie B, Greengard P 1965 The effect of the nerve sheath on the action of local anaesthetics. Journal of Pharmacology and Experimental Therapeutics 150: 160–164

Scott D B, Jebson P J R, Braid D P, Ortengren B, Frisch P 1972 Factors affecting plasma levels of lignocaine and prilocaine. British Journal of Anaesthesia 44: 1040–1049

Strichartz G 1976 Molecular mechanisms of nerve block by local anesthetics. Anesthesiology 45: 421–441

Tucker G T, Mather L E 1975 Pharmacokinetics of local anaesthetic agents. British Journal of Anaesthesia 47: 213–224

Usubiaga J E, Wikinski J, Ferrero R, Usubiaga L E, Wikinski R 1966 Local anesthetic-induced convulsions in man: an electroencephalographic study. Anesthesia and Analgesia, Current Researches 45: 611–620

Wagman I H, de Jong R H, Prince D A 1967 Effects of lidocaine on the central nervous system. Anesthesiology 28: 155–172

Wang B C, Hillman D E, Spielholz N I, Turndorf H 1984 Chronic neurological deficits and nesacaine-CE – an effect of the anesthetic, 2-chloroprocaine, or the antioxidant, sodium bisulfite? Anesthesia and Analgesia 63: 445–447

18. Neuromuscular blocking agents

R. S. J. Clarke   A. R. Hunter

Apart from the agents acting at the neuromuscular junction, relaxation of the skeletal musculature can be produced by many pharmacological mechanisms. For example, it can arise as a result of the effect of a sedative drug on the brain, especially if that drug acts as a hypnotic and causes the patient to sleep. Other drugs produce muscle relaxation by acting on the internuncial neurons of the spinal cord. These cells normally relay messages up or down the cord for a few segments. The classic example of this type of relaxant is mephenesin — which had some currency in the late 1940s. Diazepam has a similar effect. Neither of these agents will, however, relax the abdominal muscles to the point at which the reflex contraction elicited by pulling on the parietal peritoneum of the upper abdomen is eliminated.

Muscle relaxation is also obtained when a local anaesthetic drug interrupts conduction in a motor nerve fibre anywhere between the spinal cord and the myoneural junction. Muscular relaxation is produced by drugs which block conduction at this junction. There may also be drugs other than local anaesthetics which actually prevent contraction of the muscle fibre itself, but none of these has found a place in anaesthesia so far — except for the agent (dantrolene) which reverses the contracture of muscle in malignant hyperthermia, or baclofen which relieves the muscle spasm of spinal cord transection. In general, therefore, the muscle relaxants which are used by anaesthetists exert their actions at the myoneural junction.

History

In 1492 Columbus sailed from Europe to discover America. He and his immediate successors brought back from the New World a tale of the use by the native Indians of arrows tipped with poison which paralysed animals they desired to kill. Sir Walter Raleigh sailed to the New World in the early part of the seventeenth century. On his return he also made reference to poisoned arrows, and to the fact that immediate wound excision

carried out on the part of the body injured by the poisoned arrow would avoid the worst results of such a wound (Thomas 1964). It may, however, have been that the value of wound excision lay not in the removal of the material which was on the point of the arrow (for it can be calculated that the amount of crude curare which would be carried by an arrow could not possibly cause the death of a man, though it might cause the death of a small animal) but in the removal of small organisms or spores which found their way on to the arrow point during the preparation of the crude broth. The knowledge of the existence of curare as a drug which would produce generalized muscle paralysis was widespread in western Europe from the early Jacobean period onwards, though there was some argument about the plant from which the drug was derived.

The surgeon, Benjamin Brodie, in the early decades of the nineteenth century, experimented with curare (Thomas 1964). He noted that the heart continued to beat after cessation of respiration (which was in that era synonymous with death). He attempted unsuccessfully to resuscitate a curare-poisoned rabbit by tracheostomy and artificial ventilation, but later succeeded with a cat. The most dramatic intervention of this kind relates to a she-ass which was curarized and ventilated artificially until the effect of the curare wore off. She survived. There is some doubt whether this was Brodie's experiment, and about the invovement of another flamboyant personality of the times, Charles Waterton (1825). At least there is no doubt that Waterton supplied the curare, and it is he who tells the tale how the ass was named Wouralia and sent out to pasture for the remainder of her life with the following instructions: She 'shall be sheltered from the wintry storm: and when summer comes she shall feed in the finest pasture. No burden shall be placed upon her and she shall end her days in peace.'

The demonstration that curare acted at the myoneural junction is owed to Claude Bernard (Thomas 1964). He prepared a solution of curare, immersed a frog nerve muscle preparation in it and showed that the response to stimulation of the nerve was eliminated: but when a rather more prolonged and intense direct current was applied to the muscle belly itself, it would still contract. If the nerve only were immersed in the curare solution, the muscle continued to respond to the stimulation. It was thus apparent that the 'lesion' produced by curare did not affect the nerve, nor did it diminish the ability of the muscle to contract when directly stimulated. It was concluded that the drug must act at the junction of the nerve and the muscle. Further, when curare was given to a frog, one of whose legs had been isolated from the general circulation by previous arterial ligation, stimulation of the sciatic nerve to this limb still elicited a muscle contraction even after the rest of the animal's muscles had become paralysed.

In 1912 Lawen attempted to utilize curare for producing muscle relaxation for surgical purposes (Thomas 1964), but found it to be unreliable. The drug was, however, given by subcutaneous or intramuscular injection and not intravenously, so that the rate of absorption was variable. At that time modification of dosage in terms of body weight was also not practised. In addition, artificial ventilation of the anaesthetized patient by the then current Sylvester method involved external thoracic compression. It could be performed only at the expense of interrupting the surgical procedure completely — should the curare cause respiratory insufficiency. Finally the potency of the preparation of the crude curare then available was far too variable to allow consistent results to be obtained.

In 1935 King prepared an alkaloid which possessed the muscle-paralysing power of the original substance, from a specimen of crude curare in the British Museum. His tubocurarine was isolated from the plant *Chondrodendron tomentosum*, whose long flat strap-like leaves hang down from the branches of the trees in the tropical forests of the Amazon, rather than from the usual source of curare, *Strychnos toxifera*. The isolation of this alkaloid, however, was simply a piece of academic research. No use was made of the product save in the physiological laboratory, though an attempt was made to assess its clinical usefulness in conditions characterized by muscle spasm (West 1936), and indeed it was from the Physiology Department of the University of Liverpool that Gray & Halton (1946) obtained the specimen of curare whose usefulness in anaesthesia they demonstrated 9 years later.

During 1942 Dr H. R. Griffith of the Homeopathic (now Queen Elizabeth) Hospital in Montreal was persuaded by the traveller of a commercial firm which made Intocostrin, an extract containing all the curare alkaloids for use in electrical convulsive therapy, to try this drug in anaesthesia. He found it to be satisfactory, and at the end of the year he published the classical paper on the subject (Griffith & Johnson 1942) at a time at which some 3000 doses of the drug had already been given for 'softening up' of therapeutically induced convulsions.

The subsequent history of tubocurarine involves the use of the alkaloid itself by Gray & Halton (1946). Perhaps the most important feature of the whole story, however, is the fact that anaesthetists, finding that it was rather difficult to determine a dose of tubocurarine which would produce abdominal relaxation without at the same time causing respiratory insufficiency, began to ventilate patients manually when they were curarized. Had it not been for this innovation curare would still have remained a scientific curiosity, or at best a drug whose action was capricious, unreliable and potentially lethal.

The myoneural junction

The myoneural junction has two components, the expanded ending of the nerve and the adjacent receptor area of the muscle fibre. There is a gap between the two, the junctional cleft — across which the chemical transmitter at the junction passes. The membrane which covers the proximal (neural) side of the cleft is called the axolemma and that covering the muscle fibre proper, the sarcolemma. The axolemma is an investing membrane through which acetylcholine passes when it is released. Inside there are mitochondria which presumably supply the energy required for the synthesis of the transmitter acetylcholine. Between the axolemma and the mitochondria there are many small vesicles which contain acetylcholine held ready for release when physiological activity occurs (Fig. 18.1).

The adjacent sarcolemma is profoundly convoluted, and many little tubules run from it into the substance of the muscle fibre. The acetylcholine receptors, which can be identified with the aid of the snake venom α-bungarotoxin, are located in the walls of these tubules close to their origin from the main junctional cleft. The receptors first recognize the transmitter (acetylcholine) and then open up the ionic channel which allows the change in ionic balance during contraction (Dreyer 1982).

Physiology of the myoneural junction

A nerve impulse arising in an anterior horn cell of the spinal cord passes down an axon to the periphery. Very near its termination the axon breaks up into a series of branches, each of which goes to a motor nerve fibre.

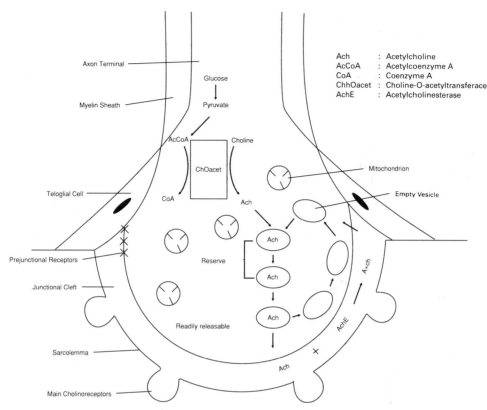

Fig. 18.1 Diagrammatic representation of the pharmacology of the neuromuscular junction.

The number of branches varies between five and 300, and the smaller the number, the more sensitive the control which can be achieved.

In the axon terminal acetylcholine is synthesized from choline and acetylcoenzyme A, a reaction catalysed by the enzyme choline *O*-acetyltransferase (formerly known as choline acetylase). Approximately 50% of the choline is derived from previously released and hydrolysed acetylcholine and in practical terms deficiency of choline, glucose or the acetyltransferase is not a problem. The enzyme can, however, be inhibited and the transport of choline within the nerve terminal can be blocked by a variety of drugs such as hemicholinium and other similar compounds (MacIntosh & Collier 1976). Acetylcholine is largely stored in many thousands of vesicles in a reserve position in the centre of the terminal, to be mobilized and moved up to the terminal membrane as the readily available material there is used up. Approximately 20% of the acetylcholine is not in vesicles and is probably used to replenish the vesicular stores.

In the absence of nerve impulses miniature endplate potentials of about 0.5–1.0 mV occur at the terminal membrane and appear to result from spontaneous release of quanta of acetylcholine, perhaps the contents of one vesicle randomly colliding with the inside of the terminal membrane, though this hypothesis is disputed — see Bowman (1980). When a nerve impulse reaches the nerve terminal many quanta of acetylcholine are released, the number being well in excess of the minimum required to depolarize the membrane. Calcium ions play an essential role in the release of acetylcholine while magnesium ions antagonize this effect (Standaert 1982).

It has been suggested (Standaert et al 1976) that a nerve action potential activates adenyl cyclase in the terminal membrane of the nerve ending converting ATP to cAMP (cyclic adenosine monophosphate). This acts on a protein kinase which opens up calcium channels, thus providing the calcium for acetylcholine release. The cAMP is degraded to AMP by a phosphodiesterase.

If this thesis is true, adenylcyclase activators such as sodium fluoride and prostaglandin E should facilitate neuromuscular transmission as does the diffusible analogue of cAMP, dibutyryl cAMP. Inhibitors such as alloxan should block the transmission and antagonize activators but not dibutyryl cAMP. Phosphodiesterase inhibitors such as theophylline and azathioprine should increase transmission whereas phosphodiesterase activators should produce block. Adenosine, which inhibits protein kinases and verapamil, which blocks calcium channels, should also cause block. In fact these relationships are true, and the role of adenylcyclase and cyclic AMP now seems to be established.

Many substances act to block acetylcholine release prejunctionally at the neuromuscular junction, the most important being the toxin of *Clostridium botulinum* (Ball et al 1979). It is thought to act within the nerve ending by reducing the sensitivity of the acetylcholine release mechanism to intracellular Ca^{2+}, and 4-aminopyridine by augmenting calcium flux has been found to have at least a short-term benefit.

The acetylcholine passes across the synaptic cleft, becomes attached to the specialized receptor area of the sarcolemma and penetrates it. Here the positively charged ion of the acetylcholine partially neutralizes the 90 mV negative potential which is there in the resting state. In an electrical record of what is happening this is seen as the endplate potential. If the endplate potential exceeds a threshold value of 45 mV an electrical impulse is propagated centrifugally towards both ends of the muscle fibre, the membrane potential falls to zero and in fact swings to the positive side. These last electrical changes are accompanied by ionic movements. Potassium ions flow outward from the inside of the fibre and sodium ions move in, the sodium pump mechanism being temporarily in abeyance. Simultaneously with these changes the actin and myosin in the muscle fibre itself undergo the changes associated with muscle contraction.

Once the membrane potential has collapsed and contraction has occurred, return to normal begins. The sodium is expelled from the muscle fibre. The membrane potential is re-established as the acetylcholine is removed from the endplate region by the enzyme acetylcholinesterase, (also known as true cholinesterase to distinguish it from plasma, pseudo- or butyryl cholinesterase, which is responsible for the breakdown of suxamethonium). Reparative changes also occur in the nerve ending, where with the help of choline acetyl transferase, acetyl groups are transferred to choline from co-enzyme A.

Neuromuscular block

The generally accepted belief is that myoneural blocking agents act by substituting incompletely for acetylcholine at the muscle endplate. Once these drugs have become bound to the endplate, unlike acetylcholine they are not hydrolysed by (true) cholinesterase and produce conduction block which persists as long as they remain in situ.

In addition to these primary blocking effects, which involve prevention of the access of acetylcholine to the postjunctional membrane or muscle endplate, tubocurarine, dimethyl tubocurarine and pancuronium diminish the rate of refilling of the acetylcholine stores in the nerve endings (Blaber 1973, Su et al 1979). Because of this effect it has been suggested that some of the myoneural blocking activity of the relaxant drugs is prejunctional. Bowman & Webb (1976) consider that the depression of twitch tension by a non-depolarizing blocker is a postsynaptic effect, whereas tetanic fade is presynaptic in origin. They have suggested that whereas tubocurarine acts both pre- and postsynaptically, pancuronium acts principally at the postsynaptic site. Such effects are also present when acetylcholine and similar substances act at the nerve endings (see Riker 1975 for a review).

Depolarizing and non-depolarizing block

As anaesthetists and pharmacologists became more familiar with the phenomena of myoneural block it became apparent that there were two separate physiological entities — depolarizing and non-depolarizing block. Essentially those drugs which have a close similarity to acetylcholine tend to produce depolarizing block. Presumably their active quaternary groupings are able to enter closely into the endplate receptors — while other drugs with a more elaborate molecular structure such as tubocurarine or gallamine are unable to attain such a close relationship with the receptors, and in consequence are unable to produce any direct changes in the muscle fibres themselves. The characteristic of depolarizing block is that if the drug is injected into an artery going directly to a muscle — so-called close intra-arterial injection — it gives rise to a contraction of the muscle, followed by a persistent depolarization of the endplate region. This prevents the centrifugal movement of the impulse which would normally lead to a muscle contraction (see Waud & Waud 1975). When depolarizing drugs are injected into chicks they produce an intense contracture of the muscles to the back of the neck, and the bird is thrown into an almost opisthotonic state. By contrast when non-depolarizing relaxants are administered to these animals the onset of paralysis is uneventful and unassociated with spontaneous muscle movement.

Comparable differences are observed in man when myoneural blocking drugs are given. When a non-depolarizing drug is given to the point of partial paralysis, and a record made of the mechanical response to supra-maximal electrical stimulation of a nerve, the response to repeated stimuli becomes progressively less (fades). The degree of block can be expressed as the percentage of the particular twitch height of the control. When the repeated stimuli are applied at a rate of some 50 Hz the response fades rapidly. If the muscle is then allowed to rest for some 5s and a single stimulus applied, the amplitude of the response is very much greater than had been the response to the initial stimulus. This phenomenon is called 'post-tetanic facilitation', and along with 'fade' constitutes the main characteristic of a non-depolarizing block.

Another method of demonstrating a non-depolarizing block is by the use of the train-of-four (TOF) stimulation (Ali et al 1971). In this, four supramaximal stimuli are applied at 2 Hz. In humans the nerve usually involved is the ulnar nerve at the wrist, and the muscle whose contractions are recorded is the adductor pollicis in the hand. In these circumstances, in non-depolarizing block, fade occurs between the first and fourth response and the ratio of the fourth to the first is a measure of the amount of non-depolarizing block present (Fig. 18.2). In clinical practice TOF stimulation is often used in preference to a single twitch because it can be assessed without reference to a control twitch height. When the block increases to 75% the fourth twitch is lost, at 80% the third twitch, at 90% the second twitch and at 100% block there are no detectable twitches. During the period of 0–75% block the TOF ratio declines in parallel with the height of T_1, though the two figures do not always correspond exactly (Lee 1975, Viby-Morgensen 1985).

In the case of depolarizing block, the response to tetanic stimulation at 50 Hz, though reduced in size, is well sustained. The response to stimulation following an interval of 5s is no greater than the first response to the tetanus. In other words, there is no post-tetanic facilitation. If TOF stimulation is used, the first and fourth responses are nearly equal, the ratio of the height of the fourth to the first response being more than 0.7.

The main pharmacological difference between depolarizing and non-depolarising block is that the latter can be antagonized with neostigmine while the former cannot. Neostigmine and the other anticholinesterase drugs are discussed in Chapter 20, but their principal mode of action is by inhibiting the enzyme acetylcholinesterase, allowing the concentration of acetylcholine at the endplate to rise and thus displace the remaining molecules of the non-depolarizing blocker.

Comparison of muscle relaxants

There is now such a range of non-depolarizing neuro-muscular blocking drugs available that it is important to be able to express the differences in numerical terms. Since these differ from the indices used for other drugs some definitions will be given here, and an outline of techniques for their determination.

Potency. This is usually expressed as the dose required to produce 50% or 95% block of the twitch response of a particular muscle (ED_{50} or ED_{95}), usually the adductor pollicis. Ideally, groups of patients are given a range of doses, a log-dose response graph is constructed and the ED_{50} or ED_{95} read off. However, this

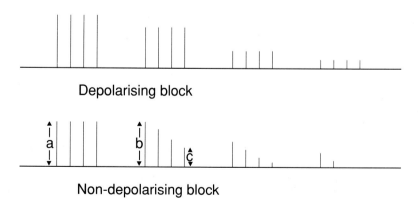

Fig. 18.2 Response of the adductor pollicis muscle to train-of-four stimulation showing fade with the non-depolarizing block and sustained response with the depolarizing block. The ratios *b/a* in both types are measures of the degree of block. The ratio *c/b* (or T_4/T_1) measures the degree of fade and is less than 0.7 in non-depolarizing block.

single-dose method requires a large number of patients, and it is more convenient to construct a cumulative dose–response curve by giving small incremental doses to the same patient until complete block is achieved. This takes longer for each subject, but is satisfactory except for drugs of short duration of action.

Speed of onset. This can be expressed as the time from injection to achieve (say) 95% block.

Duration of action. For assessment purposes, this may be regarded as the time taken for return of a single twitch to 25% of the control height, or for the return of the fourth twitch of the TOF.

Recovery index. This is a measure of the rate of recovery rather than the time of beginning or end of recovery. It is defined as the time taken from 25% to 75% recovery.

Dual or phase II block

After decamethonium had been in use for a short period as a muscle relaxant it was noted that repeated doses exerted a progressively diminishing effect (tachyphylaxis). When suxamethonium came to be used in anaesthesia, one technique, now largely forgotten, was by intravenous infusion. It was found that when considerable quantities of the drug, usually in excess of 0.5 g, had been given, the response of the partially paralysed muscles to a nerve stimulator was altered so that it became non-depolarizing in character — and in the hands of some workers at least, neostigmine reversible.

Hunter (1970), who used tetrahydroaminacrine (tacrine) to extend suxamethonium block for muscular relaxation for abdominal surgery, found that dual block regularly occurred in patients managed in this way. This was often apparent after two or three repeat doses of the drug, or after a period of $\frac{1}{2}$ h paralysis. In contradistinction to other workers, however, Hunter found that the development of dual block did not in fact prolong the action of an incremental dose of suxamethonium. It is, however, becoming more generally accepted that dual block is only an accompaniment of prolonged suxamethonium action, not the cause of it.

Chemical concepts

It has already been indicated that acetylcholine is the transmitter at the receptors in the muscle endplates. This substance alone is capable of producing total collapse of the potential difference at the endplate and the centrifugal spread of a propagated impulse throughout the muscle fibres with vigorous contraction of the muscle. However, any substance with a quaternary nitrogen atom in its structure is liable to become attached to the receptors at the muscle endplate. The firmness of the attachment depends on the remainder of the molecular structure. The more closely a substance resembles an ester of choline the more likely it is to act like acetylcholine at the endplate and to produce some depolarization of the muscle fibre. On the other hand, substances with quaternary nitrogen atoms built into a complex molecule are more likely simply to adhere to the receptors without causing depolarization.

This concept was elaborated by Bovet and others (1949), who spoke of leptocurares (smooth curares), that is drugs which have a long single chain like decamethonium and suxamethonium and pachycurares (rough curares) like tubocurarine where the quaternary nitrogen is built into a complex molecule within a structure which looks like a raspberry (p. 303). It had been suggested that those substances which have 14 Å (Ångstrom units) between the quaternary groups are the most effective myoneural blockers. The assumption was that the receptor points on the endplates are 1.4 nm apart. This theory has, however, been abandoned with the revision of the formula for tubocurarine (Everett et al 1970), and vecuronium in fact has only one quaternary group (Savage et al 1980). In addition, some bisquaternaries have a different interonium distance. Such theories should be regarded with some reserve in any case, for simple quaternary compounds like trimethylammonium bromide have no myoneural blocking activity. On the other hand, studies with radioactive tubocurarine certainly support the idea that large molecules do not readily penetrate into the substance of the muscle fibres. Also other double-ended quaternary compounds with shorter polymethylene chains, such as hexamethonium and pentamethonium, are virtually without curarizing activity, but they do block the cholinergic transmission of impulses through the autonomic ganglia of the sympathetic chain.

Even atropine, whose primary blocking effect is on the muscarinic receptors of the parasympathetic, will produce myoneural block in concentrations something like 1000 times those which produce the classical pharmacological effect on muscarinic receptors.

Protein binding

All relaxants have their own pattern of protein binding, but in general the binding of neuromuscular blocking drugs to serum proteins is relatively small in comparison with many other drugs used in anaesthetic practice, the protein binding of which often exceeds 75%. Duvaldestin & Henzel (1982) showed that in normal patients 56% of tubocurarine was bound, 51% of fazadinium, 29% of pancuronium and 30% of vecuronium. Foldes & Deery (1983) found higher bound fractions for all these drugs (77–91%) with atracurium in the middle of the range. Surprisingly, a similar pattern of protein binding was noted in cirrhotic patients who might have been expected to be hypoproteinaemic. The extent of the binding of tubocurarine and fazadinium to albumin is the same as to whole serum, suggesting that most of the binding occurs with albumin.

It has been shown that patients with liver disease require larger doses of tubocurarine than other patients, and an increased volume of distribution in such patients has been given as the explanation (Duvaldestin & Henzel (1982).

Pharmacokinetics

The accurate study of plasma levels of the neuromuscular blocking agents has only progressed during the past 10 years with improvements in analytical methods. It must still be stressed that what matters pharmacologically is the concentration of a drug at the receptor, and plasma levels only indirectly reflect receptor levels. There is a sharp difference in interpretation of dynamics between Feldman (1981), who views the duration of action as determined by the rate at which the drug dissociates from the individual receptor, and Hull (1982), who sees it as closely related to plasma concentration though the relationship is multifactorial and non-linear. However, the standard pharmacokinetic parameters measured under various circumstances do give quantitative information about drug handling under different circumstances.

In general suxamethonium is broken down rather than excreted through the kidney, and is therefore the drug least influenced by renal failure. It does, however, cause an acute rise in the serum potassium which may be undesirable in the uraemic patient. The non-depolarizing drugs range in order from minimal renal excretion with atracurium and vecuronium through tubocurarine and fazadinium to metocurine, pancuronium and gallamine, the last of these being almost totally excreted by the kidney.

Termination of the action of non-depolarizing neuromuscular blocking drugs is largely dependent not on elimination, but on redistribution of the drug to inactive sites, especially during the first hour after administration. The role of the liver in their elimination has been less extensively studied, but for pancuronium at least there is a prolonged elimination half-life, reduced clearance and larger volume of distribution in patients with a variety of liver disease (Somogyi et al 1977, Duvaldestin et al 1978a, Westra et al 1981).

Both renal and hepatic function are progressively impaired with age, and these may be the cause of the prolonged elimination half-life and of neuromuscular blockade with pancuronium outside the age range 25–55 years. Anaesthesia does not appear to influence the pharmacokinetic handling of non-depolarizing relaxant drugs (Stanski et al 1979) though it is well known that most inhalation agents potentiate the resultant block.

Despite being highly ionized there is evidence that non-depolarizing muscle relaxants enter both the cerebrospinal fluid and the circulation of the fetus in utero (Matteo et al 1977). The placental transfer of gallamine and alcuronium (Thomas et al 1969) is slightly greater than that of tubocurarine or suxamethonium. However, it has not been possible to prove that crossing the blood–brain barrier has any significant central effect, and the observed reduction in halothane anaesthetic requirement of 25% by pancuronium (Forbes et al 1979) may well be due to a reduction of muscle spindle afferent input. Likewise no clinical effect on the neonate has been demonstrated from the passage of pancuronium across the placenta (Duvaldestin et al 1980).

Factors influencing the neuromuscular block

Acid–base effects. In 1958 Payne showed that respiratory acidosis produced by the inhalation of carbon dioxide intensified the paralysis produced by tubocurarine and suxamethonium and antagonized that caused by gallamine. Attempts to explain these differing responses in terms of the effect of pH on protein binding have not been entirely convincing, for the pKa of gallamine is greater than 13, and the pH changes which would result from the administration of carbon dioxide must then be small. Payne's work has been confirmed by others showing that acidosis of any kind prolongs curarization produced by tubocurarine. The effect of pancuronium is also modified by acid–base change in that during recovery from paralysis respiratory acidosis reduces, and respiratory alkalosis increases, the speed of recovery (Norman et al 1970). However, the clinical importance of these effects is doubtful.

Body temperature. Low body temperature increases both the magnitude and duration of action of depolarizing drugs in man (Cannard & Zaimis 1959). On the other hand tubocurarine is less potent as a myoneural blocker in the hypothermic patient. These effects can be explained by an increase in depolarization and a slowing up of repolarization, inhibition of acetylcholinesterase and an increase in the evoked release of acetylcholine, when the temperature is lowered. There should therefore be an appreciable risk of recurarization as a hypothermic and curarized patient is warmed, and in fact this has been described.

Antibiotics. It has been known for 30 years that neomycin can produce myoneural block and that neostigmine antagonizes the block. Polymyxin B produces a similar effect (Lee & de Silva 1979a) whereas streptomycin exerts a prejunctional effect at the myoneural junction (Lee & de Silva 1979b, Burkett et al 1979). In a comprehensive study by Caputy and his colleagues (1981) it was found that tetracycline, penicillin G, erythromycin, vancomycin and clindamycin had negligible effects on neuromuscular transmission. Kanamycin, lincomycin, streptomycin, tobramycin and amikacin had moderate effects while netilmycin, neomycin and colistin had the most severe effects on myoneural conduction. In addition metronidazole has been shown to prolong vecuronium block. (See also pp 564–5)

Unwanted effects

Histamine liberation. This is an effect of a wide range of drugs if the dose is large enough, but is a particular problem with the neuromuscular blockers. Amongst these tubocurarine is the most potent histamine liberator (Basta et al 1983), causing urticaria, itching, hypotension and, more rarely, bronchospasm. Plasma histamine levels are difficult to measure so that the attribution of these effects to release of histamine rather than to other mechanisms of vasodilation is not always certain, but with tubocurarine at least the plasma histamine level is directly related to the dose of the drug (Moss et al 1981). It does appear that, even when given together, H_1 and H_2 blocking drugs do not prevent all these manifestations. Metocurine, atracurium, gallamine, decamethonium and suxamethonium cause less histamine liberation. Vecuronium and pancuronium are probably the least active of the clinically used drugs in this respect.

Ganglion block. Tubocurarine is also the most potent in this action, and the effect is seen particularly in blockade of sympathetic vasoconstrictor tone leading to hypotension. This is, however, a property of many neuromuscular blocking drugs though their potency at the desired site may be so high that the effect at the ganglia is not seen with the doses commonly used (e.g. fazadinium) (Bowman & Webb 1972).

The short-chain drugs of the methonium series, pentamethonium and hexamethonium, have this property to a marked extent with minimal myoneural blocking activity, but suxamethonium has no action on sympathetic ganglia.

Muscarinic receptor block. Unwanted effects on cholinergic muscarinic receptors are virtually confined to those in the heart, and the drug most noted for this action is gallamine. However, the problem is seen also with pancuronium, fazadinium and alcuronium, though not with tubocurarine, metocurine, vecuronium and atracurium. The effect on the heart is not due to blockade of the sympathetic ganglia there since the action of methacholine, which directly stimulates the muscarinic receptors, is also blocked. It is, however, now evident that other actions on the heart can contribute to the tachycardia induced by gallamine and pancuronium. These include:

1. facilitation of the release of noradrenaline at the cardiac sympathetics by blocking the controlling influence of the vagus (Shepherd et al 1978);
2. facilitation of transmission through the sympathetic ganglia by removing the inhibitory modulating influence of dopaminergic interneurons (Gardier et al 1978).

Anticholinesterase activity. This property of neuromuscular blocking drugs is not unexpected, since acetylcholine combines with both cholinergic receptors and cholinesterases. Most of the commonly used non-depolarizers inhibit both acetylcholinesterase and butyrylcholinesterase (Bowman 1980). Though pancuronium has this action on butyrylcholinesterase in relevant concentrations this is not of any practical importance (Stovner et al 1975). However, an action on acetylcholinesterase, as seen with benzoquinonium, could cause autonomic side-effects and, more important, could render ineffective the reversing action of neostigmine. Although it also inhibits its own block by the anticholinesterase effect, once this is overcome by a high enough dose, recovery cannot be accelerated by neostigmine. In consequence benzoquinonium was withdrawn at an early stage of its studies.

Noradrenaline uptake block. A blocking action on the re-uptake of noradrenaline into sympathetic nerve endings both in cardiac and smooth muscle has been noted with pancuronium in several species (Marshall & Ojewole 1979). It is also seen with fazadinium but not with tubocurarine, gallamine and vecuronium. Its practical significance is that, by prolonging the action of noradrenaline at the receptor site, it could contribute to the sympathetic overactivity seen with pancuronium and fazadinium.

Tubocurarine chloride

d-tubocurarine chloride (known loosely as 'curare') is an alkaloid derived from the leaves of *Chondrodendron tomentosum*. It was originally regarded as bis-quaternary but it is now considered that the second nitrogen atom

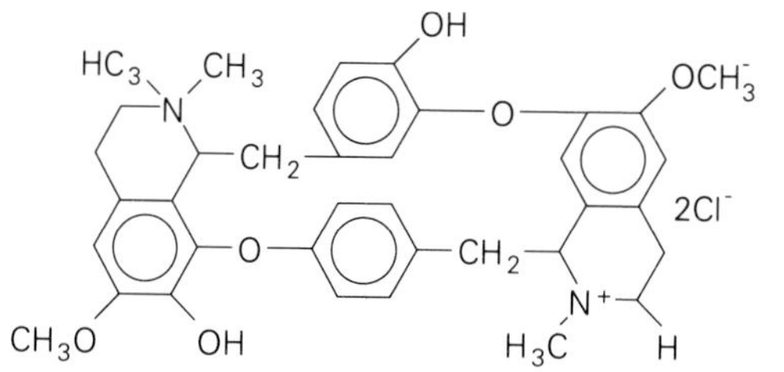

Tubocurarine

is tertiary except at low H^+ ion concentrations (Everett et al 1970).

Pharmacology

Cardiovascular system. Tubocurarine is generally said to have no direct action on the heart and does not affect the cardiac output, though its administration may be followed by tachycardia secondary to histamine release and hypotension (Coleman et al 1972). It has some blocking action on the sympathetic ganglia, causing peripheral vasodilatation and a fall in arterial blood pressure. Liberation of histamine also contributes to this. The preservative used in its storage in the USA was incriminated in a negative inotropic effect, and Johnstone and his colleagues (1978) have shown that it can inhibit calcium transport within cardiac muscle.

Histamine liberation. Tubocurarine has the highest histamine-liberating potential in humans, out of the available neuromuscular blocking agents. This effect is mainly seen in cutaneous flushing but also contributes to the hypotension and tachycardia associated with its use. More rarely it leads to bronchospasm and there may not be accompanying erythema, so that, clearly, different individuals vary in their sensitivity and clinical manifestations. While evidence is confused, the drug is probably contra-indicated in asthmatics and other atopic patients, as well as in phaeochromocytoma. There have been incidents resembling anaphylactoid collapse but these appear to be episodes of more generalized histamine liberation (Lim & Churchill-Davidson 1981).

Pharmacokinetics

Tubocurarine is strongly bound to plasma proteins, amounting to 56% which is the highest amongst the muscle relaxants studied (Duvaldestin & Henzel 1982). The drug is distributed rapidly throughout the extracellular fluid and about 45% is excreted by the kidneys in 24 h with a further 11% in the bile and some in the saliva (Meijer et al 1979). It is redistributed to inert sites

and most of the remainder is excreted over the next 24 h. Metabolism plays a minimal role in the terminator of tubocurarine's action. The terminal half-life is approximately 119 min in normal patients and is considerably prolonged in those with renal failure (Stanski et al 1979). However, because of the redistribution it does appear to be clinically safe in renal failure except in large or prolonged dosage.

Dosage and administration

The usual dose is 0.5 mg kg^{-1} and, as with other similar drugs, the block is potentiated by the volatile anaesthetics. The practice of giving smaller doses of tubocurarine or other non-depolarizing muscle relaxants to produce a 'lissive effect' is acceptable only if respiration is carefully monitored and assisted. The duration of action of the drug after full block is not of practical importance, since the safest practice is always to reverse its action with an anticholinesterase (plus atropine or glycopyrrolate) well before full recovery occurs.

Metocurine

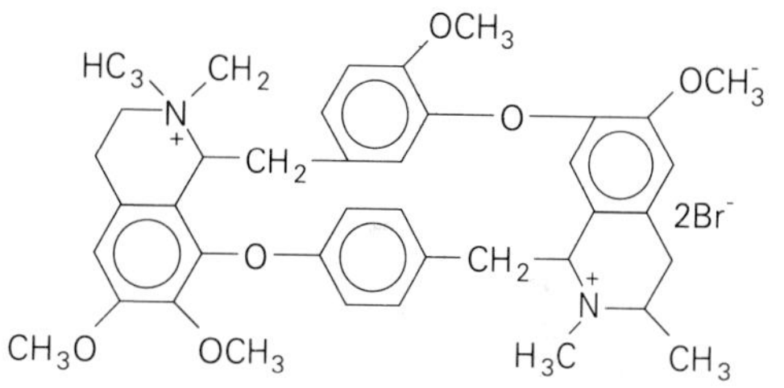

Metocurine was originally prepared by King (1935) at the time of his isolation and investigation of the properties of tubocurarine, but the drug received no further attention until 1950 when its pharmacology was investigated by Collier & Hall. It was originally known as dimethyl tubocurarine but is now regarded as trimethylated (Everett et al 1970).

Pharmacology

It is approximately twice as potent as tubocurarine (Savarese et al 1977) and it appears that an equipotent dose has a similar duration of action to that of tubocurarine. The drug has less effect on the heart rate and blood pressure than the parent substance, and histamine release is also substantially less (Basta et al 1983). The cardiovascular stability may be related to its weaker blocking action both on the sympathetic and on the vagus. The usual clinical dose is 0.25–0.3 mg kg^{-1}.

Pharmacokinetics

Metocurine is about 25% bound to plasma protein, i.e. less than tubocurarine, about 48% being excreted via the kidney in 24 h but only 2% in the bile (Meijer et al 1979). Its terminal half-life of 217 min and its routes of elimination makes it unsuitable for use in patients with renal failure.

Gallamine triethiodide

This is a synthetic non-depolarizing neuromuscular blocking drug which was first prepared and described by Bovet and his colleagues in 1949. Its clinical properties were demonstrated by Mushin and others (1949). It differs from the other muscle relaxants in containing three quaternary nitrogen atoms in its structure. It is readily soluble in water.

Pharmacology

Cardiovascular system. The most striking effect of gallamine on the circulation is an increase in heart rate of the order of 20–30 beats per minute following a dose sufficient to produce abdominal relaxation. This increase in heart rate develops simultaneously with myoneural block, but with large doses may outlast it. A dose of atropine produces a further cardiac acceleration, suggesting that even in large doses it does not produce total vagal block. Cardiac output is increased, as is wound bleeding.

Histamine liberation. Gallamine liberates less histamine than does tubocurarine.

Pharmacokinetics

Gallamine is excreted to the extent of 90–100% by the kidney (Agoston et al 1978). If it is given to a patient with impaired renal function the myoneural block will be more intense and its duration longer. Reversal of myoneural block may be followed by recurarization if

neostigmine is given to such a patient, though the half life of anticholinesterase agents is also prolonged in renal failure.

Dosage and administration

Gallamine is a myoneural blocking agent of about one-sixth the potency and a similar duration to that of tubocurarine. In general its pattern of action is like that of tubocurarine in that it affects the muscles of the face and the throat before it affects the muscles of respiration and the limb muscles. The interval from intravenous injection of the drug until maximum effect is 2–3 min. The usual clinical dose is 3 mg kg^{-1}.

Laudexium methylsulphate

This compound, whose chemical structure is intermediate between the pachycuraries and the long methylene chain leptocurares, is a non-depolarizing relaxant (Collier & Macauley 1952). The dose to produce abdominal relaxation is approximately 40 mg. The arterial blood pressure is usually stable but occasionally shows sharp falls. The main drawback to the drug was that its neostigmine reversibility, though completely satisfactory in experimental animals, was not reliable in the human subject.

C-toxiferine I

Tubocurarine is by no means the only alkaloid with myoneural blocking properties which can be extracted from crude curare. King (1935) refers to an alkaloid named curine and another named berberin. None of those substances, however, has become available for clinical use, though the earliest preparation of curare used successfully in anaesthesia was an extract of all the alkaloids of commercial curare, called Intocostrin, a reflection of the idea that it paralysed the intercostal muscles but not the diaphragm. The curare alkaloid C-toxiferine I was investigated in the 1960s as a potential drug for relaxation in anaesthesia.

Alcuronium

The diallyl derivative of C-toxiferine I has properties which make it clinically useful as a muscle relaxant.

Pharmacology

Cardiovascular system. Muscle paralysing doses are without effect on the synapses of the autonomic nervous

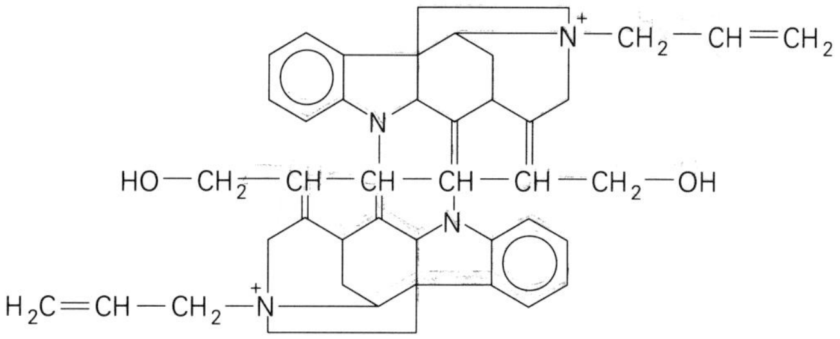

Alcuronium

system, though the heart rate is raised some 15% in humans (Kennedy & Kelman 1970). The effect of alcuronium on blood pressure in humans is dose-dependent, and some workers have found, with doses of $0.2–0.25$ mg kg^{-1}, that the hypotension was indistinguishable from that following tubocurarine. Hunter's (1964) early observations also suggested that hypotension was important at a dose level of 0.16 mg kg^{-1}. Later, however, to exclude the circulatory disturbance associated with a change from spontaneous breathing to IPPV and other influences, he repeated his observations on patients already rendered apnoeic with fentanyl, and found that alcuronium in the same dose caused no significant alteration in blood pressure, while tubocurarine 0.32 mg kg^{-1} caused a fall (Hunter 1968).

Histamine release. Alcuronium does not release histamine to the same extent as tubocurarine. Nonetheless some anaphylactoid reactions to this drug have been reported, including some in patients who were sensitive to other drugs (Lim & Churchill-Davidson 1981, Fisher & Munro 1983).

Pharmacokinetics

The elimination of radioactive alcuronium has been studied in normal patients and those who had renal failure. Over a 24 h period 80–85% of the radioactive material was recovered from the urine in healthy patients. The remaining 15% was more slowly excreted in the bile or in the faeces. The elimination half-life of radioactivity was 200 min in healthy individuals and 165 in anuric patients. However, where alcuronium has been used to produce relaxation in patients in renal failure its duration of action has been prolonged, and smaller doses have been effective.

Alcuronium is mainly bound to albumin. There is therefore a positive correlation between the dose of alcuronium required by any individual patient and the serum albumin.

Dosage and administration

Various clinical studies give information about the relative potency of tubocurarine and alcuronium. It has been found that $0.2–0.25$ mg kg^{-1} of alcuronium would immobilize the cords prior to intubation and largely abolish the succeeding bucking, compared with $0.3–0.4$ mg kg^{-1} of tubocurarine. The onset of relaxation is rapid with alcuronium, provided a large enough dose is given (0.3 mg kg^{-1}), and may be sufficiently rapid to allow a safe endotracheal intubation in a patient with a full stomach (Hey 1973). Older children are less sensitive to alcuronium than adults when doses are calculated on a body weight basis, requiring approximately 0.5 mg kg^{-1} (Bush 1964). The recommended initial dose in neonates, who are relatively sensitive to the drug, is 0.25 mg kg^{-1} (Bush 1964).

Pancuronium bromide

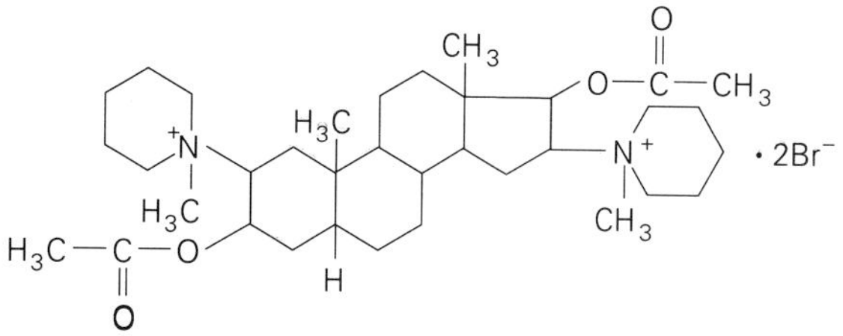

Pancuronium is a synthetic bis-quaternary aminosteroid which produces non-depolarizing neuromuscular block but is devoid of hormonal activity (Baird & Reid 1967).

Pharmacology

Cardiovascular system. In doses of approximately 0.1 mg kg^{-1} it causes a 20% rise in both heart rate and arterial blood pressure (Kelman & Kennedy 1971, Coleman et al 1972). There is no change in peripheral vascular resistance. Atropinization prevents the effect, indicating that it is due to a muscarinic blocking action (Miller et al 1975). It has also been shown that pancuronium blocks the re-uptake of noradrenaline (Marshall & Ojewole 1979) and increased sympathetic activity may result from this effect.

Histamine liberation. This is minimal with this drug, being intermediate between tubocurarine and vecuronium (Booij et al 1980). However, like other muscle relaxants it has been occasionally associated with anaphylactoid reactions (Lim & Churchill-Davidson 1981).

Pharmacokinetics

The extent of protein binding of pancuronium has been estimated by many workers with widely differing estimates, but the figure of 29% given by Duvaldestin & Henzel (1982) appears to be the most reliable. The drug is largely excreted unchanged, 46% appearing in the urine and 5–10% in the bile over the first 24 h. A further 5–10% is excreted in the urine after deacetylation in the form of the 3-hydroxy metabolite which has half the potency for neuromuscular block. Further excretion of unchanged pancuronium and both its active and inactive metabolites occurs after 24 h. Figures for elimination half-life in normal patients range from 108 to 147 min (Agoston et al 1973), but it is considerably prolonged in patients with renal and hepatic failure (Duvaldestin et al 1978a). However, as with gallamine, single low doses of pancuronium may be used safely in patients with poor renal function because of the importance of redistribution in determining early return of neuromuscular function.

Dosage and administration

Pancuronium is usually given in a dosage of 0.1 mg kg^{-1}, and early work suggested that it was about four times as potent as tubocurarine. However, this only applies to 50% depression of grip strength as measured by Lund & Stovner (1970). At 90% depression the ratio is 5 : 1 and at the supramaximal block commonly employed in the operating theatre the ratio is probably 7 : 1.

Fazadinium bromide

Fazadinium is a bis-quaternary yellow azo dye with a pH in solution of 3.2–4.3. It has a shorter interonium

Fazadinium

distance than pancuronium (0.75 nm compared with 1.11 nm).

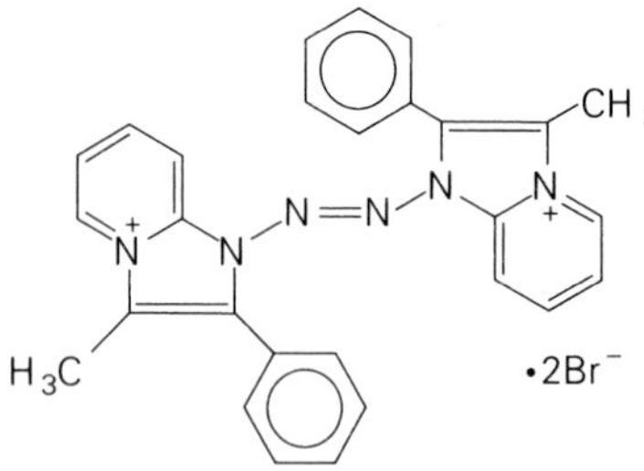

Pharmacology

Cardiovascular system. The most notable feature of the drug is the marked tachycardia (52%) which appears to be produced by blockade of the cardiac vagal endings and by blocking the re-uptake of liberated noradrenaline (Marshall & Ojewole 1979). Cardiac output is also increased by about 40%, but the peripheral resistance falls and arterial blood pressure is little affected (Savege et al 1973).

Histamine release. There is evidence of only minimal histamine release, but some episodes of anaphylactoid collapse have been reported following the drug (Rowlands & Fidler 1978, Alexander 1979).

Dosage and administration

Fazadinium has approximately 0.8 the potency of tubocurarine and a dose of 0.75 mg kg^{-1} is usually given to permit tracheal intubation. Intubating conditions, even with doses of 1.25 mg kg^{-1}, are not as good as those following suxamethonium 1 mg kg^{-1}, and the earliest time for satisfactory intubation is 75–90s (Young et al 1975). In view of its undesirable side-effects it has now been withdrawn from clinical use.

Vecuronium bromide

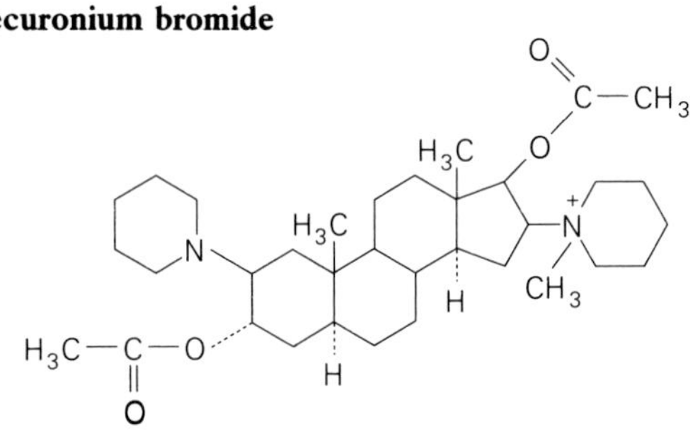

Vecuronium

Vecuronium is a steroid with one quaternary and one tertiary N group, closely related to pancuronium, which was developed in a specific attempt to produce a short-acting, non-depolarizing blocker with no cardiovascular effects (Savage et al 1980). It had been found that one of the quaternary groups in pancuronium was responsible for the block and the other for the muscarinic and nicotinic actions. Substitution of the latter group by a tertiary N in the 2 position has eliminated the cardiovascular effects seen with pancuronium. The molecule is unstable in aqueous solution, being liable to deacetylate in position 3 of the steroid molecule, so it is normally prepared as a buffered lyophilized cake which can be dissolved readily before administration. The cake is stable for a least 3 years and the aqueous solution for at least 24 h at room temperature (several days if stored at 4°C).

Pharmacology

Cardiovascular system. Studies in humans have shown that vecuronium is associated with none of the cardiovascular changes associated with so many other neuromuscular blocking agents (Morris et al 1983). Heart rate, mean arterial pressure, cardiac index and pulmonary wedge pressure are unchanged following its administration in the range 0.1–0.3 mg kg^{-1} (Lienhart et al 1983). Several workers (Salmenpera et al 1983) have reported a fall in heart rate in clinical situations where fentanyl has been used to maintain anaesthesia.

Histamine liberation. Histamine liberation is minimal with vecuronium but anaphylactoid reactions have been reported (Lavery et al 1985b, Treuren & Buckley 1990).

Pharmacokinetics

Vecuronium is 30% bound to plasma proteins, a similar figure to that with pancuronium (Duvaldestin & Henzel 1982). Its elimination half-life is 62–80 min or approximately half that of pancuronium (Fahey et al 1981,

Cronnelly et al 1982), which is in accordance with its shorter duration of action. Urinary excretion of vecuronium is only 15% during the first 24 h and this relatively low percentage means that it is a more satisfactory drug to use in patients with renal failure than is pancuronium. This is also supported by pharmacokinetic studies in patients with renal disease (Fahey et al 1981). The plasma clearance was 4.30 ml min^{-1} kg^{-1} in patients with normal hepatic function, reduced to 2.36 ml min^{-1} kg^{-1} in patients with cholestasis and the elimination half life was similarly prolonged in the latter. In conjuction with this recovery to 75% of twitch height was 111 min in cirrhotics compared with 74 min in normal patients (Lebrault et al 1986).

Dosage and administration

Vecuronium is approximately equipotent with pancuronium in humans and the usual clinical dose is 0.1 mg kg^{-1}. Doses up to 0.3 mg kg^{-1} have been given, but while 0.15 mg kg^{-1} has some advantages for early tracheal intubation (1 min after administration of the drug), there is nothing to be gained from using larger doses. The duration of action to 25% recovery is dose-dependent over the range 0.1–0.2 mg kg^{-1}, and is also significantly longer when halothane or enflurane are used for maintenance, compared with fentanyl (Mirakhur et al 1983). The duration of action of vecuronium 0.1 mg kg^{-1} to 25% recovery is 23 min or approximately half that of the same dose of pancuronium (Kerr & Baird 1982). No evidence of cumulation has been seen when 25% of the initial dose has been given repeatedly over a prolonged operation.

Atracurium besylate

Atracurium is a synthetic bis-quaternary compound which has resulted from a new approach to termination of action — that of spontaneous inactivation by Hofmann elimination. In this the quaternary amine

Atracurium

group is converted into a tertiary amine — a reaction enhanced by raising the blood pH, for instance by hyperventilation, and inhibited totally at a pH of 3.5 at which figure the solution is stored in vitro. The reaction is also temperature-dependent, being inhibited by refrigeration in vitro or clinical hypothermia. A second reaction involved in the breakdown of atracurium is ester hydrolysis in which the long chain joining the N-groups is split, this reaction being catalysed by both acid and base shifts in pH (Stenlake et al 1983). Ester hydrolysis is, in fact, the major metabolic pathway but Hofmann elimination does provide a 'safety net' in patients with hepatic or renal failure (Stiller et al 1985).

Pharmacology

Cardiovascular system. As in the case of vecuronium, one of the primary objectives was to produce a drug without cardiovascular side-effects, and this has largely been successful. However, as with vecuronium, bradycardia in the presence of fentanyl can occur.

Histamine liberation. A rise in plasma histamine level has been by observed following intravenous injection of atracurium 0.6 mg kg^{-1}, by Basta and colleagues (1983), the increase being approximately one-third of that produced by tubocurarine. Some workers have noted cutaneous erythema under clinical conditions but there is no firm indication as to predisposing factors in this effect. There have also been reports of more severe collapse (Aldrete 1985, Lavery et al 1985a).

Properties of the metabolites. The principal end-products of the metabolism are laudanosine and a quaternary monoacrylate. The former has no neuromuscular blocking properties in the cat up to a dose of 4 mg kg^{-1}, but the monoacrylate does produce a dose-dependent neuromuscular block as well as a vagal block within this dose range (Chapple & Clark 1983). Laudanosine is known to produce seizure activity in dogs, but studies with long-term infusions in patients have shown that the level reached in patients is well below the seizure threshold and no side-effects attributable to it have been seen (Yate et al 1987).

Pharmacokinetics

Atracurium is broken down in the body by Hofmann elimination and ester hydrolysis as described above. At the products of these reactions excreted in the bile approximately 55% of the injected dose with 35% ine (Neill et al 1983). Since metabolism plays t in termination of clinical action, and since independent of renal function, the drug is table for use in patients with renal failure

(Hunter et al 1983). The elimination half-life is approximately 20 min (Ward & Wright 1983) which is shorter than that of any of the other non-depolarizing blocking agents.

Dosage and administration

Atracurium is usually administered in a dose of 0.5 mg kg^{-1}, and while the speed of onset of block increases with dose, the incidence of histaminoid effects also rises. The duration of action is similar to that of vecuronium and shorter than that of pancuronium. It is increased by the comcomitant administration of inhalational anaesthetics. As with vecuronium there is no evidence of cumulation with repeated doses (Ali et al 1983).

Pipecuronium bromide

Pipecuronium is a synthetic bis-quaternary aminosteroid closely related to pancuronium. It was first used clinically in Hungary but has now been used extensively in the UK and western Europe generally (Boros et al 1980).

Pharmacology

In doses up to 0.1 mg kg^{-1} the drug has no effect on heart rate, blood pressure and cardiac output (Larijani et al 1989). As would be expected from a drug of this chemical configuration, there is no evidence of histamine liberation.

Pharmacokinetics

The protein binding of pipecuronium appears to be very low — approximately 2%. Like pancuronium, it is largely excreted unchanged through the kidneys. The elimination half-life is approximately 120 min and is significantly longer in patients with renal failure (Caldwell et al 1989).

Dosage and administration

Pipecuronium is approximately 30% more potent than

pancuronium, with an ED$_{95}$ of 49 μg kg^{-1} compared with 60 μg kg^{-1} for the latter, based on cumulative dose–response studies (Stanley & Mirakhur 1989). A dose of 70 μg kg^{-1} of pipecuronium provides satisfactory intubating conditions within 3 min but if the operation is long enough to justify a higher dose, 100 μg kg^{-1} may be used. Its duration and recovery characteristics are very similar to those of the older drug (Wierda et al 1989, Larijani et al 1989) but with its lack of cardiovascular side-effects it should have a wide application in major surgery.

Mivacurium

This is a new non-depolarising neuromuscular blocking agent with a shorter duration of action than that of the currently available drugs. It was developed under the code BW B1090U as a bis-benzylisoquinolinium diester compound which would undergo hydrolysis in vivo by plasma cholinesterase. Early studies in humans (Savarese et al 1988, From et al 1990) have confirmed that it has an ED$_{95}$ of approximately 0.1 mg kg^{-1} with an onset time similar to that of atracurium but with more rapid recovery. As with atracurium, there is cutaneous evidence of histamine liberation but no effect on heart rate or blood pressure has been noted.

Doxacurium

This is another new non-depolarising neuromuscular blocking agent developed by Burroughs Wellcome as an alternative to pancuronium or pipecuronium. The ED$_{95}$ is approximately 0.03 mg kg^{-1} and it has a minimal effect on the cardiovascular system (Basta et al 1988). The main route of elimination of the drug appears to be renal and its duration of action is approximately doubled in anephric patients (Cashman et al 1990).

Decamethonium

The drug decamethonium was chosen from a large group of compounds which sufficiently resembled acetylcholine to block the myoneural junction (Paton & Zaimis 1948) but not to block cholinergic transmission at the autonomic ganglia of the sympathetic chain.

Pharmacology

Neuromuscular system. Studies of the effect of the drug on close intra-arterial injection confirm that it is a depolarizing agent. Decamethonium spares the respiratory muscles of the cat, and especially the diaphragm, more than do other muscle relaxants. It also affects the soleus more than the tibialis anterior, that is to say it affects white muscle more than red. When patients were allowed to breathe spontaneously this sparing effect had clinical significance. Today, however, it is of academic importance only. The myoneural block produced by decamethonium is reversed by hexamethonium, presumably by some form of competitive antagonism. Decamethonium manifests the phenomenon of tachyphylaxis and with repeated doses progressively larger amounts are required to maintain relaxation, and in addition is frequently followed by dual block.

Cardiovascular system. It has no significant circulatory side-effects.

Pharmacokinetics

Decamethonium is eliminated by urinary excretion.

Dosage and administration

The onset of muscle paralysis following a dose of 3–4 mg in humans is rapid, being complete in 3–4 min, and is effective for about 20 min.

Suxamethonium

Suxamethonium has been known since the early years of this century. It was prepared by Hunt & Taveau (1906), who were investigating the actions of drugs with a similarity to acetylcholine in an attempt to elucidate the muscarinic actions of this latter agent. These authors did not comment on its myoneural blocking activity. This property was investigated subsequently, and in 1951 the drug was introduced into anaesthesia (Scurr 1951).

Chemistry

Suxamethonium is essentially a condensation of two molecules of acetylcholine, the attachment being by the

$$CH_3-\underset{\underset{CH_3}{|}}{\overset{\overset{CH_3}{|}}{N}}-CH_2-CH_2-CH_2-CH_2-CH_2-CH_2-CH_2-CH_2-CH_2-CH_2-\underset{\underset{CH_3}{|}}{\overset{\overset{CH_3}{|}}{N}}-CH_3$$

Decamethonium

$$CH_3-N(CH_3)(CH_3)-CH_2-CH_2-O-C(=O)-CH_2-CH_2-C(=O)-O-CH_2-CH_2-N(CH_3)(CH_3)-CH_3$$

Suxamethonium

terminal methyl groups of the acetyl radicals. Like decamethonium it has 10 atoms between the terminal quaternary groups of the molecule.

Suxamethonium is supplied either as the chloride or bromide, as a white crystalline solid with a melting point of 160°C. It is freely soluble in water and solutions are sufficiently stable to allow the supply of the drug in 5% solution for clinical use. Some degree of spontaneous hydrolysis does occur, especially in warm surroundings, and it is desirable to keep ampoules of this solution in a refrigerator. When added to a solution of thiopentone a white precipitate forms which redissolves, though probably both drugs retain their potency.

Pharmacology

Neuromuscular system. The primary action of suxamethonium is to produce a depolarizing block. The onset of paralysis is indicated in many patients by muscle fasciculation. This is noticed first in the face and neck, then as the drug is carried more peripherally, twitching will affect the muscles of the trunk and of the limbs. The twitching is relatively evanescent, lasting some 30–60 s. Fasciculation is prevented by hexafluorenium (Foldes et al 1960) and less reliably by the previous administration of a small dose of non-depolarizing relaxants (see below).

Electromyographic studies in humans show that suxamethonium causes the development of action potentials, which are independent of nervous impulse, as it takes effect (Standaert & Adams 1965). In experimental animals, especially the cat, the muscle twitching and the electrical activity seem both to be direct effects of suxamethonium on the muscle endplate, but the effect in humans may be related to increases in spindle activity and antidromic motor nerve discharges (Kato & Fujimori 1965).

Myoneural block produced by suxamethonium has all the characteristics of a depolarizing effect on the end plate which is related to the initial muscle fasciculation. When the patient is partly paralysed a recording of muscle contraction shows no tendency to fade on repeated stimulation; that is to say, a tetanus is well sustained and post-tetanic facilitation of the response. with myotonia congenita a generalized

marked increase in muscle tone may be produced by suxamethonium. It is possible that patients with dystrophia myotonica may show a similar response.

Tachyphylaxis develops to repeated doses of suxamethonium but not to a continuous infusion, though some patients managed in this way are slow to recover from the myoneural block.

Cardiovascular system. The action of suxamethonium on the circulation varies from species to species. In the earlier studies nicotinic stimulation of the autonomic ganglia was the most outstanding feature, especially in atropinized animals. A classic paper on the action of suxamethonium on the circulation in humans (Lupprian & Churchill-Davidson 1960) drew attention to the occurrence of vagal bradycardia and also the appearance of ventricular extrasystoles which were presumably an escape phenomenon. Particularly severe bradycardia can occur after a second and subsequent dose of suxamethonium. This can be prevented by the prior administration of atropine and most non-depolarizing drugs, for example tubocurarine, alcuronium and pancuronium (Mathias et al 1970) in a quarter or less of the myoneural blocking dose. Bradycardia after even a single dose of suxamethonium is common in children.

Histamine liberation. Suxamethonium is apparently capable of releasing histamine. Further, this property can be independent of an allergic response, for it has occurred in cases where there was no sensitivity on subsequent skin testing. In other instances, however, testing has revealed definite evidence of allergy (Laxenaire et al 1982).

Metabolism of suxamethonium

Suxamethonium or succinyldicholine is hydrolysed by plasma cholinesterase and also breaks down spontaneously in simple alkaline solution. At pH 9.5 there is a 50% loss of activity in just under 3 h. At 100°C there is 50% loss of activity in 30 min (Fraser 1954). The hydrolysis is a two-stage process, being initially (and rapidly) to succinyl monocholine and subsequently and more slowly to succinic acid and choline. Succinylmonocholine has about one-twentieth the neuromuscular blocking activity of succinyldicholine (Lehmann & Silk 1953).

Patients suffering from malnutrition or cachexia may

have low cholinesterase and the action of suxamethonium is liable to be prolonged. Its action is also prolonged in some patients undergoing chemotherapy for cancer, and patients in liver failure.

The local anaesthetic procaine is, like suxamethonium, broken down by plasma cholinesterase. It therefore competes at the groupings of the enzyme where both these drugs become attached. For this reason intravenously administered procaine will potentiate the action of suxamethonium. Trimetaphan is also broken down in this way and may therefore prolong the effect of suxamethonium.

Suxamethonium apnoea

Some patients exhibiting a prolonged suxamethonium action have proved to have relatively normal plasma cholinesterase levels. Kalow & Genest (1957) showed that these patients' cholinesterase had a lowered affinity for suxamethonium. This type of enzyme also had a smaller than normal inhibition of its activity by dubicaine, and Kalow & Genest (1957) suggested that quantification of this inhibition could be used to define those with abnormal, or as they called it, 'atypical', cholinesterase. They also demonstrated that the nature of the patient's plasma cholinesterase was genetically determined. In the vast majority of the population, approximately 80% of the enzymatic activity was inhibited by 10^{-5} M dibucaine. These were homozygotes for normal cholinesterase. In 0.05% of the population dibucaine inhibited only some 20% of the activity of the cholinesterase. These were homozygotes for atypical cholinesterase. In a third group, the heterozygotes, 45–70% of the enzymatic activity was inhibited by dibucaine. These constituted 4% of the population.

Subsequently two other forms of genetically determined abnormality of cholinesterase were demonstrated. First some patients with a prolonged action of the drug had cholinesterase which was scarcely inhibited by 5×10^{-5} M sodium fluoride (Harris & Whittaker 1961). These were homozygotes for this abnormality. There were heterozygotes also, who showed some 25–45% inhibition of cholinesterase by fluoride in comparison with the normal figure of 50–70% inhibition, that is to say heterozygotes for the fluoride abnormality had fluoride numbers of 25–45, while the normal figure was 50–70.

The recognition of these heterozygotes is complicated by the fact that heterozygotes for atypical cholinesterase also have lowered fluoride numbers, so that it requires detailed family studies of the relatives of such patients to elucidate the genetic position. The use of propranolol as a specific inhibitor may allow a sharper distinction between heterozygous atypical and fluoride-resistant patients (Whittaker et al 1981).

There is another quite different abnormality of plasma cholinesterase, the so-called 'silent' gene (Rubinstein et al 1970). Such patients have an inherited absence of cholinesterase. Because the plasma has no cholinesterase activity it is in such cases impossible in the homozygotes to quantify the degree of inhibition of activity by specific inhibitors, and the fluoride and dibucaine numbers cannot be determined. Heterozygotes, however, have normal dibucaine and fluoride numbers but reduced total cholinesterase activity.

The other feature of prolonged apnoea following suxamethonium is the development of dual block. The changes in the motor endplate sensitivities leading to this have been discussed already. Here it is only necessary to stress that dual block is an accompaniment of prolonged apnoea, and not its cause. Dual block is not necessarily neostigmine reversible and it is far better to manage the patient by ventilation until spontaneous respiration returns than to confuse the pharmacological situation by giving further drugs.

Dosage and administration

The usual clinical dose is 0.8–1.0 mg kg^{-1}. This produces visible fasciculations in 15–30 s followed immediately by paralysis. At this stage the vocal cords are wide open, respiration has ceased and, unless there is some anatomical impediment, tracheal intubation is easy. Up to the present no other neuromuscular blocking drug has predictably produced such conditions within 30 s, and for this reason suxamethonium remains the drug of choice when rapid and certain intubation is essential.

Return of neuromuscular function is usually in 3–5 min unless the patient has a low or abnormal pseudocholinesterase.

Unwanted effects

Muscarinic actions. These have been discussed above, with the pharmacology of suxamethonium.

Potassium release. The initial depolarization caused by suxamethonium releases substances normally retained within muscle cells — including potassium, myoglobin, and creatine phosphokinase (Bali et al 1975). As a result the serum potassium rises by an average of 0.5 mmol l^{-1} over the next 10 min but with some patients showing much larger rises. The administration of suxamethonium to burned patients and those following severe trauma has been associated with a high incidence of cardiac arrest which was traced to a potassium rise of

several mmol l⁻¹. Uraemic patients are often hyperkal-
aemic and the additional rise caused by suxamethonium
can raise the serum potassium to a dangerous level.

The most severe and dangerous rises in plasma
potassium level of 3–7 mmol l⁻¹ have been noted when
suxamethonium has been given to patients with large
areas of denervated muscle, for example those with a
spinal cord transection. This abnormal response appears
within a day or two of the neurological damage and may
persist up to 3 months (Tobey 1970). Those with other
diseases of the nervous system, including upper motor
neuron lesions and tetanus, are also at risk. Hyperkalaemia
may also arise after the giving of suxamethonium to a
patient whose muscles have been wasted because of
chronic arterial insufficiency (Rao & Shanmugam 1979).

The substances which minimize fasciculation after
suxamethonium also reduce the rise in serum potassium
— in particular the non-depolarizing neuromuscular
blocking drugs. Hexafluorenium, used to reduce the
dose of suxamethonium required to produce muscle paralysis, also reduces the incidence of fasciculation and the
rise in plasma potassium (Radway et al 1979)

Intragastric pressure.   The muscle twitching which
results from the action of suxamethonium on voluntary
muscles can raise intragastric pressure, particularly if the
contractions affect the abdominal muscles, though in
fact the lower oesophageal pressure rises also, and in
only a small proportion of patients is the pressure increase sufficient to cause passive regurgitation. The
preliminary administration of a non-depolarizing relaxant prevents this rise in intragastric pressure, but of
course in clinical anaesthesia it gives rise to a short
period during which the patient is under the influence
of relaxant plus thiopentone and liable to regurgitate and
inhale gastric contents. The use of the preliminary dose
of a non-depolarizer is therefore incompatible with a
rapid sequence induction.

Intraocular pressure.   Suxamethonium also raises
the intra-ocular pressure during the period of fasciculations (Dillon et al 1957). The rise in intra-ocular
tension may be due partly to contractions of the extra-
ocular muscles brought about by suxamethonium
directly. There is, however, an alternative explanation.
The muscles of the orbit have fibres in them which are
involuntary, contracting clonically, like the muscles in
the walls of the arteriole. A similar sheet of muscles extends across the inferior orbital fissure. All these fibres
are innervated by the sympathetic, and the neuromuscular junction is probably cholinergic. Suxamethonium
sufficiently resembles acetylcholine in its chemical structure to be able to initiate contraction of the muscle (Katz
& Eakins 1969).

Unlike some other undesired effects of
suxamethonium, those on the intra-ocular tension cannot be prevented by the preliminary injection of a
non-depolarizing relaxant. However, acetazolamide,
which itself lowers intra-ocular tension, usually prevents
the rise (Holloway 1980).

Myalgia.   Patients who have received suxamethonium for muscular relaxation very often complain of pain
in the postanaesthetic period. This usually begins on the
morning following the anaesthetic and may last for anything up to a week, though it usually disappears within
48 h. The pain is characteristic in its distribution, affecting the back of the neck, the back of the shoulders
and the area of the lower ribs.

These pains are more likely in the young and in
women, and are less frequent at the extremes of life.
They are much more common in those who are mobilized immediately after operation, or who undergo a
simple diagnostic procedure, for example bronchoscopy.
They are believed to be produced by the inco-ordinated
contraction of individual muscle fibres during the initial
twitching period. When a muscle contracts in response
to an impulse arising from activity of the motor unit all
the fibres contract simultaneously and there is no movement on one fibre or the other. When muscles contract
in response to the drug brought to them by the circulation, as is the situation when suxamethonium is given,
they contract in a different sequence and individual fibres move on each other and tear the fibrous septa
between them (Waters & Mapleson 1971).

The pains can be largely prevented by a preliminary
injection of a non-depolarizing relaxant 1–2 min before
administration of the suxamethonium (Ferres et al
1983), but the dose of suxamethonium must be increased by approximately 50%.

Drug interactions.

Any substance which is capable of inhibiting pseudocholinesterase will prolong the action of suxamethonium.
Neostigmine and pyridostigmine exert such an effect,
but their intense muscarinic activity makes them unsuitable for use in clinical anaesthesia. The substance
tacrine, a derivative of amino acridine, has a powerful
anticholinesterase effect and relatively little muscarinic
activity (Hunter 1970). It has been used quite widely to
potentiate and prolong the action of suxamethonium.
The administration of 0.3 mg atropine will prevent what
little muscarinic activity does occur. This form of
suxamethonium relaxation is associated with less muscle
pain than occurs when repeated intermittent doses of the
relaxant alone are given.

Another drug with anticholinesterase properties was originally itself introduced as a relaxant. This is hexafluorenium, which prevents muscular twitching produced by suxamethonium and has relatively little muscarinic effect, though tachycardia reversible with propanolol has been described (van Hemert & Pearce 1965). The administration of hexafluorenium prior to suxamethonium leads to a 5–7 fold decrease in the amount of drug required for an operation (Foldes et al 1960).

Propanidid. The now-abandoned intravenous anaesthetic propanidid prolongs the action of suxamethonium (Clarke et al 1964) by approximately 100%. This was thought to be related to the hydrolysis of both drugs by pseudocholinesterase, but since propanidid is probably broken down in the liver competition for the same enzyme cannot be the explanation.

Ecothiopate. Ecothiopate iodide is sometimes used in the treatment of glaucoma, and one of its effects is to cause destruction both of true and plasma-cholinesterase within a few days, reaching a peak in 3 weeks. It then takes 3 weeks from discontinuing the drug until the plasma cholinesterase returns to normal. If suxamethonium is given to a patient under the influence of ecothiopate prolonged apnoea may result (Gesztes 1966). However, except where other drugs have been given, the duration of the apnoea it still less than an hour.

REFERENCES

Agoston S, Vermeer G A, Kersten V W, Meijer D K F 1973 The fate of pancuronium bromide in man. Acta Anaesthesiologica Scandinavica 17: 267–275

Agoston S, Vermeer G A, Kersten V W, Scaf A H J 1978 A preliminary investigation of the renal and hepatic excretion of gallamine triethiodide in man. British Journal of Anaesthesia 50: 345–349

Aldrete J A 1985 Allergic reaction after atracurium. British Journal of Anaesthesia 57: 929–930

Alexander J P 1979 Adverse reactions following fazadinium-thiopentone induction. Anaesthesia 34: 661–665

Ali H H, Utting J E, Gray T C 1971 Quantitative assessment of myoneural block. British Journal of Anaesthesia 43: 473–477

Ali H H, Savarese J J, Basta S J, Sunder N, Gionfriddo M 1983 Evaluation of cumulative properties of three new non-depolarising neuromuscular blocking drugs, BW A444U, atracurium and vecuronium. British Journal of Anaesthesia 55: 107S–112S

Baird W L M, Reid A M 1967 The neuromuscular blocking properties of a new steroid compound pancuronium bromide. British Journal of Anaesthesia 39: 775–780

Bali I M, Dundee J W, Doggart J R 1975 The source of increased plasma potassium following succinylcholine. Anesthesia and Analgesia, Current Researches 54: 680–686

Ball A P, Hopkinson R B, Farrell I D et al 1979 Human botulism caused by *Clostridium botulinium* type E: the Birmingham outbreak. Quarterly Journal of Medicine 48: 473–491

Basta S J, Savarese J J, Ali H H, Embree P B, Schwartz A F, Rudd G D, Wastila W B 1988 Clinical pharmacology of doxacurium chloride, a new long-acting non-depolarizing muscle relaxant. Anesthesiology 69: 478–486

Basta S J, Savarese J J, Ali H H, Moss J, Gionfriddo M 1983 Histamine-releasing potencies of atracurium, dimethyltubocurarine and tubocurarine. British Journal of Anaesthesia 55: 105S–106S

Blaber L C 1973 The prejunctional actions of some non-depolarizing drugs. British Journal of Pharmacology 47: 109–116

Booij L H D, Krieg N, Crul J F 1980 Intradermal histamine releasing effect caused by Org NC 45: a comparison with pancuronium, metocurine and d-tubocurarine. Acta Anaesthesiologica Scandinavica 24: 393–394

Boros M, Szenohradsky J, Marosi G, Toth I 1980 Comparative clinical study of pipecuronium bromide and pancuronium bromide. Drug Research 30: 389–393

Bovet P, Bovet-Nitti F, Guarino S, Longov G, Marotta M 1949 Proprieta farmacodinamicho di alensia derivati della zuccinilcholina dota di azione curarica. Rendiconti Istituto Superiore di Sanita 12: 106–137

Bowman W C 1980 Pharmacology of neuromuscular function. John Wright, Bristol

Bowman W C, Webb S N 1972 Neuromuscular blocking and ganglion blocking activities of some acetylcholine antagonists in the cat. Journal of Pharmacy and Pharmacology 24: 762–772

Bowman W C, Webb S N 1976 Tetanic fade during partial transmission failure produced by non-depolarizing neuromuscular blocking drugs in the cat. Clinical and Experimental Pharmacology and Physiology 3: 545–555

Boyce J R, Wright F J, Cervenko F W, Pietak S P, Faulkner S 1986 Prolongation of anaesthetic action by BNPP (bis-[P-nitrophenyl] phosphate). Anesthesiology 45: 629–634

Burkett L, Bikhazi G B, Thomas K G 1979 Mutual potentiation of the neuromuscular effects of antibiotic relaxants. Anesthesia and Analgesia 58: 107–115

Burns B D, Paton W D M 1951 Depolarisation of the motor end-plate by decamethonium and acetylcholine. Journal of Physiology (London) 115: 41–73

Bush G H 1964 Clinical experiences with diallyl nortoxiferine in children. British Journal of Anaesthesia 36: 787–792

Caldwell J E, Canfell P C, Castagnoli K P, Lynam D P, Fahey M R, Fisher D M, Miller R D 1989 The influence of renal failure on the pharmacokinetics and duration of action of pipecuronium bromide in patients anesthetized with halothane and nitrous oxide. Anesthesiology 70: 7–12

Cannard T H, Zaimis E J 1959 The effect of lowered muscle temperature on the action of neuromuscular blocking drugs in man. Journal of Physiology (London) 149: 112–119

Caputy A J, Kim Y I, Sanders D B 1981 The neuromuscular blocking effects of therapeutic concentrations of various antibiotics on normal rat skeletal muscle: a quantitative comparison. Journal of Pharmacology and Experimental Therapeutics 217: 369–378

Cashman J N, Luke J J, Jones R M 1990 Neuromuscular block with doxacurium (BW A938U) in patients with normal or absent renal function. British Journal of Anaesthesia 64: 186–192.

Chapple D J, Clark J S 1983 Pharmacological action of breakdown products of atracurium and drugs used in anaesthesia. British Journal of Anaesthesia 55: 11S–16S

Clarke R S J, Dundee J W, Daw R H 1964 Clinical studies of induction agents. XI: The influence of some intravenous anaesthetics on the respiratory effects and sequelae of suxamethonium. British Journal of Anaesthesia 36: 307–313

Coleman A J, Downing J W, Leary W P, Moyes D G, Styles M 1972 The immediate cardiovascular effects of pancuronium, alcuronium and tubocurarine in man. Anaesthesia 27: 415–422

Collier H O J, Hall R S 1950 Pharmacology of dimethyl tubocurarine iodide in relation to its clinical use. British Medical Journal 1: 1293–1295

Collier H O J, Macauley B 1952 The pharmacological properties of Laudolissin, a long-acting curarising agent. British Journal of Pharmacology 7: 398–408

Cronnelly R, Gencarelli P, Miller R D, Fisher D M, Nguyen L 1982 Pharmacokinetics of pancuronium and Org NC45 (Norcuron). Anesthesia and Analgesia, Current Researches 61: 176–177

Dillon J B, Sabawala P, Taylor D B, Gunter R 1957 Action of succinylcholine on extraocular muscle and intraocular pressure. Anesthesiology 18: 44–49

Dreyer F 1982 Acetyl choline receptor. British Journal of Anaesthesia 54: 115–130

Duvaldestin P, Henzel D 1982 Binding of tubocurarine, fazadinium, pancuronium and Org NC 45 to serum proteins in normal man and in patients with cirrhosis. British Journal of Anaesthesia 54: 513–516

Duvaldestin P, Agoston S, Henzel D, Kersten V W, Desmonts J M 1978a Pancuronium pharmacokinetics in patients with liver cirrhosis. British Journal of Anaesthesia 50: 1131–1136

Duvaldestin P, Henzel D, Demetriou M, Desmonts J M 1978b Pharmacokinetics of fazadinium in man. British Journal of Anaesthesia 50: 773–777

Duvaldestin P, Demetriou M, Henzel D, Desmonts J M 1980 The placental transfer of pancuronium and its pharmacokinetics during Caesarean section. Acta Anaesthesiologica Scandinavica 22: 327–333

Everett A J, Lowe L A, Wilkinson S 1970 Revision of the structures of (+)-tubocurarine chloride and (+)-chondrocurine. Journal of the Chemical Society D: 1020–1021

Fahey M R, Morris R B, Miller R D, Nguyen T L, Upton R A 1981 Pharmacokinetics of Org NC 45 (Norcuron) in patients with and without renal failure. British Journal of Anaesthesia 53: 1049–1053

Feldman S A 1981 Partition coefficient v. dissociation rate constant as determinants of duration of neuromuscular blockade. Anesthesiology 54: 350–351

Ferres C J, Mirakhur R K, Craig H J L, Browne E S,

Clarke R S J 1983 Pretreatment with vecuronium as a prophylactic against post-suxamethonium muscle pain. British Journal of Anaesthesia 55: 735–741

Fisher M M, Munro I 1983 Life threatening anaphylactoid reactions to muscle relaxants. Anesthesia and Analgesia 62: 559–564

Foldes F F, Deery A 1983 Protein binding of atracurium Journal of Pharmacology 9: 429–436

Foldes F F, Deery A 1983 Protein binding of atracurium and other short-acting neuromuscular blocking agents and their interaction with human cholinesterases. British Journal of Anaesthesia 55: 31–34S

Foldes F F, Hilmer W R, Molloy R E, Monte A P 1960 Potentiation of the neuromuscular effect of succinylcholine by hexaflurenium. Anesthesiology 21: 50–58

Forbes A R, Cohen N H, Eger E I 1979 Pancuronium reduces halothane requirements in man. Anesthesia and Analgesia, Current Researches 58: 497–499

Fraser P J 1954 Hydrolysis of succinylcholine salts. British Journal of Pharmacology 9: 429–436

From R P, Pearson K S, Choi W W, Abou-Donia M, Sokol M D 1990 Neuromuscular and cardiovascular effects of mivacurium chloride (BW B1090U) during nitrous oxide-fentanyl-thiopentone and nitrous oxide-halothane anaesthesia. British Journal of Anaesthesia 64: 193–198.

Gardier R W, Tseudos E J, Jackson D R 1978 The effect of pancuronium and gallamine on muscarinic transmission in the superior cervical ganglion. Journal of Pharmacology and Experimental Therapeutics 204: 46–53

Gesztes T 1966 Prolonged apnoea after suxamethonium injection associated with eye drops containing an anticholinesterase agent. British Journal of Anaesthesia 38: 408–410

Gray T C, Halton J 1946 A milestone in anaesthesia? (d-tubocurarine chloride). Proceedings of the Royal Society of Medicine 39: 400–410

Griffith H R, Johnson G E 1942 Use of curare in general anesthesia. Anesthesiology 3: 418–420

Harris H, Whittaker M 1961 Differential inhibition of human serum cholinesterase with fluoride: recognition of two new phenotypes. Nature, London 191: 496–498

Hey V M 1973 Relaxants for endotracheal intubation. A comparison of depolarising and non-depolarising neuromuscular blocking drugs. Anaesthesia 28: 31–36

Holloway K B 1980 Control of the eye during general anaesthesia for intraocular surgery. British Journal of Anaesthesia 52: 671–679

Hull C J 1982 Pharmacodynamics of nondepolarising neuromuscular blocking agents. British Journal of Anaesthesia 54: 169–182

Hunt R, Taveau R de M 1906 On the physiological action of certain cholin derivatives and new methods for detecting cholin. British Medical Journal 2: 1788–1791

Hunter A R 1964 Diallyltoxiferine. British Journal of Anaesthesia 36: 466–470

Hunter A R 1968 Current therapeutics — alcuronium. Practitioner 200: 590–593

Hunter A R 1970 An appraisal of tacrine extended suxamethonium. British Journal of Anaesthesia 42: 155–162

Hunter J M, Jones R S, Utting J E 1983 Atracurium and renal failure. British Journal of Anaesthesia 55: 129S–130S

Johnstone M, Hahmoud A A, Mrozinski R A 1978 Cardiovascular effects of tubocurarine in man. Anaesthesia 33: 587–593

Kalow W, Genest K 1957 A method for the detection of atypical forms of human serum cholinesterase: determination of dibucaine numbers. Canadian Journal of Biochemistry 35: 339

Kato M, Fujimori B 1965 On the mechanisam of fascicular twitching following the administration of succinylcholine chloride. Journal of Pharmacology 149: 124–130

Katz R L, Eakins K E 1969 The actions of neuromuscular blocking agents on extraocular muscle and intraocular pressure. Proceedings of the Royal Society of Medicine 62: 1217–1220

Kelman G R, Kennedy B R 1971 Cardiovascular effects of pancuronium in man. British Journal of Anaesthesia 43: 335–338

Kennedy B R, Kelman G R 1970 Cardiovascular effects of alcuronium in man. British Journal of Anaesthesia 42: 625–630

Kerr W J, Baird W L M 1982 Clinical studies on Org NC 45: comparison with pancuronium. British Journal of Anaesthesia 54: 1159–1164

King H 1935 Curare alkaloids, Part I: tubocurarine. Journal of the Chemical Society 1381–1389

Larijani G E, Bartkowski R R, Azad S S et al 1989 Clinical pharmacology of pipecuronium bromide. Anesthesia and Analgesia 68: 734–739

Lavery G G, Bovle M M, Mirakhur R K 1985a Probable histamine liberation from atracurium. British Journal of Anaesthesia 57: 811–813

Lavery G G, Hewitt A J, Kenny N T 1985b Possible histamine release after vecuronium. Anaesthesia 40: 389–390

Laxenaire M C, Moneret-Vautrin D A, Boileau S 1982 Choc anaphylactique au suxamethonium. A propos de 18 cas. Annales Francaises d'Anesthesie et de Reanimation 1: 29–36

Lebrault C, Duvaldestin P, Henzel D, Chauvin M, Guesnon P 1986 Pharmacokinetics and pharmacodynamics of vecuronium in patients with cholestasis. British Journal of Anaesthesia 58: 983–987

Lee C 1975 Train-of-four quantitation of competitive neuromuscular block. Anesthesia and Analgesia 54: 649–653

Lee C, de Silva A J C 1979a Situation of neuromuscular blocking effects of neomycin and polymyxin B. Anesthesiology 50: 218–220

Lee C, de Silva A J C 1979b Acute and subchronic neuromuscular blocking characteristic of streptomycin. A comparison with neomycin. British Journal of Anaesthesia 51: 431–434

Lehmann H, Silk E 1953 Succinyl monocholine. British Medical Journal 1: 767–768

Lienhart A, Guggiari M, Maneglia R, Cousin M T, Viars P 1983 Cardiovascular effects of vecuronium in man. In: Agoston S, Bowman W C, Miller R D, Viby-Morgensen J (eds) Clinical experiences with Norcuron. Excerpta Medica, Amsterdam, pp 150–155

Lim M, Churchill-Davidson H G 1981 Adverse reactions of neuromuscular blocking drugs. In: Thornton J A (ed) Adverse reactions to anaesthetic drugs. Elsevier, Amsterdam.

Lund I, Stovner J 1970 Dose response curves for tubocurarine, alcuronium and pancuronium. Acta Anaesthesiologica Scandinavica Suppl. XXXVII: 238–242

Lupprian R G, Churchill-Davidson H G 1960 Effect of suxamethonium on cardiac rhythm. British Medical Journal 2: 1774–1777

MacIntosh F C, Collier B 1976 Neurochemistry of cholinergic terminals. In: Zaimis E (ed) Neuromuscular junction. Handbook of experimental pharmacology, vol 42. Springer-Verlag, Berlin, pp 99–228

Marshall R J, Ojewole J A O 1979 Comparison of the autonomic effects of some currently used neuromuscular blocking agents. British Journal of Pharmacology 66: 77–78P

Mathias J A, Evans-Prosser C D G, Churchill-Davidson H G 1970 The role of non-depolarising drugs in the prevention of suxamethonium bradycardia. British Journal of Anaesthesia 42: 609–613

Matteo R S, Pua E K, Khambatta H K, Spector S 1977 Cerebrospinal fluid levels of d-tubocurarine in man. Anesthesiology 46: 396–399

Meijer D K F, Weitering J G, Vermeer G A, Scaf A H J 1979 Comparative pharmacokinetics of d-tubocurarine and metocurine in man. Anesthesiology 51: 402–407

Miller R D, Eger E I (II), Stevens W C, Gibbons R 1975 Pancuronium-induced tachycardia in relation to alveolar halothane, dose of pancuronium and prior atropine. Anesthesiology 42: 352–355

Mirakhur R K, Ferres C J, Clarke R S J, Bali I M, Dundee J W 1983 Clinical evaluation of Org NC 45. British Journal of Anaesthesia 55: 119–124

Morris R B, Cahalan M K, Miller R D, Wilkinson P L, Quasha A L, Robinson S L 1983 The cardiovascular effects of vecuronium (Org NC 45) and pancuronium in patients undergoing coronary artery bypass grafting. Anesthesiology 58: 438–440

Moss J, Rosow C E, Savarese J J, Philbin D M, Kniffen K J 1981 Role of histamine in the hypotensive action of d-tubocurarine in humans. Anesthesiology 55: 19–25

Mushin W W, Wien R, Mason D F J, Langston G T 1949 Curare-like actions of tri (diethylamino-ethoxy) benzene triethiodide. Lancet i: 726–728

Neill E A M, Chapple D J, Thompson C W 1983 Metabolism and kinetics of atracurium: an overview. British Journal of Anaesthesia 55: 17S–22S

Norman J, Katz R L, Seed R F 1970 The neuromuscular blocking action of pancuronium in man during anaesthesia. British Journal of Anaesthesia 42: 702–710

Paton W D M, Zaimis E J 1948 Curare-like action of polymethylene bis quaternary ammonium salts. Nature 161: 718–719

Payne J P 1958 The influence of carbon dioxide on the neuromuscular blocking activity of relaxant drugs in the cat. British Journal of Anaesthesia 30: 206–216

Radway P A, Badola R P, Dalsinia A, El-Gaweet E I, Duncalf D 1979 Prevention of suxamethonium induced changes in serum potassium concentration of hexaflurenium. British Journal of Anaesthesia 51: 447–452

Rao T L K, Shanmugam M 1979 Succinylcholine administration — another contra-indication? Anesthesia and Analgesia, Current Researches 58: 61–62

Riker W F 1975 Prejunctional effects of neuromuscular

blocking and facilitatry drugs. In: Katz R L (ed) Muscle relaxants. Elsevier North Holland, Amsterdam, pp 59–102

Rowlands D E, Fidler K 1978 Fazadinium in anaesthesia. British Journal of Anaesthesia 50: 289–293

Rubinstein H M, Dietz A A, Hodges L K, Lubrano T, Czebotar V 1970 Silent cholinesterase gene: variations in the properties of serum enzyme in apparent homozygotes. Journal of Clinical Investigation 49: 479

Salmenpera M, Petola K, Takkunen O, Heinonen J 1983 Cardiovascular effects during high-dose fentanyl anesthesia. Anesthesia and Analgesia 62: 1059–1064

Savage D S, Sleigh T, Carlyle I 1980 The emergence of Org NC 45, 1-[2β,3α,5α,16β,17-β)-3,17-bis (acetyloxy)-2-(1-piperidinyl)-androstan-16-yl]-1-methylpiperidinium bromide, from the pancuronium series. British Journal of Anaesthesia 52: 3S–9S

Savarese J J, Ali H H, Antonio R P 1977 The clinical pharmacology of metocurine: dimethyltubocurarine revisited. Anesthesiology 47: 277–284

Savarese J J, Ali H H, Basta S J, Embree P B, Scott R P F, Sunder N, Weakly J N, Wastila W B, El-Sayad H A 1988 The clinical neuromuscular pharmacology of mivacurium chloride (BW B1090U). Anesthesiology 68: 723–732

Savege T M, Blogg C E, Ross L, Lang M, Simpson B R 1973 The cardiovascular effects of AH 8165: a new nondepolarizing muscle relaxant. Anaesthesia 28: 253–261

Scurr C F 1951 A relaxant of very brief action. British Medical Journal 2: 831

Shepherd J T, Lorenz R R, Tyce G M, Vanhoutte P M 1978 Acetylcholine-inhibition of transmitter release from adrenergic nerve terminals mediated by muscarinic receptors. Federation Proceedings 37: 191–194

Somogyi A A, Shanks C A, Triggs E J 1977 Disposition kinetics of pancuronium bromide in patients with total biliary obstruction. British Journal of Anaesthesia 49: 1103–1108

Standaert F G 1982 Release of transmitter at the neuromuscular junction. British Journal of Anaesthesia 54: 131–145

Standaert F G, Adams J E 1965 The actions of succinylcholine on the mammalian motor nerve terminal. Journal of Pharmacology 149: 113–123

Standaert F G, Dretchen K L, Skirboll L R, Morgenroth V H 1976 The role of cyclic nucleotides in neuromuscular transmission. Journal of Pharmacology and Experimental Therapeutics 199: 553–564

Stanley J C, Mirakhur R K 1989 Comparative potency of pipecuronium bromide and pancuronium bromide. British Journal of Anaesthesia 63: 754–755

Stanski D R, Ham J, Miller R D, Sheiner L B 1979 Pharmacokinetics and pharmacodynamics of d-tubocurarine during nitrous oxide-narcotic and halothane anesthesia in man. Anesthesiology 51: 235–241

Stenlake J B, Waigh R D, Urwin J, Dewar G H, Coker G G 1983 Atracurium: conception and inception. British Journal of Anaesthesia 55: 3S–10S

Stiller R L, Cook D R, Chakravorti S 1985 In vitro degradation of atracurium in human plasma. British Journal of Anaesthesia 57: 1085–1088

Stovner J, Oftedal N, Holmboe J 1975 The inhibition of cholinesterases by pancuronium. British Journal of Anaesthesia 47: 949–954

Su P C, Wen-Huey L S, Rosen A D 1979 Pre- and post-synaptic effects of pancuronium at the myoneural junction of the mouse. Anesthesiology 50: 199–204

Thomas J, Climie C R, Mather L E 1969 Placental transfer of alcuronium. British Journal of Anaesthesia 41: 297–302

Thomas K B 1964 Curare — its history and usage. Pitman, London.

Tobey R E 1970 Paraplegia, succinylcholine and cardiac arrest. Anesthesiology 32: 359–364

Treuren B C, Buckley D H F 1990 Anaphylactoid reaction to vecuronium. British Journal of Anaesthesia 64: 125–126

van Hemert V R, Pearce C 1965 Hexafluorenium extension of suxamethonium block. British Journal of Anaesthesia 37: 585–590

Viby-Morgensen J 1985 Interaction of other drugs with muscle relaxants. Seminars in Anesthesia 4: 52–64

Ward S, Wright D 1983 Combined pharmacokinetics and pharmacodynamic study of a single bolus dose of atracurium. British Journal of Anaesthesia 1983; 55: 35S–38S

Waters D J, Mapleson W W 1971 Suxamenthonium pains: hypothesis and observation. Anaesthesia 26: 127–141

Waterton C 1825 Wanderings in South America. J Mawman, London

Waud B E, Waud D R 1975 Physiology and pharmacology of neuromuscular blocking agents. In: Katz R L (ed) Muscle relaxants. Elsevier, North Holland, Amsterdam, pp 1–58

West R 1936 Intravenous curarine in the treatment of tetanus. Lancet i: 12–16

Westra P, Houwertjes M C, Wesseling H, Meijer D K F 1981 Hepatic and renal disposition of pancuronium and gallamine in patients with extrahepatic cholestasis. British Journal of Anaesthesia 53: 331–338

White R D, de Weerd J H, Dawson B 1971 Gallamine in anesthesia for patients with chronic renal failure undergoing bilateral nephrectomy. Anesthesia and Analgesia, Current Researches 50: 11

Whittaker M, Britten J J, Wicks R J 1981 Inhibition of plasma cholinesterase variants by propranolol. British Journal of Anaesthesia 53: 511–516

Wierda J M K H, Richardson F J, Agoston S 1989 Dose–response relation and time course of action of pipecuronium bromide in humans anesthetized with nitrous oxide and isoflurane, halothane or droperidol and fentanyl. Anesthesia and Analgesia 68: 208–213

Yate P M, Flynn P J, Arnold R W, Weatherly B C, Simmonds R J, Dopson T 1987 Clinical experience and plasma laudanosine concentrations during the infusion of atracurium in the intensive therapy unit. British Journal of Anaesthesia 59: 211–217

Young H S A, Clarke R S J, Dundee J W 1975 A comparison of tracheal intubating conditions with AH 8165 and suxamethonium. Anaesthesia 30: 30–33

19. Anticholinergic (Antimuscarinic) drugs

R. K. Mirakhur

The term 'anticholinergic' is rather broad, and in the true sense encompasses agents which block both nicotinic and muscarinic actions of acetylcholine. Nicotinic actions of acetylcholine involve ganglionic and neuromuscular transmission and these are more specifically blocked by ganglionic blocking agents and neuromuscular blocking agents respectively. This chapter deals with agents whose actions are generally selective at muscarinic receptors. The classical representative of this group of drugs is atropine. The actions of other drugs of this class are similar to those of atropine, with quantitative differences, and the whole group is collectively known as antimuscarinic, or simply atropine-like, drugs.

History

The intoxicating properties of Datura, Atropa and Scopola have been known since ancient times (Johnson 1967). These agents have probably been referred to in old Chinese and Sanskrit writings and in Homer's *Iliad* and *Odyssey* (Shader & Greenblatt 1972). Belladonna has been used for hundreds of years in the magical and religious rites of many ancient tribes. Deadly nightshade was used to cause prolonged poisoning of obscure origin, and Linnaeus called it Atropa after Atropos, the eldest of the three fates, the one who cuts the 'thread of life'.

The therapeutic use of the belladonna alkaloids dates back perhaps to the Middle Ages, but any attempts at understanding the rationale behind their use began in the nineteenth century. The action of the extract from belladonna leaves on the eye was accidentally discovered in 1776 by Davies, a drug clerk in Hamburg, who inadvertently rubbed some of the extract into his eye. Pure atropine was isolated by Mein in 1831 but samples of pure hyoscine (scopolamine, *l*-hyoscine) became available only in this century (Cannon & Long 1967). The blocking of the cardiac effects of vagal stimulation by atropine was shown in 1867 by Bezold and Bloebaum, and soon afterwards Heidenhain discovered its antisalivary action.

It was Dale who, in 1914, showed that atropine antagonized all the muscarinic actions of acetylcholine.

Although the earliest suggestions of the use of atropine in anaesthesia came from Harley in 1868 and Schafer in 1880, it was Dastre in 1890 who first described his 20 years experience of using atropine and morphine in dogs prior to chloroform anaesthesia for the dual purposes of preventing chloroform-induced cardiac arrests believed to be due to vagal stimulation at that time, and for counteracting respiratory depression and vomiting produced by morphine (Shearer 1960). Deaths under chloroform anaesthesia, however, continued until it was shown that the cause of such deaths was ventricular fibrillation (Levy & Lewis 1911). The early users of atropine in premedication in humans included Aubert and Smith in the last decades of the nineteeth century (Shearer 1960), although its use as an antispasmodic in the treatment of asthma had been described in the 1850s (Shutt & Bowes 1979).

The concept of premedication using morphine and scopolamine was introduced by Buxton (1909). The years 1910–11 saw a great upsurge in the use of premedication as ether was used commonly and secretions were being described as a problem with it. The routine administration of atropine before anaesthesia was suggested by Blumfeld in 1915, but in less than 50 years the routine use of anticholinergic drugs in premedication has been questioned.

Owing to the widespread actions of atropine and hyoscine, many synthetic and semi-synthetic derivatives of belladonna alkaloids have been prepared with a view to more selective action. This has mostly centred on quaternary ammonium derivatives. Such agents have been found to possess only few advantages and in spite of these and more rational understanding, atropine and hyoscine still form the mainstay of anticholinergic drugs widely used in anaesthetic practice (Mirakhur et al 1978).

Source

Atropine and hyoscine are natural alkaloids produced mainly by Solanaceae or potato plants. The alkaloid atropine, a mixture of equal parts of *d-* and *l*-hyoscyamine, is derived mainly from the plant *Atropa belladonna* (the deadly nightshade). The name of the plant Bella Donna (meaning beautiful woman) originates from the use of belladonna alkaloid by women to produce mydriasis for cosmetic purposes. *Datura stramonium* (Jimson weed, spink weed, thorn-apple) is another source of the atropine alkaloid. It is doubtful whether atropine itself is present in the plant or is formed during the process of extraction by racemisation of its isomer *l*-hyoscyamine. The alkaloid hyoscine (*l*-hyoscine, scopolamine) is derived chiefly from the plants *Hyoscyamus niger* (black henbane) and *Scopola carniolica* though some can be derived from *Atropa belladonna* as well. A third alkaloid, *l*-hyoscyamine (bellafoline) is also extracted from the plant belladonna. Being wholly composed of the *l*-fraction, it is nearly twice as potent as atropine, but is not much used due to instability of the solution.

Atropa belladonna and *Hyoscyamus* are found in England and central Europe, and *Datura Stramonium* grows mainly in the eastern United States (Krantz & Carr 1961), *A. belladonna* on the whole being a richer source of the alkaloids. The alkaloids can also be synthesized, but this is not economical. The main source of these drugs is the plant *Duboisia myoporoides* (Tyler et al 1981).

Chemistry and structure–activity relationship

Belladonna alkaloids are esters of complex organic bases with tropic acid. Atropine is an ester of tropic acid and the organic base tropine, whereas the base is scopine in the case of hyoscine. The two drugs differ in having an oxygen bridge across carbon atoms 6 and 7 in the case of hyoscine (Fig. 19.1). The compounds contain an asymmetric carbon atom in the tropic acid molecule which is responsible for their optical activity.

The antimuscarinic action of atropine was believed not to be in the tropine base but due to the aromatic ring in the tropic acid (Ing et al 1945, Stoll, 1948). The nitrogen group is believed by others to be the specifically active component joining to the anionic site of the receptor protein (Shutt & Bowes 1979). According to

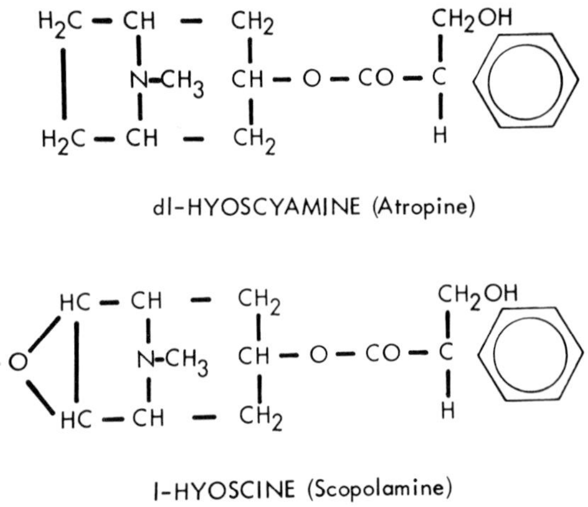

Fig. 19.1 Structural formula of atropine and hyoscine.

Weiner (1980) the intact ester of tropine and tropic acid, and the presence of a free OH group in the acid portion, are also essential for antimuscarinic activity.

Atropine is a mixture of equal parts of *d-* and *l*-hyoscyamine though the *d*-form does not contribute to its antimuscarinic activity (Oettingen & Marshall 1934, Domino & Hudson 1959). Hence atropine is less potent than hyoscine, which is almost pure *l*-hyoscine. This is supported by the fact that 0.6 mg of racemic atropine contains 250 μg of the active base in comparison to 277 μg of the active base in 0.4 mg of hyoscine (Shutt & Bowes 1979). The physicochemical properties of atropine and hyoscine are shown in Table 19.1.

Table 19.1 Physicochemical properties of atropine and hyoscine

	Atropine sulphate	Hyoscine hydrobromide
Physical appearance	Colourless or white crystals or powder	Clear or white crystals or white granular powder
Molecular weight	289.4	303.4
Melting point (°C)	191–196	195–198
Solubility of the base (1 g in each)	400 ml water 3 ml alcohol 60 ml ether 1 ml chloroform	10 ml water Freely soluble in alcohol, ether and chloroform
pKa	9.8	7.9

Atropine and hyoscine are both tertiary compounds. Their quaternary ammonium derivatives, and indeed most other quaternary ammonium antimuscarinic drugs, are in general more potent. They also lack central nervous system activity and are poorly absorbed after oral administration.

Mechanism of action

Atropine-like drugs act mainly by competitive antagonism to the actions of acetylcholine at the muscarinic receptor sites. The effectiveness is greater against injected cholinergic drugs than to the stimulation of postganglionic cholinergic nerves (Weiner 1980). The antagonism can be overcome by the administration of acetylcholine or anticholinesterase agents. Antimuscarinic agents neither undergo any chemical reaction with acetylcholine nor affect its rate of release or hydrolysis (Ambache 1955). Furthermore these drugs do not produce any blockade of transmission of impulses along the nerve fibres (Ambache 1955, Egami 1955), and most have a highly selective action at muscarinic receptors. Larger doses, particularly of the quaternary ammonium drugs, may lead to effects on ganglionic and neuromuscular transmission (Luco & Altamirano 1943, Tum-Suden 1958, Brimblecome 1974).

Muscarinic receptors in different organs differ in their sensitivity to the effects of atropine and hyoscine. Suppression of salivation and sweating occurs with the lowest doses, cardiac effects requiring higher doses while gastrointestinal effects are seen only with the highest doses (Weiner 1980). In addition there is some considerable delay for effects to be apparent on certain organs such as the eye (Herxheimer 1958, Mirakhur 1978). These differences may be due to the release of the chemical mediator in some areas in close proximity to the receptors. According to Eger (1962) the apparent selectivity of the effect of atropine at the muscarinic sites may be dose-related and probably due to other factors such as selective destruction of the drug at some receptor sites, formation of atropine-resistant agents or a true atropine resistance at some receptors. Under appropriate conditions and at high doses, atropine may partially block the response to histamine, 5-hydroxytryptamine and norepinephrine (Weiner 1980). In addition there is atropine resistance in different species (Ambache 1955), within the same species (Ursillo 1961) and within the same animal at different nerve endings (Stoll 1948, Herxheimer 1958).

The structure–activity studies of these drugs suggest the formation of a three-point attachment to the receptors on the -onium nitrogen, tropyl hydroxyl group and the benzene ring (Westfall 1976). The competition with muscarinic agonists is for identical binding sites on the receptors (Birdsall et al 1978).

The effects of anticholinergic drugs often appear to mimic those of sympathetic stimulation.

Atropine

Cardiovascular effects

All the cardiac effects of acetylcholine and vagal stimulation — such as prolongation of P–R interval, decreased conduction and cardiac output — are reversed by atropine. The most noticeable effect is on heart rate and the effect may be biphasic. The effects may also be different in awake and anaesthetized subjects. Doses of 0.3–0.6 mg are often associated with an initial slowing of the heart rate (McGuigan 1921, Gravenstein 1968). A dose of 0.5 mg administered intramuscularly or orally often results only in a decrease in heart rate (Mirakhur 1978).

Following intravenous administration maximum slowing occurs with 0.2–0.3 mg doses (Morton & Thomas 1958). The initial bradycardia is likely after slow injections (Thomas 1965). This is believed to be due to a central stimulating effect of the drug on the medullary vagal centre (Heinekamp 1922) and has been demonstrated by ablation experiments (Goth 1976). Others, however, consider this to be peripherally mediated as initial slowing has been demonstrated with smaller doses of quaternary ammonium derivatives of atropine which cross poorly into the central nervous system (Kottmeier & Gravenstein 1968, Lonnerholm & Widerlov 1975). The response of the SA node itself to atropine is thought to be bimodal, showing slowing of the rate with lower doses and acceleration with higher doses (Das et al 1975). According to Bowman & Rand (1980) small doses of antagonist drugs such as atropine often exert agonist activity on receptors before exerting the antagonistic effect.

The main effect of atropine, however, is production of a progressive and dose-related increase in heart rate (Gravenstein et al 1969, Dauchot & Gravenstein 1971, Das et al 1975, Mirakhur & Jones 1982). Although the main vagolytic action of atropine is on the sinus node, it also exerts direct effects at the AV junction and the subjunctional conduction tissue (Schwartz & de Sola Pool 1950, Averill and Lamb 1959). The amount of atropine necessary for complete vagal blockade is 2 mg according to Kahler et al (1962), but as much as 3–6 mg according to Jose (1966) and Chamberlain et al (1967). The rise in heart rate is most marked in healthy young adults whose vagal tone is high, whereas less tachycardia occurs in the very young or elderly (Dauchot & Gravenstein 1971). The degree of tachycardia following atropine administration is not, however, consistently predictable even if given on a weight-related basis, but there is a negative correlation between the initial heart rate and the rise following its administration (Boba 1976).

Negroes are relatively resistant to the cardioacceleratory effects of atropine (McGuigan 1921) due to genetic variation, and this may also be so with diabetic patients with neuropathy (Wheeler & Watkins 1973), uraemic patients (Lowenthal & Reidenberg 1972) and those who are well digitalized (Kaufman & Yapchai 1968). Though atropine administration to patients on long-term therapy with propranolol results in a significant increase in heart rate, the effects are greatly attenuated (Flessas & Ryan 1983). The effect of atropine on the cardiac vagus is sufficient to prevent vagal inhibition produced by strong electrical stimulation (Krantz & Carr 1961) and Dobkin (1959) has shown its protective effect in patients undergoing electroshock treatment. Atrial fibrillation induced by acetylcholine during vagal stimulation is frequently terminated by atropine (Westfall 1976). De Elio (1948) and Lomax (1976) have attributed quinidine-like and local anaesthetic properties to atropine when used in large doses.

As in the case of conscious humans, atropine produces a dose-related increase in heart rate in anaesthetized subjects (Mirakhur et al 1981). The chronotropic effects are, however, greater in anaesthetized adults (Jones et al 1961, Eger 1962) and more so during halothane than enflurane anaesthesia (Yamaguchi et al 1988). This is believed by Eger to be due to depression of vagal centres by anaesthetics. This is similar to what is observed in children (Samra & Cohen 1980) although in another study no difference was observed between awake and anaesthetized children (Mirakhur & Jones 1982). Reflex vagal cardiac slowing due to inhalation of irritant vapours, stimulation of the carotid sinus, pressure on the eyeballs, pulling on the extra-ocular muscles, peritoneal stimulation, etc., can all be abolished by atropine (Mirakhur 1979). Administration of atropine to children anaesthetized with halothane or isoflurane shows some increase in cardiac output; this is mainly due to an increase in heart rate, which increases to a greater extent in those anaesthetized with halothane (Murray et al 1989).

Cardiac arrhythmias such as nodal rhythm, A–V dissociation and ventricular premature beats occur frequently after atropine administration (Averill & Lamb 1959, Dauchot & Gravenstein 1971). The P–R interval diminishes with increasing doses of atropine (Gravenstein et al 1969). A–V dissociation occurs with doses of atropine around 175 μg kg^{-1} (Hayes et al 1971). Arrhythmias associated with hypotension can reduce coronary blood flow (Corday et al 1959). When used in the treatment of brady-arrhythmias associated with coronary thrombosis, ventricular fibrillation may occur with doses of atropine as small as 0.5–1.0 mg (Massumi et al 1972, Lunde 1976).

Arrhythmias occur more frequently under anaesthesia. The incidence is low during thiopentone, nitrous oxide/oxygen anaesthesia, but increases when halothane is the anaesthetic agent (Farman 1967, Eikard & Sorensen 1976, Eikard & Andersen 1977). Ventricular fibrillation may follow such ventricular arrhythmias (Jones et al 1961, Morikawa & Masuko 1968). The incidence is, however, highest under cyclopropane anaesthesia (Eger 1962). The incidence of arrhythmias during tracheal intubation or during dental surgery is increased by atropine administration (Thurlow 1972, Mirakhur et al 1978).

Cardiac output is increased by administration of atropine (Berry et al 1959, Gorten et al 1961). There is a slight decrease in right atrial and pulmonary artery pressures (Daly et al 1963). Under halothane anaesthesia Farman (1967) reported a 48% increase in cardiac output and a 17% reduction in stroke volume with atropine.

The effect of atropine on arterial pressure in humans is small because of the limited cholinergic innervation of the blood vessels (Goth 1976). However, it counteracts hypotension caused by choline esters. Farman (1967) observed a 24% increase in mean arterial pressure with 0.6 mg atropine administered during halothane anaesthesia. There may, however, be some fall in diastolic pressure (Cullumbine et al 1955).

Vasodilation of cutaneous vessels as a direct effect, and unrelated to its muscarinic actions, is produced by large doses of atropine (Westfall 1976). Flushing, which is observed many times following atropine administration, is regarded by Bowman & Rand (1980) as a sign of relative overdose.

Nervous system

The effects of anticholinergic drugs on the central nervous system (CNS) are unpredictable and variable (Shader & Greenblatt 1972). Atropine in normal doses produces no effect or mild CNS stimulation, although Longo (1966) observed a tendency towards sleep, and reduction in ability to concentrate. There is a short-term memory deficit even with the doses used in anaesthesia (Simpson et al 1987). The effects are, however, usually observed with dosages of atropine in excess of 2–3 mg which rarely produce central toxicity (Cullumbine et al 1955). Higher doses produce more pronounced effects such as restlessness, irritability, disorientation, hallucinations and even delirium (Ketchum et al 1973). Doses of atropine in the range 5–10 mg are associated with significant central effects (Shader & Greenblatt 1972). Such doses may produce what is called a 'central anticholinergic syndrome' with a bizarre and fluctuating picture of both CNS excitation and depression ultimately resulting in coma (Longo 1966, Gravenstein 1968).

Interference with central anticholinergic mechanisms is involved since physostigmine can reverse these effects (Rumack 1973, Granacher et al 1976). Both atropine and hyoscine depress the reticular activating system (Rinaldi & Himwich 1955), an effect which is again antagonized by physostigmine (Exley et al 1958).

Atropine reduces the voltage and frequency of the alpha rhythm in the electroencephalogram (EEG), a pattern like that seen in drowsiness. However, there is no established correlation between the EEG and the behavioural changes (Longo 1966).

Gastrointestinal tract

The smooth muscle tone and activity in the gastrointestinal tract following stimulation of cholinergic nerves, as well as administration of muscarinic drugs, is antagonized by atropine, but the antagonism to the former is incomplete (Weiner 1980). The frequency and amplitude of peristalsis of all segments of the gastrointestinal tract is decreased by atropine (Adler et al 1942, Atkinson et al 1943, Andrew 1954). Excessive motility and hypertonus are also inhibited. In addition gastric acidity and total gastric secretion are reduced, though larger doses manifesting most other antimuscarinic effects are necessary and there are species variations. The duration of this effect is, however, brief. Atropine abolishes or prevents the increased motility and gastric secretion induced by parasympathomimetic drugs and anticholinesterase agents.

Atropine has a mild antispasmodic action on the gall bladder and bile ducts. On the whole the effect is weak. The increased absorption of water and chloride ion from the dog ileum is believed to be not only due to smooth muscle relaxation and increase in the available surface for absorption, but also due partly to increased blood flow to the gut (Eger 1962).

Atropine reduces the opening pressure of the lower oesophageal sphincter (Lind et al 1968, Skinner & Camp 1968, Cotton & Smith 1981), although Fell et al (1983) showed minimal effect following 0.6 mg given i.m. Following i.v. administration the effect is apparent within

3 min and lasts at least 40 min (Cotton & Smith 1981). The frequency of the reflux as shown by the presence of acid gastric contents in the lower oesophagus is also increased by atropine (Brock-Utne et al 1977). There is some controversy about the effects of administration of metoclopramide on lower oesophageal sphincter pressure changes induced by atropine. In animal studies using consecutive administration of atropine and metoclopramide Laitinen et al (1978) showed that the effect of whichever drug was administered first predominated. However, in humans Cotton & Smith (1981) showed that the effects of atropine predominated in whatever order of consecutive administration atropine or metoclopramide were given. This effect of anticholinergic drugs is observed when administered with neostigmine for the antagonism of neuromuscular block, and is not prevented by use of prokinetic agents such as cisapride (Turner & Smith 1985, Derrington et al 1987, Jones et al 1989).

Atropine and hyoscine both possess anti-emetic action (Clarke 1984) but the effects are short-lasting.

Respiratory system

Respiratory stimulant properties have been attributed to antimuscarinic drugs (Wangeman & Hawk 1942) but this has been refuted by others (Steinberg et al 1957).

Atropine relaxes the smooth muscles of bronchi and bronchioles with apparently greater effect on larger airways (Ingram et al 1977). The effects may last for 3–4 h. The increase in dead space is not associated with any increase in carbon dioxide tension, (Smith et al 1967). Inhaled atropine, even in doses of 0.13–0.26 mg, is able to inhibit the effect of methacholine on specific airway resistance completely, although higher doses are required to inhibit vagally mediated bronchoconstriction such as that induced by inhalation of cold air (Sheppard et al 1982). Hypoxaemia observed by Tomlin et al (1964) following atropine premedication was not confirmed by other workers (Nunn & Bergman 1964, Taylor et al 1964).

The secretions from bronchial glands are inhibited by atropine. The reduced frequency of respiratory complications during anaesthesia following premedication with these drugs (Clarke et al 1964) is perhaps due to a reduction of secretions. The incidence of laryngospasm is also lowered by atropine (Eger et al 1961) due to the same mechanisms rather than to a direct action of these drugs on laryngeal muscles (Rosen 1960, Rex 1971). The sputum production in asthmatic and bronchitic patients is reduced by atropine but may increase in viscosity (Lopez-Vidriero et al 1975). The drug also reduces the ciliary action and the velocity of tracheal mucus (Blair & Woods 1969, Annis et al 1976).

Secretions. The reduction of salivary secretions is one of the earliest effects of antimuscarinic drugs, being observed even with the lowest doses (Herxheimer 1958, Mirakhur 1978). The salivary secretions are reduced following stimulation with carbachol or lemon juice (Eger 1962). There are, however, great individual variations (Mushin et al 1953). Subjective dryness of the mouth following atropine administration is perceptible within 15–20 min (Cullumbine et al 1955); the mouth becomes progressively dry, and swallowing and talking may be rendered difficult.

The activity of eccrine sweat glands (innervated by cholinergic sympathetic nerve fibres) again seems to be very prone to inhibition by atropine (Herxheimer 1958). It is observed even in the presence of the vasodilation these drugs may produce. Atropine readily inhibits the sweating induced by muscarinic agents. The skin may become dry and hot. The activity of the apocrine sweat glands (found in the axilla, around the nipples and labia majora and mons pubis), however, is not blocked (Westfall 1976). Lacrimation is reduced by atropine, which can cause conjunctival drying in exposed eyes, but the secretion of milk, urine and bile is not believed to be affected.

Effects on the eye

The mydriatic action of belladonna alkaloids was one of their first recognized effects. This is produced by blocking the responses of the sphincter muscle of the iris to acetylcholine, leaving the radial fibres unopposed. Paralysis of the ciliary muscle of the lens leads to paralysis of accommodation. Pupils enlarge in size and the visual near point recedes. The reaction to light may also be lost. These effects are produced by both local application and systemic administration. The ocular effects set in much later than effects on salivary secretion or heart rate, and also last longer (Herxheimer 1958, Mirakhur 1978). Larger doses may shorten the time to onset of ocular effects. The reasons for the delayed onset of ocular effects include the presence of aqueous humour acting as a reservoir, first accumulating the drug and then releasing it slowly (Herxheimer 1958), and slow release of the bound drug from the pigment of the iris (Salazar & Patil 1976). The eyes of black people are more resistant to the action of atropine (Garde et al 1978).

Systemically administered atropine in doses commonly used in premedication has no effect on intra-ocular pressure in healthy subjects (Cozanitis et al 1979). The pressure may rise on topical administration in eyes with narrow-angle glaucoma, and particularly in those with mongolism (Stoll 1948, Berg et al 1959). However, Schwartz and his colleagues (1957) have shown that atropine in doses used in premedication does not raise the intra-ocular pressure even in glaucomatous patients. Topical instillation of pilocarpine may be used as a safeguard in highly susceptible individuals.

Body temperature

Atropine in healthy normothermic volunteers does not raise body temperature (Mirakhur 1978). A rise in body temperature is, however, often seen, particularly in small children after administration of large doses of atropine or following overdosage (Mackenzie & Pigott 1971, Gillick 1974), but average doses of atropine in normothermic children even in the tropics produce no dangerous increase in temperature (Magbagbeola 1973). Suppression of sweating in high environmental temperatures is considered a contributing factor (Cullumbine & Miles 1956) but large doses may also have a central effect on temperature-regulating mechanisms (Stoll 1948).

Genitourinary tract

Atropine decreases the normal tone of the genitourinary tract and induces a state of relaxation all along from the renal pelvis down to the bladder, as shown by urographic studies (Loman et al 1938). A tendency towards urinary retention may develop (Cullumbine et al 1955). The amplitude of the contractions of the ureter and the drug-induced increase in ureteric tone can be diminished by atropine. The visibility of the renal tract is often improved on radiographs.

The human uterus is little affected by the usual doses of atropine.

Other effects

The effects on metabolism are not certain. Atropine produces no great change in oxygen utilisation (Cavanaugh 1950). The decrease in oxygen consumption observed in animal preparations stimulated with acetylcholine is not observed in man (Stoll 1948). The threshold for renal glycosuria is raised along with a sustained elevation of blood sugar following glucose administration (Cullumbine et al 1955). There is also a loss of beat-to-beat variation in the fetal heart (Taylor 1977).

Pharmacokinetics

Absorption and distribution. Atropine is well absorbed from the gastrointestinal tract except the stomach (Tonnesen 1948, Moller & Rosen 1968, Beermann et al 1971). With a pKa of 9.8 atropine is nearly totally ionized in the acid stomach environment and thus absorption from here is poor. Duodenum and jejunum are the main sites of absorption (Beerman et al 1971).

Absorption of atropine following intramuscular administration is rapid (Schriftman & Kondritzer 1957, Berghem et al 1980). The absorption is inversely related to the volume and concentration of the solution used, the addition of hyaluronidase increasing four times the initial clearance from the muscle (Schriftman & Kondritzer 1957).

Following oral administration, atropine needs to be administered in larger doses. Murrin (1973) and Mirakhur (1978) showed, by measuring salivary secretions and effects on heart rate, that atropine by the oral route is about half as effective as when given intramuscularly. In children, however, Unna et al (1950) showed that three times the parenteral dose of atropine is needed by the oral route for an equivalent effect. Some detoxication may be taking place on its passage through the liver following absorption in the gut, thus accounting for a loss of potency following oral administration (Eger 1962). The absorption from intact skin is only limited (Westfall 1976). Quaternary ammonium derivatives of atropine are only minimally absorbed following oral administration (Moller & Rosen 1968).

Between a quarter and half of the atropine in blood is bound to plasma proteins (Eger 1962, Virtanen et al 1982). Distribution occurs throughout the body and across the blood–brain and placental barriers (Kivalo & Saarikoski 1977, Proakis & Harris 1978). The transfer across the placenta is quite rapid (Kivalo & Saarikoski 1977). However, the spread into cerebrospinal fluid (CSF) may not be as rapid. Virtanen and colleagues (1982) were unable to find any atropine in CSF following a rapid intravenous injection of 0.01 mg kg^{-1}, but found a peak CSF/serum ratio of 0.5 at 45 min after administration of 0.015 mg kg^{-1} atropine intramuscularly. Proakis & Harris (1978), however, found CSF/serum ratios of 0.87 in dogs administered 0.1 mg kg^{-1} atropine intravenously.

Following intravenous administration atropine is characterized by a fast distribution phase and rapid elimination (Berghem et al 1980, Virtanen et al 1982). The peak plasma levels after 1 mg atropine intramuscularly are attained at 30 min with slow decrease over the next 4 h (Berghem et al 1980). The elimination half-life has been reported to be 3 h in adults but is prolonged in the very young and elderly to nearly 5 and 10 h respectively (Virtanen et al 1982). Brown & Geha (1975) observed biphasic plasma levels in their studies with a secondary rise 12–38 h later.

Metabolism and excretion. There is some species variation in the metabolism of atropine (Brown & Geha 1975). Enzymatic hydrolysis in liver is thought to be the main metabolic pathway (Greene 1968). According to Gosselin et al (1960), Greene (1968) and Kalser (1971) only about 30–50% of atropine is metabolized, whereas Tonneson (1950) and Brown & Geha (1975) report more extensive metabolism.

The kidney is the main channel of excretion (Kalser 1971) and over 90% of a given dose is excreted within 24 h, with up to 80% being excreted in the first 8 h. A small amount is lost in the faeces (Gosselin et al 1960).

Overdose

Overdose or poisoning may result from accidental ingestion or administration of an erroneously high dose. Infants and young children are particularly prone to it (Mackenzie & Pigott 1971, Gillick 1974). Toxicity may ensue even from topical application in the eye. The main features include dry mouth and throat, blurred vision, photophobia and hot, dry and flushed skin. The body temperature rises particularly in infants, mostly due to inhibition of sweating. Tachycardia and palpitations may be present. Pupils are dilated and react very sluggishly. Signs of central nervous system toxicity include delirium, excitement, ataxic gait, hallucinations, disorientation and disturbed speech. In very severe poisoning, clouding of consciousness, circulatory collapse and coma supervene. Death may ensue, although fatalities are rare even after large doses (Alexander et al 1946, Mackenzie & Pigott 1971).

Drugs such as the phenothiazines and tricyclic antidepressants may also produce signs and symptoms resembling those of belladonna drugs.

Treatment, apart from gastric lavage in cases of oral ingestion, is mainly symptomatic and is aimed at treating hyperpyrexia and dehydration. Occasionally sedation may be required and small amounts of diazepam are used. Physostigmine in doses of 1–2 mg, repeated if necessary, is the specific antidote, particularly where signs of CNS toxicity are present, since it has both central and peripheral actions.

Hyoscine (scopolamine)

Most of the peripheral actions of hyoscine are qualitatively similar to those of atropine although these differ quantitatively. The effects are, however, different on the central nervous system.

Cardiovascular effects

The effects of hyoscine on heart rate have been considered relatively weak (Orkin et al 1956). However Stephen and colleagues (1956) observed an increase in heart rate with it, and Gravenstein et al (1964) observed similar peak effects on heart rate with equal doses of atropine and hyoscine. The effect is usually short-lasting and followed by secondary bradycardia (List & Gravenstein 1965, Domino & Corssen 1967). Heart rate under anaesthesia is higher following premedication with atropine in comparison to hyoscine (Eger 1962). Like atropine, cardiac output is increased by hyoscine (Gravenstein et al 1964, List & Gravenstein 1965).

Central nervous system effects

The central potency of hyoscine is eight to ten times that of atropine (Longo 1966, Westfall 1976). The usual therapeutic doses produce drowsiness, amnesia, fatigue and sleep. The incidence of amnesia produced by diazepam is increased by concurrent administration of hyoscine (Frumin et al 1976). The toxic effects on CNS in higher doses are similar to those seen with atropine, and the mechanism and treatment are also similar. Elderly people may show symptoms such as restlessness and confusion even at lower doses. Although hyoscine exerts greater effects on EEG it does not produce physiological sleep (Sagales et al 1969). For pre-anaesthetic medication the sedative effect of hyoscine is considered an additional advantage (Eger et al 1961, Clarke et al 1964).

Gastrointestinal effects

The effects of hyoscine on the gastrointestinal tract are similar to those of atropine. Like atropine, it lowers the opening pressure of the lower oesophageal sphincter (Brock-Utne et al 1977). The anti-emetic effect of hyoscine is superior to that of atropine (Clarke 1984), perhaps due to its greater central effects.

Effects on respiratory system and secretions

The smooth muscles of the bronchioles are relaxed but the effect is less potent than that of atropine. The secretions from bronchial glands are inhibited and premedication with hyoscine is associated with a low incidence of laryngospasm (Eger et al 1961).

Hyoscine is more potent than atropine in reducing the salivary secretions and is longer-lasting (Wyant & Dobkin 1957, Herxheimer 1958, Domino & Corssen 1967, Mirakhur 1978). Inhibition of sweat secretion occurs fairly early after hyoscine administration (Frumin & Papper 1951).

Eye

Hyoscine is more potent than atropine with regard to effects on the eye (Herxheimer 1958, Mirakhur 1978) but like atropine these appear later than those on the heart rate or secretions and last longer. There is pupillary dilatation and loss of accommodation, particularly with larger doses. Routine premedicant doses have no effect on intra-ocular pressure (Schwartz et al 1957).

Other effects

Hyoscine is perhaps more potent than atropine in raising the body temperature in susceptible patients (Eger et al 1961). The effects are similar to those of atropine in reducing the tone of the genitourinary tract but the presence of central effects has not popularized its use in such situations. Hyoscine used in labour for producing 'twilight' sleep does not interfere with uterine contractions.

Absorption, distribution and excretion

Hyoscine is rapidly taken up following intramuscular administration but the absorption following oral administration is not as good as following atropine (Lomholt 1946, Mirakhur 1978). With a pKa of 7.9 the absorption from stomach is absent due to near complete ionization. The drug is broken down in the liver; less than 1% of an administered dose of hyoscine is recovered unaltered from urine, indicating extensive metabolism. Very little is known about the pharmacokinetics of hyoscine.

The usual dose of hyoscine in premedication is 0.2–0.4 mg. The drug has been shown not to be of any use in mixture with anticholinesterases for antagonism of non-depolarizing neuromuscular block, due to its weak and transient cardiac effects (Bali & Mirakhur 1980).

Other anticholinergic agents

Although atropine and hyoscine have been the mainstay of anticholinergic agents, particularly in anaesthetic practice, other agents have been synthesized and studied particularly from the point of view of controlling gastric acid secretion without producing other effects.

The substitutes for atropine and hyoscine can be divided into tertiary amines and quaternary ammonium compounds. Tertiary amines are further divided into two broad groups. One group includes agents such as homatropine, cyclopentolate and tropicamide, used for their mydriatic and cycloplegic effects. Homatropine is used topically in a 0.5–5% solution. It acts quickly but is shorter-acting than atropine. Children may be resistant to its effects. Cyclopentolate is used in 0.5–2.0% concentration: it acts rapidly and is short-acting. It is commonly used for fundal examination and has replaced homatropine in routine use. Tropicamide is used as a 1% solution and its effects wear off very rapidly.

The second subgroup of tertiary amines are those possessing antispasmodic properties. The agents comprising this group include oxyphencyclimine, piperidolate and dicyclomine, used in dosages of 10 mg, 50 mg and 20 mg respectively, on average. The antispasmodic action is due to possession of a papaverine-like action of these agents. Being tertiary amines, these agents are absorbed when administered orally, and they cross the blood-brain barrier producing undesirable central effects, although other antimuscarinic actions are minimal.

Another tertiary compound, bellafoline (l-hyoscyamine), was reported by Galloon (1956) and Wyant and Dobkin (1957) as an antisialogogue agent superior to atropine. It is twice as potent as atropine but produces side-effects such as dizziness, excessive tachycardia and arrhythmia.

The quaternary ammonium compounds are poorly and unreliably absorbed from the gastrointestinal tract and penetration across the blood–brain barrier is also poor. The antimuscarinic activity on the gut is relatively more specific with these agents. Their ganglion blocking action is also relatively greater. While this may contribute to their action on the gut, it may also be the reason for side-effects such as impotence and postural hypotension found with some of these agents when used for a considerable length of time. This group comprises synthetic and semi-synthetic compounds including quaternary ammonium derivatives of atropine and hyoscine.

Hyoscine butylbromide has been found to give rise to an excessive increase in heart rate (Moller & Rosen, 1968). Methantheline (Banthine), propantheline (Probanthine) and oxyphenonium (Antrenyl) have been the most widely used drugs. All are more potent and longer-lasting than atropine but also have greater ganglion blocking or neuromuscular blocking effects. All have found favour with clinicians for the management of peptic ulcer but have been replaced by more specific agents like cimetidine and ranitidine. The agents have no overall advantages over atropine and hyoscine as far as their use in anaesthetic practice is concerned (Stephen et al 1956, Wyant & Dobkin 1958).

Glycopyrrolate

Glycopyrrolate (Fig. 19.2), a quaternary ammonium compound, has been evaluated extensively in anaesthetic practice, although the drug has been used in the treatment of peptic ulcer disease for a number of years and, like other anticholinergic drugs, is no longer popular there. The major advantage of the drug is its selectivity of action (Fig. 19.3) and cardiostability (Oduro 1975, Mirakhur et al 1978, McCubbin et al 1979). The drug is a superior antisialogogue and does not cross the blood–brain barrier; it thus lacks central and ocular effects including any effects on short-term memory (Simpson et al 1987). The incidence of arrhythmias and the degree of tachycardia are less with this agent when given intramuscularly in premedication or intravenously at induction of anaesthesia (Mirakhur et al 1978, Greenan 1984). The greatest advantage of the drug is apparent when it is used in a combination with neostigmine for the antagonism of neuromuscular block. This is discussed more fully in the chapter on anticholinesterases (Ch. 20). The drug is about twice as potent as atropine regarding effects on heart rate in anaesthetized patients (Mirakhur et al 1981). The pharmacology of glycopyrrolate has recently been reviewed by Mirakhur and Dundee (1983).

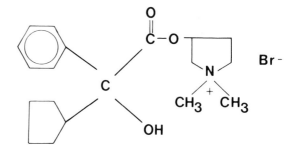

Fig. 19.2 Structural formula of glycopyrrolate bromide.

Clinical uses of anticholinergic agents

The clinical uses of atropine-like agents are found both in medical fields and in anaesthesia.

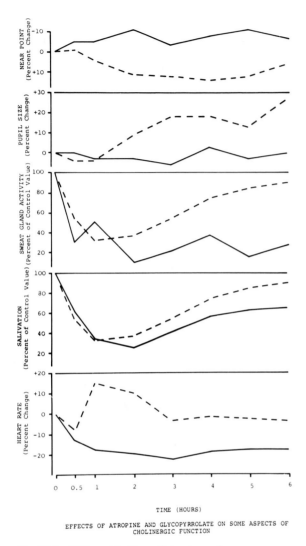

EFFECTS OF ATROPINE AND GLYCOPYRROLATE ON SOME ASPECTS OF
CHOLINERGIC FUNCTION

Fig. 19.3 Differential effects of atropine and
glycopyrrolate. Atropine – –; glycopyrrolate —— (from
Journal of the Royal Society of Medicine).

Medical uses

Although the use of anticholinergic drugs was widespread in the treatment of peptic ulcer disease at one
time, these agents are not popular due to their side-
effects, even in the case of quaternary ammonium drugs,
as well as the availability of specific H_2 receptor antagonists. Other indications pertaining to their use in gastrointestinal conditions include colic and intestinal
hypermotility. Atropine may be of value in the treatment of bradyarrhythmias associated with acute
myocardial infarction. Hyoscine is used in the manage-

ment of labour pains and as a prophylactic against
motion sickness. Anticholinergic drugs have been used
in the treatment of parkinsonism, and though replaced
by levodopa as a drug of choice, are still used sometimes
in combination with it. The main indications nowadays,
apart from anaesthesia, are in ophthalmology for mydriasis and cycloplegia, and for the treatment of
organophosphorus poisoning (due to *Amanita muscaria*).

Uses in anaesthesia

Antimuscarinic drugs are used preoperatively in premedication, during operation for treating bradycardia
and at the end of surgery in a mixture with anticholinesterase agents for antagonizing residual non-
depolarizing neuromuscular block. The main reasons for
using these drugs in premedication are for drying up of
secretions and protection against vagal reflexes
(Mirakhur 1979). Modern anaesthetic agents and techniques, with the exception of ether, rarely cause
problems with secretions and any intraoperative bradycardia is treated more effectively and predictably with
the anticholinergic agents administered intravenously.
Omitting anticholinergic drugs in premedication has
been shown to have no adverse effects and may even be
advantageous (Kessell 1974, Leighton & Sanders 1976;
Mirakhur et al 1978, 1979, Madej & Paasuke 1987). The
possible adverse effects have been discussed previously.
In addition, the drying effect of these drugs is subjec-
tively very unpleasant. Their routine use has been
questioned even in obstetric anaesthetic practice
(Mirakhur 1979 May et al 1988). It is thus not surprising to find that the use of anticholinergic drugs is no
longer routine in premedication. (Mirakhur et al 1978).
Although glycopyrrolate shares many of the disadvantages of atropine and hyoscine when used in routine
premedication, it has the advantage of cardio-stability if
one intends using an anticholinergic premedicant. Anticholinergic drug administration, either preoperatively by
the i.m. or i.v. routes or during operation, may still be
required in infants and children (Leigh et al 1957,
Mirakhur 1982), when suxamethonium is administered
repeatedly (Lupprian & Churchill-Davidson 1960), when
an ether anaesthetic is used, for intraoperative bradycardia and in cases of oropharyngeal or airway
instrumentation. Oral atropine administration preoperatively appears to attenuate cardiovascular depression
observed in infants during halothane anaesthesia (Miller
& Friesen 1988). The usual premedicant dose of atropine
is about 10 μg kg^{-1} i.m. For intravenous use the dose
is 0.2–0.6 mg. Glycopyrrolate is used intramuscularly in
a dose of about 5 μg kg^{-1} and intraoperatively in doses
of 0.1–0.2 mg.

There is no debate as to their need when neostigmine or other anticholinesterases are used to antagonize non-depolarizing neuromuscular block. The only debate is with regard to whether the anticholinergic drug should be given before or in a mixture with the anticholinesterase agent. According to the available evidence it is preferable to administer the two together for greater cardiovascular stability (Ovassapian 1969, Cozanitis et al 1980, Clarke & Mirakhur 1982). Glycopyrrolate has perhaps its best use in this situation because of greater cardiovascular stability and better antisialogogue effect (Ramamurthy et al 1972, Ostheimer 1977, Mirakhur et al 1977) and early recovery of consciousness based on lack of central effects (Baraka et al 1980, Heinonen et al 1982). It is of particular advantage in patients with cardiovascular disease (Cozanitis et al 1980, Bali & Mirakhur 1980) and has been discussed in a recent review (Mirakhur & Dundee 1983). The dosage of atropine in this situation is 20–25 μg kg^{-1} and that of glycopyrrolate 10 μg kg^{-1}.

REFERENCES

Adler H F, Atkinson A J, Ivy A C 1942 Effect of morphine and dilaudid on the ileum and of morphine, dilaudid and atropine on the colon of man. Archives of Internal Medicine 69: 974–985

Alexander E, Morris D P, Eslick R L 1946 Atropine poisoning: report of a case with recovery after ingestion of one gram. New England Journal of Medicine 234: 258–259

Ambache N 1955 The use and limitations of atropine for pharmacological studies on autonomic effectors. Pharmacological Reviews 7: 467–494

Andrew R 1954 Gastric and intestinal motility studies with morphine, atropine, hexamethonium bromide and Banthine. Australian Annals of Medicine 3: 305–311

Annis P, Landa J, Lichtiger M 1976 Effects of atropine on velocity of tracheal mucus in anesthetized patients. Anesthesiology 44: 74–77

Atkinson A J, Adler H F, Ivy A C 1943 Motility of the human colon: the normal pattern, dyskinesia and the effect of drugs. Journal of the American Medical Association 121: 646–652

Averill K H, Lamb L E 1959 Less commonly recognised actions of atropine on cardiac rhythm. American Journal of Medical Sciences 237: 304–318

Bali I M, Mirakhur R K 1980 Comparison of glycopyrrolate, atropine and hyoscine in mixture with neostigmine for reversal of neuromuscular block following closed mitral valvotomy. Acta Anaesthesiologica Scandinavica 24: 331–335

Baraka A, Yared J, Karam A M, Winnie A 1980 Glycopyrrolate — neostigmine and atropine — neostigmine mixtures affect post-anesthetic arousal times differently. Anesthesia and Analgesia 59: 431–434

Beermann B, Hellstrom K, Rosen A 1971 The gastrointestinal absorption of anticholinergic drugs: comparison between individuals. Acta Pharmacologica et Toxicologica 29 (Suppl 3): 98–102

Berg J M, Brandon M W S, Kirman B H 1959 Atropine in mongolism. Lancet ii: 441–442.

Berghem L, Bergman U, Schildt B, Sorbo B 1980 Plasma atropine concentrations determined by radioimmunoassay after single-dose i.v. and i.m. administration. British Journal of Anaesthesia 52: 597–601

Berry J N, Thompson H K, Miller D E, McIntosh H D 1959 Changes in cardiac output, stroke volume and central venous pressure induced by atropine in man. American Heart Journal 58: 204–213

Birdsall N J M, Burgen A S V, Hulme E C 1978 Correlation between the binding properties and pharmacological responses of muscarinic receptors. In: Jenden D J (ed) Cholinergic mechanisms and phychopharmacology, vol 24. Plenum Press, New York, pp 25–33

Blair A M, Woods A 1969 The effects of isoprenaline, atropine and disodium cromoglycate on ciliary motility and mucus flow measured in vivo in cats. British Journal of Pharmacology 35: 379–380

Blumfeld J 1915 The influence of preliminary narcotics on the induction, maintenance and after effects of anaesthesia. Proceedings of the Royal Society of Medicine 8: 15–17

Boba A 1976 The effects of atropine on the heart rate. Canadian Anaesthetists' Society Journal 23: 92–98

Bowman W C, Rand M J 1980 Textbook of pharmacology. Blackwell Scientific Publications, Oxford. pp 10.11–10.17

Brimblecome R W 1974 Neuromuscular effects of some antimuscarinic drugs. Macmillan, London, pp 47–50

Brock-Utne J G, Rubin J, McAravey R, Dow T G B, Welman S, Dimopoulos G E, Moshal M G 1977 The effect of hyoscine and atropine on the lower oesophageal sphincter. Anaesthesia and Intensive Care 5: 223–225

Brown B R Jr, Geha D G 1975 Biotransformation of drugs used as premedication agents. International Anesthesiology Clinics 13: 61–77

Buxton D 1909 Discussion on the treatment of shock during anaesthesia. Proceedings of the Royal Society of Medicine 2: 55–70

Cannon J G, Long P J 1967 Postganglionic parasympathetic depressants. In: Burger A (ed) Drugs affecting the peripheral nervous system, vol I. Marcel Dekker, New York, pp 133–148

Cavanaugh D J 1950 Effects of atropine on brain respiration. Proceedings of the Society for Experimental Biology and Medicine 75: 607–610

Chamberlain D A, Turner P, Sneddon J M 1967 Effects of atropine on heart rate in healthy man. Lancet ii: 12–15

Clarke R S J 1984 Nausea and vomiting. British Journal of Anaesthesia 56: 19–27

Clarke R S J, Mirakhur R K 1982 Antagonism of neuromuscular block. British Journal of Anaesthesia 54: 793–794

Clarke R S J, Dundee J W, Moore J 1964 Studies of drugs given before anaesthesia. IV: Atropine and hyoscine. British Journal of Anaesthesia 36: 648–654

Corday E, Gold H, DeVera L B, Williams J H, Fields J 1959 Effects of cardiac arrhythmias on coronary circulation. Annals of Internal Medicine 50: 535–553

Cotton B R, Smith G 1981 Single and combined effects of

atropine and metoclopramide on the lower oesophageal sphincter pressure. British Journal of Anaesthesia 53: 869–874

Cozanitis D A, Dundee, J W, Buchanan T A S, Archer D B 1979 Atropine versus glycopyrrolate. A study of intraocular pressure and pupil size in man. Anaesthesia 34: 236–238

Cozanitis D A, Dundee J W, Merrett J D, Jones C J, Mirakhur R K 1980 Evaluation of glycopyrrolate and atropine as adjuncts to reversal of nondepolarising neuromuscular blocking agents in a 'true-to-life' situation. British Journal of Anaesthesia 52: 85–89

Cullumbine H, Miles S 1956 The effect of atropine sulphate on men exposed to warm environments. Quarterly Journal of Experimental Physiology 41: 162–179

Cullumbine H, McKee W H E, Creasy N H 1955 The effects of atropine sulphate upon healthy male subjects. Quarterly Journal of Experimental Physiology 40: 309–319

Dale H H 1914 The action of certain esters and ethers of choline, and their relation to muscarine. Journal of Pharmacology and Experimental Therapeutics 6: 147–190

Daly W J, Ross J C, Behnke R H 1963 The effect of changes in the pulmonary vascular bed produced by atropine, pulmonary engorgement, and positive-pressure breathing on diffusing and mechanical properties of the lung. Journal of Clinical Investigation 42: 1083–1094

Das G, Talmers F N, Weissler A M 1975 New observations on the effects of atropine on the sinoatrial and atrioventricular nodes in man. American Journal of Cardiology 36: 281–285

Dauchot P J, Gravenstein J S 1971 Effects of atropine on the electrocardio-gram in different age groups. Clinical Pharmacology and Therapeutics 12: 274–280

De Elio F J 1948 Acetylcholine antagonists: a comparison of their action in different tissues. British Journal of Pharmacology 3: 108–112

Derrington M C, Hindocha N, Smith G 1987 Evaluation of the combined effects of glycopyrrolate and neostigmine on the lower oesophageal sphincter. British Journal of Anaesthesia 59: 545–547

Dobkin A B 1959 The effect of anticholinergic drugs on the cardiac vagus. I: clinical observations in patients undergoing electroshock treatment. Canadian Anaesthetists' Society Journal 6: 51–61

Domino E F, Corssen G 1967 Central and peripheral effects of muscarinic cholinergic blocking agents in man. Anesthesiology 28: 568–574

Domino E F, Hudson R D 1959 observations on the pharmacological actions of the isomers of atropine. Journal of Pharmacology and Experimental Therapeutics 127: 305–312

Egami M 1955 Susceptibility of afferent mesenteric impulses to procaine, dibucaine etc. Japanese Journal of Pharmacology 4: 155–159

Eger E I 1962 Atropine, scopolamine and related compounds. Anesthesiology 23: 365–383

Eger E I, Kraft I D, Keasling H H 1961 Comparison of atropine or scopolamine plus pentobarbital, meperidine or morphine as pediatric preanesthetic medication. Anesthesiology 22: 962–969

Eikard B, Andersen J R 1977 Arrhythmias during halothane anaesthesia. II: The influence of atropine. Acta Anaesthesiologica Scandinavica 21: 245–251

Eikard B, Sorensen B 1976 Arrhythmias during halothane anaesthesia. I: The influence of atropine during induction with intubation. Acta Anaesthesiologica Scandinadvica 20: 296–306

Exley K A, Fleming M C, Espelien A D 1958 Effects of drugs which depress the peripheral nervous system on the reticular activating system of the cat. British Journal of Pharmacology and Chemotherapy 13: 485–492

Farman J V 1967 Circulatory effects of atropine during halothane anaesthesia. British Journal of Anaesthesia 39: 226–235

Fell D, Cotton B R, Smith G 1983 I.M. atropine and regurgitation. British Journal of Anaesthesia 55: 256–257

Flessas A P, Ryan T J 1983 Atropine-induced cardioacceleration in patients on chronic propranolol therapy: comparison with the positive chronotropic effect of isometric exercise. American Heart Journal 105: 230–232

Frumin M J, Papper E M 1951 The inhibition of sweating in man by scopolamine. Anesthesiology 12: 627–632

Frumin M J, Herekar V R, Jarvik M E 1976 Amnesic actions of diazepam and scopolamine in man. Anesthesiology 45: 406–412

Galloon S 1956 A comparison of the antisialogogue action of atropine and hyoscyamine. British Journal of Anaesthesia 28: 113–117

Garde J F, Aston R, Endler G C, Sison O S 1978 Racial mydriatic response to belladonna premedication. Anesthesia and Analgesia 57: 572–576

Gillick J S 1974 Atropine toxicity in a neonate. British Journal of Anaesthesia 46: 793–794

Gorten R, Gunnells J C, Weissler A M, Stead E A 1961 Effects of atropine and isoproterenol on cardiac output, central venous pressure and mean transit time of indicators placed at three different sites in the venous system. Circulation Research 9: 979–983

Gosselin R E, Gabourel J D, Wills J H 1960 The fate of atropine in man. Clinical Pharmacology and Therapeutics 1: 597–603

Goth A 1976 Medical pharmacology: principles and concepts. C V Mosby Co, St Louis, pp 115–128

Granacher R P, Baldessarini R J, Messner E 1976 Physostigmine treatment of delirium induced by anticholinergics. American Family Physician 13: 99–103

Gravenstein J S 1968 The belladonna drugs. International Anesthesiology Clinics 6: 33–40

Gravenstein J S, Andersen T W, De Padua E B 1964 Effects of atropine and scopolamine on the cardiovascular system in man. Anesthesiology 25: 123–130

Gravenstein J S, Ariet M, Thornby J I 1969 Atropine on the electrocardiogram. Clinical Pharmacology and Therapeutics 10: 660–666

Greenan J 1984 Cardiac dysrhythmias and heart rate changes at induction of anaesthesia: a comparison of two intravenous anticholinergics. Acta Anaesthesiologica Scandinavica 28: 182–184

Greene N M 1968 The metabolism of drugs employed in anaesthesia. II. Anesthesiology 29: 327–360

Hayes A H, Copelan H W, Ketchom I S 1971 Effects of large intramuscular doses of atropine on cardiac rhythm. Clinical Pharmacology and Therapeutics 12: 482–486

Heinekamp W J R 1922 The central influence of atropine

and hyoscine on heart rate. Journal of Laboratory and Clinical Medicine 8: 104–111

Heinonen J, Salmenperra M, Takkunen O 1982 Advantages of glycopyrrolate over atropine during reversal of pancuronium block. Acta Anaesthesiologica Scandinavica 26: 147–150

Herxheimer A 1958 A comparison of some atropine-like drugs in man, with particularly reference to their end-organ specificity. British Journal of Pharmacology 13: 184–192

Ing H R, Dawes G S, Wajda I 1945 Synthetic substitutes for atropine. Journal of Pharmacology and Experimental Therapeutics 85: 85–102

Ingram R H J, Wellman J J, McFadden E R, Mead J 1977 Relative contribution of large and small airways to flow limitation in normal subjects before and after atropine and isoproterenol. Journal of Clinical Investigation 59: 696–703

Johnson C B 1967 Mystical force of the nightshade. International Journal of Neuropsychiatry 3: 268–275

Jones M J, Mitchell R W D, Hindocha N 1989 Effects on the lower oesophageal sphincter of cisapride given before the combined administration of atropine and neostigmine. British Journal of Anaesthesia 62: 124–128

Jones R E, Deutsch S, Turndorf H 1961 Effects of atropine on cardiac rhythm in conscious and anesthetised man. Anesthesiology 22: 67–73

Jose A D 1966 The effect of combined sympathetic and parasympathetic blockade on heart rate and cardiac function in man. American Journal of Cardiology 18: 476–478

Kahler R L, Gaffney T E, Braunwald E 1962 The effect of autonomous nervous system inhibition on the circulatory response to muscular exercise. Journal of Clinical Investigation 41: 198–207

Kalser S C 1971 The fate of atropine in man. Annals of the New York Academy of Sciences 179: 667–683

Kaufman J M, Yapchai R 1968 Atropine–digitalis tolerance test. Geriatrics 23: 112–116

Kessell J 1974 Atropine premedication. Anaesthesia and Intensive Care 2: 77–80

Ketchum J S, Sidell F R, Crowell E B Jr, Aghajanian G K, Hayes A H J 1973 Atropine, scopolamine and ditran: comparative pharmacology and antagonists in man. Psychopharmacologia 28: 121–145

Kivalo I, Saarikoski S 1977 Placental transmission of atropine at full term pregnancy. British Journal of Anaesthesia 49: 1017–1021

Kottmeier C A, Gravenstein J S 1968 The parasympathomimetic activity of atropine and atropine methylbromide. Anesthesiology 29: 1125–1133

Krantz J C, Carr C J 1961 The pharmacological principles of medical practice, 5th edn. Baillière, Tindall and Cox, London, pp 916–953

Laitinen S, Mokka R E M, Valanne J U I, Larmi T K I 1978 Anaesthesia induction and lower oesophageal sphincter pressure. Acta Anaesthesiologica Scandinavica 22: 16–20

Leigh M D, McCoy D D, Belton M K, Lewis G B 1957 Bradycardia following intravenous administration of succinylcholine chloride to infants and children. Anesthesiology 18: 698–702

Leighton K M, Sanders M D 1976 Anticholinergic

premedication. Canadian Anaesthetists' Society Journal 23: 563–566

Levy A G, Lewis T 1911 Heart irregularities resulting from the inhalation of low percentages of chloroform vapour and their relationship to ventricular fibrillation. Heart 3: 99–111

Lind J F, Crispin J S, McIver D K 1968 The effect of atropine on the gastroesophageal sphincter. Canadian Journal of Physiology and Pharmacology 46: 233–238

List W F, Gravenstein J S 1965 Effects of atropine and scopolamine on the cardiovascular system in man. 2: Secondary bradycardia after scopolamine. Anesthesiology 26: 299–304

Loman J, Greenberg B, Myerson A 1938 Human autonomic pharmacology: effect of mecholyl, prostigmin, benzedrine and atropine on the urinary tract: urographic studies. New England Journal of Medicine 219: 655–660

Lomax P 1976 Local anaesthetics. In: Bevan J A (ed) Essentials of pharmacology, 2nd edn. Harper & Row, London, pp 170–174

Lomholt S 1946 Difference in the effect of scopolamine on peroral and subcutaneous administration. British Medical Journal 1: 682–683

Longo V G 1966 Behavioral and electroencephalographic effects of atropine and related compounds. Pharmacological Reviews 18: 965–996

Lonnerholm G, Widerlov E 1975 Effect of intravenous atropine and methyl- atropine on heart rate and secretion of saliva in man. European Journal of Clinical Pharmacology 8: 233–240

Lopez-Vidriero M-T, Costello J, Clark T J H, Das I, Keal E E, Reid L 1975 Effect of atropine on sputum production. Thorax 30: 543–547

Lowenthal D T, Reidenberg M M 1972 The heart rate response to atropine in uremic patients, obese subjects before and during fasting and patients with other chronic illnesses. Proceedings of the Society for Experimental Biology and Medicine 139: 390–393

Luco J V, Altamirano M 1943 Comparison of atropine and curare as antagonists of acetylcholine. American Journal of Physiology 139: 520–524

Lunde P 1976 Ventricular fibrillation after intravenous atropine for treatment of sinus bradycardia. Acta Medica Scandinavica 199: 369–371

Lupprian K G, Churchill-Davidson H C 1960 Effect of suxamethonium on cardiac rhythm. British Medical Journal 2: 1774–1777

McCubbin T D, Brown J H, Dewar K M S, Jones C J, Spence A A 1979 Glycopyrrolate as a premedicant: comparison with atropine. British Journal of Anaesthesia 51: 885–889

McGuigan H 1921 Effect of small doses of atropine on heart rate. Journal of the American Medical Association 76: 1338–1340

Mackenzie A L, Pigott J F G 1971 Atropine overdose in three children. British Journal of Anaesthesia 43: 1088–1090

Madej T H, Paasuke R T 1987 Anaesthetic premedication: aims, assessment and methods. Canadian Journal of Anaesthesia 34: 259–273

Magbagbeola J A O 1973 The effect of atropine premedication on body temperature of children in the tropics. British Journal of Anaesthesia 45: 1139–1142

Massumi R A, Mason D T, Amsterdam E A, De Maria A, Miller R R, Scheinman M M, Zelis R 1972 Ventricular fibrillation and tachycardia after intravenous atropine for treatment of bradycardia. New England Journal of Medicine 287: 336–338

May A E, Theophilus S W, James R H 1988 Routine use of atropine in obstetric anaesthesia. British Journal of Anaesthesia 60: 243–244

Miller B R, Friesen R H 1988 Oral atropine premedication in infants attenuates cardiovascular depression during halothane anaesthesia. Anesthesia and Analgesia 67: 180–185

Mirakhur R K 1978 Comparative study of the effects of oral and i.m. atropine and hyoscine in volunteers. British Journal of Anaesthesia 50: 591–598

Mirakhur R K 1979 Anticholinergic drugs. British Journal of Anaesthesia 51: 671–679

Mirakhur R K 1982 Premedication with atropine or glycopyrrolate in children. Effects on heart rate and rhythm during induction and maintenance of anaesthesia. Anaesthesia 37: 1032–1036

Mirakhur R K, Clarke R S J, Dundee J W, McDonald J R 1978 Anticholinergic drugs in anaesthesia: a survey of their present position. Anaesthesia 33: 133–138

Mirakhur R K, Clarke R S J, Elliott J, Dundee J W 1978 Atropine and glycopyrronium premedication: a comparison of the effects on cardiac rate and rhythm during induction of anaesthesia. Anaesthesia 33: 906–912

Mirakhur R K, Dundee J W 1983 Glycopyrrolate: pharmacology and clinical use. Anaesthesia 38: 1195–1204

Mirakhur R K, Dundee J W, Clarke R S J 1977 Glycopyrrolate –neostigmine mixture for antagonism of neuromuscular block: comparison with atropine–neostigmine mixture. British Journal of Anaesthesia 49: 825–829

Mirakhur R K, Dundee J W, Connolly J D R 1979 Studies of drugs given before anaesthesia. XVII: Anticholinergic premedicants. British Journal of Anaesthesia 51: 339–345

Mirakhur R K, Jones C J 1982 Atropine and glycopyrrolate: changes in cardiac rate and rhythm in conscious and anaesthetised children. Anaesthesia and Intensive Care 10: 328–332

Mirakhur R K, Jones C J, Dundee J W 1981 Effects of intravenous administration of glycopyrrolate and atropine in anaesthetised patients. Anaesthesia 36: 277–281

Moller J, Rosen A 1968 Comparative studies on intramuscular and oral effective doses of some anticholinergic drugs. Acta Medica Scandinavica 184: 201–209

Morikawa M, Masuko K 1968 ventricular fibrillation ascribed to i.v. atropine during nitrous oxide–halothane anaesthesia. Japanese Journal of Anesthesiology 17: 479–481

Morton H J, Thomas E T 1958 Effect of atropine on the heart rate. Lancet ii:1313–1315

Murray D J, Forbes R B, Dillman J B, Mahoney L T, Dull D L 1989 Haemodynamic effects of atropine during halothane or isoflurane anaesthesia in infants and small children. Canadian Journal of Anaesthesia 36: 295–300

Murrin K R 1973 A study of oral atropine in healthy adult subjects. British Journal of Anaesthesia 45: 475–480

Mushin W W, Galloon S, Lewis-Faning E 1953 Antisialogogue and other aspects of atropine mucate. British Medical Journal 2: 652–655

Nunn J F, Bergman N A 1964 The effect of atropine on pulmonary gas exchange. British Journal of Anaesthesia 36: 68–73

Oduro K A 1975 Glycopyrrolate methobromide. 2. Comparison with atropine sulphate in anaesthesia. Canadian Anaesthetists' Society Journal 22: 466–473

Oettingen W F von, Marshall I H 1934 Comparison of the pharmacological action of atropine and its optical isomers, levo and dextro-hyoscyamine. Journal of Pharmacology and Experimental Therapeutics 50: 15–20

Orkin L R, Bergman P S, Nathanson M 1956 Effect of atropine, scopolamine and meperidine on man. Anesthesiology 17: 30–37

Ostheimer G W 1977 A comparison of glycopyrrolate and atropine during reversal of nondepolarizing neuromuscular block with neostigmine. Anesthesia and Analgesia 56: 182–186

Ovassapian A 1969 Effects of administration of atropine and neostigmine in man. Anesthesia and Analgesia, Current Researches 48: 219–223

Proakis A G, Harris G B 1978 Comparative penetration of glycopyrrolate and atropine across the blood–brain and placental barriers in anesthetised dogs. Anesthesiology 48: 339–344

Ramamurthy S, Shaker M M, Winnie A P 1972 Glycopyrrolate as a substitute for atropine in neostigmine reversal of muscle relaxant drugs. Canadian Anaesthetists' Society Journal 19: 399–411

Rex M A E 1971 The effect of other drugs on the stimulation of laryngospasm in the cat: atropine; thiopentone; suxamethonium; local analgesics. British Journal of Anaesthesia 43: 117–121

Rinaldi F, Himwich H E 1955 Cholinergic mechanism involved in function of mesodiencephalic activating system. AMA Archives of Neurology and Psychiatry 73: 396–402

Rosen M 1960 Atropine in the treatment of laryngeal spasm. British Journal of Anaesthesia 32: 190–191

Rumack B H 1973 Anticholinergic poisoning: treatment with physostigmine. Pediatrics 52: 449–451

Sagales T, Erill S, Domino E F 1969 Differential effects of scopolamine and chlorpromazine on REM and NREM sleep in normal male subjects. Clinical Pharmacology and Therapeutics 10: 522–529

Salazar M, Patil P N 1976 An explanation for the long duration of mydriatic effect of atropine in eye. Investigative Ophthalmology 15: 671–673

Samra S K, Cohen P J 1980 Modification of chronotropic response to anticholinergics by halogenated anaesthetics in children. Canadian Anaesthetists' Society Journal 27: 540–545

Schriftman H, Kondritzer A A 1957 Absorption of atropine from muscle. American Journal of Physiology 191: 591–594

Schwartz H, De Roetth A Jr, Papper E M 1957 Preanesthetic use of atropine and scopolamine in patients with glaucoma. Journal of American Medical Association 165: 144–146

Schwartz S P, de Sola Pool N 1950 Transient ventricular fibrillation. III: The effect of bodily rest, atropine sulfate and exercise on patients with transient ventricular fibrillation during established auriculoventricular dissociation. A study of the influence of the extrinsic nerves on the idioventricular pacemaker of the heart. American Heart Journal 39: 361–386

Shader R I, Greenblatt D J 1972 Belladonna alkaloids and synthetic anti-cholinergics: uses and toxicity. In: Shader R I (ed) Psychiatric complications of medical drugs. Raven Press, New York, pp 103–147

Shearer W M 1960 The evolution of premedication. British Journal of Anaesthesia 32: 554–562

Sheppard D, Epstein J, Holtzman M J, Nadel J A, Boushey H A 1982 Dose-dependent inhibition of cold air-induced bronchoconstriction by atropine. Journal of Applied Physiology 53: 169–174

Shutt L E, Bowes J B 1979 Atropine and hyoscine. Anaesthesia 34: 476–490

Simpson K H, Smith R J, Davies L F 1987 Comparison of the effects of atropine and glycopyrrolate on cognitive function following general anaesthesia. British Journal of Anaesthesia 59: 966–969

Skinner D B, Camp T F 1968 Relation of esophageal reflux to lower esophageal sphincter pressures decreased by atropine. Gastroenterology 54: 543–551

Smith T C, Stephen G W, Zeigler L, Wollman H 1967 Effects of premedicant drugs on respiration and gas exchange in man. Anesthesiology 28: 883–890

Steinberg S S, Bellville J W, Seed J C 1957 The effect of atropine and morphine on respiration. Journal of Pharmacology and Experimental Therapeutics 121: 71–77

Stephen C R, Bowers M A, Nowill W K, Martin R C 1956 Anticholinergic drugs in preanesthetic medication. Anesthesiology 17: 303–313

Stoll H C 1948 Pharmacodynamic consideration of atropine and related compounds. American Journal of Medical Sciences 215: 577–592

Taylor A B W 1977 Foetal heart rate monitoring during Caesarean section. British Journal of Obstetrics and Gynaecology 84: 281–284

Taylor S H, Scott D B, Donald K W 1964 Respiratory effects of general anaesthesia. Lancet i: 841–843

Thomas E T 1965 The effect of atropine on the pulse. Anaesthesia 20: 340–344

Thurlow A C 1972 Cardiac dysrhythmias in outpatient dental anaesthesia in children: the effect of prophylactic intravenous atropine. Anaesthesia 27: 429–435

Tomlin P J, Conway C M, Payne J P 1964 Hypoxaemia due to atropine. Lancet i: 14–16

Tonnesen M 1948 The absorption and distribution of atropine in rats. Acta Pharmacologica et Toxicologica 4: 367–378

Tonnesen M 1950 The excretion of atropine and allied alkaloids in urine. Acta Pharmacologica et Toxicologica 6: 147–164

Tum-Suden C 1958 Effect of atropine upon mammalian striated muscle. Journal of Pharmacology and Experimental Therapeutics 124: 135–141

Turner D A B, Smith G 1985 Evaluation of the combined effects of atropine and neostigmine on the lower oesophageal sphincter. British Journal of Anaesthesia 57: 956–959

Tyler V E, Brady L R, Robbers J E 1981 Tropane alkaloids. In: Pharmacology, 8th edn. Lea & Febiger, Philadelphia, pp 201–212

Unna K R, Glaser K, Lipton E, Patterson P R 1950 Dosage of drugs in infants and children. I: Atropine. Paediatrics 6: 197–207

Ursillo R C 1961 Investigation of certain aspects of atropine-resistant nerve effects. Journal of Pharmacology and Experimental Therapeutics 131: 231–236

Virtanen R, Kanto J, Iisalo E, Iisalo E U M, Salo M, Sjovall S 1982 Pharmacokinetic studies on atropine with special reference to age. Acta Anaesthesiologica Scandinavica 26: 297–300

Wangeman C P, Hawk M H 1942 The effects of morphine, atropine and scopolamine on human subjects. Anesthesiology 3: 24–36

Weiner N 1980 Atropine, scopolamine and related antimuscarinic drugs. In: Gilman A G, Goodman L, Gilman S (eds) The pharmacological basis of therapeutics, 6th edn. Baillière Tindall, London, pp 120–137

Westfall T C 1976 Antimuscarinic agents. In: Bevan J A (ed) Essentials of pharmacology, 2nd edn. Harper & Row, London, pp 128–134

Wheeler T, Watkins P J 1973 Cardiac denervation in diabetes. British Medical Journal 4: 584–586

Wyant G M, Dobkin A B 1957 Antisialogogue drugs in man: comparison of atropine, scopolamine (l-hyoscine) and l-hyoscyamine (bellafoline). Anaesthesia 12: 203–314

Wyant G M, Dobkin A B 1958 Further studies of antisialogogue drugs in man. Anaesthesia 13: 173–178

Yamaguchi H, Dohi S, Sato S, Naito H 1988 Heart rate response to atropine in humans anaesthetised with five different techniques. Canadian Journal of Anaesthesia 35: 451–456

20. Anticholinesterase drugs

R. K. Mirakhur

This class of drugs inhibits cholinesterase and thus enzymatic hydrolysis of acetylcholine. The effects are equivalent to those of enhanced stimulation of cholinergic receptors. Their actions are widespread due to widespread distribution of cholinergic receptors. Many of these agents act on both acetylcholinesterase and plasma cholinesterase, but the beneficial therapeutic effects are based on the inhibition of acetylcholinesterase. The agents can be broadly divided into two main classes: the reversible or the shorter-acting type, and the longer-acting, so-called 'irreversible' type. The agents used in therapeutics are of the reversible type, whereas the longer-acting ones represented by the organophosphorus compounds are commonly used as insecticides in agriculture and some have been developed for use in chemical warfare as 'nerve gas'.

History

The early investigations of the pharmacology of the Calabar bean were carried out by Christison in 1855, and Fraser in 1863 noted its miotic action (Taylor 1985). Physostigmine obtained from the Calabar bean was isolated as a pure alkaloid by Jobst & Hesse in 1864 and by Vee & Leven in 1865 who called it eserine (Holmstedt 1972). The agent was first used in the treatment of glaucoma in 1877. Engelhardt & Loewi (1930) were the first to report on the preservation of acetylcholine with physostigmine. The drug was synthesized in 1935. Neostigmine was introduced in 1931 for intestinal atony and was used the following year for the symptomatic treatment of myasthenia gravis. Although the first organophosphorus compound was synthesized in the middle of the last century, their potential as insecticides and later as nerve gas was realized and studied only in the 1930s.

Mechanism of action

Acetylcholinesterase has two binding sites at the active

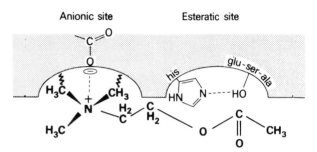

Fig. 20.1 Site of action of anticholinesterase drugs.

centre of the enzyme, an anionic and an esteratic site. The anionic site forms an ionic bond with the positively charged cationic head of acetylcholine. The esteratic site combines with the ester group.

Quaternary ammonium compounds such as neostigmine and edrophonium inhibit the enzyme by combining at the active centre by interaction of their quaternary nitrogen at the anionic site and by hydrogen bonding (Fig. 20.1). At body pH physostigmine combines with the anionic site in a similar way. The ester grouping of the compounds such as neostigmine interacts with the esteratic site of the enzyme. The inhibition occurs in a competitive manner. The interactions between anticholinesterase drugs and the enzyme occur more slowly than those of acetylcholine and remain bound to the enzyme longer. Edrophonium is not hydrolysed but dissociates intact from the enzyme.

Most of the organophosphorus compounds combine with the enzyme at the esteratic site, although quaternary agents like ecothiopate interact at both anionic and esteratic subsites. The resultant complexes are extremely stable.

Chemistry and structure–activity relationship

The structure of physostigmine (Fig. 20.2) was elucidated by Stedman & Barger (1925). The activity

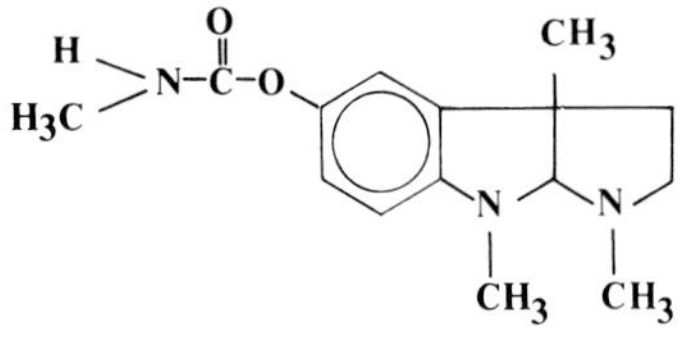

Fig. 20.2 Structural formulae of commonly used anticholinesterase agents.

of the physostigmine molecule is based in the carbamyl group. Neostigmine is a quaternary ammonium compound in contrast to physostigmine which is a tertiary amine. Although the quaternary nitrogen atom is not essential for anticholinesterase activity, it confers increased potency and greater stability. At the same time the absorption following oral administration and penetration across the blood–brain barrier is poor. Neostigmine also possesses some direct cholinergic stimulating action which is not present in physostigmine. Pyridostigmine is a closely allied compound. Neostigmine and pyridostigmine are carbamated compounds. Edrophonium, which lacks the carbamyl group, is less potent but more rapid and short-acting. Bisquaternary compounds like distigmine (two pyridostigmine molecules connected by six methylene groups) and demecarium (two neostigmine molecules connected by 10 methylene groups) are more potent and long-acting. The stability of the interaction with the enzyme is also enhanced.

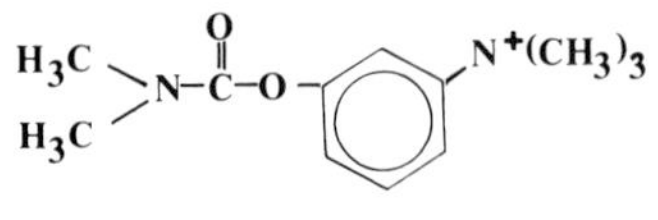

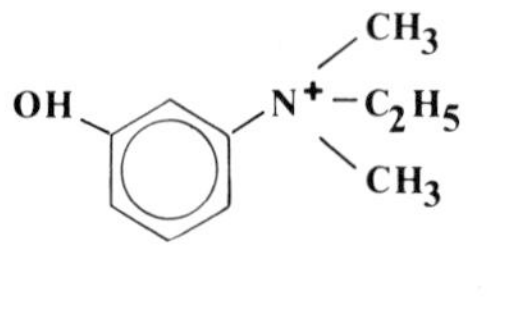

Diisopropylfluorophosphonate (dyflos, DFP), a prototype of organophosphorus compounds, and its analogues are highly lipid-soluble, thus penetrating the blood–brain barrier quite easily and producing serious toxicity in the central nervous system. Ecothiopate is a quaternary ammonium organophosphorus compound which is used clinically for the treatment of glaucoma.

Neostigmine

Neostigmine is a quaternary ammonium agent introduced in 1931 as a miotic.

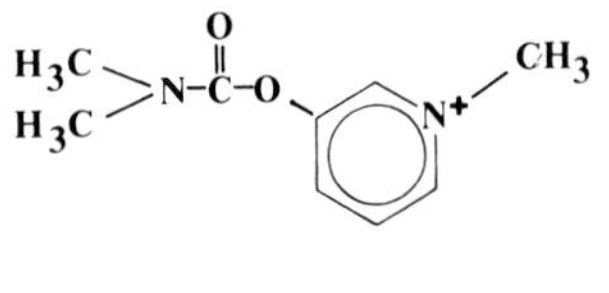

Pharmacological effects

Cardiovascular system. The effects are complex and based on muscarinic and nicotonic actions of accumulated acetylcholine. There is a decrease in heart rate, vasodilation and a fall in cardiac output. With very large doses the blood pressure and heart rate may rise due to ganglionic stimulation and release of catecholamines. The effects on parasympathetic ganglia, on the other hand, produce bradycardia and hypotension. The hypotension and bradycardia with average clinical doses can be prevented by simultaneous or prior administration of atropine. Arrhythmias such as A-V nodal rhythm, ventricular extrasystoles, ventricular tachycardia and even cardiac arrest were reported following administration of neostigmine given with, or preceded by, atropine, in the early days of its use for the antagonism of neuromuscular block (Macintosh 1949, Pooler 1957), but most of these could be attributed 'to inadequate dosage of atropine and hypoventilation in the presence of agents such as cyclopropane (Clarke & Mirakhur 1982).

Neuromuscular junction. In the absence of any neuromuscular blocking agent, neostigmine by itself produces a prolongation of the endplate potential. Muscle fibrillations and fasciculations develop due to loss of synchronization between endplate depolarization and the development of action potential, as well as due to effects on the axon terminal. Finally, with sufficient doses, a depolarizing type of block may ensue.

Neostigmine is used to antagonize residual non-depolarizing neuromuscular block, and the effect is mediated not only through its anticholinesterase effect allowing acetylcholine to accumulate at the endplate, but also by a direct stimulating action (Riker & Wescoe 1946), although the former predominates. The antagonism is competitive. The degree of antagonism is dependent upon the depth of the neuromuscular block present; very intense block may not be adequately reversed. Peak effect of neostigmine when administered for antagonism of neuromuscular block occurs in about 7 min (Miller et al 1974). Hypercarbia slows complete recovery following antagonism of pancuronium neuromuscular block with neostigmine (Wirtavuori et al 1982). Anaesthesia with enflurane also appears to impair the effect of neostigmine (Delisle & Bevan 1982).

Clinically employed doses of neostigmine result in prolongation of a depolarizing block produced by suxamethonium (Sunew & Hicks 1978). This may be due to an additive effect, since both suxamethonium and neostigmine produce depolarization of the postjunctional membrane or the effect may be due to inhibition of plasma cholinesterase (Mirakhur et al 1982). However, a phase II block which develops following administration of large or repetitive doses of suxamethonium would be antagonized.

Gastrointestinal tract. The contractility and secretions of the stomach are greatly increased by neostigmine. The effects are enhanced by morphine and attenuated by atropine. Bilateral vagotomy also reduces the effects of neostigmine on the stomach (Aitkenhead 1984). The motility of both small and large bowel is increased, particularly in patients with diverticular disease (Wilkins et al 1970) and this may result in breakdown of the intestinal anastomosis (Bell & Lewis 1968). Atropine when administered before or in a mixture with neostigmine, provides only partial protection, but halothane, pethidine and to some extent chlorpromazine may abolish the increased activity (Wilkins et al 1970, Watson & Davison 1984).

Neostigmine increases the tone of the lower oesophageal sphincter. The effects may be modified by the concurrent administration of anticholinergic drugs. Neostigmine 2.5 mg given with atropine 1.2 mg or glycopyrrolate 0.6 mg has no significant effect, but 5 mg neostigmine with the same doses of anticholinergic agents significantly increases the opening pressure of the sphincter (Brock-Utne 1979).

Eye. Neostigmine was first introduced for its miotic action. The sphincter pupillae and the ciliary muscles are contracted and the pupil becomes small. The penetration of neostigmine across the cornea, however, is poor.

Respiratory system. Smooth muscles of the bronchi are constricted, resulting in bronchoconstriction. The secretions from bronchial glands are also increased. Anticholinergic drugs given concurrently with neostigmine prevent any dangerous bronchospasm (Hammond et al 1983).

Other effects. The secretions from salivary glands are increased since their innervation is via the postganglionic cholinergic nerves. The secretions of sweat and lacrimal glands are similarly increased. The effects of neostigmine on the central nervous system are minimal since its penetration across the blood–brain barrier is poor.

Pharmacokinetics

Being a quaternary ammonium compound, neostigmine is poorly absorbed from the gastrointestinal tract and much larger doses are required, 15–30 mg as against 0.25–1.0 mg intravenously for the treatment of myasthenia gravis.

The distribution half-life $(t_{\frac{1}{2}}\alpha)$ of neostigmine is reported as between 0.5 and 3.5 min (Williams et al 1978, Cronnelly et al 1979). The elimination half-life $(t_{\frac{1}{2}}\beta)$ according to Williams et al (1978) and Calvey and his colleagues (1979) is 25 min, whereas Cronnelly and others (1979), using the same dose of neostigmine, calculated it to be 80 min. The volumes of distribution are large, probably due to extensive tissue localization. The clearance is reduced and the elimination half-life considerably increased in patients with no renal function (Cronnelly et al 1979). This is an advantage in such patients, since the elimination of drugs such as pancuronium and tubocurarine is diminished (Miller 1982). In fact Bevan and his colleagues (1982) were able to show no recurarization in patients in renal failure following antagonism of neuromuscular block.

The liver is the main site of metabolism of neostigmine and the main metabolite is 3-hydroxyphenyl-trimethylammonium (Roberts et al 1965). It has only about one-thousandth of the activity of neostigmine, and its contribution to antagonism of neuromuscular block is insignificant (Cronnelly & Morris 1982). Renal excretion accounts for about 50% of neostigmine in anaesthetized patients. Biliary excretion and hydrolysis by cholinesterase are other modes of elimination of the drug.

Indications and dosage

Apart from its use as an antagonist of non-depolarizing block (see below) neostigmine is employed for the treatment of myasthenia gravis and paralytic ileus and atony of the bladder. The drug is usually administered orally in myasthenia gravis starting at a dose of 15 mg three times a day and gradually increasing to 30 mg every 3–6 h. The intensity of muscarinic side-effects is reduced when given this way. The drug may be administered parenterally in acute situations such as myasthenic crisis. An overdose with neostigmine or other anticholinesterases may lead to cholinergic crisis in myasthenic patients.

Neostigmine is used subcutaneously in a dose of 0.5–1.0 mg for postoperative ileus or bladder atony. Care should be taken to ensure that there is no mechanical obstruction. The drug may also be used orally in doses of 15–20 mg.

An anticholinergic agent such as atropine may be required to control the undesirable muscarinic effects, but tolerance develops to these following prolonged treatment as in cases of myasthenia gravis.

The main use of neostigmine in anaesthesia is for the antagonism of residual neuromuscular block by non-depolarizing (competitive) muscle relaxants. In this situation the drug is usually given intravenously in a dose of 2.5 mg (40–50 μg kg^{-1}) although a dose of 1.25 mg has recently been shown to be as effective as a dose of 2.5 mg for antagonism of incomplete neuromuscular block by moderate doses of atracurium and vecuronium (Jones et al 1988). The speed of recovery is in any case dependent upon the degree of block prior to antagonism (Meistelman et al 1988). This will invariably result in profound muscarinic effects and should be accompanied by prior or simultaneous administration of an anticholinergic drug. Atropine is usually administered in a dose of 20 μg kg^{-1}. There is less tachycardia and greater cardiostability when atropine and neostigmine are administered together, provided oxygenation is well maintained (Baraka 1968a,b; Mirakhur et al 1981b). The initial reports of profound bradycardia and cardiac arrest (Macintosh 1949) were perhaps due to inadequate doses of atropine, or inadequate ventilation following administration of neostigmine, particularly in the presence of agents such as cyclopropane. The cardiac effects of atropine always precede those of neostigmine even when the two are administered mixed together.

In recent years even better cardiostability has been obtained by substituting glycopyrrolate for atropine (Ramamurthy et al 1972, Mirakhur et al 1981c, Mirakhur and Dundee 1983). There is minimal increase in heart rate (Fig. 20.3) due to both neostigmine and glycopyrrolate having similar times to onset of action based on their quaternary ammonium structure. In addition glycopyrrolate is longer-acting than atropine and is associated with a better control of secretions and absence of any undesirable central effects. The use of glycopyrrolate in the reversal mixture is particularly use-

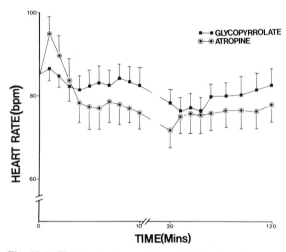

Fig. 20.3   Heart rate changes after administration of neostigmine with atropine (or glycopyrrolate from *Indian Journal of Anaesthesia*).

ful in patients with pre-existing cardiovascular disease (Cozanitis et al 1980, Bali & Mirakhur 1980). It has also been suggested that the elderly may require lower doses of anticholinergic drugs during reversal of neuromuscular block by neostigmine (Mirakhur 1985a).

Some workers have suggested that a second dose of neostigmine administered either after the first dose or after spontaneous recovery may induce neuromuscular block (Payne et al 1980, Goldhill et al 1989). Others however, have not observed such effects (Jones et al 1987).

Pyridostigmine

Pyridostigmine (Fig. 20.2) is structurally close to neostigmine but is just over five times less potent (Fogdall & Miller 1973).

As with neostigmine there is difference of opinion about the pharmacokinetics of pyridostigmine when administered intravenously for the antagonism of neuromuscular block. While Cronnelly and his colleagues (1980) found the half-lives of distribution and elimination to be 6.8 and 112 min respectively, Williams and his colleagues (1983) observed these to be about 1.0 and 46 min respectively. In spite of these large differences in terminal half-life the values of clearance (8.6 and 8.7 ml kg^{-1} min^{-1}) are quite similar. The effect of absence of any renal function is similar to that of neostigmine, elimination being prolonged many times over (Cronnelly et al 1980). About 25% of the injected drug is metabolized, mainly in the liver, to 3-hydroxy-*N*-methylpyridinium (Birtley et al 1966).

The inhibition of both acetylcholinesterase and plasma cholinesterase is much more prolonged than the actual half-life of the drug (Miller et al 1974, Mirakhur et al 1982), suggesting not only a margin of safety in enzyme inhibition but also that the time course of action of the drug may be unrelated to its clearance from the plasma (Cronnelly & Morris 1982). Pyridostigmine is preferred to neostigmine in the treatment of myasthenia gravis where it has to be administered less frequently, the usual dose being 60 mg three or four times a day. The other main use of the drug is for antagonism of non-depolarizing neuromuscular block, although it has not gained popularity for this purpose in the United Kingdom. The onset of action of pyridostigmine is slower than that of neostigmine, but the duration of action is nearly twice as long as after an equipotent dose of neostigmine (Miller et al 1974). The duration of action of both pyridostigmine and neostigmine is prolonged in the elderly (Young et al 1988).

Pyridostigmine has less muscarinic effects than neostigmine (Osserman 1955) although Fogdall & Miller (1973) were not able to substantiate this. As in the case of neostigmine, glycopyrrolate can be substituted with advantage in place of atropine as the anticholinergic component of the reversal mixture (Mirakhur et al 1981a). An initial increase in heart rate is, however, observed even with glycopyrrolate (in the same dose as with neostigmine) in a mixture with pyridostigmine. This may reflect either a much slower onset of action of pyridostigmine allowing the anticholinergic drug to exert its effect unopposed for a while, or it may simply reflect less severe muscarinic effects with this agent. The usual dose of pyridostigmine for antagonism of neuromuscular block is 0.25 mg kg^{-1} administered in a mixture with atropine or glycopyrrolate in a dose of 15–20 and 7–10 μg kg^{-1} respectively.

Edrophonium

This drug has classically been held to be too short-lasting for antagonism of residual non-depolarizing neuromuscular block (Katz 1967). This has been the case when edrophonium was used in a dose of 10 mg. However, reports by Bevan (1979) and Kopman (1979), and more recent detailed studies by Cronnelly et al (1982) have shown that, when used in a dose of 0.5–1.0 mg kg^{-1}, edrophonium induced a sustained antagonism of d-tubocurarine and pancuronium blocks. Pharmacokinetic studies with these doses have shown the half-life of elimination ($t_{\frac{1}{2}}\beta$) of edrophonium to be nearly the same as that of neostigmine (Morris et al 1981) although Cronnelly & Morris (1982) have pointed out that there is no direct relationship between the concentration of anticholinesterase agents in blood and their clinical effect.

Edrophonium is not a carbamated compound, and its binding to acetylcholinesterase is transient. Administration of edrophonium for antagonism of neuromuscular block has been shown to result in higher train-of-four ratios in comparison to neostigmine, suggesting a relatively greater presynaptic effect (Donati et al 1983, Lavery et al 1985, Mirakhur et al 1987).

The onset of action of edrophonium is significantly more rapid than that of neostigmine or pyridostigmine, and it requires only half as much atropine for blocking its muscarinic effects (Cronnelly et al 1982). In contrast to neostigmine and pyridostigmine, atropine and not glycopyrrolate appears to be the anticholinergic of choice with edrophonium (Azar et al 1983, Mirakhur 1985b) since the onset of action of edrophonium is more rapid. Edrophonium has been reported to be a better anticholinesterase than neostigmine for antagonism of neuromuscular block by the newer relaxants atracurium and vecuronium (Baird et al 1982, Jones et al 1983) and against relaxants having a greater presynaptic effect (Mirakhur 1987, Smith et al 1989). Wide experience with the agent for antagonism of neuromuscular block has, however, shown that relatively deeper blocks including those induced by atracurium and vecuronium are not adequately antagonized by it (Kopman 1979, Lavery et al 1985, Caldwell et al 1987, Mirakhur 1987, Mirakhur et al 1987).

Edrophonium is commonly used intravenously in 10 mg doses for the diagnosis of myasthenia gravis, as well as in situations where the presence of a non-depolarizing neuromuscular block is not certain. A dose of 0.5–1.0 mg kg^{-1} is considered adequate for antagonism of neuromuscular block and should be preceded by, or mixed with, 7–10 μg kg^{-1} atropine.

There has been some debate about the relative potencies of edrophonium and neostigmine. Whereas Cronnelly et al (1982) considered edrophonium to have about one-twelfth the potency of neostigmine, well-designed studies from workers in Montreal have suggested that neostigmine may be 16–20 times as potent as edrophonium, depending upon the relaxant that was being antagonized (Breen et al 1985, Smith et al 1989).

With all these anticholinesterase agents discussed so far, the antagonism of neuromuscular block attained depends upon the depth of neuromuscular block present, any acidosis and electrolyte imbalance and hypothermia.

Edrophonium does not produce any significant depression of plasma cholinesterase activity, unlike neostigmine or pyridostigmine (Mirakhur 1986).

Physostigmine

Physostigmine was the first anticholinesterase isolated from the Calabar bean. In contrast to other 'reversible' anticholinesterases, physostigmine is a tertiary compound and is able to penetrate the blood–brain barrier easily. It is readily absorbed from the gastrointestinal tract and mucous membranes. It is mostly hydrolysed in the body with renal excretion playing only a minor role.

The main application of physostigmine (eserine) is in the treatment of some forms of glaucoma where it is used in a 0.25–0.5% solution. The drug has been replaced for the treatment of myasthenia by the quaternary ammonium compounds. It is a specific antidote to atropine poisoning and is used in a 1–2 mg dose which may need to be repeated frequently. It has also been reported to be useful against other central nervous system depressants such as phenothiazines (Bernards 1973), tricyclic depressants (Chin et al 1976) and opioids (Bidwai et al 1976, Weinstock et al 1980). Some of these may be due to a general arousal effect of physostigmine rather than actions at specific receptor sites (Ghoneim 1980). There are also reports of antagonism of diazepam-induced respiratory depression (Lopez 1981, Waters & Rosenberg 1981) but Garber et al (1980) were unable to show reversal of diazepam-induced sedation. A mixture of naloxone 1.0–1.5 μg kg^{-1} and physostigmine 0.5–1.0 mg has been shown to reverse the sedation and respiratory depression induced by the use of opioids, neuroleptics and benzodiazepines in neurosurgical patients, and found to be useful clinically (Wiklund 1986). Peripheral muscarinic side-effects may need to be countered with an agent such as glycopyrrolate which does not have central effects of its own. Physostigmine may possess some analgesic effects according to Hartvig and colleagues (1986).

Physostigmine is well absorbed after both intramuscular and subcutaneous administrations, although the onset of action is slower in comparison to intravenous administration (Hartvig et al 1986). These authors also reported a short half-life ($t_{\frac{1}{2}}\beta$ 22 min) and accordingly a short duration of action.

It has been shown to be unsuitable for antagonism of neuromuscular block even in doses which exceed those required for treating the central effects of anticholinergic drugs (Baraka 1978).

Galanthamine

This anticholinesterase drug is an alkaloid from the bulbs of the Caucasian snowdrop, Galanthum nivalis.

The drug is available in Bulgaria and is supposed to have less muscarinic actions and a longer-lasting effect. It is sometimes used in the treatment of myasthenia gravis but was found to be unreliable for antagonism of neuromuscular block (Baraka & Cozanitis 1973). Cozanitis (1977) found it to be useful in treating the central effects of anticholinergic agents. The average dose of galanthamine for antagonism of neuromuscular block is in the region of 0.3–0.4 mg kg^{-1}.

Ambenonium

Ambenonium is a bisquaternary compound whose effects are more selective against acetylcholinesterase. The drug is potent and long-acting in comparison to neostigmine. It is not hydrolysed in the body and is employed in the treatment of myasthenia gravis in doses of 10–15 mg three or four times a day.

Other reversible anticholinesterase agents such as benzpyrinium (0.5 mg i.m.) and distigmine (5–10 mg orally or 1.0 mg i.m. every third day) are useful for stimulating bowel and bladder activity. Demecarium (0.25% solution), another bisquaternary agent, is used in the treatment of glaucoma.

4-Aminopyridine

4-Aminopyridine is not an anticholinesterase agent, but since the drug has been suggested as an antagonist to non-depolarizing neuromuscular blocking agents it is described here. It has widespread effects in the body at the neuromuscular junction, central nervous system, spinal cord, autonomic nervous system and directly on the muscle (Soni & Kam 1982). It acts mainly by increasing the release of acetylcholine from the motor nerve terminal (Bowman et al 1976). The drug is longer-acting and has minimal muscarinic effects (Miller et al 1979). The usual suggested dosage for antagonism of neuromuscular block is 0.3 mg kg^{-1}, but some have found inadequate antagonism even at doses in the range of 0.5 mg kg^{-1} (Booij et al 1980). It has, however, been shown to potentiate the antagonistic effect of neostigmine and pyridostigmine (Miller et al 1979) and may also be useful in neuromuscular block associated with antibiotics (Booij et al 1978).

The drug has been used for the treatment of myasthenia gravis and Eaton–Lambert syndrome (Lundh et al 1977, Agoston et al 1978), as an analeptic (Agoston et al 1980), as a respiratory stimulant (Sia & Zandstra 1981) and in botulism (Ball et al 1979).

The drug has, however, serious side-effects, mainly on the central nervous system. These include unsteadiness, restlessness, tremor, hyperexcitability and even convulsions at higher doses. In addition tachycardia and hypertension may occur due to facilitation of the sympathetic nervous system. These are serious disadvantages which limit the usefulness of the drug.

Organophosphorus compounds

The most widely known of organophorphorus anti-cholinesterases, also known as irreversible cholinesterase inhibitors, is diisopropylfluorophosphonate (DFP, dyflos). DFP and its analogues are volatile and can be absorbed through the lungs. The basic mechanism of action of reversible and irreversible anticholinesterase agents is similar, the terms only reflecting the relative durations of action. The main features of DFP are its virtually irreversible action (due to alkylphosphorylation of cholinesterase), and very marked central effects due to its very high lipid-solubility. Parathion is less volatile and more stable in aqueous solution and has gained widespread use as an insecticide. Parathion is inactive in vitro but converted in the body to paraoxon which is the active compound. Parathion is also well absorbed through intact skin. Malathion is slightly safer than parathion because it can be hydrolysed more readily. Tabun, Sarin and Soman are the most potent toxic agents used as 'nerve gases', and kill even in very minute amounts.

Amongst the organophosphorus compounds only ecothiopate is useful clinically in a 0.1–0.25% solution as a miotic in open-angle gluacoma. It is relatively stable in solution. It produces clinically important inhibition of plasma cholinesterase which may cause prolongation of suxamethonium block.

Organophosphorus poisoning

Due to widespread use of organophosphorus compounds as agricultural insecticides, accidental and suicidal intoxication from these compounds is not uncommon. The signs and symptoms are attributable to central and peripheral muscarinic and nicotinic effects. The muscarinic effects include miosis, conjunctival congestion, tightness and wheezing in the chest, excessive salivation, sweating, lacrimation, abdominal cramps, nausea and vomiting, involuntary urination and defaecation, and hypotension and bradycardia. Nicotinic effects include fatiguability and general weakness of skeletal muscles, involuntary twitching, severe fasciculations and ultimately paralysis of the respiratory muscles. Central nervous system toxicity is manifest as confusion, ataxia, slurred speech, loss of reflexes, generalized convulsions, coma and paralysis of respiratory and vasomotor centres. Death is usually due to respiratory failure compounded by severe cardiovascular depression, and can take place within 24 h.

Some organophosphorus compounds produce delayed neurotoxicity.

Treatment consists of administration of atropine, which may be required in high doses and for prolonged periods of time. Atropine antagonizes only the muscarinic effects; the dosage may be as high as 50 mg in a single day given in 2–4 mg doses at frequent intervals. In recent years pralidoxime, a cholinesterase reactivator, has been used with some success. It controls the nicotinic effects of organophosphorus compounds and is administered intravenously in doses of 1.0–2.0 g. Other supportive measures such as maintenance of airway oxygenation, artificial ventilation and cardiovascular support should be instituted at the same time.

REFERENCES

Agoston S, Van Weerden T, Westra P, Broekerg A 1978 Effects of 4-aminopyridine in Eaton–Lambert syndrome. British Journal of Anaesthesia 50: 383–385

Agoston S, Salt P J, Erdmann W, Hilkenmeijer T, Bencini A, Langrehr D 1980 Antagonism of ketamine–diazepam anaesthesia by 4-aminopyridine in human volunteers. British Journal of Anaesthesia 52: 367–370

Aitkenhead A R 1984 Anaesthesia and bowel surgery. British Journal of Anaesthesia 56: 95–101

Azar I, Pham A N, Karambelkar D J, Lear E 1983 The heart rate following edrophonium–atropine and edrophonium–glycopyrrolate mixtures. Anesthesiology 59: 139–141

Baird W L, Bowman W C, Kerr W J 1982 Some actions of Org NC 45 and of edrophonium in the anaesthetised cat and in man. British Journal of Anaesthesia 54: 375–385

Bali I M, Mirakhur R K 1980 Comparison of glycopyrrolate, atropine and hyoscine in mixture with neostigmine for reversal of neuromuscular block following closed mitral valvotomy. Acta Anaesthesiologica Scandinavica 24: 331–335

Ball A P, Hopkinson R B, Farrell I M et al 1979 Human botulism caused by Clostridium botulinium type E: the Birmingham outbreak. Quarterly Journal of Medicine 48: 473–491

Baraka A 1968a Safe reversal (1): atropine followed by neostigmine: an electrocardiographic study. British Journal of Anaesthesia 40: 27–29

Baraka A 1968b Safe reversal (2): atropine-neostigmine mixture: an electrocardiographic study. British Journal of Anaesthesia 40: 30–35

Baraka A 1978 Antagonism of neuromuscular block by physostigmine in man. British Journal of Anaesthesia 50: 1075–1077

Baraka A, Cozanitis D 1973 Galanthamine versus neostigmine for reversal of nondepolarising neuromuscular block in man. Anesthesia and Analgesia 52: 832–836

Bell C M A, Lewis C B 1968 Effect of neostigmine on integrity of ileorectal anastomoses. British Medical Journal 3: 587–588

Bernards W 1973 Reversal of phenothiazine-induced coma with physostigmine. Anesthesia and Analgesia 52: 938–941

Bevan D R 1979 Reversal of pancuronium with edrophonium. Anaesthesia 34: 614–619

Bevan D R, Archer D, Donati F, Ferguson A, Higgs B D 1982 Antagonism of pancuronium in renal failure: no recurarisation. British Journal of Anaesthesia 54: 63–68

Bidwai A, Cornelius L, Stanley T H 1976 Reversal of innovar-induced post-anaesthetic somnolence and disorientation with physostigmine. Anesthesiology 44: 249–252

Birtley R D, Roberts J B, Thomas B H, Wilson A 1966 Excretion and metabolism of ^{14}C-pyridostigmine in the rat. British Journal of Pharmacology 26: 393–402

Booij L H D J, Miller R D, Crul J F 1978 Neostigmine and 4-aminopyridine antagonism of lincomycin–pancuronium neuromuscular blockade in man. Anesthesia and Analgesia 57: 316–321

Booij L H D J, Van der Pol F, Crul J F, Miller R D 1980 Antagonism of Org NC 45 neuromuscular blockade by neostigmine, pyridostigmine and 4-aminopyridine. Anesthesia and Analgesia 59: 31–34

Bowman W C, Harvey A L, Marshal I D 1976 Facilitatory actions of aminopyridines on neuromuscular transmission. Journal of Pharmacy and Pharmacology 28: 79P

Breen P J, Doherty W G, Donati F, Bevan D R 1985 The potencies of edrophonium and neostigmine as antagonists of pancuronium. Anaesthesia 40: 844–847

Brock-Utne J G 1979 Reversal of neuromuscular blockade by glycopyrrolate and neostigmine. Anaesthesia 34: 620–623

Caldwell J E, Robertson E N, Baird W L M 1987 Antagonism of vecuronium and atracurium: comparison of neostigmine and edrophonium administered at 5% twitch height recovery. British Journal of Anaesthesia 59: 478–481

Calvey T N, Wareing M, Williams N E, Chan K 1979 Pharmacokinetics and pharmacological effects of neostigmine in man. British Journal of Clinical Pharmacology 7: 149–155

Chin L, Havill J, Rothwell R, Bishop B G 1976 Use of physostigmine in tricyclic andidepressant poisoning. Anaesthesia and Intensive Care 4: 138–140

Clarke R S J, Mirakhur R K 1982 Antagonism of neuromuscular block. British Journal of Anaesthesia 54: 793–794

Cozanitis D A 1977 Galanthamine hydrobromide, a longer acting anticholinesterase drug, in the treatment of the central effects of scopolamine (hyoscine). Anaesthesist 26: 649–650

Cozanitis D A, Dundee J W, Merrett J D, Jones C J, Mirakhur R K 1980 Evaluation of glycopyrrolate and atropine as adjuncts to reversal of nondepolarising neuromuscular blocking agents in a 'true-to-life' situation. British Journal of Anaesthesia 52: 85–89

Cronnelly R, Morris R B 1982 Antagonism of neuromuscular blockade. British Journal of Anaesthesia 54: 183–194

Cronnelly R, Stanski D R, Miller R D,Sheiner L B, Sohn Y J 1979 Renal function and the pharmacokinetics of neostigmine in anesthetised man. Anesthesiology 51: 222–226

Cronnelly R, Stanski D R, Miller R D, Sheiner L B 1980 Pyridostigmine kinetics with and without renal function. Clinical Pharmacology and Therapeutics 28: 78–81

Cronnelly R, Morris R B, Miller R D 1982 Edrophonium: duration of action and atropine requirements in humans during halothane anaesthesia. Anesthesiology 57: 261–266

Delisle S, Bevan D R 1982 Impaired neostigmine antagonism of pancuronium during enflurane anaesthesia in man. British Journal of Anaesthesia 54: 441–445

Donati F, Ferguson A, Bevan D R 1983 Twitch depression and train-of-four ratio after antagonism of pancuronium with edrophonium, neostigmine or pyridostigmine. Anesthesia and Analgesia 62: 314–316

Engelhardt E, Loewi O 1930 Fermentative acetylcholinspaltung im Blut und ihre Hemmung durch Physostigmin. Archiv für experimentelle Pathologie und Pharmakologie 150: 1–13

Fogdall R P, Miller R D 1973 Antagonism of d-tubocurarine and pancuronium-induced neuromuscular blockades by pyridostigmine in man. Anesthesiology 39: 504–509

Garber J G, Ominsky A J, Orkin F K, Quinn P 1980 Physostigmine–atropine solution fails to reverse diazepam sedation. Anesthesia and Analgesia 59: 58–60

Ghoneim M M 1980 Antagonism of diazepam by physostigmine. Anesthesiology 52: 372

Goldhill D R, Wainwright A P, Stuart C S, Flynn P J 1989 Neostigmine after spontaneous recovery from neuromuscular blockade. Effect on depth of blockade monitored with train-of-four and tetanic stimuli. Anaesthesia 44: 293–299

Hammond J, Wright D, Sale J 1983 Pattern of change of bronchomotor tone following reversal of neuromuscular blockade. British Journal of Anaesthesia 55: 955–959

Hartvig P, Wiklund L, Lundstrom B 1986 Pharmacokinetics of physostigmine after intravenous, intramuscular and subcutaneous administration to surgical patients. Acta Anaesthesiologica Scandinavica 30: 177–182

Holmstedt B 1972 The ordeal bean of Old Calabar: the pageant of Physostigma veneriosum in medicine. In: Swain T (ed) Plants in the development of modern medicine. Harvard University Press, Cambridge, Ma, pp 303–360

Jones J E, Hunter J M, Utting J E 1987 Use of neostigmine in the antagonism of residual neuromuscular blockade produced by vecuronium. British Journal of Anaesthesia 59: 1454–1458

Jones J E, Parker C J R, Hunter J M 1988 Antagonism of blockade produced by atracurium or vecuronium with low doses of neostigmine. British Journal of Anaesthesia 61: 560–564

Jones R M, Pearce A C, Williams J P 1983 Recovery characteristics following antagonism of atracurium with neostigmine or edrophonium. British Journal of Anaesthesia 56: 453–457

Katz R L 1967 Neuromuscular effects of d-tubocurarine, edrophonium and neostigmine in man. Anesthesiology 28: 327–336

Kopman A F 1979 Edrophonium antagonism of pancuronium-induced neuromuscular blockade in man. Anesthesiology 51: 139–142

Lavery G G, Mirakhur R K, Gibson F M 1985 A comparison of edrophonium and neostigmine for the antagonism of atracurium-induced neuromuscular block. Anesthesia and Analgesia 64: 867–870

Lopez J 1981 Physostigmine reversal of diazepam-induced respiratory arrest: report of case. Journal of Oral Surgery 39: 539–541

Lundh H, Nilsson D, Rosen I 1977 4-Aminopyridine — a new drug tested in the treatment of Eaton–Lambert Syndrome. Journal of Neurology, Neurosurgery and Psychiatry 40: 1109–1112

Macintosh R R 1949 Death following injection of neostigmine. British Medical Journal 1: 852

Meistelman C, Debaene B, Hollander A, Donati F, Saint-Maurice C 1988 Importance of the level of paralysis recovery for a rapid antagonism of vecuronium with neostigmine in children during halothane anesthesia. Anesthesiology 69: 97–99

Miller R D 1982 Pharmacokinetics of competitive muscle relaxants. British Journal of Anaesthesia 54: 161–167

Miller R D Van Nyhuis L S, Eger E I, Vitez T S, Way W L 1974 Comparative times to peak effect and durations of action of neostigmine and pyridostigmine. Anesthesiology 41: 27–33

Miller R D, Booij L H D, Agoston S 1979 4-Aminopyridine potentiates neostigmine and pyridostigmine in man. Anesthesiology 50: 416–420

Mirakhur R K 1985a Antagonism of neuromuscular block in the elderly: a comparison of atropine and glycopyrrolate in a mixture with neostigmine. Anaesthesia 40: 254–258

Mirakhur R K 1985b Antagonism of the muscarinic effects of edrophonium with atropine or glycopyrrolate: a comparative study. British Journal of Anaesthesia 57: 1213–1216

Mirakhur R K 1986 Edrophonium and plasma cholinesterase activity. Canadian Anaesthetists' Society Journal 33: 588–590

Mirakhur R K 1987 Antagonism of pancuronium and tubocurarine blocks by edrophonium or neostigmine: a comparative study. European Journal of Anaesthesiology 4: 411–419

Mirakhur R K, Dundee J W 1983 Glycopyrrolate: pharmacology and clinical use. Anaesthesia 38: 1195–1204

Mirakhur R K, Briggs L P, Clarke R S J, Dundee J W, Johnston H M L 1981a Comparison of atropine and glycopyrrolate in a mixture with pyridostigmine for the reversal of neuromuscular block. British Journal of Anaesthesia 53: 1315–1320

Mirakhur R K, Dundee J W, Jones C J, Coppel D L, Clarke R S J 1981b Reversal of neuromuscular blockade: dose determination studies with atropine and glycopyrrolate given before or in a mixture with neostigmine. Anesthesia and Analgesia 60: 557–562

Mirakhur R K, Jones C J, Dundee J W 1981c Heart rate changes following reversal of neuromuscular block with glycopyrrolate or atropine given before or with neostigmine. Indian Journal of Anaesthesia 29: 83–87

Mirakhur R K, Lavery T D, Briggs L P, Clarke R S J 1982 Effects of neostigmine and pyridostigmine on serum cholinesterase activity. Canadian Anaesthetists' Society Journal 29: 55–58

Mirakhur R K, Gibson F M, Lavery G G 1987 Antagonism of vecuronium-induced neuromuscular block with edrophonium or neostigmine. British Journal of Anaesthesia 59: 473–477

Morris R B, Cronnelly R, Miller R D, Stanski D R, Fahey

M R 1981 Pharmacokinetics of edrophonium and neostigmine when antagonising d-tubocurarine neuromuscular blockade in man. Anesthesiology 54: 399–402

Osserman K E 1955 Progress report on Mestinon bromide (pyridostigmine bromide). American Journal of Medicine 19: 737–739

Payne J P, Hughes R, Al-Azawi S 1980 Neuromuscular blockade by neostigmine in anaesthetized man. British Journal of Anaesthesia 52: 69–75

Pooler H E 1957 Atropine, neostigmine and sudden death. Anaesthesia 12: 198–202

Ramamurthy S, Shaker M H, Winnie A P 1972 Glycopyrrolate as a substitute for atropine in neostigmine reversal of muscle relaxant drugs. Canadian Anaesthetists' Society Journal 19: 399–411

Riker W F, Wescoe W C 1946 The direct action of prostigmin on skeletal muscle; its relationship to the choline esters. Journal of Pharmacology and Experimental Therapeutics 88: 58–66

Roberts J N, Thomas B J, Wilson A 1965 Distribution and excretion of ^{14}C-neostigmine in rat and hen. British Journal of Pharmacology 25: 234–242

Sia R L, Zandstra D F 1981 4-Aminopyridine reversal of fentanyl-induced respiratory depression in normocapnic and hypercapnic patients. British Journal of Anaesthesia 53: 373–379

Smith C E, Donati F, Bevan D R 1989 Dose–response relationships for edrophonium and neostigmine as antagonists of atracurium and vecuronium neuromuscular blockade. Anesthesiology 71: 37–43

Soni N, Kam P 1982 4-Aminopyridine — A review. Anaesthesia and Intensive Care 10: 120–126

Stedman E, Barger G 1925 Physostigmine (eserine). Part III. Journal of the Chemical Society 127: 247–258

Sunew K Y, Hicks R G 1978 Effects of neostigmine and pyridostigmine on duration of succinylcholine action and pseudocholinesterase activity. Anesthesiology 49: 188–191

Taylor P 1985 Anticholinesterase agents. In: Gilman A G, Goodman L S, Rall T W, Murad F (eds) The Pharmacological basis of therapeutics. Collier Macmillan, London pp 110–129

Waters B G, Rosenberg H 1981 Reversal of diazepam-induced apnea with physostigmine. Canadian Dental Association Journal 47: 795–797

Watson N, Davison J S 1984 The effect of anaesthetic agents on neostigmine-induced bowel activity. Canadian Anaesthetists' Society Journal 31: S67–S68

Weinstock M, Roll D, Erez E, Bahar M 1980 Physostigmine antagonises morphine-induced respiratory depression but not analgesia in dogs and rabbits. British Journal of Anaesthesia 52: 1171–1176

Wiklund L 1986 Reversal of sedation and respiratory depression after anaesthesia by the combined use of physostigmine and naloxone in neurosurgical patients. Acta Anaesthesiologica Scandinavica 30: 374–377

Wilkins J L, Hardcastle J D, Mann C V, Kaufman L 1970 Effects of neostigmine and atropine on motor activity of ileum, colon and rectum of anaesthetised subjects. British Medical Journal 1: 793–794

Williams N E, Calvey T N, Chan K 1978 Clearance of neostigmine from the circulation during the antagonism of neuromuscular block. British Journal of Anaesthesia 50: 1065–1067

Williams N E, Calvey T N, Chan K 1983 Plasma concentration of pyridostigmine during the antagonism of neuromuscular block. British Journal of Anaesthesia 55: 27–31

Wirtavuori K, Salmenpera M, Tammisto T 1982 Effect of hypocarbia and hypercarbia on the antagonism of pancuronium-induced neuromuscular blockade with neostigmine in man. British Journal of Anaesthesia 54: 57–61

Young W L, Matteo R S, Ornstein E 1988 Duration of action of neostigmine and pyridostigmine in the elderly. Anesthesia and Analgesia 67: 775–778

Drugs acting on the cardiovascular system

21. Positive inotropic drugs

S. M. Lyons   G. G. Lavery   K. G. Lowry

CARDIOVASCULAR PHYSIOLOGY

Anatomical background

The heart provides the mechanical force to drive the blood around the circulation. It is composed mainly of interlacing fibres of muscle, which have considerable similarity to skeletal muscle. They differ in that cardiac muscle cells are arranged in an interconnecting formation called a functional syncytium, so that an impulse can spread from one fibre to all others within that chamber; but are separated at their junctions by intercalated discs which slow the rate of propagation of impulses to around 0.5 m s^{-1} — one-tenth of the rate in skeletal muscle. Conducting tissue consists of specialized cardiac muscle tissue.

The atria are thin-walled structures which act as reservoirs for blood while the ventricles are contracting, and then contract during diastole, this contributing 20–30% of the volume filling the ventricles. The ventricles provide the force to circulate blood through the peripheries, and thus are thick-walled. The atria are separated from the ventricles by a ring of fibrous tissue which also supports the valves. The electrical impulse can pass this only through the band of conducting tissue which starts at the atrioventricular (AV) node.

Origin of the heart beat

The heart beat originates in the sino-atrial (SA) node (Noble 1975). Depolarization of the cardiac muscle is associated with muscle contraction and during relaxation repolarization occurs. The general cardiac muscle tissue reaches a voltage of −90 mV when fully polarized. However, in pacemaker tissue the voltage only reaches −50 mV. From then a spontaneous decay in the voltage occurs to −40 mV. At that level a rapid upstroke spike potential occurs and this is followed by muscle contraction. The pacemaker tissue of the SA node exhibits this property at a greater rate than in the pacemaker tissue

of either the AV node or the Purkinje fibres, thus giving the SA node its action of originating the heart beat.

The muscle contraction initiated by the pacemaker SA node spreads through the atrial muscle to the AV node from where, after a short delay, the impulse passes down the bundles of His and ventricular contraction ensues.

The depolarization/repolarization sequence is associated with potassium, sodium and calcium ionic shifts (see Fig. 24.1). On depolarization there is initially an increased inflow of sodium accompanied by the upstroke of the action potential. Secondly, there is a slower and smaller inward flow of current carried by calcium ions providing an important link in the excitation and contraction of cardiac muscle. Threshold excitation causes an initial fall in potassium conductance (Maylie & Morao 1984). The rapid increase in the rate of depolarization is caused by a sharp decline in the potassium current.

Acetylcholine causes an increase in the membrane conductance for potassium, hyperpolarizes the cell, reduces the action potential and may block conductance to the neighbouring atrial fibres and AV node.

Adrenaline causes an increase in the outward potassium current in atrial cells, the opposite to the effect needed to produce an increase in heart rate. However, it also augments the calcium inward current (Brown et al 1979). Thus adrenaline increases the phasic tension by increasing calcium conductance.

Peripheral vascular system

The peripheral vascular system consists of arteries, arterioles, capillaries, venules and veins. Exchange of oxygen, nutrients, hormones and drugs takes place at capillary level. All the other peripheral vessels have muscular walls, but the main site controlling the *peripheral vascular resistance*, and thus one of the main factors in controlling blood flow around the circulation, is in the arterioles. The muscle tone of the venous system controls their reservoir function.

Regulation of the cardiovascular system

The heart muscle has an intrinsic rhythm, and the peripheral vessels an intrinsic tone in their walls, but the body exerts a control over these to cope with changing demands. Nervous impulses, humoral factors, drugs and other substances can act on the heart and blood vessels through various receptors, or sometimes directly.

Receptors. Adrenergic receptors, subdivided into α_1, α_2, β_1 and β_2, occur in heart and blood vessels. These are described in more detail in chapters 16 and 22–24. The receptors vary from tissue to tissue and species to species. Both types of receptors act through the adenyl cyclase system. α_1-Receptors are mainly vasoconstrictor in function. The β-receptors are subdivided into two groups: β_1-receptors in the heart and β_2-receptors in other tissues. Stimulation of β_1-receptors causes tachycardia and an increased force of contraction of cardiac muscle, while β_2 stimulation is seen mainly as bronchospasm. The administration of a specific cardioselective β-blocking drug causes bradycardia and a decreased force of myocardial contraction, while the use of an α-blocking drug decreases vasoconstrictor effects, leading to vasodilation.

Noradrenaline produces contraction of smooth muscle and the resultant vasoconstriction causes a rise in blood pressure — the α-stimulant effect. Conversely, isoprenaline relaxes smooth muscle leading to both vasodilation and dilation of the bronchioles — the β-stimulant effect. Adrenaline has a mixed effect producing vasodilation in low or physiological concentrations by action on the β-receptors. This is an important action in skeletal muscle blood vessels. In higher concentrations the action of adrenaline is predominantly on the α-receptors producing vasoconstriction and consequent hypertension.

Autoregulation (humoral control)

Vascular control is achieved both by neural and by local chemical means. The local control involves two mechanisms — the autoregulatory control and the production of local vasodilator and constrictor substances. Autoregulation is well developed in the kidney, mesentery, skeletal muscle, brain, liver and myocardium. Two theories explain its action — the myogenic and metabolic.

In the myogenic theory, as the blood pressure rises, vascular smooth muscle contracts and so flow is unal- tered. This prevents normal blood pressure fluctuations from producing concomitant flow changes. In the metabolic theory, metabolites increase in active tissues and cause vasodilation in the vessels in these tissues and so flow is increased to meet the increased demands. These local vasodilator effects are produced by hypoxia, hypercarbia and temperature increase, but potassium, adenosine nucleotides, lactic acid and histamine are also contributory factors. The chemical vasodilation is of overwhelming importance in conditions of increasing metabolism in active tissues such as skeletal muscle. Vasoconstriction at a local level is produced by serotonin released by platelet breakdown.

In addition to these local controlling mechanisms, other vasodilator substances are released in certain regions. Notable among these are the kinins, especially bradykinin. They have actions similar to histamine, causing contraction of visceral smooth muscle and relaxation of vascular smooth muscle. This increases capillary permeability, attracts leucocytes and is associated with local pain. These kinins are formed in sweat glands, salivary glands and the exocrine portion of the pancreas, and may be responsible for the increase in blood flow in these and other tissues. The release of kinins is inhibited by adrenal glucocorticoids.

Vasoconstrictor substances include noradrenaline, adrenaline, angiotensin II and to a lesser extent serotonin. In total effect they are much less important than are the metabolites. Noradrenaline and adrenaline are released from the adrenal medulla and sympathetic system in response to stress, hypotension and exercise. These impulses are controlled from the vasomotor and other higher centres. Angiotensin II is released as a result of a fall in plasma volume leading to a release of renin from the juxtamedullary apparatus of the kidney. This acts on circulatory angiotensin I to produce angiotensin II. This, as well as having a generalized vasoconstrictor effect, acts on the adrenal cortex to increase aldosterone secretion, leading to increased reabsorption of sodium and a resultant restoration of blood volume (Guyton et al 1976, Mancia et al 1976).

Neural control

The co-ordination centre for the control of all circulatory function is the vasomotor centre in the medullary portion of the brainstem, which effectively controls the cardiovascular system to meet the varying needs of the body rather than the maintenance of the haemodynamic status quo. The vasomotor centre regulates both generalized vasomotor tone and the function of the heart, and

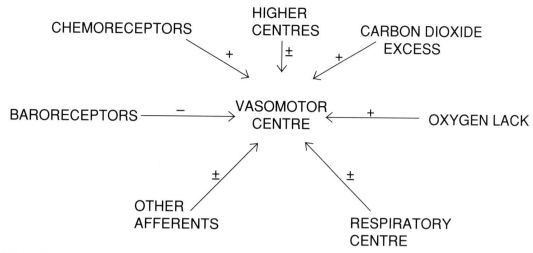

Fig. 21.1 Influences on the vasomotor centre.

is influenced by impulses reaching it from many sources (Fig. 21.1).

The baroreceptors in the carotid sinus and the wall of the aortic arch are stretch receptors. The influence of the baroreceptors on the vasomotor centre provides an example of feedback control. Stimulation of the baroreceptors by an increase in blood pressure results in reflex reduction in both vasomotor tone and heart rate, resulting in a fall in vascular resistance and cardiac output and so the blood pressure returns towards normal. The chemoreceptors respond to hypoxia and hypoperfusion and stimulate the vasomotor centre to produce vasoconstriction and a tachycardia, causing a rise in vascular resistance and cardiac output. Impulses from the skin, the muscles, the viscera and the higher centres are capable of producing either vasoconstriction or vasodilation via the vasomotor centre. The higher centres and the respiratory centre have variable effects causing both stimulation and inhibition. Vasodilation of the blood vessels in skeletal muscle in anticipation of exercise is caused by impulses from the cortex, which pass directly through the medulla.

Innervation

1. *Heart*.The heart receives innervation both from the sympathetic and the parasympathetic nervous system. The sympathetic nerve supply via the superior, middle and inferior cardiac sympathetic nerves passes to the nodal tissue in the sino-atrial (SA) and atrioventricular (AV) nodes and the muscle of the atria and ventricles. Sympathetic stimulation causes an increase in the heart rate and the force and speed of the myocardial contraction. The vagus nerves supplying the heart have their origins in the medulla. Their fibres are distributed to the SA node, the AV node and the atrial walls. There are no vagal fibres distributed to the ventricular muscle. Vagal stimulation causes a marked decrease in the rate of impulse generation at the SA node, decreases the rate of propagation of the cardiac impulse and decreases the force of atrial contraction. There is no direct effect on the ventricles. In humans the heart is normally under vagal control with a rate of about 70 beats per minute. Atropine, which causes inhibition of vagal effects upon the SA node, allows the rate to rise to 160–180 beats per minute. The completely denervated heart has a rate of about 100 beats per minute.

2. *Peripheral resistance*. The nerve fibres to the resistance vessels regulate the tissue blood flow and the arterial blood pressure, and the fibres to the venous capacitance vessels vary the volume of blood stored in the veins. Adrenergic nerve fibres from the sympathetic nervous system supply blood vessels in all parts of the body and are vasoconstrictor in character. The resistance vessels in skeletal muscle are also supplied with cholinergic vasodilator nerve fibres. At rest there is tonic vasoconstrictor tone, but no equivalent vasodilator discharge.

Mechanical function of the heart

The heart imparts both kinetic and potential energy to

the blood which it pumps: kinetic in the form of velocity, and potential in the form of pressure — the latter accounting for 96–99% of its work output. This energy is derived from metabolic reactions, and the work of the heart can be correlated with its oxygen consumption.

Blood pressure

The arterial blood pressure is a balance between the cardiac output and the resistance to flow offered by the vascular load, mainly the arterioles. Thus, it is usually stated that the blood pressure is the product of the cardiac output and the peripheral resistance. Factors which alter either the cardiac output or the peripheral resistance have the potential to change the blood pressure, though the vascular reflexes function to maintain the blood pressure close to normal levels.

In consideration of factors which affect the blood pressure, it is logical to consider those which alter the peripheral resistance and then those which alter the cardiac output. These are summarized in Fig. 21.2.

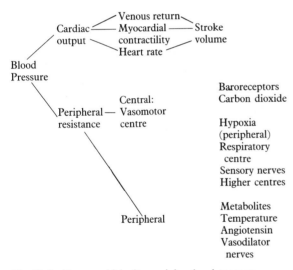

Fig. 21.2 Factors which alter peripheral resistance or cardiac output.

Cardiac output

The cardiac output is the product of the stroke volume and the heart rate. Variations of either of these indices can therefore alter the output, though a change in one will almost invariably be accompanied by a change in the other.

The stroke volume is affected by the venous return and the myocardial contractility. The heart rate is de-

creased by an increase in vagal tone and increased by an increase in sympathetic discharge.

A fall in cardiac output and consequent fall in blood pressure may be compensated by an increase in peripheral resistance leading to return of the arterial blood pressure to normal levels. Conversely, a raised cardiac output may be accommodated to some extent by a fall in peripheral resistance with only a modest rise in blood pressure as occurs in exercise.

Table 21.1 shows some of the more common ways in which the cardiac output is changed. It can be seen that the performance of the heart cannot be monitored by measuring the blood pressure alone. In studying the effects of drugs on the cardiovascular system it may be necessary to measure not only the blood pressure and heart rate but also the cardiac output and left atrial pressure or a closely related figure, the pulmonary capillary wedge pressure, so that the peripheral resistance can be calculated. Nevertheless, in a consideration of the cardiac output and the factors which affect it, it is convenient to look at the two parameters separately.

Table 21.1 Conditions affecting cardiac output

Decrease	Sitting or standing from lying
	Tachyarrhythmias
	Decreased myocardial contractility
Unaltered	Sleep
	Moderate environmental temperature change
Increase	Excitement
	Eating
	Exercise
	Major environmental temperature rise
	Pregnancy
	Alpha-adrenergic stimulant
	Histamine

Heart rate

The heart rate is altered by changes in sympathetic discharge and vagal tone affecting the sino-atrial node. Impulses pass from the vasomotor centre in response to stimuli from the higher centres, volume receptors, baroreceptors and chemoreceptors. Endogenous catecholamines may also affect the heart rate.

In tachycardia the cardiac muscle contracts and repolarizes more rapidly not only by decreasing the systolic ejection time but more especially by a decrease in the length of diastole. During diastole both ventricular filling and coronary arterial flow to the left ventricle occur, and so both may be compromised during tachycardia. In the healthy adult heart with normal coronary arteries and an adequate venous return, the cardiac output rises and is well maintained with heart rates up to 180 beats per minute. However, with rates above 180 filling is compromised, subendocardial ischaemia occurs, the cardiac output falls and heart failure supervenes. In disease states, especially coronary artery disease, such changes occur at much lower heart rates.

The heart rate is reduced by an increase in vagal tone and by certain drugs, which act on the sino-atrial node or cause slowing of conduction through the atrioventricular node — digitalis, β-adrenergic blocking drugs and some of the calcium blockers.

Stroke volume

The stroke volume is affected by changes in the preload or filling of the heart, the afterload or the peripheral resistance and by the force of contraction of the myocardium. During contraction of the normal heart at least 70% of the volume of blood in the ventricle at the end of diastole is ejected as the stroke volume (Dodge et al 1960, Rackley 1976). This is known as the ejection fraction. In disease states with poor myocardial function the heart becomes distended and is unable to empty effectively. A lesser fraction of the end-diastolic volume is expelled with each beat and thus the ejection fraction is decreased. An ejection fraction of under 50% is indicative of major myocardial dysfunction.

Preload

The venous return and subsequent atrial filling constitute the preload. An increase in venous return leads to increased atrial filling, increased ventricular end-diastolic volume, increase in stretch of the cardiac muscle and, therefore, an increase in the ensuing force of contraction of the myocardium in response to this stretch (Starling's law). This leads to an increase in the stroke volume. In myocardial failure the muscle can no longer contract fully in response to filling, there is over-distension of the muscle and pulmonary oedema or right-sided heart failure ensues (Fig. 21.3). The preload may be estimated by measurement of the central venous pressure. In patients with poor left ventricular function there may be poor correlation between preload to right and left sides of the heart, and measurement of left atrial pressure may be of clinical use.

Afterload

The greater the peripheral resistance, the more difficult it is for the heart to empty completely, and so the lower

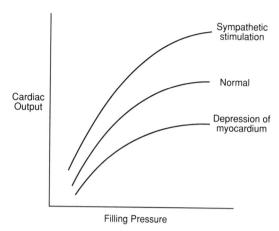

Fig. 21.3 Cardiac output changes with changes in filling pressure.

the cardiac output becomes. The heart can compensate for this by increasing the force of contraction. If the increase in peripheral resistance is sustained then left ventricular hypertrophy results. This spreads the load by increasing the total muscle mass. In myocardial failure, from whatever cause, compensatory mechanisms result in an increased peripheral resistance. This increases the work of the heart at a time when there already is decompensation. Decreasing the afterload by the use of a vasodilator drug such as sodium nitroprusside may allow the cardiac output to improve and the circulatory state to recover.

Inotropic state

The force of contraction of the heart is increased by an increase in the sympathetic discharge and catecholamine release. These factors are operative during exercise to increase the cardiac output. The infusion of dopamine, dobutamine or isoprenaline produces a similar effect. The increased force of contraction produces greater emptying of the ventricles and so an increase in stroke volume. The catecholamines act via the myocardial β-adrenergic receptors and will obviously affect the heart rate as well as the stroke volume. Figure 21.4 shows factors affecting myocardial contractile state.

Coronary blood flow

The coronary blood flow at rest is about 250 ml min^{-1}. Ventricular contraction impedes the blood flow so that the flow, especially to the left ventricle, is intermittent in character. While the autonomic control of the cor-

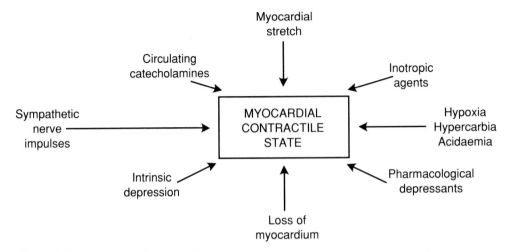

Fig. 21.4 Factors influencing myocardial contraction.

onary arteries is probably weak, sympathetic stimulation causes vasodilation, and vagal stimulation is associated with vasoconstriction. However, these effects may only be secondary to changes in myocardial metabolism, and the major factor increasing the coronary blood flow is local oxygen deficiency.

Adrenaline and noradrenaline dilate the coronary arteries while acetylcholine and 5-hydroxytryptamine also have a vasodilatory action. Nitroglycerine is the most effective drug used clinically to improve coronary blood flow. Its effects are doubly beneficial as not only does it dilate the coronary vessels but also its general venous and arterial dilating action leads to a decreased workload of the heart (Klocke & Ellis 1980).

Coronary artery steal

In this condition there is diversion of the blood flow from one area of the myocardium to another. This is intercoronary steal when it occurs from one coronary artery to another, and transmural steal when the blood is deviated from the subendocardial to the subepicardial area of the heart. When coronary artery steal occurs, there is preferential diversion of the blood from diseased vessels incapable of further vasodilation to normal vessels which can dilate. Such dilation may occur under the influence of drugs such as sodium nitroprusside, dipyridamole, papaverine and adenosine. There is also evidence that isoflurane can cause coronary steal, as opposed to halothane which does not produce such an effect (Sill et al 1987, Priebe & Foex 1987).

INOTROPES, CATECHOLAMINES AND SYMPATHOMIMETIC AGENTS

Before we consider these groups of cardiovascular drugs it would seem prudent to clarify a number of terms which are often used loosely or incorrectly. Strictly speaking the term *'inotrope'* may be used to describe any pharmacological agent which causes a change in the contractile properties of the myocardium through a direct action on the myocardial cell. The term, however, is commonly used to denote only agents which increase myocardial contractility — *positive inotropes*. Agents causing a decrease in myocardial contractility such as β-adrenoreceptor blockers and calcium channel blockers are correctly termed negative inotropes. In this chapter the term 'inotrope' will be used in its common clinical sense, i.e. to describe agents which directly increase cardiac contractility. Note that agents which are not inotropes may improve cardiac contractility indirectly, e.g. by reducing afterload. Such agents will not be considered in this chapter.

Positive inotropes may augment cardiac contractility in the following ways.

1. Increasing intracellular cyclic adenosine monophosphate (cAMP) due to activation of the adenylcyclase system (sympathomimetic agents/catecholamines).
2. Inhibiting phosphodiesterase (PDE), the enzyme responsible for cAMP breakdown (methylxanthines and derivatives).
3. Inhibiting calcium re-uptake by the sarcoplasmic reticulum (caffeine), increasing intracellular

calcium, or augmenting the response of contractile proteins to the presence of calcium.

Augmentation of myocardial contraction is most commonly due to increased activity of the sympathetic nervous system. This causes the release, at sympathetic post-ganglionic nerve endings, of the neurotransmitter noradrenaline which stimulates cardiac β-adreno-receptors (see Chapter 16). The increased sympathetic activity also causes release of additional adrenaline and noradrenaline from the adrenal medulla, resulting in further stimulation of cardiac β-adrenoreceptors.

Adrenaline and noradrenaline thus mimic the effects of the sympathetic nervous system and are an example of a group of substances termed '*sympathomimetics*'. The basic structure of the sympathomimetics is that of a benzene ring with a ethylamine side-chain — phenylethylamine. Different members of the group can be produced by substitutions on either the benzene ring, the side-chain or the terminal amino group. If —OH radicals are inserted at positions 3 and 4 of a benzene ring, the resulting compound is catechol. Thus any sympathomimetic amines which include these substitutions are termed *catecholamines*; i.e. catecholamines are a sub-group of the sympathomimetic amines.

The haemodynamic effects and pattern of receptor stimulation for the commonly used catecholamines, non-catecholamine inotropes and sympathomimetic agents are summarized in Table 21.2, (p. 359).

POSITIVE INOTROPES — CATECHOLAMINES

Dopamine

Chemical name: 3,4-Dihydroxyphenylethylamine. Hydroxylation at positions 3 and 4 of the benzene ring in phenylethamine produces dopamine (Fig. 21.6), the basic molecule of the catecholamine group and the immediate metabolic precursor of noradrenaline and adrenaline. It occurs naturally as a CNS neurotransmitter and is found in relatively high concentration in the basal ganglia.

Physical properties.   Dopamine is a water-soluble white crystalline substance which is clinically available as an aqueous solution (800 mg in 5 ml or 200 mg in 5 ml) with 1% sodium bisulphite. It is usually diluted further for intravenous infusion and is compatible with both dextrose 5% and saline 0.9% and dextrose/saline mixtures. In such solutions it is stable for at least 24 h but is inactivated rapidly if added to an alkaline solution.

Pharmacology.   The actions of dopamine can be summarized thus: it is a positive inotrope with a specific

vasodilatory effect on the renal vasculature at low dose and has a generalized peripheral vasoconstrictive effect at high dose.

Dopamine stimulates dopaminergic (DA), β_1 and α_1-adrenoreceptors with increasing dose. The β_1 and α_1, effects may be augmented by its ability to release noradrenaline from nerve endings (Nash et al 1968).

At a dose of less than 3 μg kg^{-1} min^{-1}, and possibly as low as 0.5 μg kg^{-1} min^{-1}, dopamine stimulates DA receptors in the kidney producing an increase in renal blood flow and glomerular filtration rate (GFR). This results in increased urinary output and sodium excretion (Goldberg 1972). The natriuretic effect may also be due to changes in intrarenal blood flow. There may also be similar changes in the mesenteric vascular bed. At this dose dopamine usually has no cardiac effects.

In the range 5–10 μg kg^{-1} min^{-1} dopamine stimulates cardiac β-receptors, thereby increasing stroke volume (SV) and cardiac output (CO). There is little effect on peripheral vascular beds and so no significant effect on systemic vascular resistance (SVR). Thus at this dose, dopamine increases arterial pressure, predominantly systolic pressure. Heart rate (HR) is often unchanged, although there may be a modest increase.

With doses of 10 μg kg^{-1} min^{-1} and above, α_1-adrenoreceptor stimulation becomes a more dominant effect and release of noradrenaline from nerve terminals is triggered. This produces generalized vasoconstriction and a substantial rise in systolic and diastolic arterial pressure, central venous pressure (CVP) and pulmonary artery pressures (PAP). At high dose the overall effect of dopamine may be indistinguishable from that of noradrenaline and CO may fall due to the excessive rise in SVR. Such high doses of dopamine usually produce large increases in HR with a high incidence of both supraventricular and ventricular tachyarrhythmias.

It might be expected that dopamine could have CNS effects via DA receptors within the brain. This is usually not the case, since dopamine does not easily cross the blood–brain barrier.

The pattern of receptor stimulation with differing doses of dopamine is not as clear-cut as described above (see Fig. 21.5). In any single patient, β_1-receptor stimulation may occur at doses which should only act at DA receptors. Likewise generalized vasoconstriction may occur at doses well below those known to cause α_1-receptor stimulation. In contrast, certain types of patients may show 'receptor down-regulation' and require greater doses of dopamine to produce a given effect.

Administration and pharmacokinetics.   Dopamine should be administered by slow controlled intravenous infusion into a central vein (see below). It has a plasma

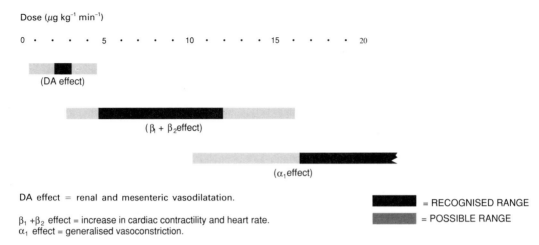

Fig. 21.5 Effects of dopamine at different doses.

half-life of approximately 2 min and so changes in infusion rate will produce haemodynamic effects within a short period. Dopamine is metabolized by both monoamine oxidase (MAO) and catechol-*o*-methyl transferase (COMT), and so is ineffective when administered via the gastrointestinal tract.

Indications. Dopamine administered at a rate of 2–3 μg kg^{-1} min^{-1} can be used to improve renal perfusion and urinary flow in oliguric patients in whom circulating fluid volume has already been restored. Often the effect is a modest, continuing increase in urinary output — not a short-lived major diuresis followed by further oliguria as may occur when loop diuretics are administered. Although it has not been proven, dopamine may reduce the incidence of acute renal failure when used prophylactically to cause renal vasodilation in high-risk groups, e.g. severe hypotension, crush syndrome.

In doses above 5 μg kg^{-1} min^{-1}, dopamine is especially indicated when an inotropic effect is required in a hypotensive patient. It is particularly useful in systemic sepsis and cardiogenic shock associated with significant hypotension. The relative merits of dopamine and dobutamine and the factors dictating the choice of inotrope are discussed below.

Side-effects and precautions. Side-effects attributed to dopamine are often those of sympathetic overactivity: nausea, vomiting, tremor, headache and cardiovascular effects — tachycardia, arrhythmias, hypertension and peripheral ischaemia due to excessive vasoconstriction.

Since it is such a potent drug it is essential to control the rate of infusion precisely, and to monitor its effects. Extravasation into the subcutaneous tissues may cause sloughing of skin and so the drug should always be ad-ministered directly into a central vein and not via a peripheral line. If extravasation does occur then local infiltration with an α-receptor blocker such as phentolamine should be tried.

As one might expect, the dose of dopamine must be radically reduced in patients on MAOI antidepressants and, to a lesser degree, in individuals on tricyclic antidepressants. As with all positive inotropes, dopamine is contra-indicated in situations of left ventricular outflow tract obstruction, e.g. idiopathic hypertrophic subaortic stenosis.

Dobutamine

Dobutamine, first introduced to clinical practice in 1978, possesses the basic dopamine structure but has a bulky aromatic ring substitution on the terminal amino group (Fig. 21.6). This synthetic catecholamine was developed specifically to have a powerful inotropic effect with no other significant haemodynamic properties (Tuttle & Mills 1975).

Physical properties. Dobutamine hydrochloride (Dobutrex) is supplied in a lyophilized form (250 mg per vial) which is reconstituted in 10 ml of either water for injection or 5% dextrose. It is usually further diluted before use, and has the same compatibilities with intravenous fluids as dopamine (see above). It is stable in solution for up to 24 h. The solution may take on a slight pink colour due to slight oxidation of the drug, but this does not effect potency over a 24 h period. Like dopamine it is rapidly inactivated under alkaline conditions. Stereoisomers exist (see below) and the commercial preparation is racemic.

Pharmacology. Dobutamine may be viewed simply

as a selective β_1-receptor agonist which produces a strong positive inotropic effect with little chronotropy, weak peripheral vascular effects and a low tendency to cause arrhythmias. There is evidence, however, that the apparent inotropic response may be due in part to α-receptor blockade and β_2-receptor stimulation causing preload and afterload reduction. The (+) isomer is responsible for the above effects and the (−) isomer is more potent as an α-receptor agonist (Ruffolo et al 1981). In theory the overall peripheral effect should be an increase in blood flow to skeletal muscle (β_2 agonism) and some reduction in skin blood flow (α_1 agonism balanced by some α-receptor blockade). However, it should be stressed that these actions are weak relative to the myocardial effects. Dobutamine does not cause release of noradrenaline from nerve endings (Robie et al 1974), nor does it have any effects on renal dopaminergic receptors (Vatner et al 1974).

Dobutamine is administered by infusion, starting at 2–3 μg kg^{-1} min^{-1} and increasing by the same amount every 10–30 min. Starting an infusion at a higher dose increases the chances of tachycardia and arrhythmias. The optimal clinical effect usually occurs between 7 and 15 μg kg^{-1} min^{-1}.

In this dose range dobutamine causes an increase in SV and CO. Since the peripheral vascular effects are relatively weak and tend to cancel each other out, SVR may be unchanged or moderately decreased. Arterial pressure therefore may rise or fall slightly, or remain unchanged.

At doses in excess of 15 μg kg^{-1} min^{-1}, tachycardia and arrythmias are more likely. When administration has continued for more than 48–72 h a reduction in clinical benefit (tolerance) may be seen (Unverferth et al 1980). It has been presumed that this is due to down-regulation of β-adrenoreceptors. Restoration of maximal effect may be obtained by increasing the infusion rate using haemodynamic improvement as a guide. In situations of receptor down-regulation, the dose required to produce toxic or side-effects seems to be increased equivalently.

Administration and pharmacokinetics.
Like dopamine, dobutamine should be administered as a precisely controlled infusion. It has little direct peripheral vascular effect and does not stimulate noradrenaline release from nerve endings. Skin necrosis/sloughing due to extravasation of dobutamine is therefore rare but has been reported (Hoff et al 1979). Since the inotropic effect may be life-saving and peripheral lines are prone to displacement or obstruction, it is prudent, where possible, to administer dobutamine via a central venous line.

Onset of action occurs within 2 min and the maximal effect associated with a given infusion rate occurs ap-

proximately 10 min after commencing the infusion. In patients with low output cardiac failure the plasma half-life is 2.37 ± 0.70 min. Most of the drug will be metabolized or eliminated approximately 10 min after cessation of the infusion (Kates & Leier 1978).

The short half-life is due to rapid redistribution and to metabolism by COMT (Murphy et al 1976). This produces 3-o-methyldobutamine and dobutamine glucuronide, which are both pharmacologically inactive and are excreted by the kidney.

Indications.
Dobutamine is very effective in increasing cardiac output and therefore systemic perfusion, but as an agent to increase arterial pressure it is relatively ineffective. It is indicated in acute myocardial failure as may occur after myocardial infarction, cardiac surgery or in association with myocarditis. It may also be valuable in the treatment of decompensated chronic congestive cardiac failure (Applefeld et al 1983). Such situations are characterized by very low cardiac output together with excessive peripheral vasoconstriction, but only modest hypotension. The use of dobutamine increases cardiac output, and reduces afterload both directly (via β_2-adrenoreceptors) and also indirectly due to its effect on cardiac output. Note that dobutamine produces no selective renal vasodilation — renal blood flow will increase, but only as a result of the global increase in cardiac output.

The inability of dobutamine to reliably increase arterial pressure may make it unsuitable as a first-line agent in the treatment of some cases of cardiogenic or septic shock. Nevertheless, it may be used in conjuction with dopamine and/or noradrenaline to maximize cardiac output and peripheral flow after perfusion pressure has been returned to acceptable levels.

Side-effects and precautions.
The side-effects of dobutamine are as for other catecholamines but are relatively uncommon (Leier & Unverferth 1983). Tachycardia and tachyarrhythmias are less frequent than with dopamine (Sonnenblick et al 1979). Since dobutamine enhances A–V conduction, it may precipitate atrial fibrillation in predisposed individuals.

Comparison of dopamine and dobutamine

Dopamine and dobutamine are by far the most widely used of all the positive inotropes. Although they both augment myocardial contractility, their other cardiovascular effects are different (Leier et al 1977). Stated simply, dopamine is an inotrope with an ability to cause systemic vasoconstriction, whereas dobutamine is an inotrope with the tendency to cause peripheral vasodilation.

In some situations dobutamine will produce a greater

increase in cardiac index than dopamine (Francis et al 1982) since it reduces left ventricular after-load rather than increasing it. It also follows, however, that dobutamine will produce no significant increase in arterial pressure (and may in fact result in a decrease) while dopamine normally produces an increase in arterial pressure — especially systolic pressure.

In addition to arteriolar vasodilation, dobutamine causes venodilation. This, coupled with improved ventricular ejection, results in a decrease in left ventricular filling pressure (preload). In contrast dopamine will cause left ventricular preload to increase or remain unchanged.

Dopamine tends to produce a greater chronotropic effect and more ventricular arrhythmias than dobutamine (Stoner et al 1977). Tissue necrosis at a site of extravasation, a well-known risk with dopamine, is much less common with dobutamine (see above). Unlike dopamine, dobutamine has no specific vasodilatory effect on the renal and splanchnic vascular beds. It may, however, improve perfusion to these areas by improving overall cardiac output.

If one considers these two agents in terms of their effect on myocardial oxygen balance one can see why dobutamine is favoured by many cardiology units. Both agents increase myocardial oxygen supply by virtue of an increased cardiac output and improved coronary artery flow. Dopamine, however, may increase myocardial oxygen demand by increasing heart rate, ventricular preload and afterload. If the chronotropic effect is excessive and diastolic filling time is severely shortened, then dopamine may actually make myocardial ischaemia worse. Such an effect would be much less common with dobutamine which tends to reduce ventricular preload and afterload.

In many situations of acute circulatory failure/myocardial insufficiency the use of either dopamine or dobutamine will be beneficial. Nevertheless, there are often aspects in the patient's condition which would suggest the use of one or other of these agents. When arterial hypotension is severe then dopamine is the agent of choice and by improving mean arterial pressure may even improve the oxygen supply/demand balance within the myocardium, despite the adverse factors outlined in the preceding paragraph. Thus in severe septicaemic or cardiogenic shock, dopamine, either alone or in combination with a vasopressor such as noradrenaline, is the inotrope of choice. When hypotension is not a major problem but cardiac output is poor then dobutamine is the more appropriate inotrope (Francis et al 1982), especially if left ventricular preload is high.

Dopamine and dobutamine have similar benefical effects on cardiac contractility while their other effects have been termed 'complementary' (Leier & Unverferth 1983). It is not surprising, therefore, that in clinical practice they are often used in combination, the proportions varying with patient's needs and responses.

Noradrenaline (norepinephrine)

Chemical name: 1β-(3,4-dihydroxyphenyl)-α-aminoethanol.

Noradrenaline is a neurotransmitter synthesized at mammalian post-ganglionic adrenergic nerve endings and in the adrenal medulla (Fig. 21.6). It is a catecholamine produced by β-hydroxylation of the side-chain of dopamine under the influence of dopamine β-oxidase. Further methylation of the terminal amino group by N-methyl transferase results in the formation of adrenaline. In the adrenal medulla about 20% of the catecholamine content is due to the presence of noradrenaline.

Physical properties. Noradrenaline bitartrate (trade name Levophed) is a water-soluble monohydrate salt. It is available as an aqueous solution containing 2 mg ml^{-1} of the salt which is equivalent to 1 mg ml^{-1} of noradrenaline base. It is usually diluted to 2–8 μg ml^{-1} for clinical use as a continuous infusion.

Pharmacology. Noradrenaline is a powerful agonist at α-adrenoreceptors; (Allwood et al 1963), has similar potency to adrenaline at β$_1$-adrenoreceptors (Goldberg et al 1960) but has no significant effect at β$_2$-receptors.

Noradrenaline causes widespread arteriolar vasoconstriction (Rose et al 1962), thus increasing both systolic and diastolic blood pressure. The β$_1$-adrenoreceptor stimulation and increased afterload produce an overall moderate reduction in cardiac output. Since arterial pressure is elevated this may cause an increase in vagal tone which produces a reflex decrease in heart rate, overcoming the direct positive chronotropic effect. Thus with a decrease in heart rate and a modest reduction in CO, SV may be well preserved despite increased afterload. There is also marked venoconstriction which produces an increase in preload as measured by CVP and PAP.

The vasoconstricting action of noradrenaline results in decreased perfusion generally — including renal, hepatic, mesenteric and skeletal muscle vascular beds. Glomerular filtration is, however, maintained unless renal blood flow is severely reduced. Coronary artery flow is often increased, due to a combination of factors. Firstly, an increase in aortic pressure improves coronary perfusion pressure. Secondly, a slowing of heart rate increases the duration of diastole. Thirdly, increased myocardial contractility results in increased myocardial oxygen consumption and causes the accumulation of vasodilatory metabolites within the myocardium.

Many of the effects of noradrenaline result from the relative balance between improved cardiac contractility and increased after-load. Normally clinically applicable doses are 2–10 μg min^{-1}. The use of excessive doses usually results in huge increases in afterload, substantial reductions in CO and organ perfusion and potentially fatal increases in myocardial oxygen requirements. Noradrenaline therapy should be accurately controlled and titrated according to information obtained by the use of a pulmonary artery flotation catheter. Such monitoring does identify a subgroup of patients, usually suffering from systemic sepsis, who are profoundly vasodilated and do not respond even to massive doses of noradrenaline. Such individuals remain in intractable shock and have a very grave prognosis.

Administration and pharmacokinetics. Noradrenaline is administered by controlled intravenous infusion via a central venous line. As with adrenaline, it is inactive when administered orally. The effect on arterial pressure lasts only 1–2 min after cessation of infusion. Like adrenaline, noradrenaline is metabolized by the enzymes MAO and COMT. The metabolites have little or no haemodynamic effects and are excreted in the urine. (Unmetabolized noradrenaline, detected in minute amounts in the urine of normal individuals, may be renally excreted at the rate of 10–15 mg per day by patients with a phaeochromocytoma.)

Indications. As a relatively weak inotrope with potent vasoconstrictor effects, noradrenaline should be used to combat hypotension due to excessive peripheral vasodilation as in systemic sepsis. On the premise that it is wrong to cause vasoconstriction without attempting to increase CO, noradrenaline should be commenced only when fluid loading and moderate-dose dopamine have failed to restore an acceptable arterial pressure. Noradrenaline, in theory, should be used in conjunction with either dopamine or dobutamine and not as a first-line drug. Used appropriately, it is certainly preferable to high-dose dopamine which produces a similar degree of vasoconstriction but also causes excessive tachycardia and cardiac arrhythmias which reduce myocardial efficiency and significantly increase myocardial oxygen demand.

Side-effects & precautions. The unwelcome effects of noradrenaline are (1) those of any catecholamine; anxiety, vomiting, headache, sweating and (2) those caused by an excessive effect on the cardiovascular system — pallor, hypertension, retrosternal pain, arrhythmias and excessive vasoconstriction with resultant ischaemia/ necrosis.

Not surprisingly, skin necrosis and sloughing is a big danger with noradrenaline. It must always be administered via a central venous line to avoid extravasation. If this does occur the use of phentolamine is recommended (see above).

Noradrenaline is an extremely potent drug which, if administered in excess, can precipitate hypertensive crisis, myocardial ischaemia and cardiac failure. It should be used only when proper arrangements for its administration and monitoring of the effect have been made. This should include a pulmonary artery flotation catheter. The infusion must be controlled using a syringe or volumetric infusion pump and the patient must have a suitable experienced person in constant attendance.

Adrenaline (epinephrine)

Adrenaline (1-β-(3,4-dihydroxy phenyl)-α-methylaminoethanol) is synthesized naturally from noradrenaline by the methylation of the terminal amino group by *N*-methyl transferase (Fig. 21.6). In adults, 80% of the total catecholamines in the adrenal medulla is present as adrenaline.

Physical properties. The base is poorly soluble in water but forms water-soluble salts with acids. It is unstable under alkaline conditions and when exposed to light for long periods. The intravenous preparation is a 1 : 1000 (1 mg ml^{-1}) or 1 : 10000 (100 μg ml^{-1}) aqueous solution of adrenaline hydrochloride.

Pharmacology. Adrenaline is a potent agonist at β_1-, β_2- and α_1-receptors. Its effects are mediated by stimulating the intracellular enzyme adenyl cyclase and thereby increasing the conversion of ATP to cyclic AMP.

Adrenaline causes very modest CNS excitation resulting in headache, tremors and agitation only at high doses.

In the bronchi and smaller airways, adrenaline causes smooth muscle relaxation and, by decreasing mucosal blood flow, a reduction in mucosal oedema and bronchial secretions.

The effect of adrenaline on the cardiovascular system is complex due to the multiple receptors at which it acts. It will cause an increase in HR and cardiac contractility (β_1) and also an increase in venoconstriction and vasoconstriction in vessels supplying skin or mucous membranes. This will be more than offset by vasodilation of the arterioles in the skeletal muscle beds, liver and splanchnic area. Therefore cardiac output increases, peripheral resistance decreases slightly and effective circulating volume and venous return increase. The nett result is an increase in systolic pressure and a reduction in diastolic pressure. At higher doses adrenaline becomes a general vasoconstrictor; then it causes an increase of both systolic and diastolic pressure and a reduction in cardiac output.

Unlike other sympathomimetics, adrenaline has widespread influences on metabolism. It tends to inhibit insulin secretion and promote glucagon — thereby decreasing the I/G ratio. Glycogenolysis is accelerated in most tissues and plasma glucose levels are increased — made worse by a reduction in peripheral glucose uptake. By stimulating triglyceride lipase, free fatty acids and glycerol are mobilized from adipose tissue and there is an increase in serum cholesterol, phospholipid and low-density lipoprotein levels. The nett result of all this is a 25% increase in oxygen consumption after moderate doses of adrenaline.

Administration and pharmacokinetics.   Oral administration produces barely detectable concentrations of adrenaline in the tissues since it is inactivated by mucosal cells of the gastrointestinal tract and by the liver. It can be administered by almost any other route although some, e.g. subcutaneous injection, result in slow absorption due to local vasoconstriction. When used for its haemodynamic effect it is given intravenously, either as repeated small bolus doses or as a controlled continuous intravenous infusion.

Adrenaline is rapidly eliminated from the body, the major degradation pathway being either oxidation by MAO and/or conjugation by COMT. Although both these enzymes are present at high concentration in the liver, they occur in many other tissues, and extrahepatic enzymatic degradation can cope when severe liver dysfunction is present. A large portion of the total dose of adrenaline administered will appear in the urine as 3-methoxy,4-hydroxy-mandelic acid, also termed vanillyl mandelic acid (VMA), although a small amount of unmetabolized adrenaline may also be present. The presence of a large amount of unchanged adrenaline in the urine is abnormal, and often denotes the presence of a phaeochromocytoma or other catecholamine-secreting tumour.

Side-effects and precautions.   Adrenaline may mimic sympathetic overactivity and produce anxiety, tremor, restlessness, weakness, dizziness, headache, pallor, hypertension, tachycardia, arrhythmias, retrosternal pain and palpitations. Pre-existing hyperthyroidism, ischaemic heart disease and hypertension predispose to these side-effects. Ventricular extrasystoles, tachycardia or fibrillation are more likely to occur when adrenaline administration coincides with hypoxaemia, hypercarbia or the use of halogenated hydrocarbon anaesthetic agents such as halothane.

Indications.   Despite potent inotropic actions, adrenaline is less frequently used nowadays as an inotrope. It may still be of use in the period immediately following cardiopulmonary bypass (Steen et al 1978), for the support of the transplanted heart and in a situation where other inotropes have failed.

Isoprenaline

This synthetically produced catecholamine (Fig. 21.6) is a powerful agonist at β_1-and β_2-receptors but has no significant effect at α-receptors.

Isoprenaline causes an increase in both cardiac contractility and heart rate with a resulting increase in cardiac output. Left ventricular afterload is reduced due to peripheral vasodilation so that, even with an increase in cardiac output, arterial blood pressure (especially diastolic pressure) tends to fall moderately. The inotropic effect occurs at infusion rates of $0.007–0.014 \ \mu g \ kg^{-1}$ min^{-1} (Leier 1986). When the rate of administration exceeds $0.020 \ \mu g \ kg^{-1} \ min^{-1}$ then tachycardia, arrhythmias and excessive vasodilation may occur.

Isoprenaline causes bronchial smooth muscle to relax and inhibits histamine liberation from passively sensitized human pulmonary mast cells. Its vasodilating effect on the lung may, however, worsen existing ventilation/perfusion mismatches.

Indications.   An indication for the use of isoprenaline is the treatment of bronchospasm, especially that associated with anaphylactoid reactions. It is rarely employed as an inotrope nowadays due to the availability of drugs with a superior inotropic effect and a greater therapeutic index. It is still of value in the treatment of resistent bradycardia or heart block where atropine has been ineffective. Isoprenaline is also of use in 'Torsade de Pointe'. In this condition ventricular fibrillation/tachycardia occurs despite large doses of anti-arryhthmics. The underlying cause is a prolongation of the Q-T interval which can be reduced by an infusion of isoprenaline.

Dopexamine

This is a relatively new synthetic catecholamine, the molecular structure having similarities with dopamine (Fig. 21.6). Work in experimental animals suggests that it is a potent agonist at B_2 adrenoreceptors, causing generalised peripheral vasodilation, and has weaker

PHENYLETHYLAMINE

DOPAMINE

NORADRENALINE

ADRENALINE

ISOPRENALINE

DOBUTAMINE

DOPEXAMINE

ENOXIMONE

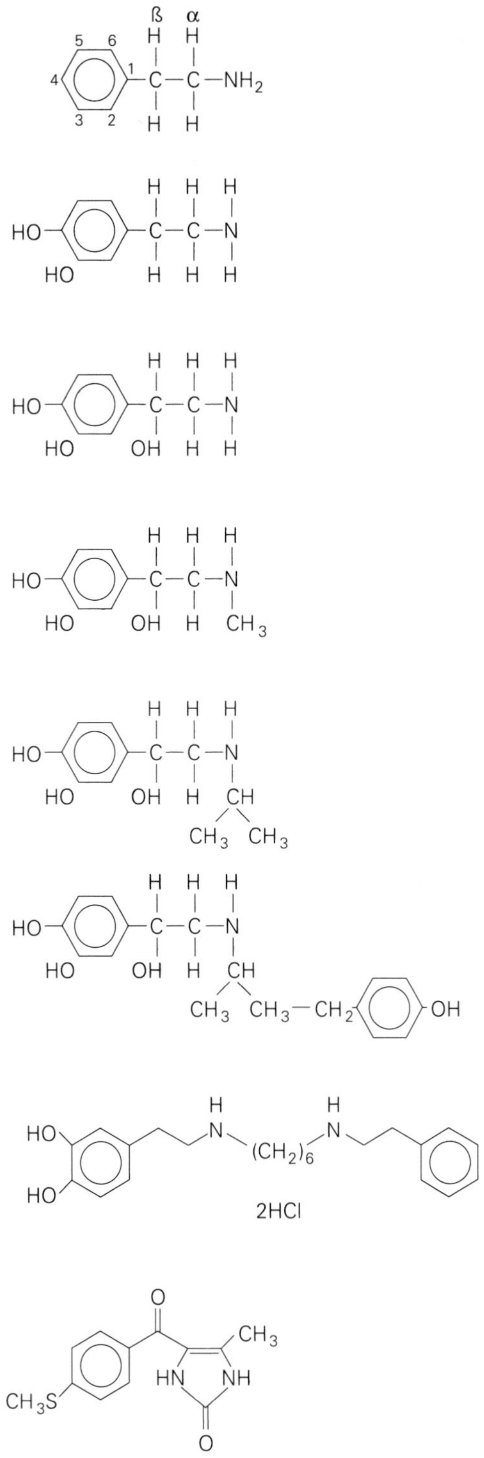

Fig. 21.6 Formulae of inotropic drugs.

agonist activity at peripheral dopamine receptors, causing renal and mesenteric vasodilation (Brown et al 1985). It is also a weak agonist at β_1 receptors, has no α-receptor activity and inhibits neuronal re-uptake of catecholamines. The overall result is an increase in cardiac index, due mostly to increased stroke volume, a moderate reduction in left ventricular afterload, a reduction in systemic blood pressure, and preferential renal and mesenteric vasodilation. In humans, this is similar to the effect of medium-dose dobutamine used in combination with low-dose dopamine. Haemodynamic effects reach their peak 6 min after intravenous administration and rapidly reverse when infusion is stopped.

In 2 ICU patients who had received liver transplants, dopexamine, when used as a renal vasodilator, was found to be more effective than low dose dopamine in preventing post-operative renal dysfunction as manifested by oliguria (Bodenham & Park 1988). When administered to a small group of patients with chronic congestive heart failure at doses ranging from $1-4$ μg kg^{-1} min^{-1}, dopexamine caused a 30% decrease in SVR, a 47% increase in CO and a 26% increase in SV (Svensson et al 1986). Heart rate increased by 14% while there was no significant change in systolic or diastolic pressure. No arrhythmias were observed at this dose range and dopexamine has been well tolerated when administered in volunteers at rates of up to 12 μg kg^{-1} min^{-1}.

POSITIVE INOTROPES — NON-CATECHOLAMINES:
Phosphodiesterase inhibitors

Another means of increasing intramyocardial cAMP is to inhibit its breakdown by phosphodiesterase (PDE). It has long been recognized that PDE inhibitors such as the methylxanthines (theophylline and caffeine) can have a beneficial effect on myocardial contractility, but only at doses which cause severe tachycardia and arrhythmias as well as neurological and gastrointestinal side-effects. Methylxanthines also inhibit calcium re-uptake by the sarcoplasmic reticulum, potentiate the effect of calcium on contractile proteins and stimulate the synthesis and release of endogenous catecholamines, so their cardiac effects may not solely be due to PDE inhibition. Nevertheless, the development of new PDE inhibitors has yielded other agents with some clinically useful inotropic action.

Bipyridine derivatives

Amrinone increases canine cardiac contractility in vitro

(Alousi et al 1979), although its mode of action is not clear. In humans, infusions of amrinone cause reductions in systemic and pulmonary vascular resistance and (potentially) decreased arterial blood pressure. There is an increase in cardiac index but opinion is divided as to whether this is due to a direct enhancement of cardiac contractility or secondary to a reduction in left ventricular afterload. It would appear that its modest inotropic effect is non-existent in patients with chronic heart failure (Wilmshurst et al 1983). Amrinone is relatively poorly tolerated at high doses, causing nausea, vomiting, anorexia, abdominal pain, fever, arthropathy, hepatic dysfunction and thrombocytopenia. It is unlikely that such a drug would be beneficial as the sole inotropic support in acute circulatory failure.

Another member of this group is **milrinone**. It has a better therapeutic index and greater potency than amrinone. It has a plasma half-life of 2 h and is excreted unchanged in the urine. Although its place as an inotrope for acute circulatory insufficency in patients without severe ischaemic heart disease is unclear, it has been claimed that it has a similar effect to dobutamine in congestive heart failure (Biddle et al 1987).

Imidazolone derivatives

Enoximone, although structurally different, has similar haemodynamic effects to the bipyridines. When administered intravenously to 24 individuals with severe refractory congestive heart failure, it was associated with a marked increase in stroke volume and cardiac output (Kereiakes et al 1984). In addition, right atrial and pulmonary capillary wedge pressures and SVR were reduced — an indication of the vasodilatory effect of the drug. This beneficial effect of enoximone on cardiac contractility has also been demonstrated in patients exhibiting low output states immediately following cardiac bypass surgery (Gonzales et al 1988) and in patients with end-stage cardiac failure requiring urgent cardiac transplantation (Dubois-Rande et al 1988). The relative contribution of increased contractility and reduced afterload to the improvement in cardiac output has yet to be determined.

Enoximone (trade name Perfan) is supplied as a clear yellow solution containing 5 mg ml^{-1} which must be diluted in 0.9% saline or water for injection before administration. If added to 5% dextrose, or allowed to come in contact with glass, crystal formation may occur. The recommended initial infusion rate is $0.5-1.0$ mg kg^{-1} over $20-30$ min. Hypotension has been associated with initial doses of 1.0 mg kg^{-1} or more. Maintenance therapy requires an infusion rate of $5-20$ μg kg^{-1} min^{-1}. The daily dose should not exceed 24 mg kg^{-1}.

Little is known at present about metabolism of enoximone in man. It undoubtedly has a long half-life and there may be a haemodynamically active metabolite. Certainly circulatory effects can persist for 8–10 h after the drug is discontinued.

Another member of this series, piroximone, has been shown to improve haemodynamic parameters in patients with refractory heart failure (Axelrod et al 1987).

At present enoximone is the most clinically useful drug in this group. It would appear to be of use in ICU primarily as an agent which improves cardiac output and (hopefully) tissue perfusion when used alone or in combination with dobutamine. It may be particularly effective in patients in whom adrenoreceptor down-regulation may have occurred due to long-term catecholamine therapy. Enoximone would also seem to be indicated in the treatment of severe congestive heart failure especially since such an agent may be suitable for oral administration. Such a development would mean an intravenous inotropic agent, administered in acute exacerbations of heart failure, could be taken orally for longer term therapy.

Other agents that have a positive inotropic effect include glucagon, calcium and digoxin.

OTHER SYMPATHOMIMETIC AGENTS

The effects of sympathomimetic agents can be due to (1) the drug itself interacting with adrenoreceptors (direct) or (2) the drug causing the release of noradrenaline from postganglionic sympathetic nerve endings (indirect). The haemodynamic effects of those sympathomimetics still to be considered in this chapter are summarized in Table 21.2. Phenylephrine, like adrenaline and noradrenaline, is an example of a direct sympathomimetic while methoxamine, ephedrine and metaraminol exert their effects by both direct and indirect mechanisms. Tyramine and amphetamines are indirectly acting agents and are not used clinically as sympathomimetics. Drugs acting with an indirect action have a reduced effect in patients with depleted noradrenaline stores, e.g. those on reserpine-like drugs. The indirectly acting sympathomimetics make use of the noradrenaline re-uptake pathways to enter the nerve endings and so they have a reduced effect where this pathway is blocked; e.g. patients on tricyclic antidepressants such as imipramine. Note that, in such patients, directly acting sympathomimetics would have an enhanced effect.

Ephedrine

Ephedrine is a naturally occurring amine which is now synthetically produced. It has both α- and β-agonist effects and acts both directly and indirectly. Its haemodynamic effects are similar to adrenaline but it has a longer duration of action and is active when administered orally. It causes an increase in cardiac contractility and heart rate. Cardiac output is thus increased. Peripheral vasoconstriction is balanced by vasodilation with little overall change in SVR. Arterial blood pressure rises — systolic more than diastolic. It may increase cardiac irritability.

Ephedrine causes relaxation of bronchial and other smooth muscle, though it is less effective than adrenaline in this regard. Unlike adrenaline, ephedrine reduces uterine muscle activity in all situations.

Side-effects are similar to those of adrenaline. It is not

Table 21.2 Effects of inotropic drugs

Drug	Receptor stimulated	Cardiac contractility	Heart rate	SVR	Renal blood flow	Arterial pressure
Dopamine	DA	–	–		↑	–
	β	↑↑	↑	–or↑	–	↑
	α	–	–	↑↑	↓	↑↑
Dobutamine	β$_1$+β$_2$	↑↑	–	↓	–	↑ or ↓
Noradrenaline	α+β (weak)	↑	↓	↑↑	↓	↑↑
Adrenaline	α+β	↑↑	↑	↑ or ↓	–or↓	↑
Isoprenaline	β	↑	↑↑	↓	–	↓
Dopexamine	DA+β$_2$+β$_1$ (weak)	–or↑	↑	↓	↑	–
Enoximone	PDE inhibitor	↑	–or↑	↓	–	–or↓
Ephedrine	α+β	↑	↑	–	–	↑
Metaraminol	α+β	↑	↓	↑	–	↑↑
Methoxamine	α+β antagonist	–	↓	↑	↓	↑
Phenylephrine	α+weakβ	–	↓	↑↑	↓	↑↑

broken down by MAO and is excreted unchanged by the kidney.

Metaraminol

Like ephedrine this agent has both direct and indirect effects and is an agonist at both α- and β-receptors.

Its cardiovascular effects are similar to ephedrine with the exception that overall peripheral resistance is increased whereas it is unchanged with ephedrine. This produces a greater increase in blood pressure — especially diastolic pressure.

Indications and dosage. It is usually administered intravenously for acute episodes of hypotension. Dosage by this route is 1–5 mg. The effect begins in 1–4 min and lasts for 20–30 min.

Methoxamine

A direct and indirect sympathomimetic agent which is an agonist at α-receptors and has a blocking effect at β-receptors. Its primary effect is peripheral vasoconstriction which will cause an increase in both systolic and diastolic arterial pressure. Heart rate will slow mostly due to the β-blocking effect of the drug, but this may be augmented by a reflex slowing due to the increase in blood pressure. There is no effect on cardiac contractility and therefore cardiac output will be decreased due to the increase in SVR.

Indications and dosage. Methoxamine may be indicated in hypotensive states caused by excessive or too-rapid vasodilation, e.g. spinal or epidural block or during hypotensive anaesthesia.

The drug is normally administered intravenously. By this route, 5–10 mg will act within 2 min and the effect will persist for around 20 mins.

Contra-indications and toxicity. Methoxamine is contra-indicated in patients on MAOI therapy, and can cause a life-threatening situation in individuals with a history of hypertension. Overdosage will cause excessive rises in blood pressure and may precipitate myocardial ischaemia. Other signs of toxicity include vomiting, headache, a desire to micturate and significant reduction in heart rate. The treatment of choice is intravenous administration of an α-blocker such as phentolamine.

Phenylephrine

An agent with similar effects to noradrenaline, but probably even shorter-acting. It is a potent α- and a weak β-receptor agonist. It causes peripheral vasoconstriction, and therefore a rise in arterial pressure – especially diastolic pressure. A reflex reduction in heart rate is also often observed. The only direct effect on the heart is to slightly increase myocardial irritability.

Indications and dosage. It may be given by infusion (10 mg/500 ml) but it has been largely replaced by the catecholamines listed earlier. Alternatively, it is given in bolus doses of 0.5 mg. For paroxysmal tachycardia 5 mg is usually given i.m. It can also be used as a mydriatic in a 5% solution.

CARDIAC GLYCOSIDES

The cardiac glycosides are a structurally similar group of compounds derived principally from vegetable sources.

Digitalis BP is the dried leaf of the purple foxglove, *Digitalis purpurea*, in which the principal glycoside is digitoxin. Other digitalis species also contain glycosides. *Digitalis lanata* is the source of digoxin, lanatoside C and also digitoxin. Ouabain is derived from *Strophanthus gratus*, a member of a different family of plants. At present, because the cardiac glycosides cannot be synthesized, the commercial source of the drugs is still the dried leaves of the plants mentioned above.

The general structure is shown below. The molecule consists of two parts, a cyclopentanophenanthrene nucleus with an attached five- or six-membered lactone ring (the aglycone) and a carbohydrate compound of up to four sugar molecules. The latter is responsible for solubilizing the drug, whilst the pharmacological action resides in the aglycone. Saturation of the lactone ring substantially reduces the potency of the glycoside while opening of the ring renders the glycoside inert.

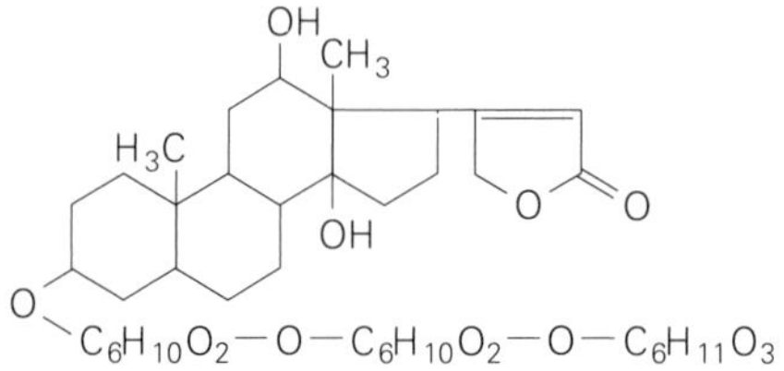

Digoxin

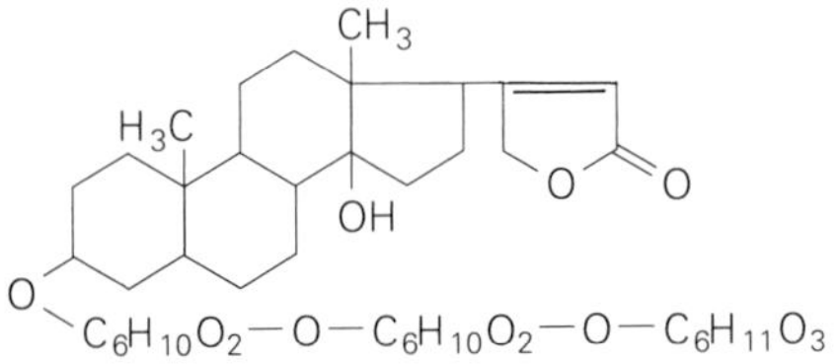

Digitoxin

Pharmacodynamics

The principal therapeutic action of digitalis is its ability to enhance the contractile function of the myocardium, and to slow conduction at the AV node. The increase in contractility is similar for both atrial and ventricular muscle and can be shown to affect isometric and isotonic contraction. The exact mechanism for this action is still a matter for debate, but the following is a summary of the current position.

Inhibition of $Na^+ K^+$ ATPase is the main mechanism involved in the action of digitalis. Specific binding of digitalis glycoside to this enzyme on the cardiac cell membrane has been demonstrated (Schwartz & Adams 1980).

This binding is reversible and is directly associated with enzyme inhibition, thus leading to an increase in the intracellular sodium concentration and a decrease in the concentration of intracellular potassium. The increase in intracellular sodium in turn reduces calcium exchange towards the exterior by reducing the transmembrane sodium gradient and depressing the $Na^+ Ca^{2+}$ ion counter transport system. The net effect of digitalis is thus an increase in intracellular sodium and calcium, the latter being thought to be responsible for the positive inotropic effect. However, current opinion is that other mechanisms, not directly involving sodium/calcium exchange, may be influencing calcium control following $Na^+ K^+$ ATPase binding (Lullman et al 1982), and that permanently elevated intracellular concentrations of sodium and calcium may in fact be associated with the toxic condition.

The picture is further complicated by studies demonstrating a positive inotropic action at concentrations of glycoside well below those associated with $Na^+ K^+$ ATPase inhibition (Noble 1980) and in fact $Na^+ K^+$ ATPase activity would appear to be enhanced at these very low glycoside levels (Hart et al 1985). It may be, however, that this increase in $Na^+ K^+$ ATPase activity, and the positive inotropic effect of very low level of glycoside are an indirect effect mediated by an increase in local catecholamine levels since it can be blocked by prior administration of β-adrenergic blocking drugs (Hougeon et al 1981). It should be noted that an increase in local release of acetylcholine also occurs at low glycoside levels, and this in itself may mask any inotropic effect. It would appear that the mechanism for the increased levels of catecholamines is decreased uptake following neuronal enzyme inhibition. Ouabain at a concentration of 10^{-8} molar has been shown to produce this effect in human myocardium (Petch & Nayler 1979). In summary it would appear that at low dose the therapeutic effects of digitalis on cardiac contractility involve a combination of direct and neurotransmitter-mediated changes in calcium ion availability at the membrane. At higher doses inhibition of $Na^+ K^+$ ATPase results in intracellular accumulation of sodium and calcium which may, if of sufficient magnitude, be linked with the development of toxic effects.

Action on cardiovascular haemodynamics. The first accounts of the use of digitalis in heart failure are of course those of William Withering (1785), though he failed to appreciate fully the cardiac actions of the drug, instead assuming that its success was due to diuretic properties. Up to the beginning of this century the use of digitalis was confined to the treatment of heart failure in association with atrial fibrillation, but in 1919 Sir Thomas Lewis wrote that digitalis could be beneficial in case of failure with sinus rhythm. Improving investigative techniques over the past 50 years have proved convincingly the increase in myocardial contractility associated with the use of digitalis, in isolated myocardium, animal models and the normal and failing heart (Hayward & Hamer 1979).

There is, of course, a difference between increased myocardial contractility and increased cardiac output or reduced left atrial diastolic pressure, and this has been reflected in the difficulty in proving clinically the effectiveness of digitalis as a positive inotrope. This can partly be explained by the fact that contractility is not the predominant factor affecting cardiac output, at least in the normal heart; instead output is linked to preload, afterload and heart rate.

In advanced myocardial disease contractility is of more importance. Clinical studies are also complicated by other therapies directed at the cardiovascular system, particularly the use of diuretics. This problem was elegantly described by Yankopoulos and colleagues (1968), who were able to demonstrate significant increases in contractility with ouabain in 20 heart failure patients in sinus rhythm, but could demonstrate clinically significant improvements in output and filling pressures in only 12. Changes in peripheral vascular resistance are perhaps most important in explaining the difficulties encountered in perceiving consistent haemodynamic benefit with digitalis. First the patients may not all be uniform in terms of vascular tone before treatment commences. Secondly digitalis may, by increasing contractility, reduce the sympathetic drive and thus produce vasodilation with resultant falls in venous pressure (Mason & Brunwald 1964). Lastly, digitalis has a direct vasoconstrictor action which can be clinically detrimental if the glycoside is given too rapidly so that resistance increases before contractility improves (DeMots et al 1978); this direct effect does not seem to be clinically important in long-term use (Arnold et al 1980).

Who then might benefit from digitalis? Most of the

evidence would suggest that digitalis is of most use in volume overloaded heart failure, and that those most likely to respond will have a third heart sound (Lee et al 1982). The presence of a third heart sound would also appear to be of value in determining which patients need to stay on long-term digitalization (Arnold et al 1980). Heart failure developing acutely as a result of myocardial infarction has been the subject of debate concerning the safety of digitalis. Principally this is because of fears that increased peripheral vascular resistance will lead to a deterioration in function and increased left ventricular work. Certainly studies where rapid injections of glycosides were used produced little benefit, and in some even precipitated angina (Balcon et al 1968). Current evidence supports the view that these deleterious effects could have been avoided by the use of slow infusions of digitalis (DeMots et al 1978). Other studies associate the use of digitalis with an increased mortality, but it is difficult to assess this work since often the use of digitalis reflects the severity of the underlying disease (Ryan et al 1983).

At present the use of digitalis post-infarction is acceptable provided the need for cautious introduction is remembered, and also the fact that in this group of hospital patients alternative therapies for acute heart failure (e.g. dobutamine) exist. Digitalis is contra-indicated in hypertrophic cardiomyopathy since it may increase outflow obstruction, and in cardiac amyloid where it has little effect and may predispose to arrhythmias. In right-sided failure, e.g. cor pulmonale, digitalis would appear to be of little use.

Effects of digitalis on heart rate and rhythm. The action of digitalis on the electrical activity of the heart is best understood by considering the effects on the Purkinje fibres. At low dose phase 2 of the action potential is prolonged and threshold potential declines, indicating increased excitability. Prolonged exposure accelerates repolarization, reducing action potential duration and refractoriness; finally the rate of spontaneous depolarization increases and this may increase the discharge rate of subsidiary pacemaker foci. The increase in rate of spontaneous depolarization is inversely proportional to the $[K^+]$, thus facilitating the emergence of ventricular arrhythmias in the presence of hypokalaemia.

Of greater importance are the indirect actions of digitalis predominantly involving the parasympathetic system. These take place at multiple levels in the vagal control system. Firstly sensitization of the afferent carotid, aortic and cardiopulmonary baroreceptors occurs (Imamura et al 1985); secondly central vagal nuclei are stimulated with an increase in efferent tone (Gillis et al

1972); thirdly cardiac sensitivity to vagal stimulation is increased (Greenspan & Lord 1973) and finally acetylcholine is released from stores within the myocardium (Hordof et al 1978). The effects occurring peripherally on the parasympathetic system are of greater importance than those occurring in the brain.

Digitalis also increases sympathetic drive. This is partly responsible for the increase in vascular tone mentioned above, though direct stimulation of α-receptors and vasoconstriction caused by inhibition of vascular smooth muscle Na^+ K^+ ATPase are also involved. CNS penetration is rapid after intravenous digitalis, and a specific area of the medulla has been identified as the centre for the increased sympathetic tone responsible for both the vasoconstriction and the development of toxic ventricular arrhythmias (Somberg & Smith 1979, Somberg et al 1981). Pretreatment with β-blockers can block the cardiac arrhythmias produced by direct injection of digitalis into the cerebral ventricles of an experimental animal, and can be clinically effective in digitalis overdose, though β-blockers may increase atrioventricular block.

The effects of digitalis on the atrioventricular node are a combination of the direct effects outlined above and direct and indirect vagal effects. Studies on transplanted hearts would suggest that these indirect effects are of major importance (Goodman et al 1978). Also of clinical importance is the fact that since some of the slowing which occurs is of vagal origin, atropine can be of benefit where bradycardia is troublesome. Digitalis is still the drug of choice for control of atrial tachyarrhythmias, though it may not provide good control during periods of exercise. It can be used in conjunction with verapamil or β-blockers to achieve greater control.

Patients with aberrant atrioventricular conduction, e.g. Wolff–Parkinson–White syndrome, may have an increased incidence of tachyarrhythmias with digitalis and care should be exercised. Finally digitalis is of proven value in the prevention of arrhythmias following intrathoracic surgery (Chee et al 1982).

Pharmacokinetics of cardiac glycosides

In long-term use the bioavailability of digitalis is of major importance, both in achieving adequate levels and in avoiding toxicity following repeated oral doses. Cardiac glycoside absorption from the gut involves first-order kinetics and is basically by passive diffusion. As a result the lipid solubility of individual glycosides determines the amount absorbed. Thus newer more lipophilic compounds such as methyl digoxin (medigoxin) achieve almost total absorption (Hayward et al 1978).

Table 21.3 Pharmacokinetics of cardiac glycosides

Drug	Route	Onset Time (min)	Peak effect (h)	$T_{\frac{1}{2}\beta}$ (h)	Percentage absorbed	Percentage bound	Elimination
Digoxin	p.o	30–120	2–6	30–40	65*	25	Renal
	i.v.	5–30	1–5				
Digitoxin	p.o.	60–240	8–12	168–190	95	95	Hepatic
	i.v	25–125	4–22				
Ouabain	i.v	5–10	0.5–2	21	–		Renal
Lanatoside C	i.v	10–30	2–3	36		25	Renal

*According to current formulation standards.

Similarly drugs which decrease or increase gut transit time will decrease or increase glycoside absorption. Absorption occurs largely in the jejunum, and surgery which leaves the jejunum intact will not affect glycoside absorption. Some agents reduce absorption by binding with digitalis in the gut lumen, for example kaolin, cholestyramine, charcoal.

Following absorption the glycosides are distributed to most tissues in the body, and have a large apparent volume of distribution due to protein binding. There is considerable variation in protein binding between the glycosides; digoxin is about 25% bound whilst digitoxin is over 90% bound, and this in part explains the difference in their respective half-lives. Concentrations of glycosides in cardiac tissue are 15–30 times those in plasma and are decreased by high intracellular levels of potassium. In view of the large volume of distribution and relatively long half-lives of these compounds steady state is not achieved quickly with repeated doses, and so where rapid digitalization is required a loading dose may be needed. By convention the loading dose is termed the 'digitalizing dose'. There may be a delay of more than an hour between peak plasma level and peak effect.

Most glycosides are eliminated as unchanged drug by the kidney both by simple filtration and tubular secretion; the exception is digitoxin, which is largely excreted by the liver following metabolism by microsomal enzymes. This metabolism may be increased by drugs such as barbiturates which induce enzyme activity.

The characteristics of the most commonly used glycosides are outlined in Table 21.3.

Clinical uses of cardiac glycosides

The principal uses of the cardiac glycosides have been discussed above in the section on pharmacodynamics, and are summarized here. The two main uses of this group of drugs are for cardiac failure, principally involving hypervolaemia, and for the control of atrial tachyarrhythmias.

In cardiac failure the benefits of digitalization are decreased where prior administration of diuretics has occurred and where there is no third heart sound. In long-term use those patients in sinus rhythm without a third heart sound can be reasonably expected to be withdrawn from therapy without compromising cardiac function.

In atrial fibrillation digitalis produces a decrease in atrioventricular conduction by a combination of direct myocardial, and direct and indirect vagal, actions. The result is a decrease in ventricular rate with improved cardiac output. In this group of patients long-term use is certainly indicated.

Toxicity

As a group the cardiac glycosides have a very low therapeutic ratio generally considered to be less than 2. The emergence of toxic effects and their duration is not improved by the long half lives of these compounds (Table 21.3). Further the incidence of toxicity is increased by potassium depletion, which is unfortunate since a large number of patients receiving digitalis will also be on potassium-depleting diuretics. Some studies have estimated that up to 25% of patients on digitalis show some signs of toxicity (Smith 1978). The therapeutic and toxic levels of digoxin and digitoxin in the adult are shown in Table 21.4. Children and infants would seem to be more tolerant of high levels of glycoside, and are thus less likely to develop toxicity.

Although the actions of digitalis are on both the contractile properties of the myocardium and cardiac rhythm, digitalis toxicity is not associated with any apparent adverse effects on contractility, but instead disorders of rhythm abound. It is important to realize

Table 21.4 Therapeutic and toxic serum levels of cardiac glycosides

Drug	Serum level(ng ml^{-1}) Therapeutic	Toxic
Digoxin	0.5–2.0	>2.5
Digitoxin	14–26	>35

that toxic effects do not necessarily mean that plasma levels are high. Firstly plasma levels are only a crude guide to cardiac tissue levels, secondly patients receiving digitalis have diseased myocardium which is prone to arrhythmia, and lastly electrolyte disturbances may also be involved. The principal arrhythmias are bradyarrhythmias involving the SA node, the atria and the AV node, and arrhythmias involving the ventricles. The bradyarrhythmias range from simple sinus bradycardia to complete heart block. Ventricular arrhythmias are principally involved with the development of ectopic foci producing bigeminy, trigeminy, ventricular ectopics, ventricular tachycardia and even fibrillation.

Other effects of toxicity include anorexia, nausea and vomiting, which may precede any cardiac effects and thus provide warning of the onset of toxicity. CNS signs include lethargy, disorientation, neuralgic pain (this can mimic the pain of trigeminal neuralgia), blurred vision and occasionally convulsions. Gynaecomastia has been reported and is thought to be due to the similarity between the structure of digitalis and the sex hormones.

Treatment of toxicity or overdose is by correction of electrolyte abnormalities (especially hypokalaemia), treatment of arrhythmias with an appropriate agent and reduction in plasma level by reducing absorption or enhancing excretion. Ventricular arrhythmias can be treated with phenytoin or lignocaine. The former is of double benefit since in addition to its anti-arrhythmic effect it opposes digitalis binding to myocardium. Bradyarrhythmias can be treated with atropine. Cholestyramine and activated charcoal are of benefit in reducing absorption from the gut. Dialysis is of no value in removing digitalis because of the large volume of distribution of the drug. Recently the use of fragmented digoxin antibodies has been described for the treatment of severe toxicity (Smith et al 1982). This topic is more fully covered in Chapter 35.

Cardiac glycosides in clinical use

The following is a short description of the currently available glycosides and the appropriate doses for each agent.

Digoxin

This is the glycoside most commonly used, and is available in both tablet and injectable forms. Intravenous injection is preferred over the intramuscular route and the use of infusions is recommended. In adults the usual dose is 125–250 μg per day for 1 week, reducing to a maintenance dose dictated by renal function, heart rate and plasma levels. Where rapid digitalization is required the digitalising dose is 750–1000 μg given over 2 h.

Lanatoside C

This drug is less well absorbed than digoxin and most is then converted to digoxin in the liver. The usual dose is 250–1000 μg per day.

Digitoxin

Digitoxin is almost completely absorbed when given orally. It differs from the other cardiac glycosides in that excretion is largely by the liver, and this route would appear to remain efficient even in hepatic failure, presumably because of enormous hepatic reserve. The usual dose is 50–200 μg daily.

Medigoxin (methyl digoxin)

Medigoxin is similar to digoxin except that absorption is almost 100%. As a result an oral dose of 300 μg is equivalent to 500 μg digoxin.

Ouabain

Ouabain is a glycoside derived from *Strophanthus*. In clinical effect it is identical to the digitalis glycosides. Its main advantage is that it has a more rapid onset of action than digoxin when given intravenously. The digitalizing dose is 120–250 μg assuming that no previous administration of glycosides has occurred. The total dose should not exceed 1 mg. Ouabain is not absorbed from the gut, and is now in limited supply in the UK.

Dosage in relation to disease and age

The above dose recommendations are for adults with normal renal and hepatic function; generally the dose should be reduced in renal impairment. In children the dose can be calculated on a weight basis, though it should be remembered that children tolerate higher levels of glycoside than adults.

REFERENCES

Allwood M J, Cobbold A F, Ginsburg J 1963 Peripheral vascular effects of noradrenaline, isopropyl-noradrenaline and dopamine. British Medical Bulletin 19: 132–136

Alousi A A, Farah A E, Lesher G Y, Opalka C J Jr 1979 Cardiotonic activity of amrinone — WIN 40680 (5-amino-3, 4'-bipyridin-6(lh)-one). Circulation Research 45: 666–667

Applefeld M M, Newman K A, Grove W R, Sutton F J, Hoffman D S, Reed W P, Linberg SE 1983 Intermittent continuous outpatient dobutamine infusion in the management of congestive heart failure. American Journal of Cardiology 51: 455–458

Arnold S B, Byrd R C, Maister W, Melmon K, Cherilin M D, Bristol J D Parmly W W, Chatterjee K 1980 Long term digitalis therapy improves left ventricular function in heart failure. New England Journal of Medicine 303: 1443–1448

Axelrod R J, de Marco T, Dae M, Botvinik E H, Chatterjee K 1987 Hemodynamic and clinical evaluation of piroximone, a new inotrope-vasodilator agent, in severe congestive heart failure. Journal of the American College of Cardiology 9: 1124–1130

Balcon R, Hoy J, Sowton E 1968 Haemodynamic effects of rapid digitalisation following acute myocardial infarction. British Heart Journal 30: 373–376

Biddle T L, Benotti J R, Creager M A et al 1987 Comparison of intravenous milrinone and dobutamine for congestive heart failure secondary to either ischaemic or dilated cardiomyopathy. American Journal of Cardiology 59: 1345–1350

Bodenham A R, Park G R 1988 Dopexamine hydrochloride, a novel drug with renal vasodilator properties: two case studies. Intensive Care Medicine 14: 663–665

Brown H F, Di Francisco D, Noble S J 1979 Adrenaline action on rabbit sino-atrial node. Journal of Physiology (London) 290: 31P–32P

Brown R A, Dixon J, Farmer J B et al 1985 Dopexamine: a novel agonist at peripheral dopamine and β-adrenoreceptors. British Journal of Pharmacology 85: 599–608

Chee T P, Prakash N A, Desser K B, Benchimol A 1982 Postoperative supraventricular arrhythmias and the role of prophylactic digoxin in cardiac surgery. American Heart Journal 104: 974–977

DeMots H, Rahimtoola S H, McAnulty J H, Porter G E 1978 Effects of ouabain on coronary and systemic vascular resistance and myocardial oxygen consumption in patients without heart failure. American Journal of Cardiology 41: 88–93

Dodge H T, Sandler H, Ballew D W, Lord J D Jr 1960 Use of biplane angiography for the measurement of left ventricular function in man. American Heart Journal 60: 762

Dubois-Rande J L, Loisance D, Duval A M et al 1988 Enoximone, a pharmacological bridge to transplantation. British Journal of Clinical Practice 42 (Suppl 64): 73–79

Francis G S, Sharma B, Hodges M 1982 Comparative hemodynamic effects of dopamine and dobutamine in patients with acute cardiogenic circulatory collapse. American Heart Journal 103: 995–1000

Gillis R A, Raines A, Sohn Y J, Levitt B, Sandaert G 1972 Neuroexcitatory effects of digitalis and their role in the development of cardiac arrhythmias. Journal of Physiology 183: 154–168

Goldberg L I 1972 Cardiovascular and renal actions of dopamine: potential clinical applications. Pharmacology Review 24: 1–29

Goldberg L I, Bloodwell R D, Braunwald E, Morrow A G 1960 The direct effect of norepinephrine, epinephrine and methoxamine on myocardial contractive force in man. Circulation 22: 1125–1132

Gonzales M, Desager J-P, Jacquemart J-L, Chenu P, Muller T, Installe E 1988 Efficacy of enoximone in the management of low output states following cardiac surgery. Journal of Cardiothoracic Anesthesia 2: 409–418

Goodman D J, Rosson R M, Cannon D S, Rider A K, Harrison D C 1978 Effect of digoxin on atrioventricular conduction. Studies in patients with and without cardiac autonomic innervation. Circulation 151: 251–256

Greenspan K, Lord T J 1973 Digitalis and vagal stimulation during atrial fibrillation, effects on atrio-ventricular conduction and ventricular arrhythmias. Cardiovascular Research 7: 241–246

Guyton A C, Cowley A W Jr, Young D B, Coleman T G, Hall J E, DeClue J W 1976 Integration and control of circulatory function. International Review of Physiology 9: 341–385

Hart G, Noble D, Shimoni Y 1985 The effects of low concentration of cardiotonic steroids on membrane currents and tension in sheep Purkinje fibres. Journal of Physiology 334: 103–131

Hayward R, Hamer J 1979 Digitalis. In: Hamer J (ed) Drugs for heart disease. Chapman & Hall, London, pp 244–317

Hayward R P, Greenwood H, Hamer J 1978 Comparison of digoxin and medigoxin in normal subjects. British Journal of Clinical Pharmacology 6: 81–86

Hoff J V, Beatty P A, Wade J L 1979 Dermal necrosis from dobutamine. New England Journal of Medicine 300: 1280

Hordof A J, Sponitz A, Mary-Radine C, Edie R N, Roson M R 1978 The cellular electrophysiological effects of digitalis on human atrial fibres. Circulation 57: 223–229

Hougeon T J, Spicer N, Smith T W 1981 Stimulation of monovalent cation active transport by low concentrations of cardiac glycosides. Role of catecholamines. Journal of Clinical Investigation 68: 1207–1214

Imamura T, Takeshita A, Ashihara T, Yammamoto K, Hoka S, Nakaura M 1985 Digitalis induced augmentation cardiopulmonary baroreflex control of forearm vascular resistance. Circulation 72: 11–16

Kates R E, Leier C V 1978 Dobutamine pharmacokinetics in severe heart failure. Clinical Pharmacology and Therapeutics 24: 537–541

Kereiakes D, Chatterjee K, Parmley W W et al 1984 Intravenous and oral MDL 17,043 (a new inotrope-vasodilator agent) in congestive heart failure: hemodynamic and clinical evaluation in 38 patients. Journal of the American College of Cardiology 4: 884–889

Klocke F J, Ellis A K 1980 Control of coronary blood flow. Annual Review of Medicine 31: 489–508

Lee D C S, Johnson R A, Bingham J B et al 1982 Heart failure in outpatients. A randomised trial of digoxin versus placebo. New England Journal of Medicine 306: 699–705

Leier C V 1986 Acute inotropic support. In: Cardiotonic drugs. Dekker, New York, Ch 3, p 67

Leier C V, Unverferth D V 1983 Dobutamine. Annals of Internal Medicine 99: 490–496

Leier C V, Heban P, Huss P, Bush C A, Lewis R P 1977 Comparative systemic and regional hemodynamic effects of dopamine and dobutamine in patients with cardiomyopathic heart failure. Circulation 58: 466–475

Lewis T 1919 On cardiac principle in cardiological practice. British Medical Journal 2: 621–625

Lullman H, Peters T, Predwer H 1982 Mechanism of action of digitalis glycosides in the light of new experimental observations. European Heart Journal 3: 45–51

Mancia G, Lorenz R R, Shephert J T 1976 Reflex control of circulation of heart and lungs. International Review of Physiology 9: 111–114

Mason D T, Brunwald E 1964 Studies of digitalis. Effect of ouabain on forearm vascular resistance and venous tone in normal subjects and patients with heart failure. Journal of Clinical Investigation 43: 532–543

Maylie J, Morao M 1984 Ionic currents responsible for the generation of pacemaker currents in the rabbit SA node. Journal of Physiology 355: 215–235

Murphy P J, Williams T L, Kau D L K 1976 Disposition of dobutamine in the dog. Journal of Pharmacology and Experimental Therapeutics 199: 423–431

Nash C W, Wolff S A, Ferguson B A 1968 Release of tritiated noradrenaline from perfused rat hearts by sympathomimetic amines. Canadian Journal of Physiology and Pharmacology 46: 35–42

Noble D 1975 The initiation of the heartbeat. Clarendon Press, Oxford

Noble D 1980 Mechanism of action of therapeutic levels of cardiac glycosides. Cardiovascular Research 14: 495–514

Petch M C, Nayler W G 1979 Concentration of catecholamines by human cardiac muscle in vitro. British Heart Journal 41: 336–339

Priebe H J, Foex P 1987 Isoflurane causes regional myocardial dysfunction in dogs with central coronary artery stenosis. Anesthesiology 66: 293–300

Rackley C E 1976 Quantitative evaluation of left ventricular function by radiographic techniques. Circulation 54: 862

Robie N W, Nutter D O, Moody C, McNay J L 1974 In vivo analysis of adrenergic receptor activity of dobutamine. Circulation Research 34: 663–671

Rose J C, Kot P A, Cohn J N, Freis E D, Eckert G E 1962 Comparison of effects of angiotensin and norepinephrine on pulmonary circulation, systemic arteries and veins, and systemic vascular capacity in the dog. Circulation 25: 247–252

Ruffolo R R Jr, Spradlin T A, Pollack G D, Waddell J E, Murphy P J 1981 Alpha and beta adrenergic effects of the stereoisomers of dobutamine. Journal of Pharmacology and Experimental Therapeutics 219: 447–452

Ryan T J, Bailey K R, McCabe C H et al 1983 The effects of digitalis on survival in high risk patients with coronary artery disease. Circulation 67: 735–742

Schwartz A, Adams R J 1980 Studies on the digitalis receptor. Circulation Research 46: 154–60

Sill J C, Bove A A, Nugent M, Blaise G A, Dewey J D, Graham C 1987 Effects of isofurane on coronary arteries and coronary arterioles in the intact dog. Anesthesiology 66: 273–279

Smith T W, 1978 Digitalis toxicity: epidemiological and clinical use of serum concentration measurements. American Journal of Medicine 58: 470–476

Smith T W, Butler V P, Haber E et al 1982 Treatment of life-threatening digitalis intoxication with digoxin specific FAB antibody fragment. New England Journal of Medicine 307: 1357–1362

Somberg J C, Smith T W 1979 Localisation of the neurally mediated arrhythmogenic properties of digitalis. Science 204: 321–323

Somberg J C, Kuhlman J E, Smith T W 1981 Localisation of the neurally mediated coronary vasoconstrictor properties of digoxin in the cat. Circulation Research 49: 226–233

Sonnenblick E H, Frishman W H, LeJemtel T H 1979 Dobutamine: a new synthetic cardiovactive sympathetic amine. New England Journal of Medicine 300: 17–22

Steen P A, Tinker J H, Pluth J R, Barnhorst D A, Tarhan S 1978 Efficiency of dopamine, dobutamine and epinephrine during emergence from cardiopulmonary bypass in man. Circulation 57: 378–384

Stoner J D 3rd, Bolen J L, Harrison D C 1977 Comparison of dobutamine and dopamine in the treatment of severe heart failure. British Heart Journal 39: 536–539

Svensson G, Sjogren A, Erhardt L 1986 Short-term haemodynamic effects of dopexamine in patients with chronic congestive heart failure. European Heart Journal 7: 697–703

Tuttle R R, Mills J 1975 Dobutamine: development of a new catecholamine to selectively increase cardiac contractility. Circulation Research 36: 185–196

Unverferth D V, Blanford M, Kates R E, Leier C V 1980 Tolerance to dobutamine after a 72 hour continuous infusion. American Journal of Medicine 69: 262–266

Vatner S F, McRitchie R J, Braunwald E 1974 Effects of dobutamine on left ventricular performance, coronary dynamics and distribution of cardiac output in conscious dogs. Journal of Clinical Investigation 53: 1265–1273

Wilmshurst P T, Thompson D S, Jenkins B S, Coltart D J, Webb-Peploe M M 1983 Haemodynamic effects of intravenous amrinone in patients with impaired left ventricular function. British Heart Journal 49: 77–82

Withering W 1785 An account of the foxglove, and some of its medical uses with practical remarks on dropsy and other diseases. In: Willius F A, Keys T E (eds) Cardiac classics. Kempton, London, 1941, pp 231–252

Yankopoulos N A, Kawai C, Frederici E E, Adler L M, Ableman W H 1968 The hemodynamic effects of ouabain on the diseased left ventricle. American Heart Journal 76: 466–480

22. Anti-arrhythmic drugs

J. P. Alexander

SITES OF ORIGIN OF ARRHYTHMIAS

Arrhythmias may arise from various sites in the heart and are classified here anatomically.

Sinus node

Sinus arrhythmia. Due to changes in the filling of the heart brought about by respiration, secondary changes occur in the cardiac output. This is sensed by the baroreceptors so that the heart rate slows on expiration.

Sinus bradycardia. This is classified as a rate of under 60 beats per minute and is common in athletes. Sinus bradycardia is also a feature of pathological conditions such as myxoedema, jaundice and raised intracranial pressure, and it occurs secondary to adrenergic blocking drugs and digitalis.

Sinus tachycardia. This is defined as a rate greater than 100 beats per minute and it occurs in exercise, anxiety and also in fever, hyperthyroidism, acute circulatory failure and cardiac failure.

Ectopic rhythms

In this instance the impulse for myocardial contraction arises somewhere other than the sinus node. The rhythm may be either regular or irregular.

Atrial

Atrial ectopics. The rhythm is basically regular with premature beats occurring.

Atrial tachycardias. These can be classified as either paroxysmal tachycardia, atrial tachycardia with AV block or atrial fibrillation.

Paroxysmal tachycardia. The rate is regular and occurs because of re-entry or due to rapidly firing ectopics. The rate can be 140–220 per minute and is best treated by an intravenous β-blocking drug, verapamil, digitalis or DC shock.

In *atrial flutter*, the atria beat at rates of 300 per minute but because of a variable AV block the ventricular rate may be 100–150 per minute.

In *atrial fibrillation* the atrial beat is chaotic and only occasional beats are conducted to the ventricle. This rhythm is classically irregularly irregular.

Ventricular

Ectopic beats occur because of ventricular escape, enhanced rate of ectopic foci and re-entry. The danger of this rhythm occurs when the ectopic beat arises close to the previous T-wave, when ventricular fibrillation may be precipitated.

Ventricular tachycardia at rates of 140–220 per minute is highly inefficient, and often leads to ventricular fibrillation.

In *ventricular fibrillation* there is chaotic movement of the ventricles with no cardiac output. If not quickly changed to normal rhythm, death supervenes due to cerebral hypoxia. Ventricular asystole may occur in patients with heart block or ischaemic damage to the conducting system. Myocardial pacing is lifesaving in these patients.

Heart block

1. Sinus node block is shown by the complete missing of one cardiac cycle.
2. Atrioventricular block. First degree heart block is defined as a situation in which the PR interval is over 0.2 s. In second degree block some impulses fail to traverse the AV node and in third degree block (complete heart block) the atrial and ventricular beats are completely dissociated.
3. Bundle branch block is evidenced by different rates of conduction in the right or left bundle of His, giving characteristic QRS patterns of the electrocardiograph.

In the treatment of these various arrhythmias it is essential to understand precisely the arrhythmia in order that the source can be attacked and either the arrhythmia suppressed or conduction to the ventricle slowed, so that efficient cardiac output may be maintained.

ELECTROPHYSIOLOGY

The heart contains two types of cells: those which fire spontaneously (automatic or type 1) and those which depolarize after they have been stimulated (type 2). Figure 22.1 shows the action potential of the left ventricular myofibre (solid line) and the dotted line is the action potential of a cell in the sino-atrial (SA) node. The cell of the sino-atrial node spontaneously depolarizes until threshold potential (TP) is reached, when the cell fires (phase 0). On the other hand, the ventricular muscle cell in phase 4 (diastole) will remain at the trans-membrane resting potential (MRP) of -90 mV until it is stimulated. Spontaneous phase 4 depolarization is called automaticity and is displayed by cells of the SA node and specialized conducting tissues. Cardiac cells also exhibit excitability and refractoriness. Excitability increases where threshold potential and transmembrane resting potential come closer together. Absolute refractoriness exists when the action potential lies above the threshold potential and as it descends in phase 3 through the threshold potential towards the transmembrane resting potential the cell is said to be relatively refractory.

Hypokalaemia, increase in catecholamines or the presence of ischaemia will increase automaticity. Increased vagal tone decreases the automaticity of the sino-atrial and atrioventricular nodes while having no effect on the His–Purkinje system. Potassium has a major influence on conduction velocity since an increase in extracellular potassium will decrease the transmembrane resting potential, the impulse generated will be of a lower magnitude, and excitability is increased.

With moderate increases in serum potassium, conduction may be increased through the atrioventricular node. With high levels, conduction is slowed and eventually block will occur.

Normally, an impulse arising in the sino-atrial node travels to the atrioventricular node where the rate of propagation is slowed. By this time the atria have contracted. In the upper and middle nodal regions, slow inward Ca^{2+}-mediated current contributes to depolarization and this is the main site of action of the calcium antagonist verapamil. The impulse then tranverses the His–Purkinje system to the ventricular muscle. The Bundle of His divides into the right and left bundles and the left bundle further divides into the left anterior fascicle and the left posterior (inferior) fascicle.

CLINICAL ASPECTS AND MECHANISM OF ARRHYTHMIAS

An arrhythmia may be due to disorder of impulse formation or of conduction. The majority of arrhythmias are innocuous, but those which result in a decrease in cardiac output or progress to cardiac standstill must obviously be considered to be serious. A simple classification is to divide them into two types — tachyarrhythmias and bradyarrhythmias.

Tachyarrhythmias

Aetiology

Tachyarrhythmias arise when the heart becomes electrically unstable due to increased automaticity and the development of re-entry. Increased automaticity refers to accelerated phase 4 spontaneous depolarization and is caused by hypokalaemia, ischaemia or hypoxia, and increased levels of catecholamines. Since the arrhythmia will depend on the area of the heart which is affected, this can explain a sinus tachycardia, atrial or ventricular premature beats and atrial and ventricular tachycardias.

Re-entry depends upon unidirectional block with slow conduction through a depressed area of the myocardium. An impulse travelling through the conducting system finds part of its pathway blocked while the other conducts normally. The impulse which conducts normally is capable of slowly depolarizing the blocked pathway in a retrograde direction. The impulse arrives back at the area which conducted normally to find it repolarized and capable of conducting another impulse

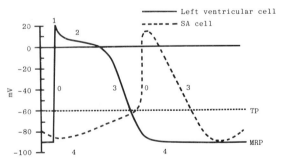

Fig. 22.1   The action potential of a left ventricular myofibre (solid line). The interrupted line depicts the action potential of a cell in the sino-atrial node. Spontaneous depolarization of the sino-atrial node cell during phase 4 is characteristic of automatic cells within the heart. TP = Threshold potential;   MRP = transmembrane resting potential.

(circus movement). Patients with ischaemic heart disease are prone to tachyarrhythmias. Electrical instability is indicated by single premature ventricular contractions (PVC), multiple PVC, multifocal PVC and ventricular tachycardia followed by ventricular fibrillation. Patients with valvular disease are likely to develop sinus tachycardia, atrial fibrillation and atrial flutter.

The Wolff–Parkinson–White syndrome

The usual version of the Wolff–Parkinson–White syndrome involves a circus movement of impulses through the atrioventricular node with retrograde conduction back along the accessory bundle of Kent, thereby again reaching the atrioventricular node. The circus movement may be initiated by either atrial or ventricular extrasystoles, and therapy is directed to prevention of supraventricular tachycardia, verapamil being the drug of choice. In a less common version of the syndrome, anterograde conduction occurs down the accessory bundle from rapid atrial fibrillation or flutter and there is a danger of ventricular fibrillation.

Drugs acting on the atrioventricular node, such as verapamil, are of no value under these circumstances but amiodarone or disopyramide may be of value. Digoxin may accelerate this anterograde conduction and is better avoided in all patients with the Wolff–Parkinson–White syndrome (Opie 1980).

Effect of anaesthetic agents

Trichlorethylene, cyclopropane and halothane strongly sensitize the myocardium to the action of adrenaline, which accelerates phase 4 depolarization and thus increases automaticity. Halothane prolongs atrioventricular nodal conduction time and can probably set up re-entry mechanisms in the atrioventricular node. The lesser effect of enflurane on atrioventricular conduction makes such disturbances less likely. Isoflurane has no demonstrable effect on atrioventricular conduction.

Hypercarbia provokes ventricular arrhythmias during cyclopropane and halothane anaesthesia, presumably due to increased endogenous secretion of adrenaline. Exogenous adrenaline will have the same effect. Specific α-adrenergic receptors are thought to exist in the heart, which respond to adrenaline in the presence of halothane (Dresel 1985). Halothane may decrease the severity of arrhythmias due to digitalis intoxication.

The muscle relaxants pancuronium, gallamine, alcuronium and fazadinium all increase heart rate. Suxamethonium frequently causes bradycardia in children or after repeated doses, but where a sudden increase in serum potassium is caused (in severe burns or patients with paralysed muscles) a variety of tachyarrhythmias occur. Sympathetic stimulation during laryngoscopy and endotracheal intubation and surgical stimulation during light anaesthesia are other frequent causes of tachyarrhythmias (Carson et al 1979).

Treatment

Generally, supraventricular tachyarrhythmias are benign while ventricular tachyarrhythmias are more likely to be malignant. This must be qualified by stating that patients with severe coronary artery disease, the elderly and the ill may tolerate any tachycardia badly.

Sinus tachycardia often responds to increasing the depth of anaesthesia. Paroxysmal supraventricular tachycardia may involve a re-entry process within the atrioventricular node or an anomalous atrioventricular connection in parallel with the node.

Termination of an attack of tachycardia may be effected by any manoeuvre which will alter autonomic tone and block atrioventricular conduction. Thus carotid sinus pressure, Valsalva's manoeuvre, digoxin or intravenous edrophonium (up to 10 mg) may all be effective but a β-adrenergic blocking drug is preferable as specific therapy for slowing atrioventricular node conduction. Verapamil may also be useful, but should not be used after β-blockade since a synergistic effect on myocardial function may precipitate heart failure. Atrial fibrillation or flutter is usually treated with intravenous digoxin with rapid short-term control by β-blockade. Premature ventricular contractions which occur singly, and which are unifocal, do not require treatment. Premature ventricular contractions which occur in salvos, more than five per minute, are multifocal, or exhibit an R on T phenomenon usually require urgent treatment as they herald ventricular tachycardia or ventricular fibrillation. Occasionally simple measures to increase the depth of anaesthesia while increasing ventilation are sufficient. Malignant ventricular ectopic beats and ventricular tachycardias are an indication for anti-arrhythmic drug therapy. Lignocaine is usually effective in 100 mg bolus (or 1 mg/kg — Table 22.4). Some arrhythmias considered to be ventricular in origin may be supraventricular and these respond best to a β-blocker, as will sinus tachycardias which cause S–T depression in patients with severe myocardial ischaemia. Ventricular fibrillation and, in many instances, ventricular tachycardia are an indication for immediate electrical direct current countershock and the anti-arrhythmic drugs are used to prevent the patient converting back to the arrhythmia.

Direct current countershock may also be indicated to terminate some episodes of supraventricular tachycardia, and to convert atrial flutter or fibrillation to normal rhythm.

In deciding which anti-arrhythmic drug to use, one appropriate to the arrhythmia and its site of origin must be selected (Tables 22.2–22.4). Thus digitalis, propranolol, intravenous potassium and bretylium suppress enhanced automaticity of the sinus node. Digitalis increases — while quinidine, procainamide and lignocaine reduce — the automaticity of the Purkinje system.

Patients are more sensitive to the hypotensive effects of calcium channel antagonists when inhalational agents are being used (Prys-Roberts 1984). Ca^{2+} infusions will reverse the haemodynamic depressive effects of calcium antagonists on the myocardium and vasculature, although a β-agonist may be required to oppose unwanted conduction effects. When deciding between a β-blocking drug or a calcium antagonist it should be appreciated that verapamil is highly efficacious (close to 90%) in the treatment of paroxysmal atrial tachycardia. Both β-blockers and verapamil will slow the ventricular response to atrial flutter and fibrillation. The β-blocking drugs are effective in treating some types of ventricular arrhythmia while the role of verapamil is somewhat unclear. The latter would be preferable in a patient with asthma or bronchospasm, although, as already mentioned, the use of β-blockers with i.v. verapamil should be avoided.

Bradyarrhythmias

Aetiology

The bradyarrhythmias are due to decreased automaticity of the sino-atrial node or to a block in the atrioventricular conduction system. A latent pacemaker may or may not assume dominance. High vagal tone slows impulse formation in the sino-atrial node and slows conduction through the atrioventricular node. The vagus nerve does not affect conduction through the His–Purkinje system. Block occurring in the His–Purkinje system (infranodal block) is usually permanent and progressive. Patients with right bundle branch block (RBBB) and left posterior hemiblock (LPH) run a high risk of developing trifascicular or complete heart block.

Sick sinus syndrome

This refers to rhythm disturbances resulting from failure of normal impulse formation in the sino-atrial node. These rhythm disturbances may include:

1. persistent sinus bradycardia,
2. intervals of sinus arrest,
3. paroxysmal or chronic atrial fibrillation,
4. tachycardia alternating with bradycardia.

The commonest cause for the sick sinus syndrome is ischaemic heart disease, and its incidence is probably underestimated at present.

Heart block

Heart block may have organic or functional causes. Reasons for organic lesions are fibrotic degenerative disease of the conduction system (Lenegre's or Lev's disease), ischaemic heart disease, cardiomyopathies, myocarditis, surgical operations or congenital abnormalities. These lesions tend to be permanent. Functional causes are increased vagal tone, and drug therapy with digitalis, quinidine, procainamide, propranolol or potassium, all of which are usually reversible. The different degrees of heart block are tabulated in Table 22.1

Table 22.1   Heart block

Type of heart block	Description
First degree	PR interval > 0.21s
Second degree Mobitz type I	Progressive lengthening of PR prior to dropping of the QRS complex (Wenckebach phenomenon)
Mobitz type II	No progressive lengthening of PR, but sudden drop of QRS — serious prognosis, often progression to third degree block
Third degree	Atrial and ventricular rate independent, may be infranodal (slow rate, QRS wide, cardiac output decreased) or AV nodal (QRS normal width, faster rate, adequate cardiac output

Effect of anaesthetic agents

Halothane and methoxyflurane depress impulse formation in the sino-atrial node and prolong the functional refractory period of the atrioventricular node. These effects may be due either to a direct action on myocardial cells or to enhanced vagal tone, the latter being antagonized by atropine. Drugs which increase vagal tone may slow the heart, as may mechanical stimulation of the airway, so that bradycardia, wandering pacemakers or junctional (nodal) rhythm are common during induction as well as during anaesthesia.

Where the atrial and ventricular contractions are occurring simultaneously, ventricular filling will be decreased so that cardiac output and arterial blood pressure may fall. Traction on ocular muscles (the oculocardiac reflex) commonly, and traction on intraperitoneal organs less commonly, may induce bradyarrhythmia and occasionally sinus arrest. The use of carbon dioxide to distend the peritoneal cavity prior to laparoscopic sterilization is a particular hazard. The muscle relaxants atracurium and vecuronium may produce unexpected, severe bradycardia in the presence of the sick sinus syndrome or vagal stimulation.

Treatment

Supraventricular bradyarrhythmias are usually benign while ventricular bradyarrhythmias may be serious. Very slow ventricular rates may compromise cardiac output. Patients with sick sinus syndrome or bifascicular block in whom there is a history of Stokes–Adams attacks or heart failure may require insertion of a temporary or permanent pacemaker prior to anaesthesia or surgery. Measurement of the AH interval (normally 30–60 ms) as determined by His bundle electrocardiography may be helpful in deciding whether a patient requires pacing or not. Some supraventricular bradycardias respond to intravenous atropine, and if not, the subsidiary pacemaker may accelerate under the influence of isoprenaline. Atropine should be used with caution in patients with bradycardia and ectopic beats due to vagal stimulation, since converting the rhythm to a tachycardia with ectopic beats may create a more hazardous arrhythmia.

Summary

The majority of arrhythmias occurring under anaesthesia are benign and disappear when pulmonary ventilation is improved or the depth of anaesthesia is appropriately adjusted. Most arrhythmias are caused by sympathetic or parasympathetic overactivity, and require only careful observation, although occasionally more serious rhythms will demand active intervention. Most serious disturbances are likely to arise in patients with pre-existing heart disease and require appropriate and aggressive therapy.

Outside the operating theatre, the first-line drugs in the treatment of ventricular arrhythmias are lignocaine and mexiletine, and therapy with the latter can be converted to oral use if required. Second-line drugs are disopyramide, procainamide and quinidine, while phenytoin can be considered to be a third-line agent except in the treatment of digitalis-induced arrhythmia. Lorcainide, encainide, flecainide and tocainide are finding their place as second- or third-line agents. Bretylium should probably be considered a 'last-resort' drug. Amiodarone is finding an increasingly important place in intensive care (Table 22.4, Lucas et al 1990).

ANTI-ARRHYTHMIC AGENTS

Classification of anti-arrhythmic agents

Compounds with anti-arrhythmic activity show considerable differences in their chemical structure; the most satisfactory classification would appear to be based on that of Vaughan Williams (1970), which is derived from electrophysiological action on isolated cardiac fibres. Four types of basic activity are recognized (Table 22.2). Although some drugs have more than one action, a dominant effect can usually be recognised.

Class I

Class I contains agents with local anaesthetic properties that have membrane stabilizing activity; depolarization of the cardiac cell membrane is slowed by restricting entry of the fast sodium current so that the maximum rise of phase 0 of the action potential is reduced, as is the rate of phase 4 diastolic depolarization. Spontaneous automaticity is reduced. A further subdivision of class I depends on the influence of the drug on the duration of the action potential, which may lengthen (group IA), shorten (group IB) or not be affected (group IC). Additional effects which help to subdivide class I are listed in Table 22.2.

Class II

Class II agents reduce the response to catecholamines. The β-adrenoceptor antagonists act as competitive antagonists and may block the potential arrhythmogenic effect of cyclic adenosine-5′-monophosphate (cyclic AMP).

Class III

Class III agents prolong the duration of the action potential so that the effective refractory period is prolonged.

Table 22.2 Classification of anti-arrhythmic agents by effects on action potential

Class	Action	Additional classification	Prototype agent	Other agents
I	Membrane stabilizing agents (fast sodium channel blockers)	IA Slows dV/dt of phase O Prolongs repolarization Prolongs PR, QRS, QT	Quinidine	Procainamide Disopyramide Cibenzoline
		IB Limited effect on dV/dt of phase O Shortens repolarization Shortens QT Elevates fibrillation threshold	Lignocaine (lidocaine)	Tocainide Mexiletine Ethmozine Phenytoin
		IC Markedly slows dV/dt Little effect on repolarization Markedly prolongs PR, QRS	Flecainide	Encainide Lorcainide Propafenone Indecainide
II	β-Adrenoceptor blockade		Propranolol	All β-Blockers
III	Prolong repolarization, alters membrane response		Amiodarone (mixed I and II)	Bretylium Sotalol (mixed II and III) N-Acetylprocain-amide
IV	Calcium channel antagonists		Verapamil	Diltiazem

Modified from Opie et al 1987, and Harrison 1986, after Vaughan Williams 1970.

Table 22.3 Classification of anti-arrhythmic drugs by site of action

Sinoatrial node
  β-Blockers
  Class IV drugs
  Cardiac glycosides
	Atrioventricular node
	  Class IC drugs
	  β-Blockers
	  Class IV drugs
	  Cardiac glycosides

Ventricles
  Class I drugs
  Class III drugs	

	Atria
	  Class IA drugs
	  Class IC drugs
	  β-Blockers
	  Class III drugs

Accessory pathways
  Class IA drugs
  Class III drugs	

After Aronson 1985.

Class IV

Class IV agents inhibit the slow inward calcium-mediated current and depress phase 2 and phase 3 of the action potential. These actions are of particular importance in the atrioventricular node where re-entry circuits can occur.

A possible *class V* has been proposed, pertaining to agents which inhibit Cl^- ion flux; no such drugs are available for clinical use. A more clinically useful classification categorizes drugs according to the cardiac tissues which each affects, as shown in Table 22.3, and may be of use when a choice of a drug has to be made to treat an arrhythmia arising from a particular part of the heart. Detailed pharmacokinetic data for each drug, where available, are shown in Table 22.5.

CLASS IA AGENTS

Quinidine

Quinidine sulphate (BP), Quinidine sulfate and gluconate (USP).

Chemical name: (8R,9S) 6-methoxycinchonan-9-ol dihydrate.

Quinidine is the prototype of class IA agents and is an isomer of the alkaloid quinine. It slows phase 0 of the action potential but leaves the resting potential unaltered. Conduction through atrial, ventricular and Purkinje fibres is slowed while its antivagal action may accelerate atrioventricular nodal conduction. Quinidine is now of limited clinical use. The lack of a suitable parenteral formulation in the UK restricts its use to prophylaxis after cardioversion or after acute administration of lignocaine. Quinidine is active against both atrial and ventricular arrhythmias (Hillis & Whiting 1983).

Pharmacokinetics

In liver disease the clearance is reduced, half-life increased and protein binding is reduced so that lower total plasma concentrations may be effective. The half-life is not affected in congestive heart failure, although the volume of distribution is reduced so that interaction with digoxin may precipitate digoxin toxicity.

Dosage and administration

The oral dose is 200–400 mg three or four times daily, or 500 mg 12-hourly by slow-release preparation.

Adverse effects

High plasma concentrations (which should be monitored) cause myocardial depression, vasodilation and hypotension. Conduction defects, prolongation of QRS and QT interval and re-entry arrhythmias may be seen. There is a risk of paroxysmal ventricular fibrillation or of *torsade de pointes* (polymorphic or atypical ventricular tachycardia). Nausea, vomiting, diarrhoea, cinchonism and hypersensitivity reactions with fever, purpura, thrombocytopenia and hepatic dysfunction may also occur (Schwartz et al 1981).

Procainamide

Procainamide hydrochloride (BP and USP).
Chemical name: *p*-amino-*N*-(2-diethylaminoethyl) benzamide hydrochloride.
Procainamide exerts similar electrophysiological effects as described for quinidine. Procainamide is closely related to procaine, the CO.O ester grouping being replaced by CO.NH. It may be effective in the treatment of atrial, junctional and ventricular arrhythmias.

Pharmacokinetics

Procainamide is metabolized to an active metabolite, *N*-acetylprocainamide. The rate of metabolism in the population has a bimodal distribution so that patients are classified as being fast or slow acetylators. The latter require smaller doses in long-term therapy. High plasma levels of the drug and its metabolite can occur in renal or cardiac failure. The response to procainamide can be used to predict the response to other conventional anti-arrhythmic agents during electrophysiological study (Waxman et al 1983).

Dosage and administration

The standard intravenous dose is 100 mg every 2 min repeating this to a total of 1000 mg over the first hour. The oral dose is 250 mg every 4–6 h or 1.0–1.5 g of a slow-release preparation 8-hourly.

Adverse effects

Rapid intravenous administration may lead to reduced cardiac output, hypotension and vasodilation. Heart block and QRS and QT prolongation may occur. Long-term use may be associated with a drug-induced lupus erythematosus syndrome, which is more likely to be seen in slow acetylators, and is usually reversible.

N-Acetylprocainamide

N-acetylprocainamide hydrochloride (BAN, USAN). *N*-acetylprocainamide is the acetylated form of procainamide and is an active metabolite of the latter. It was introduced into clinical practice (USA) in the hope of reducing the toxic effects associated with the parent drug.

The elimination half-life is prolonged in end-stage renal failure. The drug has inferior anti-arrhythmic activity when compared with the parent compound, but a longer duration of action. Therapeutic and toxic plasma concentrations overlap. *N*-acetylprocainamide may be responsible for provoking formation of antinuclear factor.

Dosage and administration

The oral dose is 500 mg 6-hourly to a maximum of 6 g daily.

Disopyramide

Disopyramide phosphate (BP, USP), Disopyramide (BP).

Chemical name: α[2- [bis (1-methylethyl) amino] -ethyl]-α-phenyl-2-pyridime acetamide.

The electrophysiological properties of disopyramide are similar to those of quinidine, with some class 3 activity. The range of activity includes action against both atrial and ventricular arrhythmias, supraventricular tachycardia and ventricular ectopics (Koch-Weser 1979).

Pharmcokinetics

Disopyramide is available as either the base compound or as the phosphate salt. The main metabolite is the *N*-dealkylated form which, like the parent compound, is excreted by the kidneys, and has some anti-arrhythmic action. Dosage is reduced in severe renal failure. Protein binding sites can be saturated by both the drug and its metabolite. This means that drug clearance will vary depending on whether it is given by mouth or by intravenous injection.

Dosage and administration

Intravenous dose is 2 mg kg^{-1} up to 150 mg administered over 5 min. A maintenance infusion of 20–30 mg h^{-1} can be given to a total dose of 800 mg in 24 h. The oral dose is 300–800 mg daily in divided doses; slow-release preparations are available.

Adverse effects

Heart failure is a contra-indication to the use of the drug. Sinus node depression and QT prolongation predisposing to ventricular re-entry arrhythmia may occur. Disopyramide may precipitate ventricular fibrillation and *torsade de pointes*. Urinary retention, dry mouth, blurred vision and precipitation of glaucoma are all related to the anticholinergic activity of the drug and one of its metabolites. In the denervated transplanted heart the drug has a markedly depressant action on myocardial contraction (Podrid et al 1980).

CLASS IB AGENTS

Lignocaine

Lignocaine hydrochloride (BP), lidocaine hydrochloride (USP).

Chemical name: *N*-diethylamino acetyl-2,6-xylidide hydrochloride.

Lignocaine has typical class 1B electrophysiological effects. It is an aminoacyl amide and a derivative of acetanilide. It is the first-line drug used for treating ventricular arrhythmias after myocardial infarction and cardiac surgery, although it is not clear if it protects against ventricular fibrillation.

Pharmacokinetics

Lignocaine is hydrolysed in the gastrointestinal tract and is subject to extensive first-pass metabolism in the liver. Absorption after intramuscular injection is erratic. Clearance is related to hepatic blood flow and hepatic function and particularly to liver microsomal activity (barbiturates enhance); clearance is prolonged in liver disease, cardiac failure, and the elderly, so that infusion rates require appropriate adjustment. Injection rate may be important in precipitating toxic reactions, which are also related to the free drug concentration, which is particularly determined by the concentration of acute phase proteins, notably α-1 acid glycoprotein.

The latter increases after myocardial infarction, so that although long-term infusion may lead to increasing total lignocaine concentrations, the free drug level may remain relatively constant. The apparent volume of distribution decreases in heart failure. Active metabolites are monoethylglycylxylidine and glycylxylidide which possess lesser anti-arrhythmic effects than lignocaine but may have more prominent central-nervous excitatory effects, while 4-hydroxyxylidine is inactive.

Dosage and administration

Lignocaine is given as an intravenous bolus of 1–2 mg kg^{-1} (100–150 mg) and then an infusion at 4 mg min^{-1} for 30 min, 2 mg min^{-1} for 2 h, and 1 mg min^{-1} thereafter will usually maintain steady therapeutic levels. Theoretically an exponential infusion rate is required to prevent plasma levels falling out of the therapeutic range.

Adverse effects

High concentration may cause bradycardia, hypotension and asystole. Apart from nausea and vomiting, central nervous system effects including paraesthesiae, twitching, and grand-mal seizures can occur. Hepatic clearance is reduced in patients receiving cimetidine, propranolol or halothane. Hypokalaemia must be corrected for maximum efficacy (as for other class 1 agents).

Mexiletine

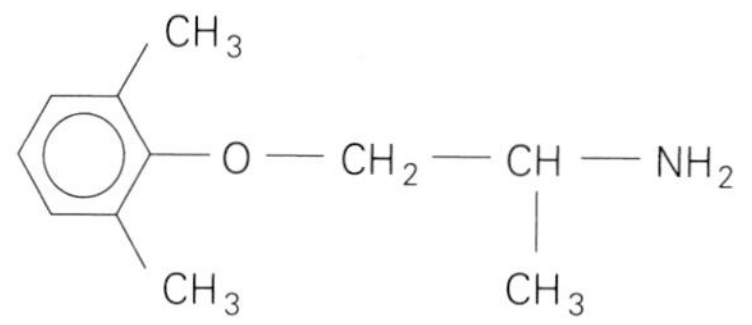

Mexiletine hydrochloride (BAN, USAN).
Chemical name: 1-methyl-2-(2,6,-xylyloxy)-
ethylamine hydrochloride.

Mexiletine is a primary amine and has similar structure and electrophysiological effects as lignocaine. It has been described as an 'oral lignocaine'. Combination with a β-adrenergic blocking agent may enhance the therapeutic efficacy (Leahey et al 1980).

Pharmacokinetics

The half-life is prolonged in heart failure and myocardial infarction. Renal clearance is reduced when the urine is alkaline. After bolus intravenous injection, plasma concentrations decrease rapidly in a manner compatible with a three-compartmental model.

Dosage and administration

The intravenous dose is 100–250 mg given slowly over 5–10 min followed by an infusion of 250 mg in the first hour, 250 mg over the next 2 h and then 0.5–1 mg min^{-1} until oral therapy is established. The oral loading dose is 400 mg followed by maintenance doses of 200 mg 6–8-hourly. A slow-release formulation is available.

Adverse effects

Hypotension, bradycardia and atrioventricular block can occur, and neurological side-effects include tremor, nystagmus, diplopia, dizziness, dysarthria, paraesthesiae, ataxia and confusion. Nausea and vomiting also occur.

Tocainide

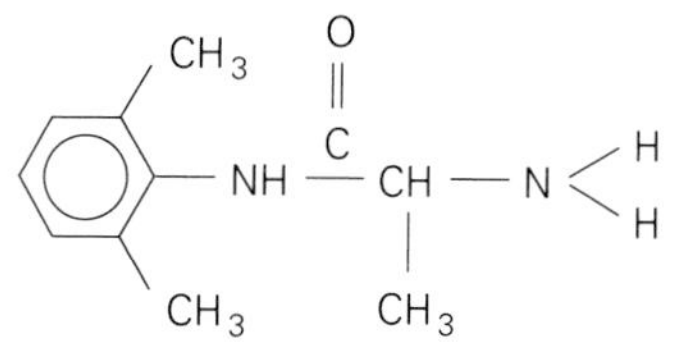

Tocainide hydrochloride (BAN, USAN).
Chemical name: 2-aminopropiono-2′, 6′-xylidide
hydrochloride

Tocainide is a primary amine with similar electrophysiological properties to those of lignocaine, and is another oral lignocaine analogue. Tocainide is used to treat acute and chronic ventricular arrhythmias.

Pharmacokinetics

Bioavailability approaches 100%. Hepatic clearance is low; about 25% is excreted as *N*-carboxytocainide. Elimination half-life is approximately doubled in severe renal failure.

Dosage and administration

Tocainide can be administered intravenously or orally. The intravenous dose is 0.5–0.75 mg kg^{-1} min^{-1} for 15 min (500–750 mg) followed immediately by 600–800 mg by mouth and then 400 mg every 8 h or 600 mg twice daily.

Adverse effects

These include anorexia, nausea, vomiting, constipation, abdominal pain, effects on the central nervous system like those with mexiletine, rashes and rarely interstitial pulmonary alveolitis. A high incidence of blood dyscrasias makes this drug unsuitable for prolonged therapy of benign arrhythmias

Phenytoin

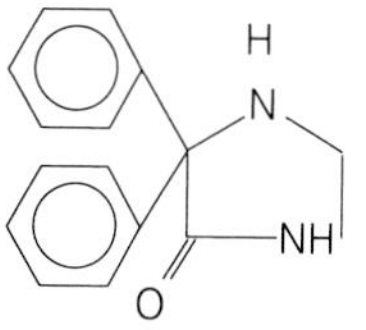

Phenytoin sodium (BP, USP).
Chemical name: sodium 5,5-diphenylhydantoin.

Phenytoin has the effect of accelerating conduction by increasing the initial rapid phase of the action potential in Purkinje fibres, especially when there is digitalis depression or hypokalaemia. Hence it is used almost exclusively in the therapy of digitalis-induced ventricular arrhythmia in the presence of hypokalaemia — it may also inhibit central sympathetic activity. The drug obeys nonlinear kinetics so that a loading dose is required to achieve therapeutic plasma levels.

Dosage and administration

The intravenous dose is 100 mg or less every 5 min until 1 g has been given or the arrhythmia is abolished or toxicity occurs. Precipitation may occur if the solution is diluted with infusion fluid. The oral loading dose is 800–1000 mg followed by maintenance doses of 200–400 mg daily.

Ethmozin

Ethmozin ethmosine moricizine (USAN).
Chemical name: ethyl [10-(3-morpholinopropionyl) phenothiazin-2-yl]-carbamate.
Ethmozin is a phenothiazine derivative synthesized in the USSR in 1964. It is a class IB anti-arrhythmic agent with lignocaine-like properties. It has been used in treating both atrial and ventricular arrhythmias, the latter requiring higher dosage.

Pharmacokinetics

Ethmozin has a short duration of action when given intravenously. Elimination half-life is prolonged in cardiac patients, and even longer (10 times) in patients with renal failure (Pratt et al 1983). Other pharmacokinetic data are not available.

Dosage and administration

Daily oral dosage is 225–600 mg divided and given 8-hourly, increasing to 800–1000 mg 8-hourly. An anti-arrhythmic effect is not seen until 24 h after initiation of therapy.

Adverse effects

Few important adverse effects have been reported with ethmozin, and none of the usual effects observed with phenothiazine therapy. Dizziness, vertigo and headache may occur after rapid intravenous injection while nausea, epigastric distress, headache and pruritis have been reported during oral therapy.

Aprindine

Aprindine is a class IB agent, effective in both ventricular and supraventricular arrhythmias, which is available in Europe and the USA but not in the UK.

CLASS IC AGENTS

Flecainide

Flecainide acetate (BAN, USAN)
Chemical name: N-(2-piperodylmethyl)-2,5 bis(2,2, 2-trifluoroethoxy) benzamide acetate.
Flecainide is the prototype of class IC agents and is used in suppressing ventricular arrhythmias. Dizziness, visual disturbances, nausea and vomiting may occur. Occasionally pro-arrhythmic effects are seen and caution should be observed in administering the drug to patients with pacemakers, since it increases endocardial pacing thresholds.

Dosage and administration

The intravenous dose is 1–2 mg kg^{-1} and oral doses of 100–300 mg twice daily are recommended (Holmes and Heel 1985).

Adverse effects

The potentially serious pro-arrhythmic effect requires that this drug is used under careful observation. Ventricular arrhythmias may be aggravated in 5–12% of patients (see under encainide). Central nervous system effects are common.

Encainide

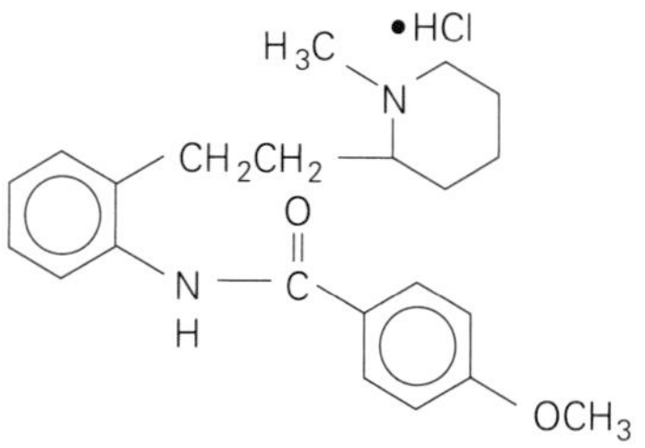

Encainide hydrochloride (BAN USAN).
Chemical name: (±)-2-[2-(1-methyl-2-piperidyl) ethyl]-p-anisanilide hydrochloride.
Encainide is a benazilide derivative and a class IC anti-arrhythmic agent, owing to its potency as a sodium-channel blocker. It is currently being used in refractory ventricular and supraventricular arrhythmias but is not available in the UK.

Pharmacokinetics

Therapeutic plasma concentrations appear to vary widely. This reflects a genetically determined deficiency in encainide metabolism, present in 7% of the population. Two major metabolites, O-desmethyl encainide (ODE) and 3-methoxy-O-desmethyl encainide (MODE), are formed and are both active. They may accumulate during prolonged therapy (Duff et al 1983, Woosley et al 1988).

Dosage and administration

Encainide may be given intravenously or orally. The intravenous dose is up to 1 mg kg^{-1} administered over 15–20 min. The oral dose is 25–60 mg every 6 or 8 h.

Adverse effects

Adverse effects include worsening of intraventricular conduction delay, neurological and visual disturbances, metallic taste, leg cramps and nausea. Pro-arrhythmic effects may be seen in up to 17% of patients.

The results of the recently published Cardiac Ar-rhythmia Suppression Trial (CAST) have challenged much of the conventional wisdom about anti-arrhythmic drugs. Although some issues are not clearly resolved, CAST has determined without question that the use of the two class IC drugs flecainide and encainide to treat asymptomatic or minimally symptomatic ventricular arrhythmias in patients after myocardial infarction is associated with a substantial increase in the sudden-death rate and total mortality, in spite of effective suppression of spontaneous ventricular premature beats. This unexpected outcome is best explained as the result of the induction of lethal ventricular arrhythmias (i.e. a pro-arrhythmic effect; Horowitz 1988, Ruskin 1989, Akhtar et al 1990).

Ajmaline

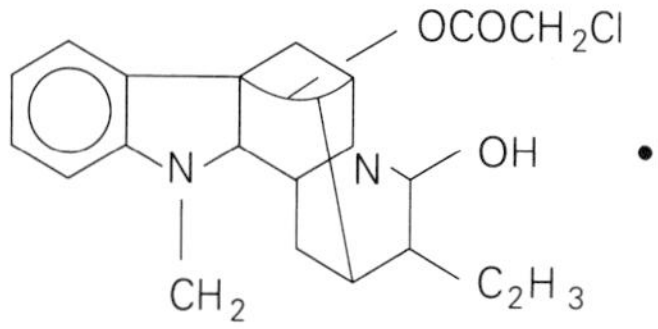

Ajmaline is an alkaloid derived from *Rauwolfia serpentina*, which has structural and pharmacological properties similar to those of quinidine. At low doses it depresses intraventricular conduction and at higher doses prolongs atrioventricular conduction time. The drug has been used in the Wolff–Parkinson–White syndrome to identify accessory pathways of conduction. At high levels it may produce complete atrio-ventricular block and even ventricular fibrillation or asystole. It is available in Europe. Prajamalium and lorajmine are derivatives of ajmaline.

Propafenone

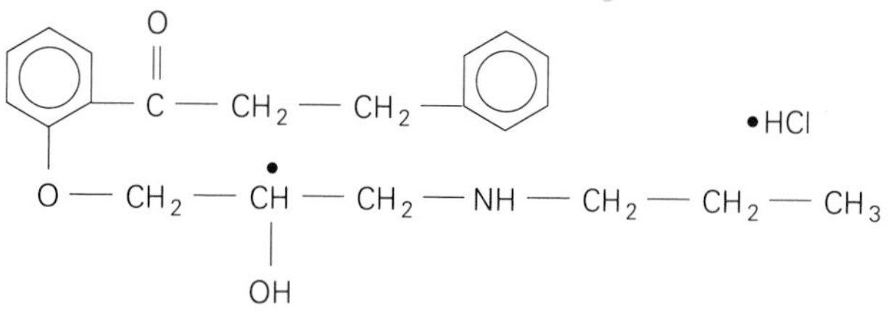

This is a new class IC agent which has been reported to be effective for the therapy of premature ventricular contractions and to prolong the PR interval. It may also have weak β-blocking and Ca^{2+} antagonistic effects. Oral dosage is 300 mg 8-hourly. It may exacerbate arrhythmias in some patients. It is available in the UK (Funck–Brentano et al 1990).

Lorcainide

Lorcainide hydrochloride (BAN USAN).
Chemical name: 4'-chloro-N-(1-isopropyl-4-piperidyl)-2-phenacetanlide hydrochloride.

Lorcainide is a class IC anti-arrhythmic compound with local anaesthetic activity, effective in suppressing ventricular ectopic activity. Intracardiac conduction times are slowed, and complete heart block may be produced in patients with pre-existing atrioventricular conduction abnormalities.

Pharmacokinetics

Lorcainide shows a first-pass effect that seems to be dose-dependent. The primary metabolite, norlorcainide, has anti-arrhythmic activity and a prolonged half-life, but appears only after oral dosage. Side-effects include heart block, hypotension and insomnia.

Dosage and administration

The intravenous dose is 2–6 mg kg^{-1} given over 15–45 min. The oral dose is 200–400 mg daily in divided doses.

CLASS II AGENTS

β-Adrenoceptor blocking compounds

β-Adrenoceptor blocking compounds (β-blockers) will be considered in detail in Chapter 24, but a brief resume of their anti-arrhythmic properties is given here. These drugs block the phase 4 depolarization which is augmented by catecholamines. The action potential is shortened and the refractory period of the atrioventricular node prolonged. Propranolol is the reference compound while practolol or metoprolol administered intravenously have usually been the first-line drugs used to reduce heart rate in atrial flutter or fibrillation and also in paroxysmal atrial tachycardia. Practolol is no longer marketed in the UK; however, the short-acting drug esmolol will be becoming available. Most β-adrenoceptor blocking drugs can be administered either by mouth or intravenously. They are particularly effective in arrhythmias caused by increased circulating catecholamines (phaeochromocytoma (with α-blockade), anxiety, exercise and anaesthesia) or by increased cardiac sensitivity to catecholamines (thyrotoxicosis) and in the arrhythmias of mitral valve prolapse. They may be used to treat the tachycardias of tricyclic antidepressant overdose. In digitalis intoxication, β-blockade may be used against paroxysmal tachycardia but the coexisting atrioventricular block usually makes phenytoin or lignocaine a better choice. Verapamil is less cardiodepressant and is usually the agent of first choice in the treatment of supraventricular tachycardias, but should not be combined with concurrent use of β-adrenoceptor blocking drugs. The anti-arrhythmic activity of the various β-blockers is reasonably uniform, and associated properties such as membrane depression (local anaesthetic action), cardioselectivity, and intrinsic sympathomimetic activity (ISA) have no major influence on the anti-arrhythmic potency. Sotalol is the only exception (additional class III effect — next section).

CLASS III AGENTS

Amiodarone

Amiodarone hydrochloride (BAN, USAN).
Chemical name: 2-butylbenzofuran-3-yl-4-(2-diethylaminoethoxy)3,5-diiodophenyl ketone hydrochloride.

Amiodarone prolongs the duration of the action potential and the refractory period in both atria and ventricles. High doses may lead to a β-blocking action and effects similar to those with quinidine. Good results are obtained with both ventricular and supraventricular arrhythmias, in the latter particularly if associated with the Wolff–Parkinson–White syndrome (aberrant atrioventricular conduction). Use of amiodarone is limited to those arrhythmias resistant to standard anti-arrhythmic compounds, but is now the drug of choice in such circumstances, and is often a first-line drug in critical care situations.

Pharmacokinetics

Onset of action is slow, taking 6 days with oral treatment. The drug is very lipid-soluble and anti-arrhythmic activity after intravenous administration is variable in onset. The drug molecule is deiodinated and leads to a rise in serum triiodothyronine levels by blocking conversion of thyroxine. Plasma concentrations of the main metabolite are similar to that of the parent drug.

Dosage and administration

The intravenous dose is 5 mg kg^{-1} administered by i.v. infusion over a period of 20 min to 2 h; in extreme emergency the drug may be given by slow injection of 150–300 mg over 1–2 min. The usual oral dose is 200–800 mg per day given 5–7 days a week.

Adverse effects

Occasionally vasodilation and hypotension or bradycardia may occur after intravenous administration, particularly after rapid infusion. Corneal microdeposits, photo-sensitization, skin discoloration (grey or blue pigmentation), hypo or hyperthyroidism, liver dysfunction, interstitial pulmonary infiltration and muscle weakness may all occur but are usually reversible. Toxicity was noted in 70% of patients after more than 1 week of treatment (Mason 1987). Simultaneous administration of amiodarone and quinidine is dangerous. Amiodarone prolongs prothrombin time and potentiates the effect of warfarin. Digoxin dosage may require reduction.

Bretylium

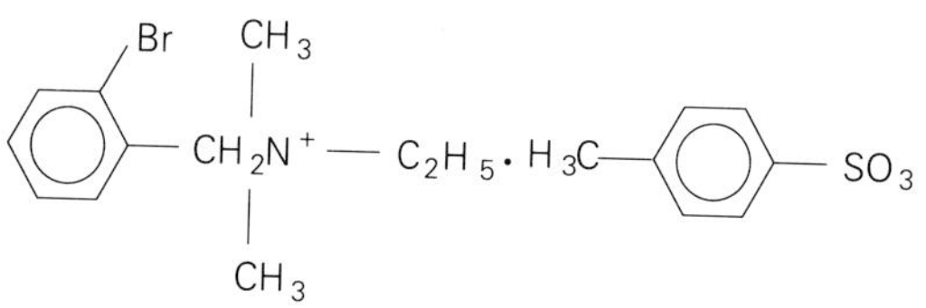

Bretylium tosylate (BAN, USAN).
Chemical name: (2-bromobenzyl)
ethyldimethylammonium
toluene-4-sulphonate.
Bretylium tosylate is effective against ventricular fibrillation refractory to lignocaine and direct current shocks. It may also be used in other ventricular arrhythmias, refractory to more conventional therapy.

Pharmacokinetics

Bretylium has adrenergic nerve-blocking properties and accumulates in sympathetic ganglia, decreases noradrenaline release and in high dosage produces a chemical sympathectomy. There may be initial sympathomimetic effect from transient discharge of noradrenaline from adrenergic postganglionic terminals. It may take 20–40 min after intramuscular injection before an action against certain ventricular arrhythmias is seen. Plasma concentrations cannot be used to guide dosage.

Dosage and administration

In the treatment of ventricular fibrillation bretylium can be given by rapid intravenous injection. In less urgent situations a 500 mg ampoule should be diluted to 50 ml or more with isotonic dextrose or saline, or intramuscular injections of 5 mg kg^{-1} can be repeated 6–8-hourly at varying sites to avoid muscle necrosis.

Adverse effects

The major side-effect is drug-induced hypotension. Nausea and vomiting are common after rapid intravenous bolus injection.

Sotalol

Sotalol is the only anti-arrhythmic drug with simple pharmacokinetics, being totally lipid-insoluble. It would appear to be safer than amiodorone, though perhaps not as effective, and combines class II and III activities. The usual contra-indications to β-blockade apply, and are joined by hypokalaemia and co-therapy with other agents likely to produce QT-prolongation. The oral anti-arrhythmic dose is 160–480 mg twice daily while the intravenous dose is 20–60 mg given over 2–3 min with ECG monitoring; this can be repeated if necessary.

CLASS IV AGENTS

Calcium channel antagonists

Verapamil and diltiazem

Verapamil is a major advance in the acute therapy of supraventricular arrhythmias (see Chapter 24). Nifedipine is devoid of this effect. Diltiazem is of similar value to verapamil.

Table 22.4 Anti-arrhythmic drug therapy

Drug	Indication	Intravenous dose regimens	Comments
Amiodarone	Atrial tachycardia Re-entrant junctional trachycardia Atrial flutter Atrial fibrillation Ventricular tachycardia	300 mg infused over 30 min followed by an infusion of up to 1000 mg over 24 h	Preferably administered through a central venous catheter because of risk of phlebitis
Bretylium	Serious ventricular tachycardia and ventricular fibrillation	5 mg kg^{-1} i.m. repeated every 6–8 h or bolus 500 mg i.v. diluted if possible	Vary i.m.site (tissue necrosis). Decrease dose in renal failure. May cause hypotension after initial sympathomimetic effects
Digoxin	Atrial flutter* Atrial fibrillation*	0.5–1.0 mg by slow i.v. injection or infusion	Maintenance dose reduction in renal failure
Disopyramide	Atrial tachycardia Re-entrant junctional tachycardia	2 mg kg^{-1} over 5 min to a maximum of 150 mg. Maintenance infusion up to 800 mg/24 h	May precipitate heart failure. May cause urinary retention. Dose reduction in renal failure
Flecainide	Atrial tachycardia Re-entrant junctional tachycardia Atrial fibrillation Ventricular tachycardia	For rapid effect, iv bolus of 2 mg kg^{-1} over 10 min. 30 min indicated in less acute states or if cardiac failure present. Maximum bolus dose is 150 mg. i.v. infusion of 1.5 mg kg^{-1} in 1st h followed by 0.25 mg h^{-1}	May precipitate heart failure Should not be administered if AV block unless pacemaker back-up available Dose reduction in renal failure
Lignocaine	Ventricular tachycardia	100 mg bolus i.v. followed by an infusion of 4 mg/min for 30 min; 50-mg bolus repeated after 15 min if required. Infusion rate reduced to 2–3 mg min^{-1} — maintenance	Should not be administered if AV block (see above). Dose reduction in heart failure.
Metoprolol	Sinus tachycardia Re-entrant junctional tachycardia. Atrial fibrillation*	5-mg bolus – repeated up to a maximum of 15 mg	May precipitate hypotension and heart falure. Concomitant verapamil therapy a relative contra-indication
Mexiletine	Ventricular arrhythmias	100–250 mg in 5–10 min then i.v. infusion of 250 mg in next hour, 250 mg in next 2 h, then 0.5 mg min^{-1}	Central nervous system and gastrointestinal side-effects, bradycardia and hypotension
Quinidine	Ventricular tachycardia	Oral only, 200–400 mg 6–8-hourly, or slow release 500 mg every 12 h	Reduce dose in liver disease. Side-effects include torsades de pointes, hypotension. conduction defects.
Tocainide	Ventricular tachycardia	250 mg i.v. in 2 min, 500 mg in 15 min, then 500 mg in every 6 h for 48 h	As with lignocaine. Dose dependent central nervous system effects (tremor) and gastrointestinal effects. Reduce dose in severe renal failure

Table 22.4 Contd

Drug	Indication	Intravenous dose regimens	Comments
Verapamil	Multifocal atrial tachycardia Re-entrant junctional tachycardia Atrial flutter* Atrial fibrillation*	5 mg bolus repeated if necessary after 5–10 min up to maximum of 15–20 mg	May precipitate hypotension and heart failure. Concomitant β-adrenoreceptor blocker therapy a relative contra-indication

*Slows ventricular response.
Modified from Rae AP, Hutton I (1986) British Journal of Anaesthesia 58: 158, with permission.

Table 22.5 Detailed pharmacokinetics and disposition for anti-arrhythmic drugs (where known)

Drug	Oral availability (fraction of dose)	Peak plasma level after oral dose (h)	Elimination half-life $t_{\frac{1}{2}}\beta$ (h)	Volume of distribution Vd_{ss} ($l\ kg^{-1}$)	Protein binding (%)	Main excretion and metabolism	Therapeutic range ($mg\ l^{-1}$)	Toxic range ($mg\ l^{-1}$)
Amiodarone	0.35	5	24 (days)	5000	95	Hepatic-desethylamiodarone a.m.	1–3	>3
Aprindine	High	—	12–66	3.7	90	Hepatic hydroxylation <1% renal	1–3	>2
Bretylium	Poor (erratic)	0.5 (after i.m.i.)	13.5 (after i.v. injection)	—	—	80–90% renal unchanged	1.3	—
Disopyramide	0.7–0.8	0.5–3	6–8	1.3	80 ↓ as plasma $conc^n$ ↑	40–60% renal unchanged a.m. Dose ↓ in s.r.f.	2–5	>5
Encainide	Variable mean 0.4	1–2	3.5	265	70	Hepatic — a.m. (O-demethyl encainide) delayed with poor metabolizers	0.03–0.17	0.14–0.5
Ethmozin	High	0.6–2	4 ↑ in c.h.f & s.r.f	—	—	Renal	0.4	—
Flecainide	0.95	3.5	15–20	7	37–58	Hepatic, 10–50% renal Dose ↓ in c.h.f., s.r.f.	0.2–1.0	>1.0
Lignocaine	0.3–0.4	–	2	1.5 ↓ in c.h.f.	60–80	Hepatic ↓ in h.d. and c.h.f. some a.m. but CNS effects	1.5–5	>5 wide range

Table 22.5   Contd

Drug	Oral availability (fraction of dose)	Peak plasma level after oral dose (h)	Elimination half-life $t\frac{1}{2}\beta$ (h)	Volume of distribution Vd_{ss} (l kg^{-1})	Protein binding (%)	Main excretion and metabolism	Therapeutic range (mg l^{-1})	Toxic range (mg l^{-1})
Lorcainide	0.3–0.75	—	7	9	85	Hepatic — a.m. (norlorcainide) 2% renal	0.1–0.4	0.5–1.2
Mexiletine	0.9	2	12–16	5	75	Hepatic –<10% renal. Clearance ↓ with alkaline urine	0.75–2	>2
N-Acetypro-cainamide	0.85	1.5–4	6.7 ↑ in s.r.f.	1.3	15	80% renal unchanged Clearance ↓ in s.r.f.	10–24	11–22
Phenytoin	1.0 or less (depends on preparation)	3–12	10–30 dose dependent	0.6	>90 ↓ in s.r.f.	Hepatic – ↓ in s.r.f.	10–20	20–40
Procainamide	0.85	1	3–5 42–70 in s.r.f.	2.7	14–23	Hepatic — acetylation (fast or slow) — a.m 50% renal unchanged accumulation in s.r.f. and c.h.f.	4–10	>10
Propafenone	0.5	2	2.5–12	—	—	Hepatic — a.m.	0.2–3.0	—
Quinidine	0.7 (0.4–0.9)	1–3	7, ↑ in h.d. ↓ in c.h.f.	3	80–90 ↓ in h.d.	Hepatic — hydroxylation 20% renal unchanged	2–5	>5
Tocainide	1.0	1–1.5	11–15	3	50	40% renal unchanged, 25% as N-carboxytocainide	6–12	>10
Verapamil	0.25	—	3–7 ↑ ×2 in h.d.	4.5	90	Hepatic — norverapamil 3–4% renal	0.02–0.15	—

Key: ↑ increased; ↓ = decreased; s.r.f. = severe renal failure; h.d. = hepatic disease; c.h.f. = congestive heart failure; a.m. = active metabolite.

Physiological anti-arrhythmics

Hypokalaemia predisposes to ventricular arrhythmias and potassium infusions may be required (McGovern 1985). Magnesium salts are reported of benefit in the therapy of torsades de pointes. Adenosine and adenosine triphosphate (ATP), given intravenously, are increasingly used to inhibit the atrioventricular node in re-entrant tachycardias (Clarke et al 1987). They are physiological 'calcium antagonists' (Belardinelli and Lerman 1990).

REFERENCES

Akhtar M, Breithardt G, Camm A T et al 1990 CAST and beyond: implications of the Cardiac Arrhythmia Suppression Trial. Circulation 81: 1123–1127

Aronson J K 1985 Cardiac arrhythmias: theory and practice. British Medical Journal 290: 487–488

Belardinelli L, Lerman B B 1990 Electrophysiological basis for the use of adenosine in the diagnosis and treatment of cardiac arrhythmias. British Heart Journal 63: 3–4

Carson I W, Lyons S M, Shanks R G 1979. Anti-arrhythmic drugs. British Journal of Anaesthesia 51: 659–670

Clarke B, Till J, Rowland E, Ward D E, Barnes P J, Shinebourne E R 1987 Rapid and safe termination of supraventricular tachycardia in children by adenosine. Lancet i: 299–301

Dresel P E 1985 Cardiac alpha receptors and arrhythmias. Anesthesiology 62: 582–583

Duff H J, Dawson A K, Roden D M, Oates J A, Smith R F, Woosley R L, 1983. Electrophysiologic actions of O-demethyl encainide: an active metabolite. Circulation 68: 385–391

Funck-Brentano C, Kroemer H K, Lee J T, Roden D M 1990 Drug therapy: propafenone. New England Journal of Medicine 322: 518–525

Harrison D C 1986. Current classification of antiarrhythmic drugs as a guide to their rational clinical use. Drugs 31: 93–95

Hillis W S, Whiting B, 1983. Antiarrhythmic drugs. British Medical Journal 286: 1332–1336

Holmes B, Heel R C 1985 Flecainide. A preliminary review of its pharmacodynamic properties and therapeutic efficacy. Drugs 29: 1–33

Horowitz L N 1988. Proarrhythmia — taking the bad with the good. New England Journal of Medicine 319: 305–306

Koch-Weser J, 1979. Drug therapy; disopyramide. New England Journal of Medicine 300: 957–962

Leahey E B, Heissenbuttel R H, Giardina E-G V 1980 Combined mexiletine and propranolol treatment of refractory ventricular tachycardia. British Medical Journal 2: 357–358

Lucas W J, Maccioli G A, Mueller R A 1990 Advances in oral anti-arrhythmic therapy: implications for the anaesthetist. Canadian Journal of Anaesthesia 37: 94–101

Mason J W 1987 Drug therapy: amiodarone. New England Journal of Medicine 316: 455–466

McGovern B 1985 Hypokalaemia and cardiac arrhythmias. Anesthesiology 63: 127–129

Opie L H 1980 Drugs and the heart. IV, Anti-arrhythmic agents. Lancet i: 861–868

Opie L H, Chatterjee K, Gersh B J et al 1987 Drugs for the heart, 2nd expanded edn. Grune & Stratton, Orlando, Ch 4, p 55

Podrid P J, Schoeneberger A, Lown B 1980 Congestive heart failure caused by oral disopyramide. New England Journal of Medicine 302: 614–617

Pratt C M, Yepsen S C, Taylor A A, Mason D T, Millar R R, Quinones M A, 1983 Ethmozine suppression of single and repetitive ventricular premature depolarisations during therapy: documentation of efficacy and long-term safety. American Heart Journal 106: 85–91

Prys-Roberts C 1984 Anaesthesia and hypertension. British Journal of Anaesthesia 56: 711–724

Ruskin J N 1989 The cardiac arrhythmia suppression trial (CAST). New England Journal of Medicine 321: 386–388

Schwartz J B, Keefe D, Harrison D C 1981 Adverse effects of antiarrhythmic drugs. Drugs 21: 23–45

Vaughan Williams E M 1970 Classification of antiarrhythmic drugs. In: Sande E, Flensted-Jensen E, Olesen K H (eds) Symposium on cardiac arrhythmias, Astra, Sodertälje, Sweden, pp 449–472

Waxman H L, Buxton A E, Sadowski L M, Josephson M E 1983 The response to procainamide during electrophysiologic study for sustained ventricular tachyarrhythmias predicts the response to other medication. Circulation 67: 30–37

Woosley R L, Wood A J J, Roden D M 1988 Drug therapy: encainide. New England Journal of Medicine 318: 1107–1115

23. Drugs used for induced hypotension

W. B. Loan

Controlled reduction in arterial blood pressure has been widely practised during surgery for many years, and has proved surprisingly free from complications. This important development was really made possible by the realization that arterial blood pressure, as an index of cardiovascular integrity, is easy to measure but is of limited physiological significance. Well-being is more dependent on tissue perfusion which can, at present, usually only be assessed clinically by monitoring indicators such as the electrocardiograph, electro-encephalograph, urinary output or acid–base status. This has certain implications for the conduct of anaesthesia and the selection of agents.

Anaesthetic technique must, of course, be impeccable. In order to maintain tissue perfusion the agents selected should have a mode of action predominantly dependent on peripheral vasodilation as opposed to cardiac depression. To permit sensitive control the hypotensive drugs used should either have rapid onset and brief duration of action or a facility for interaction with an adjuvant, such as halothane or isoflurane, which is itself capable of rapid response. Conversely, of course, the agent should be capable of providing stable conditions when the desired level of hypotension is attained. When systemic blood pressure falls, perfusion in vital organs such as brain, heart, liver and kidney is aided by local autoregulation. Ideally the hypotensive agents used should not interfere with such protective mechanisms, but if they do so, it is important that violent swings in blood pressure be avoided. Finally, it must always be remembered that, however safe induced hypotension may be under ideal circumstances, it does represent a major upset of homeostasis, and thus that undesired side-effects of drugs may assume increased significance.

The agents employed to produce controlled hypotension during surgery are widely used in other fields of medicine and the literature is consequently, in some cases, very extensive. In the interest of brevity, therefore, three constraints have been accepted in this chapter. Firstly, attention has been focused on those agents most recently adopted for intraoperative use. Also included is a brief discussion of several agents which, while little used to date, may be of potential value in the future. Secondly, consideration has been largely limited to those pharmacological actions of direct relevance to their use in the operating theatre. Thirdly, general anaesthetic agents and drugs used primarily in cardiac medicine, which can be used to produce controllable hypotension, are reviewed elsewhere in this book. It should be noted, however, that isoflurane has been widely and successfully used in this context. It does, in fact, possess many desirable attributes, notably reduction of peripheral resistance with preservation of cardiac output, reduction in oxygen consumption and relatively low toxicity. The long-term place of isoflurane in hypotensive anaesthesia may be significantly dependent on the full resolution of questions regarding its effect on myocardial blood supply.

It is improbable that a hypotensive agent which is ideal in all situations will be found. The requirements, for example, for intracranial, cardiac and middle-ear surgery differ in many respects. The individual anaesthetist can only become familiar with the pharmacology of the available drugs and select the most appropriate in the prevailing circumstances.

Conventionally, hypotensive agents have been classified in terms of their predominant mode of action, viz. directly acting vasodilator, autonomic ganglion blocker or β-adrenergic blocker. In view, however, of the complex interrelationship between the physiological components of the cardiovascular system, this is not always helpful in determining the clinical value or limitations of a drug.

In this text agents are presented in a sequence which, it is hoped, approximates to their current status in anaesthetic practice.

Sodium nitroprusside

Chemical name: $Na_2Fe_5(CN)Na2H_2O$.
Trade name: Nipride.

Sodium nitroprusside was introduced into clinical practice in 1929 (Johnson 1929) and was suggested as a suitable agent for intraoperative induced hypotension in 1962 (Moraca et al 1962).

Pharmacology

The primary action of sodium nitroprusside is to produce relaxation of smooth muscle. This effect is not mediated by the nervous system, is common to all smooth muscle and is not vasculospecific. It is a direct action of the nitroso (−NO) group, which may produce oxidation of sulphydryl groups at a common intermediate vasodilator site. The more specific mechanism may involve actions on cyclic nucleotides and arachidonate metabolism (Tsai et al 1986).

Cardiovascular system

Cardiac function.   Cardiac output is usually maintained (Casthely et al 1982, Todd et al 1982) or even increased (Luben & Hempelmann 1982). Where a significant fall has been found the dosage may have been somewhat higher than is usual, and the reduction in cardiac output attributable to reduced preload (Chamberlain et al 1980, Stanek et al 1981).

Heart rate usually rises (Wildsmith et al 1973, Vance et al 1979) to a degree comparable with that found with nitroglycerin (Kaplan & Jones 1979). Tachycardia may be controlled by the use of β-adrenergic blocking agents such as labetalol (Luben & Hempelmann 1982) but it must be remembered that an increase in heart rate may be an early sign of sodium nitroprusside toxicity. Tachycardia is not always found, possibly being masked by the presence of agents such as halothane with opposing actions (Macnab et al 1988). Neither the cardiac conducting system (Page et al 1955) nor myocardial contractility is affected.

The influence of nitroprusside-induced hypotension on myocardial blood flow is controversial. Coronary artery flow tends to increase (Tountas et al 1965) but there is evidence to suggest that myocardial oxygenation may be reduced, both in surgical patients with normal myocardial function (Fahmy 1978) and following myocardial infarction (Chiariello et al 1976). Mann et al (1978) and Haus et al (1982) reported a marked fall in myocardial tissue Po_2 in dogs even in the presence of normal arterial Po_2.

Where myocardial oxygenation is compromised several mechanisms may be involved, including cyanide-induced cytochrome-oxidase inhibition resulting in anaerobic cell metabolism, reduction in coronary perfusion pressure or failure of autoregulation. It has been suggested that sodium nitroprusside, by causing dilation of the muscularized preferential channels, may divert blood flow from functionally more important nutritive capillary channels which, being without muscle, are undilated. There is also, however, evidence to support the view that nitroprusside-induced hypotension is accompanied by a reduction in myocardial oxygen demand (Kaplan & Jones 1979, Chamberlain et al 1980), a claim supported by the absence of significant lactate production.

In summary it could be said that hypotension produced by sodium nitroprusside is accompanied by myocardial haemodynamic changes, the overall effect of which is equivocal, but that ECG abnormalities suggest that adverse effects tend to outweigh favourable factors.

Non-cardiac function.   Total peripheral resistance falls, both in man (Stanek et al 1981, Luben & Hempelmann 1982) and the dog (Vance et al 1979, Chamberlain et al 1980). A reduction in mean arterial blood pressure of between 30 and 40% could be associated with a 60% reduction in total peripheral resistance. This effect may occur despite compensatory increases in plasma levels of adrenalin, noradrenalin and renin, the possible significance of which will be discussed later. In fact there is evidence to suggest, at least in the anaesthetized dog, that reduction in total peripheral resistance is enhanced where the background total peripheral resistance is raised by elevated blood catecholamine levels (Voss et al 1985).

Central venous pressure is consistently reduced. Pulmonary artery pressure falls (Rowe & Henderson 1974) but may show a rebound increase after nitroprusside is withdrawn (Stanek et al 1981).

Arterial blood pressure falls, as might be predicted. Characteristic of the drug is, however, not only the speed with which control values of arterial pressure are regained when it is withdrawn, but also its tendency to produce subsequent undesirable rebound hypertension. It seems probable that the latter phenomenon results from raised plasma renin levels (Khambatta et al 1979). In fact this is a reaction common to many vasodilator drugs, and an essential feature in the case of nitroprusside may be its brevity of action. This could leave significant plasma renin levels at a time when the vasodilator effects of the drug have disappeared. Renin release in response to hypotension is thought to involve quite a complex feedback mechanism, which is of interest in that it suggests several points of pharmacological attack in dealing with rebound hypertension. It is believed that hypotension reflexly stimulates renal sympathetic nerves. The proteolytic enzyme, renin, thus released, produces the decapeptide angiotensin I, which is in turn cleaved by the converting enzyme to the octapeptide angiotensin II. Both angiotensins I and II act as vasoconstrictors and in addition stimulate the release of catecholamines from the adrenal glands and central nervous system, thus initiating the production of further renin (Peach 1977, Pettinger 1978). Points at which this cycle has been interrupted include sympathetic blockade by means of propranolol (Khambatta et al 1981), labetalol (Luben & Hempelmann 1982), Bunitral (Stanek et al 1981) or clonidine (Saady 1979). Alternatively converting enzyme inhibitors have been used (Miller et al 1977, Fahmy & Gauras 1985) although the safety of this combination has been questioned (Adams & Hewitt 1982).

Tissue hypoxia may occur, resulting in part from precapillary dilation with reduction in resistance, without concomitant venular dilation. This reduces the arteriolar–venular pressure gradient and functional capillary density (Endrich et al 1987). Moderate haemorrhage occurring during SNP-induced hypotension appears to have no adverse effect on cardiac output, mean arterial pressure, left cardiac work, blood flow to cerebral coronary, renal or hepatic circulations (Gustafson et al 1985).

Respiratory system

Several mechanisms may produce hypoxaemia. Dead space to tidal volume ratio is usually increased but this complication is avoided if a constant filling pressure is maintained by infusion of dextrose and Ringer's lactate solutions before and during controlled hypotension (Khambatta et al 1982).

Intrapulmonary shunting increases, possibly due to a fall in pulmonary artery pressure which permits gravity to divert more blood to dependent areas of the lung where most shunt units are situated. This mechanism may not operate in patients with chronic obstructive pulmonary disease, in which the pulmonary artery pressure is maintained (Casthely et al 1982). It has also been suggested (D'Olivera et al 1981) that sodium nitroprusside may directly inhibit compensatory vasoconstriction in underperfused areas of the lung, thus causing hypoxaemia.

Central nervous system

Cerebrovascular resistance usually falls during nitroprusside administration, the effect on cerebral blood flow probably being the resultant of this factor and changes in arterial blood pressure, and possibly of interference with the autoregulatory mechanism. The latter might, for instance, be encountered in the presence of subarachnoid haemorrhage (Fitch et al 1988). Where blood pressure falls markedly there will be a corresponding reduction in cerebral blood flow, but if blood pressure is only slightly reduced, it may actually be increased (Marsh et al 1979). Henriksen et al (1983) found no fall in cerebral blood flow in nine neurosurgical patients receiving halothane with controlled ventilation, where mean arterial blood pressure was reduced to about 55 mmHg. Pinaud et al (1989) concluded that reduction of mean arterial pressure to 40 mmHg was compatible with adequate brain perfusion, but with some reservations. Bunemann et al (1987) also found little alteration in average blood flow or oxygen metabolism, but stressed the frequency of individual variation.

Intracranial pressure tends to parallel cerebral flow where compliance is low. Under certain circumstances, however, capacitance vessels may be dilated in preference to resistance vessels, giving raised intracranial pressure without increase in cerebral blood flow (Michenfelder & Milde 1988). The rise in intracranial pressure may be reduced, but not eliminated, by hyperventilation (Turner et al 1977) and may be augmented if the drug is given as a bolus (Marsh et al 1979) or where intracranial pressure is raised prior to drug administration (Morris et al 1982). In the latter situation the increase in intracranial pressure is greatest where the initial pressure is highest. It is probably a wise precaution, in neurosurgical practice, to withhold nitroprusside until the skull has been opened. Nitroprusside may inhibit autoregulation of cerebral blood flow and consequently violent swings in systemic blood pressure are to be avoided. In summary it is probably fair to say that sodium nitroprusside is widely regarded, despite its regrettable tendency to raise intracranial pressure, as a useful agent in terms of maintaining overall brain integrity. McDowall (1980), for example, reported that both cerebral oxygenation and brain electrical activity were well maintained in the cat, even at a mean arterial pressure of 26 mmHg, and the absence of cycloplegia is an asset where cerebral function is in question.

In order to maintain perspective, however, it should be remembered that Hoffman et al (1982) found, in comparing hypotension induced with nitroglycerin, deep enflurane and sodium nitroprusside that only the latter was associated with a significant reduction in cerebral blood flow. Similarly Michenfelder & Theye (1977) concluded that sodium nitroprusside, despite maintenance of a relatively good cerebral blood flow, caused more cerebral dysfunction than either trimetaphan or halothane.

Spinal cord blood flow falls initially but returns to normotensive values after 30–40 min, even in the presence of moderate distraction, suggesting an autoregulatory mechanism (Kling et al 1985).

Renal system

Sodium nitroprusside does not appear to cause significant specific renal damage. Most investigators have reported either no change in renal function (Wang et al 1977, Norlen 1988), temporary oliguria (Michenfelder & Theye 1977) or diminished creatinine clearance (Behnia et al 1978). Urinary output may even increase slightly during nitroprusside administration (Sood et al 1987). It should, however, be remembered that toxic metabolites of sodium nitroprusside, thiocyanate and cyanide have a low renal clearance, and it may be wise to reduce dosage in the presence of renal insufficiency.

Pharmacokinetics

Onset of hypotension is within 90 s, and recovery is also very rapid. Sodium nitroprusside is broken down into nitrite and cyanide by three mechanisms:

1. rapid reaction with haemoglobin;
2. a slower reaction with sulphydryl groups, also found widely in red blood cells;
3. a very slow reaction with plasma.

Nitrite combines with haemoglobin to form methaemoglobin. One of the five cyanide radicles released combines with this methaemoglobin to form cyanmethaemoglobin. The remaining four cyanide radicles, even when dosage is within the therapeutic range, may produce a high blood level within a period of 1 h. Cyanide is converted to thiocyanate by the action of two enzymes, namely the hepatic enzyme rhodanase and β-mercaptopyruvate sulphur transferase. Rhodanase is found in large amounts in both liver and kidney. Thiosulphate, which donates the sulphur for this enzyme, is derived from cystine by way of β-mercaptopyruvate. β-Mercaptopyruvate–sulphur transferase is found in the erythrocyte, but activity in humans is low (Vesey et al 1974). The conversion of cyanide to thiocyanate is usually slow, the limiting factors being low activity of β-mercaptopyruvate–sulphur transferase and limited availability of β-mercaptopyruvate.

Toxicity of sodium nitroprusside

Toxicity may be caused by at least two metabolites of nitroprusside, namely thiocyanate and cyanide.

Thiocyanate toxicity. Conversion of cyanide to thiocyanate is, as already stated, slow, but thiocyanate excretion is by the kidney with a half-life of up to 7 days which may be prolonged in the presence of renal disease. Thus, in long-term use thiocyanate may accumulate and at levels in excess of 100 $\mu g\ ml^{-1}$ may cause symptoms such as drowsiness, lethargy, nausea and vomiting, and muscle twitching which can progress to coma or convulsions. High concentrations of thiocyanate may also affect thyroid function. It is improbable, however, that toxic levels of thiocyanate would be attained during the relatively short-term intraoperative use of sodium nitroprusside.

Cyanide toxicity. Fatalities have occurred during and after sodium nitroprusside administration which have usually been attributed to overdosage. Warning signs include resistance to hypotensive action, tachycardia, development of metabolic acidosis or elevation of venous oxygen tension. Cyanide rapidly enters the red blood cell and may affect oxygen transport or tissue oxygenation processes by blocking the actions of cytochrome oxidase and probably other enzymes. Pyruvate metabolism is therefore interrupted and lactate produced. The recommended upper limit of dosage of sodium nitroprusside is 1.5 $mg\ kg^{-1}$ or 10 $\mu g\ kg^{-1}$ min^{-1} for short-term administration (Vesey et al 1976). The minimum lethal dose of cyanide is unknown but infusion of 1.5 $mg\ kg^{-1}$ of sodium nitroprusside in 1 h (the maximum recommended dose) can produce a plasma cyanide concentration in vivo which is more than sufficient, in vitro, to reduce cytochrome oxidase activity by 50%. This cyanide concentration in vivo is accompanied by an increase in plasma lactate, indicating histotoxic anoxia.

In addition to the clinical warning signs mentioned above, biochemical monitoring has been suggested. Lactate concentrations fall during low-dose nitroprusside infusion, probably due to improved tissue perfusion (Wildsmith et al 1979). With larger doses, however, lactate levels may rise, especially if resistance is encountered. It may be preferable to monitor bicarbonate concentrations which mirror lactate changes and are more readily available. Cyanide levels in the blood or expired air have been estimated directly, but their validity as indicators of possible cyanide toxicity has been challenged (Smith & Kruszyna 1976).

If, as seems probable, toxicity of sodium nitroprusside is caused by overdosage secondary to 'resistance', the aetiology of the latter phenomenon is of fundamental importance. Unfortunately at present it is not fully understood, although similarities between nitroprusside resistance and idiopathic lactic acidosis have been noted (Strunin 1975). It has also been suggested that free plasma cyanide may be responsible (Grayling et al 1978) based on the observation that while sodium nitroprusside moves the noradrenaline dose–response curve for rabbit aortic strip to the right, this response is reduced when cyanide is also present. In fact, if contraction of the aortic strip is first caused by noradrenaline and then released by sodium nitroprusside, cyanide actually causes contraction.

A further uncertainty is introduced by Bisset et al (1981), who suggest that cyanide may not actually be released from sodium nitroprusside in vivo. These authors, using a selective electrode technique, as opposed to the usual colorimetric method, found little evidence of cyanide release. They point out that sodium nitroprusside, to which cyanide is firmly bound, is rapidly converted in light to aquapentacyanoferrate, from which cyanide is readily released in acid solution. The conversion of sodium nitroprusside to aquapentacyanoferrate is not accompanied by a colour change and will not therefore be detected on visual inspection. It is possible that observed levels of cyanide resulted from exposure to light during the lengthy colorimetric measurement procedure. While this work might suggest that doses greater than those usually recommended could be safely used, it also emphasizes the vital importance of protecting sodium nitroprusside from light. In sunlight, for example, 45% of sodium nitroprusside may be converted to aquapentacyanoferrate within 2 h, and the resulting solution will certainly release cyanide at blood pH.

Management of sodium nitroprusside toxicity. Possibly reflecting uncertainty about the precise aetiology of nitroprusside toxicity, suggested remedies are quite diverse, but can be broadly classified into attempts either to facilitate the inactivation of cyanide, or to potentiate the hypotensive effect of sodium nitroprusside, thus reducing dosage. An example of the former approach is administration of sodium thiosulphate, which is required by the enzyme rhodanase to form thiocyanate. Used at doses of 10–40 mg kg^{-1} h^{-1} it has proved effective, and is probably the treatment of choice (Cole & Vesey 1987).

Hydroxycobalamin (vitamin B_{12a}) combines with cyanide to form cyanocobalamin and is thus also a useful cyanide antagonist. Unfortunately the dose required is large (22.5 mg hydroxycobalamin per mg sodium nitroprusside) but even a relatively small dose will help

to combat cyanide toxicity (Adams & Hewitt 1982).

The alternative approach, namely potentiation of sodium nitroprusside with consequent reduction of dosage, has been quite widely used. Wildsmith et al (1983) advocate a trimetaphan/SNP combination (trimetaphan nitroprusside) in the ratio 10 : 1. This synergistic mixture retains many of the advantages of sodium nitroprusside yet permits reduction in the dosage of both agents. While confirming the finding of lower plasma and red cell cyanide levels, Sury et al (1988), however, question the overall value of trimetaphan nitroprusside. Halothane/adrenoreceptor blockers (Khambatta et al 1979), saralasin (Pertuiset et al 1980) and calcium antagonists (Muller et al 1987) have also been used with success. Excessive enthusiasm for the multiple-drug approach may, however, bring its own problems. Simpson et al (1987) reported a disturbing incidence of bradycardia among patients who had been given β-adrenoreceptor antagonists preoperatively.

It is possible that simple adherence to optimal dosage, as by use of computer-controlled administration, could be helpful (Westenskow et al 1987). Even when sodium nitroprusside dosage is within normal limits some patients are unusually vulnerable to its toxic effects. Metabolic disorders identified as potentially dangerous include Leber's optic atrophy, tobacco amblyopia and neurological deficits arising from vitamin B_{12} deficiency.

Sodium nitroprusside in pregnancy. Sodium nitroprusside crosses the placenta of the ewe and may produce fatal concentrations of cyanide in the fetus due to slow biotransformation (Donchin et al 1978). Renin release also occurs in the fetus (Zubrow et al 1988). There has been a recommendation therefore that it should not be used during pregnancy. It has subsequently been pointed out, however, that the ewe, the experimental animal employed, shows resistance to nitroprusside and that the doses used were therefore large. Several reports have been published of the successful use of sodium nitroprusside for neurosurgical emergencies during pregnancy (Rigg & McDonagh 1981) and in at least one case the child showed no abnormality at 2 years of age (Donchin et al 1978).

Platelet function. It has been found that sodium nitroprusside at doses of $\geqslant 3$ μg kg^{-1} min^{-1} was associated with dose-dependent decrease in platelet aggregation and increase in bleeding time (Hines & Barash 1989).

Dosage and administration

The preparation which is comercially available, lyophilized powder, should be diluted in a solution of 5%

dextrose immediately before use and carefully protected from light to avoid decomposition. A 0.01% solution is commonly used.

While some uncertainty exists concerning the precise nature of sodium nitroprosside toxicity it would be wise to adhere to the recommended maximum dosage of 1.5 mg kg^{-1} or 10 μg kg^{-1} min^{-1} for short-term administration. A method of infusion should be employed which permits very accurate monitoring of dosage.

Drug interactions

Nitroprusside-induced hypotension was found to be associated with prolongation of curariform blockade in dogs (Kim et al 1976). Subsequently, however, Graham & Walts (1979) were unable to detect this effect in the human, using either tubocurarine or pancuronium bromide.

Nitroglycerin

Chemical name: CH_2—O—NO_2
$\qquad\qquad\qquad$ CH_2—O—NO_2
$\qquad\qquad\qquad$ CH_2—O—NO_2

Nitroglycerin is a compound of glyceryl trinitrate. It was first used in the relief of angina pectoris in 1879 (Murrel 1879) and has been the basis of symptomatic treatment during the intervening century. Christensson et al (1969) demonstrated that it could produce steady levels of blood pressure if given intravenously, and it has subsequently been employed successfully by cardiologists in the management of congestive cardiac failure and acute myocardial ischaemia. Nitroglycerin has also been used intraoperatively, either to produce hypotension or to control reflex hypertension (Kaplan et al 1976).

Pharmacology

The fundamental action of nitroglycerin, like other nitrates, is to produce direct relaxation of smooth muscle, including that found in the walls of blood vessels. This effect is not neuronally mediated, and the affected muscle may still respond to stimulation.

Cardiovascular system

Two components have been identified in the cardiovascular actions of nitroglycerin, namely cardiac and extracardiac.

Extracardiac effects.   Nitroglycerin produces relaxation of both arterial and venous smooth muscle, but the most important site of action is on peripheral veins, producing venodilatation and increased venous capacitance (Mason & Braunwald 1965). This, in turn, results in reduced venous return, a fall in end-diastolic pressure and volume of the heart. Pulmonary venous tone is also reduced, resulting in lowered left ventricular pressure and myocardial oxygen demand (Flaherty et al 1975). Peripheral resistance and pulmonary vascular resistance are reduced. Tissue perfusion appears to be well maintained, even in the presence of significant reduction in systemic arterial pressure (Spargo et al 1987).

Cardiac effects.   Heart rate is seldom significantly altered (Bale et al 1982, Adams & Hewitt 1982). At high dose levels tachycardia may occur (Kaplan & Jones 1979) while it is also possible to find relative bradycardia (Chestnut et al 1978).

Cardiac output tends to fall (Bernstein et al 1966, Chiariello et al 1976), but the reduction is seldom great and on occasion output may actually rise (Haus et al 1982, Todd et al 1982). Where cardiac output falls to an undesirable degree it may be restored by low-dose dopamine administration without abolishing the beneficial effects of nitroglycerin on myocardial function (Bale et al 1982). Of possibly more fundamental importance is the effect of nitroglycerin on the ratio of myocardial perfusion to myocardial work. It should be remembered that the overall effect of nitroglycerin on myocardial blood flow is the resultant of several factors including:

1. direct action on myocardial blood vessels (including possible selective action on some vessels);
2. influence of coronary artery disease;
3. action on systemic circulation.

The direct action of nitroglycerin on myocardial circulation can be demonstrated by intracoronary injection. Using this technique Bernstein et al (1966) found that a dose of 0.1–0.2 mg produced a significant fall in coronary vascular resistance, with minimal alteration in mean aortic pressure, and thus an increase in myocardial blood flow of almost 40% in the presence of coronary artery disease, or over 60% without disease. However, it is probably not correct simply to equate the presence of coronary artery disease with a reduced response, in terms of myocardial blood flow, to nitroglycerin administration. Goldstein et al (1975), comparing patients with and without coronary artery occlusion during valve replacement surgery, found not only that those with coronary artery disease showed greatly increased collateral function, but also that the response to nitroglycerin may be increased in the presence of chronic coronary occlusion. Chiariello et al (1976) have suggested that nitroglycerin, in contrast to nitroprusside, dilates large coronary conductance vessels, thus producing enhanced collateral blood flow and redistributing blood to subendocardial ischaemic areas.

Systemic arterial pressure falls, but diastolic to a lesser degree than systolic, and this may assist coronary perfusion (Fahmy 1978).

Following systemic administration these apparently beneficial effects of nitroglycerin on myocardial perfusion may be obscured by reduction in systemic pressure. The overall resultant of local and systemic changes may, however, be deduced from the apparent effect of nitroglycerin on myocardial oxygenation evidenced either by electrocardiographic changes, or by direct tissue measurement. Kaplan & Jones (1979) found that nitroglycerin improved ST segment depression more consistently than did nitroprusside in patients undergoing myocardial revascularization surgery.

Fahmy (1978), studying patients without evidence of coronary artery disease, found no electrocardiographic evidence of ischaemia in cases given nitroglycerin, whereas over 30% of those receiving nitroprusside showed some ischaemic change. Direct estimation of myocardial tissue Po_2 would also suggest that nitroglycerin-induced hypotension has little adverse effect on myocardial oxygenation (Haus et al 1982).

Endocrine response to hypotension. Sudden withdrawal of nitroglycerin, in contrast to nitroprusside, is not followed by rebound hypertension, despite the finding that plasma levels of adrenaline and noradrenaline are actually higher with nitroglycerin. This discrepancy may be attributable to a prolonged action of nitroglycerin, resulting from its binding to the vessel wall and unrelated to plasma levels (Hill et al 1980). Irrespective of its causation, the absence of rebound hypertension following deliberate or inadvertent withdrawal of nitroglycerin is usually regarded as a useful attribute.

Central nervous system

Intracranial pressure usually rises due to vasodilation following nitroglycerin administration to subjects with normal cerebral function, often producing headache. Of greater interest, however, is the effect of nitroglycerin on intracranial pressure which is already raised by injury or disease. It has been suggested that further elevation is unlikely because the predominant effect of nitroglycerin is on venous as opposed to arteriolar function. There is, however, considerable clinical and experimental evidence to suggest not only that intracranial pressure rises under these circumstances, but that the level reached is related to that prior to nitroglycerin administration (Morris et al 1982).

The overall effect on intracranial pressure must, of course, be related to changes in the systemic circulation. Burt et al (1982) found that in dogs with normal intracranial pressure, nitroglycerin-induced hypotension of 35% below baseline was accompanied by elevation of intracranial pressure. Similarly, where the intracranial pressure was raised initially, a small fall in blood pressure (25% of baseline) produced a rise in intracranial pressure. However, when the mean arterial pressure was reduced by more than 25% the intracranial pressure actually fell. It is important to note that animals whose raised intracranial pressure was lowered by profound hypotension also showed a consistent tendency towards rebound increase in intracranial pressure when arterial pressure was restored. Burt et al (1982) recommended that intracranial pressure be reduced before nitroglycerin is used, to produce hypotension for neurosurgery. Despite the possibility that nitroglycerin may increase intracranial pressure there is some evidence to suggest that cerebral blood flow is relatively well maintained with this agent (Hoffman et al 1982) and that autoregulation may be unaltered (Chestnut et al 1978).

Fate in the body

Nitroglycerin, in common with other organic nitrates, undergoes biotransformation in the liver by reductive hydrolysis catalysed by the enzyme glutathione-organic-nitrate reductase. The metabolites are relatively inactive and the brief duration of action appears to be correlated with plasma concentrations of nitroglycerin.

Dosage and administration

Dosage is usually within the range 0.5–1.5 μg kg^{-1} min^{-1}, but efficacy is limited and a proportion of patients may require the use of adjuvants to produce adequate hypotension. Early intravenous solutions were produced by crushing tablets and sterilizing by filtration; but commercial preparations are now available containing 5 mg nitroglycerin in 10 ml glass ampoules. Such solutions must not come into contact with infusion bags or tubing composed of polyvinyl chloride, as nitroglycerin migrates into such materials. They can, however, be administered from rigid plastic or glass syringes or infusion sets. Onset of action is usually within

4 min and all haemodynamic effects should have disappeared within 5 min of nitroglycerin withdrawal.

Side-effects, precautions and contra-indications

There have been no reported cases of toxicity from the use of nitroglycerin by intravenous, sublingual or topical routes of administration. Excessive hypotension can be corrected using an α-adrenergic agonist such as methoxamine, and it has been claimed that low-dose dopamine may restore cardiac output without compromising the beneficial effects of nitroglycerin on myocardial blood flow. Nitroglycerin administration potentiates neuromuscular blockade produced by pancuronium in the cat, although the clinical relevance of this finding is still uncertain.

Unlike trimetaphan, nitroglycerin does not appear to augment the cardiovascular changes produced by the insertion of acrylic cement (Vazeery et al 1983).

Labetalol

Labetalol was introduced as a combined α- and β-adrenoceptor antagonist (Boakes et al 1971), and has been used extensively in the medical management of hypertension (Prichard et al 1975, Rosei et al 1975). It has been employed in association with anaesthesia during surgical removal of phaeochromocytoma (Rosei et al 1976, Kaufman 1979) and in an attempt, partially successful, to attenuate the cardiovascular response to ketamine (Dundee et al 1977). Its most widespread intraoperative application has, however, been in the induction of controlled hypotension.

Pharmacology: cardiovascular system

Labetalol exhibits a unique ability to antagonize both α- and β-adrenoceptors, the potency for β-blockade being approximately seven times that for α-blockade. Relative to propranolol, by weight, β_1 antagonism is four times less potent, and β_2 antagonism 11–17 times less potent. Angiotensin II and aldosterone levels fall during labetalol administration, especially in hypertensive patients where they may be initially raised (Trust et al 1976). Labetalol produces selective α_1-blockade but has also intrinsic α_1- and β-sympathomimetic action (Nakagawa et al 1985). Compared to phentolamine it produces seven times less α-blockade and may be similar to the actions of prazosin. It should be noted that prazosin, by selectively blocking α_1- as opposed to α_2-adrenergic receptors, allows adrenaline to produce negative feedback, thus inhibiting its own release and

consequently minimizing the tendency towards reflex tachycardia.

Cardiac effects.   Heart rate usually falls, especially if tachycardia is present prior to labetalol administration (Cope & Crawford 1979, Carswell et al 1981). This correlation between response to labetalol and the balance between autonomic influences is seen clearly in the experimental animal. Dogs, for example, anaesthetized with barbitone, show preponderance of sympathetic tone, and in these animals labetalol causes a fall in heart rate, contractility, cardiac output and work. In conscious dogs, on the other hand, or those anaesthetized with piritrimide, where parasympathetic tone predominates, labetalol increases heart rate, possibly as a reflex vagolytic response to peripheral vasodilatation (Brittain & Levy 1976, Van Aken et al 1982). It is probable that labetalol, at the dosage usually employed to induce hypotension, has a relatively small effect on cardiac output. Saarnivaara et al (1987), for example, found a maximum fall of 7% in cardiac output in patients given 0.3 mg kg^{-1}. This generalization may, however, be modified by factors such as the autonomic balance referred to above, variation in dosage, concomitant drug administration and anaesthetic technique. At the high dose level of 15 mg kg^{-1} in dogs Gustafson et al (1981) found a fall in cardiac output of 59% where fentanyl had been used to produce anaesthesia. At doses in excess of 20 mg kg^{-1} labetalol shows a significant negative inotropic effect, thought to be a manifestation of membrane stabilization Brittain & Levy 1976). When a much lower dose of 25 mg (mean 0.35 mg kg^{-1}) was given to patients receiving 1% halothane, Scott et al (1978) reported an 18% fall in cardiac output during spontaneous respiration but only a 12% reduction when respiration was controlled. The discrepancy was attributed to the fact that cardiac output was higher in the spontaneous respiration group prior to labetalol administration, but subsequently fell more markedly when the cardiovascular response to hypercarbia was blocked. It should be noted that when halothane concentration was increased from 1 to 3%, a marked further fall in cardiac output occurred, and those authors considered it unwise to exceed halothane 2% where a significant dose of labetalol had been administered.

The marked synergism between halothane and labetalol is, in fact, a recurring theme in many published studies (Cope 1979, Hunter 1979) and is widely utilized in clinical anaesthesia. The extent to which halothane contributes to the hypotensive effect is indicated by the greatly increased dose of labetalol required (2 mg kg^{-1}) when it is used in conjunction with droperidol–fentanyl anaesthesia (Kanto et al 1980).

In summary it could be said that the modest inherent depressant effect of labetalol on cardiac output may either be directly augmented by another drug such as halothane, or manifest as an inability of the myocardium to react to an additional stress such as haemorrhage (Cope & Crawford 1979); hypercapnia (Scott et al 1978), a stimulant drug (Hunter 1979); physical exercise (Edwards & Raftery 1976) or the upright position (Koch 1976).

Mean stroke volume is not usually significantly affected (Scott et al 1976, Koch, 1976). Myocardial blood flow falls during labetalol-induced hypotension but left ventricular work is reduced to a greater degree and the fraction of cardiac output going to the myocardium is maintained (Gustafson et al 1981). Pulmonary artery pressure is not greatly altered (Gustafson et al 1981, Koch 1976).

Non-cardiac actions.   Central venous pressure rises in those circumstances under which cardiac output falls. Total peripheral resistance falls (Brittain & Levy 1976, Edwards & Raftery 1976), and unlike most cardiovascular responses to labetalol administration under anaesthesia, this does not appear to be greatly influenced by the concentration of halothane employed. The extent to which total peripheral resistance is reduced by labetalol may be related to the pre-existing level of vascular tone. The observed reduction is, for example, less both in association with controlled as opposed to spontaneous respiration in the human (Scott et al 1976), and in the anaesthetized as opposed to the conscious dog (Saito et al 1986). Rebound hypertension is not usually found (Toivonen et al 1989).

Pharmacology: central nervous system

It is probable that labetalol-induced hypotension, at least in dogs, is not associated with a rise in intracranial pressure, or perhaps more importantly, with a change in intracranial compliance (Van Aken et al 1982). Cerebral blood flow may fall slightly, but the fraction of cardiac output allocated to the brain is actually increased, suggesting that cerebral autoregulation is maintained during labetalol hypotension (Gustafson et al 1981).

Little direct evidence has been found of entry into the central nervous system (Martin et al 1976) but there have been reports of drowsiness and vivid dreams which disappeared when the drug was withdrawn (Dargie et al 1976). It may also be relevant to note that the administration of propranolol to rats has been associated with the appearance of a sleep pattern in the electroencephalograph (Torbati 1986).

Pharmacology: renal system

Renal perfusion appears to be well maintained, although some reduction in creatinine clearance figures has been found in the early stages of long-term treatment of hypertension using labetalol (Joekes & Thompson 1976).

Pharmacology: hepatic system

Total liver blood flow is maintained, again by increasing its fraction of cardiac output in the presence of hypotension.

Pharmacokinetics

Labetalol is not extensively protein-bound (about 50%) and after intravenous injection is therefore rapidly transferred to the tissues. Highest levels are found in lungs, liver and kidney but very little appears to enter the brain. Labetalol is extensively metabolized by first-pass effect, 60% of the metabolites being excreted in the urine and 40% in the faeces; 5% of the dose is excreted unchanged in the urine. The principal metabolite in man is an unidentified conjugate but the *o*-phenyl glucuronide is also found. The half-life of elimination is 3.5–4.5 h determined from the intravenous clearance curve. Even when dosage is high placental transfer is minimal (Martin et al 1976).

Onset of action is within 3–5 min after intravenous injection; α and β effects persist for approximately $\frac{1}{2}$ h and 1 h respectively (Cope & Crawford 1979), although the overall hypotensive effect may last 3 h (Joekes & Thompson 1976).

Indications and clinical usage

Labetalol is used in the management of hypertension, including acute episodes, and other medical emergencies such as clonidine withdrawal (Rosei et al 1976). It has been used by anaesthetists principally in the production of controlled hypotension or to control hypertension during surgical removal of phaeochromocytoma (Rosei et al 1975, Kaufman 1979). Labetalol has been used to induce hypotension for general, orthopaedic, major ear, cardiovascular and neurosurgical procedures.

Dosage and administration

Dosage is, as already stated, greatly influenced by factors including age of patient, interaction with depressant drugs such as halothane, and whether or not respiration is controlled. In view of the fact that labetalol has a half-life of over 3 h, and also that its hypotensive action is so greatly supplemented by halothane, it is probably wise first to establish a situation of cardiovascular stability under general anaesthesia, at an inspired halothane concentration of between 1% and 2%. A small initial dose of about 10 mg of labetalol can then be given, with further increments at intervals of 5 min until an arterial pressure in the desired range is obtained. Further manipulation of the pressure can then be produced by altering the inhaled halothane concentration. Especially in those cases where ventilation is controlled using tubocurarine as muscle relaxant, the total required dose may be surprisingly small.

Where halothane is not used doses of 2.0 mg kg^{-1} may be required. When labetalol is used in conjunction with halothane, withdrawal of the latter agent will usually allow the blood pressure to reach an acceptable level within 5–10 min.

Side-effects, precautions and contra-indications

It should be remembered that combined α- and β-adrenoreceptor blockade may reduce or eliminate the cardiovascular response to haemorrhage (Cope & Crawford 1979); hypercapnia (Scott et al 1978) or β-receptor stimulants used in cardiac resuscitation (Hunter 1979).

Where substantial doses have been given to pregnant animals, significant deposition has been found in the retina of the fetus. The relevance of this finding in the context of the brief exposure characteristic of anaesthetic practice is uncertain.

As in other therapeutic situations labetalol should be used with caution in patients suffering from asthma, cardiac failure, heart block or insulin-dependent diabetes.

Trimetaphan

Trimetaphan is a sulphonium compound, evolved following experimental and clinical evaluation of the hypotensive effects of a number of quaternary and bis-quaternary ammonium ions.

Pharmacology: cardiovascular system

Trimetaphan lowers blood pressure by a permutation of at least three mechanisms. In common with the quaternary and bis-quaternary ammonium compounds, such as hexamethonium or pentolinium, it blocks sympathetic and parasympathetic ganglia competitively by occupying receptor sites, and thus preventing the stimulation of postsynaptic membranes by acetylcholine released from presynaptic nerve endings. It also has a direct dilator effect on peripheral vessels, although this may be of limited significance at the concentrations reached during controlled hypotension (Castro-Tavares 1980). Trimetaphan releases histamine from mast cells, although the extent to which this influences its haemodynamic effects in humans has been questioned (Fahmy & Soter 1985). These multiple modes of action may account for the hypotensive effect found in sympathectomized subjects. Both preload and afterload are reduced by reduction in venular and arteriolar tone.

Heart rate usually rises if existing vagal tone is high, both as a compensatory mechanism and possibly also as a result of direct parasympathetic blockade. If heart rate is initially raised, however, it may fall following trimetaphan administration. Tachycardia may be controlled by β-adrenoreceptor blockers such as practolol or propranolol, but probably at the expense of a fall in cardiac output.

Trimetaphan may exert a direct negative inotropic effect on the heart, but cardiac output also tends to fall secondary to reduction in venous return, especially if a head-up tilt is employed. Onset of action is rapid, usually within 3 min, duration being usually quoted as about 15 min, although hypotension may persist for at least 30 min on occasions.

Pharmacology: central nervous system

Trimetaphan-induced hypotension is usually accompanied by a fall in cerebral blood flow, although this is probably not significant if mean arterial blood pressure is not permitted to fall below 50 mmHg (Miletich & Ivankovitch 1978). There is, however, evidence to suggest that both cerebral blood flow and electrical activity are less well maintained under trimetaphan-induced hypotension than with sodium nitroprusside (Ishikawa & McDowall 1979). Intracranial pressure is not usually greatly altered unless it was initially raised (Turner et al 1977). This tendency to augment pre-existing raised intracranial pressure may be aggravated if hypotension is induced rapidly (Karlin et al 1988). Passage through the blood–brain barrier is limited.

Pharmacology: renal system

Renal blood flow and glomerular filtration rate are reduced and renal vascular resistance rises.

Indications and clinical usage

Trimetaphan has been used extensively to produce controlled hypotension. It has also been employed as means of improving perfusion during and after cardiac surgery, and in the management of hypertensive crises or autonomic hyperflexia. It is still regarded by some as the drug of choice in the management of pre-eclampsia on the grounds that it has less deleterious effects on cerebral blood flow and intracranial pressure than does nitroglycerin (Sosis & Leighton 1986).

Dosage and administration

The ampoule containing 250 mg is usually diluted in 250 ml with N. Saline or glucose to give a concentration of 0.1%. Solutions of 0.05% (250 mg in 500 ml) may be preferable where the patient is elderly, or 0.25% (250 mg in 100 ml) if it is desirable to limit fluid intake. Using an 0.1% (250 mg in 100 ml) it is usual to commence at a rate of about 60 drops per minute, determining the subsequent requirement by continuous monitoring of arterial blood pressure. The undiluted solution has also been used by intermittent bolus injection, usually starting with a dose of 50 mg followed by smaller increments at intervals of approximately 10 min to maintain the required blood pressure. A trimetaphan infusion should not be used as a vehicle for the administration of other substances. Trimetaphan is incompatible with thiopentone, gallamine triethiodide, strongly alkaline solutions, iodides and bromides.

Side-effects, precautions and contra-indications

Fluctuation in blood pressure may occur rapidly and there is a tendency, especially in the hands of the less experienced, to alternate between brisk haemorrhage and rather profound hypotension. The latter trend may be exaggerated in cases where histamine release is marked, with the additional possible hazard of bronchospasm. Tachyphylaxis can occur after periods of infusion, possible mechanisms being an increase in neurotransmitter release or the stimulant effect of surgery. Combination with sodium nitroprusside at a ratio of SNP : trimetaphan of 1 : 10, although advocated primarily as a means of reducing the toxicity of nitroprusside, should overcome this difficulty.

Trimetaphan may potentiate and prolong the effects of non-depolarizing muscle relaxants, and being partly metabolized by plasma cholinesterase, may also increase the duration of action of succinylcholine. It has been recommended that it should not be used in the presence of any abnormality of plasma cholinesterase whether this be of genetic, drug-induced or hepatic origin. There appears to be an interaction between trimetaphan and

acrylic cement monomer, the insertion of which produces a further fall in both stroke volume and cardiac output, which is not seen when either nitroglycerin or sodium nitroprusside have been used to induce hypotension (Vazeery et al 1983).

Hydralazine

Hydralazine is a phthalazine derivative which has been used in the treatment of hypertension of more than 30 years. Soon after its introduction it was found to be of relatively low potency, thus requiring large doses with consequent risk of side-effects, and also to show a significant fall in efficacy during chronic administration. With greater knowledge of its pharmacology, however, those difficulties have been largely overcome and hydralazine has again become a popular antihypertensive agent. More recently it has been used to produce hypotension during surgery (James & Bedford 1982).

Pharmacology

Hydralazine acts directly on vascular smooth muscle producing a fall in peripheral resistance and thus in blood pressure without affecting venous capacitance. In the anaesthetized dog this effect may be mediated through vasodilator prostaglandins (Haeusler & Gerold 1979), although the significance of this in the human subject is uncertain. It has also been found that during prolonged administration in the rat both the actomyosin content of the aortic wall and its maximum contractile response to adrenaline are reduced, although again the relevance of this to short-term intraoperative use is undetermined (Seidel et al 1980).

Heart rate and cardiac output rise. Pulmonary artery pressure is raised, in contrast to the action of nitroprusside or the organic nitrates which increase venous capacitance and thus reduce preload. Coronary autoregulation is thought to be maintained (Howe et al 1977).

Plasma renin levels are raised following hydralazine administration. Plasma catecholamine levels also rise and may be at least partly responsible for the inotropic and chronotropic effects of hydralazine. Following intravenous injection (mean dose 17 mg) during enflurane anaesthesia, a reduction of mean arterial pressure of 30% was obtained within 9 min, returning to pre-injection levels within 21 min and without rebound hypertension (James & Bedford 1982). Intracranial pressure may rise, especially in the presence of a space-occupying lesion.

Pharmacokinetics

Metabolism of hydralazine, at least in the rat, is by four major pathways, namely acetylation, hydrolysis of the hydrazine ring, ring hydroxylation and the formation of hydrazones between ketone bodies and hydralazine (McLean et al 1977). At least two of these mechanisms may play a significant role in determining duration of action. Individuals may be either fast or slow acetylators, thus affecting the plasma levels obtained, and it has also been suggested that hydrazone metabolites may either be pharmacologically active or undergo back-metabolism to hydralazine (Talseth et al 1982).

Side-effects and contra-indications

In cardiological practice it is recommended that hydralazine should be given only to patients who are already receiving a diuretic and some form of sympathetic antagonist such as a β-adrenergic blocker. This advice may not, however, be applicable when hydralazine is used during surgery, as it has been found that propranolol abolishes its acute hypotensive effect, possibly due to unmasking of an α-mediated vasoconstriction (Tsui et al 1982).

Of considerable interest to the anaesthetist are reports of serious cardiovascular depression occurring when hydralazine and diazoxide are given in sequence (Heinrich et al 1977, Romberg et al 1977, Mizroch & Yurasek 1977). The precise order of administration does not appear to be important, and it would seem to be unwise to combine drugs with such similar modes of action. A lupus syndrome may be induced in a substantial proportion of patients receiving 400 mg per day, and it is recommended that a dosage of 200 mg per day should not be exceeded except in patients who are fast acetylators or in Negroes who are relatively immune to lupus development. Where, however, the anaesthetist becomes preoccupied with the daily dose of a drug used intraoperatively, it is perhaps appropriate to discuss the duration of operations with his surgical colleagues.

Calcium antagonists

These drugs are discussed in more detail in Chapter 24.

Verapamil

Verapamil is a synthetic papaverine derivative. Originally introduced as a smooth muscle relaxant, producing peripheral and coronary vasodilation, it was subsequently found to have important cardiac actions.

Pharmacology

Verapamil selectively inhibits membrane transport of calcium ions. The slow entry of calcium into myocardial cells, following rapid depolarization by entry of sodium, appears to be of fundamental importance in the cardiac cycle. Calcium ions act as mediator in the utilization of ATP, and interference with their transport is thought to produce verapamil's negative inotropic and anti-arrhythmic actions. The atrioventricular node exhibits both reduction in conduction velocity and increase in refractory period, thus atrioventricular conduction is delayed. Calcium antagonism at vascular smooth muscle leads to coronary and peripheral vasodilation. Verapamil may also bind to postsynaptic α-adrenergic receptors. Its cardiovascular effects may be abolished by giving calcium gluconate 15 mg kg^{-1} intravenously.

Verapamil has been used during both abdominal (Zimpfer et al 1981) and coronary artery surgery (Bovill et al 1984). Doses of 0.07 mg kg^{-1}, given as a bolus, produced a fall of approximately 20% in mean arterial pressure. Onset was within 1 min and duration of hypotension 20 min (Zimpfer et al 1981). The action on conduction may, however, persist for up to 5 h. Heart rate, cardiac output and pulmonary artery pressure were unaffected. Where, however, an initial bolus dose was followed by infusion, in patients with ischaemic heart disease, pulmonary artery pressure rose, suggesting myocardial depression (Bovill et al 1984).

In the anaesthetized rat verapamil was found to compare favourably with hydralazine, diazoxide and nitroprusside, producing dose-dependent hypotension without tachycardia, tachyphylaxis or rebound hypertension (Oates et al 1979).

Side-effects and contra-indications

In the presence of heart failure the drug may cause marked reduction in cardiac output. It should also be used with great caution, if at all, in patients with atrioventricular conduction abnormalities, or in those taking digitalis glycosides or β-adrenergic blockers, as dangerous degrees of heart block may occur. Adverse interaction between verapamil and a β-blocker may be of even greater significance in the presence of halothane (Kapur et al 1987).

Nifedipine

This calcium antagonist has also been used to produce hypotension during anaesthesia, and may be preferable to verapamil in that it has a less marked negative inotropic effect (van Wezel et al 1986).

Adenine compounds

Adenine is an endogenous calcium channel blocker which modifies synaptic events throughout the nervous system.

In addition to their well-known role in intracellular metabolism, these compounds have recently excited interest by virtue of their effect on both local blood flow and cardiac function (Fukunaga et al 1982). In humans under neurolept anaesthesia adenosine has been found to produce hypotension which was stable and controllable. Neither tachycardia, tachyphylaxis nor rebound hypertension was found (Owall et al 1987). The hypotensive action appears to depend largely on a fall in systemic vascular resistance with cardiac function maintained or even enhanced (Owall et al 1988a). Postganglionic sympathetic nerve activity appears to be suppressed by inhibitors of ganglionic neurotransmission (Delle et al 1988), but may not occur in the conscious subject (Biaggioni et al 1986).

Detailed haemodynamic studies in the dog indicated that adenosine triphosphate compared favourably with sodium nitroprusside relative to tachyphylaxis, coronary blood flow, myocardial oxygen consumption, circulating catecholamine levels and lactic acid production (Bloor et al 1985).

There is also evidence to suggest that adenosine-induced hypotension may not aggravate myocardial ischaemia secondary to coronary artery stenosis (Owall et al 1988b). Tissue perfusion appears to be relatively well maintained (Eintree & Carlsson 1986).

Some of these benefits may depend on a lower tendency towards increased renin release (Lagerkranser et al 1985). It has, however, been found that adenosine-induced hypotension to a mean arterial pressure of 40–45 mmHg was accompanied by a 55–65% reduction in cerebral blood flow (Newberg et al 1985). Cerebral blood flow may be further reduced by hyperventilation (Waaben et al 1989). Conversely Stange et al (1989) found cerebral blood flow to be well maintained in the pig, and Laycock et al (1986) found no significant difference between adenosine and nitroprusside in the degree to which they reduced cerebral oxygen supply. Adenosine has been found to cause marked reduction in renal blood flow (Norlen 1988, Rooney et al 1989).

The hypotensive effects of adenosine may be antagonized by xanthine derivatives, including caffeine, apparently acting peripherally (Evoniuk et al 1987).

Dosage and administration

Adenosine has usually being given intravenously in doses between 90 and 215 μg kg^{-1} min^{-1} (Owall et al 1987, Owall et al 1988b). In view of the fact that these are physiological agents probably involved in cerebral blood flow regulation, with little inherent toxicity, they may prove to be of value. There remain, however, some uncertainties regarding their effects on renal and cerebral blood flow.

Prostaglandin E$_1$

This potent vasodilator has been used to induce controlled hypotension during surgery, and has been compared in efficacy with trimetaphan (Goto et al 1982, 1985). An initial infusion rate of 150 ng kg^{-1} min^{-1} has been suggested. Again, representing a possible trend toward physiologically derived agents, it may be of future interest.

REFERENCES

Adams A P, Hewitt P B 1982 Clinical pharmacology of hypotensive agents. International Anaesthesiology Clinics 20: 95–109

Bale R, Powles A, Wyatt R 1982 I.V. Glyceryl trinitrate: haemodynamic effects and clinical use in cardiac surgery. British Journal of Anaesthesia 54: 297–301

Behnia R, Siqueira E B, Brunner E A 1978 Sodium nitroprusside-induced hypotension: effect on renal function. Anesthesia and Analgesia 57: 521–526

Bernstein L, Friesinger G C, Lichtlen P R, Ross R S 1966 The effect of nitroglycerin on the systemic and coronary circulation in man and dogs. Circulation 33: 107–116

Biaggioni I, Onrot J, Hollister A S, Robertson D 1986 Cardiovascular effects of adenosine infusion in man and their modulations by dipyridamole. Life Science 39: 2224–2236

Bisset W I K, Butler A R, Glidewell C, Reglinski J 1981 Sodium nitroprusside and cyanide release: reasons for re-appraisal. British Journal of Anaesthesia 53: 1015–1018

Bloor B C, Fukunaga A F, Ma C et al 1985 Myocardial haemodynamics during induced hypotension: a comparison between sodium nitroprusside and adenosine triphosphate. Anesthesiology 63: 517–525

Boakes A J, Knight E J, Prichard B N C 1971 Preliminary studies of the pharmacological effects of 5-1-hydroxy-2 (1-methyl-3-phenyl propyl) amino-ethyl salicyl-amide. Clinical Science 40: 18P–19P

Bovill J G, Wezel J V, Schuller J, Hoeneveld M 1984

Comparison of nitroglycerin, verapamil and nifedipine in coronorary artery surgery. British Journal of Anaesthesia 56: 804P

Brittain R T, Levy G P 1976 A review of the animal pharmacology of labetalol, a combined α and β-adrenergic blocking drug. British Journal of Clinical Pharmacology 3, Supplement 681–694

Bunemann L, Jensen K, Thomsen L, Riisager S 1987 Cerebral blood flow and metabolism during controlled hypotension with sodium nitroprusside and general anaesthesia for total hip replacement. Acta Anaesthesiologica Scandinavica 31: 487–490

Burt D E R, Verniquet A J W, Homi J 1982 The response of canine intracranial pressure to systemic hypotension with nitroglycerin. British Journal of Anaesthesia 54: 665–671

Carswell D J, Varkey G P, Drake C G 1981 Labetalol for controlled hypotension in surgery for intracranial aneurysm. Canadian Anaesthetists' Society Journal 25: 505

Casthely P A, Lear S, Cottrell J E, Lear E 1982 Intrapulmonary shunting during induced hypotension. Anesthesia and Analgesia 61: 231–235

Castro-Tavares J 1980 Direct effect of trimetaphan on the dog mesenteric artery and saphenous vein. British Journal of Anaesthesia 52: 769–771

Chamberlain J H, Swan J C, Wedley J R 1980 Hypotension and myocardial metabolism. Anaesthesia 35: 962–971

Chestnut J S, Albin M S, Gonzales-Abola E, Maroon J C 1978 Clinical evaluation of intravenous nitroglycerin for neurosurgery. Journal of Neurosurgery 48: 704–711

Chiarello M, Gold H K, Leinbach R C, Davis M A, Maroko P R 1976 Comparison between the effects of nitroprusside and nitroglycerin on ischaemic injury during acute myocardial infarction. Circulation 54: 766–773

Christensson B, Nordenfelt I, Westling H, White T 1969 Intravenous infusion of nitroglycerin in normal subjects. Scandinavian Journal of Clinical Investigation 23: 49–53

Cole P V, Vesey C J 1987 Sodium thiosulphate decreases blood cyanide concentrations after the infusion of sodium nitroprusside. British Journal of Anaesthesia 59: 531–535

Cope D H P 1979 Use of labetalol during halothane anaesthesia. British Journal of Clinical Pharmacology 8: 223S–227S

Cope D H P, Crawford M C 1979 Labetalol in controlled hypotension. Administration of labetalol when adequate hypotension is difficult to achieve. British Journal of Anaesthesia 51: 359–364

Dargie H J, Dollery C T, Daniel J 1976 Labetalol in resistant hypertension. British Journal of Clinical Pharmacology 3, Supplement 751–755

Delle M, Ricksten S E, Delbro D 1988 Pre and postganglionic sympathetic nerve activity during induced hypotension with adenosine or sodium nitroprusside in the anaesthetised rat. Anesthesia and Analgesia 67: 307–312

D'Olivera M, Sykes M K, Chakabharti M K, Orchard C, Keslin J 1981 Depression of hypoxic pulmonary vasoconstriction by sodium nitroprusside and glyceryltrinitrate. British Journal of Anaesthesia 53: 11–17

Donchin Y, Amirav B, Sahar A, Harkoni S 1978 Sodium nitroprusside for aneurysm surgery in pregnancy. British Journal of Anaesthesia 50: 849–851

Dundee J W, Lilburn J K, Moore J 1977 Attenuation of the cardiostimulatory effects of ketamine. British Journal of Clinical Pharmacology 4: 658

Edwards R C, Raftery E B 1976 Haemodynamic effects of long-term oral labetalol. British Journal of Clinical Pharmacology 3, Supplement 733–736

Eintree C, Carlsson C 1986 Effects of hypotension induced by adenosine on brain surface oxygen pressure and cortical cerebral blood flow in the pig. Acta Physiologica Scandinavica 126: 463–469

Endrich B, Franke N, Peter K, Messmer K 1987 Induced hypotension: action of sodium nitroprusside and nitroglycerine on the microcirculation. A micropuncture investigation. Anesthesiology 66: 605–613

Evoniuk G, von Borstel R W, Wurtnam R J 1987 Antagonism of the cardiovascular effects of adenosine by caffeine or 8-(P-sulfophenyl) theophylline. Journal of Pharmacology and Experimental Therapeutics 240: 428–432

Fahmy N R 1978 Nitroglycerin as a hypotensive drug during general anesthesia. Anesthesiology 49: 17–20

Fahmy N R, Gauras H P 1985 Impact of captopril on haemodynamic and hormonal effects of nitroprusside. Cardiovascular Pharmacology 7: 869–874

Fahmy N R, Soter N A 1985 Effects of trimetaphan on arterial blood histamine and systemic haemodynamics in humans. Anesthesiology 62: 562–566

Fitch W, Pickard J D, Tamura A, Graham D I 1988 Effects of hypotension induced with sodium nitroprusside on the cerebral circulation before, and one week after, the subarachnoid injection of blood. Journal of Neurology, Neurosurgery and Psychiatry 51: 88

Flaherty J T, Reid P R, Kelly D T, Taylor D R, Weisfeldt M L, Pitt B 1975 Intravenous nitroglycerin in acute myocardial infarction. Circulation 51: 132

Fukunaga A F, Flacke W E, Bloor B C 1982 Hypotensive effects of adenosine and adenosine triphosphate compared with sodium nitroprusside. Anesthesia and Analgesia 61: 273–278

Goldstein R E, Michaelis L L, Morrow A G, Enstein S E 1975 Coronary collateral function in patients without occlusive coronary artery disease. Circulation 51: 118–125

Goto F, Otani E, Kato S, Fujita T 1982 Prostoglandin E as a hypotensive drug under general anaesthesia. Anaesthesia 37: 530–535

Goto F, Otani E, Tatsushi F 1985 Antihypertensive activity and metabolic rate of prostaglandin E, in surgical patients under general anaesthesia. Prostaglandins, Leucotrienes and Medicine 18: 359–366

Graham C W, Walts L F 1979 Nitroprusside and duration of tubocurarine and pancuronium. Anaesthesia 34: 1005–1009

Grayling G W, Miller E D, Peach M J 1978 Sodium cyanide antagonism of the vasodilator action of sodium nitroprusside in the isolated rabbit aortic strip. Anesthesiology 49: 21–25

Gustafson C, Ahlgren I, Aronsen K-F, Rosberg B 1981 Haemodynamic effects of labetalol-induced hypotension in the anaesthetised dog. British Journal of Anaesthesia 53: 585–590

Gustafson C, Aronsen K F, Rosberg B 1985 Circulatory effects of haemorrhage during nitroprusside-induced hypotension. Acta Anaesthesiologica Scandinavica 29: 502–507

Haeusler G, Gerold M 1979 Increased levels of

prostaglandin-like material in the canine blood during arterial hypotension produced by Hydralazine, Dihydralazine and Minoxidil. Naunyn-Schmiedeberg's Archives of Pharmacology 310: 155–167

Haus J, Schlonleben K, Spiegel HU, Themann H 1982 Nitroprusside and nitroglycerine-induced hypotension. Effect on haemodynamics and on the microcirculation. World Journal of the Surgery 6: 241–250

Heinrich W L, Cronin R, Miller P D, Anderson R J 1977 Hypotensive sequelae of diazoxide and hydralazine therapy. Journal of the American Medical Association 237: 264–265

Henriksen L, Thorshauge C, Harmsen A et al 1983 Controlled hypotension with sodium nitroprusside. Effects on cerebral blood flow and cerebral venous blood gases in patients operated for cerebral aneurysms. Acta Anaesthesiologica Scandinavica 27: 62–67

Hill A B, De Rosayro A M, Nahrowold M L, Tait A R 1980 Vascular uptake of nitroglycerin. Anesthesiology 53: S82

Hines R, Barash P G 1989 Infusion of sodium nitroprusside induces platelet dysfunction in vitro. Anesthesiology 70: 611–615

Hoffman W E, Bergmank S, Miletich D J, Gans B J, Albrecht R F 1982 Regional vascular changes during hypotensive anaesthesia. Journal of Cardiovascular Pharmacology 4: 310–314

Howe B B, Kopia S S, Winbury M M 1977 Comparative coronary dilator and hypotensive actions of chromonar (C), Minoxidil (M), hydralazine (H), nitroprusside (NP) and nitroglycerin (NG) in pentobarbital-anesthetised dogs. Federation Proceedings 36: 986

Hunter J M 1979 Synergism between halothane and labetalol. Anaesthesia 34: 257–259

Ishikawa T, McDowall D G 1979 Differences in cerebral blood flow and cortical electrical activity during hypotension induced by trimetaphan and nitroprusside. British Journal of Anaesthesia 51: 566P

James D J, Bedford R F 1982 Hydralazine for controlled intraoperative hypotension. Anesthesia and Analgesia 61: 192–193

Joekes A M, Thompson F D 1976 Acute haemodynamic effects of labetalol and its subsequent use as an oral hypotensive agent. British Journal of Clinical Pharmacology 3, Supplement 789–793

Johnson C C 1929 The actions and toxicity of sodium nitroprusside. Archives of International Pharmacodynamics and Therapeutics 35: 480–496

Kanto J, Pakkanen H, Allonen H, Kleimola T, Mantyla R 1980 The use of labetalol as a moderate hypotensive agent in otogical operations – plasma concentrations after intravenous administration. International Journal of Clinical Pharmacology Therapy and Toxicology 18, No 5, 191–194

Kaplan J A, Dunbar R W, Jones E L 1976 Nitroglycerine infusion during coronary artery surgery. Anesthesiology 45: 14–21

Kaplan J A, Jones E L 1979 Vasodilator therapy during coronary artery surgery. Journal of Thoracic and Cardiovascular Surgery 77: 301–309

Kapur P, Matarazzo D A, Fung D M, Sullivan K B 1987 The cardiovascular and adrenergic actions of verapamil or diltiazem in combination with propranolol during

halothane anaesthesia in the dog. Anesthesiology 66: 122–129

Karlin A, Hartung J, Cottrell J E 1988 Rate of induction of hypotension with trimetaphan modifies the intracranial pressure response in cats. British Journal of Anaesthesia 60: 161–166

Kaufman L 1979 Use of labetalol during hypotensive anaesthesia and in the management of phaeochromocytoma. British Journal of Clinical Pharmacology 8: (suppl 2), 229s–232s

Khambatta H J, Stone J G, Khan E 1979 Hypertension during anesthesia on discontinuation of sodium nitroprusside-induced hypotension. Anesthesiology 51: 127–130

Khambatta H J, Stone J G, Khan E 1981 Propranolol alters renin release during nitroprusside-induced hypotension and prevents hypertension on discontinuation of nitroprusside. Anesthesia and Analgesia 60: 569–573

Khambatta H J, Stone J G, Matteo R S 1982 Effect of sodium nitroprusside-induced hypotension on pulmonary deadspace. British Journal of Anaesthesia 54: 1197–1200

Kim K C, Patdu R, Kruszynski S 1976 Effect of induced hypotension by nitroprusside on muscular blockade. Abstract of scientific papers, 1976 Annual meeting of the American Society of Anesthesiologists, San Francisco, p 571

Kling T F, Fergusson N V, Leach A B, Hensinger R N, Lane G A, Knight P R 1985 The influence of induced hypotension and spine distraction on canine spinal cord blood flow. Spine 10: 878–883

Koch G 1976 Haemodynamic effects of combined α and β-adrenoceptor blockade after intravenous labetalol in hypertensive patients at rest and during exercise. British Journal of Clinical Pharmacology 3, Supplement 725–728

Lagerkranser M, Solleui A, Irestedt L, Tidgren B, Andreen M 1985 Renin release during controlled hypotension with sodium nitroprusside, nitroglycerin and adenosine: a comparative study in the dog. Acta Anaesthesiologica Scandinavica 29: 45–49

Laycock J R, Coakham H B, Silver I A, Walter F J 1986 Changes in brain surface oxygen tension during profound hypotension induced with sodium nitroprusside or adenosine in the sheep. British Journal of Anaesthesia 58: 1422–1466

Luben V, Hempelmann G 1982 Improved deep controlled hypotension in aneurysmal surgery. Acta Neurosurgica 60: 201–214

Macnab M S, Manninen P H, Lam A H, Gelb A W 1988 The stress response to induced hypotension for cerebral aneurysm surgery: a comparison of two hypotensive techniques. Canadian Journal of Anaesthesia 35: 111–115

McLean A J, Haegele K D, Du Souich P, McNay J L 1977 Comparative evaluation of the hypotensive activity of two major metabolites of hydralazine (1-Hydrozinophthalazine). European Journal of Drug Metabolism and Pharmacokinetics 1: 17–20

McDowall D G 1980 A comparison between sodium nitroprusside and trimetaphan-induced hypotension. Acta Anaesthesiologica Belgica 31, Supplement 73–75

Mann T, Cohn P F, Holmann L, Green L H, Markis J E, Philips D A 1978 Effect of nitroprusside on regional myocardial blood flow in coronary artery disease. Results in 25 patients and comparison with nitroglycerin. Circulation 57: 732–738

Marsh M L, Shapiro H M, Smith R W, Marshall L F 1979 Changes in neurologic status and intracranial pressure associated with sodium nitroprusside administration. Anesthesiology 51: 336–338

Martin L E, Hopkins R, Bland R 1976 Metabolism of labetalol by animals and man. British Journal of Clinical Pharmacology 3, Supplement 695–710

Mason T D, Braunwald E 1965 The effects of nitroglycerin and amylnitrite on arteriolar and venous tone in the human forearm. Circulation 32: 755

Michenfelder J D, Milde T H 1988 The interaction of sodium nitroprusside, hypotension and isoflurane in determining cerebral vascular effects. Anesthesiology 69: 870–875

Michenfelder J D, Theye R A 1977 Canine systemic and cerebral effects of hypotension induced by haemorrhage, trimetaphan, halothane or nitroprusside. Anesthesiology 46: 188–195

Miletich D J, Ivankovich A D 1978 Cardiovascular effects of ganglion blocking drugs. International Anesthesiology Clinics 16: 151–170

Miller E D, Ackerly J A, Vaughan E D, Peach M J, Epstein R M 1977 The renin–angiotensin system during controlled hypotension with sodium nitroprusside. Anesthesiology 47: 257–262

Mizroch S, Yurasek M 1977 Hypotension and bradycardia following diazoxide and hydralazine therapy. Journal of the American Medical Association 237: 2471–2472

Moraca P P, Bitte E M, Hale D E, Wasmuth C E, Pontasse E F 1962 Clinical evaluation of sodium nitroprusside as a hypotensive agent. Anesthesiology 23: 193–204

Morris P J, Todd M, Philbin D 1982 Changes in intracranial pressure in response to infusions of sodium nitroprusside and trinitroglycerin. British Journal of Anaesthesia 54: 991–995

Muller H, Mark P, Gips H, Borner U, Otto O, Adams H A, Hempelmann G 1987 Effects of the calcium antagonist nimodipine on haemodynamics, gas exchange and endocrine parameters in opiate anaesthesia. Anaesthesist 36: 561–569

Murrel W 1879 Nitroglycerin as a remedy for angina pectoris. Lancet 1: 80

Nakagawa Y, Nakahara H, Chin W P, Imai S 1985 Alpha blockade and vasodilatation induced by niprodalol, aratinalol and labetalol in pithed rats. Japanese Journal of Pharmacology 39: 481–485

Newberg L A, Milde J H, Michenfelder J D 1985 Cerebral and systemic effects of hypotension induced by adenosine or ATP in dogs. Anesthesiology 68: 429–436

Norlen K 1988 Central and regional haemodynamics during controlled hypotension produced by adenosine, sodium nitroprusside and nitroglycerine. Studies in the pig. British Journal of Anaesthesia 61: 186–193

Oates H F, Stoker L M, Stokes G S 1979 Verapamil as a hypotensive agent: a comparison in the anaesthetised rat, with hydralazine, diazoxide and nitroprusside. Clinical and Experimental Hypertension 1: 473–485

Owall A, Gordon E, Lagerkranser M, Lindquist C, Rudehill A, Solleui A 1987 Clinical experience with adenosine for controlled hypotension during cerebral aneurysm surgery. Anesthesia and Analgesia 66: 229–234

Owall A, Lagerkranser M, Solleui A 1988a Effects of adenosine-induced hypotension on myocardial hemodynamics and metabolism during cerebral aneurysm surgery. Anesthesia and Analgesia 67: 228–232

Owall A, Rudehill A, Sylven C, Solleui A 1988b Influence of adenosine-induced hypotension on the canine myocardium rendered acutely ischaemic by artificial stenosis. Acta Anaesthesiologica Scandinavica 32: 328–332

Page J H, Corcoran A C, Dustan H P, Koppany T 1955 Cardiovascular actions of sodium nitroprusside in animals and hypotensive patients. Circulation 11: 188

Peach M J 1977 Renin–angiotensin system: biochemistry and mechanism of action. Physiological Reviews 57: 313–370

Pertuiset B, Ancri D, Lienhart A, Goutorbe J, Sichez J P 1980 Electrothermic reauction and clipping of ruptured intracranial saccular aneurysms under deep hypotension (MAP 50 mmHg) induced with sodium nitroprusside with reference to vascular autoregulation (series of 377 cases). Neurological Research 2(3–4): 199–216

Pettinger W A 1978 Anesthetics and the renin–angiotensin-aldosterone axis. Anesthesiology 48: 393–396

Pinaud M, Souron R, Lelausque J N, Gazeau M F, Lajat Y, Dixneuf B 1989 Cerebral blood flow and cerebral oxygen consumption during nitroprusside-induced hypotension to less than 50 mmHg. Anesthesiology 70: 255–260

Prichard B N C, Boakes A J, Thompson F D, Joekes A M 1975 Some haemodynamic effects of compound AH 5158 compared with propranolol, propranolol plus hydralazine and diazoxide: the use of AH 5158 in the treatment of hypertension. Clinical Science and Molecular Medicine 48: 97S

Rigg D, McDonagh A 1981 Use of sodium nitroprusside for deliberate hypotension during pregnancy. British Journal of Anaesthesia 53: 985–989

Romberg G P, Lordon R E, Hall W 1977 Hypotensive sequelae of diazoxide and hydralazine therapy. Journal of the American Medical Association 238: 1025

Rooney M W, Crystal G J, Salem M R, Paulissian R 1989 Influence of nifedipine on systemic and regional hemodynamics during adenosine-induced hypotension in dogs. Anesthesia and Analgesia 68: 261–269

Rosei E A, Brown J J, Lever A F, Robertson J I S, Trust P M 1975 Intravenous labetalol in severe hypertension. Lancet ii: 1093–1094

Rosei E A, Brown J J, Lever A F, Robertson A S, Robertson J I S, Trust P M 1976 Treatment of phaeochromocytoma and of clonidine withdrawal hypertension with labetalol. British Journal of Pharmacology. Supplement: 809–815

Rowe G G. Henderson R H 1974 Systemic and coronary haemodynamic effects of sodium nitroprusside. American Heart Journal 87: 83–87

Saady A 1979 Intraoperative use of diazoxide for rebound hypertension. Anaesthesia and Intensive Care 7: 383

Saarnivaara L, Klempla U M, Lindgren L 1987 Labetalol as a hypotensive agent for middle ear surgery. Acta Anaesthesiology Scandinavica 31: 196–201

Saito D, Abe Y, Tani H et al 1986 Haemodynamic effects of labetalol in the dog. Arzneimittel-Forschung/Drug Research 36: 88–91

Scott D B, Buckley F P, Drummond G B, Littlewood D G, Macrae WR 1976 Cardiovascular effects of labetalol during halothane anaesthesia. British Journal of Clinical Pharmacology Supplement 817–821

Scott D B, Buckley F P, Littlewood D G, Macrae W R, Arthur G R, Drummond G B 1978 Circulatory effects of labetalol during halothane anaesthesia. Anaesthesia 33: 145–156

Seidel S L, Allen J C, Bowers R L 1980 Mechanical and biochemical alterations of aorta induced by hydralazine hypotension. Journal of Pharmacology and Experimental Therapeutics 213: 514–519

Simpson D L, Macrae W R, Wildsmith J A, Dale B A 1987 Acute beta-adrenoreceptor blockade and induced hypotension. Anaesthesia 42: 243–248

Smith R P, Kruszyna H 1976 Nitroprusside and cyanide. British Journal of Anaesthesia 48: 396

Sood S, Jayalaxmi T S, Wijayaraghavan S, Nundy S 1987 The use of sodium nitroprusside-induced hypotensive anaesthesia for reducing blood loss in patients undergoing lienorenal shunts for portal hypotension. British Journal of Surgery 74: 1036–1038

Sosis M, Leighton D 1986 In defence of Trimetaphan for use in pre-eclampsia. Anesthesiology 64: 657–658

Spargo P M, Tait A R, Knight P R, Kling T F 1987 The effect of nitroglycerin-induced hypotension on canine spinal cord blood flow. British Journal of Anaesthesia 59: 640–647

Stanek B, Zimpfer M, Fitzal S, Raberger G 1981 Plasma catecholamines, plasma renin activity and haemodynamics during sodium nitroprusside-induced hypotension and additional beta-blockade with Bunitrolol. European Journal of Clinical Pharmacology 19: 317–322

Stange K, Lagerkranser M, Rudehill A, Solleui A 1989 Effects of adenosine-induced hypotension on cerebral blood flow and metabolism in the pig. Acta Anaesthesiologica Scandinavica 33: 199–203

Strunin L 1975 Organ perfusion during controlled hypotension. British Journal of Anaesthesia 47: 793–798

Sury M R, Donaldson M D, Stringer M, Vesey C J, Cole P V 1988 Cardiovascular actions of trimetaphan nitroprusside. Comparison with sodium nitroprusside in greyhounds. British Journal of Anaesthesia 60: 797–802

Talseth T, McNay J L, Haegele K D 1982 Hypotensive effects of the hydralazine-acetone hydrazone in conscious rabbits: evidence for its back-conversion to hydralazine in vivo. Journal of Cardiovascular Pharmacology 4: 370–374

Todd M M, Morris P J, Moss J, Philbin D M 1982 Haemodynamic consequences of abrupt withdrawal of nitroprusside or nitroglycerin following induced hypotension. Anesthesia and Analgesia 61: 261–266

Toivonen J, Virtanen H, Kaukinens 1989 Deliberate hypotension induced by labetalol with halothane, enflurane or isoflurane for middle ear surgery. Acta Anaesthesiologica Scandinavica 33: 283–289

Torbati D 1986 Effect of propranolol on cortical electrical activity in conscious and anaesthetised rats. Neuropharmacology 25: 1251–1254

Tountas C J, Georgropolos A I, Kiyriakon K V, Marxos A A 1965 The effect of sodium nitroprusside on coronary circulation. Journal of Cardiovascular Surgery 6: 100

Trust P M, Rosei E A, Brown J J et al 1976 Effect of blood pressure, angiotensin II and aldosterone concentrations during treatment of severe hypertension with intravenous

labetalol: comparison with propranolol. British Journal of Clinical Pharmacology 3, Supplement 799–803

Tsai S C, Adamik R, Hom B E, Manganielle V C, Moss J 1986 Effects of nitroprusside on the bradykinin responsiveness of human fibroblasts. Molecular Pharmacology 30: 274–278

Tsui A, Maekawa K, Chen B, Liang C S 1982 The role of the sympathetic nervous system in hydrazaline-induced hypotension. Clinical Research 30: 227A

Turner J M, Powell D, Gibson R M, McDowall D G 1977 Intracranial pressure changes in neurosurgical patients during hypotension induced with sodium nitroprusside or trimetaphan. British Journal of Anaesthesia 48: 419–425

Van Aken H, Puchstein C, Hidding J 1982 The use of labetalol in producing deliberate hypotension and its effect on intracranial pressure in dogs. Acta Anaesthesiologica Belgica 33: 5–12

Vance J P, Brown D M, Smith G, Thorburn J 1979 Effect of hypotension induced with sodium nitroprusside on canine arterial flow. British Journal of Anaesthesia 51: 297–301

Van Wezel H B, Bovill J B, Schuller J, Gielen J, Hoeneveld M H 1986 Comparison of nitroglycerin, verapamil and nifedipine in the management of arterial pressure during coronary artery surgery. British Journal of Anaesthesia 58: 267–273

Vazeery A K, Skeie S, Anda O 1983 Changes in cardiac output and systemic arterial pressure after insertion of acrylic cement during trimetaphan, sodium nitroprusside and glycerol trinitrate-induced hypotension. British Journal of Anaesthesia 55: 783–790

Vesey C J, Cole P V, Linnell J C, Wilson J 1974 Some metabolic effects of sodium nitroprusside in man. British Medical Journal 2: 140–142

Vesey C J, Cole P V, Simpson P J 1976 Cyanide and thiocyanate concentrations following sodium nitroprusside infusion in man. British Journal of Anaesthesia 48: 651–660

Voss G I, Katona P G, Dauchot P J 1985 Effectiveness of sodium nitroprusside as a function of total peripheral resistance in the anesthetised dog. Anesthesiology 62: 130–134

Waaben J, Husum B, Hansen A J, Gjedde A 1989 Regional cerebral blood flow and glucose utilization during hypocapnic and adenosine-induced hypotension in the cat. Anesthesiology 70: 299–304

Wang H H, Lin L M P, Katz R 1977 A comparison of the cardiovascular effects of sodium nitroprusside and trimetaphan. Anesthesiology 46: 40–48

Westenskow D R, Meline L, Pace N L 1987 Controlled hypotension with sodium nitroprusside: anaesthesiologist versus computer. Journal of Clinical Monitoring 3: 80–86

Wildsmith J A W, Drummond G B, Macrae W R 1979 Metabolic effects of induced hypotension with trimetaphan and sodium nitroprusside. British Journal of Anaesthesia 51: 875–879

Wildsmith J A W, Marshall R L, Jenkinson J L, Macrae W R, Scott D B 1973 Haemodynamic effects of sodium nitroprusside during nitrous oxide–halothane anaesthesia. British Journal of Anaesthesia 45: 71–74

Wildsmith J A W, Sinclair C J, Thorn J, Macrae W R, Fagan D, Scott D B 1983 Haemodynamic effects of induced hypotension with a nitroprusside–trimetaphan mixture. British Journal of Anaesthesia 55: 381–389

Zimpfer M, Fitzal S, Tonczar L 1981 Verapamil as a hypotensive agent during neurolept anaesthesia. British Journal of Anaethesia 53: 885–889

Zubrow A B, Daniel S S, Stark R I, Husain M K, James L S 1988 Plasma vasopressin, renin and catecholamines during nitroprusside-induced maternal and fetal hypotension in sheep. Pediatric Research 24: 73–78

24. Clinical pharmacology of the β-adrenoceptor and calcium channel blocking drugs

S. M. Lyons

THE β-ADRENOCEPTOR BLOCKING DRUGS

The particular properties of this group of drugs have been of interest to pharmacologists, physicians and anaesthetists since their introduction. Their effects are demonstrable in both patients and healthy volunteers and their blood concentrations can now be readily measured.

The adrenoceptors were classified by Ahlquist (1948) into two groups designated α and β. The current concepts of the distribution and response of the receptors when activated are shown in Table 24.1 (see also chapter 16). Sympathetic or α-stimulation of the receptors in vascular smooth muscle produces vasoconstriction and a subsequent rise in the arterial blood pressure. α-Adrenergic receptors are widely distributed and are responsible for chronotropic, inotropic and dromotropic effects on the heart and also for the dilation of arterioles in skeletal muscles. The first compound shown to produce blockade of β-adrenoceptors was dichloroisoprenaline, though it was not used clinically because of its associated unacceptable tachycardia (Moran & Perkins 1958). Pronethalol was studied for a limited period in patients but propranolol was the first β-adrenoceptor blocking drug to be used widely in clinical practice, and is now the standard drug in this group against which all others are compared (Table 24.2).

Table 24.1 Distribution α- and β-receptors and their response to stimulus

Organ	Receptor	Response type
Heart		
Conduction	β_1	Increase
Contractility	β_1	Increase
A.V. Conduction	β_1	Increase
Blood vessels		
Coronary	β_2	Dilation
Skeletal Muscles	β_2	Dilation
Skin	α	Constriction
Viscera	α	Constriction
Lung		
Bronchi	β_2	Dilation
Kidney	β_1	Renin release
Eye	α	Pupil dilation
Uterus		
Contraction	α	Contraction
Relaxation	β_2	Relaxation
Adipose tissue	β_1	FFA release
Liver	β_2	Glycogenolysis
Pancreas	β_2	Insulin release

Pharmacodynamics

As well as blockade of β-receptors, some of these drugs may have additional features such as membrane-stabilizing activity, partial agonist activity and cardioselectivity. Only the cardioselectivity has been clearly demonstrated in humans, and the other properties are of little significance (Shanks 1983).

Cardioselectivity

Lands and his colleagues (1967) suggested that β-adrenoceptors could be subdivided into two groups, β_1 and β_2. The receptors mediating excitatory responses were classified as β_1, and those mediating inhibitory

Table 24.2   Available β-adrenoceptor blocking drugs and their properties

Drug	Proprietary name	Potency ratio	Intrinsic sympathetic activity	Cardio selectivity	Elimination	Half-life (h)
Acebutalol	Sectral	0.3	+	+	Non-renal	2.9
Alprenolol	Aptin	0.3	+	−	Non-renal	2.7
Atenolol	Tenormin	1	−	+	Renal 40%	6.1
Bisoprolol		4	−	+	Renal 50%	10.0
Metoprolol	Betaloc, Lopressor	1	−	+	Non-renal	3.2
Nadolol	Corgard	1	−	−	Renal 40–70%	14.1
Oxprenolol	Trasicor	0.5–1	+	−	Non-renal	1.6
Pindolol	Visken	6	+	−	Renal 50%	2.2
Practolol	Eraldin	0.3	+	+	Renal mostly	11.0
Propranolol	Inderal	1	−	−	Non-renal	2.6
Sotalol	Beta-Cardone, Sotacor	0.3	−	−	Renal 75%	14.0
Timolol	Blocadren	6	−	−	Non-renal	4.9

responses, β_2. This concept was confirmed by the introduction of the drug, practolol, which blocked the β_1 effects, but had much less effect on β_2-receptors (Dunlop & Shanks 1968). Practolol inhibited the cardiac effects of isoprenaline but had little effect on its bronchodilator or vasodilator activity (Brick et al 1968, Powles et al 1969). These actions of the β-adrenoceptor blocking drugs are summarized in Tables 24.1 and 24.6.

Examples of drugs which block both β_1- and β_2-receptors are propranolol, oxprenolol and sotalol, while cardioselective drugs are practolol, metoprolol, atenolol and bisoprolol (Pritchard 1987).

Partial agonist activity

Several of the β-adrenoceptor blocking drugs — pindolol, alprenolol and oxprenolol — have partial agonist activity, sometimes described as intrinsic sympathomimetic activity (ISA). This property is difficult to demonstrate in humans, but studies comparing the effects of a range of doses of a number of different drugs with and without agonist activity have shown a difference in resting heart rate and this gives a measure of the partial agonist activity. It is suggested that drugs with this property have a lower incidence of the undesirable side-effects of some of the β-blockers, such as

bradycardia, heart failure, cold extremities and bronchospasm (Marshall et al 1976).

Membrane-stabilizing activity

Propranolol has membrane-stabilizing activity, potent local anaesthetic properties and also demonstrates class II anti-arrhythmic properties. Drugs in this class reduce sympathetic stimulation of the heart, thereby decreasing myocardial oxygen demand and blocking the action of catecholamines on cardiac tissue.

Assessment of β-adrenoceptor blocking properties

All β-adrenoceptor blocking drugs competitively inhibit the effect of agonists such as isoprenaline at β-adrenoceptor sites, and the ability to inhibit this normal isoprenaline tachycardia can be used to assess the activity of these drugs. The disadvantage of this method is that it is non-physiological and provides no information about the effects of β-blocking drugs on endogenous sympathetic activity. However, β-adrenoceptor blocking drugs do reduce exercise tachycardia, and this can be used to give a quantitative test of the adequacy of the block and for comparison between drugs (Harron et al 1981). The inhibition of exercise tachycardia can be used only to compare the potency of non-cardioselective drugs. It has been shown that non-cardioselective β-adrenoceptor blocking drugs inhibit both isoprenaline tachycardia and an exercise-induced tachycardia, while cardioselective drugs have much less effect on isoprenaline-induced tachycardia (Brick et al 1968, de Plaen et al 1976).

General effects of β-adrenergic receptor blocking drugs

There are many potent β-receptor blocking drugs and while they differ in certain respects such as their partial agonist or intrinsic sympathomimetic activity, their membrane-stabilizing activity and the selectivity of their action at different β-receptors, they have several effects in common.

Effects on cardiovascular system

In general the β-receptor blocking drugs produce a fall in heart rate and cardiac output, with concurrent fall in systolic arterial pressure and left ventricular work. These effects are accentuated in exercise. In high concentrations propranolol has a direct membrane-stabilizing effect on the myocardium.

Effects on respiratory system

Sympathetic stimulation is associated with broncho-dilatation mediated via β₂-adrenergic receptors. The administration of non-selective β-blocking drugs may lead to a rise in airway resistance. This is particularly undesirable in patients suffering from respiratory conditions such as asthma or bronchitis. This side-effect in the earlier β-blocking drugs encouraged the development of drugs which are cardioselective, i.e. which have a relatively much greater effect on the β_1-receptors found in the myocardium than on the β_2-receptors found in the lungs and elsewhere. Practolol was the most cardioselective β-blocking drug discovered, but other drugs such as acebutalol, atenolol and metoprolol are now in use with minimal respiratory effects. If, in therapeutic doses, they do produce a significant increase in airway resistance, this can more readily be reversed by isoprenaline or a selective β_2-agonist drug such as salbutamol, as their beneficial effects on bronchial tone are relatively unaffected. Despite all the advantages of selectivity of action of these β_1-blocking drugs, all β-adrenergic blocking drugs may precipitate asthmatic attacks; β-blocking drugs are therefore contra-indicated in asthmatic patients.

Effects on the central nervous system

β-Adrenergic blocking drugs may produce effects within the brain leading to a decrease in sympathetic activity and so to a fall in blood pressure. This is most likely in drugs with a high lipid solubility such as propranolol and alprenolol which readily enter the brain tissue. Administration of propranolol, oxyprenolol and timolol may also be associated with the side-effects of vivid dreams, hallucinations, nightmares and depression. These drugs share the property of high lipid-solubility and therefore may accumulate in the brain, whereas drugs such as atenolol and sotalol with low lipid solubility rarely cause such side-effects.

Side-effects

The β-adrenergic blocking drugs have several undesirable side-effects both minor and major. They are largely typified by propranolol (Table 24.7). In certain circumstances propranolol is actively contra-indicated. The properties important in the choice of drugs that are presently available are shown in Table 24.6, from which it is possible to ascertain the most appropriate drug for different circumstances.

Pharmacokinetics of the β-adrenoceptor blocking drugs

The pharmacokinetics of these drugs will be dealt with under the headings of absorption, bioavailability, lipid solubility, protein binding, elimination and duration of action. These have been extensively reviewed by Johnsson (1976) and McDevitt (1987).

Absorption and bioavailability

Most β-adrenoceptor blocking drugs are quickly and fully absorbed by mouth with peak plasma concentrations occurring within 3 h. Nadolol and atenolol, with only 50% absorption after oral administration, are exceptions to this.

There is marked variation in the oral bioavailability of β-blocking drugs due mainly to the hepatic metabolism of the drugs before entry into the systemic circulation (Table 24.3). The greater the ability of the liver to extract the drug, the less is its subsequent bioavailability. Alprenolol and propranolol are most affected by this first-pass metabolism and their bioavailabilities are of the order of 10–30%. However, the process also affects metoprolol, oxprenolol and timolol. Atenolol and nadolol also have reduced

Table 24.3 Bioavailability

Degree	Drug	Cause
Least	Alprenolol	First-pass effect
	Propranolol	First-pass effect
Low	Metoprolol	First-pass effect
	Oxprenolol	First-pass effect
	Timolo	First-pass effect
	Atenolol	Poor absorption
High	Bisoprolol	Good absorption
	Sotalol	Good absorption
	Practolol	Slow metabolism

bioavailability due to their incomplete absorption rather than the first-pass effect. In contrast, sotalol, bisoprolol and practolol are well absorbed, are unaffected by metabolism and so have a high bioavailability. Drugs with marked first-pass effects have increased bioavailability when taken with food.

β-Adrenoceptor blocking drugs eliminated by hepatic metabolism have large variations in plasma concentration (Shand 1975). Doses of drugs which are subject to early metabolism need to be adjusted to produce the desired effect in individual patients. In the elderly, in whom the hepatic blood flow and function are decreased, the liver metabolism of propranolol is impaired so that higher plasma concentrations occur in chronic dosage (Castleden & George 1979).

Lipid solubility and plasma protein binding

As mentioned above, there is considerable variation in lipid solubility between the different drugs of this group. These differences, which are summarized in Table 24.4, are not directly related to their chemical structure or pharmacological properties (Shanks 1983).

The rank order of lipid solubility is also generally the same as that for protein binding, those with the greatest lipid solubility also having the highest degree of protein binding. However, this is not a direct influence, since metoprolol, pindolol and timolol with the same lipid solubility have markedly different protein binding.

Table 24.4 Lipid solubility and protein binding

Greatest	Least
Propranolol	Atenolol
	Sotalol
Alprenolol	Practolol
	Nadolol

Drug elimination

The method of elimination of β-adrenoceptor blocking drugs appears to be related to their degree of lipid solubility. The lipid-soluble group which undergo first-pass liver metabolism are also eliminated by this mechanism. These include alprenolol, metoprolol, propranolol and oxprenolol (Table 24.5). The non-lipid-soluble drugs practolol, atenolol and sotalol, in contrast, are unaffected by the liver and excreted unchanged by the kidneys. Acebutalol, pindolol, bisoprolol and timolol are excreted by both routes.

Table 24.5 Elimination

First-pass	Kidney	Mixed
Alprenolol	Practolol	Acebutalol
Metoprolol	Atenolol	Bisoprolol
Propranolol	Sotalol	Pindolol
Oxprenolol		Timolol

The elimination rate of the drugs from the plasma, expressed as the plasma half-life, shows that the drugs which are extensively metabolized in the liver have the shortest half-life — 2–4 h — while those which are excreted by the kidney have the longest half-life — 10–20 h. Alterations in liver and renal function interfere with drug elimination and alter these values (Berglund et al 1980, Kirch et al 1981). In disease of these organs the drug schedule must be reviewed, needing to be decreased in renal disease, while the effects of liver disease are variable (Williams & Mamelop 1980).

Duration of action

When the β-adrenoceptor blocking drugs were introduced, they were prescribed at 6–8-hourly intervals on the basis of plasma elimination half-lives of 3–4 h for propranolol and oxprenolol (Table 24.2). It has been suggested that drugs with a longer half-life should be prescribed less frequently (McDevitt & Shanks 1977). Slow, delayed, sustained release or long-acting formulations of β-blocking drugs with short half-lives have now become available to allow once- or twice-daily dosage (Leahey et al 1980, Kerr et al 1981, Harron & Shanks 1981).

To provide symptomatic control in patients with angina pectoris, drugs need to have both an adequate and sustained plasma level. Those with short half-lives should be administered every 6–8 h while the longer-acting drugs can be given once daily. However, in the treatment of hypertension the administration of the total daily dose of the short-acting drugs given once daily will control raised arterial pressure throughout the 24 h period (Douglas-Jones et al 1978, Frick & Kala 1980). The possible disadvantages of this regime are that the peak plasma level will be higher and will occur at 2–3 h after administration with an increased incidence of adverse side-effects at that time.

A recently introduced short-acting β-blocker, Esmolol, with a half-life of 9 min, has been used in anaesthesia to control tachycardia. Its use appears to be safe and it has interesting possibilities in this field (Menkhaus et al 1985).

Clinical uses of β-adrenergic blocking drugs

β-Adrenergic blocking drugs are used in the treatment of:

1. Cardiovascular disorders — hypertension, angina following myocardial infarction and a variety of arrhythmias.
2. Endocrine disorders such as hyperthyroidism and with α-blockers in the treatment of phaeochromocytoma. Propranolol enhances the stimulation of growth hormone releasing factor by dextroamphetamine.
3. Migraine.
4. Intention tremor.
5. Chronic simple glaucoma.
6. Some psychiatric disorders.

The following discussion of the particular properties of propranolol, practolol, metoprolol, acebutalol and oxprenolol as examples of the different types of β-adrenergic blocking drugs, illustrates the effects of these drugs and their indications and contra-indications.

Propranolol

$$O - CH_2 - CH\ CH_2 - NH - CH(CH_3)_2$$
$$|$$
$$OH$$

Propranolol is a non-cardioselective β-blocking drug and its use is indicated in a large number of medical conditions (Table 24.7). The dosage varies from 10 mg orally twice daily for cardiac arrhythmias to 320 mg orally per day in severe systemic hypertension and angina pectoris. Small doses, 0.25–5 mg, are used intravenously in anaesthetized patients to control hypertension, tachycardia and arrhythmias. Propranolol is contra-indicated in second- or third-degree heart block, in patients with a tendency to bronchospasm, prolonged fasting and metabolic acidosis. Propranolol should be used with special care in patients with a poor cardiac reserve. The use of the drug should be terminated gradually, otherwise there may be a rebound phenomenon of the condition under treatment. Caution must be exercised when transferring a patient who is under treatment with clonidine to a β-adrenoceptor blocking

Table 24.7 Indication for use of propranolol

Essential and renal hypertension
Angina pectoris
Prophylaxis after myocardial infarction
Cardiac arrhythmias
Migraine prophylaxis
Essential tremor
Thyrotoxicosis and thyrotoxic crisis
Hypertrophic obstructive cardiomyopathy
Phaeochromocytoma

Table 24.6 Summary of actions of β-blocking drugs

	Non-cardioselective	β_1 Selective
With intrinsic sympathetic activity–partial agonist	Oxyprenolol Alprenolol Pindolol	Acebutalol Practolol
Without intrinsic sympathetic activity	Propranolol Timolol Sotalol Nadolol	Metoprolol Atenolol

drug if the patient is receiving β-blockers and clonidine at the same time. Clonidine should be withdrawn only after the β-blockers have been stopped for several days. Patients on β-blockers should only be given class I anti-arrhythmic drugs such as disopyramide with caution, as the combination may cause unacceptable positive inotropic effects. Propranolol should also be used cautiously with drugs such as verapamil in patients with impaired left ventricular function and in patients with conduction abnormalities. The use of either drug intravenously within 48 h of stopping the other is potentially hazardous.

Anaesthesia

The use of propranolol in anaesthetized patients may cause a dangerous bradycardia, especially when agents with vagal effects are already being utilized, and notably if they also have negative chronotropic effects.

Side-effects

Propranolol is usually well tolerated. Minor side-effects include cold extremities, nausea, insomnia, lassitude, di-

Table 24.8 Propranolol side-effects

Minor	Major	Contraindication
Bradycardia Weakness	Chronic heart failure in patients with diminished cardiac reserve	Bronchial asthma Second- or third-degree heart block
Lethargy	Bronchospasm (asthmatics)	Chronic heart failure
Gastrointestinal upset	Hypoglycaemia	
	Aggravation of arterial insufficiency	Brittle diabetes mellitus
	Nightmares	
	Insomnia	
	Hallucinations	
	Depression	
	Hyperglycaemia	
	Hyperosmolar coma	

arrhoea, paraesthesia of hands and unpleasant dreams. Less acute effects include skin rashes and dry eyes. Propranolol is also available as a long-acting preparation formulated with a sustained release coating (Inderal LA).

Practolol

$$NH_2-CO-CH_3$$

$$O-CH_2-CH-CH_2-NH-CH(CH_3)_2$$
$$|$$
$$OH$$

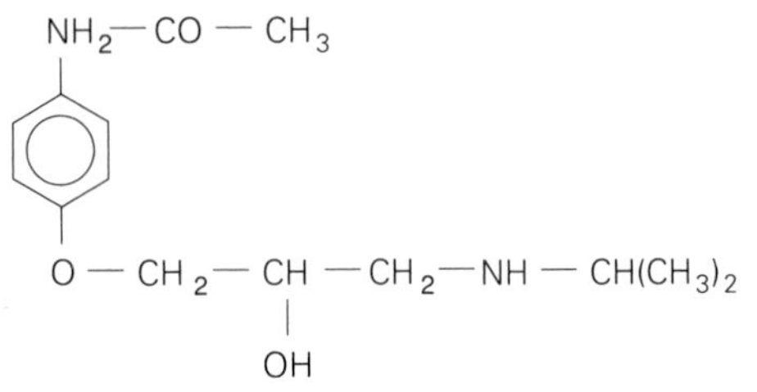

This is a cardioselective β-adrenoceetor blocking drug which unfortunately on prolonged oral therapy was found to have serious adverse effects — the practolol oculomucocutaneous syndrome. This syndrome occurred only after at least 24 months of oral therapy, but its occurrence dictated that the oral preparation of the drug should be withdrawn. The syndrome has never been reported after short-term intravenous therapy, and so the intravenous preparation has been retained for emergency use. Practolol is recommended for use in the treatment of cardiac arrhythmias caused by excessive sympathetic activity along with organic disease, especially the post-infarction arrhythmias. The dose used during general anaesthesia is 2–10 mg given slowly intravenously. Practolol is contra-indicated in patients with second- or third-degree heart block and in metabolic acidosis. It should be used with caution in patients with chronic obstructive airways disease which may be worsened with the drug. As with propranolol, practolol should be used with care in the presence of class I anti-arrhythmic drugs and in patients receiving verapamil.

Side-effects

The severe oculomucocutaneous syndrome has been referred to, but the use of the drug is also associated with nausea, sleep disturbance, paraesthesia and constipation. In a few patients there is drug intolerance as evidenced by serious bradycardia and hypotension. Overdose of the drug may be treated with either atropine or isoprenaline.

Metoprolol

$$CH_3OCH_2CH_2 \longrightarrow \bigcirc \longrightarrow OCH_2 \underset{H}{\overset{OH}{\underset{|}{\overset{|}{C}}}} CH_2NHCH \overset{CH_3}{<}_{CH_3}$$

This cardioselective drug is used in the treatment of hypertension, angina pectoris, cardiac arrhythmias, especially supraventricular tachyarrhythmias, thyrotoxicosis and post-myocardial infarction. In the latter usage it is associated with decreased infarct size, fewer arrhythmias, especially ventricular fibrillation; and pain relief. The dose of metoprolol ranges from 50 mg twice daily for arrhytmias to 400 mg daily in hypertension. Metoprolol is contra-indicated in atrioventricular block and in heart failure refractory to digitalis. It should be used with caution in the diabetic when the insulin dosage may need adjustment. It is relatively safe to use in the asthmatic patient.

Side-effects

The side-effects are usually mild, with lassitude, gastro-intestinal disturbance and sleep change being most common. Metoprolol is also available as an intravenous preparation. As Betaloc A it is also available as a long-acting preparation with slow-release properties.

Acebutalol

$$O\text{-}CH_2\text{-}CH(OH)\text{-}CH_2\text{-}NH\text{-}CH(CH_3)_2$$

$$\bigcirc \overset{C \nearrow^O}{\underset{CH_3}{}}$$

$$NHCOCH_2\text{-}CH_2\text{-}CH_3$$

Acebutalol is a cardioselective β-adrenoceptor blocking drug. It reduces exercise tachycardia, lowers the blood pressure in hypertension and has anti-arrhythmic properties. It also has partial agonist or intrinsic sympathomimetic activity which tends to balance the negative chronotropic and inotropic effects of the drug. Acebutalol also blocks the effect of excessive catecholamine stimulation in stressful situations. The dosage is

up to 20 mg given intravenously for cardiac arrhythmias, and in treatment of angina or hypertension 200–400 mg may be given orally twice a day.

Indications

Acebutalol is indicated in all grades of hypertension, angina pectoris and for the control of tachyarrhythmias.

Contra-indications

Acebutalol is absolutely contra-indicated in cardiogenic shock where there is a systolic blood pressure of less than 100 mmHg. It is also contra-indicated in atrioventricular block, marked bradycardia and uncontrolled heart failure. Acebutalol should not be used in association with verapamil, or until several days after its withdrawal. Acebutalol tends to accumulate in severe renal failure, and it should also be used carefully in chronic obstructive airways disease. The insulin dosage in the diabetic may need to be adjusted if the patient is also receiving acebutalol. This drug has a low lipid solubility and so there is less chance of sleep disturbance, depression or undesirable central nervous system effects.

Oxprenolol

$$\bigcirc \overset{O-CH_2-\overset{OH}{\underset{|}{CH}}-CH_2-NH-CH \overset{CH_3}{<}_{CH_3}}{\underset{O-CH_2-CH=CH_2}{}}$$

Oxprenolol exerts its greatest effects on the heart; causing bradycardia and thus reducing both its work and its myocardial oxygen consumption. This is particularly useful in blocking the catecholamine stimulation associated with stress. Oxprenolol has some partial agonist activity which tends to balance the negative chronotropic and inotropic effects of the drug. It also has an antihypertensive effect, although how this is produced is debatable; it is either by decreasing the cardiac output or the peripheral resistance, but effects on plasma-renin and the central nervous system may also be factors. Oxprenolol is used in the treatment of angina, hypertension, sympathetic-induced cardiac arrhythmias, in anxiety and anxiety-induced tachycardia. It may also be useful in the treatment of hypertrophic obstructive cardiomyopathy, in the treatment of thyrotoxicosis and in arrhythmias associated with anaesthesia. The dosage required is usually 40–100 mg orally three times per day. It is compatible with glyceryl trinitrate. Its sudden withdrawal may be associated with rebound angina. The slow intravenous administration of up to 2 mg has been used in the treatment of arrhythmias associated with anaesthesia.

Side-effects

Occasional dizziness, drowsiness, headache, insomnia, excitement and gastrointestinal upset have been described, and excess bradycardia and thrombocytopaenia have also occurred. Bronchospasm and ventricular failure can occur in susceptible individuals, and skin rashes and dry eyes have been described, but their incidence is low.

Contra-indications

Oxprenolol is contra-indicated in atrioventricular block, marked bradycardia, uncontrolled ventricular failure and cardiogenic shock. It should be used cautiously when there is evident ventricular decompensation, when the heart rate is below 50 and in metabolic acidosis. It may also mask the symptoms of hyperglycaemia and should not be used along with calcium-channel blocking drugs such as verapamil. Oxprenolol, when used during pregnancy, can cause the fetus to be born with a bradycardia.

Overdose

Oxprenolol overdosage may be treated with intravenous isoprenaline 2 μg intravenously. Glucagon and bronchodilators may also be required.

Esmolol

Esmolol is a recently introduced β-adrenergic blocking drug whose unusual pharmacokinetic properties should give it an essential place in anaesthesia and critical-care medicine, where a rapidly controllable effect is required.

Pharmacodynamics

Esmolol is relatively selective for β$_1$-receptors. It does have some effect on β$_2$-receptors, but much less than propranolol. There is little or no partial agonist or intrinsic sympathomimetic activity, but also little cardiac depressant or local anaesthetic action. Its cardiac electrophysiological effects are similar to other β-blockers.

The peak effects of esmolol occur rapidly, within 6–15 min, and also disappear rapidly, within about 20 min (depending on the dose) on stopping infusion (Benfield & Sorkin 1987). Effects are proportional to the logarithm of the blood concentration, and so the rapid onset and end to its effects are related to its pharmacokinetic properties, described below.

Cardiovascular system

Effects are similar to other β-adrenergic blocking drugs, but unlike these which may potentiate cardiac depressant effects of some anaesthetic and other drugs in a prolonged manner, esmolol may be safer as its effects terminate rapidly. Esmolol has been used successfully to attenuate the haemodynamic responses to laryngoscopy and tracheal intubation, and also to mediastinal and aortic dissection in cardiac surgery; several studies have shown it to be effective in reducing both tachycardia and hypertension. Other areas in which it may be used include control of tachyarrhythmias and myocardial protection following myocardial infarction.

Respiratory system

The effects of a selective β$_1$-blocker are less than a nonselective drug such as propranolol, but esmolol does cause a small increase in airways resistance in asthmatic subjects (Sheppard et al 1986), and should be used with caution.

Pharmacokinetics

Esmolol is used by intravenous infusion. It is distributed rapidly (t$_{\frac{1}{2}}$ approximately 2 min, Vd 3.5 l kg^{-1}), and also is rapidly eliminated. Its rapid clearance from the body is its major unique feature. This is due largely to rapid metabolism with a half-life of 9 min (range 5–15.8 min, Sum et al 1983). This high rate of metabolism suggests that it is mainly metabolized at extrahepatic sites, probably by an esterase in the blood (Reynolds et al 1986). Its major metabolite is excreted much more slowly, but it is relatively inactive and not likely to be of clinical importance. Only 1% of esmolol is excreted unchanged.

Dosage and administration

The range of infusion rates generally used is between 25 and 300 $\mu g\ kg^{-1}\ min^{-1}$ esmolol. In most studies there is little increase in response at above 200 $\mu g\ kg^{-1}\ min^{-1}$. The dose may be titrated; for example giving a loading infusion at a rate of 500 $\mu g\ kg^{-1}\ min^{-1}$ for 1 min, reducing to the maintenance rate. The maintenance rate is then increased in steps of 50 $\mu g\ kg^{-1}\ min^{-1}$ to a maximum of 300 $\mu g\ kg^{-1}\ min^{-1}$, each step being preceded by a further 1 min loading dose at 500 $\mu g\ kg^{-1}\ min^{-1}$.

Side-effects and precautions

These are similar to those with other β-adrenergic blockers.

THE CALCIUM CHANNEL BLOCKING DRUGS

The development of the group of drugs which interfere with the entry of calcium into cells, the calcium blockers or antagonists, has provided an opportunity for the study of the role of calcium in both pathological and non-pathological states. The drugs are a heterogeneous group of compounds with dissimilar structures and electrophysiological effects. They can be classified into several groups: papaverines, dihydropyridines, benzothiazepines, piperazines and miscellaneous. There are three main drugs clinically available with uses principally in the cardiovascular field — verapamil (papaverine group), nifedipine (dihydropyridine) and diltiazem (benzothiazepine). Other drugs which achieve their effects by action at the calcium channel are prenylamine (miscellaneous group), perhexiline maleate and lidoflazine (piperazine). Experience with these latter drugs is restricted and in some cases adverse side-effects are common.

ROLE OF CALCIUM

The intracellular calcium concentration is crucial to its actions and it needs a binding protein to regulate these actions (Cheung 1970). This binding protein, calmodulin, is folded into four matching parts, each of which has a calcium binding site of either glutamate or aspartate amino acids. Calmodulin in conjunction with calcium and cyclic AMP is interlinked in the cellular autoregulatory processes. The calmodulin calcium complexes activate adenyl cyclase and phosphodiesterase which hydrolyse both ATP and cyclic AMP, and also activates the calcium pump which returns a raised intracellular calcium to its resting level. The calcium

antagonist verapamil may act by inhibiting calmodulin (Fleckenstein 1983).

Calcium is essential for muscle contraction in the process of excitation contraction coupling. Skeletal muscle contraction is initiated by depolarization and the electrical changes in the plasma membrane of the muscle are then followed by the release of calcium from the lateral sarcoplasmic reticulum. This released calcium binds to troponin C and initiates a series of interactions among muscle proteins to cause muscle contraction. During the contraction of smooth muscle calmodulin mediates the effects of calcium rather than of troponin.

The source of activation of the calcium ions in skeletal muscle is different from that in cardiac muscle. In cardiac muscle the sarcoplasmic reticulum is sparse and highly sensitive to changes in extracellular calcium. A high proportion of intracellular calcium interchanges with extracellular calcium. The action potential of cardiac muscle is triggered from the spontaneously depolarizing sino-atrial node. The fast inward current is carried by sodium and is followed by a plateau due to a second slower inward current carried by calcium (Fig. 24.1). The outward current is carried by potassium. The stored calcium which triggers the excitation–contraction coupling is largely that which en-

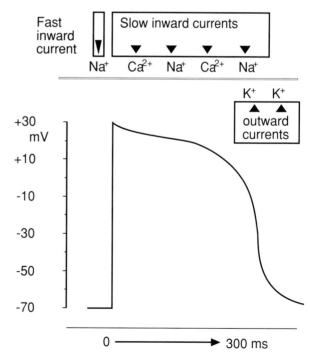

Fig. 24.1 Ventricular action potential and associated ion fluxes.

ters during the plateau phase of the previous action potential.

Calcium also plays the central role in synaptic and neuromuscular transmission. The release of acetylcholine is not a direct action but calcium is an essential intermediary. The possibility therefore exists for the potentiation of the effects of neuromuscular blocking drugs by calcium blocking drugs (see Chapter 34).

The inhibition of calcium uptake by the myocardial cells not only depresses myocardial contractility but is associated with a fall in heart rate and decreased responsiveness to sympathetic stimulation. These factors all reduce the myocardial oxygen requirements. They also cause vasodilation, mostly on the arterial side, though this is associated with only mild hypotension. The fall in peripheral resistance with the calcium blockers leads to an increase in sympathetic activity which to some extent neutralizes the negative inotropic effects of the drugs. Blockade of this compensatory mechanism releases the negative peripheral and central effects, leading to a fall in blood pressure and heart rate. These effects, along with a central amine depletion effect associated with sedation, are beneficial in angina. An increase in the size of the coronary arteries has been demonstrated in dogs, and this property has been responsible for some of the major clinical uses of nifedipine — the treatment of angina pectoris. Verapamil has a major use as an anti-arrhythmic agent when used in low doses. Thus, calcium antagonists have a place in the treatment of arterial hypertension, angina and supraventricular tachyarrhythmias. They have the same spectrum of application as β-adrenergic blockers. They are especially indicated in the treatment of hypertension in patients with Raynaud's phenomenon (Smith and McKendry 1982), asthma and cardiac conduction abnormalities, and may indeed become first-line treatment for all hypertension.

CALCIUM BLOCKERS AND ANAESTHETIC AGENTS

The most important effects of calcium for the anaesthetist are its effects on excitation–contraction coupling in heart muscle and visceral smooth muscle, its effects of sinus and atrial node activity and transmitter release and also its effect on synaptic transmission. This leads to important interaction with the volatile anaesthetic agents (Reves 1984) and possibly the neuromuscular blocking drugs.

Halothane, enflurane and isoflurane may all to some extent be regarded as calcium blockers. Their myocardial depression is due to an alteration in the calcium flux and patients exposed to both calcium blockers and inhalation agents may demonstrate additive effects. Nifedipine and isoflurane have little effect on myocardial contractility, but both cause peripheral vasodilation and potential hypotension. Verapamil impairs conduction and contractility in larger doses. Halothane also reduces myocardial contractility and conduction so the combination of verapamil and halothane may accentuate both effects (Hantler et al 1983). They also interact with neuromuscular blocking drugs because acetylcholine release is instigated by calcium ions (Carpenter & Mulroy 1983). It has been suggested that patients receiving calcium blockers require less neuromuscular blocking drugs and should have the degree of neuromuscular block carefully monitored (Jones 1984, Reves et al 1982).

Patients treated with calcium blocking drugs should continue this medication up to the time of surgery, and the patients should be monitored for possible additive effects with inhalation agents and the neuromuscular blocking drugs. Sudden withdrawal of calcium antagonists may lead to a severe worsening of anginal symptoms (Subramanian et al 1983).

Insulin secretion is controlled by the influx of calcium ions, and calcium antagonists may affect glucose tolerance.

Calcium ions also participate in platelet function and other aspects of haemostasis. They may also cause an increase in cerebral blood flow and so cause a rise in the intracranial pressure.

Verapamil

Verapamil is chemically closely related to papaverine. It is used as a racemic mixture of d- and l-optical isomers. The relative effects of the d- and l-isomers differ.

Verapamil reversibly blocks transmembrane ionic flow through calcium channels (Fleckenstein 1977, Haeusler 1972). It prolongs conduction in the atrioventricular node, making re-entry mechanisms impossible. It is therefore used in such conditions as the Wolff–Parkinson–White syndrome and its variants. Primary slowing of pacemakers also occurs, so that a serious tachycardia is reduced and there is suppression of nodal and ventricular ectopic activity. The slowing of conduction through the atrioventricular node regularizes the ventricular response to atrial flutter and fibrillation. Verapamil can be used in association with digoxin if the ventricular response is still too rapid (Klein et al 1979).

Verapamil is an anti-arrhythmic agent in low doses but in higher doses it also has negative inotropic effects which may cause rhythm disturbances. Thus it is contra-indicated in the presence of β-adrenoceptor blocking drugs because the combination may lead to cardiac failure (Kenny 1985).

Pharmacokinetics

After oral administration the drug is rapidly and almost completely absorbed (Schomerus et al 1976). It is subject to extensive first-pass hepatic extraction to leave a bioavailability of 10–20%. Most of the drug (70%) is excreted in the urine as conjugated metabolites and only 5% is eliminated unchanged. No cumulation occurs with long term usage.

Dosage

Verapamil may be given intravenously as a bolus dose of up to 10 mg (0.075–0.20 mg kg^{-1}) in 1–2 min, or orally 40–120 mg 8 hourly.

Side-effects

The action of verapamil on the conducting system, the ventricular muscles and the peripheral vascular tissue causes a slight fall in blood pressure and blockade of the atrioventricular and sino-atrial nodes. In chronic administration dizziness, headache and constipation have been reported. Massive overdose can be treated with calcium and myocardial pacing (Da Silva et al 1974).

Contra-indications

Verapamil is contra-indicated in advanced atrioventricular block, in pronounced ventricular function depression, in patients receiving anti-adrenergic drugs and in advanced hepatic dysfunction (Kieval et al 1980).

Nifedipine

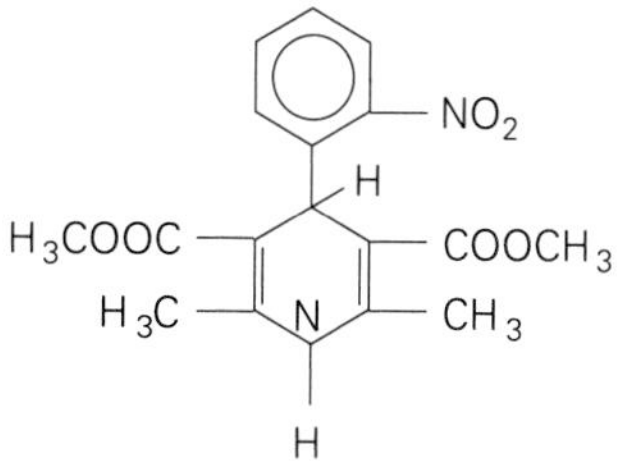

Nifedipine is a dihydropyridine derivative. It is sensitive to light.

Nifedipine is a potent inhibitor of transmembrane calcium flux in both the myocardium and vascular smooth muscle. Unlike verapamil and diltiazem it lacks local anaesthetic activity. It produces a reduction of the myocardial oxygen demands by restricting cardiac metabolism and by afterload reduction, as evidenced by a fall in blood pressure and by peripheral vasodilation. Its potent coronary vasodilator effects also increase the myocardial oxygen supply. It is therefore widely used in the prophylaxis and treatment of established and vasospastic angina pectoris and in hypertension, and it has been used in the treatment of cardiac failure and pulmonary oedema. It may also be useful in hypertrophic cardiomyopathy, acute myocardial infarction and in pulmonary hypertension.

Pharmacokinetics

Nifedipine is rapidly and almost completely absorbed after oral administration, appearing in the plasma in 2–3 min after ingestion. The first-pass liver extraction is small and the systemic bioavailability is of the order of 65%.

It is 90% bound to plasma protein. The majority of the drug (85%) is excreted in the urine and 15% from the gastrointestinal tract with an elimination half-life of about 5 h (Ebner 1976, Horster 1975) and there is no cumulation.

Dosage

The drug can be given orally in 10–20 mg doses every 6–8 h.

Side-effects

Nifedipine is well tolerated and safe (Ebner 1976). It is associated with headache in about 6% of patients and also sometimes with feelings of warmth, flushing, dizziness, palpitation and hypotension. Nausea and vomiting occur in about 3% of patients but there are no renal, hepatic, haemopoietic or immunological effects.

Diltiazem

This drug has not been as extensively studied or used as either verapamil or nifedipine. It is an antagonist of the slow calcium channel, lowers the action potential plateau, depresses the contractility of canine ventricular myocardium and has some negative inotropic effects. It has been found to increase significantly the coronary collateral blood flow in ischaemic myocardium and is also effective in preventing the coronary arterial spasm associated with alkalosis on exercise. It has also been found, like nifedipine, to be effective in the treatment of anginal symptoms and coronary spasm (Rosenthal et al 1980). It may also be effective in the treatment of patients with stable angina on exertion.

Pharmacokinetics

Diltiazem is a benzothiazepine derivative. It has rapid and complete absorption after oral administration with prominent first-pass effect (Eichizen and Eichelbaum 1986). It appears in the plasma after 15 min with a half-life of 4 h. The drug is 80% bound to the plasma proteins and much of the drug appears to be excreted unchanged.

Dosage

The drug is given orally in doses of 120–240 mg daily.

Side-effects

The drug is well tolerated but it is associated with headache, dizziness, flushing and gastrointestinal upset similar to verapamil.

Other calcium channel blocking drugs

Of the newer calcium channel blocking drugs being evaluated, most are dihydropiridine derivatives — *amlodipine, felodipine, nicardipine, nisoldipine* and *nitrendipine* — and many have increased effects on peripheral vasculature. Nicardipine and amlodipine are in clinical use at the time of writing.

Nicardipine causes coronary vasodilatation but has no appreciable effect on conduction tissue and so can be used in patients with conduction defects. It is administered in doses of 20–40 mg 8 hourly. It is closely related to nifedipine but may have less depressant effect on the compromised left ventricle (Turner, Feely and Barret 1986).

Amlodipine has a 24 hour action, so that it requires only one daily dosage regime for control of hypertension (Mroczek et al 1988) and angina (Gottlieb 1988).

Phenylalkylamines such as methoxyverapamil and teapamil, both related to verapamil, may have some advantages over verapamil (Feely et al 1988).

REFERENCES

Ahlquist R P 1948 A study of adrenoceptor receptors. American Journal of Physiology, 153: 586–600

Benfield P, Sorkin E M 1987 Esmolol: a preliminary review of its pharmacodynamic and pharmacokinetic properties, and therapeutic efficacy. Drugs 33: 392–412

Berglund G, Descamps R, Thomis J A 1980 Pharmacokinetics of sotalol after chronic administration to patients with renal insufficiency. European Journal of Clinical Pharmacology 18: 321–326

Brick I, Hutchison K J, McDevitt D G, Roddie I C, Shanks R G 1968 Comparison of the effects of ICI 50,172 and propranolol on the cardiovascular responses to adrenaline, isoprenaline and exercise. British Journal of Pharmacology 34: 127–140

Carpenter R L, Mulroy M F 1986 Lidocaine-pancuronium and verapamil-pancuronium neuromuscular blockade in cats. Anesthesiology 65: 605–610

Castleden C M, George C F 1979 The effect of ageing on the hepatic clearance of propranolol. British Journal of Clinical Pharmacology 7: 49–54

Cheung W Y 1970 Cyclic 3′,5′-nucleotide phosphodiesterase. Demonstration of an activator. Biochemical and Biophysical Research Communications 38: 533–538

Da Silva O A, De Melo R A, Filho J P 1974 Verapamil acute self poisoning. Clinical Toxicology 14 (4): 361–367

dePlaen J F, Amery A, Reybrouck T 1976 Comparative potency of atenolol and propranolol as beta adrenergic blocking agents in man. European Journal of Clinical Pharmacology 10: 297–303

Douglas-Jones A P, Baber N S, Lee A 1978 Once daily propranolol in the treatment of mild to moderate hypertension. European Journal of Clinical Pharmacology 14: 163–166

Dunlop D, Shanks R G 1968 Selective blockade of adrenoceptor beta receptors in the heart. British Journal of Pharmacology 32: 201–218

Ebner F 1976 Survey and summary of results obtained during the world-wide clinical investigations of Adalat (nifedipine). In Lochner W et al (eds) New therapy of ischaemic heart disease. Springer, Berlin, pp 348–360

Eichizen H, Eichelbaum M 1986 Clinical pharmacokinetics of verapamil, nifedipine and diltiazem. Clinical Pharmacokinetics 11: 425–429

Feely J, Pringle T, Maclean D 1988 Thrombolytic treatment and new calcium antagonists. British Medical Journal 296: 705–708

Fleckenstein A 1977 Specific pharmacology of calcium in myocardium, cardiac pacemakers and vascular smooth muscle. Annual Review of Pharmacology and Toxicology 17: 149–166

Fleckenstein A 1983 History of calcium antagonists. Circulation Research 52 (Supplement 1): 13–16

Frick M H, Kala R 1980 Once daily versus twice daily beta blockers. Effects on arrhythmias and hypertension. Lancet ii: 588

Gottlieb S O 1988 Circadian patterns of myocardial ischaemia and therapeutic considerations. Journal of Cardiovascular Pharmacology 1988 Suppl 7 s18–s21

Guarascio P, D'Amato C, Sette P, Conte A, Visco G 1984 Liver damage from verapamil. British Medical Journal 288: 362

Hantler C B, Felbeck P G, Kroll D A, Knight P R 1983 Effects of verapamil on sinus and AV nodal function in the presence of volatile anaesthetics. Anesthesiology Suppl 59: A38

Harron D W G, Shanks R G 1981 Comparison of the duration of effect of metoprolol and a sustained release formulation of metoprolol (Betaloc-SA). British Journal of Clinical Pharmacology 11: 518–520

Harron D W G, Balnave K, Kinney C D, Wilson R, Russell C J, Shanks R G 1981 Effects on exercise tachycardia during forty-eight hours of a series of doses of atenolol, sotalol and metoprolol. Clinical Pharmacology and Therapeutics 29(3): 295–302

Haeusler G 1972 Differential effect of verapamil on excitation–contraction coupling in smooth muscle and on excitation–secretion coupling in adrenergic nerve terminals. Journal of Pharmacology and Experimental Therapeutics, 180: 672–682

Horster F A 1975 Pharmacokinetics of nifedipine ^{14}C in man. In Lochner W, Braasch W, Kroneberg G. (eds) Second international Adalat symposium. Springer Verlag, New York, pp: 124–127

Johnsson G 1976 Use of beta adrenoceptor blockers in combination with beta stimulators in patients with obstructive lung disease. Drugs 11 (Supplement 1): 171–177

Johnsson G, Svedmyr N, Thiringer G 1975 Effects of intravenous propranolol and metoprolol and their interaction with isoprenaline on pulmonary function, heart rate and blood pressure in asthmatics. European Journal of Clinical Pharmacology 8: 175–180

Jones R M 1984 Calcium antagonists. Anaesthesia 39: 747–749

Kenny J 1985 calcium channel blocking agents and the heart. British Medical Journal 291: 1150–1152

Kerr M J, Harron D W G, Kinney C, Shanks R G 1981 Comparison of the beta adrenoceptor blocking activity of oxprenolol, slow release oxprenolol and a combined oxprenolol diuretic preparation. British Journal of Clinical Pharmacology 12: 869–876

Kieval J, Kirsten E B, Kessler L et al 1980 Effects of intravenous verapamil on haemodynamic states of patients receiving propranolol. Circulation 62 (Supplement 111): 87

Kirch W, Kohler H, Mutschler G, Schafer M 1981 Pharmacokinetics of atenolol in relation to renal function. European Journal of Clinical Pharmacology 19: 65–71

Klein H O, Pauzner H, Disegni E et al 1979 The beneficial effects of verapamil in chronic atrial fibrillation. Archives of Internal Medicine, 139: 747–749

Lands A M, Luduena F P, Buzzo H J 1967 Differentiation of receptor systems responsive to isoproterenol. Life Sciences 6: 2241–2249

Leahey W H, Neill J D, Varma M P S, Shanks R G 1980 Comparison of the efficacy and pharmacokinetics of conventional propranolol and a longacting preparation of propranolol. British Journal of Clinical Pharmacology 9: 33–40

Marshall A J, Roberts L J C, Barritt D W 1976 Raynaud's phenomenon as side effect of beta blockers in hypertension. British Medical Journal i: 1498–1499

Menkhaus P, Reves J, Kissen I et al 1985 Cardiovascular effects of esmolol in anaesthetised humans. Anesthesia and Analgesia 64: 327–334

McDevitt D G, Shanks R G 1977 Evaluation of once daily sotalol administration in man. British Journal of Clinical Pharmacology 4: 153–156

McDevitt D G 1987 Comparison of pharmacokinetic properties of beta-adrenoceptor blocking drugs. European Heart Journal 18 (Suppl M): 9–14

Moran H C, Perkins M E 1958 Adrenergic blockade of the dichloro analogue of isoproterenol. Journal of Pharmacology and Experimental Therapeutics 124: 223–237

Mroczek W J, Burris J F, Allenby K S 1988 A double blind evaluation of the effect of amlodipine on ambulatory blood pressure in hypertensive patients. Journal of Cardiovascular Pharmacology 12 Suppl 7: s79–s84

Powles R, Shinebourne E, Hamer J 1969 Selective cardiac sympathetic blockade as an adjunct to bronchodilation therapy. Thorax 24: 616–618

Prichard B N C 1987 Bisoprolol: a new beta-adrenoceptor blocking drug. European Heart Journal 8 Suppl 4: 121–129

Reves J G 1984 The relative hemodynamic effects of Ca^{++} entry blockers. Anesthesiology 61: 3–5

Reves J G, Kissin I, Lell W A, Tosone S 1982 Calcium entry blockers: uses and implications for anesthesiologists. Anesthesiology 57: 504–518

Reynolds R D, Gorczynski R J, Quon C Y 1986 Pharmacology and pharmacokinetics of esmolol. Journal of Clinical Pharmacology 26 (Supplement A): A3–A14

Rosenthal S J, Ginsberg R, Lamb I H, Bairn D S, Schroeder J S 1980 Efficacy of diltiazem for control of symptoms of coronary artery spasm. American Journal of Cardiology 46: 1027–1032

Schomerus M, Spiegelhalder B, Stieren B et al 1976 Physiological disposition of verapamil in man. Cardiovascular Research, 10: 605–612

Shanks R G 1983 Clinical pharmacology of beta adrenoceptor blocking drugs. In: Morselli P L (ed.) Laboratories d'etudes et de recherches scientifiques. Raven Press, New York, pp: 73–78

Sheppard D, DiStefano S, Byrd R C et al 1986 Effects of esmolol on airway function in patients with asthma. Journal of Clinical Pharmacology 26: 169–174

Smith C D, McKendry R J R 1982 Controlled trial of nifedipine in treatment of Raynaud's phenomenon. Lancet, ii: 1299–1301

Subramanian V B, Bowles M J, Khurmi N S, Davies A B, O'Hare M J, Raftery E B 1983 Calcium antagonist withdrawal syndrome: objective demonstration with frequency-modulated ambulatory ST segment monitoring. British Medical Journal 286: 520–521

Sum C Y, Yacobi A, Kartzinel R, et al 1983 Kinetics of esmolol, an ultra-short-acting beta blocker, and of its major metabolite. Clinical Pharmacology and Therapeutics 34: 427–434

Turner P, Feely J, Barret J 1986 Nicardipine: a new calcium antagonist. British Journal of Clinical Pharmacology 22 Suppl 3: 191–352

Williams R L, Mamelop R D 1980 Hepatic damage and drug pharmacokinetics. Drugs 5: 528–547

25. Management of hypertension

J. P. Alexander

THE HYPERTENSIVE PATIENT

Some impression of the importance of hypertension as a cause of death can be gleaned from the fact that in the Framingham (Massachusetts) prospective study, 37% of men and 51% of women who died of cardiovascular disease had been noted previously to have had an arterial blood pressure greater than 140/90 mmHg on at least three occasions. Ninety-five per cent suffered from idiopathic or 'essential' hypertension. The mortality of these subjects was more than twice that of those with a normal arterial pressure. Most deaths occurred with no warning, and were attributed to coronary artery disease which is not so readily controlled by treatment of hypertension. There had, however, been dramatic proof in the 1950s that reduction of blood pressure in malignant hypertension was life-saving, and recent trials in the United States and in Australia indicate that the death rate from coronary disease, stroke, and heart failure in the mild hypertensive (diastolic 90–105 mmHg) can be reduced by 20%. This has important implications since it suggests that perhaps 15–20% of the adult population in developed countries might be candidates for treatment. The Medical Research Council Trial (1985) compared a diuretic to a β-blocker; although the incidence of stroke was reduced, coronary events and mortality were not affected. Many physicians adopt a less aggressive attitude in treating elderly subjects, in whom there is as yet no good controlled evidence of benefit, and in whom side-effects are common (Sleight 1983). On the other hand, a recent European trial suggested that elderly patients should be regarded as a 'high-risk group', and although overall mortality was not affected, there was a reduction of stroke and cardiac mortality (Amery et al 1985). In general, the results of the several large-scale trials are in agreement that drug treatment of mild hypertension in men and women under 80 is worth while, aiming for a diastolic blood pressure of 85–90 mmHg (Swales et al 1989). Overtreat-

ment may increase mortality (Beevers 1988) and in any case, the cumulative experience of the large trials suggests little or no decrease in coronary events (Heagerty 1988).

Attitudes towards the management of anaesthesia and surgery in the hypertensive patient have tended to sway from one extreme to another.

There was ample evidence from the first half of the century to support the idea that patients with heart disease or hypertension were poor operative risks (Prys-Roberts 1979a) and that hypertensive heart disease constituted an unjustifiable risk. When drug therapy for hypertension was introduced in the early 1950s, reports of adverse responses to anaesthetic, operation and electroconvulsive therapy in hypertensive patients began to appear. High incidences of bradycardia and hypotension were reported when anaesthesia was administered to patients receiving reserpine, and with the advent of more potent antihypertensive drugs, fears were expressed that cardiovascular homeostasis would be adversely affected during anaesthesia and operation. In the late 1960s and early 1970s, a series of elegant papers from Oxford demonstrated that the uncontrolled hypertensive is subject to considerable risk (Prys-Roberts 1979b) and the opinion that antihypertensive agents should be discontinued before elective surgery under general anaesthesia was gradually discarded (Foëx 1978). The risk of cardiovascular accidents as a result of withholding some antihypertensive agents was established and, in addition, the cardiovascular state of treated hypertensive patients was shown to be more stable during anaesthesia than that of the untreated hypertensive (Prys-Roberts et al 1971a).

Hypertensive episodes will cause a marked increase in myocardial oxygen requirement and may be a greater threat to the myocardium than hypotension (Prys-Roberts et al 1971b). It is thus illogical to discontinue antihypertensive medication, and it may be safer to treat hypertensive patients and bring the arterial pressure back to near normal before elective surgery. On the other hand, Goldman and his colleagues (1977) did not consider hypertension as a cardiac risk index, although factors such as recent myocardial infarction, congestive failure, ECG abnormalities and frequent ventricular ectopic beats could all be related to pre-existing hypertension.

The same workers (Goldman and Caldera 1979) considered that elective surgery in the absence of ideal antihypertensive therapy need not subject patients to an added clinical risk provided that the diastolic pressure is stable and not higher than 110 mmHg, and that intraoperative and recovery room blood pressure values are closely monitored and treated to prevent hypertensive or hypotensive episodes. These workers pointed to the increased risk of postoperative hypertensive crises in patients with past histories of high blood pressure. The importance of haemodynamic monitoring in the perioperative period has been emphasized (Goldman 1983).

The sympathetic reflex provoked by stimulation of the epipharynx and laryngopharynx during intubation causes increases in blood pressure and heart rate which are usually transitory, variable and unpredictable. That this sympathetic stimulation is not necessarily benign has been confirmed by Fox and colleagues (1977), who reported two cases, one of whom developed pulmonary oedema and ultimately survived, while the other suffered fatal rupture of a cerebral aneurysm. Prys-Roberts and co-workers (1971b) recommended the prophylactic use of β-adrenergic receptor blockers to modify or prevent this reflex; Siedlecki (1975) found practolol to be ineffective. Farnon and Curran (1981) reported a case of near death following acute pretreatment with practolol prior to induction of anaesthesia. Simpson and colleagues (1987) considered that acute β-adrenoreceptor blockade for induced hypotensive anaesthesia could produce excessive bradycardia. An alternative approach would be to minimize stimulation of the pharynx and larynx. In a small number of cases, blind nasal intubation aided by 10% carbon dioxide evoked no pressor response (Prys-Roberts et al 1971a) but the induced hypercapnoea may depress the heart in the presence of β-blockade (Foëx & Prys-Roberts 1974). Treated hypertensive patients responded in a more favourable manner to lumbar or thoracic extradural anaesthesia and subsequent light general anaesthesia than did untreated hypertensive patients (Dagnino & Prys-Roberts 1984).

Further work by Stone and colleagues (1988) has confirmed the value of pretreatment with a β-adrenoreceptor blocking drug (in this case atenolol) in reducing the risk of myocardial ischaemia. It is planned to market esmolol, an ultra-short-acting β-adrenoceptor antagonist

(half-life about 9 min) in the UK in 1990 (personal communication, Du Pont). It may prove to be a valuable adjunct in the critical-care situation for treating supraventricular tachycardias, tachycardias due to surgical stimulation such as endotracheal intubation, and perhaps as a postoperative antihypertensive.

Further studies by Prys-Roberts indicated that the transient sympathetic overactivity in hypertensive patients following noxious stimuli such as laryngoscopy was accompanied by raised plasma levels of adrenaline and noradrenaline (Low et al 1986). Hypertension and ischaemic heart disease are likely to increase morbidity and mortality in patients presenting for anaesthesia and surgery, particularly if a dramatic rise in arterial pressure is allowed. A combination of tachycardia and hypertension causes a major increase in myocardial work and oxygen demand which may lead to ischaemia, particularly in the subendocardial layer of the myocardium. Suppression of noxious stimuli by the use of local anaesthetics at the site of the stimulus, high doses of analgesic drugs, use of β-receptor blocking drugs to prevent increases in myocardial work, and reduction of left ventricular ejection load by vasodilator agents are all possible therapeutic manoeuvres.

Pre-existing therapy with β-adrenoceptor antagonists, maintained up to and including the morning of surgery, has been shown to be effective in suppressing the haemodynamic response to laryngoscopy and intubation, and the subsequent responses to surgical stimulation (Prys-Roberts 1984)

The increasing use of calcium channel antagonists in the therapy of hypertension introduces another area of concern for the anaesthetist, particularly as halothane, enflurane and isoflurane may themselves be considered non-specific calcium antagonists. Volatile anaesthetics and calcium antagonists influence myocardial contractility, systemic vascular resistance and atrioventricular nodal conduction. There is similarity between the cardiovascular effects of nifedipine and isoflurane on the one hand, and verapamil and halothane on the other. Both nifedipine and isoflurane have minor influence on contractility and conduction, but markedly reduce systemic vascular resistance. Verapamil, however, significantly impairs cardiac conduction and contractility as does halothane, so that exposure to both drugs may give additive effects in terms of both myocardial depression and the risk of heart block.

Diltiazem probably has less influence on contractility and atrioventricular nodal conduction than verapamil, and less effect on systemic vascular resistance than nifedipine (Mizgala 1983).

The decrease in contractility produced by calcium antagonists is more amenable to antagonism with calcium than are the effects on the atrioventricular node and systemic vasculature (Jones 1984). As with the β-blockers, withdrawal of calcium antagonists prior to surgery may increase the number of interventions required, and also increases the risk of 'rebound' phenomena (Casson et al 1984).

The problem, then, is to choose the best anaesthetic agent or technique while maintaining drug therapy. Agents which increase sympathetic activity (cyclopropane, diethyl ether) should be avoided. Methyoxyflurane, trichlorethylene and enflurane, in combination with β-blockers, impair myocardial performance and cause a rise in peripheral vascular resistance (Saner et al 1975, Horan et al 1976; Roberts et al 1976a, Roberts et al 1976b). Halothane alone, halothane and nitrous oxide, or isoflurane in combination with beta-blockade, do not have an adverse effect on the cardiovascular system (Prys-Roberts 1975, Horan et al 1977, Foëx 1983), whereas the combination of halothane and verapamil may produce impressive myocardial depression.

ANTIHYPERTENSIVE TREATMENT

Despite advances in the understanding of the various mechanisms involved in the control of systemic blood pressure, drugs used in the treatment of hypertension have largely evolved empirically. Currently available hypotensive agents act by interfering with normal homeostatic mechanism, and this provides a useful basis for classifying drugs (Table 25.1), although the site and mechanism of action of individual drugs do not always allow for such simple classification.

Diuretics and β-adrenergic blocking agents are the first- and second-line drugs used in the treatment of hypertension, although asthma, heart failure and vascular disease are important contra-indications for the latter. For many years the only α-blockers available were phentolamine and phenoxybenzamine, which were non-specific in their effect; only phenoxybenzamine could be given by mouth and its side-effects of postural hypotension, tachycardia, drowsiness, nasal congestion and failure of ejaculation gave α-blockers a bad reputation. The newer α-blocking agents prazosin and indoramin, which act more specifically at α_1 receptors, have revived interest in their use as third-line drugs or for patients in whom β-blocking drugs are unsuitable. Other third-line agents are hydralazine, methyldopa or debrisoquine. For very resistant patients, diazoxide or minoxidil may be considered; the high incidence of induced diabetes, nausea and hypertrichosis (hirsutism) with diazoxide makes it difficult to control and

Table 25.1 Classification of antihypertensive drugs

Central adrenergic blocking agents	Methyldopa, Clonidine, Guanabenz, Guanfacine
α-Adrenergic receptor antagonists	Prazosin, Labetalol, Indoramin, Phentolamine, Phenoxybenzamine
Vasodilator drugs	Hydralazine, Endralazine, Diazoxide, Minoxidil
Adrenergic neuron-blocking agents	Guanethidine, Debrisoquine, Guanadrel, Bethanidine, Reserpine, Guancydine
Ganglion-blocking agents	Pentolinium, Trimetaphan
Angiotensin-converting enzyme (ACE) inhibitors	Captopril, Enalapril
Calcium channel antagonists	Verapamil, Nifedipine, Diltiazem, Nicardipine (Chapter 24)
Diuretics	Chapter 27
β-Adrenergic receptor antagonists	Propranolol and analogues (Chapter 24)
Serotonin antagonists	Ketanserin

minoxidil may be preferred. The latter does not cause nausea or diabetes but sodium retention and hirsutism are likely to be problems. The angiotensin converting enzyme (ACE) inhibitors, captopril and enalapril, are increasingly becoming third-line agents, while the calcium channel blockers verapamil, nifedipine and diltiazem are proving to be useful alternatives to vasodilators. Newer converting enzyme inhibitors and calcium channel blockers are being investigated or already available, and will undoubtably revolutionize this approach to therapy in the next decade. It may be some time before the precise place of ACE inhibitors and calcium channel blockers is defined in the 'stepped care' approach to the management of hypertension. What is clear is that we have entered an era in which we are capable of lowering blood pressure effectively in almost all hypertensive patients. We should now be looking at the quality of life of the treated patient. The development of untoward symptoms should not be considered acceptable but should lead to appropriate modifications of the drug regimen (Chobanian 1986, Messerli 1990).

α-ADRENERGIC RECEPTOR SUBTYPES

The past decade has been the era of β-adrenergic antagonists. Because of the side-effects of diuretics and β-blockers, as well as the growing evidence that these drugs adversely affect serum lipids, the next decade is likely to see the increased use of α-adrenergic receptor blockade (Proceedings of a symposium 1983). The demarcation between α-adrenergic and β-adrenergic receptors has long been appreciated, as has the existence of β-adrenergic receptor subtypes. Recent advances in the understanding of α-adrenergic receptors have led to the realization of the existence of subtypes of α-receptors as well. It is now recognized that there are α-receptors that regulate, in an auto-inhibitory fashion, the release of noradrenaline from the nerve ending. These α-receptors, probably localized to presynaptic sites on the nerve ending, reduce the amount of noradrenaline released by nerve impulses when stimulated by noradrenaline in the synaptic cleft. When high concentrations of noredrenaline are present, subsequent nerve impulses release less noradrenaline (Fig. 25.1). A wide variety of drugs have been found to have selectively greater potency at either presynaptic or postsynaptic α-receptors (the latter mediating smooth muscle contraction) and a nomenclature analogous to that used for β-adrenergic receptors has been adopted. However, the clear-cut division of alpha receptors comparable to that used in defining β_1- and β_2-receptors has not yet been possible. Certain α-adrenergic antagonists such as prazosin and phenoxybenazmine are considered α_1 selective, rauwolscine and its diastereoisomer yohimbine (plant alkaloids) are α_2 selective, and phentolamine non-selective. Radioactively labelled biologically active

drugs (radioligand) studies and computer modelling techniques are being used to identify drugs with affinity for one or other subtype of α-receptor (Hoffman & Lefkowitz 1980).

Pharmacological studies indicate that α_1 and α_2 receptors exist at both pre- and postsynaptic peripheral sites, and a similar situation probably exists in the central nervous system (Kobinger 1983). Methyldopa and clonidine stimulate central α_2-receptors, and it has been claimed that these are postsynaptic. Centrally acting drugs tend to produce a high incidence of central nervous system side-effects, particularly drowsiness.

ANTIHYPERTENSIVE AGENTS

CENTRAL ADRENERGIC BLOCKING AGENTS

Methyldopa

Methyldopa (BP, USP), Methyldopate hydrochloride (BP, USP).
Chemical name: 3-(3,4-dihydroxyphenyl)-2-
                methyl-1-alanine sesquihydrate.
Methyldopa (α-methyldopa). The hypotensive effect of methyldopa is slightly more pronounced in the erect than in the supine position. Cardiac output falls without a change in peripheral resistance after chronic administration. There is little change in renal blood flow or glomerular filtration rate. The mechanism of action is controversial, but it is likely that central effects account for most of the hypotensive effects; methyldopa forms α-methyldopamine and α-methylnoradrenaline in central adrenergic neurons, and perfusion of animals' brains with minute doses of all these substances produces hypotension which is prevented by an α-blocker. The existing evidence suggests that methyldopa acts on postsynaptic α_2-receptors in the hind-brain, either directly or by conversion to false transmitters, thus decreasing outflow of nerve impulses from the brain, although some contribution from peripheral mechanisms cannot be excluded. Only the laevorotatory isomer is active; the dextro-isomer has no antihypertensive effect.

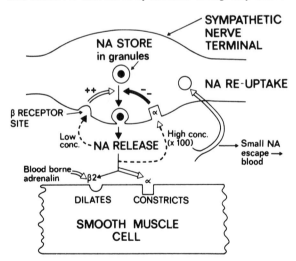

Fig. 25.1 Simplified diagram of noradrenaline (NA) release from a sympathetic nerve terminal. Feedback loops (dotted lines) control the rate of release. Low concentrations increase the rate of release while high concentrations (×100) inhibit release via the presynaptic α_2-receptor. Other feedback loops controlling noradrenaline release include angiotensin, acetylcholine, serotonin and prostaglandins. (After Langer 1976 and Sleight 1983, with permission).

Pharmacokinetics

The major metabolite is the *o*-sulphate, and its formation is dose-dependent, being greater after an oral than an intravenous dose, suggesting considerable first-pass hepatic metabolism. Unchanged drug and metabolite are excreted by the kidneys. Plasma half-life is 1.7 h, although an adequate therapeutic effect may be obtained by a single bedtime dose.

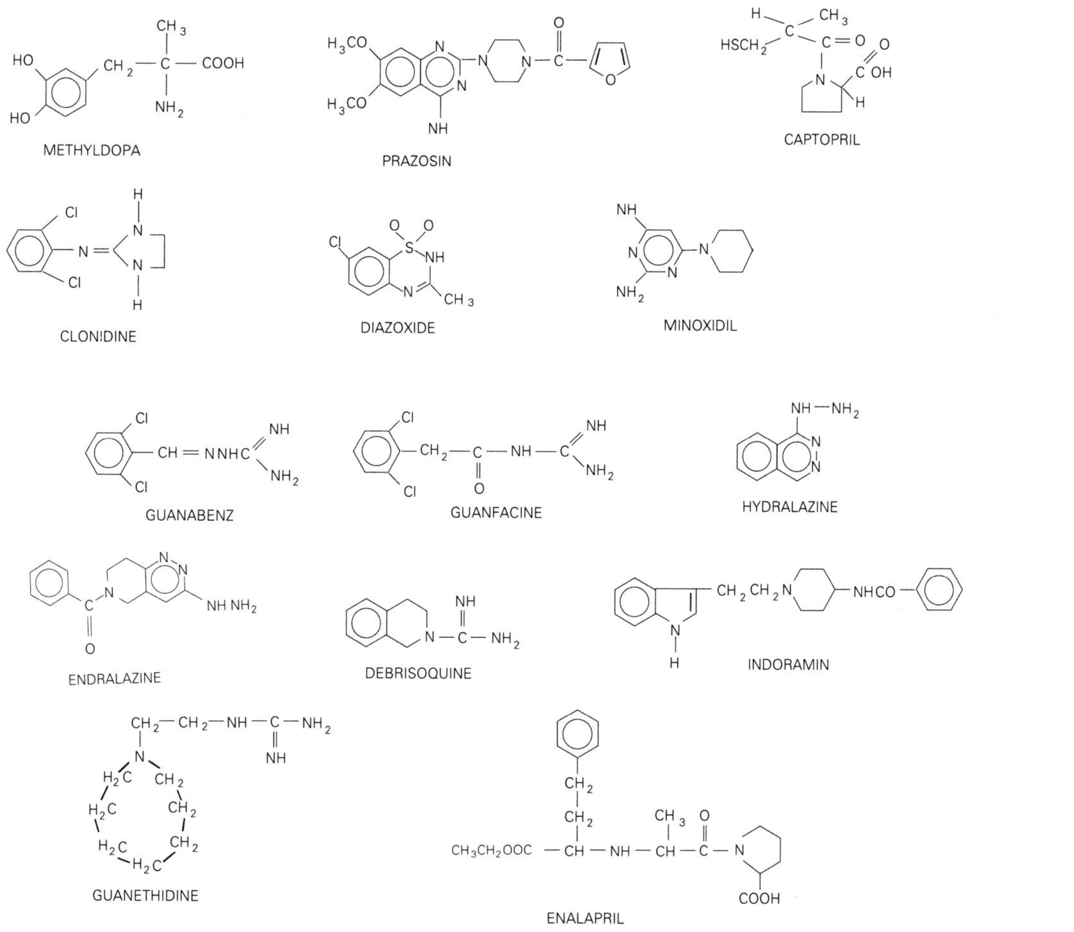

Fig. 25.2 Chemical structures of some antihypertensive drugs.

Dosage and administration

One-half to two-thirds of hypertensive patients are controlled by methyldopa in divided daily oral doses of 0.75–4 g, although the effect is not necessarily increased when daily doses exceed 1.5 g. An intravenous preparation is available for infusion in the treatment of hypertensive crises (250–500 mg 6-hourly).

Adverse effects

The decreasing popularity of methyldopa is due to the numerous side-effects it produces. These include central nervous system disturbances, sexual dysfunction, liver damage and positive Coombs' test due to production of IgG which may interfere with blood cross-matching or cause haemolytic anaemia; leucopenia, thrombocytopenia and drug fever may occur. Fluid retention can cause heart failure and there may be a mild rebound

hypertension following drug withdrawal. It might be wise to avoid the use of halothane in these patients because of the potential hepatotoxic properties of both drugs.

Clonidine

Clonidine hydrochloride (BP, USAN).
Chemical name: dichlorophenylamino-imidazoline hydrochloride.
Clonidine is a potent antihypertensive drug closely related chemically to tolazoline (an α-adrenergic blocking compound). Clonidine produces a fall in blood pressure and heart rate associated with a decreased cardiac output but unchanged peripheral resistance. It has little effect on renal blood flow or glomerular filtration rate. Renin release is decreased through a central action. Some of the cardiovascular effects of clonidine result from its

central α-agonist properties. There is a centrally mediated reduction in sympathetic activity due to its agonist effect on postsynaptic α_2-receptors in the vasomotor centre of the medulla. In dogs, administration of clonidine decreased the required anaesthetic concentration of halothane by almost 50%, an effect presumably mediated through central α-receptors.

A similar effect in humans was shown to reduce the concentration of isoflurane required to induce hypotension (Woodcock et al 1988). Both morphine and clonidine induce similar EEG behavioural and autonomic effects in dogs, probably through actions upon different receptors on the same or parallel neural pathways. Analgesia is produced in animals and humans by intravenous, intrathecal and extradural administration (Yaksh & Collins 1989).

Pharmacokinetics

Maximum effect develops at about 2 h after an oral dose or an injection, perhaps when circulating noradrenaline levels fall to a new steady state. The plasma half-life varies from 6–11 h. Sixty per cent of plasma clearance is due to renal excretion of the unchanged drug.

Dosage and administration

Clonidine is a potent drug and dosage is started at 0.05–0.1 mg 8-hourly. The dose is increased until the desired therapeutic effect is obtained, and it may be used with a diuretic or a β-blocker. An intravenous preparation is available for use in hypertensive crises, 0.15 mg by slow injection usually being effective within 30 min and the effect lasting 3–6 h. A clonidine transdermal therapeutic system is available; three strengths of clonidine patch will release either 0.1, 0.2 or 0.3 mg daily for at least a week (Anonymous 1987); these appear, however, to be accompanied by a high frequency of local allergic skin reactions.

Adverse effects

Clonidine does not produce postural hypotension or sexual difficulties. Other side-effects are common and include central nervous system effects (mainly drowsiness) dryness of the mouth, and constipation. A potentially lethal effect may occur when clonidine therapy is abruptly withdrawn. There is rebound hypertension and other symptoms associated with high levels of circulating catecholamines (anxiety, sweating, tachycardia and extrasystoles). Clonidine may increase catecholamine storage in nerve terminals by stimulating

presynaptic α-receptors, which inhibit neurotransmitter release, and when clonidine is withdrawn these stored catecholamines are released. Hypertensive crises during anaesthesia have been attributed to temporary withdrawal of clonidine. If elective surgery is required, other antihypertensive drugs should be substituted for clonidine well in advance of the procedure. Tricyclic antidepressants can nullify the effects of clonidine.

Guanabenz

Guanabenz (BAN, USAN).
Chemical name: 1-(2,6-dichlorobenzylideneamino)
                guanidine acetate.
Guanabenz is an orally active central α_2-adrenoceptor agonist with some structural similarities to clonidine. In addition to stimulation of central α-adrenoceptors, there would also appear to be a peripheral adrenergic blocking action which reduces peripheral resistance. In hypertensive patients heart rate is decreased without significant change in left ventricular stroke volume, cardiac output or ejection fraction.

Pharmacokinetics

Maximum concentrations of guanabenz in plasma (1.2–5.2 μgl^{-1}) are reached 2–5 h after administration. The drug is extensively metabolized and large amounts of metabolites are recovered in the urine in the first 24 h after a single oral dose. Guanabenz is 90% bound to plasma proteins and less than 1% excreted unchanged. The main (inactive) metabolite is (E)-p-hydroxyguanabenz.

Dosage and administration

Oral dosage begins with 4 mg twice a day increasing to a maximum of 64 mg daily.

Side-effects

The most frequent side-effects are drowsiness, dry mouth, dizziness and weakness. A withdrawal syndrome compatible with sympathetic overactivity has been described but not confirmed. Although side-effects with guanabenz are as common as with methyldopa or clonidine, major troublesome effects such as sodium retention, depression and sexual dysfunction have not been reported.

Guanfacine

Guanfacine hydrochloride (FDA approved).

Chemical name: *N*-Amidino-2-(2,6-dichlorophenyl) acetamide hydrochloride.

Guanfacine is an orally active central α_2-adrenoceptor agonist with structural similarities to guanabenz. It may be more specific then clonidine for the α_2-receptors and decreases central sympathetic tone in a similar manner. It stimulates postsynaptic α-receptors in peripheral blood vessels, so that the overall effect on mean arterial pressure is the summation of these contrary peripheral and central effects. Single-dose guanfacine administration leads to mild peripheral vasodilation and reduction in pulmonary artery pressure with little change in cardiac index.

Pharmacokinetics

The pharmacokinetic properties of guanfacine differ markedly from those of clonidine and methyldopa. Maximum concentrations in plasma ($3–12$ μgl^{-1}) are reached $1–4$ h after oral doses of $1–4$ mg. Bioavailability is 100%, the volume of distribution is large, 64% is bound to plasma proteins, and the major route of excretion involves biotransformation by the liver. Elimination half-life is $12–22$ h. Only $24–37\%$ is excreted from the kidneys. The main metabolite, 3-hydroxyguanfacine, is practically devoid of antihypertensive activity.

Dosage an administration

The initial oral dose is $0.5–1.0$ mg daily, increasing in increments of $0.5–1.0$ mg per day after 2 weeks. An average daily dose of 2 mg ($1–3$ mg) is usually adequate.

Side-effects

Since guanfacine is predominantly a centrally acting drug, the principal side-effects are dry mouth and sedation. Sudden withdrawal of the drug does not appear to lead to withdrawal syndrome or blood pressure crisis, as is described with clonidine. The reason is unclear but this may be due to the longer half-life of guanfacine (Sorkin & Heel, 1986).

α-ADRENERGIC RECEPTOR ANTAGONISTS

Prazosin

Prazosin hydrochloride (BAN, USAN).
Chemical name: (1-[4-amino-6,7-dimethoxy-2-quinazoline]-4-[2-furoxl]-piperazine.

Prazosin hydrochloride is a phosphodiesterase inhibitor which appears to act predominantly as a selective blocking agent at postsynaptic α-adrenergic receptors on vascular smooth muscle; it is thought to have relatively low affinity for presynaptic α_2-receptors. Prazosin inhibits the vasoconstriction produced by noradrenaline while the relative lack of effect on α_2-receptors allows noradrenaline to exert negative feedback control of its own release, thus reducing, though not abolishing, the cardiac stimulation that follows non-selective α-adrenergic blockade. Peripheral vascular resistance is reduced without secondary reflex tachycardia or increase in renin activity. The effect is similar, although the mechanism of action may be different, to that of nitroprusside.

Pharmacokinetics

The plasma half-life is 4 h, but blood pressure control is adequate with twice-daily dosage. The drug may be concentrated in blood vessel walls. More than 99% of the drug is metabolized and there may be a substantial first-pass effect. About $50–70\%$ of an oral dose reaches the systemic circulation. Dosage is reduced in heart failure but not in renal failure. More than 95% is protein bound; hypoalbuminaemia will increase the concentration of unbound and therefore active drug.

Administration and dosage

Treatment is started with a low dose of 0.5 mg daily increasing to a maximum of 10 mg twice daily, often in conjunction with diuretics or β-blockers.

Adverse effects

Severe hypotension, tachycardia and collapse may occur with the first dose if larger than 0.5 mg, particularly if the patient is sodium-depleted. Angina may be exacerbated, while skin rash and positive antinuclear factor occasionally occur. It appears to be less satisfactory than an ACE inhibitor in patients with chronic heart failure, probably due to fluid retention, but otherwise is a satisfactory third-line drug in the treatment of hypertension. Of all the antihypertensive drugs studied, this has produced the most consistently favourable results with respect to blood lipids and lipoproteins (many thiazide-type diuretics raise total cholesterol, triglycerides and low and very-low density lipoprotein cholesterol).

Terazosin

Terazosin is a post-synaptic α_1-adrenoceptor antagonist with a similar pharmacodynamic profile to prazosin.

The elimination half-life is 2–3 times that of prazosin, allowing once daily administration. Dosage is 1–40 mg daily.

Doxazosin

Doxazosin is another 'look alike' drug which is structurally related to prazosin, as it is to terazosin. Daily dosage is 1–16 mg.

Labetalol

Labetalol is discussed in greater detail in Chapter 24. It is primarily a β-adrenoceptor antagonist with modest α-blocking activity. The α_1-blocking properties give it a mild vasodilating action. It undergoes an extensive first-pass metabolism. Adverse reactions are similar to those of the non-selective β-blockers. It cannot be given to asthmatics without the risk of precipitating bronchospasm. The oral dose is 100 mg 8-hourly initially, increasing to 300–3000 mg daily to control blood pressure. It can be given intravenously to control hypertensive crises (see later).

Indoramin

Indoramin hydrochloride (BAN, USAN).
Chemical name: N-[-1-(2-indol-3-ylethyl)-4-piperidyl] benzamide.
Indoramin is a postsynaptic selective α_1-adrenoceptor antagonist; a 4-benz-amidopiperidine derivative, its chemical structure incorporates part of the structure of procainamide within it. Its blood pressure lowering effect results from relaxation of peripheral arterioles which is rarely associated with reflex tachycardia or postural hypotension. Best clinical response is seen when combined with a thiazide diuretic and in severe hypertension with a β-blocker.

Pharmacokinetics

Plasma concentrations of 23–126 μgl^{-1} were obtained with long-term oral therapy, depending on dosage. The bioavailability is 0.31, and since the total metabolite concentration in plasma is 10 times that of unchanged drug, there must be extensive first-pass metabolism. About 90% is plasma protein bound. Approximately one-third of the drug and metabolites can be recovered from urine. The elimination half-life is 5.5 h after oral administration.

Administration and dosage

The initial oral dose is 25 mg twice daily, and this can be increased to 200 mg daily in two or three divided doses.

Adverse effects

The most frequent side-effects are sedation, dry mouth and dizziness. Tachycardia and postural hypotension are rare. Failure of ejaculation in males is more frequently associated with higher initial doses of the drug.

Phentolamine

Phentolamine mesylate (BP, USP).
Chemical name: (3-N-(2-imidazolin-2-ylmethyl)-p-toluidine phenol-methane-sulphonate).
Phentolamine is an α-adrenergic receptor blocker, equipotent at both α_1- and α_2-receptors, with a short action. It can be used by intravenous injection in the treatment of acute left ventricular failure, in the paroxysmal hypertension associated with phaeochromocytoma, or interaction of foodstuffs with monoamine oxidase inhibitors. The dose is 5–60 mg over a period of 10–30 min or an infusion of 0.1–2 mg min^{-1} A bolus of 5 mg intravenously is used as a diagnostic test for phaeochromocytoma. Its effect on α_2-receptors in the heart probably leads to increased release of noradrenaline, with positive inotropic and chronotrophic effects which reduce its value.

Phenoxybenzamine

Phenoxybenzamine (BP, USP).
Chemical name: benzyl(2-chloroethyl)(1-methyl-2-phenoxyethyl) ammonium chloride.
Phenoxybenzamine is a long-acting α-adrenergic receptor antagonist acting mainly on α_1-receptors but with some effect on α_2-receptors, especially if the dose is large, which is used in the management of hypertensive episodes associated with phaeochromocytoma. The usual starting dose is 10 mg twice daily intravenously or intramuscularly, and this dose can be increased until the hypertensive crises of phaeochromocytoma are controlled. Concomitant β-adrenergic blockade may be necessary to control tachycardia and arrhythmias, particularly if the tumour is secreting adrenaline in addition to noradrenaline. Phenoxybenzamine is an alkylating agent, and the α-receptor blockade produced is irreversible.

VASODILATOR DRUGS

Hypertension is characterized by an increase in total peripheral resistance. Drugs acting on vascular smooth muscle will relax resistance vessels. Compensatory sympathetic outflow accompanying vasodilation leads to tachycardia and an increase in cardiac output which may be controlled by beta antagonists.

Hydralazine

Hydralazine hydrochloride (BP, USP).
Chemical name: 1-hydrazinophthalazine hydrochloride.

Hydralazine exerts its hypotensive action by reducing arterial resistance (by up to 75%) through a direct relaxation of arteriolar smooth muscle, mainly in renal, cerebral, splanchnic and coronary precapillary vessels. Heart rate, stroke volume and cardiac output are increased. Plasma renin activity is increased. There is no direct effect on the heart or circulatory reflexes, and postural hypotension is not a feature. The effects of hydralazine alone are limited by reflex tachycardia and it is best combined with a β-blocker. Its most appropriate use is therefore in patients whose response to therapy with β-blockade and thiazide diuretic is inadequate; i.e. as a third-line drug.

Pharmacokinetics

Hydralazine is rapidly and almost completely absorbed after oral administration, with peak levels occurring after 1 h. It distributes in about 50% of body water and 85% is protein-bound in plasma. Tissue binding also occurs in arterial walls so that although the plasma half-life is only 1.5–4 h, the therapeutic effect lasts for 30–140 hours after termination of treatment.

Metabolism occurs by hepatic acetylation, the rate of which is dependent upon the genetically determined activity of N-acetyl transferase. There is a moderate first-pass effect. Fast acetylators show a much-reduced therapeutic effect until the acetylating system is saturated. Acetylation is affected by uraemia, and although renal elimination of hydralazine is negligible, dosage needs to be reduced in renal failure. The main metabolites of hydralazine are pyruvate hydrazone and α-ketoglutarate hydrazone, which are also active. The drug may be effective in the treatment of primary pulmonary hypertension since it dilates pulmonary arterioles.

Dosage and administration

Hydralazine is given orally in doses of less than 200 mg daily (increased to 300 mg daily in fast acetylators) either in 6- or 12-hourly dosage. Rapid (15–20 min) reduction of severe hypertension can be achieved by intravenous administration of doses not exceeding 20 mg.

Adverse effects

These include effects due to vasodilation such as flushing, nasal congestion, headache, dizziness, palpitations, angina, oedema and weight gain, which are reduced by β-blockers and diuretics.

The incidence of drug-induced lupus erythematosus was thought to be rare when dosage is less than 200 mg daily. It has now been shown that in women the incidence of hydralazine-related lupus may be as high as 20% at a daily dose of 200 mg and 8% when the daily dose is 100 mg. Men are less vulnerable to this adverse reaction. At dosages of 400 mg daily about 15% of patients develop a rheumatoid state with LE cells and antinuclear factor in the blood, and this is commoner in those with the slow acetylator phenotype. A dose-related peripheral neuropathy due to formation of a pyridoxine–hydralazine complex is corrected by pyridoxine supplements.

Endralazine

Endralazine (BAN, USAN).
Chemical name: 6-benzoyl-3-hydrazino-5,6,7,8-tetrahydropyrido (4,3-c-)-pyridazine mesylate.

Endralazine is a new peripheral vasodilator drug, which acts by direct relaxation of the smooth muscle fibres of the peripheral arterial vessels. The drug is active in doses approximately one-fifth of the usual dosage of hydralazine and it has a 1.7 times higher molecular weight than hydralazine, so that the formation of immunologically active complexes is less likely. Bioavailability is about 75%. Metabolism may be independent of acetylation. The drug is undergoing clinical trials in Europe.

Diazoxide

Diazoxide (BP, USP).
Chemical name: 7-chloro-3-methyl-2H benzo-1,2,4-thiadiazine 1,1-dioxide.

Diazoxide is an analogue of the thiazide diuretics but paradoxically has sodium-retaining properties. It dilates arteries by a direct action on arterial smooth muscle. It has no direct cardiac effects, nor does it impair cardiovascular reflexes, so that as blood pressure falls, a reflex tachycardia and increase in cardiac output occur. Catecholamines are released by a direct action and the resulting tachycardia may be controlled by β-blockade.

Pharmacokinetics

The main elimination is via the kidneys, although there is some hepatic metabolism. Most (90%) of the drug is protein-bound and the plasma half-life is 20–30 h. The half-life is three times longer than the hypotensive action, and with the normal dosage interval of 4–12 h there is extensive accumulation in the body. There is no correlation between total plasma concentration and hypotensive effect, since the latter depends on the initial concentration in the resistance vessels. Rapid intravenous injection temporarily overpowers albumin drug-binding capacity, so that high levels of unbound drug are free to act with the arterial smooth muscle. Drug binding is reduced in renal failure and the dosage should be reduced.

Dosage and administration

Diazoxide is now only occasionally used as the i.v. preparation in hypertensive crises, and even there its use is being replaced by i.v. labetalol or sublingual nifedipine. An i.v. bolus of 300 mg acts too quickly. Smaller doses are preferable and safer (mini-bolus doses of 50 mg, which can be repeated as necessary, or controlled infusion of 5 mg kg^{-1} at 15 mg min^{-1}).

Adverse effects

Sodium retention, hyperglycaemia, hypersensitivity manifestations (as with thiazide diuretics with which there is a cross-reaction) and reduction in anticoagulant dosage requirements due to plasma binding have been reported. It is not suitable for use in pregnant patients since it inhibits contraction of uterine muscle and delays labour. Blindness has been caused by emergency blood pressure reduction.

Minoxidil

Minoxidil (BAN, USAN).
Chemical name: 2,6-diamino-4-piperidino-
pyrimidine 1-oxide.

Minoxidil is a piperidino-pyrimidine derivative. It is a potent vasodilator acting primarily on the systemic arterioles in a manner similar to hydralazine. There is a reflex activation of the peripheral sympathetic nervous system resulting in release of renin, rise in heart rate and cardiac output, and increased release of noradrenaline from sympathetic nerve endings. There is retention of sodium and water and high doses of diuretic may be required to prevent fluid retention. Increase in cardiac rate and output is suppressed by β-blockade. Small doses of clonidine may be substituted for the β-blocker.

Pharmacokinetics

Minoxidil is nearly completely absorbed after oral administration. Peak concentrations are reached within 1 h. Maximum therapeutic response may be expected in 4 h. Plasma half-life is 4.2 h, but the antihypertensive effect lasts for several days, probably due to high-affinity binding to vascular smooth muscle. Minoxidil is rapidly cleared from plasma by hepatic metabolism, while 10% appears unchanged in the urine. Little dosage adjustment is required in renal failure.

Dosage and administration

The initial daily dose is 5–10 mg increasing to a maximum of 100 mg daily in divided doses. Usually 40 mg daily is sufficient. Only oral preparations are available.

Adverse effects

Systemic toxicity is uncommon. Fluid retention may be severe and acute pulmonary oedema has been reported. Acute myocardial necrosis has occurred and introduction of this drug into clinical practice was delayed 10 years because similar lesions were found in minoxidil-treated dogs and rats. Hypertrichosis is common and may be a serious drawback to use of the drug in women. Concomitant β-blockade is required to reduce tachycardia, and diuretics are required to avoid fluid retention when minoxidil is used for hypertension.

ADRENERGIC NEURONE BLOCKING AGENTS

These drugs are taken up by adrenergic nerve terminals in a similar manner to noradrenaline. Inside the terminal they inhibit noradrenaline release by interfering with Ca^{2+} ions involved in coupling action potentials in the terminal membrane with neurotransmitter secretion. All these drugs are taken up into cardiac muscle against a concentration gradient. In renal failure, renal blood flow is further reduced. As with ganglion-blocking drugs, maximum effect is achieved in the upright position. Compensatory venoconstriction is blocked and postural hypotension is a feature of blood pressure control with these agents, particularly in the presence of dehydration, vasodilation, alcohol and anaesthetic agents. Sexual difficulties, nasal stuffiness and intestinal upset from unopposed parasympathetic activity and fluid retention also occur. Drugs which inhibit the amine uptake of adrenergic neurons (tricyclic anti-depressants and phenothiazines) prevent uptake of these drugs and inhibit their action. Amphetamines and ephedrine, which are found in over-the-counter cold remedies, may cause discharge of guanethidine from the neuron. Noradrenaline, adrenaline, amphetamines and appetite-suppressants cause marked effects, since adrenergic neurons are inhibited from exerting their normal uptake function. Central nervous system effects are not seen. Guanethidine is a guanidine derivative; debrisoquine, bethanidine, guancydine (USA), guanoxan and guanoclor are analogues. The latter three are not marketed in the UK.

Guanethidine

Guanethidine monosulphate (BP, USP).
Chemical name: 1-(2 guanidinoethyl)azacyclo-octane
monosulphate.
Guanethidine is the prototype of the adrenergic neuron-blocking agents. In addition to its action in causing vasodilation by inhibiting noradrenaline release, and unlike other members of the group, it causes gross depletion of noradrenaline from adrenergic terminals in blood vessels and the myocardium.

Pharmacokinetics

Individual pharmacokinetic differences are unpredictable. Absorption from the gastrointestinal tract is slow and incomplete, and there is a variable first-pass effect. About 3–45% is absorbed from the gut — the amount is fairly constant for any one individual. Hepatic and renal clearances are high but the apparent volume of distribution is large and the plasma half-life is several days. Hepatic metabolites are inactive. Adequate control takes several weeks, but only once-daily dosage is required.

Dosage and administration

The initial dose is 10 mg increasing by 10 mg every 4–5 days to a maintenance of 30–100 mg daily, but dosage requirements vary widely. The drug has found a useful place in the treatment of reflex sympathetic dystrophy (Sudeck's atrophy) and causalgia. Guanethidine in a dose of 20 mg diluted with isotonic saline (40 ml) is injected into a suitable vein in the affected limb which has been isolated by a tourniquet.

Guanethidine displaces noradrenaline from sympathetic nerve endings and produces a sympathetic blockade which lasts from several days to 3 weeks (Hannington-Kiff 1982, see also chapter 16). On release of the tourniquet (after 20–30 min) the arterial pressure may rise (displaced noradrenaline effect) or fall (systemic drug effect).

Side-effects

These have been discussed. Intravenous injection may exacerbate hypertension by sudden catecholamine release which could be particularly hazardous in patients with phaeochromocytoma.

Debrisoquine

Debrisoquine (BP, USAN).
Chemical name: 2-amidino-1,2,3,4-tetrahydro-
isoquinoline sulphate.
Debrisoquine, like guanethidine, shows a wide (40-fold) variation in individual dosage requirements. Over 75% is absorbed when given orally, and the variation in response is due to differences in hepatic metabolism. Extensive metabolism is genetically determined. About one in 10 persons is virtually unable to effect the first-passage metabolism of debrisoquine, and this applies to many other drugs, in particular the calcium antagonists. Patients who inherit this poor metabolizer phenotype due to absence of a particular form of cytochrome P-450 can be thought of as being compromised by their drug treatment when the drug accumulates to too high concentrations. The calcium antagonist perhexiline is one such drug which has a very long half-life in poor metabolizers; the very variable response to nifedipine suggests that it may be similarly affected. Part of debrisoquine metabolism is a first-pass effect which can be saturated by increasing the dose. Plasma half-life is long (11–26 h). The principal metabolite is 4-hydroxydebrisoquine. Dosage is similar to that of guanethidine to a maximum of 40–120 mg daily.

Guanadrel

Guanadrel sulphate.
Chemical name: (cyclohexanespiro-2'-
[1',3']dioxolan-4'-ylmethyl)
guanidine sulphate.
Guanadrel sulphate is an orally active postganglionic sympathetic inhibitor (adrenergic neuron-blocking drug). The antihypertensive effect of guanadrel, like that of guanethidine, derives from its ability to block the release of noradrenaline at sympathetic nerve terminals.

Pharmacokinetics

Since the drug action starts and dissipates quickly, and

since drug accumulation is limited, rapid titration and drug withdrawal are easily accomplished. Peak plasma concentrations are reached within 1.5–2 h after oral administration, and urinary excretion is approximately 85% complete within 24 h. The elimination half-life is about 10 h. Less than 20% binds to plasma proteins.

Dosage and administration

Guanadrel (available as 10 and 25 mg tablets) is employed as an adjunct to diuretic therapy. The starting dose is 10 mg/day and in most patients control of blood pressure is achieved with dosages of 20–75 mg/day. The maximum daily dose is 400 mg; this should be divided and taken morning and evening.

Side-effects

Side-effects are mild and there is less orthostatic dizziness with guanadrel than with guanethidine. Sexual dysfunction may occur in men.

Bethanidine

Bethanidine sulphate (BP, USAN).
Chemical name: 1-benzyl-2.3-dimethylguanidine
sulphate.
The range of individual dosage is much smaller than with either guanethidine or debrisoquine. It is well absorbed (60%) and has a faster onset and shorter duration of action than guanethidine. Peak effect occurs at 4 h and has disappeared by 8–12 h. The half-life is 8–15 h. Dosage starts at 5 mg twice daily, rising to 30–100 mg daily in divided doses.

Reserpine

Reserpine (BP, USP, Eur P).
Chemical name: methyl 18-O-(3,4,5-trimethoxy-
benzoyl) reserpate.
Reserpine is derived from an Indian plant, *Rauwolfia*, and is the prototype of purified rauwolfia alkaloids. It depletes stored catecholamines and 5-hydroxytryptamine in the brain, heart, blood vessels and adrenal medulla. There is specific inhibition of formation of storage complexes of catecholamines with ATP, so that the free amine is destroyed by monoamine oxidase. Only 30% of an oral dose is absorbed. The half-life is 2–4.5 h.

Both central and peripheral effects may contribute to its antihypertensive effect. Central effects include sedation and increased parasympathetic outflow. Peripheral effects depress responses to adrenergic nerve activity so that bradycardia is a feature. Its clinical antihypertensive use has declined as a result of its unacceptable side-effects.

Dosage and administration

Daily oral doses are 0.25–0.5 mg. The hypotensive effect is of slow onset, appearing after 2–3 weeks, and takes up to 6 weeks to wear off after stopping the drug. Paradoxically, as the interest in reserpine for treatment of hypertension has waned, its use by injection in various vasospastic states has increased. It may be used in the treatment of reflex sympathetic dystrophy using a Bier block technique as described for guanethidine, which is not available in the United States in injectable form (Benson et al 1980). The dose of reserpine is 2.5 mg. It has also been used in the treatment of Raynaud's phenomenon by intra-arterial injection. Injectable reserpine 0.5–1.25 mg diluted with isotonic saline is injected into the proximal artery of the affected limb. Improvement in the cutaneous microcirculation of the limb should appear within 1 h, usually lasts 1–3 weeks, and occasionally much longer (Nilsen & Jayson 1980). Since reserpine is barely soluble in water, a special preparation is necessary.

Adverse effects

Parasympathetic effects lead to nasal stuffiness and abdominal symptoms. Central effects include sedation, nightmares and suicidal depression. An alleged association between reserpine therapy and increased incidence of breast cancer was probably illusory, due to faulty statistical methods and an increase in both hypertension and breast cancer in the older patient. Side-effects of intra-arterial injection include generalized vasodilation, hypotension, tachycardia and headache, but are usually mild and do not last more than 24 h. Cardiac arrhythmias may be provoked by doses of 2.5 mg or more.

Ganglion-blocking agents

These drugs block autonomic ganglia by competitive antagonism of nicotinic cholinergic receptors. Postural hypotension is severe. Although they were the first effective antihypertensive agents, and were used extensively for hypotensive anaesthesia, their use is now of historical interest only. Pentolinium is still available in the United Kingdom for induced hypotensive anaesthesia.

Adverse effects

These resulted from parasympathetic blockade (which causes constipation, paralytic ileus, urinary retention, dry mouth, blurred vision and impotence) and sympathetic blockade (which inhibits ejaculation). Severe postural effects and tachyphylaxis were common.

Trimetaphan

Trimetaphan camsylate (BP, USP).
Chemical name: 1,3-dibenzyldecahydro-2-
                  oxoimidazo-[4,5-c]thieno
                  [1,2-a]thiolium(+)camphor-10-
                  sulphonate.

Trimetaphan has a swift onset of action and a single dose lasts only a few minutes, so that it is given either as an intravenous infusion at 3–4 mg min^{-1} or by intermittent injections of 10 mg. It relaxes arteriolar smooth muscle and also releases histamine and can reduce both cardiac output and stroke volume.

THE RENIN–ANGIOTENSIN SYSTEM

Investigation of renovascular hypertension has resulted in new ideas about the pathophysiology of essential hypertension. An important factor controlling arterial pressure is the circulating renin level. Renin is an enzyme released by renal glomerular afferent arterial juxtaglomerular cells which splits a circulating α_2-globulin substrate of hepatic origin to produce a decapeptide angiotensin I. Angiotensin I is inactive but is converted by converting enzyme in the lungs to angiotensin II, an octapeptide, which is the most powerful vasoconstrictor known. Angiotensin II also releases aldosterone, so that sodium retention and volume expansion induce a slow rise in blood pressure. Converting enzyme also inactivates bradykinin inhibition so that its antagonism leads to bradykinin-induced hypotension (Vidt et al 1982) Normally, renin activity is controlled by a feedback mechanism whereby a rise in pressure shuts off renin release. For practical purposes, patients with essential hypertension can be divided into subgroups according to their renin–sodium profile, and about 15% have high renin activity, 55% have normal activity, and 30% have low renin activity. High-renin patients are particularly sensitive to β-blocker therapy, while low-renin patients respond better to diuretic therapy even though the latter tends to elevate renin levels. Renin release is decreased by blockade of β-adrenoceptors, although this is probably not the main mechanism of action of these drugs.

ANGIOTENSIN-CONVERTING ENZYME (ACE) INHIBITORS

Captopril

Captopril (BAN, USAN).
Chemical name: D-3-mercapto-2
                  methylpropranoyl-L-proline.

Captopril inhibits converting enzyme which is found in many sites in the body and is responsible for activating angiotensin I to angiotensin II. The first drugs developed which were inhibitors of the renin–angiotensin system were saralsin and teprotide, which had to be given intravenously.

Captopril lowers blood pressure in both hypertensive and normotensive subjects and the effect lasts for 6–8 h. Normally there is no tachycardia. Increased plasma renin activity — as in sodium restriction, diuretic therapy or renovascular disease — enhances the hypotensive effect. Arteriolar resistance falls and venous capacitance vessels may be affected. The drug is particularly useful in hypertension associated with renal artery stenosis where plasma renin is high and secondary hyperaldosteronism is pronounced. Captopril does not impair intellectual or sexual function, neither does it cause fatigue, so that it compares favourably with other antihypertensives by preserving the 'quality of life'. It is increasingly becoming a 'first-line' drug in the treatment of hypertension (MacGregor et al 1987, Gavras 1990).

Pharmacokinetics

Captopril is well absorbed after oral administration. Peak levels occur in 30–90 min. Thirty per cent is protein-bound and the half-life is less than 2 h. There is hepatic metabolism, and renal excretion accounts for more than 50% of a single dose, but data on drug disposition are limited. In hypertension its biological half-life is long enough to allow twice-daily dosage. Dosage is reduced in renal failure.

Dosage and administration

The starting dose is 12.5 mg twice daily by mouth, increased to 50 mg twice daily. A single dose of 100 mg may be effective in hypertension. Larger doses are used in congestive heart failure. When given sublingually, 25 mg (chewed) may relieve severe hypertension.

Adverse effects

Skin rashes and gastrointestinal symptoms were common (more than 5%) when higher dosage regimes were used. Serious adverse effects are rare but include proteinuria, bone marrow depression and taste disturbances, which may be due to the sulphydryl group on the molecule. Reversible captopril-induced renal failure has been reported in kidney-transplant recipients with graft-artery stenosis, and this is a problem common to all ACE inhibitors where hypotension may cause renal failure in the presence of pre-existing renal impairment.

Enalapril

Enalapril maleate (BAN).
Chemical name: (N-[2 (S)-1-carboxy-3 phenyl propyl] L-ala pro)ethyl ester.
Enalapril maleate is an orally active ACE inhibitor which lowers peripheral vascular resistance without causing an increase in heart rate. Enalapril is a prodrug which is hydrolysed after absorption to form the active agent enalaprilat. Its effects are similar to captopril with, however, a longer half-life and slower onset of effect because the therapeutic effect depends on hepatic metabolism. The absence of the SH group from the structure theoretically lessens the risk of immune-based side-effects.

Pharmacokinetics

Enalapril maleate was designed as a prodrug to improve the systemic availability of the active ACE inhibitor enalaprilat, which is poorly absorbed. About 60% of enalapril is absorbed, giving peak serum concentrations in 1 h. Peak serum concentrations of enalaprilat are reached in 3–4 h. The bioavailability of enalapril as enalaprilat is about 40%. Enalaprilat is less than 50% protein-bound and both enalapril and enalaprilat are excreted unchanged, mainly by the kidney. Enalaprilat has polyphasic elimination kinetics due to strong binding to serum ACE, and the terminal half-life is 30–35 h. The drug accumulates in renal failure but can be removed by haemodialysis. In patients with hepatic dysfunction conversion of enalapril to enalaprilat may be delayed.

Dosage and administration

The initial dose is 5 mg daily, reduced to 2.5 mg daily if there is renal impairment or the patient is over 65 years of age. The maximum dosage is 40 mg/day.

Adverse effects

Side-effects are mild and include headache, dizziness, fatigue, nausea, rash, hypotension and angioneurotic oedema, but are generally less than those seen with captopril. In a few cases hypotension, renal failure and angioneurotic oedema were life-threatening, and indeed fatal. It is recommended that the dose of any diuretic being given concurrently should be reduced before initiating therapy, and that renal function should be monitored. Since ACE inhibitors spare potassium, potassium supplements and potassium-sparing diuretics should be used with caution.

Mechanism of action of ACE inhibitors

ACE inhibitors appear to lower blood pressure by four mechanisms. They inhibit the normal conversion of angiotensin I to the vasoconstrictor angiotensin II. They reduce the secretion of aldosterone to induce a natriuresis. Inactivation of vasodilatory bradykinins is reduced. Finally, specific renal vasodilation may enhance natriuresis. ACE inhibitors are also finding a useful place in the treatment of heart failure associated with decreased cardiac output and increased systemic vascular resistance. There is some correlation between the severity of heart failure and plasma renin activity, and use of these drugs reduces systemic vascular resistance and reverses the secondary neurohumoral changes found in severe heart failure. Their use requires considerable care (Opie et al 1987), but has a beneficial effect on mortality (CONSENSUS Trial Study Group 1987).

Cough is a common side-effect of ACE inhibitors. The reason is not understood.

New ACE and renin inhibitors

Some 20 compounds that have a similar pharmacological activity are under investigation. Lisinopril is a long-acting lysine derivative of enalapril, although not a prodrug. The following are all prodrugs; zofenopril, fosenopril, perindopril, pentopril, ramipril and alacepril. In addition, a modified analogue of angiotensinogen has been developed which has specific renin inhibition properties and which acts on the renin–angiotensin–aldosterone axis at a different site from the ACE inhibitors (Williams 1988, Breckenridge 1988).

Atrial natriuretic hormone

It has been known for 30 years that distension of the cardiac atria can cause a diuresis. It is now known that the atrial gene codes for a preprohormone with 152 amino acids. This produces a 126-amino acid pro-hormone (atriopeptigen) which is stored as granules in the atrial myocytes. The atrial natriuretic hormone or factor atriopeptin, is released into the circulation as a 28-amino acid sequence, although other low-molecular-weight peptides isolated from atrial extracts are also biologically active. Atriopeptin has a half-life of 3 min in the circulation. It is a potent diuretic, natriuretic and vasodilator, as well as inhibiting aldosterone secretion. It is more than 1000 times more potent than frusemide as a diuretic. Although the full implications of this discovery are as yet unclear, it seems more than coincidental that atrial peptides have four discrete actions that may oppose the four levels of operation of the renin–angiotensin–aldosterone axis. The implications for the treatment of hypertension, and heart and renal failure are speculative as yet, but it seems likely that the discovery and characterization of atriopeptin heralds a unique opportunity for the development of new pharmacological agents for the therapeutic manipulation of circulatory, volume and salt homeostasis (Laragh 1985, Needleman and Greenwald 1986). The possible existence of an endogenous digitalis-like factor which may be involved in the pathogenesis of low-renin essential hypertension is being investigated (Haddy 1987).

Treatment modalities in the critically ill, such as PEEP, may be shown to alter the secretion of this hormone and have a profound effect on renal function (Kharasch et al 1988)

Calcium channel antagonists

Clinically, each of the 'first-generation' calcium antagonists–verapamil, nifedipine and diltiazem — has a slightly different spectrum of clinical activity. Their common denominator is their ability to block the calcium channel, which results in their vasodilatory effect. Verapamil has been in use for almost 25 years and had such a dramatic effect in the treatment of supraventricular arrhythmias that only recently has the wide therapeutic potential of the drug come to be appreciated.

All three drugs are discussed in detail in Chapter 24, but each has a hypotensive action in addition to anti-arrhythmic actions (verapamil and diltiazem) and effect on coronary spasm (verapamil, diltiazem and nifedipine). All three agents may be used either as monotherapy or in combination with diuretics or ACE inhibitors. Only nifedipine has been well studied in combination with β-blockers; caution is required when combining α-blockers such as prazosin with calcium antagonists, for fear of excess hypotension. Comparable daily doses in the treatment of mild or moderate hypertension are verapamil 360–480 mg daily, nifedipine 40–120 mg daily and diltiazem 120–360 mg daily.

New dihydropyridines under investigation or already in clinical practice are nitredipine (in Europe for hypertension), nicardipine (in the UK for hypertension), nimodipine (for cerebral ischaemia), nisoldipine and felodipine. Other mixed sodium-calcium channel blockers include bepridil and tiapamil, while flumarizine is a mixed antihistaminic with cerebral vasodilator effect.

Diuretics

Many diuretics have antihypertensive properties, although their mode of action is incompletely understood. There is a correlation between their natriuretic and hypotensive effects, but the weaker thiazide diuretics are often more effective hypotensive agents than the very powerful diuretics such as frusemide. Potassium-sparing diuretics may also be effective. Plasma and extracellular fluid volumes decrease early in treatment, and there may be release of renin and hyperaldosteronism. With prolonged treatment the plasma volume returns towards normal, although the hypotensive action persists. Excessive salt intake or a low glomerular filtration rate will interfere with the anti-hypertensive effect and thiazides are ineffective in anephric patients. Addition of β-adrenoceptor blocking agents or vasodilators enhances the effect of thiazide diuretics. Because of the 'wrong-way' blood biochemical changes that occur, the time-honoured role of diuretics as first-line therapy in hypertension is increasingly being challenged. In addition to the volume effects noted above, these include hypokalaemia and metabolic alkalosis, hyperuricaemia and gout, hyponatraemia, carbohydrate intolerance rarely leading to diabetes or hyperosmolar diabetic coma, and 'atherogenic' blood lipid changes with rise in triglycerides and cholesterol and a fall in high-density lipoprotein. Diuretics are discussed in detail in Chapter 27.

β-adrenergic receptor antagonists

Undesirable consequences may follow the sudden withdrawal of β-adrenergic receptor blocking drugs in patients suffering from ischaemic heart disease, hypertension and arrhythmias. The optimal management of patients receiving β-blocking drugs prior to surgery has been controversial. In animal experiments, Craythorne

& Huffington (1966) observed that 200 mg kg^{-1} propranolol produced only a 10% decrease in heart rate in dogs during halothane anaesthesia, with no change in cardiac output or myocardial contractility. Roberts and co-workers (1976b) found that chronic pretreatment of dogs with propranolol produced a circulatory depression equivalent to that produced by 0.5% halothane. Kopriva and colleagues (1978) studied patients scheduled for coronary artery bypass graft. When the daily dose of propranolol averaged 140 mg, and the last dose was given 6 h before surgery, there were no unusual haemodynamic changes during thiopentone/suxamethonium/nitrous oxide/halothane and pancuronium anaesthesia.

Excessive β-adrenergic blockade can be overcome by i.v. atropine 1–2 mg. Alternatively, transvenous pacing or an infusion of glucagon, amrinone, dobutamine or isoprenaline may be used.

Detailed discussion of individual β-blocking drugs can be found in Chapter 24.

SERONTONIN ANTAGONIST

Ketanserin

Ketanserin tartrate.
Chemical name: 3-[2-(4-[4 flurobenzoyl]
1-piperidinyl) ethyl] 2,4-(1 H,
3H)-quinazolinedione.

Ketanserin, a quinazoline derivative, has been shown to be a selective blocker of 5-hydroxytryptamine type 2 receptors, and has been characterized as a highly specific serotonin antagonist, although it may also have α$_1$-adrenolytic activity (Reimann & Frölick 1983). When used acutely, ketanserin has a hypotensive action in man. Intravenous use (10 mg) in hypertensive patients causes a fall in arterial blood pressure, pulmonary artery pressure, pulmonary wedge pressure and right atrial pressure. Total peripheral resistance falls despite increases in plasma noradrenaline and renin. A bolus injection of 0.15 mg kg^{-1} followed by a continuous infusion of 4 mg/h resulted in steady-state mean plasma ketanserin concentrations of 88 μg l^{-1}. Other pharmacokinetic data are not available. The drug appears to have a relatively short duration of action (0.5–2 h). Its value in the treatment of hypertensive crises is not yet evaluated. There is one favourable report of its use during surgery for the carcinoid syndrome (Fischler et al 1983). Ketanserin has also been used successfully in the short-term control of pre-eclamptic hypertension. Griffiths & Whitwam (1986a), considered that the drug caused α$_1$-adrenoceptor blockade in addition to serotonin antagonism. The same workers showed that the drug

produced a more desirable haemodynamic profile following coronary artery surgery, and it has also been shown to modify the pressor response to sternotomy (Griffiths & Whitwam 1986b, Cashman et al 1986).

Other workers have confirmed its potential value in treating hypertension after coronary artery surgery since it does not produce a reflex tachycardia (Hodsman et al 1989), and in the treatment of essential hypertension (Breckenridge 1986). It has also been used to treat Raynaud's disease. Oral doses of 40 mg twice daily and intravenous bolus doses of 10 mg have been used.

EMERGENCY REDUCTION OF BLOOD PRESSURE

In the majority of patients with severe hypertension it is safest to lower the blood pressure gradually over an hour or so, using oral medication. Occasionally, in the perioperative period or intensive-care situation, it may be deemed necessary to lower the arterial pressure within minutes where life is threatened by hypertensive encephalopathy, dissecting aneurysm of the aorta, continuing cerebral or subarachnoid haemorrhage, acute pulmonary oedema due to severe hypertension, or eclampsia. Both sodium nitroprusside and glyceryl trinitrate by constant infusion pump are the most controllable of the emergency hypotensive drugs. Their use is more fully discussed in Chapter 23. They have largely replaced trimetaphan for control of blood pressure. Fetal cyanide poisoning has been described in animals following sodium nitroprusside.

Nifedipine

Sublingual nifedipine is now almost standard therapy. It consistently reduces systolic and diastolic pressures by about 20% within 20–30 min. Although the agents described below can still be used, when the ideal rate of reduction of hypertension requiring urgent therapy is not known, the simplicity of sublingual nifedipine (10 mg) is increasingly seen as seemingly safe therapy, provided there is no clinical evidence of cerebral or myocardial ischaemia or of renal failure. An intravenous preparation of nifedipine (not available everywhere and very unstable in light) has been shown to be a suitable vasodilator for use in the perioperative period in patients following coronary artery bypass graft surgery (Van Wezel et al 1986). Nasal administration has also been described (Kiuchi et al 1986).

Diazoxide

Diazoxide is given by a single mini bolus of 30 or 50 mg

and acts within minutes. It is the simplest to administer but least controllable of the drugs discussed here. Its use in labour in the presence of severe uncontrolled hypertension is justified, and under these circumstances a bolus of 100 mg can be repeated once. It can also be given by infusion. It interferes with uterine muscle activity.

Hydralazine

Hydralazine in increments of 5 mg to a total dose of 20 mg causes a greater rise in cardiac output and tachycardia than diazoxide, and may precipitate angina. Excessive hypotension is rarer than with diazoxide, but it takes 20 min to act. It is probably safer given as an infusion.

Labetalol

Intravenous labetalol injection reduces blood pressure within 10 min. It can be given repeatedly by bolus injections of 10–50 mg or by infusion at a rate of 2 mg min^{-1}, and the fall in blood pressure is dose-related. It reduces heart rate and may precipitate bronchospasm.

Other drugs

Parenteral preparations of methyldopa, clonidine and guanethidine are available. The hypotensive effect of methyldopa is slow, while guanethidine and clonidine are not suitable as they may cause an initial rise in blood pressure when given as a bolus. In less urgent cases, blood pressure may be controlled within a few hours with oral labetalol, bethanidine or methyldopa. In the intensive-care unit, drugs which do not rely on the upright posture for effect should be chosen. β-Adrenergic blocking agents, labetalol and methyldopa, supplemented as necessary by thiazide diuretics, are appropriate, and may be given parenterally if required. Parenteral magnesium sulphate is the drug of choice in the USA for preventing impending eclamptic convulsions (Chun et al 1990).

REFERENCES

Amery A, Birkenhager W. Brixko P et al 1985 Mortality and morbidity results from the European Working Party on high blood pressure in the elderly trial. Lancet i: 1349–1354

Anonymous 1987 Transdermal antihypertensive drugs. Lancet i: 79–80

Beevers D G 1988 Overtreating hypertension. Mortality from coronary artery disease may be increased if pressures are dropped too low. British Medical Journal 297: 1212

Benson H T, Chomka C M, Brunner E A 1980 Treatment of reflex sympathetic dystrophy with regional intravenous reserpine. Anesthesia and Analgesia 59: 500–502

Breckenridge A 1986 Ketanserin — a new antihypertensive agent. Journal of Hypertension 4 (Suppl 1): 513–516

Breckenridge A 1988 Angiotensin converting enzyme inhibitors. British Medical Journal 296: 618–620

Cashman J N, Thompson M A, Bennett A 1986 Influence of ketanserin pretreatment on the haemodynamic responses to sternotomy. Anaesthesia 41: 505–510

Casson W R, Jones RM, Parsons R S 1984 Nifedipine and cardiopulmonary bypass: Post-bypass management after continuation or withdrawal of therapy. Anaesthesia 39: 1197–1201

Chobanian A V 1986 Antihypertensive therapy in evolution. New England Journal of Medicine 314: 1701–1702

Chun G, Frishman W H 1990 Rapid-acting parenteral antihypertensive agents. Journal of Clinical Pharmacology 30: 195–209

CONSENSUS Trial Study Group 1987 Effects of enalapril on mortality in severe congestive heart failure: results of the co-operative North Scandinavian Enalapril Survival Study (CONSENSUS). New England Journal of Medicine 316: 1429–1435

Craythorne N W B, Huffington P 1966 Effects of propranolol on the cardiovascular response to cyclopropane and halothane. Anesthesiology 27: 580–583

Dagnino J, Prys-Roberts C 1984 Studies of anaesthesia in relation to hypertension. VI: Cardiovascular responses to extradural blockade of treated and untreated hypertensive patients. British Journal of Anaesthesia 56: 1065–1073

Farnon D, Curran J 1981 Beta-receptor blockade and tracheal intubation. Anaesthesia 36: 803–805

Fischler M, Dentan M, Westerman M N, Vourc'h G, Freitag B 1983 Prophylactic use of ketanserin in a patient with carcinoid syndrome British Journal of Anaesthesia 55: 920

Foëx P 1978 Preoperative assessment of patients with cardiac disease. British Journal of Anaesthesia 50: 15–23

Foëx P 1983 Beta-blockade in anaesthesia. Journal of Clinical and Hospital Pharmacy 8: 183–190

Foëx P, Prys-Roberts C 1974 Interactions of beta-receptor blockade and Pco$_2$ levels in the anaesthetized dog. British Journal of Anaesthesia 46: 397–404

Fox E J, Sklar G S, Hill C H, Villanueva R, King B D 1977 Complications related to the pressor response to endotracheal intubation. Anesthesiology 47: 524–525

Gavras H 1990 Angiotensin converting enzyme inhibition and its impact on cardiovascular disease. Circulation 81: 381–388

Goldman L 1983 Cardiac risks and complications of non-cardiac surgery. Annals of Internal Medicine 98: 504–513

Goldman L, Caldera D L, 1979 Risks of general anesthesia and elective operation in the hypertensive patient. Anesthesiology 50: 285–292

Goldman, L, Caldera D L, Nussbaum S E et al 1977 Multifactorial index of cardiac risk in non-cardiac surgical procedures. New England Journal of Medicine 297: 845–850

Griffiths H B A, Whitwam J G 1986a Ketanserin and the

cardiovascular system. 1. Modification of the effects of pressor amines in patients undergoing myocardial revascularisation. Anaesthesia 41: 708–711

Griffiths H B A, Whitwam J G 1986b Ketanserin and the cardiovascular system. 2. A study of its effects in patients undergoing myocardial revascularisation. Anaesthesia 41: 712–716

Haddy F J 1987 Endogenous digitalis-like factor or factors. New England Journal of Medicine 316: 621–622

Hannington-Kiff J G 1982 Hyperadrenergic-effected limb causalgia: relief by pharmacological norepinephrine blockade. American Heart Journal 103: 152–153

Heagerty A M 1988 Recent advances in therapy for hypertension. British Journal of Anaesthesia 61: 360–364

Hodsman N B A, Colvin J R, Kenny G N C 1989 Effect of ketanserin on sodium nitroprusside requirements, arterial pressure control and heart rate following coronary artery bypass surgery. British Journal of Anaesthesia 62: 527–531

Hoffman B B, Lefkowitz R J 1980 Alpha-adrenergic receptor subtypes. New England Journal of Medicine 302: 1390–1396

Horan B F, Prys-Roberts C, Hamilton W K, Roberts J G 1976 Interaction of enflurane anaesthesia, beta-receptor blockade and blood loss in the dog. British Journal of Anaesthesia 48: 817

Horan B F, Prys-Roberts C Foëx P, Roberts J G 1977 Interaction of isoflurane anaesthesia. Beta-receptor blockade and blood loss in the dog. British Journal of Anaesthesia 49: 187–188

Jones R M 1984 Calcium antagonists. Anaesthesia 39: 747–749

Kharasch E D, Yeo K-T, Kenny M A, Buffington C W 1988 Atrial natriuretic factor may mediate the renal effects of PEEP ventilation; Anesthesiology 69: 862–869

Kiuchi A, Kodama M, Sakai T, Yoshikawa K 1986 Nasal administration of nifedipine to hypertensive patients during anaesthesia. Abstracts of 7th Asian Australasian Congress of Anaesthesiologists, p 228

Kobinger W, 1983 Central blood pressure regulation. Involvement of presynaptic or postsynaptic, α_1 or α_2-adrenoceptors. Chest 83 (Suppl): 296–299

Kopriva C J, Brown A C D, Pappas G 1978 Haemodynamics during general anaesthesia in patients receiving propranolol. Anesthesiology 48: 28–33

Langer S Z, 1976 The role of α- and β-presynaptic receptors in the regulation of noradrenaline release elicited by nerve stimulation. Clinical Science and Molecular Medicine 51: 423s–426s

Laragh J H 1985 Atrial natriuretic hormone, the renin-aldosterone axis and blood pressure-electrolyte homeostasis. New England Journal of Medicine 313: 1330–1340

Low J M, Harvey J T, Prys-Roberts C, Dagnino J 1986 Studies of anaesthesia in relation to hypertension. VII: Adrenergic responses to largyngoscopy. British Journal of Anaesthesia 58: 471–477

MacGregor G A, Markandu N D, Singer D R J, Cappuccio F P, Shore A C, Sagnella G A 1987 Moderate sodium restriction with angiotensin converting enzyme inhibitor in essential hypertension: a double blind study. British Medical Journal 294: 531–534

Medical Research Council Working Party 1985 MRC trial of treatment of mild hypertension. Principal results. British Medical Journal 291: 97–104

Messerli F H 1990 Antihypertensive therapy — going to the heart of the matter. Circulation 81: 1128–1135

Mizgala H F 1983. The calcium channel blockers: pharmacology and clinical applications. Canadian Anesthetists' Society Journal 30: 3 (Suppl): S5–10

Needlemen P, Greenwald J E, 1986 Atriopeptin: a cardiac hormone intimately involved in fluid, electrolyte, and blood-pressure homeostasis. New England Journal of Medicine 314: 828–834

Nilsen K H, Jayson M I V 1980 Cutaneous microcirculation in systemic sclerosis and response to intra-arterial reserpine. British Medical Journal 1: 1408–1411

Opie L H, Chatterjee K, Gersh B T et al 1987 Drugs for the heart, 2nd expanded ed. Grune & Stratton, Orlando, Ch 8, p 155

Proceedings of a Symposium 1983 Initial therapy in hypertension. American Journal of Cardiology 51(4): 619–660

Prys-Roberts C 1975 Beta-receptor blockers in anaesthesia. Anaesthesia Round No 7. Imperial Chemical Industries Ltd, Macclesfield

Prys-Roberts C 1979a Hypertension and anaesthesia — fifty years on. Anesthesiology 50: 281–284

Prys-Roberts C 1979b Anaesthesia for the hypertensive patient. Lancet ii: 529

Prys-Roberts C 1984 Anaesthesia and hypertension. British Journal of Anaesthesia 56: 711–724

Prys-Roberts C Greene L T, Meloche R, Foëx 1971a Studies of anaesthesia in relation to hypertension. II: Haemodynamic consequences of induction and endotracheal intubation. British Journal of Anaesthesia 43: 531–547

Prys-Roberts C, Meloche R, Foëx P 1971b Studies of anaesthesia in relation to hypertension. I: Cardiovascular responses of treated and untreated patients. British Journal of Anaesthesia 43: 122–137

Reimann I W, Frölich J C 1983 Mechanism of antihypertensive action of ketanserin in man. British Medical Journal 287: 381–383

Roberts J G, Foëx P, Clarke T N S, Bennett M J, Saner C A 1976a Haemodynamic interations of high-dose propranolol pre-treatment and anaesthesia in the dog. III: The effects of haemorrhage during halothane and trichlorethylene anaesthesia. British Journal of Anaesthesia 48: 411–418

Roberts J G, Foëx P, Clarke T N S, Bennett M J 1976b Haemodynamic interactions of high dose propranolol and anaesthesia in the dog. I: Halothane dose response studies. British Journal of Anaesthesia 48: 315–325

Saner C A, Foëx P, Roberts J G, Bennett J M 1975 Methoxyflurane and practolol: a dangerous combination. British Journal of Anaesthesia 47: 1025

Siedlecki J, 1975 Disturbances in the function of cardiovascular system in patients following endotracheal intubation and attempts of their prevention by pharmacological blockade of sympathetic system. Anaesthesia, Resuscitation and Intensive Therapy 3: 107–123

Simpson D L, McCrae W R, Wildsmith J A W, Dale B A B 1987 Acute beta-adrenoreceptor blockade and induced hypotension. Anaesthesia 42: 243–248

Sleight P 1983 Hypertension. In: Weatherall D J, Ledingham J G G, Warrell D A (eds) Oxford textbook of medicine. Oxford University Press, Oxford, Ch 13, p 272

Sorkin E M, Heel R C 1986 Guanfacine. A review of its
pharmacodynamic and pharmacokinetic properties, and
therapeutic efficacy in the treatment of hypertension.
Drugs 31: 301–336

Stone J G, Foëx P, Sear J W, Johnson L L, Khambatta
H J, Triner L 1988 Risk of myocardial ischaemia during
anaesthesia in treated and untreated hypertensive patients.
British Journal of Anaesthesia 61: 675–79

Swales J D, Ramsey L E, Coope J R et al 1989 Treating
mild hypertension. Agreement from the large trials.
Report of the British Hypertension Society working party.
British Medical Journal 298: 694–698

Van Wezel H B, Bovill J G, Schuller J, Gielen J, Hoeneveld
M H 1986 Comparison of nitroglycerine, verapamil and
nifedipine in the management of arterial pressure during
coronary surgery. British Journal of Anaesthesia
58: 267–273

Vidt D G, Bravo E L, Fouad F M 1982 Drug therapy:
captopril. New England Journal of Medicine 306: 214–219

Williams G H 1988 Drug therapy: converting-enzyme
inhibitors in the treatment of hypertension. New England
Journal of England 319: 1517–1525

Woodcock T E, Millord R K, Dixon J, Prys-Roberts C
1988 Clonidine premedication for isoflurane induced
hypotension. Sympathoadrenal responses and a
computer-controlled assessment of the vapour
requirement. British Journal of Anaesthesia 60: 388–394

Yaksh T L, Collins J G 1989 Studies in animals should
precede human use of spinally administered drugs.
Anesthesiology 70: 4–6

26. Drugs affecting haemostasis

S. D. Nelson

INTRODUCTION: THE HAEMOSTATIC SYSTEM

Haemostasis is a complex interplay between processes which activate clotting and other reactions which inhibit it. On occasions the anaesthetist may wish to manipulate this haemostatic equilibrium. If he is to do this safely, an understanding of the fundamentals of haemostasis is essential.

Five important systems are involved in haemostasis; These are: the blood vessels, the platelets, the plasma coagulation proteins, the protease inhibitors and the fibrinolytic system.

Blood vessels (endothelial cells and tissue fibrils)

Intact endothelial cells are probably the source of part of the body's plasma factor VIII (Bloom et al 1973, Hoyer et al 1973, review article Bloom 1979). They also contain a platelet inhibitor and vasodilator, prostacyclin (PGI_2). Damage to a blood vessel exposes tissue fibres and releases a procoagulant tissue factor 'thromboplastin'. Prostacyclin activity is overcome and the haemostatic balance shifts towards coagulation.

Platelets

Platelets adhere to injured endothelial cells and tissue fibrils where they generate prostaglandins and thromboxanes (Smith et al 1983, Myers et al 1980). These encourage the aggregation of platelets (adherence to each other). Platelet aggregates release arachidonic acid from membrane phospholipids, with subsequent production of cyclic (prostaglandin) endoperoxides which further encourage platelet aggregation and are a source of thromboxane A_2. The balance between endothelial cell PGI_2 and platelet prostaglandin activity determines whether platelet aggregates disperse or extend. If the latter, clot-promoting factors (especially 'platelet factor 3') are released. These promote activation

of plasma factor X to Xa and prothrombin (II) to thrombin (IIa). Other platelet factors encourage activation of factors XII, and XI.

Plasma coagulation proteins

These are designated by roman numerals I to XIII (VI is not used). Three other factors, Fletcher factor (prekallikrein), Fitzgerald factor (high molecular weight kininogen) and protein C have not yet been assigned numbers. Most of the coagulation proteins are produced in the liver and circulate in an inactive zymogen form. When clotting is activated, one factor activates the next in the chain by an enzymatic process until ultimately thrombin is produced. This enzyme cleaves the fibrinogen molecule releasing fibrinopeptides A and B; the remainder of the molecule is fibrin monomer which rapidly polymerizes to form a clot and is then stabilized by factor XIII.

Protease inhibitors

The most important of these is antithrombin III (ATIII) which antagonizes thrombin and also has important inhibitory activity against factors IXa, Xa, XIa and XIIa. In some centres it is colloquially known as 'Anti-Xa'. In the presence of heparin, ATIII inactivates the factors mentioned very rapidly. There are numerous other protease inhibitors in the plasma including α_1-antitrypsin, α_1 anti-chymotrypsin, α_2-macroglobulin and complement C inhibitor. Of these the most important is $\alpha 2$-macroglobulin, which complexes with thrombin, plasma and kallikrein; however it accounts for less than 30% of the plasma antithrombin activity.

Fibrinolysis

This is a complex system which induces clot lysis, and like the coagulation process it involves a sequence of activation reactions. The major factor circulates as plasminogen and can be activated to plasmin, a serine protease, by several activators including urokinase, streptokinase, kallikrein and extrinsic activators which are found in the vessel wall (Collen 1980). Plasminogen activation occurs at almost the same time as clotting starts, and the fact that a clot forms at all reflects that coagulation is activated more quickly than fibrinolysis.

DRUGS WHICH AFFECT HAEMOSTASIS

Drugs affecting haemostasis often have a major effect on one aspect of the coagulation process, with a less important effect at another point of the chain. In this chapter drugs are considered in relation to the major site of their activity.

Drugs affecting the vessel wall

On rare occasions drug-induced vascular damage may result in clinical purpura. This is usually associated with increased local fibrinolytic activity and on most occasions represents a drug idiosyncrasy. There are no drugs which regularly cause haemorrhage primarily by an effect on the vessel wall. On the other hand, procoagulant activity associated with the endothelium can be increased by administration of antidiuretic hormone (ADH) analogues. In particular, desmopressin (DDAVP) has been shown to increase the plasma factor VIII activity both in the normal and in patients with mild haemophilia. Its use is recommended as an adjunct in the treatment of haemorrhage in haemophilia, whether spontaneous or following surgery (Mannucci et al 1977).

Desmopressin

(1-deamino-8-D-arginine) vasopressin, DDAVP.
Desmopressin is primarily used in the diagnosis and treatment of diabetes insipidus, its action being mainly on the renal collecting tubule. Its pressor effect is minimal. In the body it is degraded by proteolytic enzymes, the products being excreted in the urine. When used for its haemostatic effect it is given in a dose of 0.4 μg kg^{-1} at the time of surgery, and repeated 6-hourly. This regime has the effect of improving the factor VIII activity in patients with mild haemophilia, in whom factor VIII may achieve haemostatic levels for a sufficient time to cover minor (e.g. dental) surgery, etc. DDAVP may also be used as an adjunct to fresh-frozen plasma or fresh blood in multi-transfused patients.

DDAVP may cause significant water retention, but this can usually be managed purely by restriction of water intake.

It should be noted that elective operations on patients with haemophilia and Von Willebrand's disease should be carried out only in consultation with (and preferably in the care of) the local haemophilia treatment centre.

Ethamsylate

Chemical name: diethylammonium 2,5-dihydroxybenzene sulphonate.
Ethamsylate (Dicynene) is a white crystalline powder, freely soluble in water. It is readily absorbed from the gastrointestinal tract, and is excreted mainly in the urine. A small proportion appears in the bile and faeces.

It is used as a systemic haemostatic agent. Its mode of action (if any!) is unclear, but it is thought to reduce blood loss due to a capillary oozing following tonsillectomy. The evidence as to whether ethamsylate has any effect at all is very slender, and conflicting reports have been produced (see review by Verstraete 1977).

Ethamsylate may be given orally or by i.m. or i.v. injection. For prophylaxis of haemorrhage during or after anaesthesia, 750–1000 mg may be given with the premedication, or 1000 mg i.v. at the time of induction. Following operation, 750–1000 mg is given i.m., followed by 500 mg every 4–6 h.

Adverse effects include nausea, headache, skin rashes and occasionally hypotension. Note that high molecular weight plasma expanders should be given after, rather than before, ethamsylate.

Drugs affecting the platelets

The usual platelet count in the blood is 150–400 $\times$ 10^9 l^{-1}. A reduction below 80 $\times$ 10^9 l^{-1} is frequently associated with purpura (and haemorrhage following surgery). A moderate increase (up to 800–1000 $\times$ 10^9 l^{-1}) may be associated with an increased tendency to clot. Very large increases (greater than about 2000 $\times$ 10^9 l^{-1}) may be associated with haemorrhage. This effect is a complex one, but the end-result of an excess of platelets is failure to deposit a stable fibrin plug in a vascular wound.

Almost any drug can cause thrombocytopenia as an indiosyncratic reaction; and there are many drugs which very frequently cause thrombocytopenia. Those most often implicated are listed in Table 26.1. An effect analogous to thrombocytopenia (i.e. an anticoagulant activity) is produced by drugs which interfere with platelet function — the antiplatelet drugs. The most important of these are acetylsalicylic acid (aspirin), dipyridamole, sulphinpyrazone and dextran. Heparin (discussed below) also interferes with platelet function, as does synthetic prostacyclin (epoprostenol).

Table 26.1 Drugs which frequently cause thrombocytopenia by (a) immune mechanisms and (b) non-immune mechanisms.

A. IMMUNE MECHANISMS	B. NON-IMMUNE MECHANISMS
Quinine	Marrow suppressants
Quinidine	Metals, eg., Gold, Bismuth, Arsenic and Arsenical components
Digitoxin	
Thiazidine diuretics	Antibiotics including Sulphonamides, Aminoglycosides, Cephalosporins, Tetracyclines
Sedormid	
Alpha methyl dopa	Acetazolamide
Aspirin	Anticonvulsants
Carbamazepine	Antimalarials
Desipramine	Alcohol
Rifampicin	Non-steroid anti-inflammatory agents
Cephalothin	Heparin

Salicylates

Aspirin (acetylsalicylic acid), soluble aspirin (sodium salicylate)

The primary uses of salicylate are as an analgesic, anti-inflammatory and antipyretic.

Aspirin is readily absorbed from the stomach and upper small intestine. It is transported 80–90% bound to plasma proteins, especially albumin. Salicylates are excreted by the kidney, mainly after conjugation with glycine in the liver, but up to 85% of the ingested drug may be excreted unchanged in an alkaline urine. The plasma half-life for aspirin is of the order of 15–30 min.

A single bolus of aspirin as small as 0.3 g can considerably prolong the bleeding time in healthy people. Platelet cyclo-oxygenase undergoes acetylation, preventing the synthesis of endoperoxides and thromboxane A_2. This effect lasts for the lifetime of the platelet and may be manifest for 4–6 days. The antiplatelet activity of aspirin is thought to be of value in preventing thrombosis on cardiac implants. It may have a place in the prevention of myocardial infarction and in the treatment of deep venous thrombosis. The usual dose of aspirin as anticoagulant is 300–600 mg orally three or more times weekly. Long-continued aspirin administration also interferes with the synthesis of many of the plasma clotting factors, especially II, VII, IX and X, although this effect is relatively minor. If the platelet defect due to aspirin must be reversed this can be achieved by platelet transfusion.

The major side-effects of aspirin include gastrointestinal upsets; and significant blood loss associated with gastric erosions is not uncommon. Aspirin hypersensitivity is rare but may be manifest by angio-oedema, bronchospasm, etc., and a history of previous blood loss from peptic ulcer or diverticulitis should be viewed as a partial contra-indication to its use.

Dipyridamole

Chemical name: (2,6-bi-(diethanolamino)-4-8-dipiperidinopyrimido-(5,4 d) pyrimidine).

Dipyridamole is absorbed rapidly from the small intestine, being concentrated in the liver, and excreted mainly in the faeces.

It has a potent vasodilator effect and has been used (without great effect) in angina pectoris. By itself it does not induce clinical signs of platelet dysfunction, although it does undoubtedly inhibit platelet aggregation in vitro. This activity may be due to potentiation of the effects of PGI_2 or to an increase in the intracellular cyclic AMP (Moncada & Korbut 1978). Dipyridamole is used in combination with other anticoagulants. Together with warfarin it is used to prevent thromboembolism from cardiac implants. In combination with aspirin it has been shown to lengthen the shortened platelet survival associated with venous thrombosis, cardiac implants, arteriovenous shunts and prosthetic arterial grafts (Harker & Slichter 1973, Ritchie & Harker 1977). The antiplatelet effect is not significant with doses less than 200 mg daily, but 400 mg daily appears to achieve a clinical effect.

There are no absolute contra-indications and dipyridamole is relatively free from side-effects. Sometimes the vasodilator activity is prominent and this may give rise to troublesome headaches.

Sulphinpyrazone

Chemical name: sulphoxyphenylphrazolidine.

Sulphinpyrazone is readily absorbed from the gastrointestinal tract, becoming nearly all bound to plasma proteins. It has a biological half-life of about 3 h. After an intravenous injection up to 50% of the dose is excreted unchanged in the urine within 24 h.

Sulphinpyrazone is a potent uricosuric agent, and its primary value is in the treatment of gout. However, it also inhibits platelet function in a reversible manner, probably by antagonizing platelet cyclo-oxygenase (Ali & McDonald 1977). This action takes several days to develop, and it is probable that the thioether metabolite of sulphinpyrazone is responsible for most of its recorded antiplatelet activity (Pay et al 1981). The drug does not prolong the bleeding time, although it lengthens platelet survival in patients with prosthetic heart valves (Weily & Genton 1970), and with transient cerebral ischaemia (Steele et al 1977). The drug has no value as a short-term anticoagulant, but may be of some use in preventing myocardial reinfarction, and in the prevention of recurrent venous thrombosis; definitive data are as yet not available. Sulphinpyrazone is administered in a dose of 100 mg daily, increasing to 200–300 mg daily. It may cause gastrointestinal disturbances and may lead to activation of a quiescent peptic ulcer. Blood dyscrasias have been reported. Finally, it potentiates the oral anticoagulants and the sulphonylureas, and should be used with caution in their presence.

Dextran 70 and dextran 75

The dextrans are polysaccharides extracted from the bacterium *Leuconostoc mesenteroides*. Dextran 70 with a molecular weight of around 70 000, and dextran 75 (MW 75 000) are used as plasma expanders. Many workers use dextrans to prevent venous thromboembolism, especially in surgical patients. Their mode of action is complex, but certainly includes an inhibitory effect on platelet aggregation (Bygdeman & Eliasson 1967). The dextrans are discussed in more detail in Chapter 34.

Epoprostenol

Prostaglandin I_2, PGI_2, prostacyclin.
This is a prostaglandin which causes vasodilation and prevents platelet aggregation (Szczeklik et al 1978). It has a very short half-life (minutes) in the blood, the major breakdown product being 6-ketoprostaglandin F1. Following cessation of infusion the cardiovascular effects cease rapidly, while inhibition of platelet aggregation continues for up to 2 h.

The use of PGI_2 is still largely experimental, although it has been used to prevent platelet aggregation during haemodialysis and other procedures involving extracorporeal circulation.

Drugs affecting the coagulation proteins

Production of the plasma coagulation proteins depends on adequate nutrition, liver function and vitamin K. Oestrogen administration (either alone or in combination with progestogens in the oral contraceptives) encourages their synthesis (Thomson & Poller 1965). Production may be inhibited by the oral administration of members of two groups of compounds, the coumarins and the indanediones. A very large number of anticoagulants based on the parent compounds are available, and for brevity only warfarin and phenindione will be discussed. Both agents interfere with the action of vitamin K in the synthesis of factors II, VII, IX and X by preventing gammacarboxylation of glutamic acid (Stenflo & Suttie 1977) in the precursor molecules. In these circumstances inactive forms of the clotting factors are produced (demonstrated by immunological means) and they interfere with the clotting process. This phenomenon is referred to as the PIVKA effect — protein formed in vitamin K absence (Hemker et al 1968).

Coagulation may also be inhibited by heparin and related compounds which act at several points of the coagulation chain, inhibiting especially factor Xa, but also in higher dosage inhibiting the action of thrombin on fibrinogen and the platelet aggregating activity of thrombin (Eika 1971).

Warfarin sodium

The sodium salt of 4-hydroxy-3(3-oxo-1-phenyl-butyl) coumarin
Warfarin sodium is rapidly absorbed from the intestine and peak concentrations are reached 1–2 h after ingestion. It is largely bound to plasma albumin and this inhibits (incompletely) its diffusion into red cells, CSF, urine and breast milk. Warfarin is metabolized in the liver, degradation products being conjugated with glucuronic acid; excretion is via the faeces and urine.

The main indications for its use are deep venous thrombosis and pulmonary embolism. It is also used to prevent embolism in atrial fibrillation and following arterial and open-heart surgery. The usual treatment protocol is to administer 10 mg of warfarin on day 1 and again on day 2. Maintenance treatment, usually in the range 3–7 mg daily is started on day 3. Dosage is controlled by the prothrombin clotting time, nowadays reported as a British (or International) comparative ratio — the therapeutic range being 2.0–4.5.

The major risk of warfarin treatment is, of course, haemorrhage, but hypersensitivity reactions have been reported, as have alopecia, fever, nausea and diarrhoea. Skin reactions, including epidermal necrosis, are sometimes seen. Drug interactions are frequent and it is particularly important to avoid aspirin compounds. These strongly and dangerously potentiate warfarin in addition to interfering with platelet function. The nonsteroidal anti-inflammatory agents also potentiate warfarin, as do metronidazole and trimethoprim-sulphamethoxazole. Congestive cardiac failure, liver disease, alcoholism and hypermetabolic states increase the hypoprothrombinaemic response to a standard dose of warfarin, and there is a positive correlation between the patient's age and his or her warfarin response.

Barbiturates and glutethimide inhibit (often markedly) the effect of warfarin.

Warfarin should be given only with caution to hypertensive patients and those with a history of peptic ulcer or diverticulitis should receive oral anticoagulants only under the closest supervision. Haemorhage due to overdosage often gives rise to concern. In mild cases, stopping warfarin for 48 h may suffice to arrest bleeding. In more severe cases, blood transfusion may be required. The deficient clotting factors may be restored with fresh-frozen plasma or with a concentrate such as factor IX concentrate (NBTS). The action of warfarin can be reversed in 24–36 h by the administration of synthetic vitamin K (acetomenaphthone) in a dose of 5–10 mg. Larger doses may render the patient refractory to warfarin for up to 3 weeks, so that if the indication for anticoagulant therapy continues, heparin must then be used.

Phenindione

Chemical name: 2-phenylindanedione.
The absorption, distribution, mode of action and indications are similar to those of warfarin sodium. Phenindione is, however, more frequently associated with hypersensitivity reactions which can be extremely severe (Hargreaves & Howell 1965). It should be used only in patients who cannot tolerate warfarin. The usual dose is 200 mg in divided doses on the first day, 100 mg on the second, and maintenance thereafter with 25–150 mg in divided doses at 12 h intervals.

Drug interactions are similar to those of warfarin, although phenindione is less readily displaced from its albumin-bound state by phenylbutazone, and so is less strongly potentiated by this drug.

Heparin

This is not a single substance but a complex of sulphated mucopolysaccharides prepared from either beef lung or porcine intestinal mucosa (it was originally prepared from the liver). It is usually prepared as the sodium salt for injection; the calcium salt is also available. Commercial preparations have a molecular weight of 5000–35 000; dosage is expressed in international units.

When injected intravenously it is active at once, interfering with coagulation by enhancing the effect of antithrombin III (ATIII) on factor Xa, and also by preventing the formation of thrombin from prothrombin and fibrin from fibrinogen. In low doses its main activity is in potentiating ATIII. It is nearly all protein-bound in the circulation, but is rapidly broken down and metabolized, having a half-life of 1–2 h in the blood.

The indications for its use are many and varied. Its main application is in the treatment of venous thrombosis and pulmonary embolism; but it is also widely used as a prophylactic against these conditions, and as the anticoagulant for procedures involving extracorporeal circulation.

In established thrombosis the usual practice is to inject a loading dose of 7500–10 000 units, followed by a constant infusion for 7–10 days. The daily dose may be 20 000–40 000 units depending on the laboratory monitoring tests. Heparin treatment is monitored by means of the activated partial thromboplastin time (APTT, PTTK), and treatment is deemed adequate when this test is prolonged to 60–120 seconds. A markedly prolonged PTTK need not give rise to anxiety unless the patient is bleeding overtly, and it is usually sufficient merely to reduce the heparin dosage. If necessary circulating heparin can be antagonized within a few minutes by protamine sulphate (50 mg) given intravenously. This dose may be repeated in 2 h if the PTTK is still not satisfactory. It is customary following heparin treatment for deep venous thrombosis, etc., to change to oral anticoagulants for several weeks, if this option is available.

Heparin may also be used in smaller doses ('Minihep') as a prophylaxis against thrombosis in patients at risk. The usual dose is 5000 units given subcutaneously 2 h before operation and repeated every 8–12 h until the patient is mobile. At this dosage level, laboratory control is not of value.

The complications of therapy are mainly related to bleeding. However, alopecia, thrombocytopenia and osteoporosis also occur, albeit infrequently. Contra-indications are relative, rather than absolute, although severe hypertension is considered by many to constitute a very significant hazard.

As with the oral anticoagulants, drug interactions are important: heparin has many significant incompatibilities. The most important of these are the aminoglycoside antibiotics, erythromycin, and many of the cephalosporins.

Dextran sulphate and sodium pentosan sulphate have heparin-like activity; however, they are not widely used for this purpose, and they will not be further considered here.

The molecular structure of heparin is that of a

polydisperse glycosaminoglycan with a molecular weight range from 5000–30 000 daltons. The active antithrombin binding region has a pentasaccharide structure in which several sulphate groups are prominent (Bjork & Lindahl 1982). Considerable research effort has been devoted to the preparation of various low molecular weight heparin fractions, discarding the molecular fragments deemed to be undesirable (Casu 1984). Animal experiments and clinical trials are still ongoing; some fractions have been shown to have very marked Xa activity, although in clinical trials they are less effective in clot prevention than unpurified heparin (Thomas et al 1981, Thomas, Merton, Barrowcliffe et al 1982). Satisfactory dosage schedules for the low molecular weight heparins have not been developed, and these promising drugs are therefore not yet in clinical use.

Drugs affecting protease inhibitors

The most active of the protease inhibitors is antithrombin III. A reduction in this enzyme may, at least in theory, lead to hypercoagulability. Patients congenitally deficient in ATIII suffer from frequent thrombotic episodes (Egeberg 1965) and the concept of the hypercoagulable state seems also to be valid in pregnancy and in women taking oral contraceptives (Tsakok et al 1980).

Laboratory tests of coagulation status provide information analogous to the results of examining a single frame of a movie film; the results are relevant to the blood only at the time when the sample was taken. Even using a wide variety of tests it is not possible accurately to predict morbidity from haemostatic disorders in every patient (Mammen 1982, Rapaport 1983). However, groups of patients at increased risk can be identified. Women who have been on oral contraceptives and who require operations constitute such a group, and their management remains a cause for concern. Only general advice can be given, and each case must be managed individually. Recent use of oral contraceptives does not by itself constitute a reason for delaying an operation in an otherwise healthy woman. The patient's medical history must be considered, as must the proposed surgical procedure; whether the patient is likely to remain well hydrated and if she will be mobilized early after operation etc. The laboratory may provide some assistance; if prothrombin, PTTK, fibrinogen and ATIII levels are normal, and if the haematocrit is less than 0.45, the decision to proceed to operation would be encouraged. The use of 'Minihep' is scarcely, if ever, contraindicated, while full heparinization may be advisable

postoperatively, especially if ambulation is likely to be delayed. Where the anaesthetist feels that risk factors are increased, laboratory tests sometimes provide objective evidence that this is so. Frequently the prothrombin time and PTTK are shortened by the contraceptive pill (Brakman et al 1967) and often the ATIII is reduced (Sabra & Bonnar 1983). These changes may be manifest even up to 6 weeks after changing to another method of contraception; after this repeat tests often demonstrate a return to normal, and the risks of postoperative thrombosis will have abated. The action ATIII is, of course, encouraged by heparin (discussed above). ATIII concentrates can be obtained from the National Blood Transfusion Service for use in patients who are deficient in this enzyme — this will be considered below with the other blood products.

Drugs affecting the fibrinolytic system

Fluidity of the blood is maintained by an equilibrium between the processes of coagulation and fibrinolysis. Normally both sides of the equilibrium are at a low level of activity. It is possible to increase fibrinolytic activity to a minor degree by the administration of drugs such as phenformin and stanozolol (Fossard et al 1974, Dodman et al 1973) and active hepatocellular disease may also be accompanied by active fibrinolysis.

Frequently, increased fibrinolytic activity is matched by a rise in coagulant activity, manifest by a shortening of platelet life; the net result is a 'no-change' state. Strong activation of fibrinolysis resulting in anticoagulation of clinical significance can be induced by several currently available agents, described below.

Inhibitors are also available, the most frequently used being aminocaproic acid, tranexamic acid and an enzyme, aprotinin (Trasylol).

Fibrinolytic activators

Streptokinase

Streptokinase is a partly purified extract from cultures of group C haemolytic streptococci.

Streptokinase causes lysis of blood clots by activation of plasminogen, and is of value in the treatment of embolism and severe thrombotic occlusion of arteries and veins. The indications for its use have been reviewed by Bell and Meek (1979). Since high (neutralizing) antibody titres occur after a streptococcal infection a streptokinase resistance test may be necessary before the effective dose can be calculated. The initial antibody-neutralizing dose is then given intravenously over

30–60 min followed by maintenance of 100 000 international units hourly for 3–5 days. Most authorities recommend administration of hydrocortisone 100 mg with the initial dose to avoid allergic reactions. The effect of streptokinase is monitored by the plasma thrombin clotting time, which should be prolonged to approximately twice normal. The anticoagulant effect disappears rapidly after cessation of treatment, and if rethrombosis is to be avoided, treatment must be continued with heparin after only a very short delay.

The major side-effects of streptokinase are haemorrhage and allergy. Haemorrhage may be controlled by administration of blood, fresh frozen plasma, and if necesssary tranexamic acid or aprotinin. Allergic manifestation may be minimized with corticosteroids, particularly hydrocortisone.

Streptokinase is contra-indicated in patients with severe hypertension, coagulation defects, cerebral metastases or peptic ulcer, and it must be avoided in patients who have undergone surgery in the previous 3 weeks. It should also be avoided in patients with carotid or vertebral artery occlusion.

Urokinase

Urokinase is an enzyme extracted from human urine or from cultures of human kidney cells.

Urokinase directly converts plasminogen to plasmin. It has been used to lyse clots in the eye in patients suffering from vitreous haemorrhages; and in the treatment of pulmonary embolism. It is also of value in unblocking AV shunts and intravenous cannulae.

For local use in hyphaemia 5000 units dissolved in 2 ml of saline may be introduced into the anterior chamber through a small incision just within the temporal limbus. If necessary the dose may be increased to 25 000 units; this dosage is also recommended for use in cases of vitreous haemorrhage. For clotted AV shunts, 5000–25 000 units dissolved in 5 ml of saline have been instilled into the affected limb of the shunt which is then clamped off for 2–4 h. For systemic anticoagulation the usual initial dosage is of the order of 4400 international units per kg body weight, followed by 4400 i.u. kg^{-1} by constant infusion for 12–24 h.

Side-effects, precautions and contra-indications are as for streptokinase. Allergic reactions are rare since urokinase is of human origin. Although the theoretical attractions of inducing solution of a thrombus within a blood vessel are obvious, urokinase has not been very widely used. This may be due in part to its expense, but more obviously to the fact that it can exert its action only on the tip of a thrombus in an obstructed blood vessel. Many workers believe that urokinase (and streptokinase) have little advantage over more conventional anticoagulants (especially heparin).

Alteplase

Alteplase (Actilyse) is a recombinant DNA-derived version of a naturally occurring plasminogen activator which is secreted by human endothelial cells. It is thought to be relatively specific for fibrin-bound plasminogen, converting this to plasmin which then induces lysis of the fibrin clot. Thus it appears to have a selective local action, and in theory causes minimal activation of plasminogen in the systemic circulation.

Following an intravenous bolus, Alteplase is cleared rapidly from the circulation and is catabolised mainly by the liver, with a half life of approximately 5 minutes.

Alteplase is still undergoing trials in the early treatment of myocardial infarction, and its use has not, as yet, been widely extended to the treatment of thrombosis elsewhere. Studies reported to date, (e.g. O'Rouke et al 1988, TIMI studygroup 1987) suggest that the beneficial effect of Alteplase in early myocardial infarction is similar to that of Streptokinase.

Alteplase is administered intravenously in a dose of 100 mg (58×10^6 units) over a period of 3 hours, giving 10% of the dose within 1–2 minutes, 50% over 1 hour, and the remainder in the next 2 hours.

Side effects of this regime appear to be minor, and since Alteplase is of human origin, allergic/anaphylactic manifestations are unlikely to occur.

Contraindications to Alteplase are the same as those for Streptokinase.

Anistreplase

Chemical name: p-anisoylated (human lys-plasminogen — streptokinase activator complex (APSAC)

Anistreplase (Eminase) is a thrombolytic enzyme complex in which the catalytic centre is 'masked' by an anisoyl group. After injection, deacylation takes place and the complex becomes enzymatically and biologically active with a half-life of approximately 90 minutes.

Like Alteplase, Anistreplase is undergoing clinical trials in early myocardial infarction.

In this application it appears to be slightly superior to streptokinase in its efficacy (AIMS Trial study group 1988, 1990).

Contraindications and adverse side effects are similar to those of streptokinase.

As yet, neither Actilyse nor Anistreplase have been extensively used for thrombotic problems occurring at sites other than the coronary tree. Both agents are still very expensive, a factor which cannot be ignored. For the moment streptokinase should be viewed as the thrombotic agent of choice in early myocardial infarction, and especially where thrombolysis is required at extra cardiac sites.

Russell Viper Venom

Trade name: Ancrod.
A glycoprotein enzyme derived from snake venom, Ancrod has a molecular weight of about 30 000. Following injection, it becomes partially bound to plasma proteins. It has a plasma half-life of 3–5 h. It is not clear how Ancrod is metabolized.

When injected it reduces the concentration of blood fibrinogen, by forming unstable microparticles of fibrin which are easily destroyed by plasmin. Other clotting factors are not affected, and it does not activate factor XIII, nor does it digest fully crosslinked fibrin formed by the action of thrombin. It is used in the treatment of thrombotic disorders (including retinal vein thrombosis), and as a prophylactic after surgery. The usual initial dose is 2–3 i.u. kg^{-1} body weight in saline given intravenously over about 6 h followed by maintenance of 2 i.u. kg^{-1} every 12 h for up to 7 days. For prophylaxis following surgery (particularly hip surgery) Ancrod may be given as 4 i.u. kg^{-1} subcutaneously followed by 1 i.u. kg^{-1} daily for 4 days.

Adverse side-effects include localized oedema pain, and haemorrhage, occasionally from recent surgical wounds. Precautions are as for heparin. In addition, Ancrod should not be given to patients with severe thrombocytopenia, severe infections or disseminated intravascular coagulation, or during pregnancy. It should not be used together with dextrans or aminocaproic acid.

Haemorrhage occurring during Ancrod treatment may be managed by stopping this therapy; fibrinogen levels usually return to normal in a few hours. If necessary a neutralizing serum is available, which can be given intramuscularly or intravenously providing a test dose has failed to produce untoward reactions. If antiserum is required, it should be given with 1 litre of blood or fresh frozen plasma to restore the fibrinogen.

Fibrinolytic inhibitors

Aminocaproic acid

6-Aminohexanoic acid.
Aminocaproic acid (Epsikapron) is readily absorbed from the gastrointestinal tract, and becomes widely distributed throughout the body fluids; excretion is by the kidneys, mainly unchanged, and most of a single dose is excreted within 12 h. It acts as an antifibrinolytic agent by inhibiting plasminogen activation and to a lesser degree by inhibiting plasmin. Its use is indicated in severe haemorrhage associated with excessive fibrinolysis, and it can be of considerable value in haemorrhage following surgery of the lower urinary tract. It may also be used in severe haemorrhage following administration of fibrinolytic activators.

Aminocaproic acid may be given orally or by intravenous injection. Orally the dose is 3–6 g four or six times daily. By intravenous infusion, 4–5 g are given in the first hour, followed by 1 g every 8 h until bleeding has been controlled.

Adverse effects include diarrhoea, headaches, rash, muscle pain and weakness, and it may stabilize thrombi once they have been formed, so that a venous thrombus may heal by fibrosis rather than by recanalization.

It should be used with caution in patients with renal impairment, and is contra-indicated in patients with disseminated intravascular coagulation with predominant activation of the coagulation phase.

Tranexamic acid

(Trans-4 aminomethyl) cyclohexane carboxylic acid. Tranexamic acid (Cyclokapron) has the actions of aminocaproic acid, but is 10 times more potent. It too is absorbed from the gastrointestinal tract and is excreted in the urine. The indications are as for aminocaproic acid. The usual dosage is 1–1.5 g orally two or three times daily or 0.5–1.0 g by slow intravenous injection two or three times daily. The injection is incompatible with penicillin. Adverse effects, etc., are similar to those of aminocaproic acid, although the incidence of side-effects is said to be much lower.

Aprotinin

This is straight-chain polypeptide proteinase inhibitor from lung tissue, molecular weight about 6500.

Aprotinin (Trasylol) may be given intravenously and is excreted in the urine with a plasma half life of $2\frac{1}{2}$–3 h. It acts as an inhibitor of proteolytic enzymes; chymotrypsin, trypsin and kallidinogenase, as well as plasmin and some plasminogen activators, are all important substrates for its activity. It has been used in acute pancreatitis (when it is of doubtful value) and in hyperfibrinolytic states. For hyperfibrinolysis a dose of 500 000 units is given intravenously slowly, followed by a continuous infusion of up to 50 000 units hourly.

Occasionally it may cause nausea, vomiting and diarrhoea. Allergic reactions including urticaria, bronchospasm and even anaphylaxis have occurred. There are no absolute contra-indications to its use, but it is pharmacologically incompatible with corticosteroids and with nutrient solutions containing amino acids or fat emulsions. Other uses of aprotinin are discussed in Chapter 31.

Blood and blood products

No discussion of haemostasis would be complete without mention of blood and blood products. The introduction of plastic containers has permitted the development of techniques for fractionation of whole blood with minimal risk of contamination. Freshly drawn whole blood contains red cells, white cells, platelets and all the clotting factors of plasma. It also contains immunoglobulins, as a general rule not of relevance to coagulation, and the anticoagulant fluid citrate–phosphate–dextrose with adenine. The anticoagulant (100 ml) in each bag contains 18 millimoles of sodium, and the addition of adenine has permitted red cell storage up to 45 days. Blood can be considered safe for use only after the full serology tests have been carried out, usually 48 h after the blood has been drawn. On storage labile elements disappear from the blood.

There are virtually no viable platelets in blood after 4 days storage; and coagulation factor VIII reaches low levels very quickly, although the other clotting factors are much less markedly reduced (Nilsson et al 1983). Obviously, a large transfusion of bank blood may by dilution reduce the recipient's platelets and factor VIII to sub-haemostatic levels. These deficiencies may easily be corrected without risk of hypervolaemic difficulty by use of suitable blood products, but not by the use of further bank blood. The indications for the use of the various products are discussed below.

Whole blood

The value of whole blood lies in the fact that it can increase intravascular volume and oxygen-carrying capacity. Only if both these functions are needed should whole blood be given, i.e. in oligaemia due to haemorrhage whether internal, traumatic, surgical or obstetric. The average adult blood volume is in excess of 5 litres, and a loss of 20% (1 litre) can be adequately treated by volume expansion alone; the marrow will quite quickly manufacture enough red cells to rectify the deficiency. Losses significantly greater than 1 litre will usually justify the use of whole blood.

Red cells

Concentrated red cell preparations (packed cells) are indicated when a normovolaemic patient requires augmentation of the oxygen-carrying capacity of his blood, and when medical treatment is inappropriate. 'Packed cells' are prepared by sedimentation (centrifuging) and removal of the supernatant. This may be carried out in a closed system. Such red cell preparations contain insignificant amounts of clotting factors, but they do contain microaggregates or clots containing leucocytes and platelet debris which may cause alloimmunization. Frequently this is of little importance, but if the patient is given multiple transfusions over a prolonged period, leucocyte and plasma alloimmunity may result in transfusion-associated pyrexia. In these circumstances washed red cells may be considered, or if necessary reconstituted frozen red cells can be used.

Leucocyte concentrates

These are usually prepared from special donations taken with the help of one of the cell separation machines which have become available in recent years. Their value is in the treatment of patients in whom functioning granulocytes are deficient; they have no major haemostatic function and they therefore fall outside the relevance of this chapter.

Platelets

In general, platelet preparations are obtained from freshly drawn single-unit donations. For special purposes, single-donor concentrates may be required; large numbers of platelets may be obtained from a single donor by use of the cell separator. Platelet transfusions are indicated when the patient's platelet count is markedly reduced and there is evidence of bleeding. Most authorities advocate giving platelets 'prophylactically' when the platelet count is less than 20×10^9 1^{-1} even if evidence of bleeding is confined to skin purpura. Platelet concentrates may also be used when platelet function is grossly abnormal — the deficiency may be congenital or acquired — and there is associated blood loss. A significant improvement in the platelet count is usually achieved in the adult by administration of the pooled platelet concentrates from four to six (preferably six) donors ABO identical with the patient. If the platelet count is to be maintained, in the absence of autologous production, the patient will require platelets at least twice weekly, more frequently in the presence of fever, infection, splenomegaly or platelet antibodies.

Prolonged platelet support using random donors quite

quickly results in refractoriness — the transfusions become ineffective; indeed clinical experience suggests that multiple platelet transfusions may delay the resumption of production by the patient's own marrow. Refractoriness may be managed by using HLA-compatible donors, related or unrelated, and by using larger numbers of platelets (3–4×10^9 as compared with 2.0–2.4×10^9).

Storage of platelets remains a problem; even under optimum storage conditions, platelet function is much reduced after 48 h; and it is doubtful whether platelets stored more than 72 h should be used for transfusion purposes. It is now accepted that platelets function better if stored at room temperature (18–20°C) than at 4°C, although if platelet concentrates are kept at ambient temperatures the risk of bacterial growth in the (occasional) contaminated donation is increased.

Plasma and plasma fractions

Fresh-frozen plasma (FFP)

This contains all the plasma coagulation factors and is of value as a plasma expander, when coagulation factors have been diluted or destroyed. It may also be used in the management of haemophilia, although for this purpose FFP has been superseded by preparations of factor VIII concentrate.

Freeze-dried (outdated) plasma

By virtue of storage this has lost any labile coagulation factor (VIII and V) activity. Its only use is as a volume expander and its major advantage is that of extremely long shelf-life. It has been very largely superseded by purified protein fraction (PPF).

Purified protein fraction (PPF)

This is a preparation of plasma proteins (more than 90% albumin). It is supplied in 400 ml amounts in liquid form so that reconstitution is not required. It is pasteurized during preparation, and so is free from hepatitis B antigen, and from the human immune deficiency viruses (HIV).

Albumin

Salt-free concentrates of albumin are available in various strengths (up to 20%) from commercial sources and from the National Blood Transfusion Service. They should be reserved for those cases where albumin is in-

dicated to ameliorate the (osmotic) effects of severe protein deficiency.

Coagulation factors

Fibrinogen. This cannot be prepared free of hepatitis virus, and is no longer available (but see Cryoprecipitate, below).

Factor VIII concentrates. Three types of factor VIII concentrates are available: cryoprecipitate, intermediate-purity concentrates and high-purity concentrates.

Cryoprecipitate is prepared by freezing the plasma from freshly drawn donor blood. The frozen plasma is then thawed at 4°C, factor VIII and fibrinogen fail to go into solution and remain as a precipitate. The plasma supernatant can be withdrawn leaving the individual bag with 80 ± 10 i.u. of factor VIII and 250–300 mg of fibrinogen, together with sufficient supernatant to act as a vehicle when the cryoprecipitate is needed. The cryoprecipitate is stored deep-frozen. When needed, it is thawed rapidly at 37°C and the precipitate dissolved by gently kneading the bag. Several units (usually 4–10) are pooled for use, the amount being calculated as follows: Number of i.u. factor VIII required = Body weight (kg) × 0.4 × percentage increase in factor VIII required. The factor VIII blood level necessary for haemostasis depends on the site of bleeding. Tissue bleeds in haemophilic patients require a level of 15%; severe bleeds or haemarthrosis 30% and surgery at least 50–60%.

Intermediate-purity preparations are prepared by Al(OH)$_3$ adsorption of cryoprecipitate, followed by cold precipitation of factor VIII. The factor VIII is prepared from a pool of plasma and is lyophilized for storage. It is good practice when possible to ensure that as far as possible each individual patient is treated with factor VIII from a small number of batches — if possible one batch should be used for one patient over as long a period as possible, to reduce the risk of hepatitis.

High purity concentrates are prepared by special extraction techniques which remove most of the fibrinogen and contaminating protein from the factor VIII. High-purity concentrates are most frequently used in patients who develop allergic reactions to cruder concentrates.

Factor IX complex concentrates

These preparations are sometimes called prothrombin complex concentrates, since they contain not only factor IX but also factors II, VII and X. During preparation, factors VII and X may be activated, and factor IX concentrates usually contain added heparin to prevent intravascular coagulation following administration.

The levels of factor IX required for haemostasis in Christmas disease can be achieved by a single infusion of 20–25 units kg^{-1} body weight. For surgery, twice this amount is adequate, and dosage every 48 h will maintain a satisfactory level. Factor IX concentrates may also be used in the treatment of overdosage with the coumarin drugs. For this purpose, the effect is obtained with 15 units kg^{-1} of factor IX. Owing to the presence of activated factors VII and X, factor IX concentrates may be used to bypass the deficiency of factor VIII in haemophilia; factor IX is particularly useful, although expensive, in patients whose blood contains an inhibitor to factor VIII.

Other blood products

Factor XIII (fibrin stabilising factor) also has a role in wound healing. Concentrates are available commercially, but factor XIII is present in fresh-frozen plasma, which is preferable for use, since factor XIII has a biological half-life of about 12 days.

Antithrombin III (ATIII) concentrates

These preparations have been used in congenital (and acquired) ATIII deficiency states to prevent thrombo-embolism. A dose of 1.2–5.0 units kg^{-1} will raise the ATIII level to about 0.6 units ml^{-1}, which is sufficient to attain normal antithrombin activity. The biological half-life is about 2 days, so that ATIII treatment must be given at intervals suitably calculated to maintain circulating antithrombic levels.

ATIII preparations may transmit hepatitis and AIDS but they can be pasteurized to destroy these and other viruses.

Immunoglobulins

The various immunoglobulin preparations are worthy of mention. Normal human immunoglobulin has been used (with considerable effect) in a daily dose of 0.2. i.u. kg^{-1} for 5 days in the treatment of childhood idiopathic thrombocytopenic purpura. The availability of specific immunoglobulins for the prophylaxis of infectious disease should be borne in mind by the anaesthetist; and those involved in obstetrics may have occasion to administer anti-D immunoglobulin in the prophylaxis of rhesus haemolytic disease.

ACKNOWLEDGEMENT

I am grateful to Miss Marian Kelly, who transcribed the manuscript to 'floppy disc', thereby easing the rewrite burden.

REFERENCES

AIMS Trial Study Group 1988 Effect of intravenous APSAC on mortality after acute myocardial infarction: preliminary report of a placebo controlled clinical trial. Lancet i: 545–549

AIMS Trial Study Group 1990 Long term effects of intravenous Anistreplase in acute myocardial infarction: final report of the AIMS study. Lancet i: 427–431

Ali M, McDonald J W D 1977 Effects of sulfinpyrazone on platelet prostaglandin synthesis and platelet release of serotonin. Journal of Laboratory and Clinical Medicine 89: 868–875

Bell W R, Meek A G 1979 Guidelines for the use of thrombolytic agents. New England Journal of Medicine 301:1266–1276

Bjork I, Lindahl U 1982 Mechanism of the Anticoagulant action of Heparin. Molecular and Cellular Biochemistry 48: 161–182

Bloom A L 1979 The biosynthesis of factor VIII. Clinics in Haematology 8: 53–7

Bloom A L, Gaddings J C, Wilks C J 1973 Factor VIII on the vascular intima: possible importance in haemostasis and thrombosis. Nature, New Biology 241: 217–219

Brakman P, Albrechtsen O K, Astrup T 1967 Blood coagulation, fibrinolysis and contraceptive hormones. Journal of the American Medical Association 69: 199–201

Bygdeman S, Eliasson R 1967 Effect of dextrans on platelet adhesiveness and aggregation. Scandinavian Journal of Clinical and Laboratory Investigation 20: 17–23

Casu B 1984 Structure of heparins and their fragments. Nouvelle Revue Française d'Hématologie 26: 211–219

Collen D 1980 On the regulation and control of fibrinolysis. Thrombosis and Haemostasis 43 :77–89

Dodman B, Cunliffe W J, Roberts B E et al 1973 Clinical and laboratory double blind investigation on effect of fibrinolysis therapy in patients with cutaneous vasculitis. British Medical Journal 2: 82–84

Egeberg O 1965 Inherited antithrombin deficiency causing thrombophilia. Thrombosis et Diathesis Haemorrhagica 13: 516–530

Eika C 1971 Inhibition of thrombin induced aggregation of human platelets by heparin. Scandinavian Journal of Haematology 8: 216–222

Fossard D P, Field E S, Kakkar V V, Friend J R, Corrigan T P, Flute P T 1974 Fibrinolytic activity and postoperative deep-vein thrombosis. Lancet i: 9–11

Ganz W, Geft I, Shah P K et al 1984 Intravenous streptokinase in evolving acute myocardial infarction. American Journal of Cardiology 53: 1209–1216

Hargreaves T, Howell M 1965 Phenindione jaundice. British Heart Journal 27: 932–936

Harker L A, Slichter S J, 1972 Platelet and fibrinogen consumption in man. New England Journal of Medicine 287: 999–1005

Hemker H C, Veltkamp J J, Loeliger E A 1968 Kinetic aspects of the interaction of blood clotting enzymes. III. Demonstration of the existence of an inhibitor of prothrombin conversion in vitamin K deficiency. Thrombosis et Diathesis Haemorrhagica 19: 346–363

Hoyer L W, De Los Santos R P, Hoyer J R 1973 Antihemophilic factor antigen: localisation in endothelial cells by immunofluorescent microscopy. Journal of Clinical Investigation 52: 2737–2744

Mammen E F 1982 Oral contraceptives and blood coagulation: a critical review. American Journal of Obstetrics and Gynecology 142: 781–790

Mannucci P M, Pareti F I, Ruggeri Z M, Capitano A 1977 1-deamino-8-D-arginine vasopressin; a new pharmacological approach to the management of haemophilia and von Willebrand's disease. Lancet i: 869–872

Moncada S, Korbut R 1978 Dipyridamole and other phosphodiesterase inhibitors act as antithrombotic agents by potentiating endogenous prostacyclin. Lancet i: 1286–1289

Myers K M, Seachord C L, Holmsen H, Smith J B, Prieur D J 1980 A dominant role of thromboxane formation in secondary aggregation of platelets. Nature 282: 331–333

Nilsson L, Hedner U, Nilsson I M, Robertson B 1983 Shelf life of bank blood and stored plasma with special reference to coagulation factors. Transfusion 23: 377–381

O'Rourke M F, Baron D, Keogh A et al 1988 Limitation of myocardial infarction by early infusion of recombinant tissue type plasminogen activator. Circulation 77: 1311–1315

Pay G F, Wallis R B, Zelaschi D 1981 The effect of sulphinpyrazone and its metabolites on platelet function in vitro and ex vivo. Haemostasis 10: 165–175

Rapaport S 1983 Pre-operative haemostatic evaluations; which tests, if any? Blood 61: 229–231

Ritchie J L, Harker L A 1977 Platelet and fibrinogen survival in coronary atherosclerosis. American Journal of Cardiology 39: 595–598

Sabra A, Bonnar J M 1983 Hemostatic system changes induced by $50\mu g$ and $30\mu g$ estrogen/progesterone oral contraceptives. Journal of Reproductive Medicine 28: 1 (Supplement): 85–91

Smith J B, Ingerman C M, Kogsis J J, Silver M J 1983 Formation of prostaglandins during the aggregation of human platelets. Journal of Clinical Investigation 52: 965–969

Steele P, Carroll J, Overfield D, Genton E 1977 Effect of sulfinpyrazone on platelet survival time in patients with transient cerebral ischaemic attacks. Stroke 8: 396–398

Stenflo J, Suttie J W 1977 Vitamin K dependent formation of carboxyglutamic acid. Annual Review of Biochemistry 46: 157–172

Szczeklik A, Gryglewski R J, Nizankowski R, Musial J, Pieton R, Mruk J 1978 Circulatory and anti-platelet effects of intravenous prostacyclin in healthy man. Pharmacological Research Communications 13: 389–399

Thomas D P, Merton R E, Lewis W E, Barrowcliffe T W 1981 Studies in man and experimental animals of a low molecular weight heparin fraction. Thrombosis and Haemostasis 45: 214–218

Thomas D P, Merton R E, Barrowcliffe T W, Thumberg L, Lindahl U 1982 Effects of heparin oligosaccharides with high affinity for anti-thrombin III in experimental venous thrombosis. Thrombosis and Haemostasis 47: 244–248

Thomson C, Poller L 1965 Oral contraceptive hormones and blood coagulability. British Medical Journal 2: 270–273

TIMI Study Group 1987 Thrombolysis in myocardial infarction (TIMI) trial, Phase 1: a comparison between intravenous tissue plasminogen activator and intravenous streptokinase. Circulation 76: 142–154

Tsakok F H, Ho L M, Koh S, Ratnam S S 1980 The effect of long term steroid contraception on coagulation in Asian women. Singapore Medical Journal 21: 612–619

Verstraete M 1977 In: Haemostatic drugs: a critical appraisal. Martinus Nijhoff Medical Division, The Hague, pp 26–39

Weily H S, Genton E 1970 Altered platelet function in patients with prosthetic mitral valves. Effects of sulphinpyrazone therapy. Circulation 42: 967–972

Drugs acting on other systems

27. Diuretics

C. C. Doherty

INTRODUCTION

Diuretics are among the most widely prescribed drugs in clinical practice worldwide. The physiological basis of diuretic therapy involves interruption of the pathophysiological hormonal systems underlying sodium retention and blockade of electrolyte transport in discrete nephron segments. From a historical point of view the first diuretics were antisyphilitic mercury compounds which were introduced into clinical usage in 1920. The evolution of acetazolamide (1950) and chlorothiazide (1957) from the sulphonamides began the modern era of therapy which has revolutionized the treatment of congestive cardiac failure, brought alleviation of suffering to countless numbers of patients with oedematous conditions, and brought new insights into the basic sciences relating to nephrology and membrane transport of ions. Diuretics are now used in a diversity of disorders, but their principal application remains that of conditions associated with excessive extracellular fluid, where the object of treatment is to produce a decrease in oedema without compromising the circulating blood volume. The proper use of diuretics requires not only knowledge of their pharmacology, but also an understanding of the fundamental role which the kidney plays in body salt and water homeostasis.

PHYSIOLOGICAL BACKGROUND

Renal blood flow is approximately one-quarter of the total cardiac output and therefore approximately 1250 ml min^{-1}, with a corresponding plasma flow of 700 ml min^{-1} and glomerular filtrate formation of 120 ml min^{-1}, or 170 litres per 24 h. The glomerular filtrate is similar in composition to plasma, with the exception that, due to the molecular size-selective and charge-selective properties of the glomerulus, virtually no protein is present. Of the 170 litres of glomerular filtrate, 99% is reabsorbed in the renal tubules and only

1.5 litres are excreted as urine. This conservation of volume is achieved by salt transport out of the tubular fluid which leads to passive water reabsorption; pharmacological interference with this process is the principal mechanism for increasing urinary volume.

Knowledge of the transport functions and characteristics of the different segments of the nephron is critical for understanding the renal action, clinical use, and complications of diuretics. Nephron function may be discussed in terms of four major segments: the proximal tubule, loop of Henle, distal tubule and collecting system. In addition, changes in intravascular volume and circulatory capacity are perceived by a variety of volume-sensitive receptors within the heart, liver, kidneys and the great vessels. Appropriate signals are transmitted neurally so as to effect alterations in sympathetic tone of the peripheral vascular bed or in release of antidiuretic hormone (ADH), while, within the kidney itself, neurohumoral influences affect tubular salt and fluid exchange.

The proximal tubule

The fluid entering the proximal tubule is essentially a protein-free ultrafiltrate of plasma. Micropuncture studies indicate that approximately 70% of filtered sodium, as well as potassium and bicarbonate, is reabsorbed in the proximal tubule. The mechanism of reabsorption of sodium chloride and water in the proximal tubule occurs through a complex process of active and passive components, with the result that fluid entering the loop of Henle is isotonic. Active sodium transport proceeds via one of three pathways: first there is cotransport of sodium with neutral organic solutes (glucose, amino acids); second, sodium is cotransported with non-chloride anions (phosphate, acetate, lactate); and third (quantitatively most important) is the reabsorption of sodium bicarbonate. The reabsorption of sodium and bicarbonate is linked in a complex fashion. The proximal tubular cells synthesize carbonic acid which dissociates to form HCO_3^- ions and H^+ ions, a reaction influenced by the brush-border enzyme, carbonic anhydrase. The H^+ ions pass into the tubular lumen; the HCO_3^- ions, reabsorbed Na^+ ions and water enter the spaces between the proximal tubular cells, and are transferred to the peritubular capillary lumen when hydrostatic and colloid oncotic pressures therein are favourable. Intravascular volume expansion raises the capillary hydrostatic pressure and lowers the colloid oncotic pressure, thus impeding uptake of reabsorbate into the capillary lumen. Intravascular volume contraction has the opposite effect and increases reabsorption in the proximal tubule. This simple principle is important for understanding some of the effects and side-effects of diuretics.

Loop of Henle

Urine concentration is achieved by a counter current multiplier system created by the specialized microvascular anatomy of the kidney, the variation in water permeability of the tubular membrane, and the generation of a hypertonic medullary interstitium by active transport of sodium and chloride ions. In the thin descending limb of Henle's loop the tubular fluid becomes osmotically concentrated by abstraction of water; in the thick ascending limb, which is water-impermeable, active sodium transport provides the driving force for reabsorption. A steep electrochemical sodium gradient across the luminal cell membrane is maintained by a sodium extrusion mechanism, the sodium–potassium pump located in the peritubular cell membrane. The luminal sodium gradient provides a driving force for the coupled entry of chloride and potassium. Potassium ions recycle across the luminal cell membrane, which is highly permeable to potassium, and thereby generate the positive potential in the tubule lumen. This transport of chloride and sodium without water in the ascending limb creates medullary hypertonicity and a dilute tubular fluid. Only 20% of the filtered water and 10% of the filtered sodium enter the distal convoluted tubule.

The distal convoluted tubule

Sodium reabsorption in this part of the nephron is also an active process and may be accompanied by chloride reabsorption or alternatively coupled with potassium and hydrogen ion secretion. The action of these distal tubule exchange mechanisms is controlled to a large extent by aldosterone. Active sodium reabsorption results in a negatively charged lumen and passive entry of pot-

assium into the tubular fluid. Active sodium transport is driven by a sodium–potassium ATPase pump located in the peritubular cell membranes. Cellular potassium content and tubular fluid flow rate are important factors, in addition to luminal negativity, which determine potassium secretion. In common with most other cells, distal tubular cells are rich in potassium, and cellular potassium is in turn a function of total body potassium stores and the blood pH.

The collecting system

This consists of the collecting tubules and papillary collecting ducts. Sodium is actively absorbed and this is influenced by aldosterone. Potassium is passively secreted into the electronegative lumen and hydrogen ion is also secreted. Epithelial permeability to water in the cortical part of the collecting duct is increased by ADH and this allows urine concentration to occur in states of dehydration. Exchange of sodium, potassium and hydrogen in the distal nephron allows fine adjustments to the metabolic needs of the body, and when there is a need to conserve sodium this distal mechanism is so efficient that the urine is virtually sodium free.

Renal mechanisms involved in salt and water balance

There are five main mechanisms involved in the control of salt and fluid homeostasis by the kidney:

1. Intrarenal distribution of blood flow

In humans, approximately 80–85% of the million nephrons in each kidney lie in the outer cortex, have short loops of Henle and a relatively low reabsorptive capacity for sodium. The remaining 20% are juxtamedullary, possess long loops of Henle and are largely responsible for creating the hyperosmotic interstitium in the medulla which mediates the process of urine concentration. Redistribution of blood flow from outer cortical to juxtamedullary nephrons may contribute to abnormal salt and fluid retention, while a predominance of the effect of outer cortical nephrons leads to excretion of a greater fraction of filtered salt and fluid.

2. Haemodynamic factors

The peritubular capillary bed is concerned with the uptake of reabsorbed salt and fluid from the tubular lumen, and is connected in series with the glomerular capillary network via the efferent arteriole. The prevailing hydrostatic and oncotic pressures acting across and along the peritubular capillaries are therefore dependent on saluretic and fluid exchanges taking place at the glomerulus. Available evidence indicates that changes in physical forces which alter transcapillary pressure achieve their effects on net tubular reabsorption of salt and fluid by altering the resistance of lateral intercellular channels through which the tubular reabsorbate passes to reach the peritubular capillaries.

3. Neurogenic factors

Renal denervation leads to a substantial increase in urinary salt and fluid output. Selective adrenergic neural stimulation enhances tubular reabsorption of salt and fluid which persists despite blockade of the local actions of renin, angiotensin II or prostaglandins.

4. Circulating and intrarenal humoral factors.

(a) **Renin–angiotensin–aldosterone system.** This humoral system plays a major role in renal salt and fluid regulation and is not limited to the action of aldosterone on the collecting duct as angiotensin II itself may affect tubular salt and fluid reabsorption. In fact a major component of the enhanced proximal tubular reabsorption of salt and fluid which characterizes oedematous states results from the haemodynamic changes induced by angiotensin II and catecholamines upon the renal microvasculature; angiotensin-stimulated hyperaldosteronism may play only a subsidiary role. A fall in renal perfusion pressure or administration of potent diuretics may all be stimulatory either through activation of vascular or intrarenal volume sensors or through the macula densa mechanism. This humoral system can be blocked at the step of conversion of angiotensin I to angiotensin II (converting enzyme inhibition), at receptors for angiotensin II (competitive inhibitors, e.g. saralasin), or at the step where aldosterone binds to its receptor on the collecting tubule (spironolactone). Converting enzyme inhibitors prevent conversion of angiotensin I to angiotensin II, reducing peripheral angiotensin II levels and decreasing aldosterone secretion. Converting enzyme inhibitors may also have other renal and extrarenal effects that influence sodium and potassium excretion directly and indirectly.

(b) **Atrial natriuretic peptide.** ANP is a polypeptide hormone secreted by the heart that causes diuresis, natriuresis, vasodilation and suppression of the renin–angiotensin–aldosterone system (Espiner & Richards 1989). Recent evidence indicates that subtle changes in plasma levels of ANP have an important role in regula-

tion of extracellular fluid volume and blood pressure. ANP is eliminated from the circulation by many organs, especially the kidneys. A peptidase (atriopeptidase) has been identified in renal tubular preparations which degrades ANP, and preliminary studies of a specific atriopeptidase inhibitor have indicated a renal and cardiovascular effect similar to low-dose ANP infusion (Northridge et al 1989).

Renal tissue has the capacity to generate *prostaglandins and kinins*. Prostalandins play a major role in protecting the renal circulation in circumstances where intrinsic renal function might be jeopardized — for example, when intravascular volume is contracted and circulating catecholamine concentrations are high. The interrelationships between the prostaglandin and kinin systems with respect to sodium and volume homeostasis are complex, and many aspects remain to be unravelled.

5. Intrarenal feedback mechanisms

All nephrons are anatomically arranged so that each ascending limb of Henle's loop passes close to the glomerulus of the same nephron unit. The macula densa cells of the ascending limb are thus in close contact with the afferent and efferent arterioles, providing the anatomical framework for an intrarenal feedback system which regulates glomerular filtration rate and proximal tubular reabsorption in response to changes occurring in distal solute fluid delivery. Thus alterations in the rate of delivery of the filtrate to the macula densa region of the distal nephron result in reciprocal changes in glomerular filtration (GFR).

GENERAL CONSIDERATIONS REGARDING DIURETICS

Actions on the kidney

Diuretics vary not only in chemical structure but also in potency, in site and mechanism of action in the nephron, and even in their ion selectivity. The most powerful natriuretic agents are frusemide and ethacrynic acid; the thiazides are of moderate strength, while acetazolamide, amiloride, triamterene and spironolactone are weak diuretics. The currently available compounds can be divided into five groups on the basis of their preferential effects on different segments of the nephron involved in tubular reabsorption of sodium chloride and water (Lant 1985). First are the loop diuretics — a heterogeneous group of agents which act on the thick ascending limb of Henle's loop and have a powerful short-lived diuretic effect complete within 4–6 h. The second group are the benzothiadiazines and related variants, which localize their effects to the early portion of the distal tubule. The third group comprise the potassium-sparing diuretics which act exclusively on the sodium–potassium/hydrogen exchange mechanism in the late distal tubule and cortical collecting duct. The action of drugs in groups 2 and 3 is prolonged to between 12 and 24 h. The fourth group consists of diuretics chemically related to ethacrynic acid, but with the unusual property of combining within the same molecule the property of saluresis and uricosuria. These compounds have actions to different individual extents in the proximal tubule, thick ascending limb and early distal tubule and are known as 'polyvalent' diuretics. Finally there is a mixed group of weak or adjunctive diuretics which includes the vasodilator xanthines such as aminophylline, and the osmotically active compounds such as mannitol (Fig. 27.1).

Diuretics may also be classified according to mechanism of action rather than site of action. Thus some diuretics may be classified as *transport inhibitors* as they inhibit ionic transport processes for sodium, chloride and bicarbonate ions in the renal tubule; they are the most important group in clinical usage. The mechanisms of inhibition involved vary; thus thiazides interfere with sodium chloride uptake across the luminal membrane, acetazolamide affects the rate-limiting step of the carbonic anhydrase-catalysed conversion of carbonic acid to carbon dioxide, and loop diuretics inhibit the carrier-mediated process driven by the sodium/potassium pump. Spironolactone competitively inhibits aldosterone binding to its cell receptor. Various salts and crystalloids, e.g. urea and mannitol, are non-absorbable and act as *osmotic agents*. Such agents may induce a diuresis despite the maximal operation of pituitary ADH, and these substances will therefore prevent the usual postoperative oliguria which occurs due to release of this hormone (Morris et al 1959, Thomas & Morgan 1979). Agents such as digitalis and aminophylline, when given to subjects with congestive heart failure, may improve the blood supply to the kidneys and increase the GFR, hence the term *filtration diuretics* may be applied. Lithium carbonate and demeclocycline are not true diuretics but are known to block the effect of ADH on the collecting duct, thus promoting loss of water without significant loss of solute, an effect utilized to treat states of inappropriate ADH release. Such agents have been termed *aquaretics*, and other small peptide antagonists of vasopressin with aquaretic activity may be clinically available in the near future.

In addition to the effects of diuretics on monovalent ion excretion by the kidney, there are also important effects on divalent ion excretion (calcium, phosphate, magnesium), acid–base balance and uric acid excretion.

Clinical use of diuretics

The following discussion on clinical use of diuretics is centred on disorders which are common in anaesthetic practice; other conditions in which diuretic therapy is of value (nephrolithiasis, hypercalcaemia, etc.) are not considered here (Table 27.1).

Oedematous disorders

Cardiac failure.   The pathophysiological response of

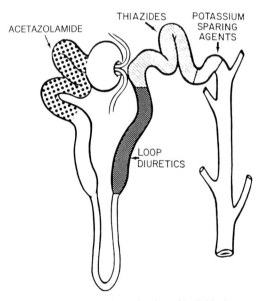

Fig. 27.1 Nephron sites of action of individual groups of diuretics.

Table 27.1 Indications for diuretics

Oedematous disorders	Non-oedematous disorders
Cardiac failure	Hypertension
Liver disease	Recurrent nephrolithiasis
Renal disease	Nephrogenic diabetes insipidus
	Hypercalcaemia
	Acute dilutional hyponatraemia
	Acid–base disorders
	Forced diuresis in poisoning
	Glaucoma
	Mountain sickness

the kidneys to heart failure closely resembles the physiological response to hypovolaemia. In both states, baroreceptors sense a fall in pressure which results in release of ADH, an increase in sympathetic nervous tone and activation of the renin–angiotensin system. In hypovolaemia the resulting salt and water retention ceases when venous volume is restored. By contrast, in heart failure, salt and water retention may continue, despite adequate filling of the venous system, so long as the cardiac output remains inadequate. The extent to which increasing venous return can increase stroke volume (via the Frank–Starling mechanism) is limited, however, and knowledge of the configuration of the Frank–Starling curve is an important consideration before diuretics are administered for preload reduction. If the heart is on the flat portion of the Frank–Starling curve, relatively little change in stroke volume will occur as left ventricular end-diastolic pressure (LVEDP) falls; conversely, on the ascending limb of the Frank–Starling curve, large changes in cardiac index may accompany small decreases in preload (Fig. 27.2). The filling pressure at which the Frank–Starling curve flattens is influenced by ventricular compliance; thus in the stiff failing ventricle, a fall in LVEDP results in a much greater decrease in stroke volume than a similar fall in LVEDP in the failing ventricle with normal compliance. In conditions of left ventricular hypertrophy such as hypertension, aortic stenosis and hypertrophic cardiomyopathy, the hearts are operating at end-diastolic dimensions on the steep segment of their Frank–Starling

curves, and attempts to reduce elevated filling pressures in these situations may result in important decreases in cardiac index. In this setting, afterload reduction (hydralazine, nitroprusside) and inotropes take precedence over diuretics, and in addition to the disorders mentioned above this is an important issue in patients with acute right ventricular infarction (Caplin 1989).

Most of the available data on the acute haemodynamic response to i.v. diuretic administration come from studies on i.v. frusemide during acute myocardial infarction. These studies showed that treatment of acute pulmonary oedema with frusemide provided relief of pulmonary congestion several hours before the onset of diuresis, and that within 15 min of administration of i.v. frusemide there is a fall in pulmonary capillary pressure and an increase in venous capacitance. The initial fall in preload following i.v. frusemide is therefore due to venodilation rather than diuresis.

The optimal left atrial pressure for any given patient with heart failure depends in part on the underlying aetiology of the heart disease. Vigorous diuretic therapy is recommended in cases of dilated cardiomyopathy to reduce heart size and prevent further dilation. Such patients are likely to have flat Frank–Starling curves and therefore tolerate diuresis without a large fall in cardiac index. Diuretics should be used with caution, if at all, in heart failure associated with abnormalities in diastolic filling, such as in constrictive pericarditis, hypertrophic cardiomyopathy or aortic stenosis.

Diuretics remain the first-line treatment for the congestive symptoms of heart failure, with thiazides the initial choice for mild heart failure, while for severe heart failure loop diuretics are indicated. Spironolactone may be a useful additional drug in patients refractory to loop diuretic therapy. Diuretics can interact adversely with other drugs commonly used in heart failure, especially digitalis, as diuretic-induced hypokalaemia and hypomagnesaemia potentiate digoxin toxicity and cardiac arrhythmias. The initiation of therapy with an ACE inhibitor drug (captopril, enalapril) in patients taking diuretics may precipitate severe hypotension, and for this reason diuretics should be withheld for several days before starting an ACE inhibitor for congestive heart failure.

Although diuretics correct the fluid retention that is one of the consequences of heart failure, they do not improve the primary myocardial dysfunction. Inotropic agents or vasodilators are necessary when symptoms of forward failure predominate, or when congestive symptoms become refractory to diuretic therapy.

Liver disease. Despite anatomical normality, the kidney exhibits a wide spectrum of functional derange-

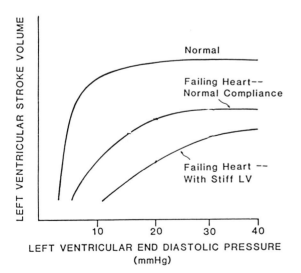

Fig. 27.2 The Frank-Starling curve in the normal heart and in heart failure.

ments in patients with liver disease, including decreased GFR and impaired renal sodium handling.

Treatment of ascites in cirrhotic patients is associated with a high incidence of diuretic-induced complications, including azotaemia, hyponatraemia, hypokalaemia, hyperuricaemia, metabolic acidosis and metabolic alkalosis. Initial therapy must include rigid dietary sodium restriction (10–20 mmol per day) and fluid restriction to avoid dilutional hyponatraemia. A distal potassium-sparing agent, e.g. spironolactone 100 mg b.d., is the drug of first choice, and if no natriuresis occurs with maximum dosage of spironolactone, frusemide 40–80 mg daily should be added. Diuretic combinations in cirrhotic patients are particularly likely to produce a wide array of complications including massive fluid/-electrolyte losses, profound circulatory collapse, hepatorenal syndrome, acute renal failure and hepatic encephalopathy. Patients with liver disease and severe hypoalbuminaemia (less than 2 gdl^{-1}) in whom there is evidence of marked intravascular volume depletion (orthostatic hypotension) may benefit from i.v. administration of albumin concentrate (20% salt-poor, 100–200 ml daily) as part of the treatment regime. In patients with massive ascites where i.v. diuretic therapy is considered necessary for rapid diuresis, the administration of i.v. albumin prior to the i.v. diuretic may enhance its efficacy and prevent circulatory complications.

Renal disease. (a) *Nephrotic syndrome.* The ideal diuresis is a slow one resulting in a gradual loss of oedema of about 0.5–1.0 kg per day in an adult patient. Only in certain circumstances is rapid diuresis with i.v. frusemide or bumetamide, usually in association with infusion of volume expanders, indicated. Indications for such treatment include severe hypertension, congestive heart failure, anasarca with respiratory embarrassment and skin complications. In patients who fail to respond to dietary salt/fluid restriction and oral combined diuretic treatment, the following possible explanations should be considered: inadequate dosage, insufficient bedrest, inappropriate corticosteroid therapy, renal failure and occult salt intake (antacids, antibiotics, effervescent analgesics, i.v. infusions).

(b) *Chronic renal failure* (CRF). In the presence of renal insufficiency, diuretic access to the tubular lumen is limited by the decrease in GFR and, probably more importantly, by impaired tubular secretion. It is appropriate to consider separately the indications, benefits and risks of diuretic therapy in patients with CRF and those with acute renal failure (ARF).

The common indications for diuretics in patients with CRF are hypertension, cardiac failure and nephrotic oedema. The benzothiadiazide diuretics may be effective until the GFR falls below 20 ml min^{-1}. Below this level of GFR, or in the event of unresponsiveness, loop diuretics are necessary and in some instances high doses of frusemide may be required (40–360 mg daily). In view of the risks of potentially lethal metabolic acidosis and hyperkalaemia, potassium-sparing drugs should be avoided in CRF patients. Neurosensory hearing loss is a well-recognized complication of the potent loop-acting diuretics and is particularly likely to occur in patients with severely impaired renal function, usually in conjunction with high doses. If diuretic therapy causes sufficient depletion of total body sodium, intravascular volume falls; as a result renal blood flow and GFR may fall, causing exacerbation of renal failure. In the volume-contracted state urea clearance by the kidney is impaired to a greater degree than that of creatinine, and changes in the latter are a more reliable index of adverse diuretic effect on renal function.

(c) *Acute renal failure.* The term acute renal failure (ARF) encompasses a number of clinical conditions associated with an abrupt deterioration in GFR. These conditions include acute tubular necrosis (ATN), severe prerenal azotaemia, acute urinary tract obstruction, acute interstitial nephritis and acute glomerulonephritis. In acute glomerulonephritis which is characterized by sodium retention, oedema and hypertension, diuretics may be of considerable value in control of hypertension and pulmonary congestion when present. The use of diuretics in ATN is more controversial.

The reduction in GFR that occurs in ATN may result from a variety of pathophysiological events including renal vasoconstriction, back-leak of filtrate across damaged tubular epithelia or obstruction of tubular flow by intraluminal precipitation of tubular debris. The relationship between these tubular events and renal haemodynamics is incompletely understood. However, the ability of diuretics such as frusemide and mannitol to induce renal vasodilation and increase tubular flow rate has led investigators to attempt prevention or alteration of the course of ATN by intervention with diuretics. Despite many studies, the therapeutic efficacy of diuretics in *established ARF* is unproven; in particular there is no evidence that conversion of oliguric to nonoliguric ARF with use of high-dose frusemide has any influence on the mortality of this syndrome. The uncritical use of i.v. frusemide when oliguria develops in diverse clinical situations is to be deprecated; if such patients are concurrently receiving aminoglycoside or cephalosporin antibiotics, diuretics may potentiate nephrotoxicity and ototoxicity. A different issue is the prophylactic use of diuretics in *patients at high risk of ARF* (patients undergoing open-heart surgery, with extracorporeal perfusion, biliary surgery in jaundiced patients, abdominal aortic aneurysm repair, trauma especially with rhabdomyolysis, and exposure to known nephrotoxins). Prophylactic mannitol given before abdominal surgery in jaundiced patients, or to patients with severe crush injuries, appears to lessen the severity of renal failure in these two settings only. The evidence of a beneficial effect is less compelling in the other disorders mentioned (Reineck 1986). Where incipient ARF is due to hypovolaemia, and volume repletion with central venous pressure measurement has failed to restore a normal urine flow rate, a trial of i.v. mannitol (50–100 ml of a 25% solution) is reasonable. In other instances where a disorder which can cause ARF is known to be present (e.g. acute intravascular haemolysis with haemoglobinuria due to incompatible blood transfusion, rhabdomyolysis with myoglobinuria) prophylactic administration of mannitol is reasonable if acute oliguria develops.

Non-oedematous disorders

Hypertension. The precise mechanism by which diuretics lower blood pressure remains uncertain. Contraction of the plasma and ECF volume appears to play an important role in the initial lowering of BP, but there is also a long-term action associated with a lowering of peripheral vascular resistance. A liberal salt intake can overcome the antihypertensive effect of thiazide therapy. The effect of thiazides on the metabolic profile (hyperlipidaemia, hyperglycaemia, hyperuricaemia) is a cause of concern with respect to their long-term usage in hypertension, as it is undesirable that an antihypertensive drug should induce other coronary risk factors (Medical Research Working Party on Mild to Moderate Hypertension 1981).

Although loop diuretics are more potent in terms of natriuresis than the thiazides, their antihypertensive effects are inferior to the former. Loop diuretics, however, have a role in the management of hypertension in the following clinical situations: (a) hypertension that is primarily volume-dependent (e.g. patients with chronic renal failure); (b) hypertensive crises; (c) in combination with antihypertensive drugs which cause fluid retention, e.g. minoxidil, hydralazine.

Acute dilutional hyponatraemia. Diuretics have a role in the treatment of some instances of acute hyponatraemia of dilutional origin. Acute symptomatic hyponatraemia ($Na^+ < 120$ mmol^{-1}) is a medical emergency with a high risk of seizures and brain damage. Frusemide and hypertonic saline can be used to acutely correct severe hyponatraemia if it occurs in the syndrome of inappropriate ADH secretion (SIADH) or the acute dilutional hyponatraemia which may follow transurethral resection of prostate due to absorption of irrigating fluid.

Acid–base disorders. (a) Severe metabolic acidosis. Patients who suffer severe metabolic acidosis (e.g. lactic acidosis) require large amounts of sodium bicarbonate administration over a short period of time. As they are often oliguric and hypotensive, sodium administration may be associated with hypernatraemia; concomitant administration of a potent diuretic such as frusemide may therefore be helpful in the prevention of severe hypernatraemia as long as fluid losses are replaced.

(b) Metabolic alkalosis. This is a frequent complication of a variety of medical conditions. In severe metabolic alkalosis, e.g. due to pyloric stenosis, the respiratory compensation may cause significant hypercapnia and hypoxia. Failure to achieve appropriate respiratory compensation for metabolic alkalosis (Pco_2 should increase by 6 mmHg for each 10 mEq l^{-1} increment in serum bicarbonate) should stimulate a search for a concomitant primary cause of respiratory acid–base disturbance, such as pneumonia or heart failure.

Posthypercapnic metabolic alkalosis is most commonly encountered in patients with chronic respiratory acidosis who suffer an acute worsening of lung disease requiring hospitalization and respiratory assistance. The compensation for the respiratory acidosis is achieved by increased renal tubular reabsorption of bicarbonate in such patients. During mechanical ventilation, if a decline in the Pco_2 achieved is faster than the capacity of the kidney to excrete bicarbonate, posthypercapnic metabolic alkalosis ensues, and the reduction in ventilatory drive may impede efforts to wean the patient from the ventilator. Prior diuretic therapy makes such patients especially sensitive to the alkalosis, and severe degrees of the disorder can induce neuromuscular irritability, seizures, coma and myocardial irritability (Rotheram et al 1964). Judicious use of potassium chloride and careful lowering of Pco_2 can usually avoid this complicating alkalosis, but patients with serum bicarbonate concentrations in excess of 35 mEq l^{-1} may benefit from small doses (125–500 mg) of the carbonic anhydrase inhibitor acetazolamide as an additional preventative measure.

Failure to respond

Cardiac oedema may require a combination of diuretic agents that act at different parts of the renal tubule, e.g. use of a loop diuretic with a distal tubule aldosterone antagonist. In resistant heart failure it is rational to combine diuretics with a low dose of an angiotensin-converting enzyme inhibitor (e.g. enalapril 2.5 mg) to block synthesis of angiotensin II and break the vicious cycle of increasing vascular resistance and falling cardiac output. In severe cases of nephrotic syndrome failure to respond to oral diuretic therapy may occur, and dramatic improvement may follow a change to intravenous administration. Intravascular volume depletion may exist in some instances of oedematous disorders associated with hypoalbuminaemia (cirrhosis, nephrotic syndrome) — such hypovolaemia causes a decrease in GFR and the consequent increase in proximal tubular reabsorption reduces the amount of sodium delivered downstream to the site of diuretic action; increased aldosterone secretion may also contribute to the blunting of natriuretic effect. In this situation, infusion of 100 ml of 20% salt-poor albumin prior to diuretic administration may restore diuretic responsiveness. In chronic renal failure, when the GFR falls below 25 ml min^{-1}, thiazide diuretics are ineffective and loop diuretics are required. The uraemic patient may, however, require dosages exceeding those used in patients with normal renal function; thus in chronic uraemia 500 mg to 1000 mg frusemide may be necessary to induce diuresis.

Complications of diuretic therapy

Some complications may occur even when diuretics are judiciously used; others occur due to injudicious use. Diuretics are the commonest cause of adverse drug reactions in old age, which is not surprising as around one-fifth of people over 65 take diuretics. Some complications are common to all diuretics, while others may be encountered with one diuretic but not with others (Table 27.2).

Extracellular fluid volume

Diuretics invariably result in some degree of extracellular fluid volume (ECF) reduction, which will initiate a sequence of compensatory haemodynamic and hormonal alterations. The haemodynamic changes result in reduced stroke volume and a fall in arterial blood pressure, which causes an increase in heart rate. If cardiac output is not maintained orthostatic hypotension, dizziness and syncope will be the presenting complaints. The compensatory hormonal changes that occur are an increase in the circulating levels of aldosterone and antidiuretic hormone. The primary purpose of the compensatory changes is to correct the compromised ECF volume by enhancing renal salt and water retention; they will also, however, aggravate several other side-effects of diuretics by reducing the excretion of urea, uric acid, calcium and free water, while increasing the excretion of potassium.

Hypokalaemia

Next to ECF volume depletion, hypokalaemia is the commonest complication of diuretic therapy. Three main factors regulate distal potassium secretion; the first is the intracellular potassium content, the second intratubular fluid volume and rate of flow, and third the intraluminal negativity that develops consequent to the reabsorption of sodium. By affecting these three mech-

Table 27.2 Complications of diuretics

Thiazides	Loop diuretics	Potassium-sparing diuretics	Carbonic anhydrase inhibitors
Hyperlipidaemia	Urinary retention	Hyperkalaemia	Metabolic acidosis
Hypercalcaemia	Ototoxicity	Gastrointestinal upset	Nephrolithiasis
Impotence		Nephrolithiasis	
	(Common to both)	Metabolic acidosis	
Hypovolaemia, hypotension, uraemia			
Hypokalaemia			
Hyponatraemia, hypernatraemia			
Metabolic alkalosis			
Hyperuricaemia			
Hyperglycaemia			
Induction of hepatic encephalopathy			
Hypersensitivity reactions			

anisms, diuretics augment the urinary excretion of potassium. Two additional side-effects of diuretic therapy which also promote distal potassium wasting are diuretic-induced volume depletion (resulting in secondary hyperaldosteronism) and metabolic alkalosis (increases intracellular potassium). The frequency with which hypokalaemia will develop, and its severity, depend on several factors; namely: the dosage and duration of action of the diuretic agent, dietary potassium and salt intake, the age of the patient and the level of circulating mineralocorticoid activity. (Oedematous patients may have a pre-existing state of secondary aldosteronism which may be aggravated by diuretic-induced volume contraction.) Finally, the acid–base status of the patient will alter potassium secretion, which is increased by alkalosis. The major symptoms of potassium depletion are fatigue, muscular weakness and ultimately paralytic ileus.

Serious side-effects of hypokalaemia result from the myocardial irritability that develops, predisposing to ventricular arrhythmias, especially in the setting of acute myocardial infarction or concurrent digitalis therapy. However, the clinical importance of the diuretic effect on potassium balance is a subject for some debate. Diuretics do not usually cause important reduction in total body potassium and the majority of patients probably do not need routine prophylaxis against hypokalaemia. A noticeable decrease in serum potassium concentration occurs in 30–50% of patients but it is generally mild and values less than 3 mmol l^{-1} are uncommon. Available evidence suggests that hypokalaemia requires correction only when the plasma potassium falls below 3 mmol l^{-1} (Morgan & Davidson 1980). Contrary to universal belief loop diuretics are less likely than the thiazides to cause important hypokalaemia.

Potassium supplements have certain risks which must be taken into account when considering replacement therapy in patients; these include hyperkalaemia and small bowel ulceration. The practice of giving potassium supplements with diuretics is based mainly on the possibility that hypokalaemia may increase the risk of cardiac arrhythmias. However, the risk in patients with uncomplicated hypertension is minimal, and it is not conclusively established that the association between diuretics and arrhythmias is due to hypokalaemia per se; other metabolic effects may be implicated (e.g. hypomagnesaemia).

Potassium-sparing agents such as amiloride, triamterene or spironolactone reduce potassium loss by their action on the distal tubule, and may induce dangerous hyperkalaemia when given to: (1) patients with reduced GFR (less than 30 ml min^{-1}) (2) diabetic patients who may have hyporeninism (3) patients taking potassium supplements or potassium-containing salt substitutes and (4) elderly patients with age-related reduction in GFR.

Azotaemia and renal failure

Diuretic administration can result in decreased renal function. Initially, the rise in blood urea is consequent to the tubular compensatory mechanisms mediated by ECF volume depletion (increased tubular reabsorption of salt and water is accompanied by increased absorption of urea). The subsequent reduction in the rate of urine flow further reduces the excretion of urea, since the clearance of urea is a function of urine flow rate. This results in a rise in blood urea at a time when the GFR is still close to normal; hence the clearance of creatinine, which depends on filtration, remains normal. Consequently, the ratio of urea concentration to that of creatinine rises disproportionately, giving the classical findings of prerenal azotaemia.

Hyponatraemia

This is a common complication of diuretic therapy which may develop acutely in oedematous states, especially if a loop diuretic is used, or insidiously when a thiazide is used. In general, the degree of hyponatraemia is modest and the patient is asymptomatic. Severe hyponatraemia ($Na^+ < 120$ mmol l^{-1}) is rare, and may produce symptoms ranging from muscle cramps, apathy and altered mental status to coma. The principal mechanism by which diuretics cause hyponatraemia is impairment of the ability to dilute the urine appropriately. The loop diuretics interfere with sodium reabsorption in the ascending limb of Henle's loop and thus limit the amount of solute-free water that the kidneys can generate. The thiazides act in the distal convoluted tubule and also interfere with urinary dilution.

Treatment of diuretic-induced hyponatraemia depends on the aetiology and severity of the disorder. Mild asymptomatic hyponatraemia will usually respond to a reduction in, or discontinuation of, diuretic therapy combined with fluid restriction. Severe symptomatic hyponatraemia, on the other hand, is a medical emergency with significant risk of death or neurological morbidity. Acute symptomatic, severe hyponatraemia of any aetiology should be corrected to mildly hyponatraemic levels (125–130 mmol l^{-1}) within 24 h using hypertonic saline. It is important to avoid rapid overcorrection to eunatraemic levels as this may result in a specific central nervous system lesion of pontine myelinolysis (Laureno & Karp 1988). Paradoxically, the loop diuretics, specifically frusemide, are used in therapy of acute severe hyponatraemia of dilutional type (e.g. the TURP syndrome). In this situation frusemide is administered in conjunction with i.v. hypertonic saline.

Hypernatraemia

The urine elaborated by all diuretic agents is relatively hypotonic to plasma, at least until the compensatory mechanisms result in the preservation of free water and elaboration of a concentrated urine. As such, the initial response is one of increased free-water clearance as urine flow rates increase, an event that is particularly evident with osmotic diuretics such as mannitol. If, at this stage of diuresis, the ability of the patient to drink or express thirst is impaired, as in stroke victims, then hypernatraemia will ensue. If undetected and uncorrected this may progress to hyperosmolar coma, and such coma may erroneously be attributed to the cerebrovascular accident rather than the electrolyte disorder.

Metabolic alkalosis

This is a common complication of diuretic therapy. Three main mechanisms are involved in the generation and maintenance of diuretic-induced metabolic alkalosis: (1) volume depletion, (2) mineralocorticoid excess, (3) potassium depletion. Elevation in circulating aldosterone levels may result in increased exchange of sodium for hydrogen ion and increased bicarbonate reabsorption by the distal nephron. Potassium depletion can result in intracellular acidosis, thus stimulating secretion of hydrogen ion by the renal tubule and therefore the absolute amount of bicarbonate reabsorption. Correction of diuretic-induced metabolic alkalosis requires normalization of ECF volume with normal saline solutions and correction of potassium depletion.

Metabolic acidosis

This acid–base disorder will invariably develop with the use of carbonic anhydrase inhibitors and often, although to a lesser degree, with potassium-sparing diuretics. The most common use of carbonic anhydrase inhibitors (e.g. acetazolamide) is in the treatment of chronic glaucoma and the observation of unexplained metabolic acidosis in elderly patients should always prompt a query for ophthalmic medications. The potassium-sparing diuretics, by blocking distal sodium reabsorption, will interfere with the ability of the distal tubule to secrete hydrogen, thus reducing the ability of the kidney to generate bicarbonate. Spironolactone is particularly prone to induce acidosis because of its specific anti-aldosterone effect.

Miscellaneous complications

Hypersensitivity reactions which have been reported with diuretics include skin rash, acute pancreatitis, acute interstitial nephritis, vasculitis, pulmonary oedema and haematological disorders. Deafness, occasionally irreversible, has been reported with frusemide and ethacrynic acid given in large doses. Gastrointestinal disturbances may occur with any of the diuretic agents, but are especially common with spironolactone. Urinary retention may be precipitated by vigorous diuresis in elderly male patients with partial prostatic obstruction. Triamterene may induce nephrolithiasis with stones which contain triamterene. Chronic spironolactone administration has been associated with a variety of endocrine disorders including impotence, gynaecomastia and irregular menstruation. This is most likely the result of the anti-androgenic effect of spironolactone.

Volume depletion induced by diuretics has been associated with an increased incidence of venous thrombosis and pulmonary embolism, particularly in the paediatric age group and in patients with severe nephrotic syndrome.

Important drug interactions

The combination of frusemide and cephalosporin is nephrotoxic, and is one of the commonest causes of drug-induced acute renal failure. Thiazides, because they decrease sodium reabsorption in the proximal tubules, indirectly may increase reabsorption of lithium and induce lithium toxicity in those with mania receiving long-term treatment with lithium. The hypokalaemia which may result in combination with steroids and carbenoxolone has already been referred to. Nonsteroidal anti-inflammatory drugs (NSAID) such as indomethacin may inhibit the diuretic response to frusemide; this may occur because prostaglandins have an effect on salt transport at the site of action of frusemide. In elderly patients the combination of diuretic therapy with NSAID or ACE inhibitor drugs is a common cause of acute renal failure. The loop diuretics displace warfarin from its binding site to albumin, resulting in the acute availability of the free anticoagulant to exert its effect. Hence the intermittent tendency to increase the prothrombin time when these agents are used together.

INDIVIDUAL DIURETICS

BENZOTHIADIAZINES (THIAZIDES AND HYDROTHIAZIDES)

Pharmacology

Chlorothiazide, the prototype of the thiazide diuretics, was discovered in 1957 during systematic study of various sulphonamides possessing carbonic anhydrase inhibitory activity (Table 27.3). All benzothiadiazines possess a chlorine or pseudohalogen group at position 6 and a sulphamoyl group at position 7. They are highly protein-bound and like the loop diuretics are thought to gain access to their renal locus of action via the probenecid-sensitive organic acid secretion pathway. They depress sodium chloride transport in the distal tubule just proximal to the site of potassium exchange and cause moderate natriuresis equivalent to 5–10% of the filtered sodium. No satisfactory biochemical mechanism has yet been proposed to explain their natriuretic action. The major difference between the various benzothiadiazines lies in the time course of their biological activity; whereas, for example, bendrofluazide has an elimination half-life of only 3 h, the half-life of hydroflumethiazide is 17 h and that of polythiazide is approximately 26 h. These differences reflect variations in lipid solubility, volumes of distribution and renal clearances.

Heterocyclic variants of benzothiadiazines

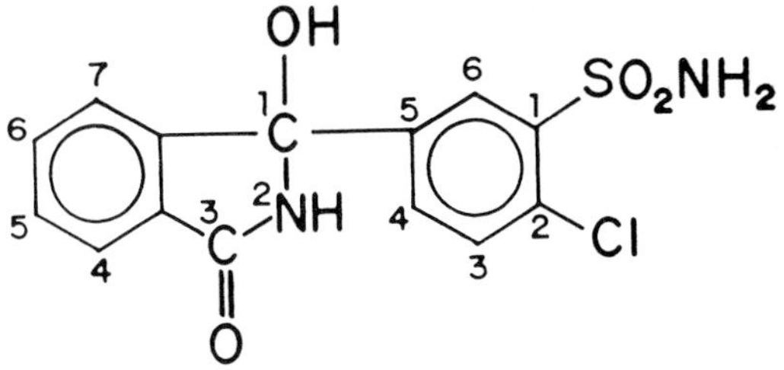

Chlorthalidone

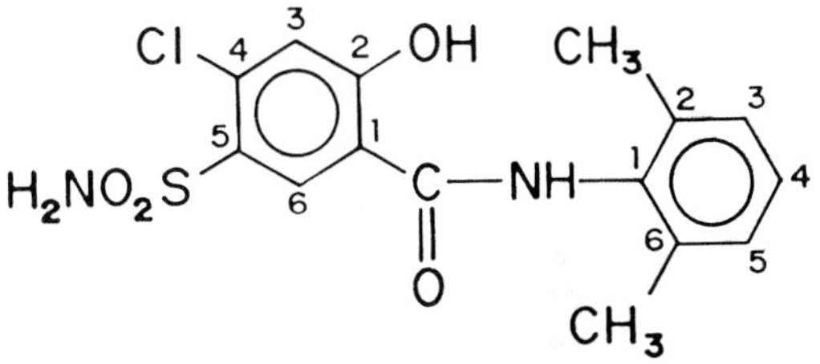

Xipamide

Chlorthalidone and clorexolone are members of the pthalimidine group and both possess prolonged biologi-

Table 27.3 Comparisons of commercially available thiazide diuretics

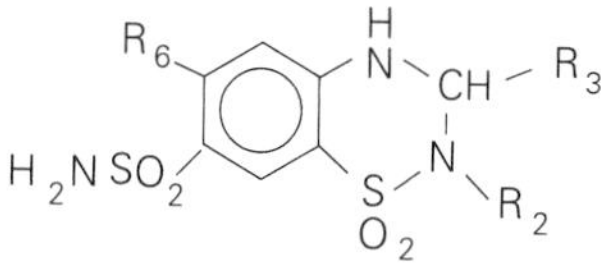

Generic name	R_2	R_3	R_6	Clinical Dose (mg/day)
Bendroflumethiazide	H	$CH_2C_6H_5$	CF_3	2.5–15
Benzthiazide*	H	$CH_2SCH_2C_6H_5$	Cl	50–200
Chlorothiazide*	H	H	Cl	500–2000
Cyclothiazide	H	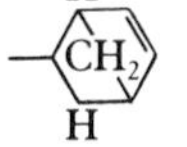 $-\!\langle CH_2 \rangle$	Cl	1–6
Hydrochlorothiazide	H	H	Cl	25–100
Hydroflumethiazide	H	H	CF_3	25–50
Methyclothiazide	CH_3	CH_2Cl	Cl	2.5–10
Polythiazide	CH_3	$CH_2SCH_2CF_3$	CL	1–4
Trichlormethiazide	H	$CHCl_2$	Cl	2–8

cal activity with elimination half-life of approximately 40–50 h. The quinazolinones, in particular metolazone, have been the subject of much study as it appears they have some distinctive features not shared with conventional benzothiadiazines. In particular, metolazone is able to retain its natriuretic potency in advanced renal insufficiency, resembling in this respect the loop diuretics. Mefruside is a representative of the benzene sulphonamide class, and although its name suggests that it bears a close biological relationship to frusemide, the profile of diuretic activity displayed, in fact, places it clearly in the benzothiadiazine class.

The chlorobenzamides — clopamide, indapamide and xipamide — may be considered together. Clopamide and indapamide have been introduced as diuretics, but indapamide is unusual in being marketed as a fixed-dose single-drug therapy specifically for the treatment of hypertension. At low dosage it exerts negligible saluretic effects, yet effectively lowers blood pressure by reducing vascular smooth muscle tone. At higher doses indapamide shares with the other two compounds the classic renal locus of action of the benzothiadiazines — the cortical diluting site. The elimination half-life of clopamide is about 6 h, that of xipamide is about 14 h and that of indapamide is about 15–20 h.

Indications

Benzothiadiazines are used mainly to relieve oedema due to moderate heart failure when the patient is not desperately ill and severe pulmonary oedema is not present. They are also used in small doses to lower blood pressure, either alone or in combination with other antihypertensive drugs, and their hypotensive effect is probably due to reduction of plasma volume combined with reduced peripheral vascular resistance.

Side-effects

Benzothiadiazines have a number of adverse effects and,

in addition to those listed in Table 27.2, they have been reported to cause neonatal thrombocytopenia when given in late pregnancy. Mild hypokalaemia occurs commonly, but only certain patients are at sufficient risk to require measures to correct this. Prevention of hypokalaemia in such patients may be achieved by addition of potassium supplements (e.g. Slow-K or Sando-K tablets which contain 8 and 12 mmol of potassium respectively) or a potassium-sparing diuretic, to maintain the plasma potassium at 3.5 mmol^{-1} or above.

Dosage

The thiazides differ in potency on a weight-for-weight basis and are usually given as an oral daily dosage, e.g. cyclopenthiazide (Navidrex) 0.5–1.0 mg or chlorthalidone 50–100 mg. It has recently been shown that cyclopenthiazide 125 μg (one quarter of the conventional dose) produces a similar hypotensive effect to 500 μg of the drug without adversely affecting the biochemical profile (McVeigh et al 1988).

LOOP DIURETICS (frusemide, bumetanide, ethacrynic acid)

Because the major effects of frusemide and ethacrynic acid lie in the medullary portion of the ascending limb of Henle's loop, the term 'loop' diuretics evolved to encompass other similarly active compounds.

Frusemide (Furosemide)

Table 27.4

Thiazides	Related compounds
Bendrofluazide (Aprinox, Centyl, Neo-naclex)	Chlorthalidone (Hygroton)
Cyclopenthiazide (Navidrex)	Clorexolone
Chlorothiazide (Saluric)	Clopamide (Brinaldix)
Hydrochlorothiazide(Hydrosaluric, Esidrex)	Quinethazone (Aquamox)
Hydroflumethazide(Hydrenox)	Mefruside (Baycaron); Metolazone (Metinix 5)
Methyclothiazide (Enduron)	Indapamide (Natrilix)
Polythiazide (Nephril)	Xipamide (Diurexan)

Pharmacology

Frusemide is a sulphonamide derivative of anthranilic acid but differs chemically and pharmacologically from the thiazides. Frusemide has both haemodynamic and renal tubular effects; the haemodynamic response involves: (a) increased renal blood flow with redistribution of flow from outer to mid-cortical zones and (b) reduction in systemic venous capacitance. These effects are probably mediated via the renin–angiotensin system and vasodilatory prostaglandins. Due to the haemodynamic effects, frusemide improves pulmonary congestion and reduces left ventricular filling pressures before any measurable increase in urinary output occurs. Frusemide-induced renal vasodilation is thought to play only a minor role in the natriuretic response. Frusemide gains access to its site of action by being transported through non-specific secretory pathways for organic acids in the proximal tubule; it subsequently acts to inhibit the active transport of sodium in the thick ascending limb of Henle's loop, and as a direct result the passive absorption of calcium and magnesium are also inhibited. Inhibition of solute absorption in the thick ascending limb markedly inhibits both renal diluting and concentrating ability. The urine tends to be isotonic with plasma or slightly dilute, bicarbonate excretion is increased and urinary pH rises. Potassium loss occurs to a lesser extent than with the thiazides, as the duration of action is shorter and the ion-exchange mechanism in the distal tubule is not directly affected. The mechanism of increased potassium excretion in the urine with loop diuretics involves both the indirect effects of increased flow rate and the inhibition of the common transport system for sodium, chloride and potassium in the luminal cell membrane. The natriuresis amounts to 30% of filtered sodium.

Frusemide has a very steep dose–response relationship, which has led to the label 'high ceiling diuretic'. It has a pKa of 3.80, possesses low lipid solubility and is extensively bound to plasma protein. The onset of action with oral therapy produces a peak diuresis within 20–30 min and the major effect of the drug is complete in 3–4 h. Bioavailability of oral frusemide is approximately 50–60% and the kinetic disposition of the drug fits most closely an open two-compartment model with an elimination half-life ranging from 19 to 100 min. The response to intravenous administration occurs within 2–3 min. The drug is chiefly excreted in the urine and faeces; only a little is metabolized. The molecular mechanism underlying the saluretic effect of loop diuretics remains inadequately explained, but it is unlikely to be due to interference with processes of cellular energetics.

Indications

Frusemide is used in patients with pulmonary oedema and is of particular value by intravenous injection in the emergency situation; it not only induces a vigorous diuresis but also reduces the preload on the heart. Oral therapy is used in patients with long-standing cardiac, renal or hepatic oedema who no longer respond to thiazide diuretics. Frusemide can be used with blood transfusion in severe anaemia where cardiac failure is imminent; it allows transfusion without increasing blood volume which would precipitate heart failure.

Dosage

In oedematous disorders the initial dose is usually 40–80 mg and this may be increased to 160 mg daily; in treatment of heart failure, if patients require more than 40–80 mg a day of frusemide, it may be appropriate to add a converting enzyme inhibitor (e.g. captopril 12.5 mg or enalapril 2.5 mg) rather than further increase diuretic dosage. In patients with advanced renal failure, very large doses may have to be given (250–1000 mg daily) but deafness is an attendant risk.

Side-effects

The response to loop diuretics may be torrential (e.g. 10 litres in 24 h) and care must be taken to avoid hypotension and vascular collapse. Other side-effects are as listed in Table 27.2.

Ethacrynic acid

Ethacrynic acid was discovered in the early 1960s as a result of systematic study of organomercurial derivatives in an attempt to produce a high efficacy diuretic lacking the toxic potential of the mercurials. The drug is an aryloxyacetic acid derivative and its pharmacological actions closely resemble those of frusemide. The peak diuretic response usually occurs within 15–20 min and results in excretion of 15–25% of the filtered load of salt. Ethacrynic acid-induced saluresis is generally accompanied by a fall in urinary pH with no bicarbonate in the urine; titratable acidity and ammonium excretion are both increased. Intravenous ethacrynic acid can cause acute uricosuria. Ethacrynic acid has a pKa of 3.50, possesses good lipid solubility and is extensively bound to plasma protein. Metabolism of the drug involves degradation in both the liver and proximal tubular cells of the nephron. The renal site of action of ethacrynic acid is the thick ascending limb of Henle's loop, where microperfusion studies have shown that it acts by inhibiting active chloride transport. As with other loop diuretics, it is not clear how much of the diuretic response is due solely to direct interference with transport systems at specific membrane sites, and how much to secondary effects resulting from a release of intrarenal mediators and the associated redistribution of blood flow within different zones of the kidney. The conventional oral dosage of ethacrynic acid is 50–200 mg daily or 50 mg by intravenous injection in emergencies.

During studies of ethacrynic acid analogues, compounds were discovered which surprisingly displayed combined saluretic and uricosuric properties (uricosuric saluretics or polyvalent diuretics). Indacrinone is a loop diuretic possessing these dual activities, and this is thought to reflect different renal activities of the constituent enantiomers. Tienilic acid has similar properties.

Bumetanide

Systematic alteration of the basic sulphamoyl-benzoic acid structure led to the development of bumetanide in 1975. This powerful loop diuretic is similar to frusemide with the exception of a phenoxy group in position 4 for the pseudohalogen CF_3 normally situated there, and a butylamino substitution at position 3. Bumetanide has a pKa of 3.60, is highly bound to plasma protein, and is rapidly and completely absorbed from the gastrointestinal tract. The elimination half-life is between 60 and 90 min. The main renal site of action is the thick ascending limb of Henle's loop, where it inhibits sodium chloride absorption and the alterations in renal haemodynamics evoked are also similar to those of frusemide. It differs from frusemide in its milligram potency, 1 mg having the equivalent effect to 40 mg of frusemide.

Piretanide

Piretanide differs from bumetanide in that the butylamino at position 3 has been replaced by a saturated pyrrolidine ring. It is a similar high ceiling diuretic with a pharmacokinetic profile resembling that of frusemide.

Azosemide

Azosemide is a halogenated monosulphamoyl diuretic, also with a similar pharmacokinetic profile to frusemide, though with a slower onset of effect. There are other miscellaneous and chemically dissimilar loop diuretics, e.g. muzolimine and etozoline.

POTASSIUM-SPARING DIURETICS (Amiloride, Triamterene, Spirolactone, Potassium Canrenoate)

There are four commercially available potassium-sparing diuretics. All act on the distal nephron to cause a modest natriuresis (less than 5% of the filtered sodium load) while conserving potassium. Two are steroidal compounds, spironolactone and potassium canrenoate, and their action is to abolish the aldosterone-dependent portion of distal sodium reabsorption. The other two agents, triamterene and amiloride, are non-steroidal in structure and they act on luminal transepithelial sodium reabsorption independently of the presence of mineralocorticoids.

Spironolactone

Pharmacology

Aldosterone enters cells of target organs by diffusion across the plasma membrane, following which it combines with a cytoplasmic receptor protein, and is then translocated as a steroid–receptor complex into the nucleus. This causes enhanced transcription of the mRNA which is then translated into new proteins within the cytoplasm and also the plasma membranes. The manner in which these mineralocorticoid-induced proteins activate transepithelial sodium transport remains uncertain, but induction of mitochondrial tricarboxylic acid cycle enzymes has been implicated. Spironolactone is a synthetic steroid lactone with structural resemblances to the natural hormone aldosterone, resulting in competition with the mineralocorticoid for binding to its receptor protein in the distal nephron, thereby preventing reabsorption of sodium chloride and increasing potassium reabsorption. It is relatively ineffective when given alone, and is usually given with a thiazide or loop diuretic to obtain added diuretic effect or prevent hypokalaemia.

Indications

Spironolactone is most useful in states where excessive secretion of aldosterone contributes to oedema formation, e.g. cirrhosis. It may also help in oedema of cardiac failure which is resistant to therapy. In Conn's syndrome of hypertension due to an aldosterone-secreting adrenal tumour, spironolactone may be useful in both treatment and diagnosis.

Dosage

Spironolactone is readily absorbed from the intestinal tract and is given in tablet form, 25 mg four times a day. Maximum diuresis is delayed for up to 4 days, and if the response is inadequate 200 mg total daily dosage may be given.

Side-effects

As spironolactone reduces renal potassium loss, there is a risk of dangerous hyperkalaemia if given with potassium supplements or to patients with impaired renal function. An important point to remember in this context is that commercial salt substitutes, e.g. 'Selora' consist of potassium chloride. Drowsiness, mental confusion and gynaecomastia are other adverse effects in addition to those listed in Table 27.2.

Potassium canrenoate

This is the potassium salt of one of the important metabolites of spironolactone, and as it is freely water-soluble it is available for intravenous use. It has

a relative potency, compared with spironolactone, of about 0.30:1.

Triamterene

Triamterene is a pteridine derivative and is not chemically related to other diuretics. It has a pKa of 6.20, is bound approximately 50% to plasma protein and the elimination half-life is between 2 and 4 h. It acts on the distal tubule to depress cell membrane permeability to sodium and indirectly decrease potassium loss. It also increases uric acid excretion (thiazides reduce it). It is not a very effective diuretic (maximal natriuresis 2–3% of filtered sodium) and is normally used in combination with other diuretics which inhibit sodium reabsorption in the proximal tubule of loop of Henle. It is well absorbed after oral administration, is excreted partly unchanged and partly in metabolite form, and its effect lasts up to 24 h.

Indications

Triamterene may be used in cardiac failure, cirrhosis and nephrotic syndrome.

Dosage

The oral dose is 50 mg twice daily but up to 300 mg may be required.

Amiloride

This is a pyrazine carboxamide derivative with a pKa of 8.70, oral bioavailability of about 50% and elimination half-life of about 6–9 h. There is no evidence that it undergoes metabolic degradation in humans. Stop-flow, micropuncture, microperfusion and microelectrode studies have localized the action of amiloride to the distal nephron and in particular the cortical collecting duct. It causes modest saluresis with decreased excretion of potassium and a rise in urine pH. It is used in oedematous states and for potassium conservation with thiazide or loop diuretics. The oral dosage is 5–20 mg daily.

OSMOTIC DIURETICS (Mannitol, Urea)

Mannitol

Mannitol is a polyhydric alcohol which is filtered across the glomerulus but not reabsorbed to any significant extent in the tubules, and is therefore excreted with its isosmotic equivalent of water. If given orally it will cause osmotic diarrhoea. Because transport processes in the thick ascending limb and more distal nephron remain intact, however, the major diuresis is water, and to a considerably lesser extent, salt.

Indications

Mannitol is most commonly used in cerebral oedema to reduce brain volume and lower intracranial pressure by shrinkage of brain cells. A further application is based on the observation that infusion of hypertonic mannitol causes intravascular volume expansion, dilation of the afferent renal arteriole with increased renal plasma flow and intratubular pressure. These properties have led to its widespread use in preventing acute renal failure in conditions which predispose to development of acute tubular necrosis, e.g. aortic aneurysm surgery or jaundiced patients undergoing surgery. Mannitol has also been advocated in the early stages of acute oliguria following trauma, major surgery or other circulatory insult, the intention of such treatment being to 'open up' the kidney and thereby prevent acute renal failure or convert it from the oliguric to the non-oliguric form. Patients with decreased renal function, however, have diminished ability to eliminate mannitol, with potentially disastrous consequences. Retained mannitol draws water into the intravascular space by osmosis, resulting in hyponatraemia and sudden increase in intravascular volume which may precipitate pulmonary oedema (Borges et al 1982).

Dosage

Mannitol is given by intravenous infusion of 10 or 20% solution, 50–200 g over 24 h preceded by a test dose of 200 mg kg^{-1} by slow intravenous injection.

Side-effects

Chills, fever and thrombophlebitis may occur. Tissue necrosis has resulted from extravasation. The acute expansion of blood volume which occurs with mannitol may precipitate pulmonary oedema. Hyperkalaemia may be worsened in renal failure as movement of water out of the intracellular compartment creates a chemical gradient favouring potassium exit from cells.

Urea

This is also an effective osmotic diuretic but has side-effects which render it inferior to mannitol. These include arrhythmias, haemolysis and a bleeding tendency.

CARBONIC ANHYDRASE INHIBITORS (Acetazolamide, Dichlorphenamide)

Acetazolamide

$$CH_3CONH \underset{\substack{4 \\ N}}{\overset{5}{\underset{\|}{}}} \overset{1}{S} \underset{\substack{3 \\ N}}{\overset{2}{\underset{\|}{}}} SO_2NH_2$$

Pharmacology

Acetazolamide acts in the proximal tubule to inhibit the action of carbonic anhydrase. This enzyme facilitates the formation of carbonic acid in the tubular cells, which in turn dissociates to produce hydrogen and bicarbonate ions. The hydrogen ions are exchanged for sodium in the glomerular filtrate so that body sodium is conserved. This reabsorption of sodium in exchange for hydrogen ions requires a supply of hydrogen ions, and this depends on the action of carbonic anhydrase. Inhibition of the enzyme reduces the supply of hydrogen ions, with the result that sodium and bicarbonate remain in the lumen of the tubule. Thus, an alkaline urine with a high sodium bicarbonate content results and the increase in sodium excretion leads to a diuresis.

Potassium excretion is also increased because it normally competes with hydrogen ions in the exchange with sodium, and when hydrogen ion excretion is reduced more potassium will be lost. The excretion of persistently alkaline urine produces a metabolic acidosis, resulting in respiratory compensation by the elimination of carbon dioxide and a reduction in plasma bicarbonate. This in turn inhibits the diuretic effect by reducing the amount of sodium bicarbonate presented to the renal tubules, and drug tolerance develops.

Indications

Acetazolamide and dichlorphenamide are only weak diuretics and have their main application in treatment of glaucoma (they inhibit the formation of aqueous humour and therefore lower intra-ocular pressure). Acetazolamide has also been used to increase bicarbonate excretion in patients with severe alkalosis (e.g. gastric alkalosis, post-hypercapnic alkalosis) and to alkalinize the urine in order to solubilize certain compounds (e.g. uric acid in myeloproliferative disorders). Acetazolamide may prevent mountain sickness by causing metabolic acidosis, which stimulates respiration and therefore minimizes hypoxaemia.

Dosage

Acetazolamide is usually given orally, 250 mg g^{-1} per 24 h and the duration of action is about 12 h.

Side-effects

Hyperchloraemic metabolic acidosis may occur and rarely may be associated with nephrocalcinosis and formation of renal calculi in patients on long-term therapy.

XANTHINE DIURETICS (Theophylline, Caffeine)

These compounds are weak diuretics and produce a small diuresis by inhibiting absorption of sodium chloride and water in the renal tubules. Theophylline (as aminophylline) increases glomerular filtration by its cardiac action, which increases renal blood flow.

MERCURIAL DIURETICS

Mersalyl is an organic mercury compound which acts through the nephron to reduce sodium and chloride reabsorption. It is no longer used, due to its nephrotoxicity and requirement for intramuscular administration. Intravenous use may cause hypotension and sudden death.

COMBINED DIURETICS

The debate on preventing potassium depletion has yet to be resolved. In old age a daily dose of at least 24 mmol potassium is required to prevent or correct depletion. An alternative is to give potassium-sparing agents; if given combined with thiazide or loop diuretics they are easier to take and at least as effective as potassium supplements. Against this must be weighed their tendency to cause hyponatraemia and uraemia in patients with impaired renal function. The use of combined diuretics does not eliminate the need to check serum electrolyte concentration. Some patients go on to develop hyperkalaemia, which is more likely to cause cardiac arrhythmias and sudden death than is potassium depletion.

REFERENCES

Borges H F, Hocks J, Kjellstrand C M 1982 Mannitol intoxication in patients with renal failure. Archives of Internal Medicine 142: 63–66
Caplin J L 1989 Acute right ventricular infarction. British Medical Journal 299: 69–70
Espiner E A, Richards A M 1989 Atrial natriuretic peptide: an important factor in sodium and blood pressure regulation. Lancet ii: 707–710
Lant A 1985 Diuretics: clinical pharmacology and therapeutic use (Part II). Drugs 19: 162–168
Laureno R, Karp B I 1988 Pontine and extrapontine myelinolysis following rapid correction of hyponatraemia. Lancet i: 1439–1440
McVeigh G, Galloway D, Johnston D 1988 The case for low dose diuretics in hypertension: comparison of low and conventional doses of cyclopenthiazide. British Medical Journal 297: 95–98
Medical Research Council Working Party on Mild to Moderate Hypertension 1981 Adverse reactions to bendrofluazide and propranolol for the treatment of mild hypertension. Lancet ii: 360–362
Morgan D B, Davidson C 1980 Hypokalaemia and diuretics: an analysis of publications. British Medical Journal 281: 905–908
Morris G C, Keats A S, Moyer J H, Debakey M E 1959 Renal function during anesthesia for cardiovascular surgery. Anesthesiology 20: 608
Northridge D B, Jardine A G, Alabaster C T, Barclay P L, Connell J M C, Dargie H J, Dilly S G, Findlay I N, Lever A F, Samuels G M R 1989 Effects of UK 69 578: a novel atriopeptidase inhibitor. Lancet iii: 591–593
Reineck H J 1986 Diuretic use in renal failure. In: Eknoyan G, Martinez-Maldonado M (eds) The physiological basis of diuretic therapy in clinical medicine. Grune & Stratton, New York, pp 277–291
Rotherham E B, Safar P, Robin E D 1964 CNS disorder during mechanical ventilation in chronic pulmonary disease. Journal of the American Medical Association 189: 993
Thomas T H, Morgan D B 1979 Post-surgical hyponatraemia: the role of intravenous fluid and arginine vasopressin. British Journal of Surgery 66: 540–542

28. Drugs acting on the respiratory system

W. McCaughey

INTRODUCTION

The factors which may adversely affect the function of the respiratory system are many. They include disease of, drug action on, or trauma to the central nervous system, peripheral nerves, neuromuscular junction, muscles, skeletal structures, the upper airways or the lungs themselves. This chapter will be confined rather strictly to drugs used in management of obstructive airways disease — that is the drugs of use in treating reduced airway calibre, and drugs which stimulate respiration.

Factors influencing calibre of airways

The tone of bronchial smooth muscle is regulated to a large extent by the intracellular nucleotides cyclic 3′,5′-adenosine monophosphate (cAMP) and cyclic 3′,5′-guanosine monophosphate (cGMP), which are converted from the respective triphosphates by adenylate cyclase and guanyl cyclase. At cellular level,

sympathetic activity or β_2-adrenergic stimulation increases adenylate cyclase activity and cAMP function, leading to sequestration of intracellular calcium and reduced bronchial smooth muscle contractility, and also to inhibition of antigen-induced release from mast cells of chemical mediators of hypersensitivity (described below) (Austen 1974). Inhaled calcium antagonist drugs can also cause relaxation of bronchial muscle (Ahmed & Abraham 1985). Parasympathetic activity or cholinergic stimulation increases guanylate cyclase activity and cGMP formation, leading to release of mediators and also to bronchial constriction. Thus drugs which increase cAMP formation, whether by β_2-receptor activation or by another pathway, and drugs which reduce cGMP, will act to reduce airway constriction.

Drugs administered by inhalation may be nebulized, but more commonly now are given from pressurized inhalers. Of the dose administered in this way, only a fraction — about 11–12%, reaches the lungs, and of this about two-thirds is deposited in the more central parts of the lungs, i.e. trachea and bronchi, while one-third

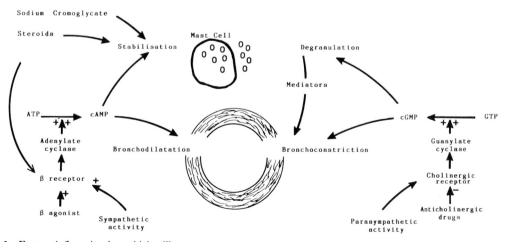

Fig. 28.1 Factors influencing bronchial calibre.

reaches the alveoli (Spiro et al 1984). There seems to be no difference in the pattern of deposition between normal subjects and patients with obstructive airways disease, nor does the size of the particle delivered influence distribution (Spiro et al 1984, Newman et al 1983). The remaining 90% or so of the dose administered is deposited in the mouth and upper airways, and subsequently swallowed, and so is effectively an oral dose — though some may be absorbed directly through the mucosa and thus avoid exposure to the possibility of hepatic first-pass metabolism.

Drugs administered by inhalation generally exert a local action rather than depending on absorption and distribution via the circulation. However, absorption will occur and systemic effects may be seen. Because of the smaller doses used, these are generally considerably less than when the drug is used systemically. Systemic effects may in some cases be reduced because first-pass metabolism occurs in the lungs — for example isoprenaline may be partly metabolized by COMT in this situation.

BRONCHODILATOR DRUGS

Three groups of drugs fall into this category. These are the symphathomimetic amines, the methylxanthines, and the anticholinergic drugs. Of these, selective β_2-adrenergic agonists, usually given by aerosol inhalation, are normally the drugs of first choice, and may be used in combination with drugs of the other two groups for additive effect on bronchial calibre. In appropriate cases cromoglycate may be used for its prophylactic effect, and inhaled steroids may also be appropriate.

SYMPATHOMIMETIC DRUGS

As described above, β_2-adrenergic receptors mediate relaxation of bronchial smooth muscle. Formerly isoprenaline, a powerful but non-selective β_2-agonist was used, as were adrenaline and ephedrine, but cardiovascular effects mediated by β_1-receptors are a major disadvantage. Selective β_2-agonists such as salbutamol or terbutaline are now preferred. Unfortunately none of these acts solely on β_2 receptors, i.e. their selectivity is relative rather than absolute, so that effects due to β_2 activity may still be seen at higher dosage. These include tremor, tachycardia or other arrhythmias, and metabolic effects: rise in plasma glucose, free fatty acids and insulin, and fall in serum potassium level, and the last might be exacerbated by concurrent use of steroids.

Salbutamol: albuterol

Salbutamol is a selective β_2-agonist, and as such causes dilation of bronchi, together with other effects as described above. It and some other β_2-agonists are also used in obstetric practice to inhibit uterine contractions.

In managing the asthmatic patient, inhalation is the preferred route, using one or two puffs of pressurized inhaler (100–200 μg). This effect lasts for about 3–5 h. Nebulized solution may also be used, by face mask or in the ventilated patient, 2.5 mg (2.5 ml of solution containing 1 mg ml^{-1}) repeated up to four times daily. Intravenously, an infusion of 5 μg min^{-1} adjusted according to response, and usually in the range 3–20 μg min^{-1} is used, or a slow intravenous injection of 250 μg may be given. Subcutaneous or intramuscular injection may also be used.

Metabolism and excretion. Salbutamol is conjugated in the liver, and eliminated both in the urine as unchanged drug and metabolites, and in the faeces. The pattern of elimination varies between parenteral and oral or inhalational administration, because of the effect of presystemic elimination. Its pharmacokinetics are reviewed in detail by Price and Clissold (1989).

Terbutaline

Effects are similar to salbutamol. (There is little β_2 specificity when given parenterally.)

Dosage: aerosol inhalation: 250–500 μg (one or two puffs); nebulized: 5–10 mg two to four times daily; i.v. infusion: 1.5–5 μg min^{-1} of solution containing 3–5 μg ml^{-1}; i.v., i.m. or s.c. injection: 250–500 μg two to four times daily.

Other β_2 agonists in use include: Fenoterol, Reproterol, Rimiterol and others.

XANTHINES

The three methylated xanthine derivatives, or methylxanthines; theophylline, theobromine and caffeine are plant alkaloids. Theophylline is used therapeutically while caffeine is more often encountered as a constituent of beverages.

Caffeine

Theophylline

Theobromine

Theophylline

Mode of action. Three main modes of action are proposed;

1. Theophylline and caffeine prevent enzymatic degradation of cyclic AMP by phosphodiesterase, leading to raised cAMP levels and possibly potentiation of action of other drugs such as catecholamines which stimulate cAMP production. Caffeine and theophylline are widely different in potency for inhibiting cyclic nucleotide hydrolysis, but are not selective as inhibitors of the major isoenzyme forms of phosphodiesterase (Wells & Miller 1988).
2. Calcium release from the sarcoplasmic reticulum. This is caused by caffeine, though theophylline is probably less potent, and this leads to augmentation of the force of muscular contraction.
3. Competitive antagonism of adenosine receptors. Xanthines are potent inhibitors at adenosine A_1 (R_1) and A_2 (R_a) receptors (Choi et al 1988). These receptors may stimulate or inhibit cAMP, and may also influence Ca^{2+} influx. This mechanism is currently thought to be the most likely to account for most of the therapeutic

actions of theophylline, with the possible exception of its anti-asthmatic effects (Fredholm 1985).

Therapeutic actions. These will be summarized.

Central nervous system. The methylxanthines are CNS stimulants — the effects of caffeine are well known. In toxic doses arousal proceeds to restlessness, insomnia, etc., and focal convulsive activity may occur. These may occur occasionally with plasma concentrations only 50% above the accepted therapeutic level.

Cardiovascular system. These may be summarized as an increase in cardiac rate and contractility (probably augmented by increased release of catecholamines), decreased peripheral resistance due to smooth muscle relaxation, and in higher doses a tendency to premature ventricular contractions or other tachyarrhythmias.

Respiratory system. Respiration is stimulated by higher doses of theophylline, and even low doses of this or of caffeine may give significant stimulation after administration of opioid drugs.

Theophylline is given mainly for its bronchodilator effect, and for maximal effect needs to be given in carefully controlled dosage with appropriate estimation of plasma levels. Bronchial dilation leads to decreased work of breathing, and the augmentation of skeletal muscle contractility is also beneficial. Plasma levels above 10 μg ml^{-1} increase the force of contraction of the diaphragm and reduce fatigue — a sustained improvement in diaphragmatic strength of 20% has been shown (Murciano et al 1984).

Other effects of benefit in treating patients with chronic obstructive airways disease include reduction in pulmonary artery hypertension, stimulation of hypoxic ventilatory drive, and enhancement of mucociliary clearance.

Other effects. The methylxanthines also cause diuresis, inhibit uterine contractions and stimulate gastric secretion of acid and pepsin.

Pharmacokinetics. Theophylline is rapidly, consistently and completely absorbed from liquid preparations and plain tablets, but its rapid elimination leads to fluctuations in plasma levels. Absorption from sustained-release preparations or by rectal suppositories is more erratic. There is 40% binding to protein, and the volume of distribution is approximately 0.5 l kg^{-1}; slightly larger in acidaemia and cirrhosis because of reduced binding. About 10% of theophylline (and 1% of caffeine) is excreted unchanged by the kidneys, while 90% is metabolized by cytochrome P450 pathways in the liver. After intravenous administration the plasma half life is approximately 4–5 h in adults and 3–6 h in children.

Clearance is reduced in cirrhosis, acute hepatitis, cardiac failure or cor pulmonale, but is not affected by cholestasis or chronic obstructive airways disease. It is increased in smokers. Drug interactions may also influence it: clearance is reduced by cimetidine (but not by ranitidine), by erythromycin or by oral contraceptives. It is increased by drugs such as phenobarbitone, phenytoin or rifampicin.

CALCIUM ANTAGONISTS

Many of the pathogenic mechanisms of asthma are calcium-dependent — these include mast cell release of mediators, mucous gland secretion, smooth muscle contraction, vagus nerve activity and inflammatory cell infiltration (Russi & Ahmed 1984). A number of studies have shown some, often considerable, benefit from use of sublingual or inhaled calcium channel blocking drugs, but they have not yet become an established part of clinical management of bronchospasm. However, a corollary is that calcium antagonists may be used for management of hypertension or angina in a patient with obstructive airways disease, where β-blockers are contra-indicated (Massey & Hendeles 1987).

STEROIDS

The glucocorticoid actions of steroid drugs may be of use in treatment of patients with bronchial asthma. Steroids are lipid-soluble and enter cells directly, to attach to their receptor sites, where a series of steps leads to gene activation, RNA synthesis, and thence synthesis of specific proteins to mediate the steroid's actions. Because of the time involved, there is a delay before most of the actions of the steroids come into play, although some actions may occur more rapidly, perhaps by activation of preformed proteins or mobilization of membrane-bound calcium.

Several mechanisms of action may be quoted; and are reviewed by Morris (1985).

1. An anti-inflammatory action.
2. Influence on mediators of pulmonary disease. A large number of substances may be involved in causing inflammation, bronchoconstriction, pulmonary vascular constriction or increased vascular permeability; and glucocorticoids can inhibit either the synthesis or release, or block the actions of some of these. Among others these include:
   (a) Arachidonic acid metabolites. Arachidonic acid is cleaved from cell membrane phospholipid, of which it is a normal constituent. It is a precursor of a large number of active products — prostaglandins, thromboxanes and prostacyclin are synthesized by the cyclo-oxygenase pathway and leukotrienes by the lipo-oxygenase pathway.
   (b) Platelet activating factor, which has potent inflammatory actions, and also causes bronchoconstriction.
   (c) Histamine. This is released both by IgE-mediated mechanisms in allergic reactions and also by non-IgE mechanisms, e.g. exposure to toxins.

Glucocorticoids may inhibit synthesis of arachidonic acid metabolites, although effects on histamine release are less consistent. They may also modify the response of the tissues to these substances. Administration of glucocorticoids potentiates the effects of β₂-adrenergic agonists and may cause unresponsive patients to respond. This appears to be due to externalization of receptors to the surface of the cell membrane, increased binding affinity for β-agonists, and enhanced coupling to adenylate cyclase, as well as increased synthesis of β-receptors.

Mechanisms of other effects are less well studied. These include improvement in ventilation–perfusion ratios, reduction in airway hypersensitivity and, of course, an anti-inflammatory action.

Steroids are generally more effective and with fewer side-effects when given by inhalation, mainly because doses required and doses absorbed are much smaller. However, inhaled steroids are ineffective for the management of acute processes in the airway, and the systemic route is used until the acute attack subsides.

Beclomethasone propionate

This is available as a pressurized aerosol and also as a suspension for nebulization. The standard dosage is 200 μg (four puffs of nebulized aerosol), three or four times daily for prophylaxis. A β₂-agonist is often given 10 min before this to try to assist penetration of the steroid to smaller airways.

Due to the small dose used, there is little systemic absorption and the associated problems are unlikely to be encountered.

ANTICHOLINERGIC DRUGS

Ipratropium

Chemical name: N-isopropylatropine bromide. Historically, anticholinergic agents were introduced for treatment of asthma-like conditions as early as the

Ipratropium bromide

seventeenth century, when travellers to India noted the beneficial effects of inhaling smoke from burning *Stramonium* leaves (Hertz 1979).

Ipratropium produces competitive inhibition of cholinergic receptors on bronchial smooth muscle, and possibly may also block cholinergic receptors on the surface of mast cells. It is used in management of both asthmatic and chronic bronchitic patients.

Ipratropium is administered by aerosol inhalation, the recommended dose being 20–40 μg (one or two puffs of metered aerosol), three or four times daily. Bronchodilation occurs fairly rapidly but does not reach a maximum for 1.5–2 h, with a duration of effect of 4–6 h, so that it may be more appropriate for prophylaxis rather than treatment of acute attacks (Massey & Gotz 1985). The amount of systemic absorption is minimal, and occurs mainly from the 90% of the dose which is deposited orally. About 70% of this is unabsorbed and excreted in the faeces, while the absorbed fraction is metabolized in the liver with a plasma half-life of 3.2–3.8 h, to largely inactive metabolites (Adlung et al 1976).

Ipratropium may be combined with other bronchodilator therapy. Additive effects have been shown with β-adrenergic agents, cromolyn sodium, theophylline and with steroids.

Adverse effects are relatively rare, mainly because of its minimal absorption. However, if given by mask rather than inhaler, some may reach the eyes, and precipitation of closed-angle glaucoma has been reported (Packe et al 1984).

OTHER DRUGS

Disodium cromoglycate: cromolyn sodium

Cromoglycate does not have any bronchodilator effect, but does have a protective effect against bronchospasm induced by allergic and other mechanisms. This effect seems to be due to inhibition of release of mediators from mast cells, and although the mechanism of this is incompletely understood it may be due to closing of the calcium channel, thus preventing entry of calcium ions into the mast cell. It may also inhibit some reflex nervous pathways which cause bronchoconstriction.

Cromoglycate is administered by inhalation of powder or of nebulized solution, at a dose of 20 mg.

As with other drugs described in this section, about 10% is deposited in the airways. The small quantity absorbed is excreted unchanged in bile and urine, with a plasma half-life of 46–99 min (Fisons Corporation 1973, Shapiro & Konig 1985).

RESPIRATORY STIMULANTS

Drugs which stimulate respiration find a place in anaesthetic practice, although they must not be used when mechanical support of ventilation is the appropriate treatment. They may be used as an alternative to opioid antagonists in managing respiratory depression, especially when this follows use of buprenorphine, which is not readily antagonized by naloxone because of its high receptor affinity. An advantage of non-specific respiratory stimulants is that they do not antagonize analgesic effects of the opioids. They may also find a use in other aspects of anaesthetic practice, but their most widespread, though still limited, use is in medical management of the patient with respiratory failure from long-standing chronic obstructive airways disease, especially if respiratory failure has been aggravated by injudicious use of oxygen or hypnotics.

Analeptic drugs which stimulate the central nervous system are a large and heterogeneous group. Most are of historical interest only, mainly because of their spectrum of toxic side-effects. They are reviewed by Wang

Disodium cromoglycate: Cromolyn sodium

& Ward (1977). No common mode of action can be described. Some of the older drugs such as strychnine or picrotoxin act by blocking central inhibitory pathways, in the latter case by direct antagonism of the inhibitory neurotransmitter GABA. Doxapram and nikethamide, however, seem to cause excitation rather than block of central inhibitory pathways. Analeptics have in the past been used to antagonize CNS depression due to drug overdose, but intensive supportive management has proved more successful.

The main adverse side-effects are on the CNS – restlessness, disorientation, headache, etc., and eventually convulsions. If used to treat CNS depression, convulsions may occur before any clinically detectable reversal of depression has occurred. Respiratory effects include cough, sneezing and hyperventilation. Cardiac arrhythmias often occur, and in high doses there is hypotension, although doxapram is unusual in causing a prolonged pressor effect (Wang & Ward 1977).

Doxapram

Doxapram is chemically a pyrrolidinone. It is unusual in that it stimulates respiration more than it activates cortical or spinal areas, and has a higher therapeutic ratio than other analeptic drugs. There is a selective effect on respiration, related to an action on peripheral chemoreceptors in the carotid sinus (Hirsh & Wang 1974, Wang & Ward 1977).

Doxapram has been used to improve respiration following anaesthesia, or as a 'pharmacological sigh' in the postoperative period when deep breathing is inhibited by pain or by opioid analgesics (Winnie 1973).

It has also been used to facilitate blind nasal intubation (Davies 1968). It may be used to antagonize the respiratory depressant effects of opioids (Gupta et al 1974), including buprenorphine as noted above. A further possible use is in low doses to reduce the incidence of apnoeic episodes in premature infants (Bairam & Vert 1986), but it should be noted that respiratory stimulants have no place in treatment of neonatal asphyxia.

Doxapram may be given in single or divided doses of 0.5–1.5 mg kg^{-1}. This causes transient respiratory stimulation for 5–10 min. Alternatively an intravenous infusion may be used at an initial rate of 2 mg min^{-1}.

Nikethamide

Ethamivan

Nikethamide and ethamivan are structurally related acid amines. Both cause stimulation of the respiratory centre, but claims that they act on the carotid chemoreceptors have not been confirmed. Indications are similar to doxapram, but the therapeutic ratio is less.

The dose of nikethamide is 0.5–1 g intravenously, repeated at 15–30 min as necessary, and of ethamivan 100 mg, repeated as necessary.

Nikethamide is absorbed readily by all routes, though usually given intravenously. It is metabolized to nicotinamide and excreted as n-methyl nicotinamide, with a plasma half-life of about 100 min.

Side-effects are as described above.

REFERENCES

Adlung J, Gohle K D, Zeren S, Wahl D 1976 Studies of pharmacokinetics and biotransformation of ipratropium in man. Arzneimittelforsch 26: 1005–1010
Ahmed T, Abraham W M 1985 Role of calcium channel blockers in obstructive airways disease. Chest 88: 142s–151s
Austen K F 1974 Reaction mechanisms in the release of mediators of immediate hypersensitivity from human lung tissue. Federation Proceedings 33: 2256–2262

Bairam A, Vert P 1986 Low dose doxapram for apnoea of prematurity. Lancet 1: 793–794
Choi O H, Shamim M T, Padgett W L, Daly J W 1988 Caffeine and theophylline analogues: correlation of behavioral effects with activity as adenosine receptor antagonists and as phosphodiesterase inhibitors. Life Sciences 43: 387–398
Davies J A H 1968 Blind nasal intubation using doxapram hydrochloride. British Journal of Anaesthesia 40: 361–364
Fisons Corporation 1973 Intal-cromolyn sodium: a monograph. Bedford, Ma: Fisons Corporation

Fredholm B B 1985 On the mechanism of action of theophylline and caffeine. Acta Medica Scandinavica 217: 149–153

Gupta P K, Dundee J W Jones C J 1974 Clinical trial of doxapram hydrochloride. Proceedings of the IV Asian and Australasian Congress of Anaesthesiologists 384–387

Hertz C W 1979 Historical aspects of anticholinergic treatment of obstructive airways disease. Scandinavian Journal of Respiratory Disease 60 (Suppl 103), 105–109

Hirsch K, Wang S C 1974 Selective respiratory stimulating action of doxapram compared to pentylenetetrazol. Journal of Pharmacology and Experimental Therapeutics 198: 1–11

Massey K L Gotz V P 1985 Ipratropium bromide. Drug Intelligence and Clinical Pharmacy 19: 5–19

Massey K L, Hendeles L 1987 Calcium antagonists in the management of asthma: breakthrough or ballyhoo. Drug Intelligence and Clinical Pharmacy 21: 505–509

Morris H G 1985 Mechanisms of glucocorticoid action in pulmonary disease. Chest 88: 133s–141s

Murciano D, Aubier M, Lecocguic Y, Pariente R 1984 Effects of theophylline on diaphragmatic strength and fatigue in patients with chronic obstructive pulmonary disease. New England Journal of Medicine 311: 349–353

Newman S P, Killip M, Pavia D, Moren F, Clarke S W 1983 Do particle size and airway obstruction affect the deposition of pressurised inhalation aerosols. Thorax 38: 233

Packe G E, Cayton R M, Mashoudi N 1984 Nebulised ipratropium and salbutamol causing closed angle glaucoma. Lancet 2: 691

Price A H, Clissold S P 1989 Salbutamol in the 1980's: A reappraisal of its clinical efficacy. Drugs 38: 77–122

Russi E W, Ahmed T 1984 Calcium and calcium antagonists in airways disease: a review. Chest 86: 475–482

Shapiro G G, Konig P 1985 Cromolyn sodium: a review. Pharmacotherapy 5: 156–170

Spiro S G Singh C A, Tolfree S E J, Partridge M R, Short M D 1984 Direct labelling of ipratropium bromide aerosol and its deposition pattern in normal subjects and patients with chronic bronchitis. Thorax 39: 432–435

Wang S C, Ward J W 1977 Analeptics. Pharmacology and Therapeutics 3: 123–165

Wells J N, Miller J R 1988 Methylxanthine inhibitors of phosphodiesterase. Methods in Enzymology 159: 489–496

Winnie A P 1973 Chemical respirogenesis: a comparative study. Acta Anaesthesiologica Scandinavica Suppl 51: 1–32

29. Antimicrobial drugs

T. S. Wilson

INTRODUCTION

Anaesthetists working in intensive care units require some knowledge of the commonly used antimicrobial drugs, including their spectrum of activity, pharmacokinetics, indications for use and possible harmful effects. This chapter gives a brief general account of the modes of action of these agents and the mechanisms of bacterial resistance, followed by descriptions of individual drugs or groups of drugs. Space limitations necessitate that major emphasis is placed on those agents most likely to be encountered in modern anaesthetic practice. Drugs which are seldom used or have been superseded are mentioned only briefly, and some have been entirely omitted. Similarly, antibiotics restricted to topical use or to specific indications which are of little importance to anaesthetists have been excluded, as have antiviral, antiprotozoal and anthelminthic agents.

HISTORICAL REVIEW

Modern chemotherapy dates from the time of Paul Ehrlich, whose discovery in 1909 of the effectiveness of arsenical compounds in the treatment of syphilis was followed by the production of other synthetic drugs with antiprotozoal activity. Further progress did not occur until the introduction of the sulphonamides in 1935 and then penicillin during the 1940s, the latter being developed for clinical use 10 years after the possibility had first been suggested by Fleming. The search for new and better antimicrobial agents continues unabated, either by systematic testing of thousands of natural substances or by laboratory development of novel synthetic compounds. Other advances have resulted from chemical modification of existing drugs, sometimes producing only minor changes in pharmacokinetics or reduced toxicity, but occasionally creating major improvements in antibacterial spectrum or activity. Unfortunately, many new drugs have been introduced in recent years with only minimal differences from others already available,

their appearance owing more to marketing considerations than to any therapeutic superiority over existing agents.

MECHANISMS OF ACTION OF ANTIMICROBIAL DRUGS

Ideal antimicrobial agents possess 'selective toxicity', interfering with a metabolic or synthetic process of the micro-organism without affecting the host. However, apart from the penicillins and cephalosporins this 'selective toxicity' is usually dose-related, and at increased concentrations many drugs may have harmful effects on some host tissues.

Antibacterial mechanisms

There are four main methods by which antibiotics kill bacteria or inhibit their growth.

1. Inhibition of cell wall synthesis

Unlike animal cells, bacteria possess a rigid outer cell wall surrounding the cell membrane, which protects the organism from its external environment, particularly from osmotic effects. Cell wall damage or inhibition of cell wall synthesis usually leads to rupture and death of the cell.

The penicillins and cephalosporins are the prime examples of antimicrobial drugs which act by inhibiting cell wall synthesis; since mammalian cells do not have any comparable structure these antibiotics are virtually non-toxic to mammalian tissues, except when hypersensitivity develops.

2. Inhibition of cell membrane function

In common with other living cells, bacteria possess a limiting cytoplasmic or cell membrane situated beneath the bacterial cell wall. This membrane acts as a selective permeability barrier and has active transport functions, thus controlling the internal composition of the cell. Agents such as polymyxin B and colistin (polymyxin E) which interfere with cell membrane function can cause leakage of internal constituents and cell death in many Gram-negative bacteria.

3. Inhibition of protein synthesis

Many antibiotics, such as the aminoglycosides, tetracyclines, chloramphenicol and erythromycin, exert their antibacterial effect by inhibiting bacterial protein synthesis. The synthetic process is complex, the final stage involving ribosomal linkage of amino acids in a genetically determined sequence, and antibiotics can act at various points. Bacterial and mammalian ribosomes differ sufficiently to allow agents to interfere with bacterial protein production without significantly affecting mammalian cells.

4. Inhibition of nucleic acids

Some antimicrobial drugs, including the sulphonamides, trimethoprim, rifampicin and the quinolones, act by interfering with the synthesis or replication of nucleic acids, which are essential constituents of living cells.

The discovery of the antibacterial activity of the first sulphonamides in the 1930s led to the elucidation of their mode of action. Bacterial cells require para-amino-benzoic acid (PABA) for synthesis of folic acid and ultimately DNA. Sulphonamides closely resemble PABA and by competitive inhibition they interfere with one stage of folic acid synthesis, while trimethoprim interrupts a later stage of this process. Combining them in preparations such as co-trimoxazole produces a synergistic antibacterial effect. Mammalian cells are generally unaffected by these drugs as they do not synthesize folic acid but must obtain it from external sources.

The mode of action of rifampicin is by inhibition of bacterial RNA polymerase, while the quinolone drugs inhibit the enzyme DNA gyrase.

Antifungal mechanisms

There are still comparatively few effective antifungal drugs which are sufficiently non-toxic to allow their use in systemic therapy; their modes of action are generally similar to those of the antibacterial agents. For example, the polyene antifungals nystatin and amphotericin B act on sterol groups in fungal cell membranes, while the imidazoles (miconazole and ketoconazole) interfere with synthesis of membrane sterols. Flucytosine and griseofulvin both inhibit nucleic acid synthesis.

Antiviral mechanisms

Viruses differ from bacteria and fungi in their structure and mode of replication, and are not affected by antibacterial and antifungal agents. Most antiviral drugs inhibit viral nucleic acid synthesis, but amantadine acts against influenza A viruses by preventing penetration of the virus into susceptible host cells.

RESISTANCE TO ANTIMICROBIAL DRUGS.

Most microbial species are sensitive to some antimicrobial drugs but resistant to others, due to variable factors such as differences in cell permeability, lack of drug binding sites, production of drug-inactivating enzymes, or absence of particular metabolic pathways. These micro-organisms have a natural or innate resistance to the drugs concerned. Other species which were originally susceptible to certain drugs have become resistant to them by acquiring some of these mechanisms.

The origin of acquired drug resistance may be either genetic or non-genetic; most drug-resistant bacteria arise from genetic change followed by a process of selection of the resistant organism. Chromosomal resistance occurs as a result of spontaneous mutation, while non-chromosomal resistance involves changes in the extrachromosomal plasmids. Genetic material which controls drug resistance can often be transferred from resistant organisms to sensitive organisms of the same species, or sometimes of different species, thus promoting the spread of resistance.

The production of drug-inactivating enzymes is a well-understood example of a drug resistance mechanism which is genetically controlled and can be transferable. Many bacteria produce β-lactamase (penicillinase) enzymes which cleave the β-lactam ring of the penicillins and cephalosporins and render them inactive. In turn, β-lactamase stable drugs have been developed which are largely unaffected by these enzymes and retain their activity against enzyme-producing strains. Similarly, an important form of resistance to the aminoglycoside group of antibiotics is by means of other drug-inactivating enzymes produced by some bacteria, although the later aminoglycosides are more enzyme-stable.

Resistance to an antibiotic may develop rapidly, even during the treatment of an individual patient, or more slowly following widespread use of a drug over a long period. Cross-resistance is common, organisms which become resistant to one drug often being resistant to other similar drugs. The development of antibiotic resistance can be minimized by restricting the use of certain agents, by adequate dosage to ensure high tissue levels, and sometimes by using two drugs simultaneously to prevent the emergence of resistant mutants.

ANTIMICROBIAL DRUGS

Space does not permit a full description of all available antimicrobial drugs. Some which have been superseded by newer drugs have been omitted, while others which are seldom encountered in anaesthetic practice are discussed only briefly.

Sulphonamides

The first of these agents, sulphanilamide (para-aminobenzene sulphonamide) was introduced in 1935, and later modifications of the basic molecule produced a series of drugs with greater antibacterial activity and improved physical and pharmacological properties.

Antibacterial activity. Sulphonamides inhibit the enzyme dihydropteroate synthetase, thus interfering with the conversion of para-aminobenzoic acid as the first stage of folic acid synthesis.

They are 'broad-spectrum' in their activity, being effective against a wide range of both Gram-positive and Gram-negative bacteria, as well as chlamydias and some protozoa. However, many groups of organisms which were previously sensitive have now developed sulphonamide resistance, including most strains of gonococci and many meningococci and enterobacteria.

Pharmacokinetics. Three main groups of sulphonamides can be recognized:

1. absorbable, short-acting, rapidly excreted;
2. absorbable, long-acting, slowly excreted;
3. non-absorbable.

Peak blood levels are usually reached 2–3 h after oral administration. The sulphonamides are to varying degrees conjugated and/or protein bound, affecting drug activity and tissue distribution. Free drug diffuses readily into most tissues and into the cerebrospinal fluid. Excretion of both free and conjugated forms is mainly via the kidneys.

Indications and clinical usage. The sulphonamides have been successfully used in many infections, including streptococcal, pneumococcal, meningococcal and gonococcal, and for infections of the urinary tract. Increasing sulphonamide resistance and the availability of more effective and less toxic antibiotics have reduced the indications for sulphonamide therapy but they may still be used in the following situations:

1. Urinary tract infections (due to sensitive organisms).
2. Treatment or prophylaxis of meningococcal meningitis (again when the causative organism is sensitive).
3. Sulphasalazine is useful in acute attacks of ulcerative colitis and Crohn's disease, and for maintenance therapy.
4. In combination with trimethoprim (q.v.).

Dosage and administration. The absorbable sulphonamides used for systemic therapy are normally given by mouth; parenteral preparations are available but tend to be irritant. Details of the various preparations and dosages are given in Table 29.1.

Side-effects, precautions and contra-indications. Minor gastrointestinal side-effects and skin rashes are not uncommon. Crystalluria and renal damage can occur with the less soluble sulphonamides. Stevens–Johnson syndrome (erythema multiforme) and blood dyscrasias such as agranulocytosis are rare but serious complications. Haemolytic anaemia may occur in patients with glucose 6-phosphate dehydrogenase deficiency. Pulmonary complications such as fibrosing alveolitis have been associated with sulphasalazine therapy. Sulphonamides are contra-indicated in the last 2 weeks of pregnancy and in the newborn, as they may compete with bilirubin for protein-binding sites and cause kernicterus.

Trimethoprim and sulphonamide — trimethoprim combinations

Trimethoprim was synthesized in 1956 and first marketed in 1969 as co-trimoxazole, a combination of trimethoprim and sulphamethoxazole. It only became available in the UK as a single agent in 1980.

Antibacterial activity. Trimethoprim inhibits the enzyme dihydrofolate reductase, preventing the conversion of folic acid to folinic acid and ultimately nucleic acid. It has a broad antibacterial spectrum but it is not active against *Pseudomonas* or *Neisseria* species, or against most anaerobic bacteria. Some organisms readily develop trimethoprim resistance in vitro. In co-trimoxazole (5 parts sulphamethoxazole to 1 part trimethoprim) the combined effects of trimethoprim and the sulphonamide on different stages of nucleic acid synthesis result in synergistic antibacterial activity, and the drug is bactericidal against a wide range of aerobic Gram-positive and Gram-negative organisms and some

Table 29.1 Sulphonamides: preparations, dosage and administration

Preparations	Dosage and administration
Short-acting	
Sulphadimidine	2 g initially, then 1 g 6-hourly orally or by i.m. or i.v. injection
Sulphadiazine	1–1.5 g 4-hourly by i.m. or i.v. injection, then orally
Long-acting	
Sulfametopyrazine	2 g orally once weekly
Non-absorbable	
Sulphasalazine	1–2 g orally 6-hourly

Other proprietary non-absorbable sulphonamides are marketed for the treatment of intestinal infections, but are of doubtful efficacy.

anaerobes. Bacterial resistance is thought to be less likely to develop than when either agent is used alone.

Pharmacokinetics. Trimethoprim is well absorbed after oral administration and is widely distributed in most body fluids. The serum half-life is 8–12 h and excretion is mainly via the kidneys, producing high urinary concentrations. The pharmacokinetics of sulphamethoxazole are broadly similar, and the 1 : 5 ratio of trimethoprim : sulphamethoxazole results in a serum ratio about 1 : 20, the optimum for antibacterial synergy. However, the drug ratios vary considerably in different tissues and in urine, and the clinical relevance of this synergistic effect has been questioned.

Indications and clinical usage. Co-trimoxazole has been used successfully in a wide variety of infections, particularly of the respiratory and urinary tracts. It is also effective in invasive salmonella infections (including typhoid fever) and in brucellosis, and is the treatment of choice in *Pneumocystis carinii* pneumonia. Trimethoprim has been increasingly used alone since 1980 for treating respiratory and urinary tract infections, being apparently equally effective and producing fewer side-effects. Bacterial resistance to trimethoprim has not shown any marked increase since its introduction as a single agent.

Dosage and administration. Trimethoprim: acute infections: 200 mg 12-hourly by mouth, or by slow intravenous injection. Chronic infections and prophylaxis: 100 mg nightly, by mouth. Co-trimoxazole: tablets and suspension: 960 mg 12-hourly by mouth. Intramuscular or intravenous injection: 960–1440 mg 12-hourly. Larger doses are recommended in some infections, such as brucellosis and *Pneumocystis carinii* pneumonia.

Side-effects, precautions and contra-indications. Minor gastrointestinal upsets and skin rashes can occur,

more frequently with co-trimoxazole. Caution is necessary in elderly and potentially folate-deficient patients, and folate supplement may be required during long-term therapy. Serious blood dyscrasias occasionally follow co-trimoxazole therapy, probably associated with the sulphonamide component. Dosages should be reduced if renal function is impaired, and both trimethoprim and co-trimoxazole are best avoided in severe renal failure, during pregnancy and in neonates.

Penicillins

More than 20 different penicillins are now available. They can conveniently be classified into five main groups: 'standard' penicillins, penicillinase-resistant penicillins, broad-spectrum penicillins, antipseudomonal penicillins, and other penicillin-like agents (including combinations).

Standard penicillins

These include benzylpenicillin, procaine penicillin, benethamine penicillin, and the acid-stable penicillins: phenoxymethylpenicillin and phenethicillin.

Benzylpenicillin (penicillin G)

This was the first of the penicillins, and all the later derivatives share a common 'penicillin nucleus' of 6-aminopenicillanic acid with different side-chains attached.

Antibacterial activity. The penicillins act by interfering with bacterial cell wall synthesis. Benzylpenicillin is effective against various groups of Gram-positive and Gram-negative cocci, Gram-positive bacilli and spirochaetes, but it is not active against most Gram-negative bacilli. Staphylococci were originally usually penicillin-sensitive but the majority are now penicillin-resistant due to β-lactamase production. Some other previously sensitive bacteria such as gonococci are becoming increasingly resistant for the same reason.

Pharmacokinetics. Benzylpenicillin is inactivated by gastric acid and is therefore ineffective orally. High blood levels are rapidly achieved following intramuscular or intravenous injection, and the drug diffuses readily into most body tissues and fluids, although cerebrospinal fluid levels are low unless the meninges are inflamed. Excretion via the kidneys is very rapid, giving a short serum half-life of about 20 min and negligible levels after 6 h. Probenecid delays tubular excretion and prolongs the half-life.

Indications and clinical usage. After 40 years benzylpenicillin remains a valuable antibiotic and is still the drug of first choice for many infections, including most streptococcal, pneumococcal and meningococcal infections, syphilis and gonorrhoea (due to penicillin-sensitive strains). It is also effective in some less common infections such as anthrax, gas gangrene and actinomycosis.

Dosage and administration. Benzylpenicillin is almost non-toxic, and dosage can vary enormously depending on clinical requirements. Administration is by intramuscular or intravenous injection every 4–6 h, or more frequently in serious infections. Details are given in Table 29.2.

Side-effects, precautions and contra-indications. Benzylpenicillin has few side-effects in normal dosage. Large doses in patients with renal failure may produce high CSF levels of the drug, causing direct neurotoxicity with convulsions and coma; for this reason also, intrathecal administration of penicillin is usually best avoided. Nephritis and haemolytic anaemia are other rare complications of high-dosage penicillin therapy, and sodium or potassium overload may follow large intravenous doses in patients with renal impairment.

Penicillin hypersensitivity (allergy) is an important complication and may present in one of two ways: immediate reactions, fortunately rare, occurring within 30 min and varying from an urticarial rash to fatal anaphylactic shock, and the commoner delayed reactions, characterized by fever, skin rash and joint pains.

Table 29.2 'Standard' penicillins: preparations, dosage and administration

Preparations	Dosage and administration
	Dosage of penicillins can be varied according to clinical requirement
Benzylpenicillin	Mild infections: 300 mg every 4–6 h by i.m. or i.v. injection. Severe infections: Up to 18 g (30 mega-units) daily in divided doses, by i.m. or i.v. injection
Procaine penicillin	300–600 mg once or twice daily by i.m. injection
Benethamine penicillin	475 mg once every 2–3 days by i.m. injection (in Triplopen combined with 300 mg benzylpenicillin and 250 mg procaine penicillin)
Phenoxymethyl penicillin (penicillin V)	250–500 mg orally 6-hourly, taken before food
Phenethicillin	250 mg orally 6-hourly, taken before food

There are no reliable tests for predicting which allergic patients will develop anaphylactic shock, so penicillins should not be administered to patients with a history of any penicillin allergy except the delayed maculopapular rash associated with ampicillin (q.v.), and adrenalin should always be available when penicillin injections are being given.

Other 'standard' penicillins

Other penicillins with similar antibacterial activity to benzylpenicillin but different pharmacokinetics have been developed to overcome some of its disadvantages. These include:

Procaine penicillin, a less soluble salt of benzlpenicillin, gives therapeutic blood levels for up to 24 h after intramuscular injection. It is often used in treatment of syphilis and gonorrhoea.

Benethamine penicillin is another benzylpenicillin salt with low solubility which gives a prolonged action after intramuscular injection.

Phenoxymethylpenicillin (penicillin V) and phenethicillin are acid-stable penicillins which can be given orally in mild penicillin-sensitive infections, or for prophylaxis. Absorption may be unreliable, so they should not be used in serious infections.

Penicillinase-resistant penicillins

During the 1950s increasing numbers of *Staphylococcus aureus* infections, including many hospital outbreaks, were caused by penicillinase-producing organisms, and the development of the penicillinase-resistant penicillins was a major therapeutic advance. Several of these penicillins have been marketed in different parts of the world, including methicillin, cloxacillin, and flucloxacillin, which are presently available in Britain.

Methicillin

Antibacterial activity. Methicillin is highly resistant to staphylococcal penicillinase and is active against most strains of staphylococci. Recently some methicillin-resistant strains of *Staph. aureus* have emerged, but their prevalence varies greatly from area to area.

Pharmacokinetics. Methicillin is not acid-stable, and must be administered parenterally. It is rapidly excreted in the urine. About 40% of the drug in the serum is protein-bound.

Cloxacillin and flucloxacillin

Antibacterial activity. These two similar agents are

more active than methicillin against sensitive staphylococci, but are less stable to staphylococcal penicillinase. Like methicillin, they are less active than benzylpenicillin against other penicillin-sensitive organisms.

Pharmacokinetics. Cloxacillin and flucloxacillin are both acid-stable and can therefore be given either parenterally or orally, flucloxacillin giving higher blood levels than cloxacillin by the oral route. Both drugs are highly protein-bound, and excretion is mainly via the urine.

Indications and clinical usage. The only indications for administering a penicillinase-resistant penicillin are infections due to penicillinase-producing *Staph. aureus*, or serious infections with sensitive strains of *Staph. epidermidis*. Infections with other penicillin-sensitive organisms should be treated with the more active benzylpenicillin. Opinions differ regarding the drug of choice amongst this group; flucloxacillin is generally favoured for oral therapy in mild infections, while for parenteral therapy cloxacillin and flucloxacillin seem equally effective, and less toxic than methicillin.

Dosage and administration. See Table 29.3.

Side-effects, precautions and contra-indications. As with benzylpenicillin, toxicity is rare, but methicillin has been implicated with bone marrow depression and nephritis. These drugs should be avoided in patients with a history of penicillin allergy.

Broad-spectrum penicillins

This group includes ampicillin, bacampicillin, pivampicillin, talampicillin, amoxycillin and ciclacillin. These have almost identical antibacterial activity but they differ in their pharmacokinetics.

Antibacterial activity. These agents are active against most organisms which are sensitive to benzylpenicillin but the activity is generally lower, apart from enterococci (*Streptococcus faecalis*) and *Listeria monocytogenes*. They are also active against a number of penicillin-resistant bacteria including *Haemophilus influenzae*, many strains of *Escherichia coli* and some other enterobacteria. Penicillinase-producing strains of bacteria are resistant, as are *Pseudomonas* species.

Pharmacokinetics. Ampicillin can be given parenterally or orally, although absorption is poor, especially after food. It is excreted in both urine and bile. The ampicillin esters (bacampicillin, pivampicillin and talampicillin) are hydrolysed after absorption, liberating free ampicillin; they and the ampicillin analogues (amoxycillin and ciclacillin) all give much higher blood levels after oral administration than ampicillin itself.

Indications and clinical usage. Many infections due to susceptible organisms can be treated with these agents, including urinary tract infections, chronic bronchitis, otitis media, enterococcal endocarditis, haemophilus meningitis, and typhoid fever (amoxycillin being more effective than ampicillin for the latter). One of the better-absorbed analogues or esters should be used for oral therapy.

Dosage and administration. See Table 29.4.

Side-effects, precautions and contra-indications. Like other penicillins, ampicillin and the related drugs are remarkably free of major toxic effects. Diarrhoea may occur in about 5% of patients receiving ampicillin, and less often with the other agents. Antibiotic-associated colitis is a rare but serious complication.

Table 29.3 Penicillinase-resistant penicillins: preparations, dosage and administration

Preparations	Dosage and administration
Methicillin	1 g every 4–6 h by i.m. injection or slow i.v. infusion
Cloxacillin	By mouth, 500 mg 6-hourly, taken before food. By i.m. or i.v. injection, 250–500 mg every 4–6 h
Flucloxacillin	By mouth, 250 mg 6-hourly, taken before food. By i.m. or i.v. injection, 250–500 mg every 6 h

Table 29.4 Broad-spectrum penicillins: preparations, dosage and administration

Preparations	Dosage and administration
Ampicillin	By mouth, 250–500 mg 6-hourly taken before food By i.m or i.v. injection, 0.5–1 g every 4–6 h; larger doses can be given in serious infections
Bacampicillin	By mouth, 400 mg two or three times daily
Pivampicillin	By mouth, 500 mg every 12 h
Talampicillin	By mouth, 250–500 mg every 8 h
Amoxycillin	By mouth, 250–500 mg every 8 h By i.m. injection, 500 mg every 8 h By i.v. injection (in severe infections), 0.5–1 g every 6 h
Ciclacillin	By mouth, 250–500 mg every 6 h

Skin-rashes develop in about 7% of patients, and two different types are recognized: an urticarial rash, indicative of true penicillin hypersensitivity, and a much commoner maculopapular erythematous rash, specifically associated with ampicillin and its derivatives. This 'ampicillin rash' is particularly common in patients with glandular fever, and does not indicate true penicillin hypersensitivity; it is therefore not a contra-indication to later treatment with penicillin drugs, although ampicillin itself should be avoided.

Antipseudomonal penicillins

This group consists of carbenicillin, ticarcillin and the three ureidopenicillins: mezlocillin, azlocillin and piperacillin. They broadly resemble ampicillin and are inactivated by β-lactamases, but have a wider antibacterial spectrum which includes antipseudomonal activity.

Antibacterial activity. Carbenicillin is similar to ampicillin, with the addition of moderate antipseudomonal activity, but it is less active against some other bacteria. Ticarcillin closely resembles carbenicillin but has better antipseudomonal activity. Mezlocillin, azlocillin and piperacillin (the ureidopenicillins) have similar antibacterial spectra with minor variations. They are more active against *Strept. faecalis* than carbenicillin or ticarcillin, and azlocillin and piperacillin have greater antipseudomonal activity. Some anaerobic bacteria are also sensitive to these agents.

Pharmacokinetics. These drugs are not acid-stable and must therefore be given parenterally, usually intravenously. The drugs diffuse readily into most body fluids and tissues and are excreted mainly via the kidneys, with an average serum half-life of about 1 h.

Indications and clinical usage. Carbenicillin was the first penicillin with useful antipseudomonal activity, but it has largely been replaced by more active antipseudomonal drugs such as ticarcillin, the ureidopenicillins, and some of the new cephalosporins; ticarcillin in turn is being superseded by newer drugs.

The ureidopenicillins have an important role in the management of patients with serious Gram-negative sepsis or with mixed infections, because of their high antibacterial activity, broad spectrum and generally low toxicity. Their ineffectiveness against some pathogens such as penicillinase-producing staphylococci or anaerobes is usually overcome by combining them with other appropriate antibiotics. Drug selection in individual cases depends on laboratory identification and sensitivity testing of the infecting organisms. When urgent treatment is needed before bacteriological results are available, empirical therapy with an ureidopenicillin and an aminoglycoside is widely favoured, although opinions differ regarding the most effective combination.

Dosage and administration. See Table 29.5.

Side-effects, precautions and contra-indications. Side-effects are similar to those experienced with other penicillins, and these drugs are contra-indicated in patients with known penicillin hypersensitivity. Spontaneous bleeding due to impaired platelet function has occasionally been reported. Electrolyte disturbance can arise from the high sodium content of these agents, especially carbenicillin and ticarcillin.

Other penicillins and related agents (including combinations)

Mecillinam and pivmecillinam

Antibacterial activity. Mecillinam interferes with bacterial cell wall synthesis but acts on a different target site to other penicillins, accounting for its unusual antibacterial spectrum. It has poor activity against Gram-positive bacteria, but is highly active against most Gram-negative bacilli, apart from *Pseudomonas*. It may be synergistic with other β-lactam antibiotics.

Pharmacokinetics. Following intramuscular or intravenous injection of mecillinam, high serum levels are achieved, and the drug is rapidly excreted both in bile and urine. It is not absorbed when given by mouth, but oral administration of its ester pivmecillinam produces good blood levels of the drug.

Indications and clinical usage. Mecillinam is effec-

Table 29.5 Broad-spectrum antipseudomonal penicillins: preparations, dosage and administration

Preparations	Dosage and administration
Carbenicillin	By i.m. injection, 2 g every 6 h
	By i.v. injection, 2–5 g every 4–6 h
Ticarcillin	By i.m. injection, 1 g every 6 h
	By i.v. injection or infusion, 15–20 g daily in divided doses
Mezlocillin	By i.m. injection, 0.5–2 g every 6–8 h
	By i.v. injection or infusion, 2–5 g every 6–8 h
Azlocillin	By i.v. injection or infusion, 2–5 g every 8 h
Piperacillin	By i.m. injection, 2 g every 8 h
	By i.v. injection or infusion, 2–4 g every 6–8 h

tive in urinary tract infections due to sensitive organisms. It has also been used successfully in typhoid fever and for treating salmonella carriers, and may be a useful alternative to established drugs for these infections.

Dosage and administration. See Table 29.6.

Side-effects, precautions and contra-indications. Side-effects are similar to those found with other penicillins. These drugs should not be used in patients with a history of penicillin allergy.

Ampicillin/cloxacillin (Ampiclox) and
Ampicillin/flucloxacillin (Magnapen)

These proprietary preparations contain mixtures of ampicillin with cloxacillin and flucloxacillin respectively, in an early attempt to provide a broad-spectrum drug with activity against penicillinase-producing staphylococci. They have been used for the treatment of mixed infections where one organism is a penicillin-resistant staphylococcus, and for blind therapy in serious infections. Magnapen was also widely used for antibiotic prophylaxis, especially in orthopaedic surgery. Both preparations are largely replaced by newer broad-spectrum drugs with antistaphylococcal activity.

Dosage and administration. See Table 29.6.

Amoxycillin/clavulanic acid (Augmentin)

Clavulanic acid is a β-lactamase inhibitor which itself has no significant antibacterial activity. In this combination it protects amoxycillin from the effect of β-lactamases produced by some resistant organisms, such as *Staph. aureus*, *E. coli*, and *Bacteroides fragilis*. The antibacterial spectrum of amoxycillin is therefore extended to include a wider range of aerobic and anaerobic bacteria.

Pharmacokinetics. Clavulanic acid has similar pharmacokinetics to amoxycillin, both being well absorbed following oral administration and mainly excreted in urine, with serum half-lives of about 1 h.

Indications and clinical usage. Augmentin can be used for oral treatment of mild infections due to susceptible organisms, including soft tissue, respiratory and urinary tract infections. The recent introduction of an intravenous preparation permits its use as a single agent in more severe mixed infections, but its role here is not yet fully evaluated.

Dosage and administration. See Table 29.6.

Side-effects, precautions and contra-indications. These are as for amoxycillin and are usually mild. Augmentin is contra-indicated in penicillin allergy.

Ticarcillin/clavulanic acid (Timentin)

This is a more recently introduced combination of clavulanic acid and ticarcillin, in which the broad antibacterial spectrum of the latter is further improved by the addition of β-lactamase stability. The preparation is bactericidal against a wide range of Gram-positive and Gram-negative aerobes, including *Pseudomonas*, and many anaerobes. Synergy with aminoglycosides has been demonstrated. Being available only in parenteral form, Timentin is indicated in the treatment of severe infections in hospitalized patients, either alone or in conjunction with other agents. Its effectiveness in these infections is not yet fully evaluated. Toxicity and contra-indications are as for ticarcillin.

Dosage and administration. See Table 29.6.

Cephalosporins and cephamycins

The cephalosporins and cephamycins comprise a large group of antibiotics which share many common features with the penicillins, including a similar chemical structure and mode of action. Substitutions of the side-chains on the original cephalosporin nucleus have produced a range of drugs with broader antibacterial spectra, greater activity and improved pharmacokinetics. New cephalosporins continue to be developed and marketed, many having only minor differences from one another.

Antibacterial activity. The cephalosporins are broad-spectrum bactericidal antibiotics which act by inhi-

Table 29.6 Miscellaneous penicillins and combinations of drugs: preparations, dosage and administration

Preparations	Dosage and administration
Mecillinam	5–15 mg/kg by i.m. or i.v. injection every 6–8 h
Pivmecillinam	1.2–2.4 g daily by mouth in three or four divided doses
Ampiclox (ampicillin 250 mg and cloxacillin 250 mg).	0.5–1 g by i.m. or i.v. injection every 4–6 h
Magnapen (ampicillin 250 mg and flucloxacillin 250 mg).	500 mg orally every 6 h *or* 0.5–1 g by i.m. or i.v. injection every 6 h
Augmentin tablets (amoxycillin 250 mg and clavulanic acid 125 mg)	375–750 mg orally every 8 h
Augmentin injection (amoxycillin 500 mg and clavulanic acid 100 mg)	1.2 g by i.v. injection or infusion every 6–8 h
Timentin injection (ticarcillin 1.5 g and clavulanic acid 100 mg)	3.2 g by i.v. infusion every 6–8 h

bition of bacterial cell wall synthesis. In general terms the antibacterial spectrum of the earlier 'first-generation' cephalosporins resembled that of the broad-spectrum penicillins such as ampicillin, with added β-lactamase stability. They are therefore effective against penicillinase-producing staphylococci, most streptococci (except *Strept. faecalis*), *Neisseria*, and some Gram-negative bacilli including *E. coli*. The 'second-generation' agents retain their β-lactamase stability and display a wider range of activity against enterobacteria, and some also against anaerobes. The 'third-generation' drugs have higher activity and a broader spectrum, sometimes including *Pseudomonas* and other usually resistant Gram-negative organisms, but this has been accompanied by a reduction in activity against staphylococci and other Gram-positive bacteria. The major antibacterial activities of the various cephalosporins are summarized in Tables 29.7 and 29.8.

Pharmacokinetics. There are many similarities between the cephalosporins in their pharmacokinetic properties. A few can be given by mouth, being well absorbed and producing adequate blood levels, but the others require parenteral administration. Like the penicillins, most are well distributed throughout the body and are rapidly excreted in the urine, with short serum half-lives, which are often less than 1 h, although some third-generation agents are more slowly eliminated. A minority, including cefotaxime, are significantly metabolized. The degree of protein-binding is very variable, but many of the drugs achieve useful levels in bile, sputum and cerebrospinal fluid. Serum half-lives are given in Table 29.7 and 29.8.

Indications and clinical usage. There are few indications where cephalosporins are drugs of first choice, but they are used to treat a wide variety of infections. These include:

1. Urinary and respiratory tract infections due to sensitive organisms.
2. Intra-abdominal sepsis and other mixed infections.
3. Bacterial meningitis. Several cephalosporins have been successfully used in meningococcal, pneumococcal and haemophilus meningitis, for example in penicillin-allergic patients.
   Third-generation agents including cefotaxime and ceftazidime are effective in Gram-negative bacillary meningitis and neonatal meningitis.
4. Life-threatening infections such as Gram-negative septicaemia, mixed infections and infections of unknown aetiology. Third-generation cephalosporins, with their broad spectrum, high activity and relative lack of toxicity, are frequently prescribed, either alone or in combination with an aminoglycoside.
5. In penicillin-allergic patients (see below).

The role of the cephalosporins for some of these indications awaits full assessment, with many trials still in progress. Choice of agent may depend on factors such as site of infection, organisms involved and their sensitivities, and the pharmacokinetics of the drugs concerned.

Dosage and administration. Most of the oral preparations are given in a dose of 250–500 mg four times daily, while average dosage of the parenteral preparations is 0.5–1 g every 6–8 h. Details for the individual drugs are given in Tables 29.7 and 29.8.

Side effects, precautions and contra-indications. Like the penicillins, the cephalosporins are generally relatively non-toxic agents. They may cause pain on intramuscular injection. Some of the earlier cephalosporins, especially cephaloridine (now withdrawn) and to a lesser degree cephalothin, were nephrotoxic but the

Table 29.7 Oral cephalosporins: preparations, antibacterial activity, serum half-life, dosage and administration

Preparations	Antibacterial activity, S	E	P	B	Serum half-life(h)	Dosage and administration
Oral agents						
Cephalexin	+	+	−	−	0.9	By mouth, 250–500 mg 6-hourly
Cephradine	+	+	−	−	0.9	By mouth, 250–500 mg 6-hourly
Cefaclor	+	+	−	−	0.6	By mouth, 250–500 mg 8-hourly
Cefadroxil	+	+	−	−	1.6	By mouth, 500 mg-1 g 12-hourly
Cefuroxime axetil	++	++	−	−	1.2	By mouth, 250–500 mg 12-hourly

S = *Staph. aureus*; E = enterobacteria; P = *Pseudomonas*; B = *Bacteroides* species
++ = Highly active, + = moderately active, − = poorly active or inactive.
There are several other cephalosporins undergoing clinical trials, some of which are in regular use in other countries.

Table 29.8 Parenteral cephalosporins and cephamycins: preparations, antibacterial activity, serum half-life, dosage and administration

| Preparations | Antibacterial activity | | | | Serum half-life (h) | Dosage and administration |
	S	E	P	B		
'First-generation' agents						
Cephalothin	++	++	−	−	0.6	i.v., 6–12 g daily in divided doses
Cephazolin	+	++	−	+	1.8	i.m., i.v., 500 mg–1 g 6–8-hourly
Cephradine	+	+	−	−	0.9	i.m., i.v., 500 mg–1 g 6-hourly
'Second-generation' agents						
Cefamandole	++	++	−	+	0.8	i.m., i.v., 500 mg–2 g 4–8- hourly
Cefoxitin	+	++	−	+	0.7	i.m., i.v., 1–2 g 8-hourly
Cefuroxime	++	++	−	−	1.4	i.m., i.v., 750 mg–1.5 g 8-hourly
'Third-generation' agents						
Cefotaxime	+	++	+	+	0.9	i.m., i.v., 1–2 g 8–12-hourly
Cefsulodin	+	−	++	−	1.5	i.m., i.v., 1–4 g daily in divided doses
Ceftazidime	+	++	++	−	1.8	i.m., i.v., 1–6 g daily in divided doses
Ceftizoxime	+	++	+	+	1.4	i.m., i.v., 500 mg–2 g 8–12-hourly.
Latamoxef	+	++	+	+	2.5	i.m., i.v., 1–6 g daily in divided doses

S = *Staph. aureus*; E = Enterobacteria; P = *Pseudomonas*; B = *Bacteroides* species
++ = Highly active, + = moderately active, − = poorly active or inactive.
There are several other cephalosporins undergoing clinical trials, some of which are in regular use in other countries.

later agents appear to be free of this hazard. Dosage of most cephalosporins must be reduced in patients with renal impairment to avoid drug accumulation. Haematological side-effects such as thrombocytopenia and hypoprothrombinaemia are occasional complications of cephalosporin therapy, most frequently with latamoxef; patients on this drug should be given supplements of vitamin K.

Cephalosporin hypersensitivity may develop in some patients, and 6–9% of penicillin-allergic patients will also react to cephalosporins. If this occurs, further use of any of these agents should be avoided.

Other β-lactam antibiotics

Aztreonam

Aztreonam is the first of a new class of β-lactam antibiotics, the monobactams. It shows high activity against a very wide range of aerobic Gram-negative bacteria, and is stable to most β-lactamase enzymes produced by these organisms, so the development of resistance is less likely. Anaerobes and Gram-positive bacteria are resistant. The drug is poorly absorbed when taken by mouth and must be administered parenterally. It is widely distributed throughout the body and mainly excreted in the urine, with a serum half-life of about 2 h.

Aztreonam is indicated in the treatment of infections due to susceptible Gram-negative organisms, such as bacteraemias and urinary tract infection, and may be a useful and less toxic alternative to agents such as the aminoglycosides. In mixed infections involving Gram-positive bacteria or anaerobes, other appropriate antibiotics would also be required. It is claimed that its restricted spectrum of activity will avoid major changes in gut flora and reduce the risk of colonization with resistant organisms. The drug is generally well tolerated but further experience with this agent is needed before its therapeutic role can be fully assessed.

Recommended dosage: 1–8 g daily in divided doses by i.m. injection or i.v. infusion, depending on site and severity of infection. Dose must be reduced in renal impairment.

Imipenem/cilastatin

This recently introduced agent is the first of a new group of β-lactam antibiotics, the thienamycins. The drug is bactericidal against an exceptionally wide range of pathogenic bacteria, Gram-positive and Gram-negative, aerobes and anaerobes. Its mode of action is by inhibition of bacterial cell-wall synthesis, and it has a high stability to β-lactamases.

Following intravenous administration, imipenem is widely distributed throughout the body, but when given alone it undergoes rapid enzymatic inactivation in the renal tubules. The concurrent administration of cilastatin, an enzyme inhibitor, prevents renal metabolism of the drug, so that elimination is mainly by urinary excretion. The serum half-life is about 1 h.

Because of its high degree of activity and broad spectrum, imipenem is indicated in a wide variety of severe infections, including mixed infections and those where the causative organism is unidentified. Experience so far with this new agent has been promising. It is generally well tolerated, but gastro-intestinal upsets, rashes and haematological side-effects have been reported.

Recommended dosage: 1–4 g daily by i.v. infusion, depending on severity of infection. Dosage should be reduced in renal impairment.

Aminoglycosides

The following aminoglycoside antibiotics are presently marketed in Britain: amikacin, framycetin, gentamicin, kanamycin, neomycin, netilmicin, streptomycin, tobramycin. A few others are available elsewhere. They have many similarities including chemical structures, antimicrobial activity, pharmacokinetics and toxic effects.

Antibacterial activity. The aminoglycosides inhibit bacterial protein synthesis by interfering with ribosome function. They are bactericidal broad-spectrum antibiotics with the newer agents having a wider range and increased activity. Sensitive organisms include some Gram-positive bacteria, particularly staphylococci, and many Gram-negative bacteria, including *Pseudomonas*. Some aminoglycosides are also active against *Mycobacterium tuberculosis*, but they have poor activity against streptococci and anaerobes. Combinations with penicillins or cephalosporins often show antibacterial synergy. Bacterial resistance to the aminoglycosides can develop in three ways: mutation, alterations in cell membrane permeability, and transferable plasmid-mediated resistance which controls production of aminoglycoside- inactivating enzymes. Amikacin and netilmicin are less affected by these enzymes than the other agents.

Pharmacokinetics. The aminoglycosides are all poorly absorbed from the gut, except in inflammatory bowel disease or liver failure, and therefore must be given parenterally in the treatment of systemic infections. After injection they are rapidly distributed through the body tissues, and excretion is mainly via the kidneys. Excretion may be delayed in the elderly and in patients with renal impairment, resulting in drug accumulation to potentially toxic levels.

Indications and clinical usage. Streptomycin, the first of the aminoglycosides, is complementary to penicillin in antibacterial spectrum, and the two agents were frequently used together therapeutically. Today the combination of a broad-spectrum penicillin (or cephalosporin) with an aminoglycoside still forms the basis for treatment of many severe infections.

There are now limited indications for clinical use of the earlier aminoglycosides. Streptomycin is almost restricted to the treatment of tuberculosis and brucellosis, while neomycin and framycetin are mainly used topically in skin, eye and ear infections. They can also be given by mouth to reduce the bowel flora in hepatic failure or in highly susceptible immunocompromised patients.

Of the newer agents, kanamycin is now seldom prescribed, but gentamicin, tobramycin, netilmicin and amikacin are all extensively used in the treatment of serious infection, either alone or in conjunction with a β-lactam antibiotic. The development of reliable and rapid serum assay methods allows these agents to be employed effectively and with minimal risk of toxicity. Specific indications include:

1. Severe Gram-negative infections.
2. Infections of unknown aetiology in neutropenic and other immunosuppressed patients.
3. Neonatal infections.
4. *Strept. faecalis* endocarditis (in combination with penicillin or ampicillin).

The choice of aminoglycoside depends on a number of factors, including sensitivity of the infecting organism (if known); potential toxicity and cost. For example, bacterial resistance is most frequent with gentamicin and least likely with amikacin; tobramycin is usually the most active against *Pseudomonas aeruginosa*; while netilmicin is claimed to be the least toxic and may be preferred when prolonged treatment is required. Often there is little to choose between these four agents and gentamicin should be prescribed for cost reasons, being by far the cheapest.

Dosage and administration. See Table 29.9.

Side-effects, precautions and contra-indications. The principal side-effects of the aminoglycosides are ototoxicity, nephrotoxicity and neurotoxicity. Ototoxicity is especially liable to occur in the elderly, in patients with renal impairment, and following prolonged

Table 29.9 Aminoglycosides: preparations, dosage and administration

Preparations	Normal dosage and administration	Comments
Neomycin	1 g orally 4-hourly	For preoperative bowel 'sterilization'
Framycetin	2–4 g orally daily	
Streptomycin	1 g daily by i.m. injection	Reduce dosage in elderly and in renal impairment
Kanamycin	1 g daily by i.m. injection in two or four divided doses	Reduce dosage in renal impairment
Gentamicin	2–5 mg/kg daily in divided doses every 8 h, by i.m. or i.v. injection; usual adult dose 80–120 mg 8-hourly	Reduce dosage in renal impairment and check serum levels (see table 29.10)
Tobramycin	3–5 mg/kg daily in divided doses every 8 h, by i.m. or i.v. injection; usual adult dose 80 mg 8-hourly	
Netilmicin	4–6 mg/kg daily in two or three divided doses, by i.m. or i.v. injection; usual adult dose 100 mg 8-hourly or 150 mg 12-hourly	
Amikacin	15 mg/kg daily in two divided doses, by i.m. or i.v. injection; usual adult dose 500 mg 12-hourly	

Table 29.10 Aminoglycosides: recommended serum concentrations

Antibiotic	Post-dose serum concentration (mg/l)*	Pre-dose serum concentration (mg/l)*
Gentamicin	<10	<2
Tobramycin	<10	<2
Netilmicin	<12	<4
Amikacin	<30	<10

*Post-dose ('peak') serum concentrations are measured 60 min after an intramuscular or intravenous injection of the antibiotic; pre-dose ('trough') concentrations are measured just before the dose.

Neuromuscular blockade with a curare-like effect can occur and may result in respiratory arrest, especially if muscle relaxants are also being used.

Quinolones

This group of antibacterials with a common chemical nucleus includes some older derivatives with a limited spectrum of activity such as nalidixic acid and cinoxacin, which are described in the section on urinary tract antiseptics; and a growing group of new agents with a broader spectrum and better activity, the first three of which, ciprofloxacin, enoxacin and ofloxacin, are discussed here.

Ciprofloxacin

Ciprofloxacin has a very broad spectrum of bactericidal activity which covers many Gram-positive organisms (although streptococci are less sensitive than staphylococci) and most Gram-negative aerobes, including *Pseudomonas*; many anaerobes including *Bacteroides* species are resistant. Its mode of action is by inhibiting the bacterial enzyme DNA-gyrase, thus interfering with nucleic acid synthesis and function. Development of bacterial resistance does not readily occur.

Pharmacokinetics. The drug is well absorbed after oral administration and is widely distributed throughout the body, undergoing concentration in some tissues. Elimination of the drug is largely via the urine, though some faecal excretion also occurs and some is metabolized. The serum half-life is about 4 h. An intravenous preparation is also available.

Indications and clinical usage. Ciprofloxacin may be indicated in a wide variety of infections due to sensitive organisms, including urinary, biliary and respiratory tract infections, intra-abdominal infections, and

therapy. Either vestibular or auditory damage can occur, their relative frequency varying with different aminoglycosides. Neomycin, kanamycin and amikacin usually cause deafness, while streptomycin and the other aminoglycosides are more liable to cause vestibular damage. The frequency of ototoxic complications can be greatly reduced, if not entirely eliminated, by regular monitoring of serum levels and dosage adjustment, particularly in the elderly and when renal function is poor. Recommended serum levels are given in Table 29.10.

Nephrotoxicity occurs more frequently with gentamicin and tobramycin than with amikacin or netilmicin. The risk of nephrotoxicity increases if aminoglycosides are given concurrently with other potentially nephrotoxic drugs such as cephalothin or vancomycin, or with potent diuretics such as frusemide. Renal damage is usually reversible if treatment is stopped.

severe Gram-negative sepsis. It has proved particularly useful in the treatment of *Pseudomonas* chest infections in patients with cystic fibrosis.

Dosage and administration. By mouth: 250–750 mg twice daily, dose depending on site and severity of infection. Intravenous: 100–200 mg twice daily. Dosage should be reduced in severe renal impairment.

Side-effects, precautions and contra-indications. Ciprofloxacin is generally well tolerated. Mild gastrointestinal disturbances may occur. Patients should be well hydrated to avoid the risk of crystalluria. The drug can cause increased levels of serum theophylline in patients receiving it. Ciprofloxacin is not recommended for use during pregnancy and in children.

Enoxacin

This recently introduced 4-quinolone antibiotic has a similar spectrum of activity to ciprofloxacin, but is generally less active against sensitive organisms. It also has similar pharmacokinetics, with a slightly longer serum half-life of 4–6 h, and is largely excreted in the urine.

This agent appears to have few, if any, advantages over ciprofloxacin and is being promoted mainly for the treatment of genito-urinary infections. Side-effects and precautions are as for ciprofloxacin.

Recommended dosage: 200 mg twice daily for 3 days (for simple urinary tract infections). See data sheet for other dosages.

Ofloxacin

This is another new 4-quinolone antibiotic with a wide spectrum of antibacterial activity against most Gram-negative and many Gram-positive aerobic organisms. It is well absorbed after oral administration and is widely distributed throughout the body, achieving high concentrations in many tissues. The serum half-life is about 6 h and most of the drug is excreted in the urine.

The antimicrobial activity and pharmacokinetics of ofloxacin suggest that it may be particularly useful in infections of the respiratory, urinary and genital tracts. Side-effects and contra-indications generally are as for other 4-quinolones, but unlike other members of the group no interactions with theophylline or warfarin have been reported.

Recommended dosage: 200–400 mg orally, once or twice daily.

Tetracyclines

The tetracyclines are a group of closely related antibiotics, very similar in their activities but with differences in their pharmacokinetics. Although they are bacteristatic rather than bactericidal, their broad spectrum of activity includes many Gram-positive and Gram-negative bacteria, as well as mycoplasmas, rickettsias and chlamydias. Some bacterial species have now developed considerable resistance to these agents.

Tetracyclines remain the treatment of choice in various chlamydial, mycoplasmal and rickettsial infections, and also in brucellosis. Most of the tetracyclines are only available in oral preparations, but tetracycline itself can be obtained in a parenteral form if required.

Side-effects commonly include minor gastrointestinal upsets, and these drugs should generally be avoided in renal failure.

Usual dosage of tetracycline: 250–500 mg 6-hourly by mouth. For dosages of other preparations, see drug data sheets.

Other miscellaneous antibiotics

Chloramphenicol

Chloramphenicol was one of the earliest broad-spectrum antibiotics, having a bacteristatic effect against a very wide range of Gram-positive and Gram-negative bacteria including anaerobes, and also rickettsias and chlamydias. The drug is well absorbed after oral administration, while a soluble salt is available for parenteral use. It diffuses freely into most body tissues and fluids, particularly into the cerebrospinal fluid, and excretion is mainly via the kidneys. The occasional occurrence of a number of potentially fatal toxic effects including aplastic anaemia and 'grey syndrome' in infants, has reduced the indications for prescribing chloramphenicol, but its use can still be justified in some life-threatening infections, such as typhoid fever and *H. influenzae* meningitis.

Dosage and administration. By mouth, 500 mg every 6 h. By i.m. or i.v. injection, 50 mg/kg daily in divided doses every 6 h.

Erythromycin

Erythromycin is the only antibiotic of the macrolide group presently available in the UK.

Antibacterial activity. Erythromycin acts by inhibition of protein synthesis. It is effective against many Gram-positive organisms, including most staphylococci and streptococci, and some Gram-negative organisms (not the enterobacteria) and anaerobes. It is also active against *Mycoplasma pneumoniae*, *Chlamydia trachomatis*, legionellas and campylobacters. Although it is bacteristatic in low concentrations, at high concentrations it may be bactericidal. Resistance to erythromycin has emerged in some bacterial species, particularly *Staph. aureus*.

Pharmacokinetics. Various erythromycin preparations are available which permit either oral or parenteral administration. Although highly protein-bound it diffuses widely throughout the body, except for the cerebrospinal fluid. There is little urinary excretion and most of the drug is probably inactivated in the liver.

Indications and clinical usage. Erythromycin is a useful alternative to benzylpenicillin in streptococcal or staphylococcal infections, especially in allergic patients. It is the antibiotic of choice in Legionnaire's disease and is effective in other atypical pneumonias. It can be used for prophylaxis of endocarditis in penicillin-allergic patients undergoing dental procedures.

Dosage and administration By mouth, 250–500 mg every 6 h. By slow i.v. injection or infusion, 0.5–1 g every 6 h.

Side-effects, precautions and contra-indications. Erythromycin is usually free of serious side-effects. Intramuscular injections are painful, and the intravenous route is preferred for parenteral therapy. Hepatotoxicity has been associated with prolonged use of erythromycin estolate. Recovery occurs on withdrawal of the drug, but this preparation should be avoided in patients with liver disease.

Fusidic acid

Antibacterial activity. Fusidic acid is effective against many Gram-positive bacteria and also the Gram-negative cocci, and is particularly active against *Staph. aureus*, including penicillinase-producing strains. Staphylococcal resistance to the drug may develop during therapy.

Pharmacokinetics. Fusidic acid in the form of sodium fusidate is well absorbed after oral administration. It is widely distributed in the body but does not enter the cerebrospinal fluid. Useful concentrations are achieved in bone. The drug is slowly eliminated, being excreted in the bile but little in the urine.

Indications and clinical usage. Fusidic acid is mainly used as an anti-staphylococcal drug in severe staphylococcal sepsis and for bone and joint infections. It is often combined with flucloxacillin or erythromycin to delay the development of bacterial resistance.

Dosage and administration. By mouth, 500 mg 8-hourly. By slow intravenous infusion, 500 mg every 6–8 h.

Side-effects, precautions and contra-indications. So-dium fusidate is usually well tolerated when given by mouth, apart from mild gastrointestinal irritation. Reversible jaundice occasionally occurs, so liver function should be checked periodically.

Lincomycin and clindamycin

Clindamycin is a derivative of lincomycin with very similar features and antibacterial activity, although clindamycin is generally the more active against susceptible organisms. These include staphylococci and the Gram-negative anaerobes such as *Bacteroides* species. The drugs can be administered either orally or parenterally and are widely distributed in the body, giving particularly good levels in bone.

The main indications for these agents have been staphylococcal sepsis, especially osteomyelitis, and severe *Bacteroides* infections. Clindamycin is usually preferred to lincomycin because of its greater activity, but usage has diminished due to the connection of these drugs with antibiotic-associated (pseudomembranous) colitis. This condition develops, usually in elderly patients, following treatment with many antibiotics but most often after lincomycin or clindamycin. Severe diarrhoea results in profound dehydration and shock, with a high mortality rate. The colitis is caused by a toxin produced by *Clostridium difficile*, a gut organism which is selected by antibiotic therapy. If colitis develops during antibiotic treatment the offending drug should be stopped, and oral vancomycin or metronidazole should be commenced immediately.

Dosage and administration. Lincomycin: by mouth, 500 mg every 6–8 h. Clindamycin: by mouth, 150–300 mg every 6 h. Parenteral preparations of both antibiotics are also available.

Metronidazole and tinidazole

Metronidazole and tinidazole are closely related imidaz-

Table 29.11 Metronidazole and tinidazole: preparations, dosage and administration

Preparation	Dosage and administration
Metronidazole*	By mouth, 400 mg 8-hourly
	By rectum, 1 g 8-hourly
	By i.v. infusion, 500 mg 8-hourly
Tinidazole*	By mouth, 2 g initially, then 1 g daily
	or 500 mg twice daily

*N.B. Above are the recommended dosages for treatment of anaerobic infections. Other dosage schedules are advised for prophylaxis, and for treatment of protozoal infections; see data sheets for further details.

ole compounds with similar antibacterial and antiprotozoal activity.

Antimicrobial activity. These agents are highly active against obligate anaerobic bacteria, but aerobic bacteria are resistant. They are also effective against various species of protozoa, including *Trichomonas vaginalis*, *Giardia lamblia*, and *Entamoeba histolytica*.

Pharmacokinetics. Metronidazole is well absorbed after oral administration and has a plasma half-life of about 8 h. It diffuses well into most tissues and body fluids, including the cerebrospinal fluid. The drug is extensively metabolized in the liver, and unchanged drug and metabolites are mainly excreted via the kidneys. It is also well absorbed when administered by rectal suppository. The pharmacokinetics of tinidazole are similar but it has a longer plasma half-life, thus allowing less frequent dosage.

Indications and clinical usage. There are two main areas of metronidazole usage:

1. Treatment and prophylaxis of anaerobic infections. Metronidazole is indicated in a wide variety of infections due to anaerobic, or mixed aerobic and anaerobic, organisms. These include postoperative surgical and gynaecological wound infections, intra-abdominal sepsis, cerebral and lung abscesses, and pseudomembranous colitis. It is also used prophylactically in abdominal and gynaecological surgery.
2. Treatment of susceptible protozoal infections. These include trichomonal vaginitis, amoebiasis and giardiasis.

Indications for tinidazole therapy are similar to those for metronidazole.

Dosage and administration. Oral or rectal administration of metronidazole is usually satisfactory; an intravenous preparation is available for use in seriously ill patients. Tinidazole can be given only by mouth.

Dosages: see Table 29.11.

Side-effects, precautions and contra-indications. Nausea, furred tongue, and a metallic taste are fairly common side-effects. Peripheral neuropathy has occasionally been reported after prolonged treatment. Metronidazole may potentiate the effect of some oral anticoagulant drugs, and alcohol should be avoided as disulfiram-like reactions may occur.

Polymyxins

The polymyxins are a group of peptide antibiotics, two of which, polymyxin B and polymyxin E (colistin), are available for clinical use. They act by interfering with

Table 29.12 Polymyxins: preparations, dosage and administration

Preparations	Dosage and administration
Polymyxin B	By slow i.v. infusion, 25 000 units/kg per day in one or two doses
Polymyxin E (Colistin)	By mouth, 1.5–3 million units 8-hourly (for bowel 'sterilization') By i.m. or i.v. injection, 3–6 million units daily in divided doses

cell membrane function, and are effective against many Gram-negative organisms; including *Pseudomonas*, while most Gram-positive bacteria are resistant. They are not absorbed following oral administration and therefore must be given parenterally. Excretion is mainly via the kidneys, so drug accumulation may occur in patients with renal impairment.

The polymyxins have been used to treat infections due to antibiotic-resistant Gram-negative bacilli, such as *Pseudomonas*, but they have largely been replaced by other effective but less toxic antibiotics. Their toxic effects include local tissue damage, neurotoxicity (paraesthesiae and neuromuscular blockade), and nephrotoxicity. Oral polymyxins are sometimes employed to suppress bowel flora in neutropenic patients, and various topical preparations are available for treatment of superficial infections.

Dosage and administration. See Table 29.12.

Rifampicin

This is the only member of the rifamycin group of antibiotics which is available at present for clinical use in the UK.

Antibacterial activity. Rifampicin is highly active against many Gram-positive bacteria, some Gram-negative bacteria and other organisms such as mycobacteria and chlamydias. Its action is bactericidal and it readily penetrates leucocytes and kills intracellular organisms. Unfortunately, resistant mutants readily emerge, and rifampicin must therefore be given in conjunction with another antibiotic to prevent resistance developing.

Pharmacokinetics. Rifampicin is well absorbed following oral administration, producing a high blood level which falls slowly. It is widely distributed throughout the body and intracellular penetration is particularly good. Excretion is partly biliary and partly in the urine.

Indications and clinical usage.

1. Tuberculosis. Because of its high activity against *Mycobacterium tuberculosis*, rifampicin is now one of the first-line antituberculous drugs, being used in conjunction with at least one other agent. It has been suggested that it should be reserved for this purpose to minimize the risk of the emergence of rifampicin-resistant strains of mycobacteria. However, its use may be justified in other situations where there is no effective alternative therapy, such as:-
2. Severe infections due to antibiotic-resistant staphylococci.
3. Chemoprophylaxis of meningococcal infection.

Dosage and administration. By mouth, 450–600 mg daily as a single dose before breakfast.

Side-effects, precautions and contra-indications. Rifampicin is generally well tolerated, although gastric disturbances and skin rashes can occur. Hepatotoxicity may develop on prolonged therapy, and especially if treatment is intermittent a flu-like syndrome is not uncommon. The drug produces a red colour in the urine and saliva of some patients.

Vancomycin

Vancomycin is a relatively toxic antibiotic with limited indications for use.

Antibacterial activity. It is bactericidal to most Gram-positive organisms, including staphylococci; streptococci and clostridia, but inactive against Gram-negative bacteria. Resistance to the antibiotic is slow to develop.

Pharmacokinetics. Vancomycin is not absorbed following oral administration. Intramuscular injections are painful and the drug must be given intravenously. It diffuses well into most tissues but little drug reaches the cerebrospinal fluid or the bile. It is mainly excreted in the urine.

Indications and clinical usage. Despite its toxicity (see below), vancomycin is a valuable drug in certain situations. These include:
1. Severe infections due to antibiotic-resistant strains of *Staph. aureus*, including staphylococcal endocarditis and septicaemia.
2. Staphylococcal and streptococcal infections in penicillin-allergic patients.
3. Prosthetic valve infections due to *Staph. epidermidis*, an organism which is often resistant to other antistaphylococcal agents.
4. Antibiotic-associated (pseudomembranous) colitis, for which oral vancomycin is the drug of choice.
5. Intra-peritoneal administration in dialysis-associated peritonitis.

Dosage and administration. By mouth (for pseudomembranous colitis), 250–500 mg every 6 h. By slow intravenous infusion, 500 mg every 6 h or 1 g every 12 h.

Side-effects, precautions and contra-indications. Vancomycin is very irritant to the tissues and must be well diluted before infusion. Thrombophlebitis and fever are common, and rashes may occur in some patients. The drug is ototoxic and nephrotoxic, and if possible should not be given concurrently with other nephrotoxic agents. It should be used with caution in patients with impaired renal function or hearing; dosage should be controlled by assay of serum levels, the aim being to obtain trough levels of 5–10 mg/l and peak levels less than 50 mg/l.

Teicoplanin

Teicoplanin is a recently marketed glycopeptide antibiotic, very similar to vancomycin in its antibacterial spectrum against most Gram-positive organisms, and generally slightly more active against sensitive bacterial species. However, the development of teicoplanin resistance in some strains of staphylococci has been reported.

The drug is well distributed throughout the body after intramuscular or intravenous administration, and is slowly eliminated in unchanged form in the urine, with the half-life of about 70 h permitting once-daily dosage.

Indications for use of teicoplanin are similar to those for vancomycin, and early reports suggest that toxic effects are less frequently encountered. Additional indications may include peritonitis associated with peritoneal dialysis and i.v. line infections.

Recommended dosage: 400 mg i.v., followed by 200 mg i.v. or i.m. once daily. Dosage can be increased in severe infections.

Antituberculous drugs

Streptomycin and rifampicin have already been discussed. Three other important antituberculous drugs — ethambutol, isoniazid and pyrazinamide — are briefly described here. Para-aminosalicylic acid (PAS), once a mainstay of antituberculous therapy, is now rarely prescribed and has been omitted, as have capreomycin, cycloserine and other second-line drugs.

Ethambutol

Ethambutol is active against human and bovine strains of *Mycobacterium tuberculosis*. Few resistant strains are found but resistance can emerge fairly rapidly if the drug is used alone. It is well absorbed after oral administration, has a long half-life of about 8 h, and is mainly excreted in the urine. Ethambutol is used in the treatment of tuberculosis in conjunction with other antituberculous drugs. Dosage must be adjusted according to body weight, the usual for adults being 15 mg/kg per day in a single oral dose.

Treatment is normally continued for 6–9 months, depending on the other drugs being given concurrently. The drug is usually well tolerated and side-effects are uncommon. The most important are visual disturbances, such as colour blindness and blurring of vision, due to the development of optic neuritis in some patients. This is usually reversible on stopping the drug, and can be prevented by careful adherence to dosage recommendations and by avoiding use of the drug in patients with renal impairment.

Isoniazid

Isoniazid was first synthesized in 1912, but its antituberculous effectiveness was not recognized until the 1950s. It has a high bactericidal activity against *Mycobacterium tuberculosis*, but has the disadvantage that resistance to it develops fairly readily. The drug is well absorbed after oral administration, and diffuses widely throughout the body, including the cerebrospinal fluid. It is inactivated by acetylation in the liver, and individuals fall into two distinct groups of fast and slow acetylators. Both the free and inactivated forms of the drug are excreted in the urine.

Isoniazid is used for the prophylaxis and treatment of tuberculosis. Prophylactically it may be given on its own to close contacts of the disease. Therapeutically it is prescribed in conjunction with other antituberculous drugs, such as rifampicin, pyrazinamide or ethambutol. Usual dosage is 300 mg daily by mouth, although an intramuscular preparation is also available. High doses can be given in the treatment of tuberculous meningitis. Toxicity is uncommon on normal dosage, but occurs more frequently on high-dose therapy, especially among slow acetylators. Toxic effects include psychotic symptoms, peripheral neuritis and hepatitis; the incidence of neuropathy can be reduced by concurrent administration of pyridoxine.

Pyrazinamide

Pyrazinamide has moderate bactericidal activity against *Mycobacterium tuberculosis*. It can be given by mouth and diffuses particularly well into the cerebrospinal fluid. Usual daily dosage is 20–30 mg/kg orally in divided doses, used in conjunction with other antituberculous drugs.

Hepatic toxicity was a common side-effect of early pyrazinamide therapy, using higher dosage schedules. Toxicity is greatly reduced at the lower dosage levels now recommended, and other side-effects are uncommon. Pyrazinamide now has a useful role in short-course regimes for treating tuberculosis, the duration of therapy with it being limited to 2–3 months.

Urinary tract antiseptics

A number of synthetic drugs are used in the treatment of urinary tract infections. The more important of these are briefly described in this section.

Nalidixic acid

Nalidixic acid is a synthetic compound of the 4-quinolone group which is active against most Gram-negative urinary tract pathogens, except for *Pseudomonas* species, but has little effect against Gram-positive bacteria. Resistant mutants of sensitive organisms occasionally emerge during treatment, but resistance amongst the enterobacteria remains uncommon. The drug is readily absorbed from the gut following oral administration and is excreted in high concentration in the urine, partly in an inactive form. Various toxic effects have been described, including gastrointestinal upsets, skin rashes and convulsions. The drug is contraindicated in young infants and in severe renal impairment.

Nalidixic acid is used for the treatment or prophylaxis of urinary tract infections due to sensitive Gram-negative organisms. Usual therapeutic dosage is 1 g four times daily by mouth; nightly doses can be taken to prevent recurrent infection.

Cinoxacin

Cinoxacin is chemically very similar to nalidixic acid, and has slightly better activity against sensitive organisms. High urinary concentrations are obtained after oral administration. Side-effects resemble those reported for nalidixic acid, and cinoxacin is similarly indicated for the treatment of urinary tract infections due to sensitive Gram-negative bacteria. Usual dosage is 500 mg twice daily by mouth.

Nitrofurantoin

This is a synthetic nitrofuran compound which is active against most of the common Gram-negative urinary tract pathogens, except *Pseudomonas* and some *Proteus* and *Klebsiella* species. Bacterial resistance can sometimes emerge during treatment. It is well absorbed when given by mouth, and high levels are quickly obtained in the urine. Gastrointestinal disturbances and skin rashes are fairly common side-effects; peripheral neuropathy and toxic pulmonary reactions occasionally occur. The drug is contra-indicated in young infants and in severe renal impairment. Nitrofurantoin is used for the prophylaxis or treatment of urinary tract infection. Usual therapeutic dosage is 100 mg orally four times daily, taken with food to minimize gastrointestinal upset; 50–100 mg at night is given for prophylaxis.

Antifungal drugs

Relatively few effective antifungal agents are available for use in the treament of systemic fungal infections. The more important of these are briefly considered in this section; drugs which are restricted to topical use in superficial fungal infections have been omitted.

Amphotericin B

Amphotericin B is a polyene antifungal antibiotic which is effective against a wide range of yeasts and other fungi, acting by interference with cell membrane function. The drug is insoluble in water and is not significantly absorbed when given by mouth. It can be given intravenously after conjugation with sodium desoxycholate. Elimination from the circulation is slow, with a serum half-life of about 24 h. Tissue concentrations are low and very little of the drug enters the cerebrospinal fluid. Urinary excretion is minimal.

Amphotericin is the most useful drug for the treatment of systemic fungal infections. It is indicated in generalized candidiasis, cryptococcal meningitis, aspergillosis, and other deep mycoses. It is administered by slow intravenous infusion, dosage increasing from an initial 0.25 mg/kg per day to a maximun of 1.0 to 1.5 mg/kg per day. Once full dosage is established treatment on alternate days may be sufficient. The manufacturers' literature should be consulted for further details. Amphotericin can also be given orally to treat gastrointestinal candidiasis, and topical preparations are available for local treatment of superficial infections.

Parenteral therapy with amphotericin is frequently accompanied by toxic effects, including local irritation and phlebitis, pyrexia, and nausea and vomiting. Anaemia, hypokalaemia and impairment of renal function also commonly occur, the latter usually being reversible when dosage is reduced.

Flucytosine

This is a synthetic pyrimidine derivative which is active against certain yeast-like fungi such as *Candida albicans* and *Cryptococcus neoformans* by interfering with nucleic acid synthesis. However, resistance in yeasts is not uncommon and can develop during treatment. Other fungi are resistant. The drug is well absorbed after oral administration, has a half-life of about 4 h, and is largely excreted in the urine. It diffuses well throughout the body and into the cerebrospinal fluid.

Flucytosine is indicated in systemic yeast infections such as generalized candidiasis or cryptococcal meningitis, but sensitivity testing of the yeast is always advisable. To avoid resistance developing during therapy, flucytosine is seldom used on its own in serious infections, but is prescribed in conjunction with another antifungal agent, usually amphotericin B.

It may be given alone in urinary candidiasis. Usual dosage is 100–200 mg/kg per day orally in four divided doses; an intravenous preparation is available if required.

Toxic effects of flucytosine include nausea, vomiting, neutropenia and thrombocytopenia. In patients with renal impairment dosage should be reduced and blood levels monitored, as toxicity can be minimized if peak levels do not exceed 80–100 mg/l.

Griseofulvin

This antifungal agent shows greatest activity against the dermatophytic fungi. It is given by mouth, and following absorption it is selectively concentrated in keratin of skin, nails and hair, where it exerts its antifungal effect. Its clinical application is confined to the therapy of dermatophyte infections of the skin, nails and scalp. Usual dosage is 0.5–1 g daily, taken by mouth after meals.

Imidazoles — miconazole and ketoconazole

The imidazole compounds have a similar broad spectrum of antifungal activity, being effective against the dermatophytes, yeasts and some other fungi. They can be used in the treatment of some systemic fungal infections; miconazole and other imidazole derivatives are also available as topical applications. Miconazole is poorly absorbed after oral administration but can be given parenterally by intravenous infusion. It diffuses well into most body tissues but not into the cerebrospinal fluid. It is rapidly metabolized in the liver and there is little urinary excretion. Ketoconazole differs in being well absorbed when given by mouth, although antacids or cimetidine inhibit absorption; otherwise its tissue distribution and elimination resemble miconazole.

These drugs have been successfully used in some systemic mycoses, but their proper therapeutic role still needs to be defined; in serious fungal infections amphotericin remains the drug of first choice.

Usual dosage: miconazole: 600 mg 8-hourly by slow intravenous infusion; ketoconazole: 200–400 mg orally once daily, taken with food.

Toxicity is low, but nausea, vomiting, pyrexia and local phlebitis can occur with intravenous miconazole administration. Ketoconazole is generally well tolerated, but endocrine effects and changes in liver function are not uncommon and fatal hepatotoxicity has been reported. The drug should therefore be used only when the potential benefits outweigh the risks, and it should be avoided in patients with liver disease.

Fluconazole

This is a recently introduced triazole antifungal with some chemical similarity to the imidazoles. It is particularly active against *Candida* species. The drug is well absorbed after oral administration, diffuses widely through the body, and is mainly excreted in the urine. The serum half-life is 24–30 h. Initial results suggest that fluconazole is effective in treating oropharyngeal and oesophageal candidiasis, particularly in immunocompromised patients. So far the drug appears to be relatively free of serious toxic effects. The recommended dosage is 50 mg daily, by mouth.

Further experience with this agent will be necessary to assess its role in other fungal infections.

Nystatin

Nystatin is a polyene antifungal agent which acts by binding to sterols in fungal cell membranes and interfering with cell membrane function. It is most active against the yeast-like fungi, particularly *Candida* species. Nystatin is poorly soluble and proved to be too toxic for parenteral therapy; little is absorbed from the intestine when nystatin suspension is taken orally. It can be given by mouth in suspension form for alimentary tract candidiasis, and also to prevent candidal colonization of the gut in immunocompromised patients. Usual oral dosage is 500 000 units three or four times daily. Various topical preparations are also available for local treatment of skin and mucosal infections.

Antiviral and antiprotozoal agents

As these agents are very rarely of direct relevance in an-aesthetic practice, they are not discussed in this chapter. If required, information about these drugs is readily available elsewhere.

ANTIBIOTIC PROPHYLAXIS OF INFECTIVE ENDOCARDITIS

Although there is no clear evidence of the value of antibiotic prophylaxis for the prevention of infective endocarditis, it seems reasonable to give antibiotic cover to at-risk patients (e.g. those with congenital heart lesions, previous rheumatic disease, or prosthetic valves) when they undergo procedures which are likely to cause bacteraemia, and it is now accepted as standard good practice to do so.

Recommendations for prophylaxis are based on the principle that at the time of a possible bacteraemic episode there should be an adequate blood concentration of an antibiotic which is effective against the most probable infecting organisms. Prolonged antibiotic administration before or after the procedure is unnecessary and may actually be harmful. The most recent recommendations of the Endocarditis Working Party of the British Society for Antimicrobial Chemotherapy (1990) are summarized in Table 29.13.

'Spear' — selective parenteral and enteral antisepsis regime

It seems appropriate to conclude the chapter with a brief consideration of this topic. Infections, either primary or secondary (unit-acquired) are an important cause of morbidity and mortality in intensive care units (ICU's), and while there have been major advances in other aspects of intensive care, little progress has been made in reducing their incidence. Unit-acquired infection is usually preceded by colonization of the oropharynx and lower gastrointestinal tract by various aerobic Gram-negative bacilli (AGNB), including *Escherichia coli* and *Proteus*, *Klebsiella*, *Enterobacter* and *Pseudomonas* species. A new approach to the control of these infections, referred to as selective decontamination of the digestive tract (SDD), attempts to prevent or reduce oropharyngeal and gut colonization with orally administered antibiotics. Agents are used which are active against AGNB and yeasts, but which have minimal effect on the normal anaerobic bowel flora.

Stoutenbeek et al (1984) reported impressive results from a trial of SDD using a mixture of tobramycin, polymyxin E (colistin) and amphotericin B, applied as a paste to the oropharynx and also instilled into the stomach through a naso-gastric tube. Concurrent parenteral cefotaxime for the first four days provided

Table 29.13   Recommended antibiotic prophylaxis of infective endocarditis

Procedure	Antibiotic, timing and adult dose.
Dental procedures under local anaesthetic Non-allergic patients	Amoxycillin, 3 g orally 1 h before procedure
Penicillin-allergic patients	Erythromycin (as stearate), 1.5 g orally 1 h before procedure and 0.5 g 6 h later, or: Clindamycin, 600 orally 1 h before procedure
Dental procedures under general anaesthetic Patients not at special risk	Amoxycillin, 1 g i.m. before induction, then 0.5 g orally 6 h later, *or:*
	Amoxycillin, 3 g orally 4 h before induction and 3 g orally as soon as possible after procedure
Patients at special risk (with prosthetic valve or history of endocarditis)	Amoxycillin, 1 g i.m. + gentamicin, 1.5 mg/kg i.m. before induction, then amoxycillin, 0.5 g orally 6 h later
Penicillin-allergic patients	Vancomycin, 1 g i.v. infusion over 60 min then gentamicin 1.5 mg/kg i.v. immediately before induction
Genito-urinary and colonic procedures Non-allergic patients	Amoxycillin, 1 g i.m. + gentamicin, 1.5 mg/kg i.m. before induction, then amoxycillin, 0.5 g orally or i.m. 6 h later
Penicillin-allergic patients	Vancomycin, 1 g i.v. infusion over 60 min, then gentamicin 1.5 mg/kg i.v. immediately before induction

Adapted from recommendations of the Endocarditis Working Party of the British Society for Antimicrobial Chemotherapy (1990)

broad-spectrum cover against early infections. This study, which was limited to a group of patients with multiple trauma and a minimum duration of four days in ICU, showed a marked reduction in oral and rectal colonization with AGNB and in the incidence of unit-acquired infections when the test patients were compared with traditionally managed controls.

A later prospective trial in Glasgow in which the combination of SDD plus parenteral cefotaxime (now called selective parenteral and enteral antisepsis regimen or 'SPEAR') was applied to both medical and surgical patients admitted to a non-specialised ICU showed similar encouraging results (Ledingham et al, 1988). Further studies are under way in other centres to confirm and extend these findings and to ensure that the widespread use of antibiotics in these regimens does not give rise to unwanted problems of increased drug resistance; preliminary results from a recent trial in Belfast have again shown a significant reduction in ICU acquired infections in the test group of patients (Webb 1990, personal communication).

REFERENCES

Endocarditis Working Party of the British Society for Antimicrobial Chemotherapy 1990 Antibiotic prophylaxis of infective endocarditis. Lancet i: 88–89

Ledingham I McA, Alcock S R, Eastaway A T, McDonald J C, McKay I C, Ramsay G 1988 Triple regimen of selective decontamination of the digestive tract, systemic cefotaxime, and microbiological surveillance for prevention of acquired infection in intensive care. Lancet i: 785–790

Stoutenbeek C P, Van Saene H K F, Miranda D R, Zandstra D F 1984 The effect of selective decontamination of the digestive tract on colonisation and infection rate in multiple trauma patients. Intensive Care Medicine 10: 185–192

GENERAL REFERENCES FOR FURTHER READING

Ball A P, Gray J A 1983 Antibacterial Drugs Today, 3rd edn. ADIS Press, Balgowlak, NSW, Australia

British National Formulary (BNF) 1990 British Medical Association and The Pharmaceutical Press, London

Garrod L P, Lambert H P, O'Grady F 1981 Antibiotic and Chemotherapy, 5th edn. Churchill Livingstone, Edinburgh

Good antimicrobial prescribing: A Lancet review 1982. Lancet, London

Kucers A, Bennett N McK 1987 The use of antibiotics, 4th edn. Heinemann, London

30. Hormones and other drugs

W. McCaughey

This chapter describes those hormones which are of particular relevance to anaesthetic practice, as well as a small number of other drugs whose use may impinge on the anaesthetist's field.

THE ENDOCRINE SYSTEM

In the past a simple picture of the endocrine system could be drawn, with the pituitary 'conducting an orchestra' of other discrete organs which each secreted one or a few related hormones with well-defined functions. However, investigation is revealing an increasing number of substances which have hormonal activity, sometimes of widespread importance, and some of these may be produced by cells in many different parts of the body, rather than in the classically recognized endocrine organs. These newcomers would include the prostaglandins, and the many hormones produced by the gut. Previously unsuspected interrelations between the different hormones are also being found — for example the common precursor molecule shared by ACTH and the endorphins, or the possible involvement of prostaglandins as an intermediate step in the action of other hormones on their receptors.

INSULIN AND ORAL HYPOGLYCAEMIC DRUGS

Diabetes is a complex syndrome in which there are abnormalities in carbohydrate and lipid metabolism. At present the most important diagnostic feature is a raised blood glucose level, due to a relative deficiency of insulin.

Insulin

Insulin is a polypeptide of molecular weight about 6000 which is synthesized and stored in the β cells of the pancreas. The basic molecular structure is common to all species, but minor differences of one or two peptide groups in bovine or porcine insulin (which are used in therapy) may lead to development of antibodies in patients on treatment.

The details of insulin's action at cellular level are still uncertain. Insulin attaches to a glycoprotein receptor on the cell plasma membrane. This activates the release of a second messenger, probably a peptide or peptides, from the plasma membrane into the cell, by a proteolytic mechanism. This then leads to changes both at the membrane and at internal structures. Glucose enters most non-epithelial cells by a process of facilitated diffusion, involving carrier proteins. In muscle and fat cells, but not in hepatocytes, this is a rate-limiting step, and it is speeded up by insulin. The influx of other substances not related to glucose — e.g. amino acids and potassium, is also increased. In the case of potassium, the mechanism may be increased activity of $Na^+ K^+$ ATPase of the sodium–potassium pump.

These actions on transport are not the whole story. Glucose transport is stimulated at the membrane, but also the activity of glycogen synthase is increased, which accounts for the high activity of the glycogen storage system.

Insulin's anabolic effect on protein metabolism is only partly due to increased amino-acid entry into cells. It also enhances protein synthesis within the cell — some of the processes of formation of peptides from amino acids, and elongation of the peptides, are defective in the absence of insulin. In the liver there is a loss in the amount of mRNA, which is restored by insulin.

The clinical features of insulin deficiency follow from these actions. In the absence of insulin, hyperglycaemia develops, due to a marked reduction of glucose transport into cells, and to an increase in gluconeogenesis from glycogen in the liver. Conversion of glucose to glycogen in other tissues is reduced, there is an abnormally high rate of conversion of proteins to glucose, there is hyperlipaemia, and ketosis develops due mainly to production of ketone bodies from fat metabolism in the liver. If unchecked, hyperglycaemia leads to an osmotic diuresis of water and electrolytes, and will result in dehydration. Excess of insulin causes hypoglycaemia.

Insulin preparations

Soluble insulin

This is a simple aqueous solution of (usually bovine) insulin. It has a half-life of minutes when given intravenously, but is usually given subcutaneously when the onset of action is in about 30 min, with maximal effect in 2–3 h and duration of 6–8 h. Flexible control of diabetes can be achieved using two or three injections of soluble insulin per day, and some unstable diabetics are routinely managed in this way. In order to reduce the need for multiple injections, depot preparations have been developed, which given alone or together with soluble insulin will often give reasonable control of diabetes with one morning injection, or occasionally one evening dose as well.

Insulin zinc suspensions (IZS)

These have a duration of 12–24 h depending on particle size — semilente is amorphous, ultralente crystalline, and lente a mixture of the two.

Protamine zinc insulin (PZI)

PZI contains protamine and zinc, and has a duration of 24–40 h. Soluble insulin should not be mixed in the syringe with PZI, as it will combine with excess protamine in the latter, but is compatible with IZS.

In the past, insulin used for therapy has been bovine or porcine, purified by crystallization. Antibodies may develop to the foreign sequences in the insulin molecule, or more often to impurities, and this leads to one form of insulin resistance. Two approaches have been taken to remedy this problem. Highly purified preparations of these insulins are now available, and should be used for all new diabetics, (or temporary 'diabetics' in intensive care units). The second approach is the development of 'human' insulin. Human insulin is available in most, but not all, of the forms described above, and is used in the same way as the older preparations.

Oral hypoglycaemic drugs

These drugs are effective only in the presence of insulin. They belong to two groups — the sulphonylureas act by stimulating the β-cells of the pancreas to produce insulin, while the biguanides do not. The mode of action of the biguanides is uncertain, but they may cause decreased absorption of carbohydrate from the gut, reduction of hepatic gluconeogenesis or increased peripheral uptake of glucose.

Sulphonylureas

Tolbutamide has a short action (half-life 5 h) so that it is given in up to four doses per day (dose 0.5–3 grams/day). It is carried bound to plasma protein, and its action may be potentiated if displaced by sulphonamide, etc. It is metabolized in the liver. *Chlorpropamide* has a longer half-life of 35 h, so is given as a single morning dose of 100–500 mg. *Glibenclamide* has a duration of action intermediate between tolbutamide and chlorpropamide, but is usually given once daily.

Biguanides

Metformin is the only available biguanide, phenformin having been discontinued because of side-effects, especially lactic acidosis, although this may also occur with metformin. It has been suggested that lactic acidosis is due to tissue anoxia, as phenformin (in vitro) inhibits oxidative phosphorylation.

Side-effects of oral hypoglycaemic drugs. These are few, and usually mild. Chlorpropamide and tolbutamide may cause facial flushing after drinking alcohol, possibly due to increased circulating met-enkephalin levels (Rees 1983).

DIABETES AND SURGERY

It is not appropriate to review the management of diabetes in this book. In general, maturity-onset diabetes, usually relatively mild, is often satisfactorily managed using diet alone, or diet plus oral drugs; while more severe diabetics, including most of the younger age group, require insulin. Stress such as infections or other illnesses, and surgery, usually increase the insulin requirement, and may make it difficult or impossible to keep up the usual oral food intake. Anaesthetic drugs have only a small effect on blood sugar — there may be a rise during ether anaesthesia (due to catecholamine in lease) while most other agents have no effect. A rise in blood sugar is of little consequence, provided that it is of short duration and does not lead to development of ketoacidosis. A number of regimes have been proposed for the management of diabetics during surgery, and these have been reviewed by Alberti & Thomas (1979).

A typical approach is described below; other regimes are discussed by Roizen et al (1989).

Diabetics controlled by diet or diet plus oral treatment

With small operations all that is required is to omit the drug on the day of operation, or the previous day in the case of long-acting preparations. For more major surgery, in patients on oral hypoglycaemics, it may be preferable to change to soluble insulin therapy. Adequate time should be given for preoperative stabilization, especially when changing from chlorpropamide which has a long duration of action due, in part, to protein binding. The insulin dose required will be variable, although 8–12 units 8-hourly may be a rough guide, and should be adjusted according to blood or urine tests. Human insulin may be preferred.

Insulin-dependent diabetics

For minor surgery, operation is best done either first thing in the morning, omitting both food and insulin preoperatively, or as the first case of the afternoon following breakfast and one-quarter to one-third of the patient's usual insulin dose. A 5% dextrose infusion is run, and blood glucose levels will be checked pre- and postoperatively.

Patients for major surgery will be more easily managed if changed to soluble insulin. One-quarter to one-half of the normal dose of insulin may be given 2 h before the operation, which is first on the list, and covered by 25 g glucose. Further glucose and insulin may be required during the operation, and both this and postoperative management should be guided by blood glucose estimations.

An alternative approach to management of diabetes during surgery is the use of a continuous infusion of glucose, insulin and potassium (Thomas et al 1984). With this regime an intravenous infusion delivers 2 units insulin, 2 mmol KCl, and 10 g glucose in 100 ml each hour. The relative amounts of the constituents may need adjustment during the postoperative period. At present there seems little to choose between the traditional methods and the use of a continuous infusion (Hall & Desborough 1988), provided of course that each is carefully managed.

Glucagon

Glucagon is one of a number of polypeptide hormones secreted by the gastrointestinal tract. Pancreatic glucagon is manufactured by the α-cells of the pancreas, while a slightly different substance, generally known as gut glucagon or enteroglucagon, is secreted by cells in the wall of the intestine. Glucagon is secreted mainly in response to hypoglycaemia, and also in response to a protein meal — intravenous infusion of amino acids, especially arginine, is a very potent stimulus to glucagon release. The details of its physiological functions, and its relation to insulin secretion and to diabetes are not fully worked out; recent work suggests that it is important in the development of ketoacidosis in diabetic patients.

The actions of glucagon are widespread. The most important may be that it acts with insulin to control blood sugar levels — glucagon controlling hepatic gluconeogenesis and glucose output while insulin controls peripheral utilization of glucose. In stress situations blood glucagon levels are increased and may contribute to the hyperglycaemia which is also found. The increase in hepatic gluconeogenesis is mediated through increased adenyl cyclase activity, and activity of this system is also stimulated in the myocardium, so that administration of glucagon may lead to an increase in myocardial contractility. This effect unlike that of isoprenaline, is not blocked by β-adrenergic blocking agents. Glucagon has been used in the treatment of heart failure, but has not achieved an established place, mainly because it causes nausea.

Glucagon has several different actions on the alimentary tract. These include inhibition of pancreatic juice and enzyme output, and glucagon has been used in the therapy of acute pancreatitis; early reports suggested a reduction in mortality when glucagon was used (Condon et al 1973). However, a more extensive double-blind trial showed no benefit from either glucagon or aprotinin (MRC 1980). Glucagon has been given in a dose of 1 mg intravenously, followed by 1–1.5 mg 4-hourly, given by infusion as it has a plasma half-life of only about 10 min in the body. A single dose of 1 mg is used to inhibit bowel motility for some radiological procedures.

THYROID AND ANTITHYROID DRUGS

The thyroid gland secretes two hormones, thyroxine and tri-iodothyronine, which control the rate of many processes in the body. It also secretes thyrocalcitonin, whose effects are unrelated.

Iodine is taken up into the thyroid gland, and concentrated 20–50-fold by an active mechanism which can be blocked by thiocyanate or perchlorate ions. Iodine then reacts with tyrosine or tyrosyl groups in a large protein, thyroglobulin; and these groups react to form thyroxine (T_4) and tri-iodothyronine (T_3), still bound as

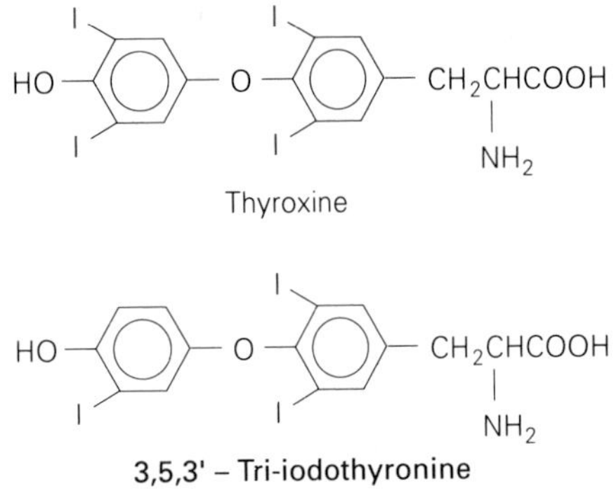

Fig. 30.1 Thyroxine and tri-iodothyronine.

part of the protein. Finally the hormones are released when the thyroglobulin is broken down by a proteolytic mechanism. Thyroxine is carried in the plasma mainly firmly bound to thyroxine-binding protein, only about 0.03% being unbound and active. Tri-iodothyronine is bound to a lesser extent and less firmly, although the free fraction is still only 0.2–0.5%. This probably accounts for the slower onset and longer action of thyroxine.

Some drugs (for example aspirin, diphenylhydantoin) can compete for binding sites, and thus lower the blood thyroxine level, whereas in pregnancy or in patients taking oestrogens the binding is increased — these effects will alter the results and significance of tests such as PBI (protein bound iodine). Specific tests which estimate the free T_3 or T_4 in plasma will give a true picture of the activity of the thyroid gland.

In normal persons, although most of the thyroid hormone present is thyroxine, about half of the thyroid hormone activity is by tri-iodothyronine, so persons who are made euthyroid by treatment with thyroxine will require higher T_4 levels since almost all their thyroid activity is due to the highly bound thyroxine.

Control of thyroid function is by the hyothalamus and pituitary. Thyroid stimulating hormone (thyrotropin) is secreted by the anterior pituitary. The main factor controlling rate of release of thyrotropin is the circulating thyroxine level, as a negative feedback.

Thyroxine

T_4 is used to treat hypothyroidism. An initial dose of 0.1 mg daily is increased gradually over a few weeks until symptoms are relieved, usually with 0.2 mg daily. In the old, or those with cardiovascular disease, treatment should start at 0.05 mg, and increase more cautiously.

Tri-iodothyronine (Liothyronine)

T_3 is not used in routine treatment of hypothyroidism, but its rapid onset of action makes it suitable for use in myxoedema coma, where L-thyroxine is too slow. In such a case the danger of its rapid action causing heart failure must be accepted. The dose is up to 100 μg, 12-hourly, depending on the condition of the patient.

Antithyroid drugs, treatment of hyperthyroidism

Thiourea derivatives block the incorporation of iodine into the organic precursors of thyroid hormone. The most commonly used drug is carbimazole. Treatment reduces the production of thyroid hormone, but this may lead to an increased TSH release and thus in turn an increase in thyroid gland size and vascularity. After about 8 weeks treatment the patient should be euthyroid, and the dose of drug (initially 40 mg daily in three divided doses for carbimazole) can be reduced to a maintenance level (5–10 mg). If a remission is not achieved in 1–2 years treatment, then surgery is considered.

Iodine

Iodine (which is necessary for production of thyroid hormone) is used in preparation for surgery. By an unknown mechanism, excess of iodide promotes involution of the thyroid, making the gland firmer and less vascular, so that surgery is easier. Potassium iodide 180 mg t.i.d. given for 10 days before operation will have this effect, or traditionally Lugol's iodine (5% iodine + 10% potassium iodide), 0.5 ml 8-hourly is often used.

Radio-iodine

Iodine is concentrated by the thyroid. A small dose of radioactive ^{125}I or ^{131}I may be given for diagnostic purposes, and the γ-radiation detected by geiger counter or scintillation scanner. Larger doses may be given therapeutically, when the β-radiation, which penetrates only 2 mm and represents most of the radioactivity, can destroy thyroid function without affecting surrounding tissues. This treatment is more suited to an older age group, and is not used in children or pregnant women.

β-Adrenergic blockade

β-Adrenergic blockade will control most of the signs and symptoms of thyrotoxicosis, without affecting the circulating levels of thyroid hormone. T_3 blockade with propranolol may be combined with the other methods, or may be used alone. The advantages of this method of treatment are that symptomatic control may be achieved much more rapidly, so that operation can be carried out in a few weeks from diagnosis; and the hyperplasia of the gland caused by carbimazole treatment is avoided. Adrenergic blockade is also the most important part of treatment of thyroid crisis, a condition which is still seen on rare occasions. This, which is due to release of large amounts of thyroid hormone, may occur following a technically difficult thyroidectomy when the gland has been much handled. Apart from use of propranolol or a similar adrenergic blocking drug, treatment of thyroid crisis includes sedation, cooling of the patient when this is necessary, and also antithyroid drugs may be given to prevent further thyroid hormone synthesis.

ADRENOCORTICAL STEROIDS

The corticosteroids are secreted by the cortex of the adrenal glands. They have many diverse physiological and pharmacological actions influencing metabolism of carbohydrate, protein, fat and purines, and the balance of water and electrolytes. They give the organism the ability to survive in a constantly changing environment, by adapting rapidly to changes in temperature, availability of food, water and salt, differing degrees of stress and so on.

Synthesis

The steroids are synthesized in the adrenal cortex from cholesterol, which is partly (20–40%) synthesized in the adrenal cortex from acetate, but mainly comes from exogenous sources. Synthesis of 21-carbon corticosteroids and 19-carbon androgenic steroids takes place through several stages. Three groups of steroids are produced: the glucocorticoids, hydrocortisone (cortisol) and corticosterone; the mineralocorticoid, aldosterone; and in small amounts, in both sexes, androgenic steroids such as testosterone. There is virtually no storage of corticosteroids, so that the rate of secretion is the rate of synthesis.

Regulation of secretion

Hydrocortisone secretion is regulated by adrenocorticotrophic hormone (ACTH). A variety of stimuli enter the brain and act on an area in the median eminence of the hypothalamus. Corticotrophin releasing factor (CRF) is secreted here, and travels in the portal venous system to the anterior pituitary where it releases ACTH. This, carried in systemic blood vessels, reaches the adrenal cortex, and stimulates the cells of the zona fasciculata to produce hydrocortisone and corticosterone. There is a 'negative feedback' of these to the hypothalamus, to inhibit secretion of ACTH.

Aldosterone secretion is controlled by the renin–angiotensin system, and to a small extent by ACTH.

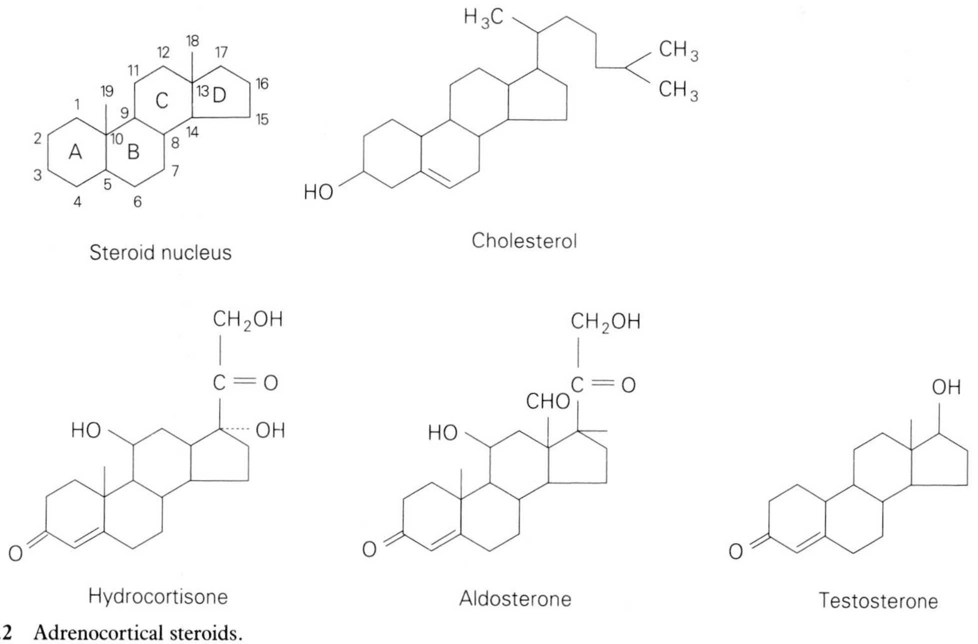

Fig. 30.2 Adrenocortical steroids.

The juxtaglomerular apparatus in the kidney, sensing a pressure–volume change, alters its secretion of renin. Renin acts on angiotensinogen to produce angiotensin I, which is then converted to active angiotensin II, which causes release of aldosterone from the zona glomerulosa of the adrenal cortex.

Physiological and pharmacological actions

There is a clear-cut distinction between the potencies of various corticosteroids in causing on the one hand sodium retention, and on the other hand effects such as increased liver glycogen deposition, anti-inflammatory effect, etc. On this basis they are traditionally classified as mineralocorticoid or glucocorticoid, although this is a classification of convenience, and most steroids have both properties in differing proportions. The overall effect of the adrenal cortex, and the corticosteroids which it secretes, is that by acting along with other hormones and enzymes, it enables the body to maintain its metabolism in the face of a changing environment and changing stresses. This ability is lost in conditions of adrenal insufficiency.

Mechanism of action

Corticosteroids, like most other hormones, interact with a specific receptor on the cell surface. The receptor–hormone complex moves to the nucleus, where it causes increased synthesis of certain enzymes. In tissues where the effect of corticosteroids is catabolic, this may be because the proteins whose synthesis is stimulated, are inhibitory in their effects.

Hydrocortisone (cortisol)

This is the important natural glucocorticoid. In the normal unstressed individual it is secreted at a rate of approximately 25 mg/day, with a clear diurnal rhythm so that secretion is maximal in the morning, and falls to a minimum after midnight. For replacement therapy, in patients lacking adrenal function, 37.5 mg is the usual dose, given as 25 mg in the morning and 12.5 mg in the evening to mimic the normal diurnal variation.

The body secretes increased amounts of hydrocortisone, up to 300 mg per day, in response to stress, and the ability to produce this response may be reduced by long-continued treatment with corticosteroids.

Effect on metabolism. In deficiency, depletion of glycogen stores and hypoglycaemia occur easily. Replacement therapy corrects this, while administration of higher doses of glucocorticoid leads to increased liver glycogen stores, raised blood glucose levels, and gluconeogenesis from protein. There is insulin resistance, so that latent diabetes may become overt, and the effect on protein metabolism leads to wasting of muscle, reduction in bone matrix with osteoporosis, skin atrophy with capillary fragility and a tendency to bruising, and reduced healing of wounds. (These unwanted effects are seen with long-term use, not after short-term, high-dose treatment as for example in the treatment of shock.) Fat metabolism is changed, and in the long term this leads to increased fat deposition on the face, shoulders and abdomen, with loss from the extremities (truncal obesity).

The inflammatory response is reduced, which may be a danger as well as a benefit. Allergic effects are suppressed, antibody production reduced, eosinophilia reduced.

The effects on the cardiovascular system are poorly understood. In the absence of corticosteroid there is increased capillary permeability, inadequate vasomotor response of the small vessels, and reduced cardiac output. The result of these changes is a decreased resistance to blood loss, with disproportionately severe hypotension developing after only moderate trauma.

Suppression of the hypothalamic–pituitary axis may be caused by long-term treatment either with corticosteroids above the normal physiological range, or with ACTH, although with the latter the adrenals can function normally. Function may be abnormal for as long as 9–12 months after steroids given for more than 2 weeks, although most have recovered much earlier (see below).

Aldosterone

Aldosterone is the main naturally occurring mineralocorticoid, causing sodium retention. This it does by acting on the distal renal tubule to cause reabsorption of sodium in exchange for potassium. In Addison's disease the ability to reabsorb sodium is reduced, and the consequent increased excretion of sodium (not only from the kidney but also from other secretory cells in salivary glands, sweat glands, etc.) leads to hyponatraemia and hypovolaemia. Replacement therapy is currently performed by using fludrocortisone, a synthetic steroid with almost exclusively mineralocorticoid effects.

Spironolactone is used as a competitive antagonist to block the sodium-retaining effect of aldosterone and other steroids.

Corticosteroids in common use

Because of their wide use and misuse, many preparations have been developed. Those most commonly encountered in anaesthesia and acute medicine are included here.

Hydrocortisone

Hydrocortisone is available as such, or as salts such as acetate, sodium phosphate and sodium succinate.

Hydrocortisone is rapidly absorbed by the oral route, as are most other synthetic and non-synthetic steroids with the exception of desoxycorticosterone (DOCA). In the plasma, hydrocortisone is carried up to 95% bound to a globulin, transcortin, while some of the remainder is loosely bound to albumin. The synthetic steroids are rather less bound to globulin.

The plasma half-life of hydrocortisone is about 90 min, although that of several of the synthetic drugs is longer. The biological (i.e. anti-inflammatory) action of all the glucocorticoids is greater than their plasma half-life.

Metabolism occurs both in the liver and at extrahepatic sites, and includes several processes involving mainly reduction, glucuronidation and sulphation. About 70% of hydrocortisone is metabolized in the liver, and metabolites and some unchanged hydrocortisone are excreted by the kidneys.

Synthetic steroids

The aim in synthesizing new compounds has been to dissociate mineralocorticoid and glucocorticoid effects, and apart from fludrocortisone the common synthetic steroids have a powerful glucocorticoid effect (Table 30.1). It has not been possible to separate anti-inflammatory effect from other glucocorticoid effects.

Prednisone, prednisolone ($\triangle'$-cortisone, $\triangle'$-hydrocortisone)

These are about four times as potent as hydrocortisone in anti-inflammatory effect, while having slightly less mineralocorticoid action. Prednisolone is widely used both orally and parenterally, mostly in long-term management of inflammatory disease, for example rheumatoid arthritis, or in treatment of exacerbations of asthma.

Methylprednisolone (6α-methylprednisolone)

6α-methylation of prednisolone leads to an increase in anti-inflammatory effect and a decrease in sodium and water retention. Methylprednisolone is available both in soluble injectable form and as a depot preparation. The latter is used by intramuscular injection for sustained treatment of various medical disorders or by direct injection for local treatment of painful conditions such as epicondylitis, bursitis, tenosynovitis, etc. The dose used is generally within the range 10–40 mg.

In high doses (up to 30 mg kg^{-1}) methylprednisolone has been the most widely used corticosteroid in treatment of the critically ill or shocked patient. This use is discussed further below.

Dexamethasone (9α-fluoro-16α-methylprednisolone)

Dexamethasone has high glucocorticoid and low mineralocorticoid activity. When used to treat the cerebral oedema associated with stroke or space-occupying lesions, a dose of 10 mg intravenously may be followed by 4 mg given 6–hourly. A high-dose schedule, 50 mg followed by 8 mg 2–hourly for 3 days and then reducing, is also used for short-term management of life-threatening cerebral oedema.

Table 30.1 Relative potencies of some adrenocorticosteroid drugs

	Approximate relative potencies		Approximate equivalent anti-inflammatory dose
	Glucocorticoid	Mineralcorticoid	
Hydrocortisone	1	1	20 mg
Cortisone	0.8	0.8	25 mg
Prednisone	4	0.25	5 mg
Prednisolone	4	0.25	5 mg
Methylprednisolone	5	±	4 mg
Dexamethasone	25	±	0.8 mg
Aldosterone	0.3	400	–
Fludrocortisone	10	300	–

Adverse effects of corticosteroids

The problems associated with withdrawal of steroid therapy have been discussed above. Prolonged use of steroids may also lead to other problems including:

1. Increased susceptibility to infections;
2. Haemorrhage from or perforation of peptic ulcers;
3. Reduced wound healing;
4. Fluid and electrolyte disturbance (rarely);
5. Growth retardation in children and 'Cushingoid' appearance in both children and adults;
6. Osteoporosis.

Clinical use in relation to anaesthesia

The indications, real and imagined, for steroids are so many that it is not useful to list them here.

Steroids and surgery. Long-continued therapy may lead to suppression of the pituitary–adrenal axis, so that the response to stress is reduced or abolished. The problem is much less than previously thought, and patients may be expected to have regained their ability to respond to stress 2 months after discontinuing treatment. Many of the cases of postoperative collapse which have in the past been attributed to adrenal insufficiency can on closer examination be seen to have been due to inadequate transfusion, etc. If treatment is continuing or has been stopped for less than 2 months, then a replacement regime will be required, except in very minor cases, but in all cases the possibility of failure of adrenal response should be kept in mind. Many regimes have been proposed. Hydrocortisone is to be preferred to cortisone acetate, and may be given in a dose of 100 mg 6-hourly or 8-hourly beginning at the time of premedication, and continuing for approximately 24 h for minor surgery or 3 days for major procedures. For the very minor cases a single dose will suffice (Plumpton et al 1969).

An alternative simple approach is to give 25 mg hydrocortisone intravenously at the induction of anaesthesia, followed in major cases only by 100 mg hydrocortisone infused intravenously over each 24 h until oral replacement therapy, if needed, can be restarted (Kehlet 1975).

Yet another method suitable for operations of intermediate severity is the use of a depot preparation steroid drug, to give an initially high glucocorticoid effect wearing off over about 5 days (Gran 1978).

High-dose steroid therapy

In contrast to the use of 'physiological' doses of steroid drugs, as described above, much larger, 'pharmacological' doses have been used to treat several conditions such as septic shock, adult respiratory distress syndrome, increased intracranial pressure, etc. The evidence for benefit in most such applications is anecdotal, and still not supported by adequate controlled clinical trials (Bihari & Tinker 1982, Bihari 1984), although many clinicians have considered that there is no major detrimental effect of high-dose steroids, and thus that the critically ill patient deserves the benefit of the doubt until these issues are resolved (Sibbald 1984). More recent work quoted below would rule out the use of high dose steroids in most of the conditions described here (Bersten and Sibbald 1989).

The dosage of corticosteroids when used in these situations is high. The drug most commonly employed is methylprednisolone, and this has been recommended at a dose of 30 mg kg^{-1}. Methylprednisolone has a slightly slower onset of effect than hydrocortisone, which has been used in doses of 1–2 g, but methylprednisolone has the advantage of less mineralocorticoid effect, and therefore less tendency to cause excessive urinary potassium loss. Dexamethasone has been the drug most commonly used in the treatment of raised intracranial pressure.

Septic shock

High-dose glucocorticoid therapy given close to the onset of septic shock does improve mortality in experimental animals. Human studies have suggested a similar effect, but to date none of these has been prospective and adequately controlled.

The mechanism of such a protective effect, if it exists, is unclear. Suggested beneficial effects (Sibbald 1984, Nicholson 1982) of pharmacological doses of steroids include:

1. Improved cellular oxygen transport
2. Protection of lysosomal membranes
3. Depression of release of lysosomal enzymes
4. Restoration of depressed reticuloendothelial function
5. Clearance of myocardial depressant factor (MDF)
6. Prevention of activation of complement C5

all of which might lead to reduction in cellular damage by bacterial toxins, reduced capillary leakage and improved myocardial performance. A further effect which has been quoted in this context is the inhibition by corticosteroids of the release of endorphins.

Unfortunately, although the question whether steroids are of use in the early stages of shock remains controversial, a recent multicentre study has shown increased mortality from secondary infection in patients receiving high-dose methylprednisolone (Bone et al 1989), and led to removal of this indication from the manufacturer's data sheet.

Acute respiratory distress syndrome (ARDS)

Steroids have been used in various forms of ARDS including septic and other shock, fat embolism, and pulmonary aspiration, with the hope of reducing damage to pulmonary capillary endothelium and also inhibiting other effects such as platelet aggregation, etc. Again evidence of a significant reproducible effect is highly equivocal, but when given very early in development of ARDS, the evidence of a beneficial effect is perhaps more convincing than in some other indications (Bihari & Tinker 1982).

The evidence for an improvement in survival from acid pulmonary aspiration is also inconclusive, and any possible benefits must be balanced against an increased likelihood of pneumonia (Wolfe et al 1979).

Increased intracranial pressure (ICP)

Steroids have been used for some years in treatment of raised ICP, from varying causes. They have been shown to be effective in patients with a space-occupying lesion, but their use in cases where raised ICP is a result of trauma is decreasing, as no convincing evidence of benefit has been shown (Bihari 1984, Jooma 1987). However there is evidence in a recent multicentre trial that early high dose methylprednisolone does improve the outcome in acute spinal cord injury (Bracken et al 1990).

Fat embolism

Here again a beneficial effect is hard to prove, but at least one recent study has seemed to show a reduction in the incidence of the fat embolism syndrome when steroids were given to patients without other complicating factors (Schonfeld et al 1983).

PROSTAGLANDINS

The prostaglandins are 20-carbon fatty acids, which are found widely distributed throughout the body. They were first recognized in the 1930s, from the ability of human semen to cause contraction of strips of uterine muscle. This is how they received their name, but recently there has been increased interest as they have been found to be widely distributed in the body, and to

have a wide range of actions, although currently their only routine clinical application is in obstetrics.

Chemistry

Prostaglandins are named as though they were derivatives of the hypothetical molecule prostanoic acid. They are subdivided according to the structure of the five-membered ring, being named by a letter, for example A, B, E and F. A subscript numeral after the letter indicates the degree of unsaturation — the number of C——C double bonds; and in the F series the position of the hydroxyl group at C_9, above or below the plane of the ring, is denoted as α or β. Thus for example prostaglandin $F_{2\alpha}$ ($PGF_{2\alpha}$).

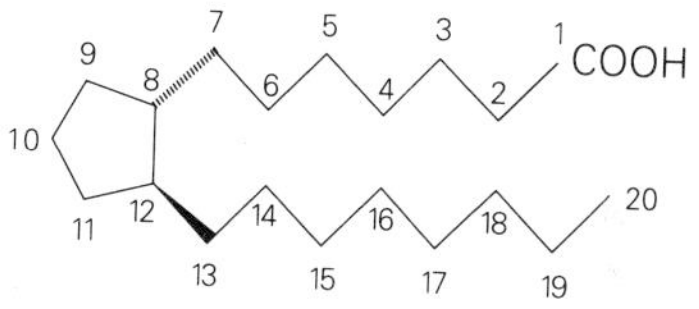

Fig. 30.3 Prostanoic acid

Prostaglandins A to F were studied most intensively initially, but more recently interest has focused on the G, H and I series, especially prostaglandin I_2 (PGI_2, epoprostenol, prostacyclin), and on the related thromboxanes, for example thromboxane A_2 (TXA_2).

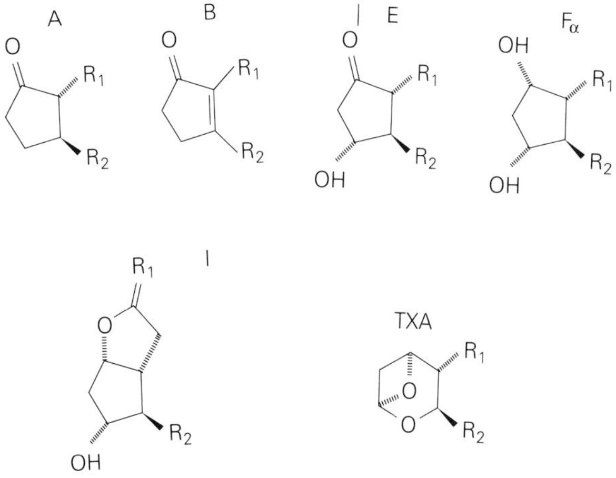

Fig. 30.4 Structures of some prostaglandins and to thromboxane A. The group indicated by ⸻▪ lie behind the plane of the cyclopentane ring, while those indicated by ⸻▶ lie in front of it.

Mode of action

The prostaglandins occur and are synthesized in many tissues, being among the active products of arachidonic acid metabolism. Their modes of action are poorly understood at present. There is evidence that they may at times act as circulating hormones — they are effective when administered intravenously, and it has been reported that they may be absorbed vaginally in amounts sufficient to stimulate smooth muscle of the reproductive tract. However, it is likely that they act mainly at local level, on the cell membrane. The experimental data are complicated, but the prostaglandins seem to be involved in the actions of many hormones and transmitters, perhaps as an intermediate step in stimulating cyclic AMP production. In platelets, substances which inhibit platelet adhesiveness, such as PGE_1, or PGI_2, cause an increase in cyclic AMP concentrations; while substances which cause platelet clumping, such as thromboxane A_2, reduce cyclic AMP activity.

The effects on a large number of organs have been studied, and the effects of different prostaglandins are usually not the same.

Reproductive system

Prostaglandins are involved in normal reproductive function at several stages, from the beginning when transvaginal absorption of seminal prostaglandins may act on the uterus and adenexae to aid transport of spermatozoa to the ovum and help conception; to the end, when at labour or during spontaneous abortion the maternal circulation contains E and F prostaglandins. The E and F prostaglandins have in general been found in vivo to cause uterine contraction, and they are used therapeutically or are being investigated for induction and conduct of labour, induction of therapeutic abortion, and contraception. Intravenous, oral, vaginal, intra-uterine and intra-amniotic routes have been used, though there is a fairly high incidence of side-effects when given intravenously, these being mainly nausea, vomiting and diarrhoea.

Cardiovascular system

Vasodilatation is the commonest response to prostaglandins, being both of peripheral vessels and also of coronary and renal beds, but there are some exceptions. Vasodilatation is accompanied by a fall in peripheral resistance and in blood pressure, and an increase in cardiac output, which is partly reflex and partly due to a weak direct inotropic effect. Prostaglandins E_2 and I_2 may be involved in maintaining patency of the ductus arteriosus. Prostaglandin E_1 (alprostadil) may be administered intravenously to neonates with congenital defects to maintain patency of the ductus pending corrective surgery. It has also been used in management of peripheral vascular disease. Thromboxane A_2 causes vasoconstriction in vitro, and it may be closely involved in the pulmonary vasoconstriction and 'vascular pruning' which occurs in severe adult respiratory distress syndrome.

In the kidney, prostaglandins appear to have a function in maintaining renal blood flow in stress situations such as congestive heart failure, hepatic disease, and during operations, when there are high levels of circulating vasoconstrictor hormones.

Blood

Thromboxane A_2 is synthesized in platelets, and its effect in causing platelet aggregation has been mentioned above. This is inhibited by low doses of aspirin. Prostacyclin (PGI_2, epoprostenol) is produced in the vessel wall, and has an anti-aggregation effect which is inhibited by higher doses of aspirin. This effect of epoprostenol may be the body's main defence against deposition of platelet aggregates (Moncada & Vane 1979).

Epoprostenol is being intensively investigated at present, and potential applications are mainly for its antiplatelet and vasodilator effects. It is given by intravenous infusion as it is chemically unstable with a half-life of only 2–3 min, and has been used experimentally in peripheral vascular disease, in coronary artery disease, in endotoxic shock, and during cardiopulmonary bypass and charcoal haemoperfusion procedures. The precise place of epoprostenol or of more stable analogues should become clear in the next few years (Vane 1983).

Respiratory system

The lungs contain and synthesize F and small amounts of E prostaglandins. They also remove 95% of circulating E prostaglandins from the blood. The effects of prostaglandins on the lungs have been found in most studies to be bronchoconstriction caused by $PGF_{2\alpha}$ and bronchodilation by PGE_2. This effect of PGE_2 is additive to that caused by α-adrenergic stimulation, and is not affected by adrenergic blockade. It has been suggested that normal bronchiolar tone may depend on a balance between E and F prostaglandins, or between PGI_2 and TXA_2.

Other effects

The inflammatory process is complicated, but has recently been found to involve prostaglandins, and the mode of action of anti-inflammatory drugs such as aspirin is now thought to be by inhibition of prostaglandin synthesis. The prostaglandins may be involved in normal and abnormal motility of the gastrointestinal tract. (Aspirin relieves experimental cholera diarrhoea.) In the central nervous system, prostaglandins are found widely, but their function is still extremely speculative.

In summary, prostaglandins seem to be intimately involved in many essential regulatory functions in the body, mainly at cellular level. It seems likely that, when these functions are more clearly elucidated, they will be found to be very important, and to have widespread therapeutic applications.

OBSTETRICS–DRUGS ACTING ON THE UTERUS

In modern obstetrics the use of drugs to initiate and to modify the course of labour is routine practice.

Uterine smooth muscle has a high degree of spontaneous electrical and contractile activity. Cell-to-cell spread of excitation occurs as in myocardium. There is both sympathetic and parasympathetic innervation, α-adrenergic receptors being stimulatory, and β inhibitory. A number of drugs which relax smooth muscle will also relax the uterus; these include some anaesthetics, in particular halothane.

Stimulation of uterine activity

Oxytocin

The posterior lobe of the pituitary secretes antidiuretic and oxytocic hormones. Both are octapeptides, with six of the eight peptides in common. As natural extracts are not purely of one or the other, a synthetic version of oxytocin is now used — Syntocinon.

Actions. Oxytocin binds to specific sites in the myometrium. The important action of oxytocin is a stimulation of contraction of the pregnant uterus. It differs from ergometrine in that contractions are less prolonged, and full relaxation occurs between them. There is little effect on the non-pregnant uterus, but sensitivity of the uterus to the action of oxytocin increases during pregnancy, being maximal at term. It also acts on the mammary gland, causing contraction of myoepithelial cells and ejection of milk. There is a transient but marked direct relaxant effect on vascular smooth muscle.

Oxytocin is inactive orally, although it is absorbed through the buccal mucosa and can be administered by this route to avoid first-pass metabolism. However, absorption is uneven and difficult to control, so that oxytocin is normally given by intravenous infusion. It is metabolized in liver and kidney.

Clinical use. Oxytocin is used to stimulate uterine activity during labour. The dose used will depend on obstetric considerations, but will often start with 1–2 units Syntocinon in 500 ml, at a rate of 10 drops/min, doubling the rate of infusion or concentration of drug until labour is established, and with generally a maximum concentration of 32 units/500 ml. If restriction of fluid is of concern, a more concentrated preparation may be given by a syringe pump.

Oxytocin has a direct vasodilator effect, mentioned above, which may lead to hypotension if oxytocin or Syntocinon is used in large doses, especially in the anaesthetized patient. Also when used in high doses, the slight antidiuretic effect which it posesses has occasionally contributed to development of water intoxication.

Ergometrine

Ergot is the product of a fungus which grows on several grain crops, of which rye is the most susceptible. A large number of alkaloids can be isolated from it, among which ergotamine and ergometrine are important. Chemically the ergot alkaloids are derived from lysergic acid.

The effects of ergot poisoning have been known for over 2000 years, but written descriptions appear first in Middle Ages. The main symptoms are gangrene of the limbs, due to vasoconstrictive effects, and abortion was also common. Although ergot was identified as the cause of these epidemics in 1670, there have been outbreaks of ergot poisoning as recently as 1953.

The important actions of the ergot alkaloids are: (1) a stimulating effect on the activity of the uterus, (2) a stimulation of vascular smooth muscle, (3) an adrenergic blocking action, which is antagonistic to the vasoconstrictor effect, but insufficient to prevent severe vasospasm. Ergometrine possesses mainly the first effect, ergotamine the second and third. There is evidence that ergot alkaloids act mainly at adrenergic, dopaminergic or tryptaminergic receptors. Central nervous effects occur, including stimulation of the vomiting centre.

Ergometrine is active after oral administration, although absorption is variable. The ergot alkaloids are mainly metabolized in the liver and excreted in the bile.

Clinical use in obstetrics. Ergometrine causes frequent contractions of the uterus superimposed on a tonic contraction, and is thus suited to use post-partum rather than in conduct of labour. When given intravenously a dose of 0.3–0.5 mg acts immediately, while after i.m. injection it acts in about 7 min. The duration of action is 3 h. For intramuscular use a preparation with oxytocin (Syntometrine; ergometrine 0.5 mg + oxytocin 5 i.u.) is available, which has a more rapid action, in 2–3 min.

Vascular effects from ergometrine do occur to a slight extent. The rise in venous pressure often seen after its use is a result of venoconstriction, more than of sudden 'transfusion' from the uterine circulation as was formerly held, but the caution advised in patients with incipient cardiac failure still holds.

Prostaglandins

These have been described earlier in this chapter.

Inhibition of uterine activity

Many drugs which relax smooth muscle will inhibit uterine contraction. This action is generally unselective and thus of no clinical use, although amyl nitrite may occasionally relax the cervix to release a retained placenta, and halothane may be introduced briefly during anaesthesia for the same purpose.

β-Adrenergic stimulation will inhibit uterine activity, and may be used in selected cases of premature labour. Other effects such as tachycardia may be troublesome. Several β-agonist drugs are used clinically, for example salbutamol and ritodrine.

DRUGS ACTING ON THE GASTROINTESTINAL SYSTEM

Antacids

The stomach usually secretes about 3000 ml per day of gastric juice, containing digestive enzymes and hydrochloric acid. The pH of the stomach contents may be as low as 1.0. When a peptic ulcer occurs, pain may be relieved and healing of the ulcer promoted by use of antacids to raise the pH to above 3.5. In pregnancy, and particularly during labour, emptying of the stomach is poor, and the pH is low, leading to the well-known dangers of regurgitation of stomach contents at anaesthesia, and of pulmonary acid burns (Mendelson's syndrome) should these contents be inhaled. The danger of this can be reduced if antacid therapy is given to increase the pH, although drug therapy is certainly not the complete answer to this clinical problem.

Drugs which act to raise the gastric pH may do so either by neutralizing acid after it has been produced, or by an action to reduce secretion of acid by the parietal cells of the stomach wall. In the first group are various alkaline compounds, often with considerable buffering capacity. Drugs which reduce acid secretion may act by blocking cholinergic or histamine receptors on the cell surface, or act on the final mechanism of acid production. Anticholinergic drugs such as atropine or glycopyrronium block the muscarinic cholinergic receptors, though their use has the disadvantage that they also reduce the tone of the lower oesophageal sphincter. In contrast, the other receptor blocking drugs, the histamine H_2 antagonists, may increase sphincter tone. The final common pathway of acid secretion is a $H^+ K^+$ ATPase which acts as a proton pump. This is inhibited by omeprazole (Figure 30.5).

Antacids are (1) systemic — that is they are absorbed and may cause metabolic alkalosis: sodium bicarbonate; or (2) non-systemic — not absorbed significantly: magnesium and aluminum salts, and others.

Sodium bicarbonate

Sodium bicarbonate reacts quickly, but with release of carbon dioxide, which causes stomach distension and belching. It is absorbed causing alkalosis, which is not usually important except in cases of renal insufficiency.

Aluminum hydroxide, magnesium trisilicate, sodium citrate

These react slowly, and do not upset the acid–base balance of the body.

In obstetric practice, all patients who are likely to require anaesthesia — and this includes all patients in labour — should receive routine antacids. The type of antacid therapy to be used is controversial. Compounds of aluminum or magnesium hydroxides, magnesium trisilicate, etc., probably can produce the best results in terms of maintaining a high pH over a long time. A widely recommended regimen is Mist Magnesium Trisilicate BP 20 ml given 2–hourly throughout labour with an additional dose immediately before induction of anaesthesia (Crawford 1978). However, there is a suspicion that these compounds, being particulate, may themselves cause lung damage, and in the case of the aluminum salts, long-term effects have been shown to be even worse than those following acid aspiration (Gibbbs et al 1979). The case against magnesium trisilicate is not proven. The non-particulate antacids, sodium citrate and bicarbonate, do not have this disadvantage, but their buffering power is less, and they are probably

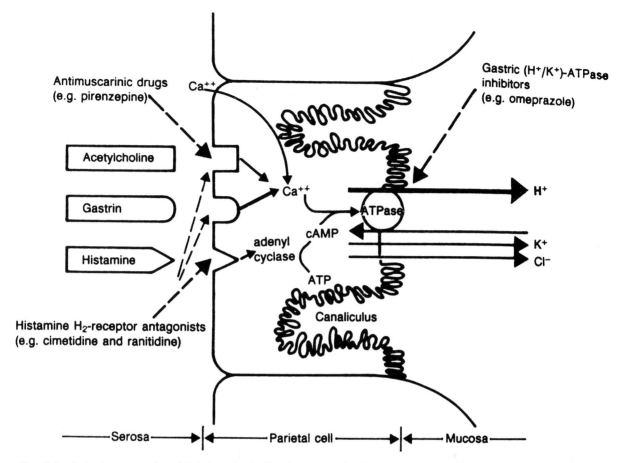

Fig. 30.5 A simple conceptual model of the parietal cell and some speculated mechanisms involved in the control and inhibition of gastric acid secretion. ➡ represents proposed mechanisms by which certain classes of anti-ulcer drugs antagonize gastric acid stimulation; → indicates other additional effects of the H₂-receptor antagonists (although it is not necessarily at the receptor level) which may contribute to their antisecretory activity. Reproduced with permission from Clissold and Campoli-Richards (1986).

best used in combination with histamine H_2 blocking therapy (see below).

Histamine H_2 blocking drugs

Histamine is widely distributed throughout the body. Effects such as contraction of smooth muscle of gut, and of the bronchi leading to bronchoconstriction, and the peripheral and cutaneous vasodilation (histamine wheal) can all be inhibited by low doses of conventional antihistamines such as mepyramine. The receptors acting and inhibited in this way have been termed H_1-receptors (Ash & Schild 1966). Histamine also stimulates gastric secretion and has other actions which cannot be blocked by conventional antihistamines. These actions are mediated by the H_2-receptor.

Histamine H_1 antagonists, the conventional antihistamines, tend to resemble histamine in possessing a charged (usually ammonium) side-chain, and are lipophilic, while the H_2 antagonists have more similarity to the imidazole ring end of the histamine molecule, and tend to be hydrophilic (Durant et al 1977). The histamine H_2 blocking drugs have been used clinically because their action on H_2 receptors in the gastric mucosa inhibits all forms of gastric secretion. However H_2 receptors exist also in other parts of the body, i.e. uterus, heart and blood vessels including the ductus arteriosus, and the lower oesophageal sphincter.

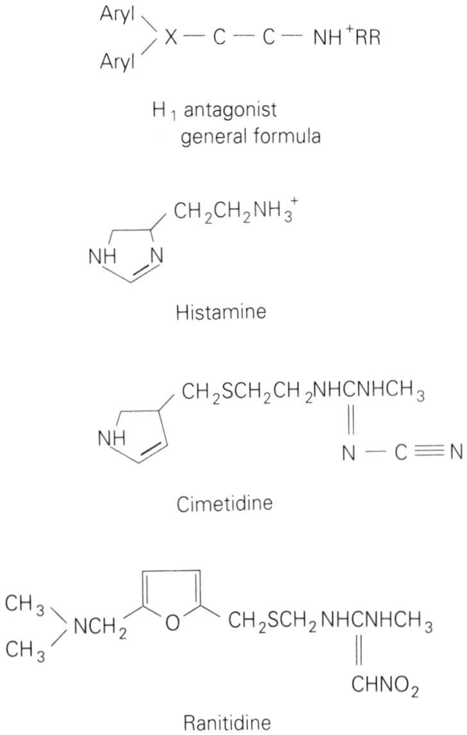

Fig. 30.6 Histamine H_2 blocking drugs.

The significance of these in man is still the subject of investigation.

Cimetidine

Cimetidine is readily absorbed after oral administration, reaching peak levels after 69–90 min, but later if given with food. It is eliminated with a plasma half-life of about 2 h, mainly (about 70%) being excreted unchanged by the kidneys. The plasma half-life is increased to about 5 h in renal failure (Canavan & Briggs 1977)

The usual oral dose of cimetidine is 200–400 mg. In treatment of duodenal ulcer total daily doses of 0.8–1.6 g are usual, or 300–400 mg at night for maintenance therapy.

In obstetric anaesthetic practice, 400 mg orally given 60–90 min before elective procedures will raise gastric pH satisfactorily. For patients in labour (Johnston et al 1982), 400 mg at commencement of labour followed by 200 mg 2-hourly gives satisfactory results (see below).

Cimetidine does have side-effects which, though not generally serious, have led to its partial replacement by

ranitidine. Arrhythmias have been reported on rare occasions after intravenous administration. There is a slight anti-androgenic effect, probably not related to its action on H_2 receptors.

Cimetidine can inhibit metabolism of other drugs both by enzyme inhibition (Henry et al 1980) and also because it causes a reduction in liver blood flow (Feely et al 1981); it binds to mitochondrial cytochrome P450 to cause the former effect.

Ranitidine

Ranitidine differs from cimetidine mainly in that it does not contain an imidazole group. It is 4–10 times more potent than cimetidine.

Ranitidine is absorbed readily, with peak plasma concentrations at 90–120 min. There is significant first-pass metabolism. The elimination half-life during oral treatment is about 2–3 h. About 30% of an intravenous dose, or 68% of an oral dose, is excreted unchanged in the urine, the remainder being cleared by the liver. As with cimetidine, the elimination half-life in renal failure is increased.

The usual intravenous dose is 50 mg, and the oral dose 150 mg. Although there is little difference in plasma half-life between cimetidine and ranitidine, at clinically used doses the duration of action of ranitidine is considerably longer.

In obstetric anaesthetic practice, 150 mg may be given 2–3 h before elective Caesarean section (McAuley et al 1983). For management of labour, 150 mg may be given at commencement of labour and 6-hourly throughout labour. As with cimetidine, this will raise the pH of the stomach satisfactorily, but not until 2 h have elapsed from the initial dose. This therapy should therefore be combined with use of a single dose of non-particulate alkali, sodium bicarbonate or citrate, given immediately before anaesthesia (Thompson et al 1984).

Side-effects of ranitidine are few, and it is free of those listed above for cimetidine.

Omeprazole

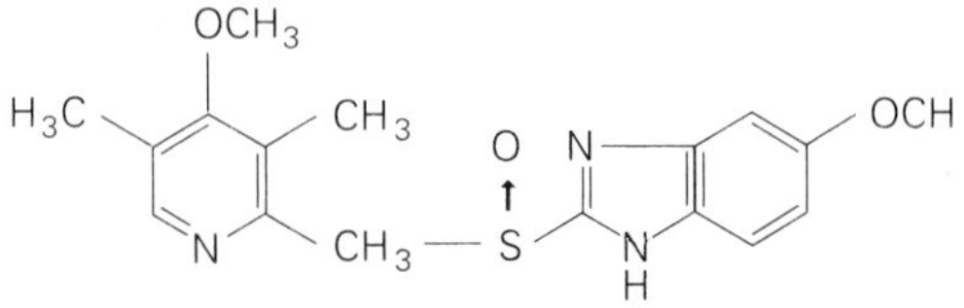

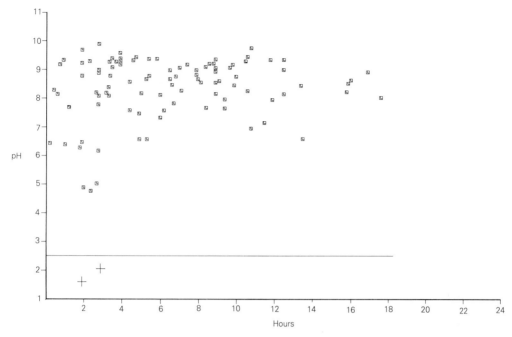

Fig. 30.7   pH of gastric contents from women who required general anaesthesia in labour who were given 150 mg ranitidine 6-hourly plus a dose of 20 ml 8.4% sodium bicarbonate orally 10 min pre-induction; + no bicarbonate. Reproduced with permission from Thompson et al (1984).

Omeprazole is a subsitituted benzimidazole. It is a weak base with a pKa of 3.97, and thus accumulates within the acid environment of the gastric mucosa. It is thought that omeprazole is activated only at low pH, and this, together with the fact that it is rapidly localized to gastric mucosa, should make its action highly selective.

Omeprazole is slightly soluble in water but highly soluble in alkaline solutions. It degrades rapidly in acid surroundings and so oral administration must be accompanied by sufficient alkaline buffer, or as an enteric-coated preparation. Peak plasma concentrations are reached about 20 min after ingestion as solution, but only 2–5 h after enteric-coated tablets. Omeprazole is 95–96% bound, mainly to serum albumin and α_1-acid glycoprotein (Regårdh et al 1985). Distribution is rapid, with a $t_{\frac{1}{2}}\alpha$ of approximately 3 min. The volume of distribution is relatively small; little crosses the blood–brain barrier, but it does cross the placenta. It is rapidly metabolized and excreted, with a terminal plasma half-life of about 0.5–1.5 h in most studies. However, there is no correlation between plasma level and antisecretory effect, which may persist long after the drug can no longer be detected in plasma. There is, however, a significant correlation of effect with area under the curve (AUC), suggesting that distribution to

the tissues — in particular the parietal cells of the stomach — is the major factor in its activity. It is believed that omeprazole may irreversibly inhibit the $H^+ \ K^+$ ATPase enzyme, blocking acid secretion until further enzyme is synthesized. Its effects increase over the first 2–3 days of administration, and then reach a plateau, perhaps because it increases its own bioavailability by reducing its degradation by stomach acid.

Most studies of its clinical use have been in ulcer therapy, where it has shown a high rate of ulcer healing. Preliminary studies of its use in anaesthetic practice are under way (Cruikshank et al 1989, Moore et al 1989).

Omeprazole has few side-effects but it has been shown, like cimetidine, to inhibit hepatic oxidative metabolism of some drugs. Long-term animal studies have shown an increased incidence of chromaffin tumours, probably related to hypergastrinaemia.

Anti-ulcer drugs

Liquorice and carbenoxolone (Biogastrone)

These promote ulcer healing. Their relevance to anaesthetic practice is their side-effect of sodium retention which may cause oedema, hypertension and heart failure. Hypokalaemia may also occur, especially if a diuretic is being used to relieve the oedema, and potassium supplements may be required.

DRUGS USED IN PANCREATITIS

Management of acute haemorrhagic pancreatitis is largely management of the associated shock. Two drugs which have been used for specific effects are glucagon (see above), and aprotinin.

Aprotinin

Proteinase inhibitors exist naturally in both plant and animal tissues. The commercially available product 'Trasylol' or aprotinin is derived from bovine organs. It is a basic polypeptide with a molecular weight of approximately 6000 and consists of 16 amino acids in a folded chain.

The enzymes subject to inhibition by aprotinin are so-called endopeptidases, which break up long protein chains into peptide fragments of greater or lesser size. Enzymes inhibited by aprotinin include trypsin, chymotrypsin, kallikrein and plasmin. Many other enzymes have been shown to be unaffected.

The enzymes affected by aprotinin appear to be active in the areas of inflammation, blood coagulation and shock. Inhibition of proteolytic reactions which occur early in the coagulation process is caused by aprotinin, and it is suggested that it will inhibit excessive activity both of the coagulation process and of the fibrinolytic system, so that it can be used in treatment of haemorrhage due to the defibrination syndrome (see Chapter 26). In shock aprotinin has been used in order to prevent kinins from producing microvascular changes and circulatory stagnation. Inhibition of damage due to kinin release is also the rationale for its use in treatment of the fat embolism syndrome.

Aprotinin is administered parenterally. It has a biological half-life of about 150 min, and is usually given by intravenous infusion. The recommended dose is 200 000 K.i.u. (Kallidinogenase inactivating units), followed by 200 000 units 4- or 6-hourly, during the acute phase of the disease (3–5 days). It appears essential in all conditions to start therapy early to obtain any benefit, and therapy should not be 'tailed off'.

Despite much study, its effectiveness in all of the above situations is still controversial. Use of aprotinin in acute pancreatitis has been widespread, as some trials have shown a small decrease in mortality in cases where aprotinin has been used in conjunction with other supportive therapy (Trapnell et al 1974). However, well-controlled double-blind studies have failed to show any benefit (MRC 1980), and its use is declining.

REFERENCES

Ahearn R S, Walker B A 1980 Diabetes in relation to anaesthesia. In: Gray T C, Nunn J F, Utting J E (eds) General anaesthesia, 4th edn. Butterworths, London, pp 797–808

Alberti G M M, Thomas D J B 1979 The management of diabetes during surgery. British Journal of Anaesthesia 51: 693–710

Ash A S F and Schild H O 1966 Receptors mediating some actions of histamine. British Journal of Pharmacology 27: 427–439

Bersten A, Sibbald W J 1989 Acute lung injury in septic shock. Critical Care Clinics 5: 49–79

Bihari D 1984 The case for steroids. Intensive Care Medicine 10: 113–114

Bihari D, Tinker J 1982 Steroids in intensive care. British Journal of Hospital Medicine 28: 323–320

Bone R C, Fisher C J Jr, Clemmer T P, Slotman G J, Metz C A, Balk R A 1989 Sepsis syndrome: a valid clinical entity. Methylprednisolone severe sepsis study group. Critical Care Medicine 17: 389–393

Bracken M B, Shepard M J, Collins W F, Holford T R, Young W, Baskin D S, Eisenberg H M, Flamm E, Leo-Summers L, Maroon J, Marshall L F, Perot P L, Piepmeier J, Sonntag V K H, Wagner F C, Wilberger J E, Winn H R 1990 A randomised, controlled trial of methylprednisolone or naloxone in the treatment of acute spinal-cord injury. New England Journal of Medicine 322: 1405–1411

Canavan J S F, Briggs J D 1977 Cimetidine clearance in renal failure. In: Burland W L, Simkins M A (eds) Cimetidine. Proceedings of the second international symposium on Histamine H$_2$-receptor antagonists. Excerpta Medica, Amsterdam, Oxford

Clissold S P, Campoli-Richards D M 1986 Omeprazole: A preliminary review of its pharmacodynamic and pharmacokinetic properties, and therapeutic potential in peptic ulcer disease and Zollinger–Ellison syndrome. Drugs 32: 15–47

Condon J R, Knight M, Day J L 1973 Glucagon therapy in acute pancreatitis. British Journal of Surgery 60: 509–511

Crawford J S 1978 Principles and practice of obstetric anaesthesia, 4th edn. Blackwell Scientific Publications, Oxford

Cruikshank R H, Morrison D A, Bamber P A, Nimmo W S 1989 Effect of IV omeprazole on the pH and volume of gastric contents before surgery. British Journal of Anaesthesia 63: 536–540

Durant G S, Emmett J C, Ganellin C R 1977 The chemical origin and properties of histamine H$_2$ receptor antagonists. In: Burland W L Simkins M A eds, Cimetidine. Proceedings of the second inernational symposium on Histamine H$_2$-receptor antagonists.

Excerpta Medica, Amsterdam, Oxford

Feely J, Wilkinson G R, Wood A J J 1981 Reduction of liver blood flow and propranolol metabolism by cimetidine. New England Journal of Medicine, 309: 692–695

Gibbs C P, Schwartz D J, Wynne J W, Hood C I, Kuck E J 1979 Antacid pulmonary aspiration in the dog. Anesthesiology 51: 380–385

Gran L 1978 Rational substitution therapy for steroid treated patients. Anaesthesia 33; 59–60

Hall G M 1984 Diabetes and anaesthesia — a promise unfulfilled? Anaesthesia 39: 627–628

Hall G M, Desborough J P 1988 Diabetes and anaesthesia — slow progress. Anaesthesia 43: 531–532

Henry D A, MacDonald I A, Kitchingman G, Bell G D, Longman M T S 1980 Cimetidine and ranitidine: comparison of effects on hepatic metabolism. British Medical Journal 281: 775–777

Johnston J R, McCaughey W, Moore J, Dundee J W 1982 A field trial of cimetidine as sole oral antacid in obstetric anaesthesia. Anaesthesia 37: 33–38

Jooma R 1987 Dexamethasone and the serious head injury. British Journal of Neurosurgery 1: 400–403

Katz R L and Katz G J 1974 Prostaglandins — basic and clinical considerations. Anesthesiology 40: 471–493

Kehlet H. 1975 A rational approach to dosage and preparation of parenteral therapy during surgical procedures. Acta Anaesthesiologica Scandinavica 19: 260–264

Levine R 1982 Insulin: the effect and mode of action of the hormone. Vitamins and Hormones 39: 145–173

M.R.C. 1980 Multicentre trial of glucagon and aprotinin. Gut 21: 334

McAuley D M, Moore J, McCaughey W, Donnelly B D, Dundee J W 1983 Ranitidine as an antacid before elective caesarian section. Anaesthesia 38: 108–114

Moncada S, Vane J R 1979 Pharmacology and endogenous roles of prostaglandin endoperoxidases, thromboxane A2 and prostacyclin. Pharmacological Reviews 30: 293–331

Moore J, Flynn R J, Sampaio M, Wilson C M, Gillon K R W 1989 Effect of single dose omeprazole on gastric acidity and volume during obstetric anaesthesia. Anaesthesia 44: 559–562

Nicholson D 1982 Glucocorticoids in the treatment of shock and the adult respiratory distress syndrome. Clinics in Chest Medicine 3: 121–132

Plumpton F S, Besser G N, Cole P V 1969 Corticosteroid treatment and surgery. 2. The management of steroid cover. Anaesthesia 24: 12–18

Rees L H 1983 The endorphins. Intensive Care Society autumn meeting, St Bartholomew's Hospital, London

Regårdh C-G, Gabrielson M, Hoffman K-J, Löfberg I, Skåberg I 1985 Pharmacokinetics and metabolism of omeprazole in animals and man — an overview. Scandinavian Journal of Gastroenterology, 20 (Suppl 108): 79–94

Roizen M F, Stevens A, Lampe G H 1989 Perioperative management of patients with endocrine disease. In: Nunn J F, Utting J E, Brown B R Jr (eds) General Anaesthesia (5th ed) Butterworths, London

Schonfeld S A, Ploysongsang Y, DiLisio R, Crissman J D, Miller E, Hammerschmidt D E, Jacob H S 1983 Fat embolism prophylaxis with corticosteroids. Annals of Internal Medicine 99: 438–443

Sibbald W J 1984 The case for steroids: another viewpoint. Intensive Care Medicine 10: 115–117

Thomas D J B, Platt H S, Alberti G M M 1984 Insulin-dependent diabetes during the peri-operative period. An assessment of continuous glucose–insulin–potassium infusion, and traditional treatment. Anaesthesia 39: 629–637

Thompson E M, Loughran P G, McAuley D M, Wilson C M, Moore J 1984 Combined treatment with ranitidine and saline antacids prior to obstetric anaesthesia. Anaesthesia 39: 1086–1090

Trapnell J E, Rigby C C, Talbot C H, Duncan E H L 1974 A controlled trial of Trasylol in the treatment of acute pancreatitis. British Journal of Surgery 61: 177–182

Vane J R 1983 Prostaglandins and the cardiovascular system. British Heart Journal 49: 405–409

Wolfe J E, Bone R C, Ruth W E 1979 Effects of corticosteroids in the treatment of patients with gastric aspiration. American Journal of Medicine 63: 719–722

Special drug problems in patient management

31. Pharmacology of drugs in pregnancy

J. Moore

The use of drugs in pregnancy is limited by their potentially harmful effect on the developing fetus or, if administered during parturition, their actions on the newborn infant. Investigations in the human to determine the potential fetal hazards of maternal drug therapy are obviously restricted and animal experiments, while valuable, sometimes fail because of special variation. The problem of dysmorphogenesis and other effects due to exposure to drugs in early pregnancy is often resolved by case reports, and emphasizes the need for central reporting of such occurrences. The dramatic changes in the cardiovascular, respiratory and temperature-regulating systems of the newborn infant at birth associated with a reduced capacity for metabolism and excretion increase its vulnerability to adverse reactions from transferred drugs. While these considerations obviously impose limitations on drug therapy in obstetrics there are many agents which provide great benefit to mother and child. It is essential therefore that the altered maternal pharmacokinetics in pregnancy, the mechanisms of placental transfer and the effects, distribution, metabolism and excretion of the transferred drug to the infant be considered.

Maternal pharmacokinetic changes

Drug absorption from the intestinal tract is altered in late pregnancy because of prolongation in gastric emptying time. This delay is further accentuated during labour by the use of opioid analgesics. The resultant decreased uptake of orally administered drugs may mean that an effective therapeutic plasma concentration is not achieved. For rapid effect, parenteral administration is best.

The volume of distribution of drugs is altered as pregnancy advances. This is due to increases in the total body water with associated expansions of blood and plasma volume. Polar drugs with a low distribution volume are most affected and their increased V_d lowers their plasma concentration and may prolong their half-life by slowing their elimination.

Drug distribution in pregnancy is further altered by the reduction in plasma protein concentration. There is a major fall in the concentration of plasma albumin to which many commonly used drugs, e.g. anticonvulsants, benzodiazepines, are bound. This fall reduces the binding capacity of a given volume of plasma and increases the apparent volume of distribution of protein-bound drug. A number of other drugs, e.g. propranolol and lignocaine, bind to α_1-acid glycoprotein, the concentration of which remains relatively unaltered.

The metabolism of drugs takes place mainly in the liver, and hepatic cells of pregnant patients show hyperplasia of the smooth endoplasmic reticulum. Such changes suggest increased metabolizing ability, possibly invoked by the high circulating levels of progesterone. Plasma concentrations of drugs known to undergo hepatic metabolism are lower in pregnancy but this is mainly due to increased plasma dilution.

During pregnancy renal plasma flow almost doubles and glomerular filtration rate increases by up to 70%. These changes enhance the renal excretion of drugs solely dependent on this route for their elimination.

The placenta contains enzyme systems for oxidation, reduction, hydrolysis and conjugation of many substances. However, information regarding their role in drug metabolism is limited. Hydrolysis in human placental fractions has been shown for pethidine, acetyl salicylic acid and procaine. The placenta also contains enzymes capable of metabolizing pharmacologically active endogenous compounds, vasoactive substances such as adrenaline, noradrenaline, serotonin, angiotensin and vasopressin, some of which are used in therapeutics and may therefore be referred to as drugs. Placental biotransformation of phencyclidine to hydroxy derivatives has been demonstrated by in vitro studies. While the pseudocholinesterase and oxidative metabolizing enzymes play a part in protecting the fetus from maternal drug administration, their capacity is readily saturated.

In late pregnancy alveolar ventilation is increased by 50% mainly due to an increase in tidal volume. There is a 20% reduction in functional residual capacity of the lungs. The resultant hypocarbia is compensated by a 20% reduction in serum bicarbonate. These respiratory changes, together with the associated increase in cardiac output, have marked effects on the uptake and elimination of inhalation anaesthetics. A more rapid equilibration of inspired and blood concentrations during induction, especially with the more soluble agents, shortens this phase of anaesthesia. The reverse pertains during elimination, and recovery is rapid. During labour pains anxiety may contribute to further increases in ventilation and minute volume may increase by 300% or more. Marked hypocapnia occurs and may be balanced by lactic acidosis due to the increased work of breathing.

The pregnant patient generally reacts as her non-pregnant counterpart with respect to drug effects, despite the above changes in pharmacokinetic parameters. However, for drugs with a relatively narrow therapeutic ratio, such factors must be considered.

The placenta

The human placenta, formed during the first 3 months of pregnancy, is a distinct organ with a maximum number of cotyledons by the 12th week. The cotyledon contains maternal blood sinuses into which protrude villi carrying the fetal capillaries. The villi are covered with a trophoblastic layer beneath which is a layer of mesenchymal tissue and finally the capillary endothelium. Maternal blood to the villous space comes from several hundred spiral arteries derived as branches from the uterine artery. This blood travels from the centre to the periphery of each lobule where it drains into the open ends of the uterine veins. The fetal circulation is derived from two umbilical arteries which successively divide into smaller vessels within the fetal villi. Capillaries traverse the tops of the fetal villi and it is here that exchange of nutrients and waste products occurs with maternal blood within the intervillous space. The fetal blood is collected into a series of tributaries of a single umbilical vein carrying it back to the fetus. The maternal surface of the placental villous system, because of its syncytial nature, is a continuous plasma membrane and this ensures its integrity to hydrophobic substances. The tissue layers between the fetal and maternal capillaries become progressively thinner with placental age,

being about 25 μm in early pregnancy and only 2 μm at term.

Approximately 10% of the maternal cardiac output at term is distributed to the uterus and of this 70–90% passes through the intervillous space. Pressure at the open end of the spiral artery is 35–50 mmHg, and at the uterine veins 3–5 mgHg. The mean pressure in the relaxed uterus is about 10 mmHg. The blood supply in the maternal side of the placenta is best described as a high-flow, low-resistance system dependent mainly on cardiac output and blood pressure. It is reduced by aortocaval occlusion, haemorrhage, vasoconstrictors of the α-adrenergic stimulating group, prostaglandin F_2 and disease processes such as pre-eclamptic toxaemia and hypertensive disorders.

The flow of blood in the umbilical vessels is less than the maternal, and in humans has been estimated at 250 ml/min. The fetal placental circulation is a high-flow, low-resistance system and there is no autoregulatory mechanism. Fifty per cent of the fetal cardiac output is directed to the placenta and as the cardiac output varies with heart rate the adequacy of the placental circulation will be jeopardized by large heart rate fluctuations.

Mechanisms of placental transfer

Drug transfer is related to blood flow rate on the maternal and fetal aspects of the placenta, the quantity of highly lipid-soluble drugs transferred being flow-dependent rather than permeability-dependent. During labour the maternal placental circulation can be altered by variations in blood volume, maternal posture (caval occlusion syndrome) hypoventilation and hyperventilation, hypotension and hypertension, and uterine contractions. Umbilical blood flow can be increased or decreased by fetal stress, asphyxia, hypotension, bradycardia and cord compression or kinking.

In a review of the transfer of naturally occurring materials Page (1957) stated that the important question is not whether a given substance does or does not pass the so-called placental barrier, but the rate and mechanism involved. Transfer processes are simple diffusion, ultrafiltration, facilitated diffusion, active transport and special mechanisms such as pinocytosis. Most drugs with a molecular weight less than 600 cross biological membranes by simple diffusion and the variables associated with this will be discussed in more detail. Ultrafiltration allows the passage of water, crystalloids and colloids of low molecular weight but blocks that of high molecular weight compounds. Facilitated diffusion differs from simple diffusion in that equilibrium across the membrane occurs much more rapidly than would be possible on physicochemical grounds, and is greatly influenced by structural and spatial characteristics of the molecule. Active transport involves temporary combination with membrane or cellular constituents, the carrier mechanism, and an expenditure of energy. Pinocytosis is the phenomenon by which microscopic invaginations of the villi engulf tiny droplets and transport them into the fetal circulation.

Diffusion of drugs is often said to be dependent on the concentration gradient between maternal and fetal blood. Reynolds (1981) challenges the accuracy of this statement in that particles in general diffuse down a pressure gradient and only those which are diffusible can be said to exert a pressure across a membrane. It is therefore more accurate to consider the pressure rather than the concentration gradient of a drug across the placenta, and this is proportional to the concentration of free unionised drug. Non-ionized drugs with high lipid-solubility are transferred rapidly, whereas lipid-insoluble drugs penetrate poorly, despite a low degree of ionization. The dissociation constant of the weakly acidic or basic drugs is important because it determines the plasma concentrations of the non-ionized portion of the drug. Variations in plasma pH affect the degree of ionization. Ionized drug is partly protein-bound and as such is not available for transfer. More detailed analyses of these factors related to membrane transfer are discussed in Chapter 3. The placental membrane is composed largely of lipoprotein and hence facilitates transfer of highly lipid-soluble drugs. The membrane carries a surface charge and the ionized moieties of a drug are either repelled or held bound by the membrane. Drugs such as succinylcholine, d-tubocurarine and THAM, which are highly ionized and of low lipid solubility, have poor membrane penetration. On the other hand thiopentone sodium, which is highly lipid-soluble and largely undissociated in the physiologic pH range, crosses easily from mother to fetus and achieves equilibrium within 1 or 2 min (Finster et al 1966).

Maternal blood concentration is related to the route of administration and to the size of the dose and number of treatments given. Highest concentrations follow intravenous administration, and there is some evidence that during labour the concentrated bolus given between contractions leads to high concentrations of drug in the fetus (Crawford & Rudofsky 1965). However Dawes (1968), commenting on this, stated that injections during contractions may facilitate transfer because of the obstruction to venous outflow from the placental villous space. Neither Finster et al (1966) investigating thiopentone sodium, nor Thomas et al (1969), studying alcuronium transfer, found evidence to substantiate that placental transfer is reduced at this time.

The fetus and transferred drugs

Early pregnancy

Drugs transferred from the mother can affect the developing fetus by causing structural defects. The period in which a dysmorphogenic agent can affect the development of the human embryo is very short, and is over by the 9th week of pregnancy. From fertilization through early post-implementation the embryo has few cells with capacity for replacement of omnipotent cells, and at this stage the result of the teratogenic insult is all or none, that is death or repair. The period from the 18th to the 60th day of gestation is that of organogenesis and represents the time of greatest likelihood of malformations (Beckman & Brent 1984). Beyond this time drugs can cause cell depletion, growth retardation and occasionally fetal death. Thalidomide is the most widely known structural teratogen, but some of the more commonly used drugs, salicylates, corticosteroids and the antimicrobial drugs tetracyclines and rifampicin, have also been implicated.

Behavioural teratogenesis is becoming increasingly recognized as a condition where a prenatally administered drug influences behaviour in the infant long after the drug has been eliminated. These effects are most commonly produced by drugs used to treat mental illness or central nervous system disorder in the mother. As the fetal nervous system is in a state of continuous development throughout pregnancy, vulnerability is ever present. It is thought that interference with neurotransmitter synthesis, release or function may interfere with the physical development of the interneuronal connections within the central nervous system.

Later pregnancy

The fetal type circulation is of considerable importance in the distribution of transferred drugs within the infant. Umbilical vein blood passes either directly via the ductus venosus to the inferior vena cava or through the liver. It is also mixed with venous blood from the lower extremities. Further mixing occurs in the right atrium but a large part of the inferior vena caval blood stream is directed via the foramen ovale to the left atrium. Superior vena caval blood, together with the remainder, enters the right ventricle and is ejected into the pulmon-ary artery where, because of high vascular resistance in the unaerated lungs, it passes to the aorta via the ductus arteriosus. Considerable dilution of transferred drug oc-curs and that portion of umbilical vein blood directed towards the liver with its metabolizing enzymes leads to further reduction in concentration. The umbilical vein drug concentration therefore does not represent that which is presented to fetal tissues.

The concentration of drug returning to the placenta in umbilical arterial blood is determined by the amount of drug transferred from the mother and the uptake by fetal tissues. The latter is related to such factors as tissue blood flow and lipid solubility, pKa and protein binding characteristics of the drug concerned.

Fetal liver enzyme activity related to drug metabolism is well developed at term, cytochrome P450 and NADPH cytochrome C being present from as early as the 14th week of gestation (Yaffe 1976). This sug-gests that even the premature fetus can metabolize nu-merous drugs. Recently, however, Morselli (1983) has stated that blood esterase activity, including acetylcholinesterase, pseudocholinesterase and aryl-esterases, is reduced in full-term infants. Of the other enzymes involved in biotransformation of drugs, N-desmethylating activity is normal but hydroxylation and glucuronidation is less efficient than in the adult. The fetus can accumulate water-soluble drugs given to the mother over a long period and hydrophilic metabolites such as conjugates which cannot readily traverse the placenta are trapped in the fetal compartment. Chronic treatment of the mother during pregnancy with hepatic enzyme-inducing agents might induce similar activity in the infant. In newborns exposed to phenobarbitone dur-ing intra-uterine life diazepam is more rapidly metab-olized than in their non-treated counterparts. Barbiturate induction of liver enzymes has been used to increase the rate of bilirubin conjugation with glucuronic acid in the management of neonatal jaundice (Maurer et al 1968).

Glomerular filtration and renal plasma flow do not reach adult values for some weeks or months after birth, and therefore result in a poor urinary excretion of drugs.

Compounds which are not extensively metabolized and dependent on renal excretion are disposed of at a very slow rate in the newborn. Such agents include the antibiotics gentamicin and kanamycin. Penicillins de-pendent on tubular secretion are also slowly excreted.

The infant has a reduced plasma protein concen-tration, and a qualitatively different albumin which shows a lower avidity for drugs. The higher concentra-tion of free fatty acids, bilirubin and other endogenous competing substrates, together with a lower blood pH, are all capable of modifying the plasma protein binding

of several compounds. The pH difference between ma-ternal and fetal blood at birth means that basic drugs are more ionized in the more acid infant blood, the con-verse being true of acidic drugs. This factor will affect the degree of binding of local anaesthetics, opioid anal-gesics, phenobarbitone, phenytoin and salicylates. The reduced binding to protein and the higher extracellular fluid volume of the infant gives a higher apparent vol-ume of distribution for highly protein-bound drugs (Levy & Garrettson 1974).

Amniotic fluid

The amniotic fluid can be regarded as an additional compartment to the fetal-maternal unit. The volume of the amniotic fluid reaches a maximum of around 1 litre at about 36 weeks and declines slowly thereafter. Up until about 20 weeks gestation the volume of amniotic fluid is closely related to fetal weight. After this, amni-otic fluid volume varies and this variation is related to fetal swallowing and urine production (Lind & Hytten 1972). Many drugs and their metabolites have been identified in amniotic fluid, and it is likely that the major avenue of access is fetal urine. However, some transfer across the amnion and chorion, fetal skin or ex-posed mucous membrane may be possible. If drugs accumulate in the amniotic fluid compartment it may become a slowly equilibrating reservoir with the charac-teristics of a deep compartment (Mirkin & Singh 1976).

The infant's condition at birth can be graded by 'Apgar-minus colour' score, as it has been shown to be more reliable than the original (Crawford 1978). Study of acid-base parameters in the umbilical artery and vein blood gives further information on the neonate's well-being but neurobehavioural examinations at fixed time intervals after birth are being increasingly used.

Sedative drugs

Phenothiazines

Phenothiazine derivatives have been used in obstetrics to augment opioid analgesia, enhance sedation and for their anti-emetic action. Chlorpromazine, promazine, promethazine and prochlorperazine have all been shown to transfer to the fetus. The pharmacokinetics of these compounds in the infant are unknown but it is likely that their elimination is slow. Serious infant side-effects are infrequent, particularly when promethazine is used.

Benzodiazepines

Diazepam and its metabolites readily cross the placenta and plasma concentrations of diazepam, desmethyldiazepam, methyloxazepam and oxazepam at birth are similar to those found in maternal plasma. The fetal plasma clearance rate of diazepam is reduced and is apparently related to the degree of maturation of metabolic activity (Nation 1983). The plasma half-life in full-term infants ranges from 20 to 50 h. Neonatal depression is prolonged after large maternal doses but small single treatments are unlikely to harm the infant. The clinical features in the neonate are hypotonia, lethargy and hypothermia.

Lorazepam, a long acting benzodiazepine with a half-life of about 12 h, is mainly metabolized to a pharmacologically inactive glucuronide. While cord plasma concentrations are generally lower than maternal concentrations at birth the neonate conjugates lorazepam to the inactive glucuronide and this metabolite is detectable in the urine for up to 7 days after birth (Whitelaw et al 1981). Oxazepam, another benzodiazepine and a metabolite of diazepam, has a half-life in the infant 3–4 times that of the mother (Tomson et al 1979). Oxazepam, lorazepam, nitrazepam and flunitrazepam appear to penetrate the human placenta more slowly than diazepam, but the clinical significance of this phenomenon remains uncertain. Repeated doses will tend to accumulate on the fetal side of the placenta because neonatal metabolism and excretion is slower than in the adult. Midazolam, a water-soluble benzodiazepine, has shown less transfer and more rapid fetal clearance than diazepam (Kanto et al 1983).

Chlormethiazole

Chlormethiazole is a sedative and anticonvulsant used in the treatment of severe pre-eclampsia and eclampsia. It is commonly given intravenously as an 0.8% solution and transfers rapidly to the fetus. Its half-life ($T_{\frac{1}{2}}$) in pregnant subjects at term is 9–10 h (Moore et al 1978). The UV/MV plasma ratio at delivery is 0.8 to 1 with approximately 65% of the drug in plasma being protein-bound in both circulations. The $T_{\frac{1}{2}}$ of chlormethiazole in neonates is usually in the range of 5–15 h and appears to be inversely related to gestational age.

Analgesics

Simple analgesics

Salicylates rapidly cross the placenta because of their high lipid solubility but slow maternal fetal equilibration occurs because of high maternal protein binding. Fetal and infant elimination of transferred drug is slow because of reduced capacity to convert the agent to glycine and glucuronic conjugates, together with the low glomerular filtration rate in the neonate (Levy 1978).

Repetitive daily intake of salicylates has been suspected of inducing congenital defects but a large prospective study carried out in the United States failed to substantiate this claim. Platelet function in the newborn may be decreased by maternal intake and minor bleeding tendencies such as petechia, purpura or cephalohaematoma can result. Rumack et al (1981) found a significantly higher incidence of intracranial haemorrhage in premature infants whose mothers had ingested aspirin during pregnancy.

Acetylsalicylic acid, as well as indomethacin and naproxen, are prostaglandin synthesis inhibitors and their administration to pregnant rats results in closure or marked constriction of the ductus arteriosus (Sharpe et al 1975). These drugs are slowly cleared by the infant and repeated maternal administration may cause prolonged pulmonary arterial hypertension in the newborn. They have been used to delay premature labour and their continued use in this respect is questionable.

Opioid analgesics

These drugs are seldom prescribed during the developmental stage of gestation. In recent times evidence from the increasing problem of addiction in pregnant patients suggests that teratogenicity is not associated with their use at this time. However, perinatal mortality is increased and both premature birth and growth retardation are common (Tylden 1973). Fetal death has been reported following maternal opioid withdrawal (Rementeria & Nunag 1973) and the neonate of the addicted mother will display signs of acute opioid abstinence which may be lethal if naloxone is given at birth. Diamorphine has been reported to accelerate the appearance of a mature L/S ratio (Gluck & Kulovich 1973) and to induce fetal hepatic enzymes (Zelsen et al 1971).

Opioid analgesics are given during the first stage of labour, and pethidine is regarded as the standard against which other drugs should be compared. It is readily transferred from mother to fetus in whom its depressant effects are recognized by low Apgar scores or upsets in neurobehavioural function. A significant correlation has been observed between infant depression and the dose and timing of maternal administration of pethidine, respiration and temperature regulation being particularly affected. Impairment of breathing is marked if the opioid is given between 1 and 3 h before birth and its duration is related to the total dose given. Peak-plateau fetal concentrations of pethidine are reached 1–5 h after maternal intramuscular administration. The metabolism of pethidine in the neonate is prolonged, being 18.1 ± 2.9 h as compared to 3–4 h in the adult (Caldwell & Notarianni 1978). The excretion of pethidine and nor-pethidine by the infant parallels the urine flow rate and 95% of transferred drug is eliminated by the 2nd or 3rd day after birth (Hogg et al 1977). Slow disappearance of pethidine is probably due to reduced N-desmethylating activity, reduced hydrolysis and conjugation, and later to low glomerular filtration rate in the infant. There is a significant increase in nor-pethidine plasma concentration for 24 to 36 h after birth (Morselli & Rovei 1980). Nor-pethidine is more polar than pethidine and therefore its tubular reabsorption will be less and its rate of renal secretion more rapid. Highest concentrations of drug occur in the infant following concentrated intravenous bolus administration to the mother and UV/MV concentrations in excess of unity are common.

Morphine is regarded as the opioid analgesic most likely to cause respiratory depression in the newborn (Way et al 1965). Animal studies have shown that the concentration of morphine and methadone in the central nervous system is two to three times that in the maternal brain. This may be due to greater permeability of the fetal blood–brain barrier. Papaveretum, a favoured obstetric analgesic, contains more than 50% of its weight as anhydrous morphine and therefore is a marked depressant of the neonate.

None of the more recently introduced opioid analgesics such as fentanyl, alphaprodine, numorphan or levorphanol have shown any advantage for the fetus, and their use has similar disadvantages to pethidine and morphine.

Analgesic drugs with both opioid agonist and antagonist properties, such as pentazocine, offer the potential advantage that the antagonist fraction limits the degree of respiratory depression especially when repetitive treatments are used. Pentazocine is transferred to a lesser extent than pethidine (Moore et al 1973). Naloxone is the only pure opioid antagonist and can be administered to the mother to counteract anticipated respiratory depression in the infant. Unlike its forerunners, levallorphan and nalorphine, which may enhance the depressant effects of opioids because of their agonist properties, naloxone is free from this danger. All three are transferred easily to the infant but their subsequent fate has not been extensively studied.

Cardiovascular drugs

Digoxin

Digoxin has not been shown to be teratogenic, and therapeutic maternal drug levels do not appear to affect the neonatal electrocardiograph. Digoxin crosses the placenta, and fetal to maternal ratios from 50% to 100% are found (Chan et al 1978). The fetus metabolizes digoxin and excretes it in the bile. The apparent plasma half-life in the healthy and sick newborn is very long, ranging from 20 to 70 h in full-term neonates.

Digoxin enters the umbilical circulation within 5 min of maternal intravenous administration (Saarikoski 1976). It has been used successfully to treat fetal tachycardia. Gross maternal overdosage can give rise to digitalis intoxication in the infant.

Methyldopa

This agent crosses the placenta, and Jones & Cummings (1978) have reported the cord to maternal plasma ratio at delivery to be 1.38 ± 0.51. Its widespread use suggests that prolonged treatment does not cause developmental abnormalities or impair the rate of fetal growth.

Hydralazine

Hydralazine is used in the management of acute hypertensive states, and in animal experiments it increases uterine artery blood flow simultaneously with a reduction in maternal blood pressure (Ring et al 1977). This drug is short-acting and its hypotensive action is readily reversed.

β-Blockers

Propranolol is transmitted to the infant and may cause fetal bradycardia, hypoglycaemia and increased perinatal mortality (Lieberman et al 1978). Prolonged treatment with β-blockers has been reported to be associated with intra-uterine growth retardation, but this did not occur in clinical trials of oxprenolol (de Swiet 1983) or atenolol (Rubin et al 1983) when used for hypertension in pregnancy. Labetalol, a combined α/β-blocker may be a superior therapy not causing fetal bradycardia and resulting in higher birth weights when compared to atenolol (Lardoux et al 1983).

Short-acting hypotensive agents

Short-acting hypotensive agents used in obstetrics include nitroprusside and nitroglycerin. Nitroprusside produced no ill-effects on the fetus when used to control the hypertension associated with tracheal intubation. Lethal fetal cyanide levels have been associated with maternal tachyphylaxis in sheep experiments. Nitroglycerin crosses the placenta and the fetal/maternal ratio of 0.04

reported in pregnant sheep experiments was not associated with heart rate or blood pressure changes in the fetus (de Rosayro et al 1980).

Diuretics

Frusemide crosses the placenta rapidly at term and UV/MV ratios attain a value of unity about 8–10 h after maternal administration (Riva et al 1978). No teratogenic effects have been reported. Ethacrynic acid and thiazide diuretics can cause deafness, hyponatraemia and thrombocytopenia in the infant. Differential binding of chlorthalidone to carbonic anhydrase in erythrocytes of maternal and fetal blood has been suggested as the mechanism responsible for the cord to maternal ratio of 0.15 found at delivery for that drug (Mulley et al 1978). Hypertension associated with pre-eclampsia is usually accompanied by plasma volume contraction which will be aggravated by further salt and water loss, so that these agents are contra-indicated.

Vasoconstrictors

Uterine blood flow, though not autoregulated, is markedly reduced by α-adrenergic stimulation. Adrenaline has significant effect on both α and β-adrenergic receptors. Low blood levels such as occur from systemic absorption during epidural anaesthesia have been shown to produce a generalized β-adrenergic response that becomes maximal 15 min from administration. The effect of this response on uterine blood flow is dependent on the presence or absence of maternal hypotension. Elevated noradrenaline levels in response to stress have been shown to markedly reduce uterine blood flow (Cosmi & Shnider 1979). Vasopressors, such as methoxamine, with a predominant α-adrenergic activity, reduce uterine blood flow, whereas ephedrine, used to reverse maternal hypotension due to autonomic blockade associated with regional anaesthesia, does not. Other vasopressor drugs — metaraminol, mephentermine and dopamine — can impair the blood supply to the pregnant uterus and induce fetal acidosis. The placenta contains enzymes capable of metabolizing adrenaline and noradrenaline. Ephedrine is transferred to the fetus but its further fate has not been reported.

Anticoagulants

Heparin has a particular advantage over other agents in that it is so strongly polar it does not cross the placenta. The coumarin series of anticoagulants is associated with a low, but definite, incidence of teratogenesis. Their use in late pregnancy can cause serious retroplacental and intracerebral fetal bleeding. The fetus has low levels of clotting factors and is likely to be excessively anticoagulated if the mother's prothrombin time is within normal therapeutic limits.

Anti-epileptic drugs

The effect of pregnancy on seizure control is variable, both from patient to patient and during different pregnancies in the same patient. Factors that are considered to be associated with a lower seizure threshold during the gestational period include water and sodium retention, hyperventilation, a rise in oestrogen levels, emotional and psychological problems and possibly altered pharmacokinetics of the anti-epileptic drugs (Perucca & Richens 1983).

The publicity given to adverse effects on the fetus can cause women either not to take, or to reduce the intake of, prescribed medication during pregnancy. Delayed uptake from the gastrointestinal tract has been reported for phenytoin, and parenteral administration is advisable for rapid pharmacological effect during labour. The increased volume and reduced binding capacity of the plasma in the mother affects the distribution of phenytoin, valproic acid and diazepam because of their extensive binding to plasma protein. For phenytoin this is moderate, but in the case of diazepam and valproic acid the increase in serum unbound fraction during the last weeks of pregnancy approaches 50% of the values in non-pregnant controls (Perucca & Richens 1983). An increase in unbound fraction occurs with phenobarbitone but not carbamazepine. This impairment in binding capacity may result in potentiation of pharmacological effect but also facilitates renal elimination. Hepatic metabolism of phenytoin is decreased but this may be compensated for by an increase in liver size (Blake et al 1978).

Anti-epileptic drugs readily diffuse across the placental barrier, are partly metabolized in the fetus and are found in the plasma of the newborn at concentrations comparable to those observed in the mother (Morselli et al 1980). Thereafter many of these compounds are eliminated at a comparatively slow rate, particularly in the premature infant, resulting in occasional prolonged toxicity.

There is now extensive evidence that newborns of epileptic mothers have increased mortality and morbidity rates. Congenital malformations associated with anticonvulsant therapy have been reported. Cleft lip and palate, congenital heart disease and digital hypoplasia occur more frequently in the offspring of drug-treated epileptic mothers. The exact role of the therapy has not been clearly defined, but almost all of the commonly used agents have been implicated. It may be that the hereditary tendency of epileptic women to produce malformed infants may play a part.

The adverse effects of maternal high-dose diazepam have already been referred to. Chronic medication with benzodiazepines can cause withdrawal effects such as paradoxical hyperactivity in the newborn (Rementeria & Bhatt 1977). An abstinence syndrome beginning at mean age 7 days and lasting up to 6 months has also been described for chronic barbiturate therapy with symptoms of overactivity, restlessness, vomiting, diarrhoea and vasomotor instability (Desmond et al 1972).

Phenytoin and phenobarbitone treatment may give rise to neonatal bleeding which usually starts within the first day of life and frequently occurs internally. Here maternal coagulation is normal, and it has been suggested that these anticonvulsant drugs stimulate the conversion of vitamin K to inactive metabolites in the fetus, thereby resulting in clinically significant vitamin K deficiency. Gingival hyperplasia following phenytoin therapy has been reported (Hill et al 1974).

Administration of phenytoin, phenobarbitone or carbamazepine to the mother results in increased hepatic mono-oxygenase activity in the fetus and newborn. One consequence of this phenomenon is that newborns of epileptic mothers have greater oxidative drug-metabolizing capacity (Rame & Wilson 1976). Hepatic glucuronidation is also increased and reduces serum bilirubin levels, providing the basis for phenobarbitone treatment in the prophylaxis of neonatal jaundice.

Antibiotics

The physiological changes associated with pregnancy alter the pharmacokinetics of antibiotics. Dosage regimens for use in the non-pregnant may not be appropriate for treating pregnant patients, as a wide variation in serum concentrations following standard doses has been demonstrated in the latter (Philipson et al 1976). Studies of the placental transfer of antibiotics at term show that all of these agents cross the placenta to some degree (Nation 1983). While fetal blood levels of most antibiotics are generally achieved rapidly after maternal administration, amniotic fluid levels increase slowly and are consistent with agents being delivered there by fetal micturition. This may be important where they are administered to prevent or treat infection associated with prolonged rupture of the membranes. Ampicillin achieves more rapid and higher levels in amniotic fluid than dicloxacillin.

There is no evidence that any of the antimicrobial drugs approved for general use are teratogenic, with the possible exception of tetracyclines and rifampicin. Metronidazole has caused mutagenesis in animals. Tetracyclines are concentrated and deposited in fetal bone and teeth where they compete with calcium, the period of risk being from the middle to the end of pregnancy. In addition a fulminating hepatic decompensation has been described in pregnant patients with pyelonephritis treated with large intravenous doses of tetracyclines. Streptomycin may cause 8th nerve dysfunction but kanamycin therapy, because of its limited transfer, seems to be free of this complication. Chloramphenicol, given in late pregnancy, causes toxic manifestations in the neonate which in extreme cases may result in circulatory collapse. Sulphonamides cause an increased incidence of kernicterus in the neonate, the suggested mechanism being competition of the drug with bilirubin for conjugation with glucuronic acid.

Gastrointestinal drugs

Anti-emetics

Anti-emetics used in pregnancy include phenothiazines (see above), antihistamines and metoclopramide. The possibility of teratogenicity following the use of the combination dicyclonine, doxylamine and pyridoxine (Debendox) has led to its withdrawal, although large prospective studies (Fleming et al 1981, Shapiro et al 1977) have not confirmed a teratogenic effect. There is some evidence that meclozine and cyclizine, while generally safe in humans, may be associated with an increased incidence of cleft palate (Lenz 1966). No deleterious effects on the fetus have been reported following the use of metoclopramide; it has also been used to hasten gastric emptying in labour. Metoclopramide rapidly crosses the placenta, fetal plasma concentrations being 60–70% of maternal (Arvela 1983).

H_2-receptor blockers

These drugs are being increasingly used to reduce gastric acid secretion during labour. Cimetidine crosses the placental barrier and following maternal intravenous administration umbilical cord blood levels during the first hour are markedly lower than maternal venous levels. Amniotic fluid levels increase with time from administration indicating fetal renal elimination (Howe et al 1981). Cimetidine has a low lipid solubility and pKa value of 6.8, indicating that the degree of ionization may be important in its transfer. The UV/MV ratio for ranitidine was shown to vary with the route of administration to the mother. Lesser transfer is associated with oral treatment, the mean ratio here being 0.38 (McAuley et al 1983). No untoward infant effects have been reported following treatment in labour with either drug, but careful screening of infant is still advisable when they are used.

β-Sympathomimetic drugs

β-Sympathomimetic drugs are used in pregnancy for the treatment of asthma and for their ability to inhibit preterm labour. The available drugs include ritodrine, fenoterol, salbutamol, terbutaline and hexoprenaline. Half-lives in maternal blood vary from 22 min for fenoterol to 6 h for salbutamol. All of these drugs cross the placenta, the fetal blood concentration of terbutaline being 55% of the maternal blood at delivery. The lowest F/M ratio is associated with ritodrine. These drugs are eliminated as sulphate or gluconate compounds and directly by renal excretion, so that elimination by the fetus may be prolonged. Effects on the fetus include increased heart rate, hyperglycaemia and acidosis.

Other drugs used in the management of asthma include aminophylline and various corticosteroids. Aminophylline crosses the placenta and the possibility of high fetal levels causing jitteriness, opisthotonus and tachycardia (Yeh & Pildes 1977). The maternal to fetal concentration of prednisolone is 10 to 1, in comparison to hydrocortisone 6 to 1 and betamethasone 3 to 1 (de Swiet 1983). Maternal steroid therapy can suppress the fetal hypothalamo–pituitary–adrenal axis, leading to collapse in the neonatal period. A higher incidence of early hypoglycaemia in infants of mothers treated with steroids to prevent respiratory distress syndrome has been reported, but others have observed no adverse effects in children up to age 4 years.

Drugs used in anaesthesia

Intravenous induction agents

The thiobarbiturates have physical and chemical characteristics which facilitate their ready transfer across the placental membrane and reported studies (Finster et al 1966, Kosaka et al 1969) confirm this. The umbilical vein/maternal vein ratio varies with the time from maternal administration but is more commonly less than unity. Umbilical arterial blood levels measured within minutes of treatment were always much less than those of umbilical vein blood and are more representative of

fetal tissue levels. Repetitive intermittent injection of barbiturates to maintain anaesthesia results in greater transfer of drug and prolonged depression of the newborn. The fetus is protected from the initial high maternal arterial concentrations of thiobarbiturates by way of dilution of umbilical vein blood and initial hepatic extraction. Following a single administration to the mother the longer the injection to delivery interval the less the likelihood of infant depression. Nevertheless elimination is greatly prolonged in the neonate as compared to the mother.

Methohexitone is about four times more potent than thiopentone. It is also less ionized at pH 7.4, and this may contribute to its greater potency and slightly more rapid elimination. While this may give a more rapid recovery in the mother, larger doses of methohexitone are associated with a high percentage of low Apgar scores (Holdcroft et al 1974).

Other intravenous anaesthetic agents, Althesin, propanidid and etomidate, have been used in obstetrics, but despite marked difference in their metabolism no marked advantage has been demonstrated for the mother or her infant. Placental transfer and pharmacokinetic data from the neonate are not available.

Ketamine rapidly crosses the placenta and the plasma concentration in mixed cord blood is similar to the maternal venous level 1.5–6.5 min after maternal administration (Ellingson et al 1977). Neonatal depression has been associated with the use of ketamine as an anaesthetic agent at the time of delivery (Little et al 1972).

Inhalational anaesthetics

The maternal uptake and elimination of inhaled anaesthetic drugs is greatly facilitated by the respiratory and cardiovascular changes associated with pregnancy. The distribution of gaseous substances in the alveolar air is enhanced, and mixing of the inspired air with the residual air more effective. Consequently higher concentrations of volatile agents may be achieved more rapidly in the alveolar air, and the diffusion rate of highly soluble substances with a respiration-linked equilibration rate may considerably increase. The increased cardiac output and pulmonary blood flow can influence the equilibration rate of volatile substances and tissue concentrations may rise more quickly in those organs with a high blood perfusion rate such as uterus and placenta. Full-term pregnancy is associated with reduced anaesthetic requirements; in one study MAC was decreased by 32% for methoxyflurane, 25% for halothane and 40% for isoflurane. Those factors are therefore of greater importance for the agents with greatest blood/gas partition coefficients, viz. diethyl ether, methoxyflurane, halothane and isoflurane. Blood is so readily saturated with the insoluble agents such as nitrous oxide that the availability of an increased amount of this anaesthetic has little effect on rate of uptake. Deep anaesthesia with the more potent agent causes myocardial depression and peripheral vasodilation, and will produce a marked reduction of the uteroplacental circulation.

Intermittent self-administration of nitrous oxide, methoxyflurane and trichloroethylene is used during labour to provide analgesia during the late first and second stage. Each inhalation with nitrous oxide–oxygen mixture is timed to coincide with a uterine contraction, and pain relief is rapid with complete recovery from effects occurring between contractions. The more lipid-soluble agents, methoxyflurane and trichloroethylene, accumulate in the maternal tissues and with prolonged use of these agents both maternal and infant depression will occur. Methoxyflurane may cause impairment of kidney function, especially with pre-existing renal disease due to the production of free fluoride ion from its metabolism. While urine and serum inorganic fluoride concentrations are increased in maternal and neonatal blood (Young et al 1976) it is unlikely that intermittent use of methoxyflurane for short periods will upset the kidney function of the mother or her infant.

All of the inhalation anaesthetic agents reach the infant when administered to the mother. The inspired concentrations, the duration of exposure, their lipid solubility and adequacy of the placental perfusion are the main factors in determining the amount transferred. High concentrations in fetal blood can produce serious central nervous and cardiovascular depression with marked impairment of its well-being. Nitrous oxide transmission is rapid and the concentration in the umbilical artery is only 70% less than the umbilical vein concentration after 19 min (Marx et al 1970). The rapid excretion of nitrous oxide into the infant's alveolar space after prolonged maternal exposure can cause diffusion hypoxemia in the infant. Methoxyflurane, used to induce anaesthesia for vaginal delivery, has been shown to cross the placenta, and cord venous to maternal arterial blood concentration ratios at delivery varied from 0.5 to 0.7. No correlation could be established between fetal levels of the drug and condition of the infants at birth (Siker et al 1968). In reports of enflurane transfer, 1.5% inspired concentrations were associated with levels in the fetus not greater than 50% of the maternal levels at delivery following a mean exposure time of 15 min (Dick et al 1979). Halothane is rapidly transferred and

cord blood concentrations varying from 6 to 78% of the mother's level following 2–17 min of maternal anaesthesia have been reported (Sheridan & Robson 1959). Halothane is also concentrated in lean tissues and uptake by fetal liver is considerable (Gibbs et al 1975). Trichloroethylene has been shown to cause marked sedation in the infant when used for maternal anaesthesia.

There is no reason to believe that the single administration of anaesthetic, analgesic or sedative drugs is capable of inducing fetal abnormality in man. However, in animal experiments continuous exposure to volatile and gaseous agents for periods in excess of 12 h produced a high incidence of skeletal and nervous system abnormalities (Basford & Fink 1968). The prolonged use of relaxants in the treatment of maternal tetanus has been followed by the delivery of an infant suffering from arthrogryposis (Jago 1970). Perhaps more pertinent is the problem of theatre pollution by inhalation agents, and its association with a higher rate of spontaneous abortion (Askrog 1970) and possibly increased incidence of congenital abnormality (Corbett et al 1974, ASA Report 1974). While exact statistical proof of such a relationship is difficult to achieve it would seem wise for theatre staff in the early stages of pregnancy to avoid such exposure, and for effective antipollution precautions to be available in all operating theatres.

Muscle relaxants

The non-depolarizing relaxants are quaternary ammonium compounds of low lipid solubility and therefore completely ionized. A small proportion crosses the placenta when used during anaesthesia for Caesarean delivery. Comparative values are shown in Table 31.1. For pancuronium the UV/MV ratio has been observed to increase with prolongation of the dose/delivery interval up to intervals of 10–30 min. Fetal uptake over this interval was indicated by considerably lower arterial than venous concentrations in the cord (Duvaldestin et al 1978). In spite of the placental transfer the neonate does not appear to suffer from obvious relaxant effects when the drugs are used in therapeutic doses. The disposition of these drugs in the newborn has not been examined.

The depolarizing relaxant succinylcholine is dependent on pseudocholinesterase for its metabolism, but despite the reduced levels associated with pregnancy, prolonged activity is only associated with abnormalities of this enzyme. Following maternal doses of 1–2 mg kg^{-1} no measurable amounts of succinylcholine were found in fetal blood (Moya & Kvisselgaard 1961). Large bolus injections given to pregnant monkeys did produce

Table 31.1 Placental transfer of muscle relaxants

Drug (ref)	Method of assay	No.of studies	Maternal dose (mg kg^{-1})	Blood levels at delivery Maternal	Cord
Tubocurarine	Spectroscopic	6	not stated	1.1–3.2 (μg ml^{-1})	0–0.1 (μg ml^{-1})
Tubocurarine	Bioassay	6	0.18–0.27	0.4–1.8 (μg ml^{-1})	0–0.1 (μg ml^{-1})
Gallamine triethiodide	Bioassay	13	0.9–1.55	1.0–8.0 (μg ml^{-1})	1.0–3.0 (μg ml^{-1})
Dimethyl tubocurarine	Liquid scintillation	18	0.005	1.74–4.42 (nCi ml^{-1})	0.14–0.21 (nCi ml^{-1})
Alcuronium	Bioassay	19	0.118–0.22	0.4–3.00 (μgml^{-1})	0–0.4 (μg ml^{-1})
Pancuronium	Chemical	10	0.092–0.095	0.20–0.47 (μg ml^{-1})	0.04–0.1 (μg ml^{-1})
Fazadinium	Bioassay	10	0.5–0.9	0.3–2.1 (μg ml^{-1})	0–0.53 (μg ml^{-1})
Suxamethonium	Bioassay	—	1.69–11.0	0–4.4 (μg ml^{-1})	0

From Moore & Dundee 1983

transfer of significant amounts to the infant (Drabkova et al 1973).

Local anaesthetics

Local anaesthetic drugs, because of their high lipid solubility, are easily transferred to the fetus. Their dissociation constants range from 7.0 to 9.0 so that at physiological pH there is considerable variation in the ionized to unionized fractions. Ionized drug is bound to protein and is not available for transfer. Bupivacaine and etidocaine are 80–90% bound to maternal proteins, whereas for prilocaine, lignocaine and mepivacaine the percentage bound is 55, 64 and 77% respectively. This would seem to indicate that in order to minimize infant effects bupivacaine could be the agent of choice. However, while the concentrations of free drug in maternal and umbilical vein blood rapidly equilibrate, the pH gradient existing between maternal and fetal blood influences the concentration at equilibrium. As these agents are weak bases the higher hydrogen ion concentration in the fetal blood increases the amount ionized and thus its binding to protein. This phenomenon of 'ion trapping' has been shown to occur, Brown et al (1976) reporting high umbilical vein to maternal vein ratios of lignocaine and mepivacaine in neonates with umbilical artery pH values of 7.03–7.23. However, other causes for the high levels may be circulatory depression, reduced liver and tissue blood flow, leading to reduced clearance of the drug in the acidotic infant.

Chloroprocaine is the most commonly used ester-type local anaesthetic in obstetrics. Its rapid breakdown by maternal plasma and placental pseudocholinesterase to 2-chloroaminobenzoic acid and 2-diethylaminoethanol limits transfer to the fetus. In vivo studies revealed insignificant amounts of chloroprocaine in fetal blood after its use for maternal analgesia (O'Brien et al 1979, Kuhnert et al 1980). Its half-life in the fetus is 43 s,

twice as long as in the mother, and is due to decreased fetal cholinesterase activity (Fox & Gertel 1980). Amethocaine and cinchocaine are used almost exclusively for spinal or subarachnoid block, so that the quantities of drug used offer no threat to fetal well-being.

In vitro investigation of the direct effects of amide-type local anaesthetics on the uterine arteries indicate that high plasma concentrations of lignocaine and mepivacaine constrict these vessels (Cibils 1976). Umbilical veins, but not arteries, constrict when exposed to high concentrations of lignocaine but not chloroprocaine (Gibbs & Noel 1976). The clinical significance of these in vitro experiments is difficult to evaluate, but investigation of placental blood flow during extradural anaesthesia has shown that it is unimpaired if maternal hypotension is avoided (Jouppila et al 1978). However, the paracervical injection of these agents may create plasma levels sufficient to constrict the uterine vessels, and may explain in part the fetal bradycardia associated with this procedure.

The human fetus can metabolize the amide local anaesthetics but there is a marked variability with different agents. Mepivacaine disappears at a much slower rate than other drugs, and this is possibly due to its dependence for clearance on the fetal kidney (Blankenbaker et al 1975). Neurobehavioural effects following the use of mepivacaine or lignocaine persisting for long periods may be related to their continued presence, their estimated half-life being 9 and 3 h respectively. Scanlon et al (1976) detected bupivacaine in only one of 20 newborns after epidural analgesia for delivery, and 4 h later the fetal concentration was one-tenth that of the umbilical vein concentration. More recent investigation has shown that both bupivacaine and its main metabolites, 2,6-pipecolylidine, can be detected in neonatal urine up to 72 h after birth (Kuhnert et al 1981). A considerable amount of bupivacaine was taken up by fetal tissue, and while the infant could metabolize it, a higher percentage of unchanged bupivacaine was excreted by the neonate than the mother. The breakdown product of prilocaine, *O*-toluidine, causes methaemoglobinaemia, and the parent drug and its metabolite by-product are transferred.

The infant effects of transferred local anaesthetics are considered less harmful than those associated with opioid analgesics. Nevertheless convulsions due to toxic plasma levels have been reported (Dodson et al 1975) while mepivacaine has been shown to have a direct negative inotropic effect on the fetal heart (Anderson et al 1970).

Anticholinergic drugs

There is little information on the placental transfer of this group. Hyoscine, atropine and glycopyrrolate are the most commonly used. Hyoscine has central nervous system depressant effects and its use during labour augments opioid-induced infant depression. Atropine given intravenously to the mother readily crosses to the infant (Kivalo & Saarikoski 1977) and umbilical vein concentrations were 93% of maternal venous levels 5 min after administration. At 30 min the umbilical artery and vein concentrations were similar. Fetal heart rate increases and the drug should not be used to treat bradycardia due to hypoxia as the cardiac output may fall and diminish umbilical blood flow. Glycopyrrolate is a quaternary ammonium compound and is highly ionized, thus making membrane penetration difficult. It is likely therefore that transfer from mother to infant, if it occurs at all, is limited (Abboud et al 1981).

Anticholinesterase drugs

Neostigmine and pyridostigmine, being quaternary ammonium compounds, are highly ionized in maternal blood and are not likely to be transferred to the fetus in significant amounts. Physostigmine, being a tertiary amine, is transferred and can cause cholinergic effects in the fetus.

Conclusion

Drug treatment in pregnancy and parturition is associated with many variations in pharmacokinetic parameters as compared to the non-pregnant state. Investigation is restricted by obvious moral and ethical considerations. Information from humans is therefore limited, particularly with regard to disposition kinetics, metabolism and elimination of transferred drug in the neonate. All new treatments required in early gestation must be regarded as potential teratogens.

REFERENCES

Abboud T K, Read J, Miller F, Chen T, Valle R, Henriksen E H 1981 Use of glycopyrrolate in the parturient: effect on the maternal and fetal heart and uterine activity. Obstetrics and Gynecology 57: 224–227

American Society of Anesthesiologists 1974 Report of an ad hoc committee on the effect of trace anesthetics on the health of operating room personnel. Occupational disease among operating room personnel: a national study. Anesthesiology 41: 321–340

Anderson K E, Gennser G, Nilsson E 1970 Influence of mepivacaine on isolated human foetal hearts at normal and low pH. Acta Physiologica Scandinavica 80: (Suppl 353): 34–47

Arvela P 1983 Placental transfer and hormonal effects of metoclopramide. European Journal of Clinical Pharmacology 24: 345–348

Askrog V F 1970 Teratogenic effects of volatile anaesthetics. 3rd European Anaesthesiology Conference 13: 1.

Basford A B, Fink B R 1968 The teratogenicity of halothane in the rat. Anesthesiology 29: 1167–1173

Beckman D A, Brent R L 1984 Mechanisms of teratogenesis. Annual Review of Pharmacology and Toxicology 24: 483–500

Blake D A, Collins J V, Miyasaki B C, Cohen F 1978 Influence of pregnancy and folic acid on phenytoin metabolism by rat liver microsomes. Drug Metabolism and Disposition 6: 246–250

Blankenbaker W L, Di Fazio C A, Berry F A Jr 1975 Lidocaine and its metabolites in the newborn. Anesthesiology 42: 325–330

Brown W V Jr, Bell G C, Alper M H 1976 Acidosis, local anesthetics, and the newborn. Obstetrics and Gynecology 48: 27–30

Caldwell J, Notarianni L F 1978 Dispositions of pethidine in childbirth. British Journal of Anaesthesia 50: 307–308

Chan V, Tse T F, Wong V 1978 Transfer of digoxin across the placenta and into breast milk. British Journal of Obstetrics and Gynaecology 85: 605–609

Cibils L A 1976 Response of human uterine arteries to local anesthetics. American Journal of Obstetrics and Gynecology 126: 202–210

Corbett T H, Cornell R G, Endres J L, Lieding K 1974 Birth defects among children of nurse anesthetists. Anesthesiology 41: 341–344

Cosmi E V, Shnider S M 1979 Obstetric anesthesia and uterine blood flow. In: Shnider S M, Levinson G (eds) Anesthesia for obstetrics. Williams & Wilkins, Baltimore/London, pp 23–41

Crawford J S 1978 Principles and practice of obstetric anaesthesia, 4th edn. Blackwell, Oxford, pp 325–330

Crawford J S, Rudofsky S 1965 The mode of administration of promazine as a factor in determining the extent of placental transmission. British Journal of Anaesthesia 37: 310–313

Dawes G S 1968 Foetal and neonatal physiology. Year Book Medical Publishers, Chicago, p 36

de Rosayro M, Nahrwold M L, Hill A B, Tah A R, Busch T, Kirsh M M 1980 Plasma levels and cardiovascular effects of nitroglycerin in pregnant sheep. Canadian Anaesthetists' Society Journal 27: 560–564

de Swiet M 1983 Therapy for asthma in pregnancy. In: Lewis P (ed) Clinical pharmacology in obstetrics, 1st edn. Wright, Bristol, p 56

Desmond M M, Schwanecke R P, Wilson G S, Yasunaga S, Bergdorff I 1972 Maternal barbiturate utilisation and neonatal withdrawal symptomatology. Journal of Pediatrics 80: 190–197

Dick W, Knoche E, Traub E 1979 Clinical investigations concerning the use of ethrane for Caesarean section. Journal of Perinatal Medicine 7: 125–133

Dodson W E, Hillman R E, Hillman L S 1975 Convulsions in fetus due to local anaesthetics. Journal of Pediatrics 86: 624–627

Drabkova J, Crul J F, van der Kleijn E 1973 Placental transfer of C-labelled succinylcholine in near term *Macaca mulatta* monkeys. British Journal of Anaesthesia 45: 1087–1095

Duvaldestin P, Demetriou M, Henzel D, Desmonts J M 1978 The placental transfer of pancuronium and its pharmacokinetics during Caesarean Section. Acta Anaesthesiologica Scandinavica 22: 327–333

Ellingson A, Haram K, Sagem M, Solheim E 1977 Transplacental passage of ketamine after intravenous administration. Acta Anaesthesiologica Scandinavica 21: 41–44

Finster M, Mark L C, Morishima H O, Moya F, Perel J M, James L S, Dayton P 1966 Plasma thiopental concentrations in the newborn following delivery under thiopental-nitrous oxide anesthesia. American Journal of Obstetrics and Gynecology 95: 621–629

Fleming D M, Knox J D E, Crombie D L 1981 Debendox in early pregnancy and fetal malformation. British Medical Journal 283: 99–101

Fox G S, Gertel M 1980 In: Marx G F, Bassell G M (eds) Obstetric analgesia and anesthesia. Elsevier/North-Holland Biomedical Press, p 230

Gibbs C P, Mumsom E S, Tham M K 1975 Anesthetic solubility coefficients for maternal and fetal blood. Anesthesiology 43: 100–103

Gibbs C P, Noel S C 1976 Human uterine artery responses to lidocaine. American Journal of Obstetrics and Gynecology 126: 313–315

Gluck L, Kulovich M V 1973 Lecithin/sphingomyelin ratios in amniotic fluid in normal and abnormal pregnancy. American Journal of Obstetrics and Gynecology 115: 539–546

Hill R M, Verniaud W M, Horning M G, McCulley L B, Morgan N F 1974 Infants exposed in utero to antiepileptic drugs. A prospective study. American Journal of Diseases of Children 127: 645–653

Hogg M I J, Wiener P C, Rosen M, Mapleson W W 1977 Urinary excretion and metabolism of pethidine and norpethidine in the newborn. British Journal of Anaesthesia 49: 891–899

Holdcroft A, Robinson M J, Gordon H, Whitwam J G 1974

Comparison of effects of two induction doses of methohexitone on infants delivered by elective Caesarean section. British Medical Journal 2: 472–475

Howe J P, McGowan W A W, Moore J, McCaughey W, Dundee J W 1981 The placental transfer of cimetidine. Anaesthesia 36: 371–375

Jago R H 1970 Arthrogryposis following treatment of maternal tetanus with muscle relaxants. A case report. Archives of Disease in Childhood 45: 277–279

Jones H M R, Cummings A J 1978 A study of the transfer of methyldopa to the human fetus and newborn infant. British Journal of Clinical Pharmacology 6: 432–434

Jouppila R, Jouppila P, Juikka J, Hollmen A 1978 Placental blood flow during Caesarean Section under lumbar extradural analgesia. British Journal of Anaesthesia 50: 275–279

Kanto J, Sjovall S, Erkkola R, Himberg J-J, Kangas L 1983 Placental transfer and maternal midazolam kinetics. Clinical Pharmacology and Therapeutics 33: 786–791

Kivalo I, Saarikoski S 1977 Placental transmission of atropine at full term pregnancy. British Journal of Anaesthesia 49: 1017–1021

Kosaka Y, Takahashi T, Mark L C 1969 Intravenous thiobarbiturate anesthesia for Cesarean section. Anesthesiology 31: 489–506

Kuhnert B R, Kuhnert P M, Prochaska A L, Gross T A 1980 Plasma levels of 2 chloroprocaine in obstetric patients and their neonates after epidural anesthesia. Anesthesiology 53: 21–25

Kuhnert P M, Kuhnert B R, Stitts J M, Gross T L 1981 The use of a selected ion monitoring technique to study the disposition of bupivacaine in mother, fetus and neonate following epidural anesthesia for Caesarean section. Anesthesiology 55: 611–617

Lardoux H, Gerard J, Blazquez G, Flouvat B 1983 Which beta-blocker in pregnancy-induced hypertension? Lancet ii: 1194

Lenz W 1966 Malformations caused by drugs in pregnancy. American Journal of Diseases of Children 112: 99–106

Levy G 1978 Clinical pharmacokinetics of aspirin. Pediatrics 62 (Suppl): 867–872

Levy G, Garrettson L K 1974 Kinetics of salicylate elimination by newborn infants of mothers who ingested aspirin before delivery. Pediatrics 53: 201–210

Lieberman B A, Stirrat G M, Cohen S L, Beard R W, Pinker G D 1978 The possible adverse effect of propanolol on the fetus in pregnancies complicated by severe hypertension. British Journal of Obstetrics and Gynaecology 85: 678–683

Lind T, Hytten F E 1972 Fetal control of fetal fluids. In: Hodari A A, Mariona F G (eds) The physiological biochemistry of the fetus. Thomas, Springfield, pp 54–65

Little B, Chang T, Chucot L, et al 1972 Study of ketamine as an obstetric anaesthetic agent. American Journal of Obstetrics and Gynecology 113: 247–260

McAuley D M, Moore J, McCaughey W, Donnelly B D, Dundee J W 1983 Ranitidine as an antacid before elective Caesarean section. Anaesthesia 38: 108–114

Marx G F, Joshi C W, Orkin L R 1970 Placental transmission of nitrous oxide. Anesthesiology 32: 429–432

Maurer H M, Wolff J A, Finster M et al 1968 Reduction in Concentration of total serum bilirubin in offspring of women treated with phenobarbitone during pregnancy. Lancet ii: 122–124

Mirkin B L, Singh S 1976 Placental transfer of pharmacologically active molecules. In: Mirkin B L (ed) Perinatal pharmacology and therapeutics. Academic Press, New York, pp 1–69

Moore J, Dundee J W 1983 Analgesia in labour. In: Lewis P (ed) Clinical pharmacology in obstetrics. Wright, Bristol, pp 337–359

Moore J, McNabb T G, Glynn J P 1973 The placental transfer of pentazocine and pethidine. British Journal of Anaesthesia 45: 798–801

Moore R G, Tischler E, Burnard E D, Thomas J 1978 Perinatal disposition of chlormethiazole used in the management of severe pre eclampsia. Clinical and Experimental Pharmacology and Physiology 5: 257–258

Morselli P L 1983 Clinical pharmacokinetics in neonates. In: Gibaldi M, Prescott L (eds). Handbook of clinical pharmacokinetics. ADIS, Auckland. pp 79–97

Morselli P L, Franco-Morselli R, Bossi L 1980 Clinical pharmacokinetics in new-borns and infants. Age-related differences and therapeutic implications. Clinical Pharmacokinetics 5: 485–527

Morselli P L, Rovei V 1980 Placental transfer of pethidine and norpethidine and their pharmacokinetics in the newborn. European Journal of Clinical Pharmacology 18: 25–30

Moya F, Kvisselgaard N 1961 The placental transmission of succinylcholine. Anesthesiology 22: 1–6

Mulley B A, Parr G D, Pau W K, Rye R M, Mould J J, Siddle N C 1978 Placental transfer of chlorthalidone and its elimination in maternal milk. European Journal of Clinical Pharmacology 26: 952–966

Nation R L 1983 Drug kinetics in childbirth. In: Gibaldi M, Prescott L (eds) Handbook of clinical pharmacokinetics, Section 2. ADIS Health Science Press, Cameron Printing Co Ltd, Hong Kong, pp 18–43

O'Brien J E, Abbey V, Hinsvark O, Perel J M, Finster M 1979 Metabolism and measurement of chloroprocaine, an ester-type local anesthetic. Journal of Pharmaceutical Sciences 68: 75–78

Page E W 1957 Transfer of material across human placenta. American Journal of Obstetrics and Gynecology 74: 705–718

Perucca E, Richens A 1983 Antiepileptic drugs, pregnancy and the newborn. In: Lewis P (ed) Clinical pharmacology in obstetrics. Wright, Bristol, pp 264–267

Philipson A, Sabath L D, Charles D 1976 Erthromycin and clindamycin absorption and elimination in pregnant women. Clinical Pharmacology and Therapeutics 19: 68–77

Rame A, Wilson J T 1976 Clinical pharmacokinetics in infants and children. Clinical Pharmacokinetics 1: 2–24

Rementeria J C, Bhatt K 1977 Withdrawal symptoms in neonates from intrauterine exposure to diazepam. Journal of Pediatrics 90: 123–126

Rementeria J L, Nunag N N 1973 Narcotic withdrawal in pregnancy. Stillbirth incidence with a case report. American Journal of Obstetrics and Gynaecology 116: 1152–1156

Reynolds F 1982 The placenta: structure, physiology and pharmacokinetics. In Scurr C, Feldman S (eds) Scientific foundations of anaesthesia, 3rd edn. Heinemann Medical, London, pp 475–487

Ring G, Krames E, Shnider S M, Wallis K L, Levinson G 1977 Comparison of nitroprusside and hydralazine in hypertensive pregnant ewes. Obstetrics and Gynecology 51: 598–602

Riva E, Farina P, Tognoni G, Bottino S, Orrico C, Pardi G 1978 Pharmacokinetics of furosemide in gestosis of pregnancy. European Journal of Clinical Pharmacology 14: 361–366

Rubin P C, Butlers L, Clark D M et al 1983 Placebo controlled trial of atenolol in treatment of pregnancy-associated hypertension. Lancet i: 431–434

Rumack C M, Guggenheim M A, Rumack B H, Peterson R G, Johnson M L, Braithwaite W R 1981 Neonatal intracranial haemorrhage and maternal use of aspirin. Obstetrics and Gynecology 58: 52S–56S

Saarikoski S 1976 Placental transfer and fetal uptake of 3H-digoxin in humans. British Journal of Obstetrics and Gynaecology 83: 879–884

Scanlon J W, Brown W V Jr, Weiss J B, Alper M H 1974 Neurobehavioural responses of newborn infants after maternal epidural anesthesia. Anesthesiology 40: 121–128

Shapiro S, Heinonen O P, Siskind V, Kaufman D W, Monson R R, Slone D 1977 Antenatal exposure to doxylamine succinate and dicyclamine hydrochloride (Bendectin) in relation to congenital malformations, perinatal mortality rate, birth weight and intelligence quotient score. American Journal of Obstetrics and Gynecology 5: 480–485

Sharpe G L, Larsson K S, Thalme B 1975 Studies on closure of ductus arteriosus. Prostaglandins 9: 585–596

Sheridan C A, Robson J C 1959 Fluothane in obstetrical anaesthesia. Canadian Anaesthetists' Society Journal 6: 365–374

Siker E S, Wolfson B, Dubnan S K Y, Fitting G M 1968 Placental transfer of methoxyflurane. British Journal of Anaesthesia 40: 588–592

Thomas J, Climie C R, Mather L E 1969 Placental transfer of alcuronium. British Journal of Anaesthesia 41: 297–302

Tomson G, Lunell H O, Sumdwall A, Rane A 1979 Placental passage of oxazepam and its metabolism in mother and newborn. Clinical Pharmacology and Therapeutics 25: 74–81

Tylden E 1973 The effects of maternal drug abuse on the fetus and infant. Adverse Drug Reactions Bulletin 38: 120–123

Way W L, Costley F C, Way E L 1965 Respiratory sensitivity of the newborn infant to meperidine and morphine. Clinical Pharmacology and Therapeutics 6: 454–461

Whitelaw A G L, Cummings A J, McFadyen I R 1981 Effect of maternal lorazepam on the neonate. British Medical Journal 282: 1106–1108

Yaffe S J 1976 Developmental factors influencing interactions of drugs. Annals of the New York Academy of Sciences 281: 90–97

Yeh T F, Pildes R S 1977 Transplacental aminophylline toxicity in a neonate. Lancet i: 910

Young S R, Stoelting R K, Bond V K, Peterson C 1976 Methoxyflurane biotransformation and renal function following methoxyflurane administration for vaginal delivery or Caesarean section. Anesthesia and Analgesia, Current Researches 55: 415–419

Zelsen L, Rubio E, Wasserman E 1971 Neonatal narcotic addiction: 10 year observation. Pediatrics 48: 178–189

32. Clinical trials

J. W. Dundee

The experimentation must be done with the human body, for the testing of a drug on a lion or a horse might not prove anything about its effects in Man.

Avicenna (980–1037)

This quotation from the Arab physician/philosopher suggests that the concept of clinical trials is nothing new, although there is no evidence that he studied drugs in animals. The first recorded, perhaps even the first ever, therapeutic trial was recorded by James Lind in the year 1747 (Bull 1959). In 1600 four ships had been sent to India by the East India Company; in one which had been provided with lemon juice as part of the ration, the crew were free from scurvy. This trial was exemplary in its design (Table 32.1) apart from the small number of subjects, and it even contained a dose–response effect since cider may contain some vitamin C. However, Lind was not convinced by his own findings

Table 32.1 Clinical trial by James Lind (1716–1794), ship's surgeon.

Constant factors	Patients (sailors)	
	Disease (scurvy)	
	Diet	
	Surroundings	
Variable factors	Supplements to the diet	

Supplement	No. of patients	Outcome
Cider	2	Slight improvement
Elixir of vitriol	2	No improvement
Vinegar	2	No improvement
Oranges and lemons	2	*Cured*
A recommended electuary	2	No improvement

and it was another 50 years before lemon juice was used regularly (L'Etang 1970). The first controlled clinical trial to match up to present-day criteria was organized by J. A. Sinton, who evaluated antimalarial drugs on a rational basis in the Punjab in the 1920s. It was in the 1930s and 1940s that the subject was really taken seriously, with the introduction of the sulphonamides, penicillin and other similar drugs.

There were relatively few new drugs introduced into anaesthesia until the early 1950s, when studies with relaxants heralded a new concept of anaesthesia and their early use was the first approach to the modern clinical trial. In 1949 H. J. V. Morton from Hillingdon Hospital, Uxbridge, published a paper entitled 'Chance in anaesthetic investigation'. This unique presentation included a consideration of variables, controls, significance levels, sample size and statistics, and paved the way for controlled clinical trials in anaesthesia. In 1955 the author described the steps involved in planning a clinical investigation, illustrated by an actual study. Most of the suggestions made in these two early papers are still applicable today. The earliest anaesthetic use of the words 'clinical trials' in British anaesthetic literature appears to have been by Dundee et al (1954) with laudexium, Jolly (1957) with prestonal and Kaufmann (1958) with bemegride. Their final acceptance by anaesthetists was evidenced by an education issue of the *British Journal of Anaesthesia* being devoted to this topic in April 1967.

Nor were our surgical colleagues unaware of these developments. The President of the Royal College of Surgeons, in a symposium 'Towards clinical knowledge', stressed their importance. 'There are many paths which might lead to the acquisition of clinical knowledge that might profitably be explored, but . . . there is only one high road to an increase in therapeutic knowledge and that is the controlled clinical trial' (Atkins 1966).

OBJECTIVES

A clinical trial is a scientific experiment in which a therapy or therapeutic procedure is studied in patients (Maxwell 1969). Its purpose should be to obtain the *maximum* amount of *unbiased* information concerning the *principal action* and *side-effects* of a drug or procedure from the *minimal* number of patients in the *shortest* time with the *least* potential hazard or inconvenience to them (Gray 1967). All the adjectives stressed in this definition are important: if one is subjecting a patient to some inconvenience it is important to obtain as much information as possible; to be meaningful this information should be unbiased and since most studies are comparative they should deal with both the therapeutic and toxic effects of therapy. If a clinical trial is prolonged it can result in boredom of the investigator, who may unwittingly 'modify the protocol' by taking short cuts.

Sir Austin Bradford Hill, who made a major contribution to the evolution of clinical trials, extends these definitions and emphasizes the importance of control. 'The clinical trial is a carefully, and ethically, designed experiment with the aim of answering some precisely framed questions. In its most rigorous form it demands equivalent groups of patients concurrently treated in different ways' (Hill 1966). This lifts the trial from the realm of clinical impression and attaches real value of the conclusions to the practising doctor. However, it is worth remembering that the more original scientific work is, the less reliable and precise it will be (Paton 1979).

Acquiring reliable knowledge (certainty) can be looked on as the precise aim of a clinical trial. Dudley (1983) has categorized various stages in this process (Fig. 32.1) and places the prospective randomized trial near the goal — probably only finishing in application of the study results to the population as a whole.

Like all scientific experiments a clinical trial deserves logical pre-thinking and a clear statement of intent — which *must* be written down. It is important that one does not lose sight of the original objectives, as it is easy to get side-tracked, and perhaps more interesting aspects of research may emerge when a pilot study is carried out. A written protocol must be prepared, not only giving objectives, but the logistics of the study. This will be discussed later.

ROLE OF THE CLINICAL TRIAL

While it is important to emphasize again that a clinical trial can involve a technique or a non-medicinal therapy (such as physiotherapy) or a combination of both, this discussion concentrates on evaluation of drugs and Figure 32.2 shows the place of the clinical trial in this process. The various clinical evaluations are referred to as phase I, II and III, phase II studies being the initial clinical trials, carried out in a limited number of centres and usually co-ordinated by a pharmaceutical company. This requires a Clinical Trials Certificate (CTC) in Britain and equivalent authorization elsewhere. At a later stage the workers can be granted a certificate of exemption (CTX) from CTC, provided supplies of the drug can be obtained.

Most clinical trials compare drugs with similar actions but with varying potency and side-effects, and very rarely does one get the opportunity of assessing the activity of a new product with a unique action or an action which is present to a unique degree. Occasionally one may use an accepted drug as 'standard' only to find that it has never been fully evaluated by modern methods. In 1965 the author and colleagues (Dundee et al 1965) compared the time course of action of equivalent doses of morphine and pethidine — a comparison that had never been made previously.

Figure 32.2 shows that clinical evaluation of drugs deals with both their therapeutic and toxic effects. The latter may require further study in volunteers and even more animal studies, and in the final evaluation one may make recommendation as to precautions and contra-indications which are necessary for the safe use of a preparation. The term 'benefit–risk' ratio has to be considered before a preparation is ultimately marketed. one is prepared to accept more side-effects from an anti-neoplasm drug than from an antisialogogue or oral

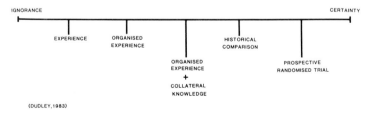

Fig. 32.1 From ignorance to certainty

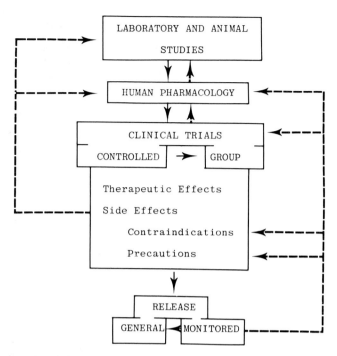

Fig. 32.2 Schematic representation of the stage in evaluation of new drugs (Dundee 1974).

contraceptive. In anaesthesia it is difficult to envisage circumstances when a more toxic preparation than the existing standard therapy would be preferred. Perhaps a drug with a unique pharmacokinetic profile would justify this.

The group trials listed in Figure 32.2 may be unique to anaesthesia — these are not to be compared with 'post-marketing surveillance' which the drug regulatory authors may request from a pharmaceutical company (Inman 1986). 'Controlled' trials are often carried out by a limited number of trained observers and demand strict elimination of variables. Ideally the group trial is organized by the same person as the initial controlled study, but in this there is less vigorous patient selection and a large number of clinically orientated observers are involved. A useful trial of this kind is particularly difficult to carry out.

STUDY POPULATION

Homo sapiens is a very variable creature, with a variable response to drugs. In clinical evaluations we study a group of subjects, aiming at obtaining knowledge of the response of the appropriate population. This is the basis of inductive reasoning, which assumes that the group findings are representative of the population findings. As most clinical studies are aimed at a specific category

of patients, it is important that the group studied must be typical of the target population. Studies of requirements of opioid in patients recovering from coronary artery operations will not provide data for the use of the same drugs in women in labour — while this is an extreme example it shows the need for carefully selecting the study population.

Dudley (1983) ascribes a different meaning to the concept of inductive reasoning. 'To generalise from those of study sample to the world at large requires a leap which some call induction and others merely a value judgment on the application of exclusions from a sample'.

TYPES OF TRIAL

This is a very complex topic (Hayward 1969) which will be simplified by restricting considerations to drugs used in anaesthesia. This excludes 'crossover' study, in which the patient receives two different medications during the course of an illness. Group comparisons are the most commonly used in anaesthesia. Here patients drawn from the same population receive either: trial therapy (new drug), standard therapy, or no therapy (where applicable), under standard conditions using the same method of study and observers, and in the case of subjective observations (e.g. premedicants) at a standard time and ideally in the same surroundings. Clearly the use of 'no therapy' is limited to pre- or postoperative studies and will be discussed later in relation to the use of placebos. The number of patients in such a trial will depend on a number of factors, and the advice of a statistician should be sought on this point. Factors to be considered include the degree of difference which one would hope for from a standard and new therapy (including side-effects), availability of suitable patients and avoidance of bias by the observer. Non-statistical considerations include financial restraints and time available for the study.

The use of 'matched pairs' is a valuable technique used in sequential trials. Here one of two therapies is given, at random, to similar patients and the observer makes a balanced judgment as to which, if any, proves more effective or satisfactory. The preferences in serial pairs are plotted on specially designed charts, such as those pioneered by Armitage (1960). Provided one does not encounter too many 'tied pairs', where no clear preference exists, this is economical as far as the number of patients is concerned. The main problem is deciding what is considered to be a significant difference between the response of a pair of patients, and for guidance one should consult standard statistical texts. In a clinical study the important point is that the difference should, in the opinion of the assessor, be of clinical relevance. Even if one does not achieve a clear decision with respect to preferences before stopping the trial, there remain data from two very well-matched series of patients which can be analysed by other means (Girvan et al 1976).

PROTOCOL

Ethical approval

Before starting the clinical trial the protocol should be submitted to the regional medical ethical research committee or its equivalent. Such applications must include the method of obtaining informed consent from the subjects, or their relatives where appropriate. It must also present a balanced justification of any invasive monitoring procedure. The potential ethical objections to studies should be borne in mind at every stage in their design. Many committees issue guidelines for investigations and some hospitals have their own committees which must also be consulted. Some journals insist on reference being made to approval by the appropriate ethical committee, but others will only consider publication of work when proof of such approval is submitted, although this may not be stated in the paper.

Guidelines for studies in volunteers have been published by the Royal College of Physicians (1986) and the precautions recommended for volunteer studies should be consulted by clinical investigators.

The preparation of a suitable protocol is the key to any successful clinical investigation. Much has been written on this topic of which the report of the Medico-pharmaceutical Forum Working Party on Clinical Trials (1973), the primer on clinical trials by Maxwell (1969), Andersen's (1976) book on the principles underlying the clinical evaluation of drugs and the aide-memoire for clinical trials prepared by the Department of Pharmacology and Therapeutics, London Hospital Medical College (1977), although seemingly outdated, are extremely valuable. It is essential also to consult basic statistical texts which deal with this subject.

The author has always worked on the assumption that a clinical trials protocol should be so complete that if the principal investigator were to drop dead the study could be carried on without interruption. This ideal is difficult to achieve, but the use of a pilot study makes it easier. As shown in Figure 32.3, after a pilot study one may have to modify the objectives but in the end it is important that the final protocol is a perfect compromise between theoretical desires and practical necessities. When complete this will often refer to the input of other specialties in the study. In the cases of anaesthetics this can include the hospital pharmacist, statistician and possibly the surgeon. A properly written protocol can be an introduction to the subsequent publication of the results, and for this reason it should be fully referenced.

The aide-memoire mentioned above lists 83 items (under 15 main headings) which should be considered in the protocol. Some of the important points of interest to the anaesthetist (Table 32.2) will be discussed.

Avoidance of bias

Failure in inductive reasoning can be due to random variation, and is most likely with small samples, or bias in that the study sample differs from the population which it is intended to represent. In a biased study sample one outcome is more likely or less likely than any other before the study begins. This is best avoided by randomization of treatments, as will be discussed later.

With assessments of subjective effects the attitude of the doctor can influence the findings and induce bias. Some practitioners who impress the patient may be placebo inductor, others non-inductor. In a study of various premedicants it was noted that patients visited at 20-minute intervals after drug administration were

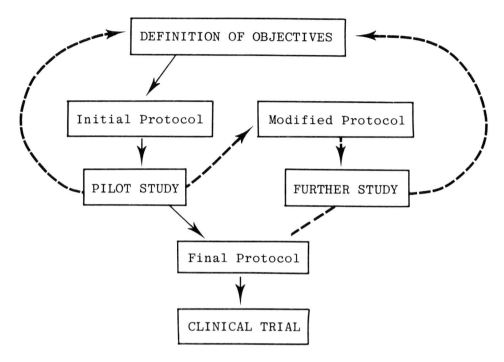

Fig. 32.3 Stages in preparation of a protocol (Dundee 1974).

Table 32.2 Factors to be considered in the protocol for a clinical trial

Aims	Dosage
Design	Dispensing
Population	Randomization
Documentation	Statistics
Assessments	Dropouts
Significance levels	

more sedated than those seen on only one occasion (Morrison et al 1968) — here the observer was acting as an inductor, with a significant effect on the findings. This emphasizes the need for consistency of observation and observers when studying the subjective effect of a medication such as anxiety or sedation. The attitude of nursing staff to clinical studies could have similar effects.

Bias due to measurement may result from the doctor's attitude to the study, and ideally the observer should not know whether the patient is in the study, or control or inert therapy group (single-blind study). This is not always possible, and the person in charge of the study must be aware that some observers can produce readings which are prejudicial to the outcome of the study. This can result from lack of interest and be an attempt to shorten the study.

The single-blind technique, in which the observer is unaware of the therapy given, is adequate for most anaesthetic studies. However, in the field of pre-medication, where it may not be advisable for patients to know whether they have received a test or standard drug (although the possibility of receiving either may be told when obtaining informed consent), a curious observer may try to 'break the key' of the study, particularly if there is a marked difference between the effects of the test and standard preparations. The likelihood of this can be minimized by keeping the period of study as short as possible. The use of multiple concurrent studies may have the same effect, but these can become very complicated.

Placebo

The use of a placebo is important when studying the subjective effect of any drug given with therapeutic or scientific intent. It works through psychological mechanisms and is independent of any pharmacological drug effects. It has been described as something which pleases the patient, a therapy which is not a therapy and also as an imitation of a therapy. Its use can assess the placebo response rate in the study population and also what part of a therapeutic response may be due to this. It is a valuable tool in blind trials but in many instances one is giving dummy medication rather than a placebo.

It is interesting to note that the placebo response is not consistently repeatable, as is the effect of genuine medication. In postoperative pain a placebo may produce relief in about one-third of patients for up to 3 hours, but will rarely work if repeated. Standards of patient care demand an 'escape clause' in any study of this nature, e.g. if pain is not adequately relieved in 1 hour, the key is broken and any patient given a placebo should immediately have a preparation of proven therapeutic value. This means that in all placebo-controlled studies the key to the medications must be readily available to nursing as well as to medical staff.

In the case of oral medication it is desirable to have the placebo and active medication as similar in appearance as possible — not because the patient is likely to be aware of this but because the person giving the medication may also be the observer. Here one could inadvertently introduce an element of bias.

Controls

This may seem simple in that one compares the effect of a new medication or therapy with the generally accepted standard. However, because of the incidence of side-effects, differing time course of action or physical dissimilarity it may be difficult to adopt a blind technique of administration and assessment. A recent example of this is the introduction of an emulsion form of propofol which was physically dissimilar from any other intravenous anaesthetic: the obvious standard is thiopentone, and it is only by the use of an independent person giving the drug that a proper comparison can be made. This is unsatisfactory clinically, and in practice physical dissimilarity is not a problem as objective observations are relatively free from bias.

There are occasions when a new medication offers such promise of lack of toxicity compared with the standard therapy that one has to consider the controversial use of historic controls. Some will condemn these outright on the grounds that circumstances change and comparisons with the past are invalid, and believe that high scientific reliability requires contemporaneous comparisons (Popper 1957). Others take a less rigid stand, Dudley (1983) has pointed out that 'we live by history and all comparisons must of necessity be with the past; transferring the results of a controlled trial into future practice implies using the result as historical evidence'. He suggests a 'rolling programme', in which the better result of a previous trial is used as the control for a subsequent study, but this is not always feasible. In scientific terms this is not as reliable as contemporaneous comparisons, but with certain caveats historical controls are appropriate (Cranberg 1979).

To give a concrete example, when studying the anti-emetic effects of acupuncture and various medications in a standard population premedicated with an opioid, the incidence of sickness in the untreated controls was so consistently high that, after a 'baseline' incidence has been established, only one control was included per ten treated cases (Dundee et al 1986). Most other examples are outside the field of anaesthesia, such as cancer chemotherapy.

Randomization

This essential step in avoidance of bias seems very simple, but can be full of pitfalls. The use of random numbers in allocating treatments or anaesthetic techniques is a well-established method. In other fields, such as obstetrics, treatments can be allocated when the patient enters hospital, knowing that not every patient may proceed along the same course — some having operative deliveries and others not even needing pain relief. Where a group of patients can have contact with each other (and perhaps compare treatments) randomization may have to be on a day-to-day basis. On any one day all patients will receive either the trial therapy, standard therapy or inert medication, but the order of these can be randomized. 'Contagious vomiting' is another problem which can be minimized, but not eliminated, by all patients in a ward having the same treatment on the same day.

Patient variables

This is the most difficult factor to control and only a few guidelines can be given. Generally speaking patients can be divided into four age groups with regard to their response to drugs — neonates, children (pre-puberty), adults and the elderly. The division between adults and elderly is difficult, as the chronological age may differ from the actual life span, e.g. a patient aged 50 may have a lower tolerance to drugs than a very fit 70-year-old. Nevertheless the response to some intravenous anaesthetics changes between the ages of 50 and 60 years, and this has to be considered in designing clinical trials.

There are few sex-related changes in response to drugs, the most important being the greater tendency of women to postoperative vomiting. It is only at extremes of weight or in gross obesity that this has to be considered as an important factor. As regards patient pathology, the well-established classification of physical status of the American Society of Anesthesiologists (Table 32.3) has proved very useful. For most studies grades 1 and 2 can be considered 'fit patients' and these are the basis for initial clinical trials, with poor-risk patients reserved for special studies.

Table 32.3 American Society of Anesthesiologists Classification of Physical Status

1. A normal healthy patient.

2. A patient with a mild systemic disease.

3. A patient with a severe systemic disease that limits activity, but is not incapacitating.

4. A patient with an incapacitating systemic disease that is a constant threat to life.

5. A moribund patient not expected to survive 24 hours with or without operation.

From *Anesthesiology*, 1963.

Drug variation

Table 32.4 lists factors that have to be considered. An example of lack of stability is the aqueous solution of diamorphine, while an important physical interaction is that between thiopentone and suxamethonium. The comparison of premedicant drugs which are given by the oral and intramuscular routes is best achieved by the 'double-dummy' technique, in which each patient gets both an injection and a tablet or capsule, the respective inert preparations have the solvent and excipient (Dundee 1974). With this, the 'placebo' consists of both the dummy tablet and injection.

Table 32.4 Drug variables which have to be standardized in clinical trials.

Stability
Interaction
Route of administration
Dosage-equivalents
Comparability

MEASUREMENT

A detailed discussion of this is outside the scope of this chapter, particularly with regard to quantitation of subjective responses. The essential basis is the assignment of numerals to things so as to represent facts and conventions about them. There is, however, an important difference between objective and subjective data. In the former there is a linear relationship between numbers (e.g. a systolic blood pressure of 120 mmHg is 30 mmHg higher than one of 90) while a sedation score of 4 allocated for a satisfactory state is not twice that of 2 allocated for only slight sedation.

While numerals can be allocated to subjective responses one has to remember that feelings are subjective responses, beyond absolute analysis (Aitken 1969). No final judgment of validity can ever be given — validity can only be relative and examined by expensive comparison. An example of allocation of numbers to a subjective experience is the use of pain scores. The concept of the 'pain chart', first introduced by Keele in 1948, has been greatly expanded, the most important addition being a concurrent estimate of pain by a trained observer, using objective signs such as the facial expression of the patients. Generally speaking the patient will overestimate the degree of pain compared with the observer, but the response to effective analgesics is similar with both (Dundee & Loan 1966).

The use of the visual analogue scale (Aitken 1969, Huskisson 1974) as an estimate of a subjective feeling is increasing in popularity, but is only applicable to a conscious, co-operative, intelligent patient. The addition of any disruptive data, except at the extremes, converts the analogue into a simple subjective scoring system and can be misleading. Variations of this are shown in Figure 32.4. The bottom example is unsatisfactory as it converts VAS into severity grading. There is no objection to patients being shown their previous estimate on the scale. For further data on the use of this, one should consult current statistical texts, particularly with reference to analyses of results. The arc sine transformation, or other similar test, may be applicable, but at the design of a clinical trial, statistical advice should be obtained in the analysis of data.

Documentation of data in an easily analysable form is essential in the design of any clinical trial — here again the advice of a statistician is essential in the planning stage. This is particularly important when one wants to do a computerized analysis of the results.

INTERPRETATION OF FINDINGS

Statistics serve as a guide to the unknown, and permit

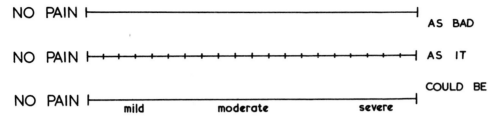

Fig.32.4 Three forms of visual analogues for testing pain severity (Dundee, 1980).

us to draw conclusions that do not vary, about phenomena that do. Observations, if selected independently at random for a well-defined patient population, with minimal variation due to the patients, the observer or the method of study, will behave as random variations and be amenable to statistical analysis. The proposed method of analysis must be included in protocol, but may be modified or altered when the study is completed.

The conclusions are subject to two types of error — the difference found could be due to chance and no true difference results (with the accepted $P = 0.05$ this could happen in 1 in 20) or 'error of the second kind' showing no difference when true differences exist. The latter error is more difficult to detect and the possibility of it occurring is often ignored. The likelihood of it occurring is dependent on the sample size and the variation within the sample, and also the true difference between treatments. Generally speaking small samples permit detection only of large differences.

Post hoc ergo propter hoc — event A is followed by event B and B is therefore caused by A. This is fallacious thinking and must be avoided, except in the simplest of circumstances, e.g. apnoea after administration of a neuromuscular blocking drug. It is in the interpretation of the findings of a clinical trial that one may have the utmost difficulty, and in their application in clinical practice. Ideally one should present findings to a well-informed group of colleagues and ask for suggestions before presenting them to a learned society. This can often prevent a wrong interpretation being put on the findings, as those closely involved in a study may be unaware of their limitations.

It is immoral to seek informed consent from a group of patients and subject them to the risk, or discomfort, no matter how small, of a clinical trial and not make the findings, whether positive or negative, available to the medical profession in general. Communications do not have to be long and intricate, but the important conclusions must be presented with a reasoned case for their validity. This could even be in the form of an abstract presented to a learned society and published in the appropriate journal. There can be few fields of endeavour which fall short of completion as often as the unpublished results of a clinical trial, and this reflects poorly on the investigators.

It has been aptly stated that 'clinical trials are easiest when they are least needed and hardest when they are most required' (Dudley 1977). There are circumstances when it is thought unlikely that a difference will be found in a clinical trial — the initial assumption being that the null hypothesis is correct — but it is necessary to convince someone that this is so. Under these circumstances it is arguable that those who need to be convinced by scientific evidence are the least capable of responding to it. To paraphrase Patrick O'Donovan (1976): all the writing on the wall of science is invisible to those who most need to read it.

Update

This chapter has dealt with "established practice" for clinical trials. There have been many publications suggesting changes in standards, ethics and design which may eventually be adopted. A list of useful references to recent work is included at the end of the bibliography.

REFERENCES

Aitken R C B 1969 Measurement of feelings using visual analogue scales. Proceedings of the Royal Society of Medicine 62: 989–993

American Society of Anesthesiologists 1963 New classification of physical status. Anesthesiology 24: 111

Andersen B 1976 The principles underlying the clinical evaluation of drugs, 2nd ed. R. Roussel Bogtryk + Offset, Denmark

Armitage P 1960 Sequential medical trials. Blackwell, Oxford

Atkins H 1966 Conduct of a controlled trial. British Medical Journal 2: 377

Bull J P 1959 The historic development of clinical therapeutic trials. Journal of Chronic Diseases 10: 218–248

Cranberg L 1979 Do retrospective controls make clinical

trials 'inherently fallacious'? British Medical Journal 2: 1265–1266

Dudley H A F 1977 Communication in medicine and biology. Churchill Livingstone, Edinburgh

Dudley H A F 1983 The controlled clinical trial and the advance of reliable knowledge: an outsider looks in. British Medical Journal 287: 957–960

Dundee J W 1974 Introduction of new drugs symposium — clinical trials in anaesthesia. Proceedings of the Royal Society of Medicine 67: 586–588

Dundee J W, Chestnutt W N, Ghaly R G, Lynas A G A, 1986 Reduction in emetic effects of opioid preanaesthetic medication by acupuncture. British Journal of Clinical Pharmacology 22: 214P–215P.

Dundee J W, Clarke R S J, Loan W B 1965 Comparison of the sedative and toxic effects of morphine and pethidine. Lancet 2: 1262–1263

Dundee J W, Gray T C, Riding J E 1954 A clinical trial of laudolissin as a relaxant in 524 cases. British Journal of Anaesthesia 26: 13–21

Dundee J W, Loan W B 1966 Clinical evaluation of analgesic drugs. Acta Anaesthesiologica Scandinavica, Suppl 25: 336–342

Girvan C B, Dundee J W, Moore J 1976 A sequential comparison of pethidine alone and combined with naloxone for the relief of labour pain. Anaesthesia 31: 144–145

Gray T C 1967 The need for clinical trials. British Journal of Anaesthesia 39: 279–282

Hayward J L 1969 Controlled clinical trials. In: Atkins H (ed) Measurement and precision in surgery. Blackwell, Oxford, p p 67–81

Hill A B 1966 Principles of medical statistics, 8th edn. Lancet, London

Huskisson E C 1974 Measurement of pain. Lancet 2: 1127–1131

Inman W H W (ed) 1986 Monitoring for drug safety, 2nd edn. MTP Press, Lancaster

Jolly C 1957 Prestonal. Clinical trial of a new muscle relaxant. Anaesthesia 12: 3–9

Kaufmann L 1958 Clinical impression and clinical trial: with a study of the evaluation of bemegride. Anaesthesia 13: 43–55

Keele K D 1948 The pain chart. Lancet 2: 6

L'Etang H J C J 1970 Historical aspects of drug evaluation. In: Harris E L, and Fitzgerald J D (eds) The principles and practice of clinical trials. E & S Livingstone, Edinburgh

London Hospital Medical College 1977 Aide-memoire for preparing clinical trial protocols. British Medical Journal 1: 1323-1324

Maxwell C 1969 Clinical trials' protocol. Stuart Phillips Publications, London

Medico-pharmaceutical Forum 1973 A report by the Forum's working party on clinical trials. Medico-Pharmaceutical Forum, London

Morrison J D, Hill G B, Dundee J W 1968 Studies of drugs given before anaesthesia. XV: Evaluation of the method of study after 10,000 observations. British Journal of Anaesthesia 40: 890–900

Morton H J V 1949 Chance in anaesthetic investigation. Anaesthesia 4: 100–107

O'Donovan P 1976 The Observer, 12 September

Paton A W 1979 Ends, means and achievements in medical research. Lancet ii: 512–516

Popper K 1957 The poverty of historicism. Routledge & Kegan Paul, London

Royal College of Physicians of London 1986 Research on healthy volunteers. Journal of the Royal College of Physicians of London 20: 243–257

ADDITIONAL READING

Baum M, Zilkha K, Houghton J 1990 Ethics of clinical research: lessons for the future. British Medical Journal 299: 251–253

Brahams D 1990 Legal Considerations. Benzadiazepams: Current Concepts. Hindmarch I, Beaumont C, Brandon S, Leonard B E, John Wiley (eds) Chichester

Cohen A T, Webster N R 1988 The computer in clinical research and anaesthesia. Bailliere's Clinical Anesthesiology 2: 213–233

Cormac R S, Montel N 1990 Doubt and certainty in statistics. Journal of the Royal Society of Medicine 83: 136–137

Furrow L, Wartman S A, Brook D W 1988 Science, ethics and the making of Clinical Decisions. Journal of the American Medicine Association 259: 3161–3167

Glynn C 1988 Clinical methods in pain relief research. Bailliere's Clinical Anaesthesiology 2: 89–105

Hoffenberg R 1990 Medicine and Ethics. Journal of the Royal College of Physicians of London 24: 6–7

Mirakhur R K 1988 Designing a clinical trial. Bailliere's Clinical Anaesthesiology 2: 151–174

Newton D E F, Webster N R (eds) 1988 Clinical Research in Anaesthesia. Clinical Anaesthesiology Vol 2 No 2 Bailliere Tindall, London

Oliver I N, Simon R M, Aisner J 1986 Antiemetic studies: A methodological discussion. Cancer treatment report 70: 555–563

Research involving patients — Summary and recommendations of a report of the Royal College of Physicians 1990. Journal of the Royal College of Physicians of London 24: 10–14

Stafford M A 1988 Statistical analysis of anaesthetic experiments. Bailliere's Clinical Anesthesiology 2: 193–212

Watt J (ed) 1988 Talking Health: Conventional and complimentary approaches. Royal Society of Medicine, London

Zelen M 1979 A new design for randomized clinical trials. New England Journal of Medicine 300: 1242–1245

33. Electrolyte balance and parenteral nutrition

W. McCaughey   R. S. J. Clarke

FLUID AND ELECTROLYTE BALANCE: BASIC CONCEPTS

Electrolytes, non-electrolytes and colloids

Many substances in solution dissociate into two or more ions carrying positive or negative charges. These substances are described as electrolytes. As described earlier in this book, the degree of ionization is dependent on other factors such as the pH of the solution. Other substances, including a majority of organic compounds, may dissolve, but do not dissociate into charged particles — these are non-electrolytes. Usually in a complex mixture, the ions which have arisen from dissociation of an electrolyte can be considered in isolation — for example a sodium ion which entered the body as part of a sodium bicarbonate molecule may be balanced by any of the other anions present, and simply becomes another member of the sodium content of the body. Many drugs are formulated as salts — e.g. penicillin-V-K, and on occasion the amount of an ion administered in this way may become important in the electrolyte balance of the body.

Larger molecules do not enter a true solution, but rather are in a suspension in the solvent. Such a solution is known as a colloidal solution, and the substances behaving in this way are colloids, while the smaller molecules, either electrolytes or non-electrolytes, which form true solution, are known as crystalloids.

Osmotic and oncotic pressures

The body is separated into many compartments by membranes which may be regarded as semipermeable — that is, whereas one substance may cross relatively easily, another may be unable to, or may cross the membrane only with difficulty. When a membrane is permeable to a solvent such as water, and impermeable (or relatively impermeable) to a solute, then solvent tends to pass through the membrane so as to equalize concentrations on each side. This is osmosis. The force causing this movement, the osmotic pressure, is related to the number of particles in solution, rather than to their nature, so that for example the potassium-rich intracellular fluid may be in osmotic balance with the sodium-rich extracellular fluid. (Such properties, related to the number of particles rather than their nature, are known as colligative properties.) The standard unit of osmotic pressure is the Osmole, which is the gram molecular weight of the substance divided by the number of ions or particles into which it dissociates in solution. The normal osmotic pressure of body fluids such as plasma is approximately 290 mOsmol.

Osmolarity is a measure of the concentration of solute per litre of solution, while osmolality is solute concentration per kilogram of water. The difference between these two measurements is not normally significant.

The osmotic pressure which colloidal solutions exert is known as oncotic pressure. In biology the main feature of colloids is that, due to their greater molecular size, they do not cross animal membranes as readily as do small crystalloid molecules. For this reason, although the osmotic (oncotic) pressure which they exert is relatively small because the number of particles in solution is small, it is important because of the way in which it is confined — for example the oncotic pressure of plasma proteins is a major factor in balancing hydrostatic pressures and preventing fluid leakage from capillaries.

Body compartments

The total body water is about 62% of body weight in men, 51% in women, the sex difference being mainly due to differing amounts of stored body fat, which is water-free. Body water is usually considered as being made up of three compartments: intracellular, extracellular and, included within the latter, the intravascular space. The volumes of these spaces are measured by dilution of substances whose distribution is limited appropriately (and which do not bind or otherwise concentrate in one compartment) — i.e. by estimating the volume of distribution (Vd) of the substance.

Water in the form of deuterium or tritium oxide will spread throughout the body water, and is used by physiologists in measuring this space. Sodium remains largely extracellular in distribution, and a substance such as sodium thiosulphate may be used. Measured in this way, the extracellular fluid (ECF) volume is 17% of body weight. This volume includes intercellular fluid as well as plasma, CSF, joint fluids, etc. Intravascular volume may be measured using a substance which remains within the vascular space, such as ^{131}I-labelled albumin, and represents about one quarter of the ECF. The intracellular fluid volume is the difference between total and ECF volumes.

Distribution of administered fluids

Plasma protein oncotic pressure is responsible for balancing hydrostatic pressure and keeping fluid within the intravascular space. Colloid solutions such as plasma protein preparations, dextrans, etc., will tend to remain within this space, whereas a solution such as 0.9% sodium chloride will have access to the whole of the ECF, and dextrose 5% (which is essentially water) will distribute throughout the body water. This concept goes a long way to defining the uses of such solutions. However, plasma proteins, especially albumin, normally leak in considerable quantities from the blood circulation through pores between cells, returning by the way of the lymph circulation. In certain pathological states this leakage is considerably increased. In such conditions where there is capillary leak, for example in septic shock or the adult respiratory distress syndrome, colloid infusions will not be retained well within the circulation, and there is current and continuing controversy over the relative amounts of colloid and crystalloid which should be used. It is apparent that extremely low serum albumin levels will result in an increased danger of pulmonary and other oedema, but also that attempts to maintain normal laboratory values of serum albumin by giving large amounts of colloid can dramatically increase mortality if they are given without sufficient regard to the rise in pulmonary artery and left atrial pressures which can follow excessive volume expansion.

Sodium is actively excluded from the intracellular space. In the critically ill patient these processes may function inefficiently, so that sodium is lost to the intracellular space, in a situation sometimes loosely called the 'sick cell syndrome'. This situation aside, sodium may be considered as confined to the extracellular space.

THE ELEMENTS IN BODY FLUIDS

The organic molecules of the body are composed mainly of carbon, hydrogen, oxygen and nitrogen. The total number of elements which have been shown to have a functional role in the body is about 20, and a number of others are under consideration or have been shown to be necessary in other species.

Sodium

In evolutionary terms the extracellular fluid (ECF) of the body is a personal supply of sea water, and thus the predominant salt in ECF is sodium chloride. It is actively extruded from the intracellular space by the Na^+ K^+ pump. The daily requirement of sodium in a healthy adult is of the order of 1 mmol kg^{-1}. Sodium balance in the body is maintained mainly by monitoring of ECF volume by several mechanisms, and by regulation of renal sodium excretion, where aldosterone is the most important controlling factor. Reduction of sodium intake will lead to a reduction in ECF and circulating volume, which may be desirable in some medical patients with poor cardiovascular performance.

Sodium administered intravenously or otherwise to a patient is excluded from cells, but will equilibrate with the ECF. A 0.9% solution of sodium chloride, 'normal saline', is isotonic with body fluids, and contains 154 mmol l^{-1} sodium and chloride. This solution, along with 5% dextrose, which may generally be regarded as an isotonic preparation of water, are the basic materials of intravenous replacement therapy. Normal saline is used widely as a replacement for deficits in ECF volume, or for minor degrees of blood loss, although other solutions such as Hartmann's solution which more closely follow the composition of ECF may be slightly more appropriate. As an approximation, one-third of the volume infused will remain within the circulation once equilibration has taken place.

In contrast, if a dextrose solution is given, the dextrose will rapidly be metabolized, and the associated water will equilibrate with the total body water, so 5% dextrose is not a good choice to treat circulating volume deficit. It provides 200 kcal $^{-1}$, which is not a useful amount of energy — higher concentrations of dextrose, 20–50%, which are hypertonic, may be used in parenteral nutrition (see below).

Depending on several factors, including cardiovascular and renal function, and the degree of catabolism going on, an adult requires 30–40 ml water and around 1 mmol sodium per kg body weight, each 24 h.

The daily maintenance requirements of sodium and

water may be given using normal saline and dextrose or other solutions such as 1/5 normal saline (31 mmol^{-1}). Proprietary mixtures and specially formulated mixtures for maintenance fluid replacement are available, which will also contain some of the other electrolytes required, such as potassium. Such solutions may also be more appropriate in patients, especially children, in whom replacement for a mixed fluid and electrolyte deficit is needed, and where the plasma sodium levels may be raised.

Hypertonic saline solutions, 1.8% or greater, may be used, with caution, to replace a gross sodium deficit where there is not an associated deficit of water.

Potassium

This is the main intracellular cation, the difference between intracellular and extracellular Na$^+$ and K$^+$ being important in maintaining the electrical function of the cell membrane. The normal plasma K$^+$ concentration is 3.5–4.5 mmol^{-1}, and levels of above 7.0 are dangerous while levels above 8.5 are frequently fatal, usually through cardiac arrest, although respiratory paralysis may occasionally occur before the heart stops.

Hyperkalaemia is most often associated with renal disease where there is failure of excretion, but it may occur more acutely where there is rapid loss of potassium from cells. This may occur in certain burned and other patients given suxamethonium (see Chapter 34), or where there is muscle damage as in crush injuries or in the malignant hyperpyrexia syndrome (see Chapter 34). As potassium must enter the ECF to gain access to the intracellular space, too rapid administration may also cause potentially fatal hyperkalaemia.

Potassium deficit is commoner in surgical and anaesthetic practice. The normal daily requirement is 0.75–1 mmol kg^{-1}, i.e. about 50–70 mmol per day, but the response of the body to operative and other trauma includes increased potassium loss. Renal conservation of potassium is not efficient, and many critically ill patients require a considerably larger intake to maintain potassium balance, frequently in excess of 200 mmol per day.

Administration

Potassium is usually added to infusion fluids as the chloride salt, and is already contained in several balanced electrolyte preparations. Due to the dangers of iatrogenic hyperkalaemia, any infusion containing more than 40 mmol^{-1} potassium should be fitted with a suitable controlling device to prevent inadvertent rapid entry of potassium into the circulation.

Emergency treatment of hyperkalaemia

A high and rising serum potassium is one of the indications for peritoneal or haemodialysis in the patient with renal failure. In the chronic renal failure patient, or if for other reasons dialysis cannot be used, then an ion exchange resin can be administered either orally or rectally. Calcium resonium is given in a dose of 15–30 g one to four times in 24 h, usually along with some form of laxative. Calcium ions are exchanged for potassium ions within the structure of the resin, and the calcium ions released into the intestine. Some of this is absorbed, which may be useful in counteracting the effects of potassium on neuromuscular activity.

Bicarbonate, glucose and insulin all promote movement of potassium from the extracellular space into cells. Thus treatment with these may be a useful temporary expedient in reducing dangerously high potassium levels. A typical regime is to give glucose and insulin — 100 ml 25% dextrose followed by 10 units soluble insulin intravenously — when the potassium level is less than 8.0 mmol^{-1}, while for higher levels bicarbonate, glucose and insulin are given; 75 mmol sodium bicarbonate, and 50 ml 50% dextrose, diluted with 5% dextrose to 300–500 ml, are given intravenously over 2 h, with 10 units insulin given 20 min after infusion is started (McGeown 1983).

This is effective only as a holding measure, and after 4–6 h the potassium level will begin to rise again as potassium comes out of the cells.

Calcium is effective immediately in antagonizing the effects of potassium, and in a life-threatening situation calcium gluconate 10% 10–20 ml may be given intravenously.

Phosphorus

Phosphate is the main intracellular anion — the adult body contains about 64 g phosphorus. The normal plasma inorganic phosphate level is 0.8–1.5 mmol l^{-1} (3.5–4.5 mg/100 ml), while the intracellular concentration is about 100 mmol l^{-1}.

Phosphorus is of great importance as a major constituent of cell membranes, and in nucleic acid generation, energy metabolism and other areas. Thus phosphate deficiency can lead to widespread disturbances. Depletion of red cell ATP and 2,3-DPG occur, with a shift of the oxygen dissociation curve, so that the P$_{50}$ of haemoglobin may be reduced by 10 mmHg. Leucocyte function is depressed. Myocardial performance is also reduced (O'Connor et al 1977), and skeletal muscle weakness may occur. Respiratory failure has been reported in alcoholic patients (Newman et al 1977).

Clinical symptoms begin to occur when plasma inorganic phosphate levels have dropped to around 0.3 mmol l^{-1}.

Phoshorus is contained in adequate quantities in almost all foods, but hypophosphataemia may be rapidly precipitated by intravenous nutrition which contains inadequate phosphate.

Dosage and administration

The normal daily requirement of phosphorus in adults is 0.5 mmol kg^{-1}. It is unnecessary to use phosphate supplementation to normal fluid and electrolyte solutions, but essential to ensure that regimes for parenteral nutrition contain an adequate amount. Some proprietary mixtures for intravenous nutrition contain adequate phosphate, but several have inadequate amounts, or none at all, so that supplementation is required.

Various phosphate salts may be used for supplementation. Dipotassium hydrogen phosphate K_2HPO_4 is often employed as it allows a useful amount of potassium supplementation. The standard preparation contains potassium 1 mmol ml^{-1}. Other compounds such as KH_2PO_4 or Na_2HPO_4 may also be used where these are more appropriate for the total electrolyte needs of the patient.

Calcium

More than 90% of body calcium is contained in the skeleton. Plasma calcium is about 50% ionized, and this is the important fraction in physiological function. The majority of the remainder is bound to plasma protein, while about 10% is complexed to anions such as citrate or phosphate. The normal total calcium level in plasma is 2.2–2.64, and of ionized calcium 1.14–1.3 mmol l^{-1}. Because so much is bound to protein, total calcium measurements must be interpreted in the light of plasma protein concentrations.

Calcium deficiency

In anaesthetic practice this is most often seen in conditions such as acute pancreatitis, where calcium may be immobilized in diseased tissues and exudates, after surgical removal of parathyroid tissue, or after massive transfusion of citrated blood. As symptoms are related to ionized rather than total calcium levels, they may also occur with a normal total calcium level, if the ionized fraction decreases. This is commonly caused by alkalosis, often respiratory alkalosis due to hysterical overbreathing. The classical symptoms of hypocalcaemia include increased neuromuscular excitability, tetany, laryngospasm, and muscle cramps.

The normal daily intake of calcium is 200–400 mg (5–10 mmol). This may be added as required to intravenous feeding fluids, although if phosphate and calcium are both required in relatively large quantities, they may have to be administered alternately to avoid precipitation in the container.

Calcium chloride BP, USP: $CaCl_2.H_2O$

This can be given intravenously but not intramuscularly. It is used intravenously mainly when required to improve myocardial contractility. A 10% solution contains 0.68 mmol ml^{-1} calcium. It should be injected slowly, as hypotension may occur.

Calcium gluconate BP, USP: $[CH_2OH(CHOH)_2—COO]_2Ca.H_2O$

Calcium gluconate 10% contains 0.22 mmol ml^{-1} calcium. It is the preparation of choice for treatment of hypocalcaemic tetany. It is normally given intravenously, but it can be given intramuscularly, although this should not be done in neonates.

It may also be used in place of the chloride, as contrary to previous opinion it is equally effective in raising the plasma ionized calcium level (Heining et al 1984), and is less toxic to local tissues should extravasation occur.

Magnesium

Magnesium is the fourth most abundant cation in the body. It is a component of several intracellular enzyme systems, especially those involved in transfer of high-energy phosphate radicals to ATP, and is important in neuronal transmission and muscle contractility. Normal plasma magnesium level is 0.7–1.2 mmol l^{-1}, of which about 35% is protein-bound, while within cells there is a concentration of about 20 mmol l^{-1}, varying between tissues.

Magnesium deficiency

Magnesium depletion can occur in malnourished patients, those with prolonged diarrhoea or fistulae, or with diuretic therapy.

Clinical symptoms of deficiency may develop with plasma levels below 0.5 mmol l^{-1}. The picture is similar to that of calcium deficiency, characterized by hyperexcitability or tetany, as well as cardiac arrhythmias and ECG changes similar to those of potassium deficiency. Hypomagnesaemia may often be associated with hypokalaemia and digitalis toxicity.

The daily requirement of magnesium is about 0.17–0.25 mmol kg^{-1} in well-nourished patients, but may be several times higher in those with chronic depletion (Schneider & Biebuyck 1983).

Magnesium sulphate BP, USP: $MgSO_4.7H_2O$

This salt is available in several concentrations. For acute treatment of hypomagnesaemia a dose of 5–10 ml of 50% solution, i.e. about 10–20 mmol, given slowly by the parenteral route, is suitable for initial correction of deficiency, and may be followed by supplemental doses.

Treatment of eclampsia

At higher plasma levels, magnesium depresses neuromuscular transmission as well as having a widespread depressant action on the central nervous system. In treatment of eclampsia, the aim is to achieve a plasma level of 3–4 mmol l^{-1} (Hibbard & Rosen 1977) using a regime, for example, of 4 g magnesium sulphate given over 5 min, followed by 1 g hourly (Flowers 1965), with monitoring of plasma levels. Hypermagnesaemia is a danger — symptoms begin at above 2 mmol l^{-1}, tendon reflexes are lost at about 5 mmol l^{-1}, and respiration may be affected at 7.5–10 mmol l^{-1}, while at lower levels the action of neuromuscular blocking drugs is prolonged; 10–20 ml of calcium gluconate 10% may be given to treat hypermagnesaemia.

TRACE ELEMENTS

The eleven elements mentioned above make up the bulk of living matter, but about seventeen others are required in small quantities, as they occupy key positions in certain molecules, often enzymes. These are known as trace elements. In humans, chromium, cobalt, copper, fluorine, iodine, iron, manganese, molybdenum, selenium, and zinc are all important, while some others have been shown to play a role in animals.

Minimum daily requirements have been established for some of these, but much of such work is based on nutritionally deprived 'third world' populations, and the figures may not always be directly applicable to the situation of the critically ill patient. Trace element deficiency may become apparent after a variable period of unsupplemented parenteral feeding, depending on many factors including the severity of disease and the degree of pre-existing malnutrition.

The most important of the trace elements, together with estimated daily requirements are shown in Table 33.1 , and some other recent estimates of requirements are referred to in the text. These minerals do not need to be given to patients on short-term intravenous treatment, but long-term parenteral nutrition should be supplemented. The concept that occasional infusions of blood and plasma can supply trace element requirements is outdated and should not be encouraged.

Chromium

The place of chromium is not well established. It forms part of an organic complex known as glucose tolerance factor (GTF), and chromium deficiency may play a part in some cases of maturity-onset diabetes, as well as in impaired glucose tolerance seen in kwashiorkor. Chromium deficiency may also occur during parenteral nutrition, where it has been characterized by glucose intolerance and neuropathy (Jeejeebhoy et al 1977, Brown et al 1986).

Cobalt

Cobalt is required in the form of vitamin B_{12}. In humans it must be supplied as this compound, although cows and other ruminants are able to utilize the inorganic element, as micro-organisms in their gut synthesize vitamin B_{12}. There is some evidence that inorganic cobalt may be important in certain other enzymes (Taylor & Marks 1978), but this is at present unproved.

Copper

Copper is a constituent of several important enzymes, including cytochrome oxidase which is a key enzyme in mitochondrial energy production for protein biosynthesis, δ-amino levulinate-dehydratase and ceruloplasmin which are important in haemoglobin formation and iron metabolism, and dopamine β-hydroxylase which is involved in synthesis of neurotransmitters such as noradrenaline and adrenaline.

Copper deficiency is rare in humans. It is characterized by anaemia, neutropenia and bone demineralization, and in Menke's syndrome by cerebral degeneration. The haematological changes have been seen in patients on total parenteral nutrition (Vilter et al 1974). Although measured plasma copper levels may not be a good indication of total body stores (Kay 1981), they were reduced in these patients. The daily requirement of copper has been set at 2 mg. There is not any greatly increased loss in critically ill patients.

Fluorine

This has been shown to be an essential trace element in animals, playing a role in haemopoiesis. In humans the only important effect of fluorine deficiency demonstrated to date has been the encouragement of dental caries.

As with other trace elements, toxicity can occur with excess dosage, in this case mainly manifest as skeletal changes. Several volatile anaesthetic agents contain fluoride atoms, which may be released during metabolism. In the case of methoxyflurane, the inorganic fluoride concentration may rise to toxic levels — above 50 mmol l^{-1}, after prolonged exposure, and toxicity is manifested by a high-output renal failure (Mazze et al 1971). With enzyme induction, high F^- levels may also occur after enflurane anaesthesia (Mazze et al 1982), but renal toxicity is unlikely as pulmonary excretion of enflurane is more rapid.

Iodine

Iodine is required for normal thyroid function, and thus the place of iodine as an essential trace element is well known. The daily requirement is about 100 μg. As it is taken up preferentially by the thyroid, radioactive iodine, ^{131}I, is used in diagnosis of thyroid disorders and treatment of thyroid cancer. Iodide is sometimes used in management of hyperthyroidism, and in particular in immediate preoperative preparation for surgery. By apparently complex and poorly understood mechanisms, release of thyroid hormone is inhibited, and the size and vascularity of the gland is reduced, with a maximal effect in 10–15 days.

Iron

Iron is required for haemoglobin formation, as well as in some enzyme systems. As the details of iron deficiency and its therapy are well known from general texts, they will not be covered at length here.

Manganese

Manganese activates a number of enzymes, including some which are involved in synthesis of polysaccharides and glycoproteins. Deficiency in young animals results in impaired skeletal and other growth. In man, there may be depression of vitamin K-dependent clotting factors.

Molybdenum

Molybdenum is an essential part of the enzymes xanthine oxidase, sulphite oxidase and aldehyde oxidase, which act in the disposal of purines and pyrimidines, cystine and methionine, and various other nitrogen-containing heterocyclic compounds.

Deficiency of molybdenum can occur, and there is also a complicated three-way interaction between copper, molybdenum and sulphur. Thus in cattle, deficiency of either metal may lead to excessive retention and toxicity of the other, but adequate dietary sulphur is also required for molybdenum to protect against copper toxicity, perhaps because it is required in the form of a thiomolybdate.

Molybdenum deficiency has been seen as a syndrome of amino-acid intolerance with tachycardia, tachypnoea and headache leading rapidly to disorientation and coma (Abumrad et al 1981). The patient described had been fed parenterally for 6 months and responded to 300 μg/day ammonium molybdate.

Selenium

Selenium has been relatively recently recognized as an essential trace element in humans. Glutathione peroxidase is a selenoprotein which has a broad role in protecting tissues from oxidative damage. Ethanol metabolism in the liver generates toxic radicals which are broken down by metalloenzymes including glutathione peroxidase; levels of this and of selenium are reduced in patients developing alcoholic cirrhosis (Ritland and Aaseth 1987).

Where the diet contains less than 30 μg selenium per day, signs of deficiency may occur. The commonest manifestation is Keshan disease, a cardiomyopathy named for the Chinese province where it was discovered. A similar picture has occurred in patients on long-term parenteral nutrition (Johnson et al 1981, Stanley et al 1982).

The toxic effects of selenium are less well known, but chronic exposure can result in pulmonary and other damage.

Zinc

Over 80 metalloenzymes require zinc for their function, and many of these occupy key roles in DNA and RNA synthesis and degradation, and in carbohydrate, protein and lipid metabolism. Zinc deficiency is thus likely to have widespread consequences, and as there is little or no functional store of zinc in the body, its effects can occur in a few days. Human zinc deficiency showing features which include retarded growth, hypogonadism and skin changes was first reported from the Middle East, but a degree of dietary deficiency can occur even in well-nourished populations, for example in middle and upper socioeconomic groups in the United States (Prasad 1979).

The distribution of zinc in the body is not uniform — pancreas, skin, prostate, liver, eye and muscle having high concentrations of the metal.

The normal plasma level is 12–20 μmol l^{-1}, but as with other mainly intracellular substances, plasma levels may not be a good guide to adequacy of body content (Fleming 1989). Normally the main route of excretion is faecal with only about 10 μmol/day urinary loss. However, in catabolic patients the loss increases by two to four times in parallel with increases in potassium and creatinine, the major source of this loss being muscle. In some critically ill patients, losses of almost 100 times normal have been seen.

Acute zinc deficiency may occur in severely ill patients on total parenteral nutrition (Kay et al 1976), especially as most preparations for parenteral nutrition contain very small quantities of zinc. The first manifestation is diarrhoea, which may occur when zinc levels are not much below normal. More severe signs occur when the plasma zinc level is below 3 mmol l^{-1}, and include inflammatory skin changes and alopecia.

The normally recommended dose for zinc supplementation is 15 mg per day for adults. However, in view of the increased losses of zinc in seriously ill patients, higher quantities may be desirable. Wolman and colleagues (1979) estimated intravenous requirements as between 2.5 and 18 mg zinc, while the cases described by Kay and colleagues responded rapidly to 80 mg zinc sulphate daily.

Zinc supplementation does appear to promote accelerated healing of burns and surgical wounds, but only in patients who are already zinc-deficient.

Zinc is relatively non-toxic as compared to other trace metals, but symptoms may occur with acute ingestion of large doses.

ACID–BASE BALANCE

In normal health the pH of the blood is maintained within a narrow range, between 7.36 and 7.44 units ($[H^+]$44–36 nmol l^{-1}). Acidity is usually described in terms of pH, and it must be remembered that this is a logarithmic scale, so that a fall in pH from 7.4 to 7.1 represents a doubling of H^+ concentration from 40 to 80 mmol l^{-1}.

Several different mechanisms in the body combine to maintain pH:

1. Buffering effect of bicarbonate ion;
2. Buffering effects of other substances — e.g. phosphate, haemoglobin, plasma proteins;
3. Ventilatory control of $P\text{CO}_2$ in response to chemoreceptor activity;
4. Changes in renal excretion of H^+.

In terms of intravenous therapy the most important of these to consider is the bicarbonate buffering system, although in terms of total buffering capacity it is not the most powerful.

Assessment of acid–base state

pH and $P\text{CO}_2$ are measured by specific electrodes. The nature of a disturbance of pH may be distinguished by considering both pH and $P\text{CO}_2$ — a rise in $P\text{CO}_2$ will result in a fall in pH, and vice-versa. $P\text{CO}_2$ may also change secondarily to a change in pH, as a compensating event. Changes in pH — acidosis or alkalosis — are defined as being respiratory or metabolic, depending on whether the primary event causing pH change was a change in ventialtion and thus $P\text{CO}_2$ (respiratory), or any other disturbance in acid–base balance (metabolic). The body will, when it is able, show compensation from one to the other; for example a metabolic acidosis will be compensated by hyperventilation and lowering of $P\text{CO}_2$, while a chronic respiratory acidosis will cause (slow) compensation by renal conservation of bicarbonate.

Indices of bicarbonate level

Bicarbonate and carbonic acid in equilibrium form a buffer system.

$$H^+ + HCO_3^- \rightleftharpoons H_2CO_3$$

The state of the equilibrium depends on the pH and $P\text{CO}_2$, and can be calculated using the Henderson–Hasselbalch equation

$$pH = pK + \log \frac{[HCO_3^-]}{[H_2CO_3]}$$

(the pK of carbonic acid is 6.10)
Such an equation is generally used in blood-gas analysers to derive plasma bicarbonate values from the measured pH and $P\text{CO}_2$.

The *plasma bicarbonate* level calculated in this way is the actual bicarbonate present, but it is usual to extrapolate further.

Standard bicarbonate is the amount of bicarbonate which would be present if the blood were equilibrated to a $P\text{CO}_2$ of 5.3 kPa at full oxygenation. The normal range is 22–26 mmol l^{-1}.

Table 33.1 Tentatively recommended daily allowances of water, energy, amino acids, carbohydrates, fat, and minerals for patients on complete intravenous nutrition. The basal allowances will cover resting metabolism, some physical activity and specific dynamic action, but no increased needs because of trauma, burns, etc. The *moderate* amounts should be used when the patient has increased losses or is in a depleted status. The *high* supply should be used in severe catabolic conditions as burns, after trauma, etc. Reproduced with permission from Wretlind (1978)

	Allowances per kg body weight for adult			Allowances per kg body weight for neonates and infants		
	Basal amounts	Moderate amounts	High supply	Basal amounts	Moderate amounts	High supply
Water	30 ml	50 ml	75–100 ml	100 ml	125 ml	125–150 ml
Energy	30 kcal = 0.13 MJ	35–40 kcal = 0.15–0.17 MJ	50–60 kcal = 0.21–0.25 MJ	90–120 kcal = 0.38–0.50 MJ	125 kcal = 0.52 MJ	125–150 kcal = 0.52–0.63 MJ
Amino acid nitrogen	90 mg (0.7 g amino acids)	0.2–0.3 g N (1.5–2 amino acids)	0.4–0.5 g N (3–3.5 g amino acids)	0.3 g (2.5 g amino acids)	0.45 g (3.5 g amino acids)	0.5 g (4.0 g amino acids)
Glucose	2 g	5 g	7 g	12–18 g	18–25 g	25–30 g
Fat	2 g	3 g	3–4 g	4 g	4–6 g	6 g
Sodium	1–1.4 mmol	2–3 mmol	3–4 mmol	1–2.5 mmol	3–4 mmol	4–5 mmol
Potassium	0.7–0.9 mmol	2 mmol	3–4 mmol	2 mmol	2–3 mmol	4–5 mmol
Calcium	0.11 mmol	0.15 mmol	0.2 mmol	0.5 mmol	1 mmol	1.5–2 mmol
Magnesium	0.04 mmol	0.15–0.20 mmol	0.3–0.4 mmol	0.15 mmol	0.15–0.5 mmol	1 mmol
Iron	0.25–1.0 μmol	1.0 μmol	1.0 μmol	2 μmol		3–4 μmol
Manganese	0.1 μmol	0.3 μmol	0.6 μmol	0.3 μmol	0.7 μmol	1 μmol
Zinc	0.7 μmol	0.7–1.5 μmol	1.5–3 μmol	0.6 μmol	1 μmol	1.5 μmol
Copper	0.07 μmol	0.3–0.4 μmol	0.4–1 μmol	0.3 μmol		
Chromium	0.015 μmol			0.01 μmol		
Selenium	0.006 μmol			0.04 μmol		
Molybdenum	0.003 μmol					
Chlorine	1.3–1.9 mmol	2–3 mmol	3–4 mmol	2–4 mmol		4.6 mmol
Phosphorus	0.15 mmol	0.4 mmol	0.6–1.0 mmol	0.4–0.8 mmol	1.3–1.5 mmol	2.5–3 mmol
Fluorine	0.7 μmol	0.7–1.5 μmol		3 μmol		
Iodine	0.015 μmol			0.04 μmol		0.1 μmol

Buffer base is an estimate of the total buffering capacity of the blood, from bicarbonate and protein (including haemoglobin). It will be dependent on the patient's haemoglobin. The buffer base may be estimated from a nomogram such as that of Siggaard-Andersen, or by an algorithm in the analyser.

Base excess is an essentially practical concept of the amount of base or acid which needs to be added to return the pH of the blood to normal — i.e. to a pH of 7.4 at a P_{CO_2} of 5.3 kPa and full oxygenation at 37°C. It is the difference between measured buffer base and the normal value for buffer base at the patient's haemoglobin level.

This is the measurement used clinically in management of metabolic derangements. It is expressed in mmol l^{-1}, a negative result representing a base deficit. The normal range is ±3. Base excess is used practically, as the formula

$$\text{Base excess} \times \text{Body weight} \times -0.3$$

is the number of millimols base required for total correction of the base deficit in adults. Usual clinical practice is to administer one-half of this calculated amount initially. In neonates a relatively greater amount of base is required: 0.45 to 0.5 instead of 0.3 mmol kg^{-1} body weight — see Chapter 4.

Sodium bicarbonate, $NaHCO_3$

This is the solution most commonly used in correction of metabolic acidosis. A preparation of 8.4% sodium bicarbonate contains 1 mmol ml^{-1} of sodium and of bicarbonate, which is convenient for administration. This concentrated solution also limits the volume administered, which may be important, for example in the coronary-care unit. However, for routine practice more dilute solutions may be preferred for several reasons. The high osmolarity of the solution can cause severe skin and tissue damage should it leak outside a vein — not an uncommon happening in the emergency situations in which it is used. Use of a concentrated solution also makes it more likely that excess may inadvertently be administered, with a danger of hypernatraemia — especially dangerous in the dehydrated child. Too rapid correction of acidosis is also to be avoided, and care must be taken to prevent the development of hypokalaemia as potassium moves into cells as the acidosis is corrected — for example in treatment of diabetic keto-acidosis.

Sodium bicarbonate may also be the solution of choice for sodium replacement in some hyponatraemic patients who are also acidotic.

Sodium lactate

One-sixth molar sodium lactate, a racemic mixture of d- and l-lactate, contains 162 mmol l^{-1} sodium and lactate, and is thus approximately isotonic. It is preferred by some clinicians for correction of acidosis where an immediate action is not required. Lactate ions are metabolized in the liver to bicarbonate. It should not therefore be used in patients with impaired hepatic function, or obviously in patients whose acidosis is already due to shock or to lactic acidosis.

PLASMA EXPANDERS

Several colloidal solutions are employed at present as substitutes for human plasma proteins, or for other properties which they possess. They are substituting largely for albumin, which has a molecular weight (MW) of 65 000. They fall into three groups — dextrans, gelatins and hydroxyethylated starch. These preparations do not have any oxygen-carrying capacity, unlike fluoro-carbon compounds, which are usually made up in combination with another plasma expander, and have now reached the stage of clinical trials.

Dextrans

Dextrans are polysaccharides made by fermentation of sucrose by a strain of *Leuconostoc mesenteroides*, and subjected to subsequent hydrolysis and fractionation to obtain compounds of differing average molecular weight:

1. Dextran 70 intravenous infusion is a 5.5–6.5% solution of average MW 70 000.

2. Dextran 40 intravenous infusion is a 10% solution of average MW 40 000.
3. Other preparations, e.g. 60 000, 110 000, 150 000 are also available in some countries.

Dextran 70 has similar colloid osmotic pressure to plasma, and therefore is effective as a plasma expander. Because of its lower molecular weight, and because it is supplied in a slightly more concentrated form, dextran 40 is more osmotically active. It will therefore temporarily attract extravascular fluid into the circulation, and give an initially greater effect than higher molecular weight preparations. However, this apparent benefit is transitory, and is more than offset by the greater incidence of renal complications with dextran 40.

About half of an infused dose of dextran 70 is excreted within 24 h, while 5–10% remains in the circulation by 7 days. Some undergoes metabolism, mainly in the liver, to CO_2 and water. Dextran 40 is eliminated more rapidly, 60% being excreted within 6 h. As well as expanding the circulating volume, dextran has other effects, which may limit the quantities infused.

Dextran has an antithrombotic effect due to a combination of several factors (Bergqvist 1982). Platelet adhesiveness is reduced, this effect being maximal 1–2 h after dextran infusion, and factor VIII activity is also reduced. However, there is no observable effect on primary haemostasis with dextran 40 or dextran 70 in the doses normally used clinically (up to 1 g kg^{-1}, Bergqvist 1982). Studies of operative blood loss in dextran-treated patients have not been entirely conclusive, but there is no important increase, and dextran can be given in doses up to 1–1.5 g kg^{-1} to normal patients. However, caution should be exercised in any patient with a congenital or acquired haematological deficit, or who is receiving heparin.

Dextran 70 has been used in the prophylaxis of post-operative deep venous thrombosis, in varying doses. A typical regime would be 500–1000 ml/day initially, reducing after 3 days to 500 ml on alternate days for 10 days (Barber et al 1977). A reduction in infusion rate is required because of gradual accumulation of higher molecular weight fractions with their slower rate of elimination, and consequent danger of circulatory overload. The effectiveness of dextran has not been proven in all trials, but most reports have been encouraging.

In the management of microcirculatory insufficiency, dextran 40 has been used more than dextran 70, although there is probably little difference in their effectiveness, and use of dextran 40 may be more likely to lead to renal or circulatory overload problems.

Sensitivity reactions can occur to dextrans, although the incidence is low — only 0.008% for life-threatening reactions (Ring & Messmer 1977). Histamine released from mast cells may react with a 'histamine receptor' on cell membranes (Moodley et al 1982), but histamine release is probably not the mechanism for the more severe reactions (Doenicke et al 1977). 'Hapten inhibition' by prior injection of very low molecular weight dextran — dextran 1, MW 1000 — appears to dramatically reduce the incidence of reactions to dextran 40 or 70 (Ljungström et al 1988).

A further complication of dextran infusion is renal failure. Dextrans with an MW of below 60 000 are filtered rapidly, and probably cause renal failure by plugging of tubules. This is more likely when renal perfusion is already reduced, as in the shocked patient. It is also much more likely to occur with dextran 40, but use of dextran 70 can also lead to this problem. Certain rules have been suggested to reduce the risks (Holti 1973):

1. Do not give more than 1 l/day;
2. Do not give if urine output is less than 1500 ml/day;
3. Stop if urine SG rises above 1045;
4. Do not give if blood urea is above 10 mmol $^{-1}$.

Gelatin solutions

These belong to three groups — oxypolygelatins, modified fluid gelatin and urea-linked gelatin (polygeline, 'Haemaccel'). They are of average MW 30 000–35 000, so that they remain in the circulation for a much shorter time than dextrans. However side-effects and effects other than those due to volume loading and dilution appear to be minimal. Anaphylactoid reactions are thought to be commoner than with dextrans, but the incidence with polygeline, which is cross-linked with hexamethylene di-isocyanate, has been reduced since excess of the latter was removed in manufacture (Schoning et al 1982). It has proved to be a safe and adequate plasma expander for resuscitation in the battlefield (Williams et al 1983).

Hydroxyethylated starch (HES)

This is prepared from amylopectin, a polymer of starch, which is resistant to the action of alpha amylase. A preparation with an MW of about 450 000 (hetastarch) is the most commonly available; pentastarch has an MW of about 200 000. Hydroxyethyl starch is broken down by alpha amylase in the blood, and smaller molecules excreted by the kidneys. The half life of hetastarch is

initially (in the first 48 hours) 1.5–3.8 days, and the terminal half life is as much as a month, so that multiple dosing may lead to accumulation (Klotz and Kroemer 1987). In general, the uses and effects of HES are similar to those of dextran. Hetastarch has little effect on coagulation, and may be used in place of albumin (Falk et al 1988), but there is a reduction in factor VIII which is greater than that simply due to dilution; this effect is less with pentastarch (Strauss et al 1988). Like the other plasma expanders, there is a low but definite incidence of anaphylactoid reactions (Doenicke et al 1977).

PARENTERAL FEEDING

The purpose of intravenous feeding is to provide the patient's energy needs together with substances needed for synthetic processes in the body.

The criterion of success in nutrition should be that the body does not have to break down any of its own structural components (i.e. proteins) in order to provide energy, and so the aim of feeding may also be defined practically as conservation of lean body mass, or the achieving of a positive nitrogen balance. In order to achieve this, three factors must be considered: the provision of components specifically to be metabolized to produce energy; provision of the amino-acid building blocks for protein syntheses, and provision of the many other minerals or trace elements, vitamins and essential fatty acids which the body cannot synthesize itself.

Various considerations, some of a commercial nature, have determined the composition of the mixtures available for parenteral nutrition. Ideally the various components should be provided in a form similar to that found in the peripheral circulation, and in proportions which will maintain the circulating concentrations at near physiological levels (Krebs 1978).

Energy sources

The basic energy currency of the body is in the form of high-energy bonds in substances such as ATP. Food molecules provide energy for formation of these bonds, as they are 'burned' in the body. Complete breakdown of carbohydrate or protein yields 4 kcal g^{-1}, and of fat, 9 kcal g^{-1}. Although administered amino acids may be utilized by the body as energy sources, they are not normally given with this intention, and energy is provided by carbohydrate or fat.

Carbohydrate

Glucose is usually considered to be the natural energy

fuel of the body, although in fact circulating fatty acids account for 50–90% of energy needs.

The carbohydrates currently in use in parenteral nutrition are glucose, fructose, sorbitol and ethanol. The pathways for metabolism of glucose, and of sorbitol and fructose are shown in Fig. 33.1

Glucose

Glucose entry into cells is by facilitated diffusion which is highly insulin-dependent, and infusion of too great a glucose load may lead to hyperglycaemia. In normal humans, up to 0.5 g kg^{-1} h^{-1} glucose can be given (Dudrick et al 1972). However, at rates above 0.3 g kg^{-1} h^{-1}, any extra glucose given may be converted into and stored as fat, rather than contributing to energy needs (Burke et al 1979). In addition, stressed patients are often insulin-resistant, and require exogenous insulin to be given. Problems of hyperglycaemia, together with the high osmolality of concentrated glucose solutions led in the past to a search for alternative carbohydrates.

Fructose

Fructose entry into cells is not insulin-dependent, and thus there is not the same danger of hyperglycaemia as with glucose. However, 30% of infused fructose is normally metabolized to lactate, and the removal of lactate from the blood is the rate-limiting step in full utilization of fructose. If the body's capacity to remove lactate is exceeded, then lactic acidosis will develop. Hypoxic conditions lead to a greater proportion of fructose following this pathway, and patients in whom these conditions occur are also those ill patients who are al-

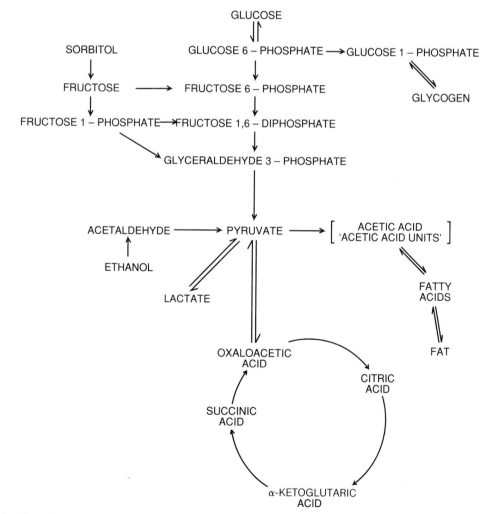

Fig. 33.1 The pathways for metabolism of glucose, sorbitol and fructose.

ready on the borderline of metabolic acidosis. Neonates also have a greater likelihood of developing lactic acidosis if fed using fructose. The maximum safe infusion rate for fructose may be quoted as 0.25 g kg^{-1} h^{-1} (Newton et al 1978).

Sorbitol

Sorbitol is a hexahydric alcoholic sugar. It is oxidized to fructose in the liver and kidney (Fig. 33.1), and thus it shares most of the advantages and disadvantages of fructose. However, the conversion of sorbitol to fructose does require energy, and may be a rate-limiting step.

Ethanol (ethyl alcohol)

Ethanol provides 7.1 kcal g^{-1}, and is normally metabolized according to zero-order kinetics at a rate of about 10 g h^{-1} in an adult. The body is well equipped to deal with alcohol, because alcohol may in nature often be encountered in decaying fruit. The euphoria which may accompany its use for parenteral feeding is probably an advantage, and high blood levels are unlikely to occur with the amounts normally infused. Its metabolism is enhanced by fructose, and for this reason the combination of fructose and ethanol is found in several proprietary mixtures. However, this is a questionable practice, as the effect of alcohol on fructose metabolism is such as to increase the chances of the development of lactic acidosis.

Fat

Fat gives 9 kcal g^{-1} and is thus an efficient energy source. The fat preparations currently available are based on soya bean oil, and are prepared as an emulsion of vegetable oil particles which are of a similar size to chylomicrons, together with an emulsifying agent, and a polyhydric alcohol to make the solution isotonic. Cottonseed oil emulsions have been found to be hepatotoxic. Fat emulsion is not hypertonic and thus avoids the problem of venous damage and reduces the total osmolar load to the patient.

Fat gives rise to free fatty acids, which are the primary fuel for many parts of the body, including muscle.

As well as acting as an energy source, fat emulsions contain linoleic and linolenic acids which are precursors of arachidonic and docosahexaenoic acids, important constituents of cell membranes. These cannot be synthesized in the body, and are thus classified as essential fatty acids. Deficiency syndromes can become apparent after some weeks of a diet deficient in essential fatty acids, but abnormal blood levels may occur as early as 3 days (Paulsrud 1972, Wene et al 1975). The administration of a half-litre of fat emulsion per week is sufficent to prevent development of essential fatty acid deficiency.

Choice of substrate for energy provision

The mainstream of thought as to energy provision has evolved gradually over the past two decades. Initially in North America, glucose was used as the main or only calorie source, while in the UK and Europe other carbohydrates such as fructose, sorbitol, ethanol and others were common, often with fat supplementation. European practice has changed in that many authorities now consider glucose to be the only carbohydrate which should be used. This is certainly so in seriously ill patients, but those who are not highly catabolic — for example those cachetic patients receiving preoperative supplementation — may do as well or better with nonglucose carbohydrates (Woolfson et al 1979), and be at less risk of hypo- or hyperglycaemia.

Fat emulsions were available later in the USA than in Europe. Traumatized or septic patients are more dependent on fat and amino acids for energy provision than is the normal, and may not be able to utilize large amounts of carbohydrate, so excessive glucose intake may result in raised oxygen consumption and fatty infiltration of the liver. For these reason the present trend is towards a balanced approach, where at least 30% of calories are provided from carbohydrate and at least 30% from fat.

Because of the complications associated with large quantities of glucose infused into hypermetabolic patients, recent data would suggest that most critically injured patients should maintain energetic balance by receiving only enough glucose calories to meet their resting metabolic requirements (30–35 kcal kg^{-1} per day). If additional calories are required, fat emulsion should be administered (Black & Wilmore 1983).

In the ill patient, insulin resistance is common, and so it is routine practice to administer insulin as required, along with infusion of glucose. As well as maintaining normoglycaemia, insulin has a positive effect in encouraging positive nitrogen balance.

Amino acids

Dietary protein is absorbed as amino acids. These are extracted by the liver or other organs and used in protein synthesis. The body maintains an amino-acid 'pool', and there is a dynamic state of movement of nitrogen as amino acids between organs as they are required. The essential amino acids (Table 33.2) are so called because they cannot be synthesized in the body and must be given exogenously. They consist of the three branched-chain amino acids, leucine, isoleucine and valine, together with threonine, methionine (which can be converted into cysteine), phenylalanine (which can be converted into tyrosine), tryptophan and lysine. Methionine is one of the most important because it is a main source of organic sulphur used for making taurine, etc. It is also an important source of biologically labile methyl (CH_3) groups used in the formation of choline, creatine and adrenaline. In addition, histidine and arginine can only be synthesized by humans in small quantities, so they are almost essential. The latter is specially valuable in liver disease in that it takes part in the Krebs urea cycle and helps to convert ammonia to urea. Thus the classification into essential and non-essential amino acids is not always clear-cut; the classification is examined by Laidlaw and Kopple (1987), and their further subdivisions indicated in Table 33.2.

Altough the normal plasma concentrations of the amino acids are known, the exact influence of disease on these, and the effects of infusing amino-acid mixtures of differing proportions, are far from clear. In deciding the formulation of an amino-acid solution for intravenous nutrition, the early principle of using the

'profile' found a first-class protein of the diet (for example egg albumen), has not yet been superseded. However, studies of protein turnover in disease are beginning to provide a better understanding. It is apparent that the three branched-chain amino acids (BCAA) leucine, isoleucine and valine, have several unique properties. These are used by the body as a peripheral calorie source during stress or starvation, and it may be that solutions enriched in BCAA may provide a better inhibition of body protein breakdown and stimulation of protein synthesis in traumatized and septic patients (Madsen 1983). Such considerations have still to make themselves felt in the formulation of commercially available preparations. The use of BCAA infusions has also been advocated in hepatic encephalopathy, but it has not yet been proven that this is more effective than conventional therapy (Alexander et al 1989).

The older solutions of amino acids were prepared by hydrolysis of proteins such as fibrin or casein. However alkaline hydrolysis degrades some of the amino acids and always results in a mixture of D- and L-forms. In general only L-forms of the amino acids can be utilized in the body, so that the D-forms are destroyed to provide energy. The exceptions are D-methionine and D-phenylalanine, as these can be used in either form. At present amino acid solutions are produced by mixing the synthetic components in a planned manner, which ensures that only the l-forms are present and that pH is controlled at a figure which will minimize venous irritation. Cost still leads some manufacturers to add a larger amount of the cheaper non-essential amino acids such as glycine, but this can be readily checked.

It might be thought that plasma was an ideal nutrient but, like other proteins, the albumin and globulin must be broken down to their constituent amino acids before use by the body. They are in fact deficient in tryptophan and isoleucine, and tracer studies have shown that it takes many weeks for significant amounts of amino acids derived from infused plasma proteins to be incorporated into body protein.

Table 33.2 Essential and non-essential amino acids

Essential amino acids	Non-essential amino acids
*Leucine[2]	Alanine
*Isoleucine[2]	Glycine
*Valine[2]	Arginine[4]
Phenylalanine[2]	Proline
Methionine[2]	Tyrosine[3,4]
Lysine[1]	Ornithine[3]
Histidine[2]	Aspartic acid
Threonine[1]	Cysteine[3,4]
Tryptophan[2]	Cystine
	Glutamic acid
	Serine

* Branched chain.
[1] Totally indispensable.
[2] Carbon skeleton indispensable
   (i.e. ketoacid or hydroxyacid analogue can be substituted).
[3] Conditionally indispensable
   (may become indispensable in absence of dietary precursor).
[4] Acquired indispensable
   (may be indispensable in immaturity — newborn, in genetic or acquired disease, or in severe stress).
See Laidlaw and Kopple (1987) for details of classification.

Vitamins

Vitamins are organic compounds of diverse composition, which are essential to normal functioning of mammals, but which cannot be synthesized in the body. They are required in small quantities for synthesis of cofactors essential to various metabolic reactions. This definition excludes the essential amino acids, which are required in much larger amounts.

Vitamins are classified into water-soluble and fat-soluble groups. Recommended dietary allowances

Table 33.3 Tentatively recommended daily amounts of vitamins in basal metabolic state and in conditions of increased need. The recommendations for *basal*, *moderate* and *high* supply are explained in the text to Table 33.1.

	Allowances per kg body weight per day for adult			Allowances per kg body weight per day for neonates and infants		
	Basal amounts	Moderate amounts	High supply	Basal amounts	Moderate amounts	High supply
Thiamin	0.02 mg	0.04 mg	0.3 mg	0.05 mg	0.1 mg	2 mg
Riboflavin	0.03 mg	0.06 mg	0.3 mg	0.1 mg	0.2 mg	0.4 mg
Nicotinamide	0.2 mg	0.4 mg	2 mg	1 mg	2 mg	4 mg
Pyridoxine	0.03 mg	0.06 mg	0.4 mg	0.1 mg	0.2 mg	0.6 mg
Folic acid	3 μg	6 μg	6–9 μg	20 μg	40 μg	50 μg
Cyanocobalamin	0.03 μg	0.06 μg	0.06 μg	0.2 μg	0.4 μg	5 μg
Pantothenic acid	0.2 mg	0.4 mg	0.4 mg	1 mg	2 mg	
Biotin	5 μg	10 μg	10 μg	30 μg	60 μg	
Ascorbic acid	0.5 mg	2 mg	25 mg	3 mg	6 mg	20 mg
Retinol	10 μg (33 IU)	10 μg (33 IU)	20 μg (67 IU)	0.1 mg (333 IU)	0.1 mg (333 IU)	0.15 mg (500 IU)
Ergocalciferol or cholecalciferol	0.04 μg (2 IU)	0.04 μg (33 IU)	0.1 μg (4 IU)	2.5 μg (100 IU)	2.5 μg(100 IU)	2.5 μg (100 IU)
Phytylmenaquinone	2 μg	2 μg	2 μg	50 μg	50 μg	150 μg
Tocopherol	0.5 IU	0.75 IU	1 IU	1 IU	1–1.5 IU	1.5 IU

(RDA) have been laid down, based arbitrarily on minimum amounts needed to prevent deficiency disease. The amount required by a critically ill patient may be different, but such information is only slowly becoming available. Some recommendations are shown in Table 33.3 (Wretlind 1978).

REFERENCES

Abumrad N N, Schneider A J, Steel D, Rogers L S 1981 Amino-acid intolerance during prolonged parenteral nutrition reversed by molybdate therapy. American Journal of Clinical Nutrition 34: 2551–2559

Alexander W F, Spindel E, Harty R F, Cerda J J 1989 The usefulness of branched chain amino acids in patients with acute or chronic hepatic encephalopathy. American Journal of Gastroenterology 84: 91–96

Barber H M, Feil E J, Galasko C S et al 1977 A comparative study of dextran 40, warfarin and low dose heparin for the prophylaxis of thromboembolism following total hip replacement. Postgraduate Medical Journal 53: 130–133

Bergqvist D 1982 Dextran and haemostasis: a review. Acta Chirurgica Scandinavica 148: 633–640

Black P R, Wilmore D W 1983 Alterations in fuel metabolism in stress. In: Johnston I D A (ed) Advances in clinical nutritine. MTP Press, Lancaster

Brown R O, Forloines-Lynn S, Cross R E, Heizer W D 1986 Chromium deficiency after long-term total parenteral nutrition. Digestive Diseases and Sciences 31: 661–664

Burke J F, Wolfe R R, Mullany C J, Mathews D E, Bier D M 1979 Parameters of optimal glucose infusion and possible hepatitis and respiratory abnormalities following excessive glucose intake. Annals of Surgery 190: 274–284

Doenicke A, Grote B, Lorenz W 1977 Blood and blood substitutes British Journal of Anaesthesia 49: 681–688

Dudrick S J, Macfadyen B V, VanBuren C T, Ruberg R L, Maynard A T 1972 Parenteral hyperalimentation.

Metabolic problems and solutions. Annals of Surgery 176: 259–264

Dunlop W M, James G W, Hume D M 1974 Anemia and neutropenia caused by copper deficiency. Annals of Internal Medicine 80: 470–476

Falk J L, Rackow E C, Astiz M E, Weil M H 1988 Effects of hetastarch and albumin on coagulation in patients with septic shock. Journal of Clinical Pharmacology 28: 412–415

Fleming C R 1989 Trace element metabolism in adult patients requiring total parenteral nutrition. American Journal of Clinical Nutrition 49: 573–579

Flowers C E 1965 Magnesium sulfate in obstetrics. American Journal of Obstetrics and Gynecology 91: 763

Heining M P, Band D M, Linton R A 1984 Choice of calcium salt. A comparison of calcium chloride and gluconate on plasma ionised calcium. Anaesthesia 39: 1079–1082

Hibbard B M, Rosen M 1977 The management of severe pre-eclampsia and eclampsia. British Jounal of Anaesthesia 49: 3–9

Holti G 1973 Intermittent low molecular weight dextran infusion in the management of ischaemic skin disorders. Bibliotheca Anatomica 11: 159–363

Jeejeebhoy K N, Chu R C, Marlissa E B, Greenberg G R, Bruce-Robertson A 1977 Chromium deficiency, glucose intolerance and neuropathy reversed by chromium supplementation, in a patient receiving long term total parenteral nutrition. American Journal of Clinical Nutrition 30: 531–538

Johnson R A, Baker S S, Fallon J T, Maynard E P, Ruskin J N, Wen Z, Cohen H J 1981 An occidental case of cardiomyopathy and selenium deficiency. New England Journal of Medicine 304: 1210–1212

Kay R G 1981 Zinc and copper in human nutrition. Journal of Human Nutrition 35: 25–36

Kay R G, Tasman-Jones C, Pybus J, Whiting R, Black H 1976 A syndrome of acute zinc deficiency during total parenteral alimentation in man. Annals of Surgery 183: 331–340

Klotz U, Kroemer H 1987 Clinical pharmacokinetic considerations in the use of plasma expanders. Clinical Pharmacokinetics 12: 123–135

Krebs H A 1978 Some general considerations concerning the use of carbohydrates in parenteral nutrition. In: Johnston I D A (ed) Advances in clinical nutrition. MTP Press, Lancaster

Laidlaw S A, Kopple J D 1987 Newer concepts of the indispensable amino acids. American Journal of Clinical Nutrition 46: 593–605

Ljungström K-G, Renck H, Hedin W, Richter W, Wiholm B-E 1988 Hapten inhibition and dextran anaphylaxis. Anaesthesia, 43: 729–732

Madsen D C 1983 Branched-chain amino-acids: metabolic roles and clinical applications. In Johnston I D A (ed) Advances in clinical nutrition. MTP Press, Lancaster

Mazze R I, Trudell J R, Cousins M J 1971 Methoxyflurane metabolism and renal dysfunction: clinical correlation in man. Anesthesiology 35: 247–252

Mazze R I, Woodruff R E, Heerdt M E 1982 Isoniazid-induced eflurane defluorination in humans. Anesthesiology 57: 5–8

McGeown M G 1983 Clinical management of electrolyte disorders. Martinus Nijhoff, Boston

Moodley I, Mongar J, Foreman J C 1982 Histamine release induced by dextran: the nature of the dextran receptor. European Journal of Pharmacology 83: 69–81

Newman J H, Neff T A, Ziporin P 1977 Acute respiratory failure associated with hypophosphatemia. New England Journal of Medicine 296: 1101–1103

Newton D, Connor H, Woods H F 1978, Metabolic pathways for carbohydrates in parenteral nutrition. In: Johnston I D A (ed) Advances in clinical nutrition. MTP Press, Lancaster

O'Connor L R, Wheeler W S, Bethune J E 1977 Effect of hypophosphatemia on myocardial performance in man. New England Journal of Medicine 297: 901–903

Paulsrud J R 1972 Essential fatty acid deficiency in infants induced by fat-free I V feeding. American Journal of Clinical Nutrition 25: 897–904

Prasad A S 1979 Clinical, biochemical and pharmacological

role of zinc. Annual Review of Pharmacology and Toxicology 20: 393–426

Ring J, Messmer K 1977 Incidence and severity of anaphylactoid reactions to colloid volume substitutes, Lancet i: 466–469

Ritland S, Aaseth J 1987 Trace elements and the liver. Journal of Hepatology 5: 118–122

Rothe K F 1982 Comparison of intra- and extracellular buffering of clinically used buffer substances: tris and bicarbonate. Acta Anaesthesiologica Scandinavica 26:194–198

Rudowski W J 1980 Evaluation of modern plasma expanders and blood substitutes. British Journal of Hospital Medicine 23: 389–399

Schneider A J L, Biebuyck J F 1983 Intraoperative management of patients receiving total parenteral nutrition. Clinics in Anaesthesiolgy 1: 647–667

Schoning B, Lorenz W, Doenicke A 1982 Prophylaxis of anaphylactoid reactions to a polypeptide plasma substitute by H_1 plus H_2-receptor antagonists: synopsis of three randomised controlled trials. Klinische Wochenschrift 60: 1048

Stanley J C, Nesbitt G, Alexander J P 1982 Selenium deficiency during total parenteral nutrition — a case report. Ulster Medical Journal 51: 130–132

Strauss R G, Stansfield C, Henriksen R A, Villhauer P J 1988 Pentastarch may cause fewer effects on coagulation than hetastarch. Transfusion 28: 257–260

Taylor A, Marks V 1978 Cobalt: a review. Journal of Human Nutrition 32: 165–167

Vilter R W, Bozian R C, Hess E V, Zellner D C, Petering H G 1974 Manifestations of copper deficiency in a patient with systemic sclerosis on intravenous hyperalimentation. New England Journal of Medicine 291: 188–192

Wene J, Connor W, DenBesten L 1975 The development of essential fatty acid deficiency in healthy men fed fat-free diets intravenously and orally. Journal of Clinical Investigation 56: 127–134

Williams J G, Riley T R D, Moody R A 1983 Resuscitation experience in the Falkland Islands campaign. British Medical Journal 286: 775–777

Wolman S L, Anderson G H, Marliss E B, Jeejeebhoy K N 1979 Zinc in total parenteral nutrition: requirements and metabolic effects. Gastroenterology 76: 458–467

Woolfson A M J, Heatley R V, Allison S P 1979 Insulin to inhibit protein catabolism after injury. New England Journal of Medicine 300: 14–17

Wretlind A 1978 Parenteral nutrition. Surgical Clinics of North America 58: 1055–1070

34. Adverse reactions and drug interaction

W. McCaughey   R. S. J. Clarke

Ehrlich's concept of the 'magic bullet' is still valid in considering today's drugs. Many of the body's functions are controlled by endogenous substances which have a specific action only at a single site, and many others by substances which, although they are capable of action in several systems, are delivered accurately only to the required site. Drugs are rarely so precise.

Adverse reactions to drugs are common, and the incidence of adverse reactions increases dramatically as a larger number of drugs is given to the patient. It has been suggested that 'one seventh of all hospital days is devoted to the care of drug toxicity' (Melmon 1971), and although this is certainly an overstatement, the problem is serious. Adverse reactions to drugs take several forms.

Overdosage

The exact control of dosage of some drugs may be both critical and difficult. Overdosage of a drug may be absolute, where more than the intended dose is given in error, or because the bioavailability has changed (as occurred some time ago with the introduction of a new preparation of digoxin) or the drug is administered by an inappropriate route (for example accidental intravenous injection of local anaesthetic). It may also be relative, due to an abnormality in the patient; for example, hypokalaemic patients are abnormally sensitive to digitalis.

Intolerance

Here the patient exhibits a qualitatively normal response to the drug, but at an abnormally low dose. This may be simply a response at the extreme of the normal range of variation. The Gaussian distribution of variation in response to drugs includes individuals who are unusually sensitive and those who are resistant. The response to some drugs shows two or more genetically determined populations — for example, the response to

suxamethonium in normal persons and those with abnormal pseudocholinesterase.

Idiosyncrasy

'Idiosyncrasy' is a response which is qualitatively different from the action of the drug in normal individuals, again often genetically determined. Of importance to anaesthetists are the abnormal responses to several drugs in patients with acute intermittent porphyria and in those susceptible to the malignant hyperpyrexia syndrome.

Allergy and hypersensitivity

Allergic and hypersensitivity responses are not closely dose-related, and are not related to the usual spectrum of effects and side-effects of the drug.

Direct organ toxicity

Some substances may directly damage cells of a particular organ or system, either because they are specifically toxic to these cells or because they are concentrated in one area. Carbon tetrachloride, for example, damages liver cells. Alternatively, a metabolite may be responsible; inorganic fluoride from metabolized methoxyflurane leads to renal damage if there is excessive exposure to the drug.

Secondary effects

The effect may be only indirectly related to the action of the drug; for example, vitamin deficiency in patients whose gut bacteria have been modified by broad-spectrum antibiotics.

Drug interaction

When more than one drug is given, one may modify the

action of the other in some manner. Predictable interactions form the basis of the drug combinations used in anaesthesia. However, with the increasing number of drugs being used in different facets of the patient's treatment, there is a considerable risk of unexpected interactions occurring before, during or after anaesthesia and surgery. A growing knowledge and understanding of the mode of action and pharmacokinetics of drugs is helping to make more of these understood and predictable. Overall, drug interactions form only a small proportion of all adverse reactions to drugs (6.9% in one large study), but some interactions are important. The number of reported interactions is enormous, and only those of specific importance in anaesthetic practice are discussed further.

Details of adverse reactions to drugs

The majority of the types of adverse reaction listed above are described in the appropriate chapters earlier in this book; indeed many of them may be anticipated by a clear knowledge and understanding of the principles underlying a drug's action, and of the pharmacokinetic principles. In the rest of this chapter allergic and hypersensitivity reactions, and interactions between drugs are discussed in more detail, as is one example of an idiosyncratic reaction, the malignant hyperpyrexia syndrome.

DRUG INTERACTION

Classification

The result of the interaction of two drugs may be an increased action of one or both, a decreased action or an effect different from either. Where possible, an interaction is described in terms both of the mechanism and site of interaction.

Where the result of interaction is an increased action, this may be of different types. An additive effect (or summation) occurs where the combined action of the drugs is simply the sum of each (2 + 2 = 4) — allowing for the fact that it is generally the *log* dose which is proportional to effect. In this case there is in fact no real interaction between the drugs. Where the combined effect is greater than this (2 + 2 = 5) the effect is synergism, and the term potentiation is used where an agent shows no appreciable effect on the biological system, but exaggerates the response of the system to the other substance (2 + 0 = 3). The more subtle aspects

of these differences are discussed by Halsey (1987) in a review article.

Where one drug opposes all, or part, of the action of another, the term antagonism is used. The concepts of competitive and non-competitive antagonism at receptor sites, and of agonist and partial agonist actions, have been discussed in Chapter 2. Non-competitive antagonism may also occur if a drug modifies the absorption, transport, biotransformation or excretion of the other. Also non-competitive are most of the interactions where the two drugs have directly opposing actions, though at different sites — physiological or functional antagonism. If the two drugs form an inactive complex this is chemical antagonism.

Drug interactions are most easily grouped according to the site at which interaction takes place. Drug interactions are also sometimes classified as kinetic or dynamic, depending on whether the influence is on the disposition of the drug affected, or on its effect at its site of action. Many interactions can be predicted from a knowledge of the principles of pharmacokinetics and of the mode of action of the drugs concerned, and so this chapter should be read in conjunction with the relevant sections of Chapters 2 and 3, which describe these principles.

PHARMACOKINETIC INTERACTIONS

Direct chemical or physical interaction

Interaction may occur even before administration, as in the case of the chemical incompatibility of thiopentone and suxamethonium. Some substances may react with the container; for example, insulin molecules will stick to the walls of a glass or plastic container. Many drugs may be incompatible with infusion fluids — penicillins lose their activity over a few hours in alkaline dextrose solutions (such as lactated Ringer's solution in dextrose), while ampicillin (which is itself alkaline) is inactivated in dextrose. With more complicated infusion fluids, incompatibilities are multiple, and additions should be kept to a minimum.

Many drugs cannot be mixed together for administration because one will partly or completely inactivate the other; for example, gentamicin and carbenicillin, though these form a useful combination if given by separate routes. Similar actions can also occur within the body — when tetanus toxoid and antitetanus serum are given together at the same site the toxoid is largely ineffective. The reversal of heparin's anticoagulant effect by protamine is a direct chemical effect.

Modified absorption

Absorption of a drug may be modified by another constituent of the preparation or by another substance given simultaneously. Parenterally injected drugs will be absorbed more slowly when mixed with a vasoconstrictor (e.g. local anaesthetics with adrenaline or felypressin). Slow absorption will also occur if the drug is bound or adsorbed to another substance as in the slow-release insulin preparations. Some water-insoluble substances may depend on organic solvents or a solubilizing agent to increase absorption; diazepam is made up with propylene glycol and alcohol for this reason.

Orally administered drugs are absorbed through the lining of the stomach and intestine, and many factors may influence absorption, as described in detail in Chapter 3.

Transport and distribution

Most drugs are carried by the circulation from their sites of absorption to their sites of action and elimination. Competition for the same protein-binding site will result in changes in the free and bound fractions of the drug, and modify the pharmacokinetics of the drug, which may occasionally be clinically important. This is described in detail in Chapter 3, and will not be repeated here. Some relevant examples of this interaction are listed in Table 34.3.

In conditions where there is hypoalbuminaemia, a greater fraction of a given dose of drug will be unbound, which effect will be increased if other bound drugs have already occupied binding sites. This can result in a greater peak intensity of pharmacological action. Tubocurarine is unusual in that it is bound to γ-globulin, and dose requirements are related to globulin levels (Stovner et al 1971). Tubocurarine resistance is seen in liver disease, in which reversed albumin/globulin ratios are common.

Modified metabolism

The action of a drug is influenced to a large extent by the rate of its metabolic degradation (generally in the liver) and excretion as unchanged drug or as active or inactive metabolite. Interference by one drug with the metabolism of another may occur by several means. Commonly enzyme induction may increase the rate of metabolism, while inhibition of enzymes, either in the liver or elsewhere, may reduce it. Changes in regional blood flow, and especially liver blood flow, lead to changes in metabolism of drugs. The rate and direction of metabolism may also be influenced by availability of substrates — for example hypoxia favours a reductive pathway for halothane breakdown.

Few examples of enzyme induction are important in anaesthetic practice, although it may be that the toxicity of pethidine is potentiated by phenobarbitone pre-treatment (Stambaugh et al 1977), and it has been suggested (though not proved) that a similar increase in hepatotoxicity of some halogenated anaesthetics such as fluroxene can occur (Reynolds et al 1972).

Enzyme inhibition is caused by a few drugs. It may be due to a depression of the activity of the enzyme system, or to competition by the second drug as an alternative substrate for the enzyme system. Two relevant examples are the inhibition of monoamine oxidase and of cholinesterase.

Modified excretion

Change in the pH of urine modifies the excretion of many drugs. Weak bases such as amphetamine or pethidine are excreted more readily in an acid urine, while weak acids such as salicylates and phenobarbitone are excreted more readily in alkaline urine. This is the rationale of the regimens of forced alkaline diuresis which are used (perhaps less energetically now than in the past) to hasten excretion of aspirin or phenobarbitone in cases of overdosage.

Drugs may compete for the same transport mechanism in the kidney tubule. Probenecid blocks the excretory transport of organic acids, and in the early days of penicillin therapy was used therapeutically to raise blood penicillin levels. Less desirable interactions may occur — chlorpropamide and phenylbutazone interact, resulting in raised levels of chlorpropamide and a danger of hypoglycaemia.

Hypokalaemia may often result from the action of diuretic drugs, so that an indirect interaction between diuretic and digitalis occurs, the hypokalaemic patient being more sensitive to digitalis. Hypokalaemia from diuretic therapy may also cause prolonged paralysis from non-depolarizing muscle relaxants and may antagonize the anti-arrhythmic action of lignocaine or quinidine.

PHARMACODYNAMIC INTERACTIONS

Interactions at receptor sites

Many drugs have their actions at a particular receptor site which has a unique chemical configuration to which the drug attaches. Some act simply by denying access to a normal physiological transmitter substance, while others actively react with the receptor. The drug inter-actions of most interest to anaesthetists almost all occur at the receptor sites associated with the various divisions of the nervous system.

Central nervous system

While noradrenaline and acetylcholine are well recog-nized as chemical transmitters in nerve and neuromuscular junctions peripherally, several other sub-stances are believed to be involved within the brain — for example, serotonin or dopamine — see Chapter 5 for details of these. Although most psychoactive drugs probably affect these processes, only a few are given with any knowledge of their possible mechanisms. Monoamine oxidase inhibitors and tricyclic antidepress-ant drugs are thought to increase the concentration of transmitter amines in the brain and so 'elevate mood'. They will also act at peripheral nerve terminals; inter-actions with them are a combination of peripheral and central actions, and are described in more detail below.

Levodopa

In Parkinson's disease the basal ganglia are depleted of dopamine. As dopamine does not cross the blood–brain barrier, its precursor levodopa (*l*-dopa), which does, is used in the treatment of parkinsonism. About 95% of orally administered levodopa is rapidly decarboxylated in the periphery to dopamine, although a dopa-carboxylase inhibitor given simultaneously reduces this effect and, therefore, the required dose of levodopa. Cardiovascular effects are due to the action of circulating dopamine on α- and β-adrenergic receptors, and at the dopamine vas-cular receptor, leading to an increase in cardiac index and reduction in systemic vascular resistance. This may be of benefit in patients with heart failure, but of more concern is the increase in myocardial irritability which is maximal at about 1 hour after taking levodopa, and which may lead to tachycardia and ventricular arrhyth-mias. These may be treated with β-blockers. Therapy with levodopa is thus a relative contra-indication to drugs such as halogenated anaesthetics or cyclopropane, which sensitize the heart to the arrhythmogenic effects of catecholamines. However, although fluctuations in blood pressure during anaesthesia have been reported in patients on levodopa, serious interactions are unlikely. Sudden withdrawal of levodopa may lead not only to reappearance of symptoms of parkinsonism, but also to development of hyperthermia and signs resembling the neuroleptic malignant syndrome (see p. 568), which

may be due to imbalance in central dopaminergic path-ways (Friedman et al 1985).

Opioid drugs

Opioid drugs act at specific receptor sites within the brain and spinal cord, as described in Chapter 13.

Problems arising from the preoperative use of potent opioid analgesics depend on the duration of administra-tion and the degree of tolerance which has developed to their effects. As with tranquillizers and sedatives, ac-quired tolerance to potent analgesics leads to cross-tolerance to other depressants, particularly intravenous barbiturates. Liver damage due to hepatitis is often seen in addicts, and this may affect the response to drugs.

Withdrawal symptoms may be encountered in the surgical patient who is deprived of his usual intake of opioids, and a serious situation can occur if a correct diagnosis is not made. The abstinence syndrome in-cludes sweating, tachypnoea, restlessness, diarrhoea and cardiovascular instability, and the purely symptomatic treatment of any of these may cause problems. An un-expected degree of benefit following a normal therapeutic dose of morphine may lead one to think of withdrawal symptoms, or a full physical examination of the patient may reveal numerous injection sites. A simi-lar situation can arise in patients on large doses of opioids for pain relief, particularly postoperatively when 'normal' doses are used. Withdrawal may also occur in the pain clinic if opioids are withdrawn after a successful nerve block and, in the intensive therapy unit, after long-term ventilator therapy. A withdrawal syndrome can be precipitated by antagonists such as nalorphine, levallorphan or naloxone, and also by agonist–antagonist drugs such as pentazocine or nalbuphine.

Autonomic nervous system

The sympathetic adrenergic nerve ending is the site of many important drug interactions, as many drugs inter-fere with different aspects of its function. These will generally alter cardiovascular performance and they are of great importance in anaesthetic practice.

1. Cardiovascular drugs

The drugs used in treatment of hypertension and their interactions with anaesthetics are described in Chapters 21–25, and will not be detailed here. As stated there, the untreated hypertensive is now thought to be at greater risk than a treated patient, but a knowledge of the actions of the drugs used is essential to avoid problems. Drugs used to control arrhythmias have also already been described (Chapters 22 and 24) and will not be further discussed here.

2. Psychoactive drugs

Monoamine oxidase inhibitors

Monoamine oxidase inhibitor (MAOI) drugs were among the earliest effective antidepressant drugs. Their use diminished partly because of side-effects, but they are now receiving renewed interest in treatment of selected cases. MAO is widely distributed throughout the body, being situated mainly on the outer membrane of mitochondria. Its main function is to inactivate monoamine substances formed in the body, many of which are, or are related to, neurotransmitters or neuromodulators. In the nervous system it, in combination with catechol-o-methyl transferase (COMT), regulates the content of neurotransmitter substances and their by-products. In other tissues such as liver, kidney and lung the function is to inactivate circulating monoamines, and in particular liver MAO will act as a first-line defence against ingested monoamines from food.

The MAO enzyme may be subdivided into MAO-A and MAO-B subtypes, which are of different molecular weight. Various tissues have differing contents of these. In the CNS the monoaminergic neurons contain mainly MAO-A, whose substrates are adrenaline, noradrenaline, metanephrine and 5-HT; extraneuronal tissues contain mainly MAO-B which metabolizes β-phenylethylamine, phenylethanolamine, o-tyramine and benzylamine (Glover & Sandler 1986), while serotonergic neurons have a mixture. Most of the MAOI drugs at present used clinically act irreversibly, and inactivate both MAO-A and MAO-B. More recently new drugs have been introduced, which are reversible and short-acting, and selective for MAO-A or -B. It remains to be seen whether the incidence of reactions to food or drugs is less with these.

MAO inhibition has been thought to act by increasing levels of transmitter substances such as noradrenaline in the brain. However the results of their administration are complex. CNS levels of monoamine do increase, but this leads to reduced rates of synthesis. By-products such as the false transmitter octopamine, accumulate, and slowly displace noradrenaline from storage vesicles. Inhibitory presynaptic α-adrenergic and dopamine receptors may be stimulated. With longer treatment there are reductions in numbers and sensitivity of α_1, α_2, and β-adrenoreceptors, $5HT_1$ and $5HT_2$ receptors but not dopamine receptors (Finsberg 1984). The overall effect

of MAO inhibition, apart from behavioural changes, is a generalized reduction in sympathetic tone, with lower resting blood pressure and a reduced ability to respond to stresses such as postural change. The effects of MAOI treatment have been reviewed recently by Wells and Bjorksten (1989) and Stack et al (1988) and there is further discussion in Chapter 16 of this book.

The reaction with MAOIs, although complex, can largely be regarded as extreme overstimulation of the sympathetic nervous system. Tyramine, one of the main culprits in the 'cheese' reaction, has been shown to act by inhibiting the inhibitory α_2-adrenergic pathways within the locus coeruleus (Oreland & Engberg 1984). Should it occur, treatment will be largely symptomatic; chlorpromazine 50–100 mg may control the central excitatory symptoms and contribute to the control of others, while more specific antihypertensive therapy may be provided by an α-adrenergic blocking drug such as phentolamine. Arrhythmias may be treated by β-blockade. Labetalol, a combined α- and β-blocker, has been used successfully (Abrams et al 1985). This is the more typical (type 1) MAOI interaction, but there is also a 'type 2' depressive response (Stack et al 1988) perhaps related to inhibition of hepatic enzymes, and accumulation of, for example, opioids. Serious interactions do not appear to occur between MAOIs and the common anaesthetic drugs, although there may be a prolongation and intensification of the action of central depressants including general anaesthetics. Indirectly acting sympathomimetics (i.e. those which work by stimulating catecholamine release, such as ephedrine) may have an augmented action. Although the incidence of reported adverse reactions is low, directly acting vasopressors are to be preferred and should be titrated carefully in reduced dosage. Most local analgesic solutions used in dental practice contain vasopressors, and although they are unlikely to cause trouble, the danger can be avoided by use of local analgesic mixtures which employ felypressin as a vasoconstrictor agent, since this does not potentiate MAO inhibitors.

Opioid analgesics present a more difficult problem. A serious hyperpyrexic reaction may occur with the use of pethidine, the mechanism of which probably involves release of 5-HT. This reaction appears to be unlikely with morphine and other opioids chemically unrelated to pethidine, but data available are insufficient to be sure of this in every case. It has been seen with dextromethorphan. Cameron (1986) reports uneventful use of pentazocine in five cases, and others have used morphine and fentanyl uneventfully. Depending on the circumstances, an increased level of monitoring should be considered. The enzyme inhibition of the older

MAOIs is irreversible, and normal function is restored only slowly as new enzyme is synthesized. It is generally advised that such therapy should be stopped 1 week before an elective operation, although a hypertensive crisis has been reported 3 weeks after stopping treatment.

Although MAOI therapy is less commonly used than formerly, there is increasing support for the opinion that these drugs may be preferentially effective for some subtypes of depressive disorder, and treatment should not be arbitrarily stopped at the risk of recurrence of serious psychiatric symptoms. An alternative approach is for the anaesthetist to avoid drugs likely to interact. This is now preferable to carrying out a sensitivity test to pethidine, as suggested by Churchill-Davidson in 1965.

Tricyclic antidepressant drugs

Tricyclic antidepressant drugs act by blocking the reuptake of noradrenaline into nerve terminals. As would be expected, they enhance the action of noradrenaline or adrenaline, or other directly acting sympathomimetics. They also commonly have anticholinergic activity, and this may summate with other atropine-like drugs and lead to tachycardia or atrial ectopic beats. Tricyclics have a high affinity for cardiac muscle, and a quinidine-like, membrane-stabilizing effect, leading to a negative inotropic effect and delayed conduction which may manifest as prolonged PR, QRS and QT_c times, the latter increasing the risks of sudden ventricular fibrillation. At therapeutic doses, orthostatic hypotension may also be seen, but severe cardiovascular side-effects generally occur only in overdose. Some of the cardiac arrhythmias produced in overdose are due to anticholinergic activity within the brain, and may be treated using physostigmine, an anticholinesterase which penetrates the blood–brain barrier, while β-adrenergic blocking drugs may be used to control tachycardia. Bradyarrhythmias are the most serious disturbances in tricyclic poisoning, and here physostigmine is contra-indicated and cardiac pacing may be required (Starkey & Lawson 1980, Broden et al 1986).

Phenothiazines

The phenothiazines were the first of the really effective tranquillizers. The preoperative use of any of them makes patients more susceptible to the hypotensive action of general anaesthetics, particularly the rapidly acting barbiturates. This may be partly due to an α-adrenergic blocking action. Patients are also rendered unduly sensitive to the effects of blood loss. These considerations apply whether patients are on short-term or long-term phenothiazine therapy. About 1 in 100 patients on long-term chlorpromazine therapy develops liver dysfunction of the cholestatic type.

Some phenothiazines (including promethazine, perphenazine, thiethylperazine and trifluoperazine) may be given preoperatively. This group has a particular effect in increasing the incidence and severity of the excitatory phenomena — tremor, spontaneous involuntary muscle movement or hypertonus — which follow induction with barbiturates, especially methohexitone.

The neuromuscular junction

The current state of knowledge of the physiology and pharmacology of the neuromuscular junction is described in Chapter 18. Prolongation of the neuromuscular blockade from a relaxant drug given during anaesthesia can occur due to interactions of several different types.

The main sites of action of the clinically used neuromuscular blocking drugs are postjunctional, where they compete with acetylcholine (Ach) for occupancy of one or both of the receptor sites on the Ach complex (Standaert 1985). Both suxamethonium and non-depolarizing drugs may also cause a channel block by plugging the ionic channel in the postjunctional membrane and thus preventing the flow of ions. Interference with prejunctional release of Ach may also be involved in the mechanism of action of some of these — e.g. tubocurarine.

Antibiotics

A large number of antibiotics have been found to possess some neuromuscular blocking activity. Most fall chemically into four groups — streptomycin and related compounds, the polymyxins, the tetracyclines and the lincosamides (lincomycin and clindamycin). Some, including the pencillins, the cephalosporins and erythromycin, have not been implicated clinically.

The actions of these groups differ. The aminoglycosides have their main site of action prejunctionally, where they compete at presynaptic sites required for evoked transmitter release (Fiekers 1983). This block is similar to the block caused by high concentrations of magnesium ion. Neomycin is more potent in this respect than is streptomycin, but both these and other aminoglycosides reduce the number of quanta of Ach released by a nerve impulse. At concentrations which are higher by at least an order of magnitude, they cause a neuromuscular block at the postsynaptic membrane. Here it seems that neomycin causes an open-channel block by plugging the ionic channel, but the action of streptomycin is different and weaker. Like neomycin, clindamycin and polymyxin-B also cause an open-channel block. In the case of the lincosamides and polymyxin this is the main site of action, although they do also have a prejunctional effect. Clindamycin is about equally active at both sites, but lincomycin requires about 20 times greater concentration to show a prejunctional effect (Fiekers et al 1983).

The tetracyclines also act postjunctionally, and their action may resemble that of classical competitive neuromuscular blocking drugs (Sanders & Sanders 1979), although they are not readily antagonized by anticholinesterases. They may have pre- as well as postjunctional effects, and there are differences between the different members of the group (Singh et al 1982). They may also have a direct action on muscle contractility, as does clindamycin. The pre- and postjunctional effects of the lincosamides appear to be dose-dependent, and this has made interpretation of their action difficult.

Although, as noted above, neither the penicillins nor erythromycin has been involved in any clinical reports, erythromycin and penicillin V (not penicillin G) have been shown in the experimental setting to cause muscle paralysis in high concentrations, outside the range used clinically (Singh et al 1978). The block produced by the streptomycin group may sometimes be antagonized by calcium and also by neostigmine if incomplete, but neostigmine may prolong the blockade produced by other antibiotics. The different features of neuromuscular block produced by the different groups are summarized in Table 34.1.

Calcium antagonists

Verapamil blocks entry of calcium ions into the nerve terminal, and thus interferes with the mechanism of release of 'quanta' of acetylcholine. At high doses it also blocks uptake of calcium into the sarcoplasmic reticulum, or may cause release of calcium from it, which may result in muscle contracture (Wali 1986). At the nicotinic receptor it has closed-channel blocking activity at low doses and causes open-channel postjunctional block at higher doses (Durant et al 1984, Edeson et al 1988).

As a result, verapamil by itself reduces the amplitude of individually elicited twitches (Wali 1986), and although this is probably not significant in the normal individual, it may well be so if muscle power has already been compromised. Acute respiratory failure has been reported, occurring immediately after verapamil was given to a 17-year-old suffering from Duchenne muscular atrophy (Zalman et al 1983). The neuromuscular block caused by both depolarizing and non-depolarizing neuromuscular blocking drugs is potentiated (Durant et al 1984).

Neuromuscular transmission may be apparently normal when as many as 70–80% of receptors are occupied. However, if more than one factor is acting to compromise function, then this safety margin may be overcome. Thus synergistic interactions between neuromuscular blocking drugs used clinically, antibiotics, or other drugs such as calcium channel blockers are to be expected, and will also be more marked in any disease state where the neuromuscular mechanism is already compromised. Potentiation of the action of non-depolarizing

Table 34.1 General features of antibiotic-induced blockade

	Aminoglycosides	Polymyxins	Tetracyclines	Lincosamides
Effect on neuromuscular blocking activity of				
Competitive agents	potentiate	potentiate	potentiate	potentiate
Depolarizing agents	potentiate	potentiate	none	none
Reversibility of antibiotic-induced blockade by				
Calcium	complete	inconsistent	inconsistent	none
Anticholinesterases	inconsistent	inconsistent (may augment)	inconsistent	partial (may augment)
3, 4 diaminopyridine	complete	partial	none	inconsistent
Presynaptic effect	yes	possible	possible	yes
Postsynaptic effect	yes	yes	yes	yes

Reproduced with permission from Sanders & Sanders (1979).

muscle relaxants by antibiotics is well known and occurs with the newer as well as the older agents. Like calcium channel blockers, as described above, antibiotics which have a neuromuscular blocking action can also aggravate weakness if transmission is already compromised, for example in myasthenia gravis (Hokkanen 1964), as can some anaesthetic agents such as methoxyflurane (Elder et al 1971).

Antagonism of neuromuscular block due to these combinations is difficult, due to the complexity of the actions and interactions. The prejunctional component of block may respond to administration of calcium to raise extracellular calcium levels. Experimentally, 75% reversal of the effects of aminoglycosides can easily be achieved, but in the clinical setting, possible adverse effects of calcium administration on other systems have to be considered. Anticholinesterases also may be useful. Wali (1986) showed edrophonium to be more potent than neostigmine in antagonizing block due to the calcium channel blocker verapamil, probably because edrophonium has a prejunctional component to its effect (Harper et al 1984). In practice it will often be safer to continue ventilation until adequate muscle power has returned.

Neuromuscular blockade by both depolarizing and non-depolarizing drugs is potentiated by quinidine, and there have been several reports of prolonged paralysis. Local anaesthetic drugs may also potentiate both types of block, in concentrations which might be reached clinically (Brückner et al 1980). The mechanism of action is not clear, though they do have both a prejunctional effect interfering with Ach release, and a postjunctional effect causing an open-channel block of the sodium channel; and procaine can also interfere with the contractile process in the muscle. Edrophonium may again be of use in antagonizing this type of combined block (Carpenter and Mulroy 1986).

Magnesium sulphate is used widely in treatment of eclampsia, and there have been clinical reports of potentiation of neuromuscular block. The mechanism has been mentioned above.

Lithium has also been implicated clinically, but Waud et al (1982) after a detailed in-vitro study consider that lithium is unlikely to have been a significant factor in the cases reported.

Inhibition of cholinesterase

The short action of suxamethonium is due to its rapid breakdown by the pseudocholinesterase normally present in the plasma. If the level of this enzyme is reduced, suxamethonium breakdown will be delayed and its action correspondingly potentiated. Even in extreme degrees

of deficiency, single moderate doses of suxamethonium are likely to be associated with only minor prolongation of action, provided the cholinesterase is qualitatively normal. Serious potentiation of suxamethonium is most likely in patients whose cholinesterase is abnormal in type rather than those in whom cholinesterase levels are reduced due to drug therapy or other reasons and, unfortunately for the anaesthetist, this abnormality causes no other symptoms from which he might ascertain that this relaxant should not be used. However, if it is known that plasma pseudocholinesterase levels are depressed (though normal in type), repeated doses or infusions of suxamethonium should be avoided and single intravenous injections kept small.

Some of the drugs which are known to lower the plasma cholinesterase are listed in Table 34.3.

Endocrine: steroids

The stress of surgery provokes a complicated endocrine response, mainly aimed at substrate mobilization, with a change in metabolism towards catabolism and a negative nitrogen balance with retention of salt and water. A part of this response is a rapid rise in plasma cortisol secondary to a rise in ACTH secretion from the pituitary.

The magnitude of the response is proportional to the severity of the surgical trauma. The significance of many elements of this response is controversial, and the common opinion is that it has 'evolved to assist survival in a more primitive environment by providing appropriate substrates to maintain the function of vital organs' (Traynor and Hall 1981), and that modern anaesthetic techniques should aim to reduce the changes.

However, the ability to respond to stress may still be needed. A basic problem arises when physiological depression of the pituitary–adrenal axis, with atrophy of the adrenal cortex, results from long-continued therapy with cortisone or its analogues. Although depression may persist for months, there is often spontaneous recovery of near-normal plasma cortisol levels within 48 hours of stopping corticosteroid therapy. In induced adrenocortical insufficiency, as in Addison's disease, patients may react to the stress of surgery and anaesthesia by hypotension (out of proportion to blood loss), respiratory depression and delay in return of consciousness. The degree of deviation of the response from normal will depend on the extent of the adrenal insufficiency and on the severity of the stress.

The interaction between preoperative steroid therapy and the patient's subsequent response is of historical interest, as it was one of the first authenticated examples of iatrogenic disease occurring in anaesthesia.

The published literature on the topic is very large, including many case reports. However, although the majority of reported cases responded dramatically to intravenous administration of cortisol or other steroids, there is an increasing tendency to believe that many cases were due to other causes — unrecognized blood loss, septicaemia, etc. — with improvement due to pharmacological actions at the steroid. In only a few cases have depressed plasma cortisol levels been demonstrated.

A study of plasma cortisol levels during surgery (Plumpton et al 1969a,b) showed no difference in response between controls and patients who had recently discontinued steroid therapy, and only slightly depressed responses in those who were still receiving prednisolone at the time of operation. On the basis of their findings, and a review of the literature, the authors suggested that, as few series have included any patient who had stopped therapy for more than 3 weeks before operation, 'collapse from adreno-cortical suppression is very unlikely to occur more than 2 months after cessation of treatment; routine cover need only be considered in patients who had received steroids since that time'. The need for steroid 'cover' may be assessed by testing the adequacy of response of the pituitary–adrenal axis to stress, using the insulin hypoglycaemia test or another test of this function (Leading article 1970). This procedure may be worthwhile in patients in whom it is particularly desirable to avoid giving steroids, or in patients likely to have repeated operations. The simpler test of adrenal function which measures the cortisol response to a synthetic ACTH analogue (cosyntropin, tetracosactin) may fail to reveal a few patients with inadequate response to stress (Cunningham et al 1983).

Many regimens of replacement therapy have been suggested. Several of these are described in Chapter 30.

Malignant hyperpyrexia

Some susceptible patients, who suffer from an inherited subclinical myopathy, may develop a fulminating and often fatal hyperpyrexic response when given certain anaesthetic drugs or non-depolarizing muscle relaxants (Denborough & Lovell 1960, Gronert 1980, Various authors, 1988). Most patients have a rapid rise in temperature, with muscle contracture, and an enormous increase in aerobic and anaerobic metabolism leads to respiratory and metabolic acidosis, and hyperkalaemia. Initial diagnosis depends on the suspicion that some of these signs, especially muscle stiffness together with rising temperature, are present.

Inheritance may not be by simple Mendelian autosomal dominance, as was originally thought, but may

perhaps involve more than one gene, so that there can be different grades of susceptibility (Kalow et al 1979). However more recently a 'halothane sensitivity' gene has been demonstrated in pigs; homozygotes show a characteristic hyperpyrexic response, while heterozygotes do not, but have demonstrable biochemical abnormalities (Gallant et al 1989). In humans the susceptibility locus for malignant hyperpyrexia has been localised in chromosome 19 (McCarthy et al 1990). An uneventful previous anaesthetic does not rule out the possibility of susceptibility.

The aetiology of malignant hyperpyrexia is unknown, although theories centre on the movement of intracellular calcium, related to a genetically determined defect in excitation–contraction coupling probably arising from a change in the protein of the calcium channel (Mickelson et al 1989). Statistically, the susceptible population shows several biochemical differences from normal, such as raised creatinine phosphokinase (CPK) levels, but variability of such measurements is too large for them to be of any value in identifying individuals. In-vitro testing of a muscle biopsy specimen from the patient is more reliable, but can be carried out at only a few centres in the world.

Malignant hyperpyrexia is triggered by exposure to certain drugs although in pigs, and perhaps rarely in humans, it may develop as a result of stress alone. Halothane and suxamethonium (succinylcholine) are the drugs which have most often been incriminated, but all the volatile anaesthetic drugs, and several other drugs, have been involved, or are suspected (see Table 34.2). Nitrous oxide, which had been suspected of belonging to this list, is now generally regarded as being safe, if provided from uncontaminated apparatus.

Mortality from the established condition is over 60%, so that a high index of suspicion, and early recognition of the development of hyperthermia, is essential. Treatment is not well defined at present, and consists mainly

Table 34.2 Malignant hyperpyrexia

Completely contra-indicated
Halothane and other anaesthetic vapours
Cyclopropane
Suxamethonium and other depolarising relaxants.

Probably contraindicated
Lignocaine and cocaine
Phenothiazines — especially trimeprazine
Tricyclic and other similar antidepressants
Monoamine oxidase inhibitors
Atropine and hyoscine
Ketamine

Ellis (1984)

of early withdrawal of the initiating drug, followed by symptomatic treatment including vigorous cooling, artificial ventilation, correction of metabolic acidosis, and in particular recognition and treatment of hyperkalaemia which often occurs early in the development of the syndrome. Other symptomatic measures may include the use of high dose steroids, or α-adrenergic blockade to promote vasodilation, but the only specific therapeutic drug known is dantrolene, although calcium channel blockade may have some influence (Foster et al 1989).

Neuroleptic malignant syndrome (NMS)

A severe and potentially fatal hyperpyrexic reaction following psychotropic medication may also be due to the NMS (Caroff 1980). This shows many resemblances to malignant hyperthermia, but the relationship between the two syndromes is not yet clearly defined. Drugs implicated in triggering this reaction include phenothiazines, butyrophenones, thioxanthines and miscellaneous antipsychotic agents such as loxapine, and a drug's potential for including NMS may parallel its anti-dopaminergic potency.

Dantrolene sodium

Dantrolene Sodium

Dantrolene, a hydantoin derivative, has a low water solubility, and for this reason a lyophilized formulation of its sodium salt is used, and reconstituted with mannitol and sodium hydroxide. It has a high lipid solubility, and thus can cross all membranes easily.

Dantrolene is a directly acting skeletal muscle relaxant which acts by dissociating excitation–contraction coupling in the muscle by inhibiting release of calcium ions from the sarcoplasmic reticulum. The site of this action may be on the transverse tubular–sarcoplasmic reticulum coupling, or on the sarcoplasmic reticulum directly, or both (Morgan & Bryant 1977, Harrison 1988).

Dosage and pharmacokinetics. A dose of 2.4 mg kg^{-1} dantrolene intravenously will cause maximal (75%) depression of twitch response of skeletal muscle (Flewellen et al 1983), and this appears to be an adequate dose

for prevention or initial treatment of malignant hyperpyrexia during anaesthesia (Kolb et al 1982, Lerman et al 1989). The dose may be infused over 10–15 min, and if necessary may be repeated at 15-min intervals until a therapeutic effect has been achieved or until a total dose of 10 mg kg^{-1} has been reached. Later treatment is not clearly defined, but a further prophylactic dose of 2.4 mg kg^{-1} after 10–12 h may be considered (Harrison 1989). In a study in healthy volunteers the blood concentration of dantrolene was found to remain relatively steady for about 5.5 h, and thereafter decline exponentially with an elimination half-life of about 12 h, but elimination may be more rapid after rapid intravenous administrations (Flewellen et al 1983).

Oral administration of dantrolene has been used for prophylaxis of malignant hyperpyrexia, in daily doses ranging from 1 to 12 mg kg^{-1}. It may be that a short course of pretreatment is preferable to a longer, and a regime of 2.2 mg kg^{-1} given half 8 h before operation, and half 4 h before has been recommended (Wingard 1983). Given orally, dantrolene is 70% absorbed, and peak blood concentrations are reached at about 4–6 h. However, the effectiveness of oral treatment is controversial, and it may be better to use the intravenous route in all cases.

Dantrolene is metabolized in the liver by both reductive and oxidative pathways, and excreted in bile and urine, 4% unchanged and the remainder as 5-hydroxydantrolene and as a reduced acetylated derivative (Leitman et al 1974, Dykes 1975).

The main side-effect of dantrolene is muscle weakness, which may be experienced for up to 48 h, but which is not clinically important. Myocardial depression is not a problem at the doses described, but if given with verapamil, then studies in animals have shown marked myocardial depression (Lynch et al 1986).

Hypersensitivity reactions

Definitions

This term may be used to cover a type of adverse reaction resembling the effects of histamine liberation ('histaminoid') rather than the effects of an overdose of the drug itself. The term 'anaphylactoid' may equally well be used to describe these reactions, meaning simply that they resemble anaphylactic reactions. The latter term is best restricted to immune-mediated phenomena involving previous sensitization of the patient. Since one does not always know the patient's history, the mechanism or even with certainty the drug involved, the more general terms are safer for descriptive purposes.

Reactions can then be classified according to their severity.

Frequency of reactions

Hypersensitivity reactions can occur with almost any substance taken into the body, but are naturally more severe when the substance is injected intravenously than when it is given intramuscularly. Reactions to oral substances are largely cutaneous, apart from those due to contaminating toxins. In general, reactions are most common with substances of high molecular weight, but smaller molecules can attach themselves to plasma proteins or polypeptides and become antigenic.

In the field of anaesthesia hypersensitivity reactions occur most commonly with induction agents, muscle relaxants, plasma substitutes and antibiotics, and it is often difficult to identify the causative drug. Twenty years ago they were regarded as very rare and even now published figures for incidence probably grossly underestimate the true number. Figures quoted for 'life-threatening' reactions are between 1 in 5000 and 1 in 20 000 for general anaesthetics as a whole (Fisher & Moore 1981) which may be broken down into 1 in 10 000 to 1 in 30 000 for the barbiturates and 1 in 1000 for Cremophor-based solutions, now withdrawn (Clarke 1988). The safest of the induction agents in this respect is probably etomidate (Watkins 1983). The incidence with muscle relaxants is thought to be higher than for the intravenous barbiturates (Fisher & Munro 1983) though this is still uncertain. The most frequently incriminated of these are suxamethonium (Laxenaire et al, 1982) and alcuronium (Fisher & Baldo 1983) and the lowest number of reactions occurs with pancuronium and vecuronium. Reactions to plasma substitutes range in incidence from 1 in 10 000 for human albumin to 1 in 700 for oxypolygelatin (Haemaccel) though the formulation of the latter has been improved since this study (Ring & Messmer 1977). Figures for reactions to penicillin are about 1 in 5000 (Idsoe et al 1968).

Clinical features

Cutaneous. The majority of clinically definite and immunologically confirmed reactions have erythema as a main feature. Erythema is, however, a common accompaniment to the administration of many drugs (e.g. tubocurarine) and it should not be regarded as part of a life-threatening reaction unless there are changes in other systems of the body. In addition most reactors have oedema, particularly of the eyelids, and when this is detectable over much of the body it must represent a circulatory loss of 1–2 l (Fisher 1977).

Cardiovascular. Hypotension is the other common feature of hypersensitivity reactions. Its basis is hypovolaemia from extravasation of protein-containing fluid through the capillary wall, together with the arteriolar and capillary vasodilation. Both these are classical features of histamine liberation. There is usually a marked tachycardia which is both histamine-induced and compensatory for the hypotension. Cardiac arrest is rare as a primary feature and many patients respond to vigorous fluid replacement though α-sympathetic stimulant drugs are often helpful.

In a small proportion of patients cutaneous pallor accompanied by oedema and severe hypotension has been seen (Clarke et al 1975). These may be described as 'cardiovascular collapse,' and although they are hard to include in the histaminoid group, they should probably be regarded as another manifestation of hypersensitivity.

Respiratory. Bronchospasm has been seen in more than half of the published descriptions of reactions, either on its own or as an accompaniment to other changes. It should, however, only be regarded as indicative of a reaction if other forms of airway obstruction and other causes of tracheal irritation have been excluded. It is a more common physical sign, as one would expect, in asthmatic patients and patients receiving muscle relaxants. However, the latter group receive manual ventilation and tracheal intubation, both of which are non-pharmacological causes of respiratory tract irritation.

Gastrointestinal disturbance. Abdominal pain, nausea or vomiting occur in about 10% of published case reports.

Course of reaction

The first event to attract attention is usually a flush within a minute of completing the intravenous drug injection and this is often followed by coughing and bronchospasm. Marked hypotension then follows within 1–2 min with an impalpable pulse, but the ECG shows a sinus tachycardia. Most patients recover spontaneously though the combination of cardiovascular collapse and bronchospasm may rapidly lead to ventricular fibrillation. In a small proportion of patients the time course is delayed and prolonged (Clarke et al 1975), but in such cases it is harder to establish a cause-and-effect relationship.

Mortality

The mortality in published reactions to thiopentone is

approximately 10% (Clarke 1988) and the same figure applies to penicillin reactions (Idsoe et al 1968). Reaction to the Cremophor-containing solutions carries a lower mortality of 2–4% (Clarke 1988).

Mechanisms

Hypersensitivity reactions have been classified as types I to IV but only type I, an immune-based phenomenon involving an antigen–antibody interaction, is of major interest to anaesthetists. The first exposure to the antigen results in the formation of specific IgE antibodies which are firmly fixed to mast cells and basophils. Subsequent exposure results in rapid degranulation of these cells and liberation of vasoactive substances, particularly histamine. This mechanism still only accounts for about 20% of all reactions to thiopentone but is important for reactions to plasma substitutes (Watkins 1983). Complement-based reactions of some type were common with the Cremophor-containing solutions but are rare with other drugs. Probably the most frequent cause of hypersensitivity reactions is histamine liberation by the drug or drug combination concerned. This is therefore related to the dose and rate of administration. It is not predictable in terms of previous exposure and is not reliably detectable by skin testing.

Histamine. This appears to be the main factor involved in all types of hypersensitivity reactions (Lorenz et al 1981) and its presence explains most of the manifestations. Plasma histamine levels are difficult to estimate, particularly in the emergency situation, but levels correlate closely with the severity of the reaction (Lorenz et al 1972, Doenicke et al 1973), figures above 10 ng ml^{-1} indicating a severe reaction and above 100 ng ml^{-1} being usually fatal.

Predisposing factors

A history of atopy (asthma, hay fever or eczema) or of allergy to any injected substance is frequently seen in patients reacting to anaesthetic drugs and this association can be confirmed statistically (Dundee et al 1978). In most of these cases there is probably a raised IgE level, but this is not an essential feature in patients having true hypersensitivity reactions. Repeated exposure to particular drugs is not a predisposing factor to reactions as judged by the drug history of thiopentone reactors and others (Fee et al 1978).

Prevention and management of reactions

This does not come within the scope of this book, but recent general accounts include those by Fisher (1984), Levy (1986) and Watkins & Levy (1988). The drugs recommended for prevention include the H$_1$ and H$_2$ receptor antagonists, chlorpheniramine and cimetidine. Those used in treatment include plasma expanders, adrenaline, aminophylline, chlorpheniramine and hydrocortisone.

Table 34.3 Drug interactions of relevance to anaesthetic practice.

Drug	Secondary drug or clinical situation	Site and pharmacology*	Management and implication in anaesthesia
Anaesthetics: inhalational			
Chloroform Cyclopropane Halothane Enflurane Methoxyflurane	Adrenaline and other sympathomimetics	(S) Anaesthetic sensitizes myocardium to adrenaline, risk of severe ventricular arrhythmias	Adrenaline solutions should be dilute and not given i.v. Avoid hypercarbia
Halothane	Previous exposure to halothane	(M) Halothane-associated hepatitis in rare cases	Avoid repeat exposure within 3 months if this is practical
Methoxyflurane Enflurane	Renal disease	(M) Renal toxicity from inorganic fluoride	Avoid prolonged exposure to methoxyflurane or to enflurane in patients with pre-existing renal disease.
	Tetracycline	(S) Increased risk of renal toxicity with concurrent tetracycline treatment	

Table 34.3 Contd

Drug	Secondary drug or clinical situation	Site and pharmacology*		Management and implication in anaesthesia
Diethyl ether	β-Adrenergic blockers		Blockade of normal sympathetic compensation for depressant effects of ether	Risk of myocardial depression and heart failure
Diethyl ether Enflurane	Epilepsy	(S)		Risk of convulsions
Halothane Enflurane	Tubocurarine	(S)	Hypotensive side effects more pronounced	Caution when used together
Halothane Ether Enflurane Isoflurane Methoxyflurane	Tubocurarine Pancuronium Gallamine	(S)	Potentiation of neuromuscular blockade	Reduction in dosage requirement
Anaesthetics: i.v. Thiopentone Methohexitone	Acute intermittent porphyria	(M)	Induction of ALA synthetase by barbiturates	Precipitation of attack
Thiopentone	Pancuronium Suxamethonium	(C)	Chemical incompatibility	Avoid mixing
Thiopentone	Renal failure Cirrhosis	(B)	Decreased binding may enhance activity of thiopentone	Care with dosage
Thiopentone Methohexitone	Allergy Asthma Eczema	(S)	Hypersensitivity	Increased risk of anaphylactic response and bronchospasm
Methohexitone	Epilepsy	(S)		Increased risk of convulsions
Ketamine	Barbiturates Diazepam	(S)		Prolonged recovery time with these premedicants
Thiopentone	Sulphonamides	(B)		Dose requirement of thiopentone may be reduced
Anaesthetics: local All local anaesthetics	Metabolic acidosis	(B)		Increased risk of toxicity
Amethocaine Procaine	Low serum cholinesterase activity	(M)		Prolonged activity
Prilocaine	Large or repeated doses		Methaemoglobinaemia	Care with dosage
Muscle relaxants	Antibiotics		See below	Prolongation of block
Suxamethonium	Severe liver disease Anticholinesterases Cyclophosphamide Phenelzine (MAOI)	(M)	Reduction of serum cholinesterase levels	Prolonged block may recur. Desirable to assess pseudocholinesterase levels before use of suxamethonium

Table 34.3   Contd

Drug	Secondary drug or clinical situation	Site and pharmacology*	Management and implication in anaesthesia
Non-depolarizing relaxants	Diuretics Hypokalaemia	(S) Neuromuscular blocking activity may be increased due to hypokalaemia	Danger of prolonged paralysis and of respiratory arrest
Suxamethonium	Trauma, burns, prolonged immobilisation, neuromuscular disorders	(S) Changes in muscle endplate, leading to rapid rise in serum potassium	Risk of cardiac arrhythmias or cardiac arrest (from about 14 days after trauma or burn)
Suxamethonium	Abnormal plasma cholinesterase	(M) Autosomal recessive inheritance of abnormal genotype	Prolonged block
Suxamethonium	Procaine	(M) Competes for plasma cholinesterase	Prolonged block
Alcohol	Metronidazole Sulphonylurea oral hypoglycaemic drugs	(M) Altered alcohol metabolism	Disulfiram (Antabuse)-like reaction
Analgesic drugs 1. Opioids Morphine, etc.	Diazepam and other CNS depressants Antagonist and agonist–antagonists	(S) Additive effect (S) Competitive antagonism	Titrate doses carefully Precipitation of abstinence syndrome in addicts
Pethidine (meperidine)	MAOI drugs	See below	Dangerous interaction: see above
Pethidine (meperidine)	Phenobarbitone and other enzyme-inducing agents	(M) Increased production of norpethidine	Increased sedation, danger of convulsions
Methadone	Enzyme-inducing agents	(M) Reduced plasma methadone levels	Increased dosage requirement in treatment of addiction
2. Aspirin and other anti-inflammatory analgesics	Surgery	Inhibition of platelet adhesiveness	Increased bleeding tendency
Antibacterial drugs Aminoglycosides (Streptomycin Neomycin Kanamicin Gentamicin, etc) Polymyxins Tetracyclines Lincomycin Clindamicin	Neuromuscular blocking drugs	(?S) Mechanism uncertain, possibly like magnesium ions, these reduce Ach release prejunctionally, and desensitize post junctionally (see text)	Prolonged neuromuscular blockade may occur when given together. Rarely, muscle weakness has been caused by antibiotic alone. Calcium may aid reversal of blockade, but mechanical assistance will usually be better management
Aminoglycosides	Frusemide (furosemide) ethacrynic acid	(?) Mechanism uncertain	Increased risk of ototoxicity
Cephalosporins	Aminoglycosides, frusemide, ethacrynic acid	(?) Probably additive toxicity (?) Possibly reduced clearance of cephalosporin	Increased risk of nephrotoxicity

Table 34.3   Contd

Drug	Secondary drug or clinical situation	Site and pharmacology*	Management and implication in anaesthesia
Metronidazole	Alcohol	(M) Probably inhibition of acetaldehyde dehydrogenase	Uncommon, disulfiram (antabuse)-like reaction to alcohol, unpleasant rather than serious
Anticoagulants Oral anticoagulants	Magnesium-containing antacids	(A) Increased rate of absorption	Theoretical risk of excessive effect
	Cholestyramine	(A) Chelation and decreased absorption	Reduced anticoagulant effect
	Chloral hydrate	(B) Competition for binding sites	Transient hypoprothrombinaemia due to displacement of warfarin
	Phenylbutazone	(B) Competition for binding sites (M) Inhibition of more active isomer of warfarin preferentially	Increased anticoagulant effect
	Enzyme-inducing agents: barbiturates	(M) Increased metabolism	Reduced anticoagulant effect
	Cimetidine	(M) Reduced metabolism	Increased anticoagulant effect
	Dichloralphenazone	(M) Enzyme inhibition and reduced metabolism	Increased anticoagulant effect
	Metronidazole	(M) Enzyme inhibition Additive hypoprothrombinaemic effect	Increased anticoagulant effect
	Quinidine	Additive hypoprothrombinaemic effect	Increased anticoagulant effect
	Salicylates, etc.	Inhibition of platelet adhesiveness	Additive effect on bleeding tendency
Heparin	Aspirin Dextran	(?) (?)	Increased bleeding tendency Increased bleeding tendency
Antidepressants Monoamine oxidase inhibitors	Pethidine (meperidine)	(?) Possibly due to increased 5-HT level in brain, a certain critical level may have to be reached	Severe potentially fatal reaction in some patients. Excitement, muscle rigidity, hyperpyrexia, flushing, sweating, unconsciousness. Respiratory depression and hypotension may occur. Other opioids, e.g. morphine are safer,
	Indirectly acting sympathomimetics (amphetamine ephedrine mephentermine, etc.,	(S) Inhibition of (M) metabolism of noradrenaline (norepinephrine) which accumulates at	Severe and potentially fatal hypertensive crisis. May be treated by alphaadrenergic blocking drug, or chlorpromazine

Table 34.3 Contd

Drug	Secondary drug or clinical situation	Site and pharmacology*	Management and implication in anaesthesia
	including some proprietary cold remedies)	sympathetic nerve endings. This is released leading to overstimulation and adrenergic crisis	
	l-Dopa	Inhibition of metabolism of dopamine and noradrenaline	Severe and potentially fatal hypertensive crisis. May be treated by alphaadrenergic blocking drug, or chlorpromazine
	Adrenaline Noradrenaline	Inhibition of metabolism of dopamine and noradrenaline	May be slight enhancement of pressor effect
	Tricyclics	(?) Possibly additive effect on brain 5-HT levels	Rare toxic reactions, but combination may be used therapeutically
Phenelzine	Suxamethonium	(M) Reduction of serum cholinesterase	Prolonged block
Tricyclics	Directly acting sympathomimetics	Tricyclics block noradrenaline re-uptake into adrenergic neuron, so concentration outside is elevated, and magnifies response to any sympathomimetic amine administered	Marked enchancement of pressor effect. Avoid these sympathomimetics and local anaesthetics containing them. Felypressin may be used.
Antihypertensive drugs Clonidine	Withdrawal of treatment	(S)	Rebound hypertension may occur. Clonidine treatment must be continued or replaced in patients for operation
Adrenergic neuron blocking drugs Guanethidine Debrisoquine Bethanidine, etc	Indirectly acting sympathomimetics (amphetamine, ephedrine, etc. Tricyclic antidepressants Chlorpromazine	(S) These drugs prevent the uptake of guanethidine, etc. into the noradrenergic neurons	Antagonism of the antihypertensive action of guanethidine-related drugs
Vasodilator drugs Diazoxide Hydrallazine	Combination therapy	(S) Probably additive effect	May be severe hypotension
β-Adrenergic blocking drugs	General anaesthetic agents: methoxyflurane ether cyclopropane	(S) Cardiovascular depressant effects are additive, but usually concurrent use is not contra-indicated With methoxyflurane, or	β-Blockade is not normally a problem during anaesthesia, but avoid drugs which are myocardial depressant

Table 34.3 Contd

Drug	Secondary drug or clinical situation	Site and pharmacology★	Management and implication in anaesthesia
		drugs which normally maintain cardiac performance by decreased sympathetic drive (ether, cyclopropane) a dangerous degree of depression may occur	
	Calcium-ion antagonists (Verapamil, nifedipine, etc)	(S) Additive negative inotropic effects on heart	Hypotension or heart failure may occur
Antiarrhythmic drugs: Disopyramide	β-Adrenergic blockers	(?)	Severe bradycardia when used together
Verapamil	β-Adrenergic blockers	(S) See above	Hypotension or heart failure may occur
Verapamil	Neuromuscular blocking drugs	(S) See text	Prolonged block may occur — see text for details
Cardiac glycosides	β-Adrenergic blockers	(S)	Propranolol used to treat tachyarrhythmias of digitalis intoxication may cause dangerous bradycardia. Atropine pretreatment may be advisable
	Suxamethonium	(S) Mechanism unclear	Ventricular arrhythmias may occur
	Potassium-depleting diuretics	(S) Probably increased loss of intracellular K^+ from myocardial cells	Increased risk of digitalis toxicity
Sympathomimetic drugs	Antihypertensive drugs	(S) See above	See above
	Antidepressant drugs	(S) See above	See above
Diuretics	Digitalis	(S) Potassium-depleting diuretics may reduce intracellular K^+	Increased risk of digitalis toxicity
	Lithium	(E) Sodium depletion leads to lithium retention	Danger of lithium toxicity
Ethacrynic acid	Cephalosporins		Increased risk of nephrotoxicity
Frusemide (furosemide)	Tetracyclines	(?) Mechanism uncertain	Increased risk of nephrotoxicity

★(C) = Chemical incompatibility, (A) = site of absorption, (B) = binding/transport, (M) = metabolism, (S) = at or near site of action, (E) = excretion.

REFERENCES

Abrams J H, Schulman P, White W B 1985 Successful treatment of a monoamine oxidase — tyramine hypertensive emergency with intravenous labetalol. New England Journal of Medicine 313: 52

Broden N J, Jackson J E, Walson P D 1986 Tricyclic antidepressant overdose. Pediatric Clinics of North America 33: 287–297

Brückner J, Thomas K C, Bikhazi G B, Foldes F F 1980 Neuromuscular drug interactions of clinical importance. Anesthesia and Analgesia 59: 678–682

Cameron A G 1986 Monoamine oxidase inhibitors and general anaesthesia. Anaesthesia and Intensive Care 14: 210

Caroff S N 1980 The neuroleptic malignant syndrome. Journal of Clinical Psychiatry 41: 79–83

Carpenter R L, Mulroy M F 1986 Edrophonium antagonises combined lignocaine–pancuronium and verapamil–pancuronium neuromuscular blockade in cats. Anaesthesiology 65: 506–510

Churchill-Davidson H C 1965 Anaesthesia and monoamine oxidase inhibitors. British Medical Journal. 1: 520

Clarke R S J 1988 Hypersensitivity to intravenous anaesthetics. In: Dundee J W, Wyant G M Intravenous anaesthesia. Churchill Livingstone, London, Ch.14

Clarke R S J, Dundee J W, Garrett R T, McArdle G K, Sutton J A 1975 Adverse reactions to intravenous anaesthetics. A survey of 100 reports. British Journal of Anaesthesia 47: 575–585

Cunningham S K, Moore A, McKenna T J 1983 Normal cortisol response to corticotrophin in patients with secondary adrenal failure. Archives of Internal Medicine 143: 2276–2279

Denborough M A, Lovell R R H 1960 Anaesthetic deaths in a family. Lancet ii: 45

Doenicke A, Lorenz W, Beigl R et al 1973 Histamine release after intravenous application of short-acting hypnotics. A comparison of Etomidate, Althesin (CT 1341) and Propanidid. British Journal of Anaesthesia 45: 1097–1104

Dundee J W, Fee J P H, McDonald J R, Clarke R S J 1978 Frequency of atopy and allergy in an anaesthetic patient population. British Journal ot Anaesthesia 50: 793–798

Durant N N, Nguyen N, Katz R L 1984 Potentiation of neuromuscular blockade by verapamil. Anesthesiology 60: 298–303

Dykes M H 1975 Evaluation of a muscle relaxant: Dantrolene sodium. Journal of the American Medical Association. 231: 862–864

Edeson R O, Madsen B W, Milne R K, Le-Dain A C 1988 Verapamil, neuromuscular transmission and the nicotinic receptor. European Journal of Pharmacology 151: 301–306

Elder B F, Beal H, de Wald W and Cobb S 1971 Exacerbation of subclinical myasthenia by occupational exposure to an anaesthetic. Anesthesia and Analgesia 50: 383–387

Ellis F R 1984 Personal Communication.

Fee J P H, McDonald J R, Clarke R S J, Dundee J W, Pal PK 1978 The incidence of atopy and allergy in 10 000 preanaesthetic patients. British Journal of Anaesthesia 50: 74

Fiekers J F 1983 Effects of the aminoglycoside antibiotics, streptomycin and neomycin, on neuromuscular transmission. Journal of Pharmacology and Experimental Therapeutics 225: 487–495, 496–502

Fiekers J F, Henderson F, Marshall I G, Parsons R L 1983 Comparative effects of clindamycin and lincomycin on end-plate currents and quantal content at the neuromuscular junction. Journal of Pharmacology and Experimental Therapeutics 227: 308–315

Finsberg J P M 1984 Pharmacology of monoamine oxidase inhibitors. Journal of Pharmacology and Pharmacy 36: Suppl. 36w

Fisher M M 1977 Blood volume replacement in acute anaphylactic cardiovascular collapse related to anaesthesia. British Journal of Anaesthesia 49: 1023–1026

Fisher M M (ed) 1984 Adverse reactions. Clinics in Anaesthesiology Series. Saunders, London

Fisher M M, Baldo B A 1983 Adverse reactions to alcuronium. An Australian disease? Medical Journal of Australia 1: 630–632

Fisher M M, Moore D G 1981 The epidemiology and clinical features of anaphylactoid reactions in anaesthesia. Anaesthesia and Intensive Care 9: 226–234

Fisher M M, Munro 1 1983 Life-threatening anaphylactoid reactions to muscle relaxants. Anesthesia and Analgesia 62: 559–564

Flewellen E H, Nelson T E, Jones W P, Arens J F, Wagner D L 1983 Dantrolene dose response in awake man: Implications for management of malignant hyperthermia. Anesthesiology 59: 275–280

Foster P S, Hopkinson K C, Denborough M A 1989 Effect of diltiazem on porcine malignant hyperthermia induced by suxamethonium and halothane. British Journal of Anaesthesia 62: 560–565

Friedman J H, Fensberg S S, Feldman R G 1985 A neuroleptic malignant-like syndrome due to levodopa therapy withdrawal. Journal of the American Medical Association 254: 2792–2795

Friedman J H, Fensberg S S, Feldman R G 1985 A neuroleptic malignant-like syndrome due to levodopa therapy withdrawal. Journal of the American Medical Association 254: 2792–2795

Gallant E M, Mickelson J R, Roggow B D, Donaldson S K, Louis C F, Rempel W E 1989 Halothane–sensitivity gene and muscle contractile properties in malignant hyperthermia. American Journal of Physiology 257: c781–c786

Glover V, Sandler M 1986 Clinical chemistry ot monoamine oxidase. Cell Biochemical Functions 4 :89–97

Gronert G A 1980 Malignant hyperthermia. Anesthesiology 53: 395–423

Halsey M J 1987 Drug interactions in anaesthesia. British Journal of Anaesthesia 59: 112–123

Harper H J N, Bradshaw E G, Healy T E J 1984 Antagonism of alcuronium with edrophonium or neostigmine. British Journal of Anaesthesia 56: 1089–1094

Harrison G C 1988 Dantrolene sodium: Pharmacodynamics and pharmacokinetics. British Journal of Anaesthesia 60: 279–286

Harrison G C 1989 Malignant Hyperthermia. In: General anaesthesia, 5th edn. Nunn J F, Utting J E Brown B R Jr (eds) Butterworths, London

Hokkanen E 1964 The aggravating effect of some antibiotics on the neuromuscular blockade in myasthenia gravis. Acta Neurologica Scandinavica 40: 346

Idsoe O, Guthe T, Willcox R R, De Weck A L 1968 Nature and extent of penicillin side-reactions with particular reference to anaphylactic shock. Bulletin of the

World Health Organisation 38: 159–188

Kalow W, Britt B A, and Chan F Y 1979 Epidemiology and inheritance of malignant hyperthermia. International Anesthesiology Clinics 17: 119–139

Kolb Mary E, Horne M L, Martz R 1982 Dantrolene in human malignant hyperthermia. Anesthesiology 56: 254–262

Laxenaire M C, Moneret-Vautran D A, Boileau S 1987 Choc anaphylactique au suxamethonium a propos de 18 cas. Annales Francais d'Anesthesie et de Reanimation 1: 29–36

Leading article 1970 Testing the hypothalamic–pituitary–adrenal axis. British Medical Journal 1: 644

Leitman P S, Haslam R H, Walcher J R 1974 Pharmacology of dantrolene sodium in children. Archives of Physical Medicine and Rehabilitation 55: 385–392

Lerman J, McLeod M E, Strong H A 1989 Pharmacokinetics of intravenous dantrolene in children. Anesthesiology 70: 625–629

Levy J M 1986 Anaphylactic reactions in anesethesia and intensive care. Butterworths, Boston

Lorenz W, Doenicke A, Meyer R et al 1972 Histamine release in man by propanidid and thiopentone: pharmacological effects and clinical consequences. British Journal of Anaesthesia 44: 355–369

Lorenz W, Doenicke A, Schoning B, Neugebauer E 1981 The role of histamine in adverse reactions to intravenous agents. In: Thornton J A (ed) Adverse reactions to anaesthetic drugs. North-Holland Biomedical, Amsterdam

Lynch C, Durbin C G JR, Fisher N A, Veselis R A, Althaus J S 1986 The effects of dantrolene and verapamil on atrioventricular conduction and cardiovascular performance in dogs. Anesthesia and Analgesia 65: 252–258

McCarthy T V, Healy J M, Heffron J J, Denfel T, Lehmann-Horn F, Farrall M, Johnson K 1990 Localization of the malignant hyperthermia susceptibility locus to human chromosome 19q 12–13.2 Nature 343: 562–564

Melmon K L 1971 Preventable drug reaction — causes and cures. New England Journal of Medicine 284: 1361–1368

Mickelson J R, Gallant E M, Rempel W E, Johnson K H, Litterer L A, Jacobson B A, Louis C F 1989 Effects of the halothane-sensitivity gene on sarcoplasmic reticulum function. American Journal of Physiology 257: c787–c794

Morgan K G, Bryant S H 1977 The mechanism of action of dantrolene sodium. Journal of Pharmacology and Experimental Therapeutics 201: 138–147

Oreland L, Engberg G 1984 Suppression of cortical noradrenergic neurons by tyramine. Journal of Pharmacology and Pharmacy 36 (Suppl) 44w

Plumpton F S, Besser G N, Cole P V 1969a Corticosteroid treatment and surgery. 1. An investigation of the indications for steroid cover. Anaesthesia 24: 3–11

Plumpton F S Besser G N, Cole P V 1969b Corticosteroid treatment and surgery. 2. The management of steroid cover. Anaesthesia 24: 12–18

Reynolds E S, Brown B R, Vandam L D 1972 Massive hepatic necrosis after fluroxene anesthesia — a case of drug interaction? New England Journal of Medicine 286: 530–531

Ring J, Messmer K 1977 Incidence and severity of anaphylactoid reactions to colloid volume substitutes. Lancet i: 466–469

Sanders W E Jr, Sanders C C 1979 Toxicity of antibacterial agents: mechanism of action on mammalian cells. Annual review of Pharmacology and Toxicology 19: 53–83

Singh Y N, Harvey A L, and Marshall I G 1978 Antibiotic-induced paralysis of the mouse phrenic nerve — hemidiaphragm preparation, and reversibility by neostigmine. Anesthesiology 48: 418–424

Singh Y N, Marshall I G, Harvey A L 1982 Pre- and postjunctional blocking efffects of aminoglycoside, polymyxin, tetracycline and lincosamide antibiotics. British Journal of Anaesthesia 54: 1295–1306

Stack C G, Rogers P, Linter S P 1988 Monoamine oxidase inhibitors and anaesthesia: a review. British Journal of Anaesthesia 60: 222–227

Stambaugh J E, Wainer I W, Hemphill D M Schwartz I 1977 A potentially toxic drug interaction between pethidine (meperidine) and phenobarbitone. Lancet I: 398–399

Standaert F G 1985 The doughnut and its hole. Clinics in Anaesthesiology 3: 243–259

Starkey I R, Lawson A A H 1980 Poisoning with tricyclic and related antidepressants — a ten-year review. Quarterly Journal of Medicine 49: 33–49

Stovner J, Theodorsen L, Bjelke E 1971 Sensitivity to tubocurarine and alcuronium with special reference to plasma protein pattern. British Journal of Anaesthesia 43: 385–391

Traynor C, Hall G 1981 Endocrine and metabolic changes during surgery: anaesthetic implications. British Journal of Anaesthesia 53: 153–160

Various authors 1988 Symposium on malignant hyperthermia. British Journal of Anaesthesia 60: 251–319

Wali F A, 1986 Interaction of verapamil with gallamine and pancuronium and reversal of combined neuromuscular blockade with neostigmine and edrophonium. European Journal of Pharmacology 3: 385–393

Watkins J 1983 Etomidate: an 'immunologically safe' anaesthetic agent. Anaesthetist 38 suppl: 34–38

Watkins J, Levy C J 1988 Guide to immediate anaesthetic reactions. Butterworth, London

Waud B E, Farrell B A, Waud D R 1982 Lithium and neuromuscular transmission. Anesthesia and Analgesia 61: 399–402

Wells D G, Bjorksten A R 1989 Monoamine oxidase revisited. Canadian Anaesthetists Society Journal 36: 64–74

Wingard D W 1983 Controversies regarding the prophylactic use of dantrolene for malignant hyperthermia. Anesthesiology 58: 489–490

Zalman F, Perloff J K, Durant N N, Campion D S 1983 Acute respiratory failure following intravenous verapamil in Duchenne muscular atrophy. American Heart Journal 105: 510–511

35. Management of drug overdose

J. R. Johnston   D. L. Coppel

INTRODUCTION

Drug overdose is one of the commonest causes of admission to hospital and encompasses the following categories.

Self-poisoning or parasuicide

This refers to the ingestion of a drug or toxic substance in response to a personal or social crisis, and accounts for approximately 10% of all medical admissions (Kessel 1985). The commonest drugs incriminated are the psychotropic drugs, benzodiazepines being the commonest individual group (Prescott & Highley 1985).

Non-accidental poisoning

This is used to describe the administration of a potentially harmful substance usually by a parent to their child.

Accidental poisoning

This describes unpremeditated poisoning and is commonest in children aged between 9 months and 5 years. The substances usually involved are drugs (60%), household cleaning products (35%) and plants (4%). Adults also become poisoned accidentally, generally by ingestion or inhalation of substances at home or at work.

GENERAL PRINCIPLES OF MANAGEMENT

The management of poisoned subjects involves carrying out an initial assessment of their vital signs followed by the appropriate interventions to support life. Measures to obtain a working diagnosis of the cause of the poisoning are also carried out at this time and from this a treatment plan can be instituted.

Life support

The vast majority of poisoning cases only require observation and do not enter a life-threatening situation. However, if the patient is unconscious the first priority is the time-honoured triad of maintenance of the airway, breathing and circulation. It should be noted that mouth-to-mouth respiration is contra-indicated with hydrogen sulphide or cyanide poisoning because of their toxic effects.

Diagnosis

The diagnosis is often made by exclusion or using circumstantial evidence. An overdose must be suspected in all patients presenting with an unexplained decrease in the level of consciousness, particularly when it is associated with depressed respiration, hypotension, flaccidity, arreflexia and absent bowel sounds.

Specific signs to be looked for during examination and investigation are summarized in Table 35.1. Laboratory investigations that are likely to provide useful information include arterial blood gases, electrolyte and urea estimations, blood glucose and in certain circumstances a toxicological screen.

TREATMENT PLAN

The first objective of a treatment plan is always to provide life support and manage any of the further consequences of the poisoning (see Table 35.1). Further management involves consideration of prevention of absorption, antidotes and promotion of excretion of the poison.

Prevention of absorption

The methods available to prevent absorption include removal from a toxic atmosphere, decontamination of

Table 35.1 Clinical effects of the common poisons

Clinical effect	Poison
Skin	
Colour	
Blue	(Cyanosis, methaemoglobinaemia)
Flushed	Carbon monoxide; anticholinergics, cyanide, alcohol
Puncture marks	Opioids
Bullae	Barbiturates, carbon monoxide, tricyclics
Sweating	Salicylates, organophosphates
Pupils	
Constricted	Opioids, organophosphates, hypoxia
Dilated	Hypothermia, tricyclics, phenothiazines, anticholinergics
Mouth	
Burns	Corrosives, caustics, paraquat
Flaccidity	Benzodiazepines, barbiturates, alcohol, β-blockers
Hyperreflexia	Tricyclics, anticholinergics, phenothiazines
Convulsions	Tricyclics, isoniazid, lithium, amphetamines, theophylline, mefenamic acid, carbon monoxide, phenothiazines, ethylene glycol
Specific organ damage	
Renal	Paracetamol, paraquat
Hepatic	Paracetamol, carbon tetrachloride
Temperature	
Pyrexia	Anticholinergics, tricyclics, carbon monoxide, salicylates
Hypothermia	Barbiturates, alcohol, opioids
Cardiac rhythm	
Bradycardia	Digoxin, β-blockers, carbamates, organophosphates
Tachycardia	Salicylates, theophylline, cyanide, carbon monoxide, anticholinergics
Arrhythmias	Digoxin, phenothiazines, quinine, tricyclics, anticholinergics
Blood pressure	
Hypotension	Sedatives, hypnotics
Hypertension	Anticholinergics, tricyclics

affected skin and, most commonly, prevention of absorption from the gastrointestinal tract. This last method involves the following techniques.

1. The stomach may be emptied by lavage or by emetics. Lavage must be performed only if a potentially harmful substance has been taken relatively recently, i.e. within 4 h. Exceptions to this rule include substances which delay gastric emptying such as salicylates and tricyclic antidepressants. If the patient is unconscious the airway must be protected using an endotracheal tube.

2. Emesis is especially useful in children but must not be used if there is a risk of aspiration into the lungs or if substances such as petroleum distillates, petrol or corrosives have been taken. The standard emetic is syrup of ipecacuanha (Vale et al 1986). This plant extract has as its active constituents the alkaloids emetine and cephaeline. Both induce vomiting by a central action, cephaeline being twice as potent as emetine and also having a direct irritant action on the gastric mucosa. This results in the initial bout of vomiting; the combined central actions causing the later vomiting. The recommended dose is given in Table 35.2. Problems that may arise with the use of ipecacuanha include prolonged vomiting from using too large a dose which can mimic symptoms of poisoning and confuse the clinical picture. It may also cause diarrhoea and lethargy again mimicking the signs and symptoms of poisoning. Serious side effects from forceful vomiting such as gastric rupture and barotrauma may occur. Emetine can also act as a myocardial depressant. Allied to these problems is the concern that using ipecacuanha may not be the most effective method for reducing drug absorption. Activated charcoal can reduce the absorption of paracetamol, aminophylline and tetracycline more effectively than by causing emesis (Neuvonen et al 1983). Emesis however remains useful in children but must not be used if there is a risk of aspiration into the lungs or if substances such as petroleum distillates, petrol or corrosives have been taken. It must be remembered that if emesis is used then administration of agents such as methonine or activated charcoal is precluded. The use of ipecacuanha in adults must be questioned especially in the growing number of poisonings for which activated charcoal appears to be effective.

3. Whole-gut lavage is reserved for the elimination of sustained-release drug formulations.

4. Administration of adsorbents such as activated charcoal, bentonite, Fuller's earth or

Table 35.2 Recommended dose of ipecacuanha

6–18 months	10 ml	
Older children	15 ml	one dose with water
Adult	30 ml	

cholestyramine bind poison in the gut. Activated charcoal is available as Medicoal or Carbomix. They have a high adsorptive capacity for a wide range of substances and should be given as an aqueous suspension as soon as possible after the ingestion of the poison. Later administration may result in binding of drug remaining within gut lumen and drug returned to the lumen by enterohepatic circulation. It should not be used simultaneously with oral emetics as both substances are rendered ineffective. The degree of adsorption to the poison depends on the degree of ionization and molecular size of the latter. Many drugs require more than double their weight of charcoal for complete adsorption; a ratio of 10:1 of charcoal:poison is recommended. Its adsorptive capacity for the following compounds is too low to be of use: ferrous sulphate, cyanides, sulphonylureas and some insecticides.

Antidotes

Specific antidotes to poisons work in a number of ways.

1. An antidote may interact with a poison to form an inert complex which is then excreted. Heavy metals (arsenic, copper, gold and mercury) are poisonous because of their ability to interact with sulphydryl groups found on organic enzymes. Dimercaprol, a chelating agent which substitutes its own sulphydryl groups, forms a complex with the heavy metal, thus releasing the enzymatic complex. An alcohol group on the dimercaprol promotes excretion by keeping the complex water-soluble. Further examples of inert complex formation are given in Table 35.3.
2. Certain antidotes may accelerate the formation of a less toxic form of the poison. The main route of

detoxification of cyanide is the formation of thiocyanate. Thiosulphate is required for this process and its administration increases the rate of cyanide metabolism.
3. An antidote can reduce the metabolism of the poison to a more toxic compound. Methanol is metabolized in the liver to formaldehyde and formic acid, which are responsible for its toxic effects. This metabolic step is inhibited by ethanol.
4. Antidotes can compete with the poison at receptor sites. Oxygen is used in the treatment of carbon monoxide poisoning because the half-life of elimination of carbon monoxide is reduced from 250 min while breathing room air to 50 min when breathing 100% oxygen at 1 atmosphere.
5. Antidotes may cause the blockade of receptor sites for action of the poisons. Organophosphorus compounds act at nicotinic and muscarinic receptor sites causing accumulation of acetylcholine. Atropine will block the effects at the muscarinic receptor and pralidoxime blocks the effects at the neuromuscular junctions.
6. An antidote may bypass the effects of a poison, e.g. oxygen following poisoning with cyanide.

Enhancement of drug elimination

There are several methods available to promote excretion of a poison, which differ in complexity and in principle. These measures have a limited role and are most effective in situations where there are high plasma concentrations of the poison (small volume of distribution). They will be ineffective where the poison is easily tissue bound (large volume of distribution) e.g. tricyclic antidepressants.

Activated charcoal

Activated charcoal is especially useful because of its adsorptive properties preventing drug absorption and because of its use in promoting increased drug elimination.

It is a fine black powder made by the distillation of certain organic materials (wood pulp, coconut shells or coal) which is activated by the action of steam or strong acids at high temperatures. This gives it a large surface area of 950–1200 sq.m/g which along with its electrostatic properties aids binding. Its absorptive capacity is 500–1000 mg of drug per gram of charcoal.

With repeated oral dosing the bowel, especially the small intestine, becomes the site of transfer of poison from circulation in the gut villi to the charcoal in the

Table 35.3 Antidotes which act by inert complex formation

Poison	Antidote
Arsenic, copper, gold, mercury	Dimercaprol
Cholinesterase inhibitors	Pralidoxime
Cyanide	Sodium nitrite, dicobalt edetate, thiosulphate
Digoxin	Fab antibody fragments
Lead, copper, mercury, zinc	Penicillamine
Thallium	Prussian blue

gut lumen, otherwise known as 'gastro-intestinal dialysis'. This is especially so for lipophilic compounds that are unionised in plasma, have a long elimination half life, a small volume of distribution and are not heavily tissue bound. Those that have an enterohepatic recirculation or are actively secreted in the bowel can be particularly easy to clear using this technique.

The technique involves instilling 50–100 g activated charcoal as soon as possible after poisoning followed by instillation of 12.5 g h^{-1} via a nasogastric tube. Precautions to protect the airway should be taken if it is at risk from aspiration. The following compounds can be eliminated using this technique — salicylates, benzodiazepines, digoxin, meprobamate, phenytoin, phenobarbitone, phenylbutazone, carbamazepine, theophylline and quinine. The cyclic antidepressants have a large volume of distribution and should theoretically not be eliminated successfully using this technique. However, patients with this type of poisoning do seem to benefit.

Apart from being unpalatable there were hazards reported with this technique. Menzies and colleagues (1988) reported a death following aspiration of gastric contents containing Medicoal (Lundbeck). A further possible hazard of hypernatremia from the sodium load has been reported (Gorchein et al 1988) (Medicoal contains 18 mmol sodium/5g sachet). Although large doses of charcoal are needed, this method of elimination is simple and cheap to perform and also relatively safe. It is practical only in those cases not associated with vomiting. It needs transport of the adsorbant through the bowel and the question of the best formulation has not been answered. It should be noted that Medicoal may cause diarrhoea while Carbomix may cause constipation.

Forced diuresis

The poison is excreted preferentially in the urine by manipulating urine pH so that the poison becomes fully ionized. The degree of ionization depends on the ionization constant (Ka) of the drug and the pH of the solution in which it is dissolved. Thus ionization of weak acids, and therefore their excretion, will be increased in an alkaline urine; basic drugs are maximally ionized in an acid urine. Alkaline diuresis is useful for poisoning with drugs with a pKa range of 3.0–7.5 where the pH of urine is maintained at 7.5–8.0, e.g. phenobarbitone, salicylates and phenoxyacetate herbicides. An acid diuresis may be used for drugs with a pKa range of 7.5–10.5 where the pH of urine is maintained at 5.5–6.5. The potential complications of this technique relate to the amount of fluid used, which may lead to pulmonary and cerebral oedema, cardiac failure and to

electrolyte disturbances. Its use has declined in recent years.

Peritoneal dialysis or haemodialysis

A drug or poison, if present in quantity in the plasma as low molecular weight particles, will diffuse through the peritoneum or dialysis membrane. Thus if it is highly tissue-bound, dialysis will not be effective. Peritoneal dialysis, although a simple technique, has practically been abandoned because of the low clearance obtained. Haemodialysis relies upon diffusion of the poison across a semipermeable cellophane membrane down a concentration gradient from blood to dialysate. Small molecules cross the membrane freely; larger molecules (MW 2000–10 000) pass with difficulty. The technique is used mainly to increase the elimination of lithium, methanol and ethylene glycol, although some barbiturates and salicylates can be removed. It requires sophisticated equipment and, because of the foreign membrane, either heparin or prostacyclin as anticoagulants.

Haemoperfusion

This technique uses broadly similar apparatus to that of haemodialysis except that the 'membrane' used is a column containing an adsorbent material such as polymer-coated activated charcoal, anion resins and uncharged resins. As with the methods outlined above it is contra-indicated if the ingested poisons have a large volume of distribution; the plasma will contain only a small proportion of the total amount of poison in the body. It is also contra-indicated if an antidote is available or if binding to a receptor site can readily be reversed. It is of particular value in treatment of poisoning with all the barbiturates, some hypnotics, carbamazepine, disopyramide, theophyllines, salicylates and paracetamol.

MANAGEMENT OF COMMON POISONINGS

Analgesics

Salicylates

Ingestion of acetylsalicylic acid (Aspirin) is the most common form of salicylate poisoning. As an acid with pKa 3.5 it is unionized in the acidic medium of the stomach and is therefore rapidly absorbed.

If taken as an overdose it may precipitate out in the stomach and coat the gastric mucosa. This may produce absorption continuing over many hours, and warrants emptying the stomach after the usually recommended time for complete absorption. It is also readily absorbed from the small intestine and is then hydrolysed to salicylic acid. The main route of excretion of salicylate is conjugation to form salicyluric acid. This step is easily saturated even within the therapeutic dose range. Elimination is slow after overdose and toxicity can arise easily.

The two main toxic effects are a direct central stimulation of the respiratory centre and uncoupling of oxidative phosphorylation. The former effect leads to a respiratory alkalosis with compensatory excretion of bicarbonate, sodium, potassium and water, leading to dehydration and hypokalaemia. The latter effect leads to interference with carbohydrate, lipid, protein and amino-acid metabolism and accumulation of organic acids. Oxygen utilization and carbon dioxide production are increased. Energy released by the uncoupling is dissipated as heat, manifesting itself as hyperpyrexia and sweating. Central stimulation also causes nausea and vomiting which, together with decreased oral intake, exacerbate fluid loss. All of these lead to a metabolic acidosis. This will tend to reduce the degree of ionization of the salicylic acid which will increase its intracellular concentration, and lead to CNS toxicity and a poorer prognosis.

These two effects usually manifest themselves at different rates depending on the age of the subject. In adults there is often a first stage of 12–24 h which, if left untreated, leads to the second stage of metabolic acidosis. In children below the age of 12 the first respiratory alkalosis stage is short or absent and the more dangerous acidotic stage predominates earlier. Glucose metabolism is also affected and there may be an increased peripheral demand leading to hypoglycaemia. However, with the increased metabolic rate and increased demand, the combined effects of adrenocortical stimulation, increased glucose 6-phosphatase activity and hepatic glycogenolysis may lead to hyperglycaemia.

Elimination of the drug relies upon the renal pathway, a urinary pH of greater than 6 leading to increased excretion. A stage of respiratory alkalosis tends to protect against serious salicylate toxicity and will also help excretion.

The clinical manifestations of salicylate overdose are summarized in Table 35.4. The therapeutic blood level of aspirin is approximately 150 mg l^{-1}; toxicity becomes apparent when the level is 250–350 mg l^{-1}. Levels between 500 and 750 mg l^{-1} give rise to moderate toxicity and levels of greater than 750 mg l^{-1} indicate severe toxicity. The levels must be interpreted in association with the plasma pH because with an acidosis intracellular levels may rise while blood levels fall. The presence of a metabolic acidosis following salicylate poisoning indicates a poor prognosis.

Table 35.4 Salicylate poisoining — clinical features

Mild to moderate (500–750 mg l^{-1})	Irritability, tremor Tinnitus, deafness Nausea, vomiting, epigastric discomfort Hyperventilation Sweating, vasodilation (hyperpyrexia in children)
Severe (750–1200 mg l^{-1})	Confusion, delirium, convulsions, coma Hypotension, cardiac arrest Hyperpyrexia Pulmonary oedema, cerebral oedema Hypoglycaemia Renal failure, liver failure Tetany Gastrointestinal haemorrhage

In patients who present within 24 h of poisoning gastric aspiration and lavage or emesis should be carried out. If presentation is early, oral activated charcoal should be given and, if clinical conditions allow, repeated. Fluid and electrolyte deficits from the vomiting, sweating and hyperventilation must be corrected; plasma pH should be treated especially if the pH is low, and temperature should be reduced using tepid sponging. Vitamin K may be given for hypoprothrombinaemia.

Forced alkaline diuresis should be carried out only in the more severely affected patients (greater than 500 mg l^{-1} in adults or 300 mg l^{-1} in children). It is most likely to cause harm in the very young, in the elderly and in those with pre-existing cardiac and renal disease. It also needs to be carried out with care in those severely poisoned (greater than 750 mg l^{-1}). In patients with an acidosis this must be corrected first. A urinary pH of greater than 7.5 is more effective than a very brisk diuresis. If there is any potassium deficit it will be difficult to obtain a suitably alkaline urine.

With very severely poisoned patients (level greater than 1000 mg l^{-1}) it may be necessary to use haemodialysis or haemoperfusion, with the former technique being preferred because it enables correction of the fluid and electrolyte deficits.

Paracetamol

This drug is now the main cause of acute liver necrosis in the UK, and is taken either as paracetamol or in compounds such as Distalgesic (dextropropoxyphene and paracetamol).

Approximately 1–4% of the dose of paracetamol is excreted as the free drug. Of the remainder the majority

(60–90%) is excreted as glucuronide and sulphate conjugates. A small proportion, however, forms an oxidative metabolite (N-acetyl-p-benzoquinone) which is either excreted as catechol derivatives (5–10%) or conjugated with glutathione and excreted as cysteine or mercapturate conjugates (5–10%).

If an overdose of paracetamol occurs, the stores of glutathione are depleted and the levels of the oxidative metabolite increase; this is free to cause hepatic and renal cell damage.

Within the first 24 h of poisoning there may only be anorexia, nausea and vomiting, abdominal pain and sweating. By 24–36 h there may be right subcostal pain due to early hepatic damage. In situations where the microsomal oxidative enzymes are induced, the hepatic and nephrotoxic effects of paracetamol are enhanced. This can occur in alcoholics and in those taking barbiturates and anticonvulsants.

Hepatic damage can occur after as little as 10–15 g of paracetamol (20–30 tablets of 500 mg). Because the circulating levels of hepatic enzymes do not rise until some days after the damage has been done, great reliance is now placed on estimation of the plasma paracetamol level and interpreting this in relation to the time since ingestion. This will indicate the expected degree of damage and may influence treatment. It is possible to produce an approximate prognosis from a zoned graph (Fig. 35.1) of drug levels against time (Prescott 1978).

Treatment initially involves gastric lavage or emesis if presentation is within 6 h of ingestion. An estimation of plasma paracetamol level must be made no sooner than 4 h after ingestion. If presentation is within 12 h and the history reliable, measures to prevent hepatic damage with either methionine or acetyl cysteine are instituted while awaiting the result.

Oral methionine increases the synthesis of hepatic glutathione. Difficulty with the oral administration of this drug may be encountered because of vomiting or because of unconsciousness. Acetylcysteine is rapidly hydrolysed to cysteine, which is a precursor of glutathione. It may also act by reducing the oxidative metabolite back to paracetamol. It can be given either by intravenous injection (Prescott et al 1979) or orally, and causes less nausea and vomiting, although its use has been associated with anaphylactoid reactions (Mant et al 1984).

Both of the above drugs must be given within 10 h of ingestion of the poison because, apart from being less effective, there is a chance that if hepatic damage has already occurred they may precipitate hepatic encephalopathy.

Forced diuresis and haemodialysis are of limited or no value in treatment of this type of poisoning, although haemoperfusion may be some value in very severe toxicity, especially if presentation is delayed.

Opioid analgesics

This group includes drugs such as morphine, diamorphine (heroin), pethidine and methadone. As potent respiratory depressants these drugs can be dangerous. Other clinical features include constricted pupils, convulsions, hypotension and coma. Severe intoxication can lead to pulmonary oedema by an unknown mechanism, cardiac arrhythmias and renal failure.

Management is initially supportive until the opioid antagonist naloxone can be administered. As this drug is a competitive antagonist the dose required for full reversal will be greater than that used to reverse therapeutic doses of morphine. Initial doses of 1.2–2.4 mg are often necessary. It also has a short duration of action (approximately 10 min) and an initial bolus dose may need to be followed by an infusion. The dose given must be titrated to effect; up to 5 mg h^{-1} may be needed. Overtreatment with naloxone can produce hyperventilation, tachycardia and hypertension, with pulmonary oedema and even cardiac arrest reported in some cases. These features are almost certainly due to a noradrenaline 'storm'. An acute withdrawal in narcotic addicts may also be produced.

Some combination analgesics contain constituents which can be reversed with naloxone. The combination of dextropropoxyphene and paracetamol (Distalgesic) requires treatment of both drug entities to be successful.

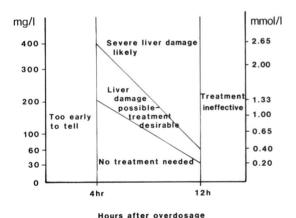

Fig. 35.1 The prediction of toxicity and treatment plan following paracetamol overdose in relation to time after ingestion and plasma paracetamol levels. (Reprinted with permission from Henry & Volans 1984)

Non-steroidal anti-inflammatory agents (NSAID)

This very broad range of compounds includes drugs such as indomethacin, phenylbutazone, ibuprofen and mefenamic acid. Overdose is infrequent but several are worthy of mention.

Mefenamic acid (Ponstan), often used for rheumatoid arthritis and dysmenorrhagic pain, if taken as an overdose will cause twitching leading to convulsions. Management includes gastric lavage and symptomatic treatment of the fits; the drug is cleared rapidly because it has a short half-life (3–4 h).

Benorylate (Benoral) an aspirin–paracetamol ester, if taken as an overdose will give rise to symptoms resembling salicylism. Treatment should be based on the levels of salicylate and paracetamol found in the blood.

The propionic acid derivatives appear to be of low toxicity even after large overdoses. In the majority of reported cases the patients have either no symptoms or mild symptoms of gastrointestinal irritation such as nausea and vomiting. Hypotension, acidosis, coma and renal dysfunction are rare results of toxicity.

Phenylbutazone has a half-life of approximately 3 days and can cause convulsions, coma, metabolic acidosis, hepatic and renal failure. Haemoperfusion has been shown on occasion to be successful (Strong et al 1979).

Psychoactive drugs

Approximately 60% of patients admitted with poisoning have taken one of these drugs. Most cause CNS depression which resolves if supportive measures are undertaken. They are also often associated with hypotension caused by direct cardiac and peripheral vascular effects and by a central action. Treatment involves restoration of the central venous pressure and the use of an inotrope.

Barbiturates

These used to be the 'overdose drug of choice', but have since been replaced by the benzodiazepines. The half-life may differ after overdose from that found with therapeutic doses, so the plasma concentrations may only be taken as a rough guide. The clinical condition of the patient must be the ruling factor in management. Usually supportive measures are all that is needed. Haemoperfusion may be used if any serious complications arise. Haemodialysis is effective for removal of phenobarbitone but is ineffective for the short-acting barbiturates.

Benzodiazepines

Benzodiazepines probably act by facilitating the inhibitory effects of the γ-aminobutyric acid (GABA) postsynaptic receptor in the CNS producing anxiolysis, muscle relaxation and seizure control (Whitwam 1987). Overdose with this group of drugs produces very few serious side-effects. Symptoms include drowsiness, ataxia, dysarthria and nystagmus. The drugs are less likely to cause respiratory depression. Management is similar to that needed for the barbiturates and active elimination measures are not warranted.

A specific benzodiazepine anatagonist, flumazenil, can reverse the effects of benzodiazepines by competitively displacing them at the benzodiazepine–GABA–chloride complex. It has a rapid onset of action in less than 1 min following intravenous injection with an effect maximal at 5 min. It should be administered in 0.1 mg aliquots to a total of 1.0 mg. It has a short duration of action, the elimination half life being 54 minutes mainly due to rapid hepatic clearance. It can reverse a comatose state and return respiratory rate and blood pressure towards normal but because of its short half-life repeat administration is required (Knudsen et al 1988). An infusion of flumazenil can be useful in reversing prolonged sedation if given by infusion at a rate of 0.5–1.0 $mg.hr^{-1}$ (Bodenham & Park 1989). Flumazenil should be used with caution both when used to reverse pure benzodiazepine depression and for a mixed drug overdose. Rapid reversal may cause ventricular fibrillation, (Short et al 1988) status epilepticus or could counteract possible beneficial effects of benzodiazepines following a mixed drug overdose (Burr et al 1989).

Chloral derivatives

These are all rapidly metabolized to the active compound, trichloroethanol. The clinical features of note are gastric irritation, profound cardiac and respiratory depression and cardiac arrhythmias. Treatment is usually supportive, but if the poisoning is severe then haemodialysis or haemoperfusion can be useful.

Chlormethiazole

This compound (Heminevrin) is used extensively as an anticonvulsant and for the management of acute alcohol withdrawal. It is metabolized mainly in the liver and as such has a short half-life. Where hepatic function is decreased, or if taken in overdose, the half-life is prolonged giving rise to effects similar to barbiturate overdose. There is increased salivation which can be treated with an anticholinergic. Other treatment is supportive.

Glutethimide

Available in the USA as Doriden, this piperidinedione derivative is a more powerful hypnotic than the barbiturates. It is more soluble in alcohol than water, and if taken as an overdose with alcohol its absorption is facilitated. It is lipid-soluble and therefore collects in the tissues. It is metabolized in the liver, forming a range of active metabolites which cause a fluctuating level of consciousness during the course of recovery from an overdose.

Sudden episodes of apnoea may occur and are probably related to rises in ICP due to cerebral oedema. Hypotension may be severe and myocardial damage may occur due to a direct toxic effect. The drug has pronounced anticholinergic properties which are manifested by dilated pupils, dry mouth and an ileus.

Treatment will require gastric lavage and intensive supportive measures. Lavage should be carried out with a 1 : 1 mixture of castor oil : water, and castor oil (50 ml) left in the stomach; this will increase the capture of this lipid-soluble drug. Of the active elimination procedures only haemoperfusion is recommended for severe cases. It must be continued for several hours following the return of consciousness, because of the continuing release of drug from fat deposits.

Phenothiazines

Chlorpromazine is the best-known member of this group of drugs which are used to quieten disturbed patients. They are thought to act by blocking dopaminergic impulses within the CNS but can also affect cholinergic, adrenergic and histamine receptors.

They may therefore give rise to extrapyramidal side-effects which require treatment with anticholinergic agents. They are well absorbed from the alimentary tract and are chiefly metabolized in the liver with a prominent enterohepatic recirculation occurring. The biological half-life of the phenothiazines is prolonged and metabolites may be excreted in the urine for months. Blood levels are correspondingly low. Poisoning with this group of drugs gives rise to irritability, lowered level of consciousness, convulsions, hypotension, tachycardia, hypothermia, ECG changes and a range of dystonic reactions. These latter problems can be alleviated by an anticholinergic drug such as benzotropine (Cogentin), orphenadrine (Disipal) or procylidine (Kemadrin). General management measures such as gastric lavage, emesis and administration of activated charcoal depend on the individual circumstances. Active elimination measures are ineffective because of the low plasma drug levels. Repeated doses of activated charcoal may bind drug excreted via the enterohepatic route.

Although hypothermia is usual in overdose, hyperthermia may occur. In rare cases it may be severe; 'neuroleptic malignant syndrome'. This requires active cooling and treatment with dantrolene (see Chapter 34).

Monoamine oxidase inhibitors

Although the use of this class of antidepressant is limited because of the serious side-effects, renewed interest has occurred because of favourable therapeutic responses in certain psychiatric conditions (Linden et al 1984). MAOIs act by inhibition of monoamine oxidase and cause an accumulation of amine neurotransmitters. However, they have inhibitory effects throughout the body, and can obstruct the first-pass metabolism of such compounds such as tyramine, resulting in severe sympathetic overactivity. They are readily absorbed from the gastrointestinal tract, metabolized in the liver and rapidly excreted as the acid metabolite, although their effect is prolonged due to irreversible inhibition of their target enzyme.

Overdose or interaction with these compounds will result in CNS excitation and sympathetic stimulation. There is a latent phase of 12–24 h before the onset of toxic symptoms. This is followed by neuromuscular excitation (muscle spasm, rigidity, facial grimacing, opisthotonus) and sympathetic hyperactivity (tremor, irritability and agitation, tachycardia and hypertension and fixed dilated pupils). The core temperature often rises, causing severe hyperpyrexia. Convulsions may occur and precede CNS depression and cardiovascular collapse.

Treatment is predominantly supportive, always remembering that there is a latent period before symptoms appear. The sympathetic overactivity should be controlled with sedatives or β-adrenergic blocking agents. Chlorpromazine can control the cerebral excitement and hyperpyrexia. If this is severe, dantrolene (1 mg kg^{-1} bolus repeated as necessary to total of 10 mg kg^{-1}), muscle relaxation and artificial ventilation may be necessary for control.

Hypertension should be controlled with a rapid, short-acting parenteral agent such as phentolamine or sodium nitroprusside. Hypotension will require volume replacement and agents that act directly on the post-synaptic receptors rather than relying on the release of intracellular amines whose kinetics may be altered by MAOIs (noradrenaline, dopamine).

The use of elimination procedures is not warranted.

Tricyclic antidepressants

These are the most commonly prescribed antidepressants and act by blocking the re-uptake of noradrenaline and/or 5-hydroxytryptamine, thus leading to increased amine concentration in certain areas of the brain. As basic compounds they are poorly absorbed from the stomach but much better from the duodenum, and as very lipophilic compounds they become extensively tissue-bound with a predilection for cardiac tissue. Overdose has wide-ranging effects on the central and peripheral nervous system, the parasympathetic system (atropine-like) and on the cardiovascular system (quinine-like). Symptoms appear within 1 h and are initially anticholinergic in character such as drowsiness, dry mouth, dilated pupils, tachycardia, blurred vision, urinary retention and a paralytic ileus. Convulsions and increased reflexes with an extensor plantar response associated with hypertension and arrhythmias herald the onset of reduced re-uptake of noradrenaline. Once the catecholamine reserves are depleted the stage of cardiorespiratory depression occurs with brainstem areflexia and coma leading to death.

The cardiac effects are varied because of the conflicting influences of the anticholinergic, sympathetic and quinidine-like actions. This latter effect probably accounts for the ECG changes and the impaired myocardial contractility.

In severe intoxication the usually slightly raised heart rate returns to normal or even slows. There may be widening of the QRS complex and decreases in the size of the P wave. There is an associated fall in blood pressure.

Severity of poisoning can be estimated from the duration of the QRS complex and from plasma levels. Severe poisoning occurs at levels of more than 1 mg l^{-1}. Treatment involves gastric lavage even up to 12 h following ingestion, as the anticholinergic effects delay gastric emptying. Activated charcoal may be useful in reducing absorption. Supportive measures are necessary and include correction of arterial pH, blood gas tensions and electrolyte levels. Arrhythmia control will be easier when these are normalized. Further treatment of the arrhythmias should be resisted if possible, but phenytoin or practolol may be needed. Treatment with disopyramide, lignocaine, quinidine or procainamide is contra-indicated, as they potentiate the cardiotoxicity. Bradycardia may be treated by cardiac pacing; ventricular fibrillation should be treated by conventional means.

Physostigmine, an anticholinesterase which can cross the blood–brain barrier, will reverse the coma and delirium, given as an infusion of $4–6 \text{ mg h}^{-1}$. Its use to reverse the arrhythmias is potentially dangerous as it can lead to bradycardia and even asystole. It should be used to treat arrhythmias only if they are life-threatening.

Tricyclic antidepressants have a large volume of distribution and as such are not readily eliminated by forced diuresis, haemodialysis or haemoperfusion.

Amoxapine

This dibenzoxazepine derivative has a tricyclic structure with a fourth ring as a side structure (Kulig 1986). Unlike other tricyclic agents it blocks dopamine receptors, perhaps resulting in neuroleptic, in addition to antidepressant, effects. Compared with other tricyclic drugs, features of overdose with amoxapine are a lack of cardiovascular toxicity but a higher incidence of convulsions and acute renal failure. The mortality rate following overdose may be higher. Treatment is supportive.

Maprotiline

This tetracyclic antidepressant, like the tricyclics, inhibits re-uptake of noradrenaline at nerve endings. It may have the advantage of fewer anticholinergic side-effects; conversely, central effects such as delirium and convulsions occur more readily than with tricyclics (Kulig 1986). Thus, maprotiline's toxicity to the CNS may exceed its peripheral anticholinergic effects. Physostigimine is therefore not likely to be useful, and indeed has been shown to precipitate seizures. Cardiac toxicity is probably similar to that found with tricyclics.

Mianserin

This tetracyclic is thought to act by increasing noradrenaline release and by inhibiting serotonin uptake. It has no anticholinergic properties and appears to be less toxic when taken as an overdose. The clinical features include a lowered level of consciousness, sinus tachycardia, dizziness and ataxia. Treatment is supportive.

Trazodone

This compound has a unique structure among antidepressants and acts by selectively inhibiting serotonin reuptake (Kulig 1986). It has no anticholinergic properties and little or no effect on noradrenaline, although it can block adrenergic receptors. It has no active metabolites and also stands out among tricyclics and tetracyclics by having a shorter half-life of 4–6 h. Its volume of distribution is thought to be smaller than tri- or tetracyclics, which have large volumes. Overdose would appear to cause only mild cardiac effects but other symptoms include drowsiness, dizziness and nausea.

Lithium

The salts of this metal are used in the treatment of mania. They have a low therapeutic index and as the main route of elimination is by the kidneys, reduced renal function can lead to accumulation. Toxicity is worsened by sodium depletion so disruption of water and electrolyte balance (diuretic therapy or water loss by vomiting or diarrhoea) can also promote poisoning. The therapeutic range is 0.6–1.2 mmol l^{-1} with poisoning occurring if levels reach 1.5 mmol l^{-1} and becoming severe at 2.0 mmol l^{-1}. Symptoms may be delayed by 12 or more hours and include apathy followed by thirst, polyuria, diarrhoea and vomiting. In severe cases depressed level of consciousness, hypertonicity and tremor, nystagmus, dysarthria, convulsions and coma occur. Further problems which may arise are oliguria leading to anuria, electrolyte disturbances, hypotension, cardiac conduction defects and arrhythmias.

In mild cases, administration of sodium and fluid may reverse toxicity. Initial management of the more severe cases includes gastric lavage, which can be useful up to 6 h after ingestion. A plasma estimation should be performed, although its interpretation should be combined with a clinical assessment of the patient. Supportive therapy including diazepam to control convulsions is indicated. In the more severe cases with renal impairment forced diuresis and saline infusions may be dangerous. Haemodialysis removes lithium easily and is the treatment of choice, especially if the plasma level is greater than 5 mmol l^{-1}. It may need to be repeated as lithium returns into the plasma from the extravascular compartment.

Agricultural and horticultural chemicals

Paraquat

This weedkiller is available either as Gramoxone (20% paraquat), Weedol (2.5% paraquat and diquat) or Pathclear (2.5% paraquat and simazine). Its herbicidal action is due to an interference with electron transfer during photosynthesis, causing superoxide and peroxide radical production. In humans these radicals are also produced in the gastrointestinal tract, kidney, liver and

lungs. In the lungs an active transport mechanism results in concentrations at least 6 times that of the concentration in other tissues. It is rapidly absorbed after ingestion, causing burns and ulceration to the mouth and oesophagus, vomiting and diarrhoea. It is rapidly distributed to tissues and at doses of less than 6 g may lead to death over a period ranging from several days to months. Hepatic, renal or pulmonary damage may appear within 24 h but is more usual after 3 days. The hepatocellular and renal tubular damage can be mild but the pulmonary damage is often severe with a chemical pneumonitis leading to progressive fibrosis and death. Ingestion of 6 g or more will lead to a rapid death within hours from circulatory failure, convulsions and metabolic acidosis.

Confirmation of paraquat poisoning is made by adding urine to an alkaline solution of sodium diathionite. A green or blue colour is confirmatory; the prognosis can then be estimated by relating the plasma paraquat level to time from ingestion (Proudfoot et al 1979).

Treatment involves gastric emptying and lavage followed by measures to absorb the poison either with Fullers earth (250 ml of a 30% solution every 4 h) or activated charcoal (50 g) followed by a purgative. Further measures such as whole-gut lavage, forced diuresis, haemodialysis or haemoperfusion are not warranted unless performed very soon after ingestion as the poison becomes tissue-bound very quickly. Other therapy is supportive, but added oxygen therapy may *increase* the toxicity of paraquat.

Organophosphates and carbamates

These substances are found in a wide range of insecticides and are all cholinesterase inhibitors. They can be absorbed through skin, respiratory tract and gastrointestinal tract and give rise to effects due to accumulation of acetylcholine at nicotinic and muscarinic receptors in autonomic ganglia, neuromuscular junctions, smooth muscle and CNS.

There are considerable differences in toxicity between different members of this group, organophosphates having a longer effect than carbamates. The organophosphate compounds phosphorylate the active site of acetylcholinesterase forming a stable complex, but the carbamates carbamylate the site forming a compound which can hydrolyse spontaneously. The earliest features seen are muscarinic effects in the body system where entry was obtained. There is miosis and blurred vision, salivation, nausea and vomiting, abdominal colic and diarrhoea, bradycardia, coughing with frothy secretions and pulmonary oedema. The nicotinic effects are manifested as progressive fasciculation, flaccidity and weakness of all muscle groups which may proceed to paralysis. In severe poisoning there are CNS effects of anxiety, irritability, and dizziness leading to lowering of the conscious level and convulsions.

Treatment initially involves removal of the poison, establishment of an airway, artificial ventilation if needed and removal of bronchial secretions. Atropine inhibits the effects of these agents at the muscarinic receptor. Full atropinization will require 2 mg repeated at 5–10-min intervals until there is evidence of dilated pupils, a dry mouth and a restored or rapid pulse. It may need to be continued for several days but has little effect at the autonomic ganglia or neuromuscular junction.

With carbamate poisoning, cholinesterase inhibition reverses spontaneously but with organophosphate poisoning treatment is needed. Pralidoxime mesylate will regenerate the cholinesterase enzyme and reverse the action of the poison at the neuromuscular junction but not at autonomic or CNS sites. It acts by forming an inert complex with the organophosphate. The antidote (15–30 mg kg^{-1} is given by slow intravenous injection, which may be repeated. If it is given too quickly it may precipitate further weakness, diplopia, dizziness, headache, nausea and tachycardia. It should be given with the atropine or as soon after as possible, and certainly within 24 h of poisoning as the organophosphate–acetylcholinesterase complex becomes resistant to regeneration. Regeneration will allow a reduction in the dose of atropine.

Phenoxyacetates (2,4-D; MCPA)

These compounds are widely used as 'hormone' weed-killers. After ingestion they cause a feeling of burning in the mouth, nausea and vomiting, pyrexia, sweating, hyperventilation leading to convulsions, and coma. An acute myopathy with pain, fasciculation, weakness and myoglobinuria may occur. Appropriate steps to empty the stomach should be made. 2,4-D and mecoprop as acidic compounds will be eliminated more rapidly with the help of a forced alkaline diuresis.

Cardiac drugs

Although uncommon, poisoning with these drugs requires an intimate knowledge of their pharmacodynamic profile for correct management. They often present with hypotension and/or arrhythmias. General management for them all includes gastric lavage or emesis, the administration of activated charcoal (5–10 times the suspected amount of overdose) and supportive care of the cardiorespiratory systems. Electrolyte concentrations must be measured and corrected urgently. Invasive measures such as the administration of positive inotropes and temporary cardiac pacing may be necessary.

β-Adrenergic blocking agents

These compounds exert their effect by competing with catecholamines for β-adrenoceptor sites, although most have no stimulatory effect on those sites. Those that do possess intrinsic sympathomimetic activity (pindolol, oxprenolol, acebutolol, alprenolol and oxprenolol) have a low-grade stimulatory effect on the β-receptor while inhibiting the much stronger effect of endogenous catecholamines (Weinstein 1984). β-Adrenoceptors exist as two subgroups and certain compounds can selectively inhibit the inotropic and chronotropic of catecholamines at the β_1-receptors in the heart. The β_1-selective agents such as practolol, atenolol and metoprolol usually do not produce bronchospasm or hypoglycaemia at therapeutic doses, but lose their selectivity at the doses achieved after an overdose; they become the same as the non-selective agents.

The clinical features found following a small overdose are usually bradycardia and hypotension. Larger overdoses can present with convulsions and coma in association with severe bradycardia and hypotension. Other features include hypoglycaemia, hallucinations and a variety of ECG changes such as first-degree heart block, prolongation of the QRS complex, absence of the P wave, conduction defects, ventricular tachycardia and fibrillation and asystole.

A patient's clinical picture will depend on the pharmacological properties of the particular agent taken. The widening of the QRS complex seen with propranolol is probably due to its membrane-stabilizing effect. Overdose with sotalol may cause prolongation of the QT interval giving rise to life-threatening ventricular arrhythmias; the prolongation is related to the drug's ability to prolong the duration of the action potential and lengthen the effective refractory period. Practolol and pindolol both possess a relatively high degree of intrinsic sympathomimetic activity (ISA) which can help to maintain heart rate and blood pressure during overdose. Both drugs also lack the membrane-stabilizing properties, making overdose-induced convulsions unlikely. On the other hand the seizures seen with propranolol overdose are related to its membrane-stabilizing effect and its high lipid solubility which allows easy access to the CNS. The capacity of the other β-blockers to cause seizures is probably in direct relation to their membrane-stabilizing effect and lipid solubility.

Management involves instituting supportive measures. Gastric lavage is perhaps preferable to emesis because of the unpredictable nature of the seizures (especially with propranolol). On the other hand, it may stimulate an overwhelming vagal discharge; lavage should be covered by the administration of atropine (0.6–1.2 mg). A nasogastric tube should be left in situ if glucagon is to be used, as it may produce vomiting.

Many treatments have been tried to reverse the adverse haemodynamic effect of a massive β-blocker overdose. The agents or treatments commonly used are atropine, isoprenaline, dobutamine, and intracardiac pacing. The most successful appears to be glucagon; the polypeptide hormone produced by the α cells of the pancreas with biological half-life of approximately 3–6 min. It promotes formation of cyclic AMP from ATP and thus exerts a direct stimulating effect on the heart that is independent of the β-adrenergic receptor. As a positive inotrope it is unaffected by β-blockade although as a chronotrope it is partially affected. Glucagon therefore increases cardiac output and decreases total peripheral resistance. It should be given as a dose of 4–10 mg over 30 s followed by an infusion of 1–3 mg h^{-1}. When administered intravenously it elevates the serum glucose and may cause severe nausea and vomiting. During the infusion the serum glucose should be monitored and after cessation of treatment rebound hypoglycaemia should be guarded against.

For those drugs with a high renal excretion, (practolol, nadolol, sotalol) promotion of a diuresis may help.

Calcium channel blockers

Calcium antagonists inhibit transmembrane calcium transport, reducing peripheral vascular resistance, myocardial contractility, sinus node automaticity and the speed of AV nodal conduction. As with β-blockers there are differences between members of this class of drug. Nifedipine reduces peripheral and coronary vascular resistance more than verapamil, which has its greatest effect on the speed of AV nodal conduction.

Overdose may produce nausea and vomiting, dizziness, bradycardia, atrioventricular block, hypotension and metabolic acidosis. Treatment is supportive along with measures to combat the cardiovascular effects. Injection of 10–20 ml of calcium chloride (10%) intravenously may shorten the intracardiac conduction time. With severe poisoning large amounts of intravenous fluids and inotropic support may be necessary to combat hypotension.

Digoxin and digitoxin

Digitalis is widely available and serious overdose is important because it is often fatal. Following doses of 15 mg the average mortality is approximately 18% and reaches 95% following ingestion of over 35 mg. Plasma concentrations become toxic at levels greater than 2.5 μg l^{-1} but serious problems only arise at levels above 10 μg l^{-1}. However, plasma levels may not correlate closely with severity of poisoning.

Digoxin overdose leads to inhibition of the sodium and potassium activated ATP-ase pump which causes an increase in the plasma potassium level. This rise is correlated strongly with the clinical course. A single ECG recording with only minor changes or only a few symptoms may be misleading, as severe deterioration in cardiac state or rhythm may occur very suddenly.

Nausea and vomiting are constant features of a toxic overdose, with diarrhoea occurring less frequently. Drowsiness, mental confusion and even a psychosis have been observed. Bradycardia and cardiac arrhythmias are common. There may be varying degrees of atrioventricular block. Supraventricular arrhythmias with or without heart block, and less commonly ventricular ectopic beats, ventricular tachycardia and ventricular fibrillation, may also occur.

Treatment is supportive. Gastric lavage, if indicated, should be carried out with care because any increase in vagal tone may lead to cardiac arrest. Bradycardia can be treated with atropine which may need to be repeated over a period of several days. In serious poisoning transvenous cardiac pacing may be required. Hyperkalaemia should be treated with intravenous glucose and insulin, although with a large overdose the potassium level may not decrease because of the severe inhibition of the Na$^+$/K$^+$ pump. In these cases treatment with Fab digoxin specific antibody fragments (Digibind — Wellcome Foundation Ltd) is warranted (see below). Hypokalaemia can occur in certain cases receiving chronic diuretic therapy. A cautious intravenous infusion of 30 mmol potassium chloride in 200 ml 5% dextrose should be given until the plasma potassium level is normal. Ventricular ectopics should be treated only if they are compromising the cardiac output; lignocaine 100 mg or mexiletine 250 mg intravenously followed by an infusion of a 0.1% solution are suitable for ventricular extrasystoles and ventricular tachyarrhythmias. Should these fail, amiodarone 5 mg kg^{-1} as a bolus over 5–10 min followed by an infusion of 900 mg over 24 h is appropriate.

Measures to increase elimination, such as forced diuresis, haemodialysis or haemoperfusion, are ineffective because the plasma is constantly being replenished from the extensive tissue compartment; the volume of distribution is large at 7 l kg^{-1}. The results of haemoperfusion with Amberlite XAD-4 resin are more encouraging. Haemoperfusion in cases of digitoxin poisoning may be more effective because of its smaller volume of distribution (0.5 1 1 kg^{-1}).

The treatment of choice for the elimination of digoxin is the administration of digoxin specific Fab antibody fragments (Wenger et al 1985). IgG antibodies to digoxin are raised in sheep and then cleaved enzymatically by papain. The Fc and other Fab fragments are separated from the drug-specific antibody by affinity chromatography. The Fab fragments lack complement-fixing activity and are not susceptible to immune degradation. They work because their affinity for digoxin is greater than that of digoxin for its receptor. Digoxin is therefore attracted away from the receptor on heart tissues. Following administration, improvements in signs and symptoms begin within 30 min. At this time the plasma digoxin concentration rises (10–20-fold), the digoxin now being plasma-bound. It is, however, protein-bound and is pharmacologically inactive. There is also a decrease in the serum potassium.

The low molecular weight of the complex (50 000 Daltons) means it is small enough to cross the glomerular basement membrane. The plasma elimination half-life after intravenous administration of Fab ranges from 16 to 34 h in patients with good renal function. Experience with the use of Fab fragments in patients with severe renal impairment is limited. Such patients might exhibit a decreased elimination of the complex which eventually would be metabolized with the subsequent release of free digoxin and a recurrence of toxicity.

After the administration of Fab fragments, most of the digoxin in serum is bound and cannot displace radiolabelled digoxin in competitive binding assays. Thus it is not possible to follow serum digoxin concentrations with routine radio-immune assays. As the Fab fragments are extremely expensive this approach must be used only when specific indications are fulfilled. They are a rising and uncontrollable potassium concentration, life-threatening cardiac arrhythmias and a serum digoxin concentration of greater than 20 μg l^{-1}. Following a dose of 2 mg to test for rare allergic reactions a therapeutic dose is given diluted in 100 ml 5% dextrose over 15 min. The dose is calculated from the amount of digoxin ingested multiplied by 0.80 to take into account incomplete absorption and by 60 (molecular weight of drug/antibody complex = 60).

As experience of this treatment is limited the side-effects are unknown. The re-exposure of animals to these fragments has led to an antibody response; in humans re-exposure could lead to severe hypersensitivity or even anaphylaxis. The immunogenic threat of Fab fragments should, however, be less than that from an intact immunoglobulin molecule. In patients therapeutically dependent on digoxin the use of Digibind could precipitate a return of heart failure or arrhythmia.

Disopyramide

This is used to control cardiac tachyarrhythmias, increasing the refractory period of both the atrial and ventricular myocardium and slowing conduction in the accessary conducting pathways. It has no α- or β-adrenergic blocking activity but anticholinergic effects are prominent. It is rapidly and almost completely absorbed, peak plasma levels being reached within 2 h; 80% of an absorbed dose is excreted through the kidney, 50% as the unchanged drug.

The main organ affected is the heart. The drug is a potent negative inotrope and can cause death from cardiac failure within 2 h. There is bradycardia and often, though not always, hypotension. With its effect on the conducting pathways there may be widening of the QRS complex and serious cardiac arrhythmias. There is often respiratory depression which may be severe, and other effects associated with the anticholinergic properties of the drug such as dry mouth, dilated pupils and blurring of vision. Glaucoma and urinary retention may also occur.

Management is supportive with particular attention being paid to correction of acidosis and hypokalaemia. Bradycardia may be corrected with atropine aided by an infusion of isoprenaline (5–50 μg min^{-1}). This drug may also be needed to treat hypotension. Other depressant drugs such as quinidine or procainamide are contraindicated. Of the elimination techniques only haemoperfusion has been shown to be effective.

Amiodarone

This drug is probably the most potent anti-arrhythmic in use for management of tachyarrhythmias of a paroxysmal nature, including supraventricular, nodal and ventricular tachycardias. Because of its association with frequent and serious side-effects it is used only when conventional therapy has failed. It has a slow onset of action; requires a loading dose period to achieve a therapeutic effect and therefore has a low acute toxicity. The terminal half-life is within the range 15–30 days so that excessive dosage can lead to toxicity within the maintenance period. Side-effects will disappear slowly as the tissue levels decline after treatment has been withdrawn.

Following an acute overdose the signs and symptoms that may be found include nausea and vomiting, headache with flushing, paraesthesia, ataxia, tremor and vertigo, bradycardia and hypotension.

Management is supportive with inotropic agents (dopamine or dobutamine infusions) being necessary to treat hypotension. Glucagon (see β-blockers) may be required.

Respiratory drugs

Poisoning with drugs used in respiratory therapy is common. In particular the slow-release form of the theophylline derivatives has become a serious and frequent problem.

Theophyllines

The mechanisms of action of this group of drugs are varied but there are three main ones. These are an increase in the levels of cyclic AMP (adenosine 5-monophosphate) by phosphodiesterase inhibition; catecholamine-related increases in cAMP and effects on calcium kinetics.

Adverse effects occur readily because theophylline has a low therapeutic index, the therapeutic range of plasma concentration being $10-20$ mg l^{-1}. There is, however, only a general relationship between the features of toxicity (Buckley et al 1983) and the plasma concentration, with toxic effects becoming evident at 25 mg l^{-1} and convulsions occurring at levels of over 50 mg l^{-1}. Levels of greater than 60 mg l^{-1} are often fatal. If a slow-release formulation has been taken serum levels may continue increasing for a prolonged period, necessitating repeated blood sampling. Drug metabolism is mainly hepatic and is reduced in cirrhosis, cardiac failure, pulmonary disease, severe renal failure, obesity, in those over 50 years of age and in neonates. Conversely the half-life is shortened by a high-protein diet, in patients who smoke or take phenobarbitone or are aged between 1 and 20 years of age.

The early clinical features are those of nausea and vomiting, abdominal pain, haematemesis and diarrhoea. With the increased myocardial stimulation and catecholamine release there may be sinus, supraventricular and ventricular tachycardias. Hypotension with a metabolic acidosis may be precipitated by the decline in peripheral resistance, or can be a result of a severe gastrointestinal haemorrhage. Stimulation of the central nervous system may produce headache, restlessness, agitation, hyperventilation with a respiratory alkalosis, tremor, hyper-reflexia and convulsions leading to coma. An important feature is the development of hypokalaemia with the sodium-potassium ATPase causing influx of potassium into the cells. This predisposes to arrhythmias and skeletal muscle damage (rhabdomyolysis).

Gastric lavage should be carried out on all those who present within 12 h of an overdose, and should be followed by the administration of oral activated charcoal. This will reduce absorption and increase enterohepatic elimination. Serum levels should be measured and repeated in order not to miss a rising drug level.

It is vital that electrolyte and acid–base disturbances are corrected early, as this may be the only aggressive treatment needed. Nausea and vomiting may not respond to anti-emetics, although the gastrointestinal haemorrhage may respond to H_2 receptor blockers. Convulsions will require intravenous diazepam. Cardiac arrhythmias should be treated only if severe, and not with β-blockers if the patient is an asthmatic. They should initially be managed by correction of pH, Po_2 and electrolytes, and if necessary by verapamil or disopyramide.

Active elimination measures such as haemodialysis and especially haemoperfusion should be reserved for those with uncontrollable severe symptoms; a serum theophylline level of greater than 60 mg l^{-1} at 4 h after ingestion (greater than 30 mg l^{-1} in the elderly; greater than 80 mg l^{-1} in a child); in high-risk groups such as those with cardiac/respiratory/hepatic disease and in the elderly.

β$_2$-Agonists

Overdose with these agents can occur with the oral, parenteral or even nebulized forms. They all, however, tend to have a wide margin of safety. At high doses β-selectivity is lost, producing agitation, excitement, headache with a tachycardia, tremor and peripheral dilation. More serious complications include ventricular tachyarrhythmias, pulmonary oedema and convulsions. Hyperglycaemia, hypokalaemia and lactic acidosis also occur.

Gastric lavage should be performed if appropriate, and especially if a slow-release compound has been taken. Hypokalaemia should be treated with an intravenous potassium infusion. Should any serious cardiac arrhythmias remain following this correction, they may be treated with a cardioselective β-blocker such as atenolol ($2.5-10$ mg).

Alcohols and ethylene glycol

Methanol, ethanol, isopropanol and ethylene glycol are the most commonly ingested aliphatic alcohols. They are rapidly absorbed from the upper gastrointestinal tract and initially oxidized mainly by hepatic alcohol dehydrogenase. With the exception of isopropanol they are further metabolized by aldehyde dehydrogenase to yield acids. Methanol and ethanol will produce a large anion gap metabolic acidosis, whereas isopropanol does not result in an acidosis.

Methanol

Otherwise known as wood alcohol or methyl alcohol, this substance can cause poisoning from an accidental ingestion or when taken in home-made beverages, varnish, paint-removers, or antifreeze. This latter compound may also contain ethanol, isopropanol or ethylene glycol. Methylated spirit contains only 5% methanol and 95% ethanol, and is toxic because of its ethanol rather than methanol content.

Methanol is much more toxic than ethanol because it is metabolized to formaldehyde and formic acid, which cause a severe metabolic acidosis by an accumulation of hydrogen ions and by inhibiting gluconeogenesis and lactate conversion.

Initially the patient is confused and ataxic. A period of restlessness is followed by impairment of consciousness. The severe metabolic acidosis which develops after a latent period of 8–12 h leads to tachypnoea. The distribution of methanol to different tissues is determined by their water content and thus a high concentration is found in the vitreous body and optic nerve. Impairment of vision is a characteristic feature of the poisoning and may progress to blindness. Methanol can produce gastric irritation resulting in epigastric pain, nausea and vomiting, and has been associated with acute pancreatitis.

The treatment of methanol poisoning should be centred on gastric lavage followed by correcting the acidosis, inhibiting its metabolism and removing methanol itself with its metabolites. The acidosis will often require large doses of sodium bicarbonate and the sodium load may lead to hypernatraemia and fluid overload. The enzymatic oxidation of methanol is inhibited by ethanol because of the saturation of the alcohol dehydrogenase by ethanol. Indeed methylated spirit drinkers seldom develop toxic effects from methanol because they are protected by the larger amounts of ethanol ingested. Ethanol treatment should be instituted only if there are large amounts of methanol still to be metabolized, and only in adults.

Ethanol should be administered orally or intravenously as a loading dose to achieve a blood level of at least 1000 mg l^{-1}. As the V_d of ethanol is 600 ml kg^{-1} the intravenous dose needed is approximately 600 mg kg^{-1} of ethanol or approximately 1 ml kg^{-1} of a 95% solution, (95% alcohol has a density of 750 mg ml^{-1}). This could conveniently be given orally as 125 ml of whisky. These should be followed by an intravenous infusion of 10–15 g ethanol per hour or orally as 25 ml per hour of whisky. By maintaining an ethanol level of 1000–2000 mg l^{-1} the metabolism of methanol will be blocked because the alcohol dehydrogenase enzyme will be 90% saturated. The plasma ethanol and methanol concentrations should be frequently measured and the infusion continued until methanol is undetectable and the patient is no longer becoming acidotic, when the infusion is stopped. It is slowly eliminated by renal excretion over a period of days.

Removal of methanol and its metabolites once its metabolism has been halted by ethanol may be prompted by haemodialysis. This should be performed if more than 30 g of methanol has been ingested; if the blood concentration is greater than 500 mg l^{-1}; if the patient has a metabolic acidosis; if mental, visual or fundoscopic complications are present or there is renal failure. Should haemodialysis be undertaken the infusion of ethanol must be increased to 17–22 g h^{-1} to allow for ethanol that will be removed by dialysis. Folinic acid 30 mg intravenously every 6 h may protect against ocular toxicity by accelerating formate metabolism.

Ethanol

Ethanol or ethyl alcohol is a primary and progressive CNS depressant and as a frequent companion to other drugs in self-poisoning, ethanol can exacerbate effects of the other drugs. High concentrations induce pylorospasm, thus retarding gastric emptying. It is rapidly absorbed once in the small intestine, and is distributed throughout the body tissues according to their water content. Five per cent is eliminated intact and the rest is oxidized to acetaldehyde and then to acetate. The fatal dose will vary because of individual tolerance but about 600 ml of pure alcohol consumed in 1 h will be fatal.

Its effects are related to its blood concentration (Table 35.5). It also produces peripheral vasodilation, hypothermia and hypotension. In children hypoglycaemia is likely to occur and in adults a lactic acidosis may develop when associated with severe liver disease, pancreatitis, sepsis or hypotension. Dehydration and hypoglycaemia may lead to a ketotic state.

Most patients require only supportive measures. If levels are greater than 7500 mg l^{-1} haemodialysis should be carried out. Those with an acidosis will require correction of the blood glucose concentration and the fluid deficit. If unresponsive to treatment, haemodialysis may be needed.

Table 35.5   Clinical effects of Ethanol

Blood ethanol concentration (mg l^{-1})	Clinical effects
0–500	Decreased inhibition, slight inco-ordination
500–1000	Slowed reaction time, emotional instability, slurred speech
1000–1500	Poor reaction time, poor co-ordination, personality and behavioural changes
1500–3000	Sensory loss, visual disturbances, ataxia
3000–4000	Hypothermia, hypoglycaemia, severe ataxia, poor recall, blurred vision, stupor
4000–7000	Hyporeflexia, convulsions, respiratory failure, death

Isopropanol

This alcohol is found in disinfectants, aftershave lotions and antifreeze. An ingestion of 20 g may produce symptoms; 150–250 g may be fatal; the toxicity being due to the compound rather than its metabolites. Ingestion of this substance does not lead to an acidosis, 20% being excreted unchanged and 15% metabolized to acetone, most of which is excreted in the urine.

The CNS effects resemble those of ethanol. There is often a haemorrhagic gastritis, renal tubular necrosis, an acute myopathy and a haemolytic anaemia. Hypotension occurs with severe intoxication.

Treatment is supportive, with haemodialysis being used to control the serious complications especially if blood concentrations are greater than 400 mg l^{-1}.

Ethylene glycol

Ethylene glycol is a colourless, odourless liquid with a pleasant taste, which is used as an antifreeze compound either alone or with other alcohols. It is metabolized to glycoaldehyde by alcohol dehydrogenase and then to glycolic acid by aldehyde dehydrogenese in a similar fashion to methanol. Glycolic acid is the major metabolite responsible for the metabolic acidosis; 3% is converted to oxalic acid. This may combine with calcium to cause renal, cardiac and cerebral oxalosis.

Three stages of ethylene glycol poisoning have been identified (Berman et al 1957). An initial period of inebriation is followed several hours later by nausea and vomiting. There may be convulsions leading to coma, and also visual disturbances culminating in optic atrophy. The second stage is manifested by a progressive metabolic acidosis with tachycardia and tachypnoea arising from cardiac failure and pulmonary oedema. A later stage occurring 1–3 days following poisoning is distinguished by acute renal failure, often with pain in the renal angle. Calcium oxalate crystals may be found in the urine and there may be hypocalcaemia from chelation by the anionic metabolites of ethylene glycol.

Treatment of ethylene glycol poisoning is similar to that of methanol poisoning, and is based on inhibiting formation of toxic metabolites with ethanol, thus preventing the acidosis. The acidosis must be controlled with sodium bicarbonate. Haemodialysis will be indicated if more than 30 g of ethylene glycol is ingested, if the plasma concentration is greater than 500 mg l^{-1} and if there are serious clinical effects of the poisoning. Hypocalcaemia will need to be treated by infusions of calcium gluconate, repeated as necessary.

Asphyxiants

Asphyxiants interfere with tissue oxygenation either by preventing delivery of oxygen to the cell (carbon monoxide) or by interfering with cellular oxygen utilization (cyanide).

Carbon monoxide

Carbon monoxide (CO) poisoning is the most common type of chemical asphyxiation, causing over 1000 deaths in England and Wales annually. It is the most common cause of death from poisoning in children (Vale & Meredith 1985). It is a colourless, odourless, tasteless, non-irritating gas produced by the incomplete combustion of carbonaceous materials.

The causes of toxicity from CO poisoning are multifactorial. CO combines avidly with haemoglobin to form carboxyhaemoglobin (COHb). The affinity of CO for Hb is 223 times as great as that of oxygen and thus oxygen is replaced by CO reducing the total oxygen carrying capacity of blood, producing an 'anaemia'. Moreover the addition of CO to a molecule of haemoglobin shifts the HbO_2 dissociation curve to the left as the affinity of the remaining oxygen for their haem groups is increased. This interferes with the unloading of oxygen at tissue level and results in a greater degree of tissue anoxia than would be expected from a simple loss of oxygen carrying capacity. There is also strong evidence that CO inhibits cellular respiration by combining with other haem-containing proteins such as myoglobin and the cytochrome system (Meredith and Vale 1988). Combining with cytochromes only occurs under hypoxic conditions because its affinity of oxygen is 9.2 times that for CO (Ball et al 1951). Tissue toxicity of CO poisoning will therefore only be significant under hypoxic conditions when CO can combine with these enzymes. Once this occurs, CO may bind tightly and be resistant to reversal by conventional oxygen therapy. This tissue toxicity may be the major cause of the clinical features of severe CO poisoning and may explain the discrepancies between clinical features and blood COHb levels.

The clinical course is directly related to the degree and duration of exposure (Table 35.6). The acute effects of CO poisoning are due to tissue hypoxia, and as the brain and heart are the organs with the highest metabolic rate, they are the organs which demonstrate the major toxic manifestations. Individuals with pre-existing coronary and cerebral artery disease, myocardial insufficiency, pulmonary disease, or anaemia are more vulnerable. The CNS, being especially vulnerable to hypoxia, tends to be the most affected and the effect ranges from lethargy to acute agitation and mental confusion to coma.

Patients in whom consciousness is maintained usually recover rapidly and completely. Those who become unconscious may continue to deteriorate clinically despite a COHb which is returning to normal. This indicates the presence of cerebral oedema and is associated with papilloedema, hypertension and increased reflexes. Some patients may recover completely only to develop days or weeks later a 'delayed post-hypoxic encephalopathy'. Myocardial ischaemia is frequent and may precipitate angina and even progress to infarction. In severe poisoning the marked degree of hypoxia initially causes stimulation of the respiratory centre with hyperventilation. Acute pulmonary oedema may occur and respiratory centre failure may follow. Visual defects including loss of vision and retinal haemorrhage may occur. Acute neuropsychiatric findings range from headache and fatigue to epilepsy and chronic cognitive and psychomotor changes which may be permanent. Many of these abnormalities may be induced at low levels of COHb.

Various types of skin lesions can occur and vary from bullous eruptions to areas of erythema and alopecia. The pink skin colour due to carboxyhaemoglobin is uncommon unless poisoning is severe. Cyanosis and skin pallor are more common. It should be noted that in cyanide, atropine and phenothiazine poisoning a pink colour is also seen. The distinction between cyanide and CO poisoning is critical because appropriate treatment for one would be inappropriate for the other. Hyperpyrexia following skin sweat gland necrosis may be a feature. Myonecrosis may occur as a compartmental symptom and may even lead to rhabdomyolytic renal failure.

The most reliable method for diagnosis of CO poisoning is a direct measurement by spectrophotometry (oximetry). The correlation between COHb concentrations and clinical effects is given in Table 35.6. It must be borne in mind that CO is very rapidly eliminated and the blood level on arrival at hospital does not necessarily reflect the true insult if a delay occurs between exposure and COHb analysis. It should be noted that the Pao_2 is usually normal in CO poisoning as it reflects dissolved oxygen content of the blood and not haemoglobin saturation.

Treatment is initiated by terminating exposure, securing the airway and administering 100% oxygen as soon as possible, using either a tightly fitting face-mask or an endotracheal tube. The half-life of COHb in room air is 5–6 h; with 100% oxygen the half-life decreases to 45–90 min; with a hyperbaric pressure of 3 atmospheres the half-life approximates to 23 min. The mechanism of action of a high inspired oxygen fraction is that the CO will be diluted and displaced by oxygen from cytochromes, myoglobin and haemoglobin by a mass action effect. Hyperbaric oxygen will also increase the amount of oxygen dissolved in the blood to a level sufficient to meet tissue needs even without functioning haemoglobin. Treatment with hyperbaric oxygen will reduce the duration of coma, the incidence of the delayed encephalopathy and the long-term morbidity to less than 5% (Meredith & Vale 1988). Unfortunately it is not widely used because of the lack of suitable facilities. Broome and his colleagues (1988) recommend that if consciousness has not been lost and there are no other symptoms apart from headache or nausea or the COHb level is less than 40%, normobaric O_2 is sufficient. If however there are other symptoms or consciousness has been lost or the COHb level is greater than 40% then HBO is the treatment of choice. HBO should be applied at 2.5–3.0 atmospheres for periods of

Table 35.6 Clinical effects of carbon monoxide poisoning

Concentration COHb (%)	Signs and symptoms
0.3–0.7	Normal range
<10	No symptoms
10–20	Slight headache, variable vasodilation
20–30	Throbbing headache, dyspnoea and angina on exertion
30–40	Severe headache, nausea, vomiting, visual disturbance, weakness, dizziness
40–50	Syncope, tachycardia, tachypnoea
50–60	Coma, convulsions, Cheyne–Stokes respiration
60–70	Cardiorespiratory failure, death

at least 90 mins and should be repeated till there is no further improvement in the level of consciousness.

Further supportive treatment should be given as required, especially if there is evidence of myocardial ischaemia or cerebral oedema.

Cyanide

Inhalation, cutaneous absorption or ingestion of cyanide can produce death from asphyxia within a few minutes, although it can be delayed for several hours. Hydrogen cyanide (hydrocyanic acid: prussic acid) or its salts are widely used in numerous industrial processes including precious metal extraction and electroplating processes. It is also used as a fumigant and in the extermination of rabbits by farmers. It arises from the combustion of polyurethane foams from furniture upholstery, which is probably a more common cause of cyanide poisoning than is generally appreciated. Cigarette smokers have been found to have mean whole blood cyanide levels of about 0.41 μg ml^{-1} (Ballantine 1983).

Cyanide causes a histotoxic (intracellular) hypoxic poisoning by the binding of the cyanide ion to the ferric (Fe^{3+}) ion of mitochondrial cytochrome oxidase. This causes inhibition of cytochrome oxidase activity paralysing the tricarboxylic acid cycle and leading to anaerobic metabolism with reduced formation of ATP and lactic acidosis. Cellular utilization of oxygen is severely depressed and the venous Po_2 is increased. Indeed the arterial and venous blood samples will demonstrate a similar Po_2. The body has major routes of cyanide detoxication (thiosulphate or rhodanese pathways) and minor routes (cysteine binding, hydroxy cobalamin binding, oxidation and excretion via the lungs). These mechanisms may be rapidly overwhelmed in the face of significant quantities of cyanide.

The speed of onset and severity of symptoms and signs depends on the quantity of cyanide absorbed. Following exposure to a small amount the initial features often mimic those of anxiety with hyperventilation and CNS stimulation. There is cyanide stimulation of the carotid chemoreceptors and the respiratory centres during this early phase. There may also be hypertension with a reflex bradycardia and various degrees of atrioventricular block. Headache, dyspnoea, palpitations, vomiting, ataxia and loss of consciousness may occur gradually. If a large amount is absorbed the features appear very rapidly and the patient becomes deeply unconscious. There is hypotension and the ECG will show changes consistent with hypoxia. The limb reflexes are absent and the pupils become dilated. A metabolic acidosis can present, as can slowing of the respiratory rate leading to profound respiratory depression. Pulmonary and cerebral oedema may arise. Since the oxygen-carrying capacity of haemoglobin is unimpaired the blood looks well oxygenated and cyanosis does not occur until the stage of circulatory collapse and respiratory depression. The odour of bitter almonds, although pathognomonic, may not necessarily be present.

Blood cyanide levels of below 1 mg l^{-1} are usually associated with the early stage of poisoning, while levels of 1–3 mg l^{-1} correlate with severe toxicity leading to death. Some cyanide binds to the ferrous (Fe^{2+}) ion of normal haemoglobin. This cyanhaemoglobin cannot transport oxygen and will lead to a discrepancy between the measured (by Co-oximeter) arterial oxygen saturation and the calculated (by nomogram) oxygen saturation. If the difference between the two values is 5 or greater it is suggestive of a poison producing an abnormal (non-oxygen-transporting) haemoglobin. Poisons which will produce this gap include carbon monoxide, hydrogen sulphide and methaemoglobin producing agents.

Once the diagnosis is suspected, therapy must be instituted rapidly. Removal of the patient from exposure to hydrogen cyanide gas in inhalational exposures, or gastric emptying after ingestion, can decrease absorption of the poison. Administration of activated charcoal has not yet been shown to be beneficial. Provision of supportive care in the form of 100% oxygen, carefully applied artificial ventilation avoiding intoxication of the resuscitator, control of seizures, correction of acidosis and cardiovascular support may be sufficient to allow survival in the less severe cases.

For the severe cases there are three specific types of antidote: thiosulphate and nitrites; dicobalt edetate and hydroxocobalamin. Some of these compounds are extremely toxic in the absence of cyanide ions and it is therefore essential to be certain that the diagnosis of cyanide toxicity is correct and that free cyanide is still circulating, before administration of the antidote.

Cyanide may be converted to the less toxic thiocyanate by rhodanese. Thiosulphate is required for this reaction and its administration increases the rate of cyanide metabolism; 50 ml of a 25% solution is administered intravenously over 10 min. It is not very effective on its own and is usually preceded by sodium nitrite (10 ml of a 30% solution intravenously over 5 min) which causes the formation of methaemoglobin. This has iron in the ferric state rather than the ferrous state. It will attach to the cytochrome oxidase–cyanide complex to form cyanmethaemoglobin, freeing the cytochrome oxidase to take up its normal activity. Methaemoglobinaemia should be reduced to levels of less that 40%. As the cyanide dissociates from the methaemoglobin it is metabolized by rhodanese to thiocyanate.

The methaemoglobin-producing agents have now been superseded by the chelating agent, dicobalt edetate (Kelocyanor). It forms inert complexes with the cyanide. An initial 600 mg is given intravenously over 1 min followed by a further 300 mg if there is no improvement within 1 min. This compound, if administered in the absence of cyanide or when cyanmethaemoglobin has already been produced by nitrite administration, may produce its own toxic effects – hypotension, tachycardia, vomiting, facial and palpebral oedema. It should not be used as a precautionary measure.

One mole of hydroxocobalamin inactivates one mole of cyanide by forming cyanocobalamin in a minor route of elimination of cyanide. This method of treatment is not practical because of the relatively large volumes of hydroxocobalamin needed, its brevity of action ($T_{\frac{1}{2}} = $ 5 min) and its high cost.

If poisoning is due to ingestion, the administration of the antidotes should be carried out as soon as possible. Gastric lavage should then be carried out and 300 ml of 25% sodium thiosulphate left in the stomach.

Anticonvulsants

Phenytoin

This is an effective broad-spectrum anticonvulsant. The metabolism is mainly hepatic and is saturable. When this occurs it causes a substantial rise in the circulating concentration leading to toxicity. Nystagmus, ataxia and dysarthria occur at levels (greater than 25 mg l^{-1}) only slightly exceeding those needed therapeutically (10–20 mg l^{-1}) and are the cardinal symptoms of poisoning. Severe overdose may result in coma with unresponsive pupils and hypotension. Treatment is supportive.

Carbamazepine

This is a first-line drug for management of grand-mal, focal and temporal lobe seizures, as well as for patients with trigeminal neuralgia. It has a tricyclic structure; it is related to the tricyclic antidepressants and has anticholinergic properties. Absorption from the gastrointestinal tract is slow and probably incomplete. It is metabolized in the liver to an active metabolite, very little unchanged drug appearing in the urine. The therapeutic range is 4–10 mg l^{-1}, although some patients tolerate 16 mg l^{-1} or above. Overdose will cause symptoms ranging from lowered level of consciousness with hyporeflexia to convulsions and coma. Bradycardia or even complete heart block may occur.

Sodium valproate

This drug can be used in a variety of types of seizures. It is rapidly absorbed so gastric emptying procedures may be non-productive. The therapeutic range is 5–100 mg l^{-1}. At plasma levels of 5–6 times the therapeutic maximum the symptoms experienced are nausea, vomiting and dizziness. Levels of 10–20 times the maximum therapeutic levels may be associated with CNS depression. Valproic acid inhibits platelet aggregation, and thrombocytopenia may occur so that bleeding may be a feature of overdose. Treatment is supportive.

Primidone

This is especially indicated for management of grand-mal and temporal lobe epilepsy. It is partially metabolized to two active metabolites, phenobarbitone and phenylethylmalonamide. Overdose will lead to ataxia, CNS depression and eventually respiratory depression and coma.

Most anticonvulsants are lipid-soluble, and although their precise mode of action is not clear they appear to halt the spread of depolarization from an epileptic focus. Overdose is more likely to have serious effects if a combination of drugs is taken.

Miscellaneous

Quinine

Quinine is an alkaloid originally extracted from the bark of the Cinchona tree. It is used therapeutically as an antimalarial and to control nocturnal cramps. It is also used as an abortifacient, and because of its bitter taste as an additive in tonic water and illicit heroin.

Overdose will give rise to the collection of symptoms known as cinchonism; headache, vertigo, tinnitus, deafness, nausea and vomiting. Severe poisoning will also lead to collapse with depressed consciousness, hyperventilation, tachycardia and hypotension. Cardiac arrhythmias and arrest may occur; quinine and quinidine are optical isomers. ECG changes that may occur include widening of the QRS complex and flattening of the T waves. Acute intravascular haemolysis and thrombocytopenia may occur.

Visual disturbances are a hallmark of quinine poisoning. Initially there may be blurring of vision and the pupils may become dilated and non-reactive. After a latent period the optic fundi show optic pallor, arteriolar constriction and a cherry-red macular spot. Progression to total blindness can occur. Return of vision is usual, although some patients may be left with a peripheral field defect and optic atrophy. The optic toxicity of quinine is caused either by retinal artery vasospasm or by a direct toxic effect on the ganglion or retinal cells or both. Visual loss appears to occur in patients with quinine concentrations greater than 10 mg l^{-1}.

Treatment is aimed at removal of the poison from the gastrointestinal tract. Because of quinine's anticholinergic properties gastric emptying may be delayed, warranting measures to empty the stomach beyond the usual 4 h period. Activated charcoal may then be given. Further treatment is supportive.

Management of the visual complications is controversial. There are many clinical reports of the efficacy of stellate ganglion block in treating the vasospasm of the retinal vessels. However, blindness often precedes any ophthalmological changes and can be associated with normal fundal appearances and normal arterial calibre. If stellate ganglion block can be carried out by an experienced operator it may be useful. Otherwise management of the visual disturbances should be expectant, as reversal often occurs without active therapy.

Acidification of the urine and forced diuresis should double the excretion of the alkaloid base by rendering it less likely to be reabsorbed by the renal tubule. As the compound is largely protein-bound the amount removed will still be limited. The other methods of increasing elimination are also unwarranted.

REFERENCES

Ball E G, Strittmatter C F, Cooper O 1951 The reaction of cytochrome oxidase with carbon monoxide. Journal of Biological Chemistry 193 (2): 635–647

Ballantine B 1983 Artifacts in the definition of toxicity of cyanides and cyanogens. Fundamental Applied Toxicology 3: 405–406

Berman L B, Schreiner G E, Feys J 1957 The nephrotoxic lesion of ethylene glycol. Annals of Internal Medicine 46: 611–619

Bodenham A, Park G R 1989 Reversal of prolonged sedation using flumazenil in critically ill patients. Anaesthesia 44: 603–605

Broome J R, Pearson R R, Skrine H 1988 Carbon monoxide poisoning: 'forgotten not gone!' British Journal of Hospital Medicine 39: 298–305

Buckley B M, Braithwaite R A, Vale J A 1983 Theophylline overdose. Lancet ii: 618

Burr W, Sandham P, Judd A 1989 Death after flumazenil. British Medical Journal 298: 1713

Gorchein A, Chong S K F, Mowat A P 1988 Hazards of oral charcoal. Lancet i: 1220

Henry J, Volans G 1984 ABC of poisoning. British Medical Journal 289: 907–908

Kessel N 1985 Patients who take overdoses. British Medical Journal 290: 1297–1298

Knudsen L, Lonka L, Sorensen B H, Kirkegaard L, Jensen O V, Jensen S 1988 Benzodiazepine intoxication treated with flumazenil (Anexate, RO 15–1788). Anaesthesia 43: 274–276

Kulig K 1986 Management of poisoning associated with 'newer' antidepressant agents. Annals of Emergency Medicine 15: 1039–1045

Linden N C H, Rumack B H, Strehlke C 1984 Monoamine oxidase inhibitor overdose. Annals of Emergency Medicine 13: 1137–1144

Mant T G K, Tempowski J H, Volans G N, Talbot J C C 1984 Adverse reactions to acetylcysteine and effects of overdose. British Medical Journal 289: 217–219

Menzies D G, Busuttil A, Prescott L F 1988 Fatal

pulmonary aspiration of oral activated charcoal. British Medical Journal 297: 459–460

Meredith T J, Vale J A 1988 Carbon monoxide poisoning. British Medical Journal 296: 77–79

Neuvonen P J, Vartiainen M, Tokola O 1983 Comparison of activated charcoal and ipecac syrup in prevention of drug absorption. European Journal of Clinical Pharmacology 24: 557–562

Prescott L F 1978 The chief scientist reports . . . Prevention of hepatic necrosis following paracetamol overdose. Health Bulletin 36: 204–212

Prescott L F, Highley M S 1985 Drugs prescribed for self poisoners. British Medical Journal 290: 1633–1636

Prescott L F, Illingworth R N, Critchley J A J H, Stewart M J, Adam A T 1979 Intravenous N-acetylcysteine: the treatment of choice for paracetamol poisoning. British Medical Journal 2: 1097–1100

Proudfoot A T, Stewart M S, Levitt T, Widdop B 1979 Paraquat poisoning: significance of plasma-paraquat concentrations. Lancet ii: 330–332

Short T G, Maline T, Galletly D L 1988 Ventricular arrhythmia precipitated by flumazenil. British Medical Journal 296: 1070–1071

Strong J E, Wilson J J, Douglas J F, Coppel D L 1979 Phenylbutazone self-poisoning treated by charcoal haemoperfusion. Anaesthesia 34: 1038–1040

Vale J A, Meredith T J 1985 A concise guide to the management of poisoning, 3rd edn. Churchill Livingstone, Edinburgh

Vale J A, Meredith T J, Proudfoot A T 1986 Syrup of ipecacuanha: is it really useful? British Medical Journal 293: 1321–1322

Weinstein R S 1984 Recognition and management of poisoning with beta-adrenergic blocking agents. Annals of Emergency Medicine 13: 1123–1131

Wenger T L, Butler V P, Haber E, Smith T W 1985 Treatment of 63 severely digitalis-toxic patients with digoxin-specific antibody fragments. Journal of the American College of Cardiology 5: 118A–123A

Whitwam J G 1987 Benzodiazepines. Anaesthesia 42: 1255–1256

36. Analytical methods

J. S. Millership

INTRODUCTION

The development of suitable methodology for the determination of the concentration of a particular drug, present in body fluids or tissues, may be considered a two-step procedure.

1 The development of a suitable separation technique for the isolation of the drug (and possible metabolites) from the endogenous compounds which might interfere with the analytical determination.
2 The choice of the most suitable analytical technique for the determination of the drug under investigation.

The choice of the analytical technique depends on a number of factors such as the therapeutic level of the drug in question and the chemical structure of that drug. Once the analytical technique has been defined, then the separation technique can be developed so as to complement the analytical technique; thus a complex isolation and clean-up procedure may be required if the drug is to be assayed by a spectroscopic technique, whereas the separation procedure may be less rigorous with a radio-immunoassay.

The scope of this chapter is such that a detailed discussion of the factors involved in analytical methods development is not possible. A brief outline of certain problems associated with methods development is presented, along with details of the most commonly used analytical techniques — gas-liquid chromatography, high-performance liquid chromatography, ultraviolet/ visible spectroscopy, fluorescence spectroscopy, radio-immunoassay and enzyme immunoassay. For a more detailed discussion of the determination of drugs in biological samples see Sadee and Beelan (1980), Lin and Sadee (1986), Moffat et al (1986) and Bye & Brown (1977).

SAMPLE PREPARATION

With samples of biological origin the sample preparation will depend upon the source of the sample, the drug under investigation and the analytical technique to be employed for the estimation. With many determinations the drug may be isolated from the matrix by means of a solvent extraction procedure. In its simplest form this procedure involves the adjustment of the sample pH, so that the ionic form of the drug is suppressed, followed by extraction of the drug into an organic solvent. Care is required with this method and precautions must be taken to ensure that there is no interference with the analytical determination due to extracted endogenous compounds. In certain cases, this single-stage solvent extraction may not be suitable, due to the presence of interfering substances, and a back-extraction technique may be required. This technique involves buffering of the sample followed by extraction into an organic solvent which is then re-extracted using a suitably buffered aqueous phase.

In certain instances the biological sample may contain proteinaceous material which, if not removed, may interfere with the analytical determination. Protein precipitation is therefore carried out, generally as the first stage in the sample clean-up procedure. To remove proteinaceous material the sample is treated either with a water-miscible organic solvent such as acetonitrile or with an acid such as trifluoroacetic acid. The precipitated protein can be removed from the sample by means of centrifugation and isolation of the supernatant.

The increasing use of chromatographic methods for the determination of drug levels has led to the development of special sample preparation techniques. These methods involve the use of Bond Elut™ or Sep-Pak™ cartridge systems. These cartridges contain small amounts of chromatographic material. After conditioning of the cartridge the sample is applied and retained on the cartridge. The sample may then be subjected to a series of washings to clean up the sample. The drug may then be eluted from the cartridge by means of an appropriate solvent system. The chromatographic materials available in the cartridge system include straight-phase and reversed-phase materials (see below) allowing a high degree of selectivity.

Chemical derivatization

In some instances the drug under investigation may not be suitable for analysis by any available technique, and the use of chemical derivatization may become necessary. Nowadays the most extensive use of chemical derivatization is in chromatography. Derivatization may be used for: (a) the improvement of the chromatographic separation (b) the reduction of the thermal instability of the drug under investigation or (c) the improvement of the sensitivity of detection. Gas–liquid chromatography (GLC) of molecules containing functional groups such as —COOH, —OH or —NH$_2$ often results in poor chromatography. This may be due to low volatility (as a result of hydrogen bonding), adsorption of the compound onto the column or thermal decomposition of the compound under the chromatographic conditions. Chemical derivatization is sometimes utilized to obviate these difficulties. The modification of chromatographic parameters in high-performance liquid chromatography (HPLC) will on many occasions allow the generation of suitable chromatograms; therefore chemical derivatization is used less for the improvement of separation but does find use in the enhancement of detection limits.

ANALYTICAL TECHNIQUES

Ultraviolet/visible spectroscopy

The ultraviolet/visible portions of the electromagnetic spectrum extend from about 200 to 400 nm and from 400 to 750 nm respectively.

Ultraviolet/visible light is capable of excitation of the electrons associated with certain bonds, functional groups or molecules. If ultraviolet/visible light is incident on a solution of a compound (active in the ultraviolet/visible spectrum) then some of the incident light will be absorbed and electrons will be promoted from the ground state to higher energy levels. The wavelength (λmax) of the light associated with a particular electronic transition is related to the energy difference between the two electronic energy levels. Ultraviolet/visible spectroscopy is generally considered unsuitable for qualitatitive work; however, it is used extensively for quantitative estimations. The basis of the quantitative measurements by means of ultraviolet/visible spectroscopy is the Beer–Lambert law which states:

$$A = \varepsilon \times c \times l$$

Where A = absorbance
    ε = molar absorptivity
    c = concentration (g mol/l)
    l = path length of the cell (cm)

In general there is a range of concentrations over which the Beer–Lambert law is obeyed. To obtain quantitative measurements of the concentration it is necessary to establish this range by means of a calibration curve.

The application of ultraviolet/visible spectroscopy to the estimation of drug concentrations in biological samples, although possible, does present a number of problems. The extraction procedures used to clean up a biological sample will often lead to the extraction of endogenous compounds which absorb in the ultraviolet region. Metabolites of drugs are often similar in structure to the parent compound and produce similar ultraviolet/visible spectra, leading to interferences in the quantitative estimation. In some cases the lack of sensitivity of the technique is considered something of a drawback. Despite the disadvantages detailed above there are many examples of the use of ultraviolet/visible spectroscopy for drug concentration measurements. The Bratton–Marshall procedure (Bratton & Marshall 1939) for the estimation of sulphonamides demonstrates the use of derivatization. The azo derivative produced in this method is determined at 545 nm, which is well away from any interfering absorbances. Several authors (Broughton 1956, Bogan & Smith 1967, and Goldbaum 1952) have investigated the use of ultraviolet spectroscopy for the determination of barbiturates in biological samples. The methods are based on absorbance measurements in buffered solutions. At a pH value of 10, barbiturates exist as the monoanion, whilst at pH 13 the dianion form predominates. These two anions produce different ultraviolet spectra and the concentration of barbiturate may be measured by determination of the absorbance differences between solutions at these pH values at a wavelength of approximately 260 nm.

Spectrofluorimetry

With ultraviolet-visible spectroscopy the phenomenon of absorbance was detailed in which an electron was promoted from a lower energy level to a higher energy level. If the electron possesses higher vibrational energy in the excited state than in the ground state then this excess vibrational energy may be lost by collision. If the electron then reverts to the ground state, the radiation associated with this transition will be of longer wavelength than the excitation wavelength. This emitted radiation is referred to as fluorescence. Measurement of the intensity of this emitted radiation allows quantitation by spectrofluorimetry. Spectrofluorimetry is more specific than ultraviolet-visible spectroscopy in that even with a number of fluorescing compounds careful choice of the excitation and emission wavelengths will lead to greater selectivity. Many compounds are not naturally fluorescent; however the use of derivatization allows many compounds to he assayed by this technique. Stewart & Williamson (1976) reported a fluorimetric assay of chlordiazepoxide in dosage forms and biological fluids. The procedure involves the acid hydrolysis of a solution containing chlordiazepoxide followed by adjustment of the pH to 9 and the addition of fluorescamine. Fluorescamine is a reagent which readily reacts with primary amines at specific pH values to produce fluorescent products. The authors reported intense fluorescence (excitation 390 nm, emission 486 nm) consistent with the fluorophor from methylamine (formed during hydrolysis of chlordiazepoxide). The authors also reported that little interference was observed from the major metabolites of chlordiazepoxide; however, some benzodiazepines did interfere.

Chromatographic methods

Chromatography is basically a technique for the separation, and in some cases quantitation, of the components of a mixture. Chromatographic separation is achieved by the continuous distribution of the components between two phases, one of which (the *mobile phase*) is moving past the other (the *stationary phase*). Perhaps the simplest form of chromatography is paper chromatography, in which the stationary phase is a strip of paper, the mobile phase is a buffer or organic solvent and separation is achieved by the differential partitioning of the components between the two phases. In this form of chromatography the components of the mixture are identified by the varying distances travelled along the paper (the R_f values). In other forms of chromatography, e.g. thin-layer chromatography, column chromatography, GLC and HPLC, a variety of materials are employed as stationary and mobile phases and the separation is brought about by means of a variety of physical properties such as partition, adsorption, size exclusion and ion exchange.

In the modern methods of GLC and HPLC the stationary phase is contained in a *column*, through which the mobile phase passes. The sample is injected into the flow of gas or liquid before passing onto the column. As the components pass through the column they are sep-

arated, and the eluting mobile phase is monitored by a detector which, as described below, may take several forms. The output from this detector, as an electrical signal, is plotted on moving graph paper, giving a trace in which each peak represents the presence of a different substance (Fig. 36.1). The substances are identified by the time they take to emerge from the column (the *retention time*) and the quantity present is proportional to the area under the peak. Both these are calibrated previously using known samples. Given ideal conditions the peaks obtained will be well resolved with a narrow base, and their retention times will also remain constant.

Many chromatographic methods are used for the investigation of drug substances in the pure state, in formulations and in extracts from biological fluids and tissues. GLC and HPLC are the two main chromato-

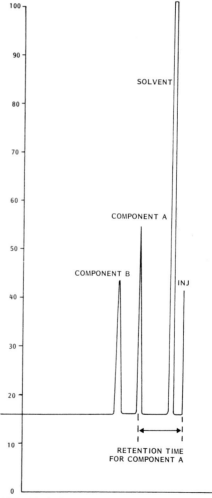

Fig 36.1 Typical gas chromatograph of a two-component mixture.

graphic methods now used for the determination of the concentrations of drugs in samples from biological sources.

Gas–liquid chromatograpy

Gas–liquid chromatography (GLC) is a chromatographic technique in which separation of the components of a mixture is achieved by the differing partition between the mobile phase (the carrier gas, e.g. argon, helium or nitrogen) and the stationary phase (silicone oil, long-chain hydrocarbon, etc.). The basic instrumentation required for GLC consists of an injection port, a column housed within a carefully controlled oven and a detector (Fig. 36.2). Sample introduction in GLC is usually carried out by syringe injection of a solution of the sample. Sample injection via the injection port introduces the components to a heated zone where solvent and solutes are volatilized. The carrier gas sweeps the injection port continuously and carries the vaporized samples onto the column. In modern GLC instruments columns may be of two types — packed columns or capillary columns. Packed columns consist of coils of glass or metal containing the column packing material. The column packing material is prepared by coating the stationary phase onto an inert support material. The stationary phase is the most important contributing factor to the separation since the effect of changing from one carrier gas to another produces only minor modifications. The choice of the most suitable stationary phase for a particular separation may often be aided by the wealth of information provided by the commercial and scientific literature. Packed columns are generally 1 or 2 m in length with internal diameters of several millimetres. Capillary columns differ from packed columns in that they contain no packing material, the stationary phase is coated onto the inner wall of the column. These columns vary in length from about 20 m to 100 m with an internal diameter of about 0.25 mm. These capillary columns are now used for complex separations. The columns are housed in ovens so that the temperature at which the separation is carried out may be carefully controlled. A variety of detectors is available for GLC, the most common being thermal conductivity detectors, flame ionization detectors, nitrogen/phosphorus detectors and electron capture detectors. Gas chromatographs may also be linked with mass spectrometers; this form of detection is very useful in drug analysis. The use of mass spectroscopy allows the identification of unknown peaks by means of the fragmentation patterns, and selected ion monitoring is useful for quantitation. Combined GLC–mass spectroscopy has proved one of the most important analytical techniques in drug analysis.

GLC may be used for both quantitative and qualitative analysis of drugs. Moffat et al (1986) and Sadee and Beelen (1980) present extensive details of the application of GLC in these areas.

High-performance liquid chromatography

High-performance liquid chromatography (HPLC, high-pressure liquid chromatography) is a development of classical liquid column chromatography, based on the applications of the theories of chromatography derived for GLC. These theories predicted that two major fac-

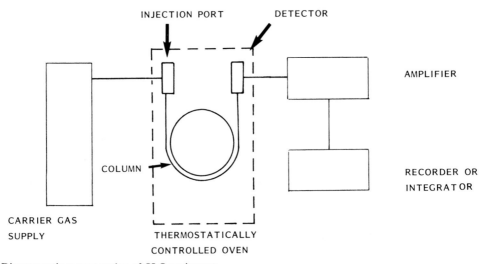

Fig. 36.2 Diagrammatic representation of GLC equipment.

tors could improve the efficiency of classical liquid chromatography. These were:

1. that the mean diameter of the column packing material would have to be smaller than conventional packing materials;
2. that the operating pressure of the system would have to be higher, due to the differences in viscosities between gases and liquids.

The implementation of these theoretical considerations has led to the production of the present-day HPLC equipment in which we use column packing materials with a mean particle diameter of 10 or 5 μ (in some cases 3 μ) with an operating pressure of between 1000 and 2000 p.s.i.

The efficiency of modern HPLC systems owes much to the development of these smaller-diameter column packings; however, improvements in systems hardware have allowed great improvements in the levels of sensitivity, especially with regard to the analysis of drugs in biological samples.

The basic set-up of a modern HPLC system (Fig. 36.3) consists of a mobile phase reservoir, a pump, a sample introduction device, a column, a detector and a recorder or integrator. Two components of the system which have a great influence on the sensitivity and efficiency are the pump and the detector. Most modern pumps deliver the mobile phase at a constant flow rate and are designed so as to minimize pulsations in flow which would lead to a loss of sensitivity. Correct choice of flow rate is necessary for the optimization of efficiency. Many detection systems are available for HPLC, including ultraviolet/visible, fluorescence, refractive index, electrochemical and radioactivity detectors. The use of ultraviolet/visible detectors is probably the most common form of detection in drug analysis, although recent publications have demonstrated increasing use of fluorescence and electrochemical detection. The development of microbore HPLC systems with flow rates of microlitres per minute allows the use of mass spectrometers as detectors. This development is extremely important for drug concentration measurement and drug metabolism studies.

The utilization of small-diameter particles has already been cited as a major contributing factor with regard to the efficiency of separation. The development of chemically bonded stationary phases, utilizing these particles, has also added greatly to the development of HPLC, especially with regard to selectivity. Conventional column chromatography used to be carried out using a polar stationary phase and a mobile phase consisting of relatively non-polar organic solvents. This type of chromatography is still carried out in HPLC, and is referred to as

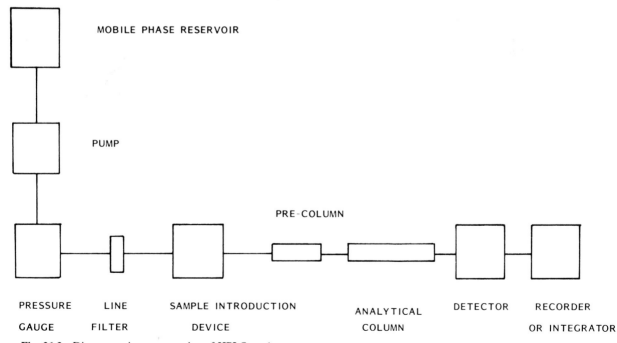

Fig. 36.3 Diagrammatic representation of HPLC equipment.

normal-phase chromatography (simply because it was the first to be used). Reversed-phase chromatography utilizes a non-polar stationary phase and a polar mobile phase. Chemically bonded stationary phases have been developed which allow both normal-phase and reversed-phase chromatography to be carried out using HPLC equipment. These chemically bonded stationary phases are prepared by a chemical reaction between silanol groups on the surface of silica and reagents such as trichloro-octadecasilane.

There are many examples of the application of HPLC to the analysis of drugs, Wessely & Zech (1979) and Pryde & Gilbert (1979) have produced excellent reviews of the topic. A more recent text (Gilbert 1987) contains many examples of drug analysis by HPLC, including a chapter describing the separation of chiral drug molecules. The previously mentioned texts (Moffat et al 1986 and Sadee & Beelan 1980) also contain specific details of drug analysis by HPLC.

Radio-immunoassay

The basic requirements for a radio-immunoassay are:

1. a sample of the biological fluid containing the drug to be determined;
2. a sample of the drug to be determined which has been radiolabelled (usually with ^{3}H, ^{14}C or ^{125}I);
3. the antibody to the drug.

The sample of the biological fluid is mixed with known amounts of the radiolabelled drug and the antibody. This mixture is then allowed to reach equilibrium, i.e. equilibrium between free drug (labelled and unlabelled) plus the antibody and the antibody–drug (labelled and unlabelled) complex. The non-complexed drug is then separated from the antibody-drug complex either by addition of charcoal or by use of the precipitating antibody technique. Measurement of the radioactivity associated with either fraction allows the determination of the drug concentration. Moffat (1976) and Stewart (1986) discuss in detail the practical aspects of radio-immunoassay, including the methods of production of the antibody required.

Radio-immunoassay methods are now widely used for the estimation of drug concentrations in biological samples. Commercial kits are available for the radio-immunoassay of a range of drugs including barbiturates, digoxin and morphine. Moffat (1976) has reviewed the use of radio-immunoassay methods for drug substances. Sensitivity levels with radio-immunoassay methods can be as low as ng/ml or pg/ml; however, the technique does suffer in some instances due to cross-reactivity with metabolites or co-administered drugs.

Enzyme immunoassay

This is similar to radio-immunoassay, but the drug used in the test is labelled with an enzyme, rather than by a radioactive isotope. Again antibody is added to the sample containing the drug to be measured, and the antibody binds to any drug it recognizes. The labelled drug is then added, and binds to any remaining sites, its enzyme being inactivated during this process. The amount of active enzyme remaining is directly related to the concentration of drug initially present in the sample, and it can be measured, for example by absorbance at a specific wavelength. This method is currently used in the assay of aminoglycoside antibiotics, phenytoin, etc.

REFERENCES

Bogan J, Smith H 1967 Analytical investigation of barbiturate poisoning–description of methods and a survey of results. Journal of the Forensic Science Society 7: 37–45

Bratton A C, Marshall E K 1939 A new coupling component for sulphanilamide determination. Journal of Biological Chemistry 128: 537–550

Broughton P M G 1956 A rapid ultraviolet spectrophotometric method for the detection, estimation and identification of barbiturates in biological material. Biochemical Journal 63: 207–213

Bye A, Brown M E 1977 An analytical approach to the quantitation of known drugs in human biological samples by HPLC. Journal of Chromatographic Science 15: 365–371

Gilbert M T, 1987 High performance liquid chromatography. Wright, Bristol

Goldbaum L R 1952 Determination of barbiturates. Analytical Chemistry 24: 1604–1607

Lin E T, Sadee W 1986 Drug level monitoring, vol2. John Wiley, New York

Moffat A C 1976 The radioimmunoassay of drugs. Analyst 101: 225–243.

Moffat A C, Jackson J V, Moss M S, Widdop D 1986 Clarke's isolation and identification of drugs in pharmaceuticals, body fluids and post-mortem material. Pharmaceutical Press, London.

Pryde A, Gilbert M T 1979 Applications of high performance liquid chromatography. Chapman & Hall, London

Sadee W, Beelen G C M 1980 Drug level monitoring. John Wiley, New York

Stewart M J 1986 Immunoassays. In: Moffat A C, Jackson J V, Moss M S, Widdop D (eds) Clarke's isolation and identification of drugs in pharmaceuticals, body fluids and post-mortem material. Pharmaceutical Press, London, pp 148–159

Stewart J T, Williamson J L 1976 Fluorometric determination of chlordiazepoxide in dosage forms and biological fluids with fluorescamine. Analytical Chemistry

48: 1182–1185

Wessely K, Zech K 1979 High performance liquid chromatography in pharmaceutical analysis. Hewlett-Packard GmbH, Boblingen.

Index